Quick Reference to Standard Protocols for All Nursing Interventions

All nursing skills must include certain basic steps for the safety and well-being of the client and the nurse. To save space and prevent repetition, *these steps are not included in each skill unless it is necessary to clarify them as applied for that skill.* Remember that these steps are essential and must be followed to deliver appropriate and responsible nursing care.

When indicated, a logo is used to identify the need for **clean gloves.** Personnel wear clean, disposable gloves before contact with mucous membranes, nonintact skin, or moist body substances. The following logo indicates clean gloves are needed:

 Gloves are changed between clients and between activities with the same client when gloves become excessively soiled (Centers for Disease Control, CDC, 1992).

EQUIPMENT

Armband for client identification
Consent form (if required by agency policy)
Clean disposable gloves (if contact with body secretions or excretions is anticipated)

Before the skill

1. Verify physician's orders if skill is a dependent or collaborative nursing intervention. Independent nursing interventions may be verified with the nursing care plan, Kardex, or primary nurse.

2. Identify client by checking armband and having client state name (if able to do so).

3. Introduce yourself to client, including both name and title or role, and explain what you plan to do.

4. Explain the procedure and the reason it is to be done in terms client can understand.

5. Assess client to determine that the intervention is still appropriate. (Each skill has an assessment section that includes appropriate specific findings.)

6. Gather equipment and complete necessary charges.

7. Wash hands for at least 10 seconds before each new client contact.

8. Adjust the bed to appropriate height and lower side rail on the side nearest you.

9. Provide privacy for client. Position and drape client as needed.

During the skill

10. Promote client involvement if possible.

11. Assess client tolerance, being alert for signs of discomfort and fatigue. Inability to tolerate a procedure is described in the nurses' notes.

Completion protocol

12. Assist client to a position of comfort, and place needed items within reach. Be certain client has a way to call for help and knows how to use it.

13. Raise the side rails and lower the bed to the lowest position.

14. Store or remove and dispose of soiled supplies and equipment.

15. Wash your hands for at least 10 seconds after client contact and after removing gloves.

16. Document client's response and expected or unexpected outcomes.

Nursing
Interventions

AND

Clinical Skills

Martha Keene Elkin, RN, MSN

Adjunct Faculty
Lincoln Land Community College
Springfield, Illinois

Anne Griffin Perry, RN, MSN, EdD

Professor, St. Louis University School of Nursing
Coordinator, Cardiopulmonary Specialty
St. Louis University Health Sciences Center
St. Louis, Missouri

Patricia A. Potter, RN, MSN

Director of Nursing Practice
Barnes and Jewish Hospitals
St. Louis, Missouri

with over 900 illustrations

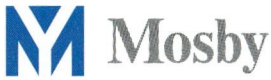

St. Louis Baltimore Boston Carlsbad Chicago Naples New York Philadelphia Portland
London Madrid Mexico City Singapore Sydney Tokyo Toronto Wiesbaden

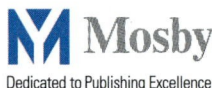

Mosby
Dedicated to Publishing Excellence

Vice President and Publisher: Nancy L. Coon
Senior Editor: Susan Epstein
Senior Developmental Editor: Beverly J. Copland
Project Manager: John Rogers
Production Editor: Lavon Wirch Peters
Designer: Renée Duenow
Manufacturing Supervisor: Linda Ierardi
Original Art: Jack Reuter
Photography: Patrick Watson, Michael Clement, M.D., Diana Kleidon

Printed in the United States of America
Composition by Graphic World, Inc.
Printing/binding by Von Hoffmann Press

Mosby-Year Book, Inc.
11830 Westline Industrial Drive
St. Louis, Missouri 63146

Library of Congress Cataloging in Publication Data

Elkin, Martha Keene.
  Nursing interventions and clinical skills / Martha Keene Elkin,
Anne Griffin Perry, Patricia A. Potter.
    p.   cm.
  Includes bibliographical references and index.
  ISBN 0-8151-3045-7 (softcover)
  1. Nursing   2. Clinical competence.   I. Perry, Anne Griffin.
II. Potter, Patricia Ann.   III. Title.
  [DNLM: 1. Nursing Process. 2. Nursing Care—methods.   WY 100
  E43n   1995]
  RT41.E39   1995
  610.73—dc20
  DNLM/DLC
  for Library of Congress   95-31361
                                                         CIP

95 96 97 98 99 / 9 8 7 6 5 4 3 2 1

Contributors

Elizabeth A. Ayello, RN, BSN, MS, PhD, CS, CETN
Clinical Assistant Professor of Nursing,
New York University,
New York, New York

V. Christine Champagne, RN, MSN(R)
Pulmonary Clinical Nurse Specialist and Director,
Cardiac and Pulmonary Rehabilitation,
St. Joseph Health Center,
St. Charles, Missouri

Julie Eddins, RN, BSN, MSN, CRNI
Staff Nurse, IV Therapy,
Barnes Hospital—Christian Health Services;
Faculty,
The Jewish College of Nursing and Allied Health,
St. Louis, Missouri

Deborah Oldenburg Erickson, RN, BSN, MSN
Instructor, School of Nursing,
Methodist Medical Center of Illinois,
Peoria, Illinois

Joan O. Ervin, RN, BSN, MN, CCRN
Adjunct Faculty,
Florence Darlington Technical College,
Florence, South Carolina

Susan A. Hauser, RN, BSN, BA, MS
Instructor,
Mansfield General Hospital School of Nursing,
Mansfield, Ohio

Carolyn Chaney Hoskins, RN, BSN, MSN
Clinical Instructor,
Rockingham Community College,
Wentworth, North Carolina

Nancy Jackson, RN, BSN, MSN(R), CCRN
Pulmonary Clinical Nurse Specialist,
St. Mary's Health Center,
St. Louis, Missouri

Antoinette Kanne Ledbetter, RN, BSN, MS, TNS
Clinical Education Coordinator,
Missouri Baptist Medical Center,
St. Louis, Missouri

Mary "Dee" Miller, RN, BSN, MS, CIC
Clinical Nursing Specialist/Infection Control and
    Epidemiology,
St. Joseph's Hospital and Medical Center;
Faculty, BSN & MSN Nursing and Business,
University of Phoenix,
Phoenix, Arizona

Rose M. Miller, RN, BSN, MSN, MPA, ACLS
Instructor,
Wallace College,
Dothan, Alabama

Kathleen Mulryan, RN, BSN, MSN
Professor,
LaGuardia Community College,
Long Island City, New York

Elaine K. Neel, RN, BSN, MSN
Instructor, School of Nursing,
Methodist Medical Center of Illinois,
Peoria, Illinois

Marsha Evans Orr, RN, MS, CNSN, CS
Site Manager, Clinical Nutrition Network,
Caremark, Inc.,
Tempe, Arizona

Paulette D. Rollant, RN, BSN, MSN, PhD, CCRN
Consultant and President,
Adult Health Clinical Specialist,
Multi-Resources, Inc.,
Grantville, Georgia

Linette M. Sarti, RN, BSN
RN Education Specialist,
Barnes Hospital,
St. Louis, Missouri

Victoria McGreevy Steelman, RN, MA, PhD(c)
Clinical Nurse Specialist,
University of Iowa Hospitals and Clinics,
Iowa City, Iowa

Pamela Becker Weilitz, RN, MSN(R), CS
Manager, Nursing Care Delivery,
Barnes and Jewish Hospital, BJC Health System,
St. Louis, Missouri

Jana L. Weindel-Dees, RN, BSN, MSN
Registered Nurse,
Barnes Hospital,
St. Louis, Missouri

Reviewers

Janice Arbour, RN, BN
Psychomotor Skills Clinician, Faculty of Nursing,
University of Calgary,
Calgary, Alberta

Meri Jayne Basti, RN, BSN, MSN, CNAA, FNS
Instructor,
Cuesta Community College,
San Luis Obispo, California

Margie E. Brown, RN, C, MS, ANP
Professor, ADN Program,
Long Beach City College,
Long Beach, California

Kathlyn Carlson, RN, BSN, MA, CPAN
Staff RN, PACU,
Abbott Northwestern Hospital,
Minneapolis, Minnesota

Patricia Castaldi, RN, BSN, MSN
Assistant Dean,
Elizabeth General Medical Center School of Nursing,
Elizabeth, New Jersey

Sheila Cunningham, RN, MSN
Assistant Professor,
Neumann College,
Aston, Pennsylvania

Lynne Dearing, RN, BSN, MSN, MA
Instructor of Nursing,
Grays Harbor College,
Aberdeen, Washington

Janet Louise Dougherty, RN, BS, MSN
Nursing Instructor,
Baptist Medical Center, School of Nursing,
Little Rock, Arkansas

Patti A. Ellison, RN, BSN, MSN, CEN
Assistant Professor of Nursing,
University of Cincinnati, Raymond Walters College,
Cincinnati, Ohio

Muriel Fairchild, RN, BSN, MPH
Nursing Instructor,
Walla Walla Community College,
Walla Walla, Washington

Linda Hobrook Freeman, RN, BSN, MSN, DNS
Associate Professor,
University of Louisville,
Louisville, Kentucky

Mary A. Hamm, RN, MEd, MSN
Professor of Nursing,
Bucks County Community College,
Newton, Pennsylvania

Renee Covey Harrison, RN, BSN, MS
Assistant Professor,
Tulsa Junior College,
Tulsa, Oklahoma

Pat Hartley, RN, BSN, MEd
Associate Dean, Health Sciences Division,
Vancouver Community College,
Vancouver, British Columbia

Susan Herman, RN, MSN
Associate Professor,
Chaffey College,
Rancho Cucamonga, California

Mary Reuther Herring, RN, BSN, MSN
Occupational Health Nurse, Motorola;
Nursing Faculty, University of Phoenix,
Phoenix, Arizona

Judith Ann Kilpatrick, RN, C, BSN, MSN
Lecturer,
Widener University School of Nursing,
Chester, Pennsylvania

E. Jacquelyn Kirkis, RN, BSN, MS, MSEd, CIC, PHN
Consultant,
ECHOES Seminars, Inc.,
Seal Beach, California

Marilee Kuhl, RN, BSN, MSN
Nursing Instructor,
Northern Nevada Community College,
Elko, Nevada

Chestine Kurth, RN, PhD, CCRN
Professor of Nursing,
Central Wyoming College,
Riverton, Wyoming

Joe R. Lacher, RN, BSN, MSN, CNA
Associate Professor,
University of Texas of Brownsville,
Brownsville, Texas

Jennifer Lemmink, RN, MSN, CCRN
Nurse Clinician, College of Nursing and Health,
University of Cincinnati,
Cincinnati, Ohio

Erma R. McNeill, RN, BSN, MNSc
Instructor,
Jefferson School of Nursing,
Pine Bluff, Arkansas

Sharon Miller, RN, BSN, MSN
Assistant Professor of Nursing,
The University of Charleston,
Charleston, West Virginia

Claudia Louth Mitchell, RN, BSN, MSN
Professor of Nursing, Assistant Director ADN Program,
Santa Barbara City College,
Santa Barbara, California

Ann Nelson Moore, RN, MSN
ADN Faculty,
Seattle Central Community College,
Seattle, Washington

Diane M. Moro, RN, MS
Nursing Arts Lab Coordinator,
St. Joseph's Hospital Health Center School of Nursing,
Syracuse, New York

Kathryn Nold, RN, BS, MSN
Instructor,
St. Charles County Community College,
St. Peters, Missouri

Catherine Libert Peterson, RN, C, MSN
Professor,
San Diego City College,
San Diego, California

Melissa Powell, RN, MSN
Assistant Professor of Nursing,
Eastern Kentucky University,
Richmond, Kentucky

Cheryl M. Prandoni, RN, BSN, MSN
Director of Learning Resources,
The Catholic University of America,
Washington, District of Columbia

Mary Reuland, RN, BSN, MS
Assistant Professor,
College of St. Catherine,
Minneapolis, Minnesota

Vanice Roberts, RN, DSN
Professor of Nursing,
Kennesaw State College,
Marietta, Georgia

Ellen Rosbach, RN, MSN
Instructor,
Lower Columbia College,
Longview, Washington

April Sieh, RN, MSN
Assistant Professor of Nursing,
Delta College,
University Center, Michigan

Thomas J. Smith, RN, C, GCNS, PhD
Associate Professor,
Nicholls State University,
Thibodaux, Louisiana

Preface

Nursing Interventions and Clinical Skills is designed to present the most current information on basic and advanced nursing skills in a unique, dynamic format that promotes learning and understanding and helps students apply their knowledge in the real world of client care. The nursing process framework; crisp, clear writing style; consistent, logical presentation; generous use of full color photographs and drawings; and functional use of color in the design combine to make this text attractive, practical, and easy to understand.

Organization

Progressing from **basic** to **advanced skills,** the first part of this text presents those procedures commonly covered in the early components of the nursing curriculum. Intermediate and advanced interventions that relate more closely to medical-surgical nursing content comprise the latter section of the text. Throughout, skills are grouped and combined to eliminate repetition and more closely reflect their actual implementation in practice.

The 5-step **nursing process** serves as the organizational framework. Each chapter begins with an overview of pertinent concepts and principles, including a discussion of the nursing diagnoses that commonly call for the interventions that follow. These diagnoses are compared and clarified, not merely listed, so students develop an understanding of the link between the diagnoses and the selection of nursing interventions. The remaining steps—assessment, planning/expected outcomes, implementation, and evaluation—are provided for each skill.

The presentation of skills is clear and consistent, beginning with a list of required equipment, appropriate assessment criteria, and expected outcomes. The actual steps of the skill—within the implementation section—are set off in a 2-column format that includes rationales for key steps. Each skill also includes sample documentation, evaluation, and unexpected outcomes with appropriate interventions.

Key Features

- Clear, concise writing style, particularly in steps of skills, makes material easy to follow and comprehend.

- Contemporary, attractive design uses color to identify related elements and concepts.
- More than 900 large, full-color photographs and drawings emphasize and clarify important concepts and actions.
- Nursing process framework provides a logical, consistent presentation that reinforces the use of the process in all aspects of care.
- Skills format clearly and concisely presents essential information to facilitate understanding and retrieval of content.
- UNIQUE! A Standard Protocol that details essential steps for the beginning and completion of skills is provided in Chapter 1 and summarized inside the front cover for quick retrieval; references to this protocol within the skills eliminates redundancy.
- A special logo alerts the student when gloves are required to ensure that proper infection control practices are observed .
- The step-by-step instructions for performing the skill are set off in a clear, 2-column format that is easy to follow and can be quickly located for later reference or review.
- Nurse Alerts remind students of conditions or situations that contraindicate or require modification of the procedure, as well as provide practical tips that can enhance the effectiveness of the intervention.
- Rationales for key steps help students understand why they must be performed.
- Closely related or similar skills are combined to reduce repetition and more closely parallel how they are actually performed in practice.
- Evaluation criteria describe how to determine whether nursing actions achieve expected outcomes.
- Unexpected outcomes and related interventions identify problems that may occur during or after performance of the skill and provide guidelines for appropriate nursing actions.
- Sample documentation shows students both what to record and how to properly phrase reports.
- Critical Thinking Exercises for each chapter help students develop problem-solving and decision-making skills.
- Numerous appendices provide sample forms, abbreviations, normal lab values, and NANDA diagnoses listed

both alphabetically and according to Functional Health Patterns.

Key Content

- A separate chapter on Pressure Ulcer Care includes the latest AHCPR guidelines for assessment, prevention, and treatment.
- Chapter on Discharge Teaching and Home Health Management highlights teaching strategies and skills frequently performed in the home.
- Unique chapter on Shift Assessment provides a quick overview of those skills normally performed at change of shift.
- Infection Control chapter includes the latest CDC guidelines and features a skill on special TB precautions.
- Coverage of lab and diagnostic tests focuses on the nurse's role in preparing for and assisting with procedures, as well as monitoring client responses.
- Chapter on Fluids, Electrolytes, and Acid-Base Balance provides skills for monitoring imbalances as well as interventions for correcting them.
- Client teaching is integrated throughout to promote compliance and self-care ability.
- Cultural considerations alert students to pertinent variations in assessment and potential modifications in care.

Teaching-Learning Package

The most comprehensive array of teaching and learning tools available, this package includes:

- Instructor's Resource Manual with performance checklists for all skills in the text.
- 54 full color transparency acetates to enhance lectures.
- A Skills Performance Checklist booklet for students that is available separately or packaged with the text.
- Answers to Critical Thinking Exercises that are provided in both the Instructor's Resource Manual and the Skills Performance Checklist booklet.
- Mosby's Nursing Skills Video Series.
- A new set of interactive videodiscs, available beginning in the fall of 1996, that helps students learn to apply critical thinking to nursing skills.

Acknowledgements

The art and science of nursing are continuously changing. A number of talented people have helped to make this text an accurate, concise, and visually appealing learning resource. We express our sincere appreciation to our nursing colleagues and nursing students, who continue to stimulate our thinking about creative ways to provide excellence in nursing education. Gratitude must also be expressed to our contributors and reviewers, whose dedication and expertise make the details of this book both practical and current.

Thanks to the professional nursing staff of Barnes Hospital, Jewish Hospital, Saint Louis University Hospital, Saint Louis University School of Nursing, and Jewish College of Nursing and Allied Health in St. Louis, Missouri; and of St. John's Hospital, Memorial Medical Center, and Lincoln Land Community College in Springfield, Illinois. We are indebted for their cooperation in providing equipment and models for realistic photographs. Thanks also to the administrative staff of these institutions for their support and cooperation in this project.

Thanks to Susan Epstein, Senior Editor, who helped develop the concept of the text and supported the process for its development. Special acknowledgement to Beverly Copland, Senior Developmental Editor, Nursing Division, who diligently and persistently helped keep us on schedule with the many details of preparation of manuscript and illustrations. Her vision of the project helped to make it a quality project.

Thank you to Lavon Peters, Production Editor, for meticulous attention to detail and thoroughness in guiding the manuscript, photos, and illustrations through the production process, and to Renée Duenow, the designer whose creativity and expertise resulted in an easy to use, colorful text.

Thanks to Pat Watson, Diana Kleidon, and Michael Clement M.D., the photographers whose careful attention to detail ensured high-quality photographic images. Thanks also to Jack Reuter, who provided meticulous attention to accuracy in line drawings.

And finally, we offer grateful appreciation to family and friends, who provided support and understanding throughout many long hours of creating, developing, improving, and refining manuscript, and participating in the details of production of the final product.

Martha "Marty" Keene Elkin
Anne Griffin Perry
Patricia A. Potter

Contents

Appendices

Nursing Interventions

AND

Clinical Skills

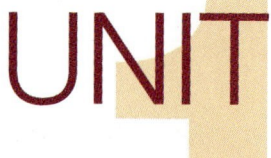

UNIT 1

Fundamental Concepts

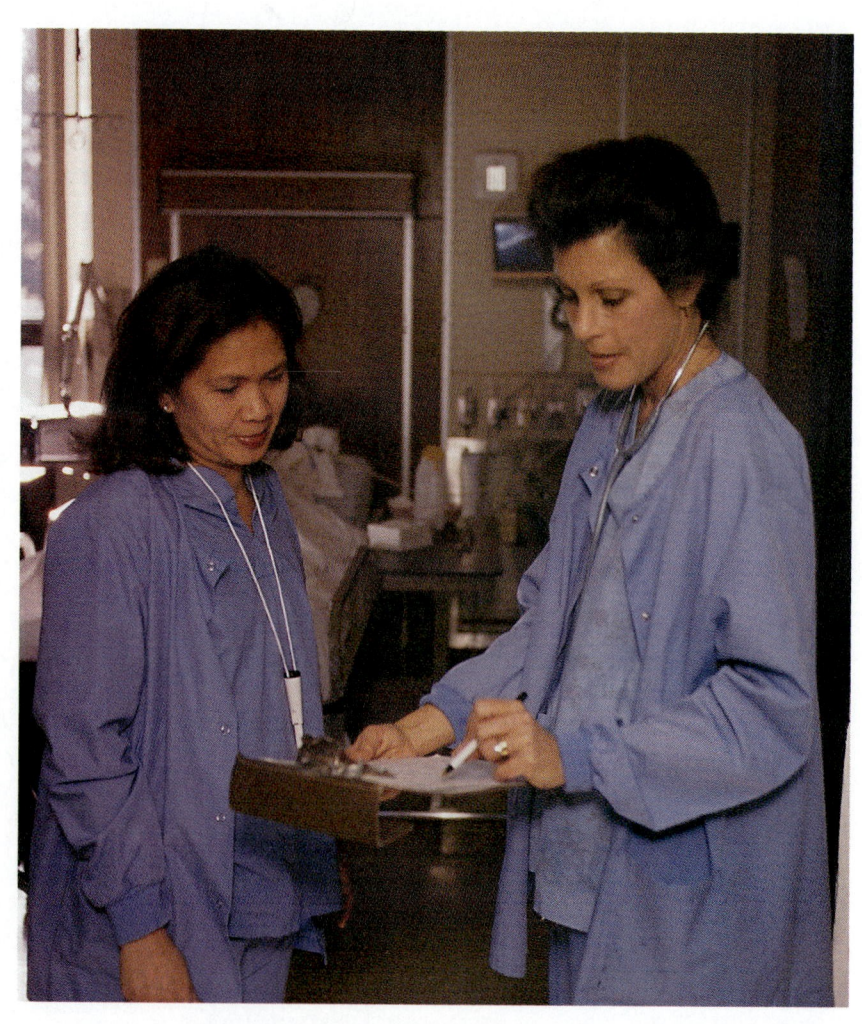

chapter 1 | # Nursing Diagnosis and Nursing Interventions

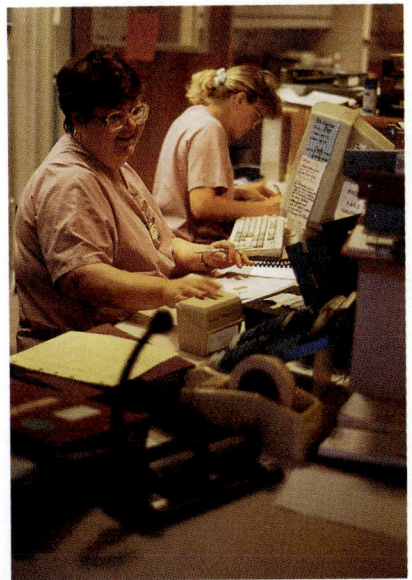

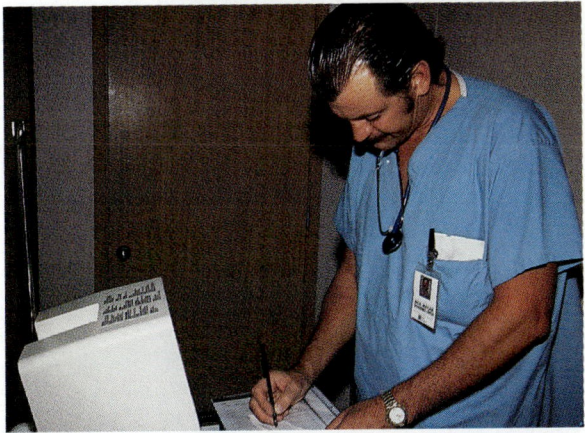

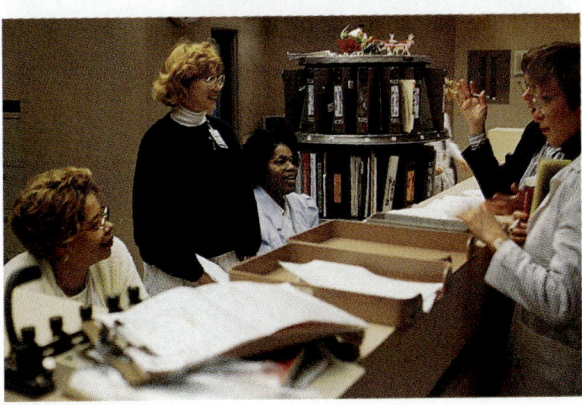

Skill 1.1
Standard Protocols

Nursing as defined in 1980 by the American Nurses Association (ANA) is the diagnosis and treatment of human responses to actual or potential health problems. This definition is implemented by the use of the nursing process. In this process, the nurse **assesses** a client's health status by obtaining specific data through communicating with the client and others, from conducting a physical assessment, and from reviewing information from the client's record. The nurse uses nursing theory to understand and analyze these data to identify one or more nursing diagnoses. A **nursing diagnosis** is a clinical judgment about individual, family, or community responses to actual or potential health concerns. **Planning** includes identifying goals and outcomes of care and setting priorities for a plan of care that can result in goal achievement. **Implementation** includes performing nursing actions to assist the client to reach a maximum state of health. **Evaluation** involves observing for changes in the client's response to determine if goals and outcomes were met. The nursing process is closely related to the *Standards of Clinical Nursing Practice* of the ANA (1973, 1980, 1991) (Figure 1-1).

Nursing interventions include actions and skills that promote health, prevent illness, relieve symptoms, or restore health. Interventions include nursing actions such as assisting, monitoring, promoting, and facilitating. Clients may need nursing interventions in the form of emotional and physical support, medication, treatments, or client and family education.

Specific skills are required for implementation of nursing interventions. The nursing role involves skills in the areas of assessment, communication, decision making, teaching, procedure, administration and leadership, documentation and reporting, and research. These skills require both knowledge and practice for the nurse to de-

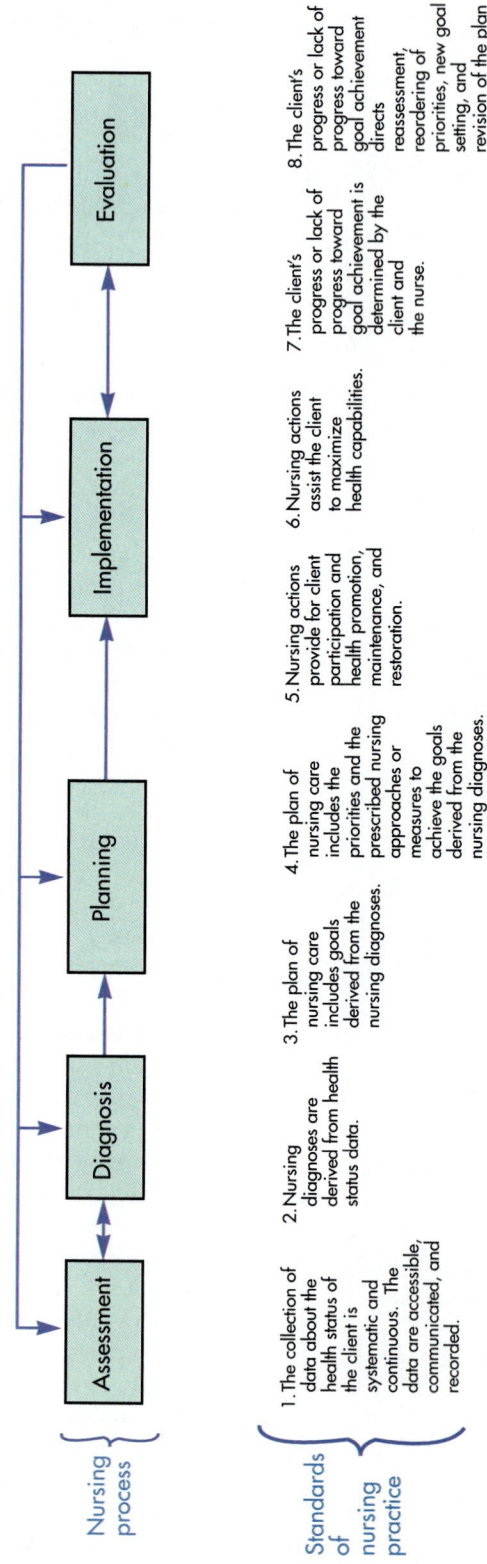

Figure 1-1 Relationship between the nursing process and the standards of nursing practice. (Modified from the American Nurses Association: *Nursing and social policy statement*, Kansas City, Mo, 1980, The Association.)

velop proficiency. Knowledge of the **rationale** for the action, as well as the ability to adapt creatively while supporting underlying principles, improves the quality of nursing care. When choosing nursing interventions, the nurse considers assessment data, priority setting, knowledge, and experience to select interventions that promote movement toward appropriate expected outcomes.

When nurses carry out medical orders, they function dependently. Examples include administration of medications and scheduling of diagnostic tests. Nurses also function autonomously, initiating independent nursing interventions. They function interdependently or collaboratively with other health professionals by communicating identified client needs to other health care professionals.

An integral relationship exists between the individualized nursing diagnosis and nursing interventions. Nurses use knowledge, experience, and intuition to determine individualized interventions for a specific client situation. Recent research is assisting nurses to develop a

nursing interventions classification system. The purpose of this classification system is to create a standardized list of the interventions that nurses perform so that it will be possible to determine which interventions work best for a specific nursing diagnosis (McCloskey and Bulechek, 1992).

The nursing diagnosis, an essential component of the nursing process, is the method by which nursing is practiced systematically. It is a means by which nurses demonstrate accountability and responsibility to clients and families (Carroll-Johnson, 1990). The North American Nursing Diagnosis Association (NANDA) is a formal organization that has developed a classification system for nursing diagnoses. A list of diagnoses as currently accepted by NANDA is found in Appendix C. The accepted diagnoses are evolving as research continues. The terminology from the NANDA list of accepted nursing diagnoses is used in this text.

THE DIAGNOSTIC PROCESS

The diagnostic process begins with the nurse collecting information about the client (see box at left). This includes interviewing the client and others significant to the situation, conducting a physical assessment, conferring with health team members, and reviewing information in the client record. Data are analyzed and organized into clusters of related cues, which then lead to the formulation of a nursing diagnosis. Clusters of subjective and objective cues support the selection of the nursing diagnosis. Numerous resources are available to assist nurses with identifying characteristics that may be included in cue clusters for a given nursing diagnosis. Many agencies have initial nursing assessment forms that facilitate identification of nursing diagnoses (see Appendix A).

A nursing diagnosis is composed of problem and etiology statements:

The problem statement describes a physiological or psychological response to a health problem.

The etiology statement describes contributing factors that influence development of the response.

Identifying the First Part of the Diagnostic Statement

The NANDA list of accepted nursing diagnoses can also be categorized into the 11 functional patterns listed in Appendix D. For each of the 11 patterns, the nurse assesses clients by organizing patterns of behavior and physiological responses that pertain to a functional pattern category. The assessment of each of the 11 patterns represents the interaction of the client and the environment, and each pattern interacts with other patterns (Gordon, 1991).

The first part of the statement, the problem or stem, may be an actual or high-risk nursing diagnosis. A high-risk nursing diagnosis indicates the client is at risk for

---

Creating a Nursing Diagnosis

STEP 1

Start with information from a client assessment.

a. Make a comprehensive list of all significant cues, such as symptoms, laboratory data, subjective data, and other information. This would *not* include medical diagnosis, physician orders, treatments, or interventions.

b. These cues are then grouped according to ways that make sense to you.

c. Each group of cues then provides supporting defining characteristics for a nursing diagnosis label.

STEP 2

Determine the etiology or contributing factors for these data. (This becomes the "*related to*" part of the statement.)

a. "What makes or maintains the client's unhealthy response?"

b. This should clearly indicate what nurses can independently do to help alleviate the problem.

c. Compare to *contributing factors* or related factors as listed in references. NOTE: Watch out for medical diagnoses that may be there and may *not* be used in this step except by using the phrase "...secondary to...."

d. This part should direct the nursing interventions and becomes the second part of the statement.

e. In some cases the contributing factors are "unknown."

STEP 3

Identify the patient *problem* or *response* from the NANDA listing.

a. This becomes the *stem* or *label* and the first part of the statement.

b. For this part you must use the exact NANDA words.

this response, although it is not yet present. Most nursing diagnosis labels can be used as either actual or high-risk nursing diagnoses. For example, a client may have a nursing diagnosis of actual **Impaired Physical Mobility** or **High Risk for Impaired Physical Mobility.**

The NANDA stem (client response) suggests possible client goals and expected outcomes. It is essential that the identified diagnosis communicates something that nurses can address within the domain of nursing practice. After a focus assessment that clarifies additional related data, specific and individualized expected outcomes can be identified.

Identifying the Second Part of the Diagnostic Statement

Etiology or contributing factors for a nursing diagnosis are the second part of the statement and are linked with a connecting phrase "related to." Interventions are selected based primarily on this part of the nursing diagnosis. The contributing factors would be validated with the client when possible. For example, the diagnosis **Impaired Physical Mobility** could be related to "pain, weakness, or lack of balance." One can understand that interventions for pain are very different than those for weakness or lack of balance. In some cases the contributing factors are unknown. The statement could read, "...related to unknown factors," and interventions involve assessment for contributing factors. More than one contributing factor may be identified for a single nursing diagnosis.

When the primary nursing focus needs to be client teaching, the second part of the nursing diagnosis is "lack of knowledge of (specific topic)." Example: **High Risk for Injury** related to lack of knowledge of safe transfer and crutch-walking techniques.

When assessment reveals that a client has significant risk factors that could contribute to a nursing diagnosis, the second part of the statement includes identified risk factors, and the focus becomes prevention. Example: **High Risk for Impaired Skin Integrity** related to immobility and diaphoresis. In this case, interventions are directed toward promoting mobility, positioning, and dry skin, all of which prevent skin breakdown.

Since physicians are responsible for the treatment related to the medical diagnosis, it is not appropriate to use a medical diagnosis in a nursing diagnosis statement. When it is difficult to identify an etiology or contributing factor different from the medical diagnosis, the identified client response may be the contributing factor. For example, the nursing diagnosis **Pain** used as a contributing factor suggests asking, "What is this client's response to the pain?" Possible responses may include **Sleep Pattern Disturbance, Anxiety,** and **Impaired Physical Mobility.**

It is also ineffective to repeat the same concept in different words for the first and second parts of the nursing diagnosis, for example, **Fluid Volume Deficit** related to dehydration. This statement does not identify contributing factors, which could include either increased losses or decreased intake. Knowing the contributing factors directs the nurse toward identifying appropriate interventions. Table 1-1 provides an example of the diagnostic process.

This text includes information in each chapter that identifies nursing diagnoses that are related to the interventions and skills for that chapter. This information includes a description of the diagnostic statement, related factors that may be pertinent, and the focus for related nursing care. By reviewing this information, the reader is able to compare applicable data and determine which diagnosis would best communicate a client's particular needs.

Table 1-1 **Example of the Diagnostic Process**

Inspection of skin	Open lesion on sacrum 1 × 1 cm	Pressure on coccyx	
	Red area 3 × 3 cm around coccyx		
Palpation of skin	Skin moist from diaphoresis	Skin moisture promotes breakdown	
	Tenderness noted around lesion		**Impaired Skin Integrity** related to immobility secondary to traction manifested by 1 × 1 cm tender lesion, redness on coccyx, and moist skin with diaphoresis
Historical data	Fractured left leg on 5/3	Immobility	
	Positioned on back for traction to leg for 2 weeks; anticipate 4 more weeks minimum		

GOALS AND EXPECTED OUTCOMES

Goals and expected outcomes are specific statements of client behaviors or responses that the nurse anticipates from nursing care. Each must be realistic, observable, client centered, and mutually set with the client. Goals reflect the client's highest level of wellness. Expected outcomes are specific, step-by-step achievements that help the client achieve the goals of care and resolution of the etiology for the nursing diagnosis. Expected outcomes must be measurable and specify a time frame. An example of an expected outcome is as follows: Client will demonstrate insulin self-injection by 3/20. At the time specified, progress toward achievement is evaluated, and if necessary, the plan of care is revised. For the purpose of this text, outcomes will be described behaviorally; to avoid redundancy, expected time frames will not be included.

NURSING INTERVENTIONS

Interventions need to be individualized to the client's needs. These include what, when, how much, how far, how long, how often, where, by whom, and with what. For example, "Encourage ambulation" is not adequate. Acceptable nursing interventions may include "Assist to walk to bathroom two times on 5/9"; "Assist to ambulate in hall at least 20 feet two times on 5/9"; and "Assist to ambulate 50 feet three times on 5/10."

EVALUATION

The nursing process is dynamic and continuous. Whether or not outcomes were achieved by the target date should be well documented. If not achieved, the interventions or expected outcomes should be revised. Often, changing the target date is all that is required. When expected outcomes are achieved, the goals of care are met and the nursing diagnosis can be documented as "resolved." Evidence of systematic evaluation of the nursing process is one of the standards of the Joint Commission on Accreditation of Healthcare Organizations (JCAHO, 1993).

Skill 1.1 | Standard Protocols for All Nursing Interventions

All nursing skills must include certain basic steps for the safety and well-being of the client and the nurse. To save space and prevent repetition, *these steps are not included in each skill unless it is necessary to clarify them as applied for that skill.* Remember that these steps are essential and must be followed to deliver appropriate and responsible nursing care.

When indicated, a logo is used to identify the need for **clean gloves.** Personnel wear clean, disposable gloves before contact with mucous membranes, nonintact skin, or moist body substances. The following logo indicates clean gloves are needed:

 Gloves are changed between clients and between activities with the same client when gloves become excessively soiled (Centers for Disease Control, CDC, 1992).

EQUIPMENT

Armband for client identification
Consent form (if required by agency policy)
Clean disposable gloves (if contact with body secretions or excretions is anticipated)

Implementation

Steps	Rationale
Before the skill	
1. Verify physician's orders if skill is a dependent or collaborative nursing intervention. Independent nursing interventions may be verified with the nursing care plan, Kardex, or primary nurse.	Dependent and collaborative interventions include most invasive procedures, such as medications and urinary catheterization. Check agency policy.
2. Identify client by checking armband and having client state name (if able to do so).	Armbands are standard for client identification in most agencies. Clients who have difficulty hearing or have an altered level of consciousness may answer to a name other than their own. Some agencies use arm-

Steps	Rationale
	bands to communicate special safety concerns, such as allergies.
3. Introduce yourself to client, including both name and title or role, and explain what you plan to do.	Clients have the right to know what will be done and by whom, as well as when those involved are students (*A Patient's Bill of Rights,* 1992; see box on pp. 7-8).
4. Explain the procedure and the reason it is to be done in terms client can understand.	Understanding what is being done enhances client's ability and willingness to cooperate. Client has the right to relevant, current, and understandable information (*A Patient's Bill of Rights,* 1992).
5. Assess client to determine that the intervention is still appropriate. (Each skill has an assessment section that includes appropriate specific findings.)	Clients have the right to make decisions about the plan of care before and during the course of treatment (*A Patient's Bill of Rights,* 1992).
6. Gather equipment and complete necessary charges.	Some equipment is reusable and is kept at the bedside. Some equipment is disposable and charged to the client as used. Check agency policy.
7. Wash hands for at least 10 seconds before each new client contact (see Skill 3.1 on p. 28).	Handwashing is the most important technique in prevention and control of the transmission of microorganisms (CDC, 1992).
8. Adjust the bed to appropriate height and lower side rail on the side nearest you.	This minimizes muscle strain on care givers and helps prevent injury and fatigue.
9. Provide privacy for client. Position and drape client as needed.	Respect for privacy is basic for preserving human dignity. Clients have the right to privacy (*A Patient's Bill of Rights,* 1992).
During the skill	
10. Promote client involvement if possible.	Participation enhances client motivation and cooperation.
11. Assess client tolerance, being alert for signs of discomfort and fatigue. Inability to tolerate a procedure is described in the nurses' notes.	Clients' ability to tolerate interventions varies depending on severity of illness and disability. Nurses need to use judgment in providing the opportunity for rest and comfort measures.
Completion protocol	
12. Assist client to a position of comfort, and place needed items within reach. Be certain client has a way to call for help and knows how to use it.	Clients may attempt to reach items and risk falling or injury.
13. Raise the side rails and lower the bed to the lowest position.	This minimizes the risk of clients getting out of bed unattended. Nursing judgment may allow alert cooperative clients to have side rails down during the day without risking injury. (See Chapter 4.)
14. Store or remove and dispose of soiled supplies and equipment.	See CDC guidelines for handling and disposal of contaminated supplies/equipment (see Chapter 3).
15. Wash your hands for at least 10 seconds after client contact and after removing gloves.	Wearing gloves does not eliminate the need to wash hands. Handwashing is the most important technique in prevention and control of the transmission of microorganisms (CDC, 1988).
16. Document client's response and expected or unexpected outcomes.	Quality documentation enhances continuity of nursing care.

A Patient's Bill of Rights

INTRODUCTION

Effective health care requires collaboration between patients and physicians and other health care professionals. Open and honest communication, respect for personal and professional values, and sensitivity to differences are integral to optimal patient care. As the setting for the provision of health services, hospitals must provide a foundation for understanding and respecting the rights and responsibilities of patients, their families, physicians, and other caregivers. Hospitals must ensure a health care ethic that respects the role of patients in decision making about treatment choices and other aspects of their care. Hospitals must be sensitive to cultural, racial, linguistic, religious, age, gender, and other differences, as well as the needs of persons with disabilities.

The American Hospital Association presents *A Patient's Bill of Rights* with the expectation that it will contribute to more effective patient care and be supported by the hospital on behalf of the institution, its medical staff, employees, and patients. The American Hospital Association encourages health care institutions to tailor this bill of rights to their patient community by translating and/or simplifying the language of this bill of rights as may be necessary to ensure that patients and their families understand their rights and responsibilities.

BILL OF RIGHTS*

1. The patient has the right to considerate and respectful care.

2. The patient has the right to and is encouraged to obtain from physicians and other direct caregivers relevant, current, and understandable information concerning diagnosis, treatment, and prognosis.

   Except in emergencies when the patient lacks decision-making capacity and the need for treatment is urgent, the patient is entitled to the opportunity to discuss and request information related to the specific procedures and/or treatments, the risks involved, the possible length of recuperation, and the medically reasonable alternatives and their accompanying risks and benefits.

   Patients have the right to know the identity of physicians, nurses, and others involved in their care, as well as when those involved are students, residents, or other trainees. The patient also has the right to know the immediate and long-term financial implications of treatment choices, insofar as they are known.

3. The patient has the right to make decisions about the plan of care prior to and during the course of treatment and to refuse a recommended treatment or plan of care to the extent permitted by law and hospital policy and to be informed of the medical consequences of this action. In case of such refusal, the patient is entitled to other appropriate care and services that the hospital provides or transfer to another hospital. The hospital should notify patients of any policy that might affect patient choice within the institution.

4. The patient has the right to have an advance directive (such as a living will, health care proxy, or durable power of attorney for health care) concerning treatment or designating a surrogate decision maker with the expectation that the hospital will honor the intent of that directive to the extent permitted by law and hospital policy.

   Health care institutions must advise patients of their rights under the state law and hospital policy to make informed medical choices, ask if the patient has an advance directive, and include that information in patient records. The patient has the right to timely information about hospital policy that may limit the hospital's ability to implement fully a legally valid advance directive.

5. The patient has the right to every consideration of privacy. Case discussion, consultation, examination, and treatment should be conducted so as to protect each patient's privacy.

6. The patient has the right to expect that all communications and records pertaining to care will be treated as confidential by the hospital, except in cases such as suspected abuse and public health hazards when reporting is permitted or required by law. The patient has the right to expect that the hospital will emphasize the confidentiality of this information when it releases it to any other parties entitled to review information in these records.

7. The patient has the right to review the records pertaining to medical care and to have the information explained or interpreted as necessary, except when restricted by law.

8. The patient has the right to expect that, within its capacity and policies, a hospital will make reasonable response to the request of a patient for appropriate and medically indicated care and services. The hospital must provide evaluation, service, and/or referral as indicated by the urgency of the case. When medically appropriate and legally permissible, or when a patient has so requested, a patient may be transferred to another facility. The institution to which the patient is to be transferred must first have accepted the patient for transfer. The patient must also have the benefit of complete information and explanation concerning the need for, risks, benefits, and alternatives to such a transfer.

9. The patient has the right to ask and be informed of the existence of business relationships among the hospital, educational institutions, other health care providers, or payors that may influence the patient's treatment and care.

10. The patient has the right to consent to or decline to participate in proposed research studies or human experimentation affecting care and treatment or requiring direct patient involvement, and to have those studies fully

---

A Patient's Bill of Rights was first adopted by the American Hospital Association (AHA) in 1973. This revision was approved by the AHA Board of Trustees on Oct. 21, 1992.

*These rights can be exercised on the patient's behalf by a designated surrogate or proxy decision maker if the patient lacks decision-making capacity, is legally incompetent, or is a minor.

Continued.

A Patient's Bill of Rights—cont'd

explained prior to consent. A patient who declines to participate in research or experimentation is entitled to the most effective care that the hospital can otherwise provide.

11. The patient has the right to expect reasonable continuity of care when appropriate and to be informed by physicians and other caregivers of available and realistic patient care options when hospital care is no longer appropriate.

12. The patient has the right to be informed of hospital policies and practices that relate to patient care, treatment, and responsibilities. The patient has the right to be informed of available resources for resolving disputes, grievances, and conflicts, such as ethics committees, patient representatives, or other mechanisms available in the institution. The patient has the right to be informed of the hospital's charges for services and available payment methods.

The collaborative nature of health care requires that patients, or their families/ surrogates, participate in their care. The effectiveness of care and patient satisfaction with the course of treatment depend, in part, on the patient fulfilling certain responsibilities. Patients are responsible for providing information about past illnesses, hospitalizations, medications, and other matters related to health status. To participate effectively in decision making, patients must be encouraged to take responsibility for requesting additional information or clarification about their health status or treatment

when they do not fully understand information and instructions. Patients are also responsible for ensuring that the health care institution has a copy of their written advance directive if they have one. Patients are responsible for informing their physicians and other caregivers if they anticipate problems in following prescribed treatment.

Patients should also be aware of the hospital's obligation to be reasonably efficient and equitable in providing care to other patients and the community. The hospital's rules and regulations are designed to help the hospital meet this obligation. Patients and their families are responsible for making reasonable accommodations to the needs of the hospital, other patients, medical staff, and hospital employees. Patients are responsible for providing necessary information for insurance claims and for working with the hospital to make payment arrangements, when necessary.

A person's health depends on much more than health care services. Patients are responsible for recognizing the impact of their life-style on their personal health.

CONCLUSION

Hospitals have many functions to perform, including the enhancement of health status, health promotion, and the prevention and treatment of injury and disease; the immediate and ongoing care and rehabilitation of patients; the education of health professionals, patients, and the community; and research. All these activities must be conducted with an overriding concern for the values and dignity of patients.

Evaluation

Evaluation involves comparing the client's actual behavior after the nursing intervention with the behavior or response identified in each expected outcome using the specified time frame.

UNEXPECTED OUTCOMES AND RELATED INTERVENTIONS

In some instances the client may not achieve expected outcomes. Each intervention or skill describes common unexpected outcomes and possible interventions to initiate in response to that response or failure to respond.

SAMPLE DOCUMENTATION

Each skill includes guidelines for evaluation and information about unexpected outcomes. Sample documentation gives examples of subjective or objective data. Some routine skills are recorded on a flow sheet using a symbol or check mark. Sample flow sheets are shown in the Physical Care/Activity form in Appendix A.

DOCUMENTATION GUIDELINES

Clients depend on care givers to communicate with one another to ensure that the best quality of care is delivered. All health care team members need certain information about clients to ensure a caring, organized, and effective plan of care (see Plan of Care [POC], Appendix A). Unless the client's needs are communicated effectively, care becomes fragmented and tasks can be repeated, delayed, or omitted. Records and reports communicate specific information about a client's health care so that interventions are directed toward the client's maximum recovery (Figure 1-2).

Documentation and reporting by nurses must meet standards of quality to ensure that information is accurate, thorough, and complete. Regulatory agencies such as departments of health and the JCAHO establish standards for nurses and other health care providers to monitor and evaluate the quality and appropriateness of client care. These standards often can be measured only by the content of written records. Thus, nurses must

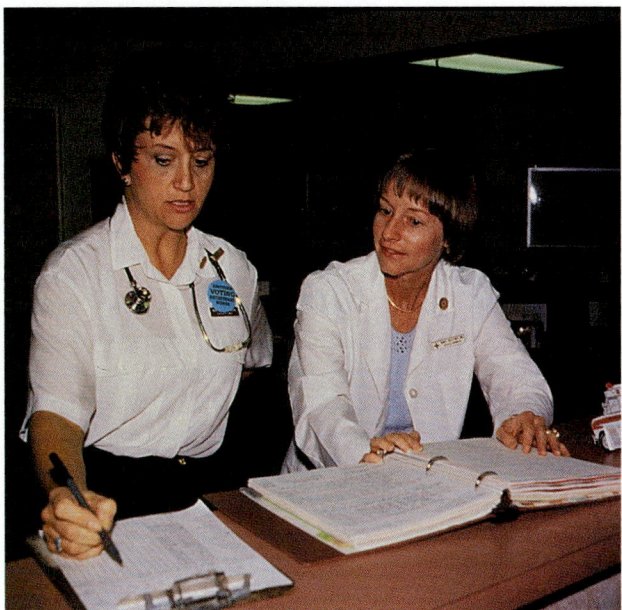

Figure 1-2 Accurate communication between nurses is essential.

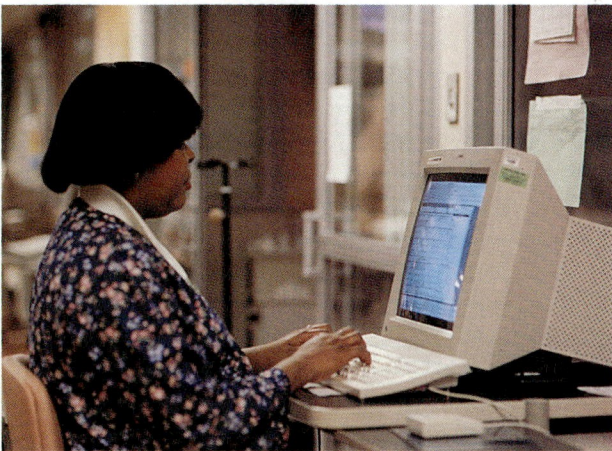

Figure 1-3 Data entry using computer keyboard.

learn to document information following the recommendations of various regulatory groups. Under the prospective payment system, hospitals are reimbursed a set dollar amount by Medicare for each diagnosis-related group (DRG). This same payment system is used by other third party payors. For hospitals to validate the costs involved in the care of clients, it is important for nurses to document accurately any procedures or therapies performed. Finally, the medical record is a legal document. Nurses are accountable for their actions, and as a result, information in the record must be clear and logical, exactly describing all care delivered.

COORDINATING NURSING INTERVENTIONS

The nurse spends more time with clients than most other members of the health care team and therefore has the best perspective for a holistic approach needed in a client's health care. The nurse coordinates the many resources required to ensure a smooth transition from the hospital to the home. The processes of admission and discharge involve simultaneous and continuous planning. The nurse identifies the client's health care needs and physical and psychological deficits that have implications for resuming normal activities, involves family members in a plan of care, provides for health education, and assists in having health care resources made available both in the hospital and at home. Ultimately, the client and family need to be prepared to assume the responsibilities for continued care in the home setting.

Discharge planning conferences often involve mem-

bers of several disciplines (e.g., nursing, social work, physical therapy) meeting to discuss the client's progress toward discharge goals. Consultations are a form of discussion whereby one professional care giver provides another with formal advice about the care of a client. For example, a dietitian may consult with the nurse on the best foods to meet a client's preferences and dietary restrictions. Consultations and conferences are documented in a client's record so that all care givers benefit from the information and can plan the client's care accordingly.

THE MEDICAL RECORD

A medical record is a permanent written description of a client's health status and needs, as well as information relevant to a client's care management. Good documentation reflects not only quality of care, but also evidence of each health care team member's accountability in giving care. The purpose of a record is to provide information for communication, education, assessment, research, financial billing, auditing, and legal accountability.

COMPUTERIZED DOCUMENTATION

The computerization of charting has become one of the strongest trends in nursing documentation (Iyer and Camp, 1991) (Figure 1-3). Data can be entered into the computer using a light pen, a touch-sensitive screen, a keyboard, or a mouse. Technology is being developed that utilizes voice recognition and enters data in response to the spoken word. Data may be entered by filling in blanks, constructing sentences, or selecting from a menu. Computer terminals may be at the nurses' station, at the bedside, or in both locations. The ideal system would permit the following functions:

- Automatic entry of information from intravenous pumps and cardiac monitors

> ## Guidelines for Effective Documentation
>
> Factual: includes descriptive, objective, and pertinent subjective data
> Accurate: uses precise terms that facilitate comparisons
> Complete: includes significant data and describes progress toward wellness
> Concise: eliminates unnecessary words and repeating information
> Current: entries are made as soon as possible after completed
> Organized: sequence of events is readily apparent

- Documentation of vital signs, intake and output, and medications
- Integrated flow sheets, care plans, progress notes, and physician's orders
- Patient acuity, classification, and quality assurance activities
- Information for client education

Because the nursing process shapes a nurse's approach and direction of care, good documentation reflects the nursing process. Assessment results are recorded to offer to all health care members a data base from which to draw conclusions about the client's problems. Information describing the client's concerns or condition assists care givers to choose an appropriate care plan. Evaluation of client responses to nursing care determines the client's success in achieving expected outcomes of care.

Nurses involved in the direct care of clients are responsible for recording thorough assessments of a client's condition, descriptions of changes in a client's condition, a detailed accounting of nursing interventions, and an evaluation of the client's response to care. Various methods are used for nursing progress notes. Regardless of the method, certain basic guidelines must be followed (see box above).

GUIDELINES FOR EFFECTIVE DOCUMENTATION AND REPORTING

Factual information is **objective** information about what a nurse sees, hears, feels, and smells. An objective description (e.g., "Respirations 14 per minute, regular, with clear breath sounds bilaterally") is the result of direct observation and measurement. Words that are only meaningful within a specific frame of reference, such as good, adequate, fair, or poor, are subject to interpretation and should be avoided. **Inferences** are conclusions based on data. For example, an inference might be, "The client has a poor appetite." The factual data is, "The client ate only two bites of dessert and the bread from the supper tray."

Suppose that in one case the client was nauseated, whereas in another case the client was hungry but did not like the food on the tray. If nurses document inferences or conclusions without supportive factual data, misinterpretations about the client's health status occur.

Subjective data include clients' perceptions about their health problems. Documentation using the client's words in quotes, for example: The client states she is "nauseated" or The client states she "does not like the food choices," is factual and acceptable. In both cases, it would be helpful to document the actual food intake as well as the subjective data.

Accurate documentation uses reliable, precise measurements as a means to determine when a client's condition has changed. Charting that an "abdominal wound is 5 cm in length, without redness or edema" is more accurate and descriptive than "large abdominal wound is healing well." To avoid misunderstandings, use only approved agency abbreviations and write out all terms that may be confusing. For example, o.d. (once daily) could be misinterpreted to mean OD (right eye). Correct spelling is essential, since terms can easily be misinterpreted (e.g., accept or except, dysphagia or dysphasia). When observations are reported to another care giver and interventions are performed by someone else, clearly indicate that fact (e.g., "Surgical dressings removed by Dr. Kline. Pulse of 104 reported to J. Kemp, R.N."). End each entry with first name or first initial, last name, and title. Nursing students include the approved abbreviation for the school and level.

Complete and concise information is essential. Consider the following example.

A nurse does not document or report the teaching session about giving insulin injections. During the next shift, another nurse spends time assessing Mrs. Blake's learning needs because the previous teaching was not communicated. Time is wasted, and Mrs. Blake becomes frustrated with the unnecessary repetition.

A comparison of a concise and lengthy note follows:

Concise, factual entry	Lengthy entry using vague terms
0900 L toes cool and pale; capillary return > 5 sec; L pedal pulse 1+; R pedal pulse 4+. Describes pain as dull, aching 4 (scale 0-10).	0900 The client's left toes are cool with color pale. There is no inflammation. There is slow capillary return present exceeding 5 seconds. Dorsalis pedis pulse in left foot is weak, and the client complains of some discomfort. The pain is described as aching at a level of 4 on a scale of 0-10.

To be current, the following activities or findings need to be communicated at the time of occurrence:

1. Critical changes in vital signs
2. Administration of medications and treatments

Table 1-2 **Comparison of Military and Civilian Times**

Military	Civilian
0100	1:00 AM
0200	2:00 AM
0415	4:15 AM
1200	Noon
1420	2:20 PM
1800	6:00 PM
2400	Midnight
0001	12:01 AM

3. Preparation for diagnostic tests or surgery
4. Critical change in status
5. Admission, transfer, discharge, or death of a client

Refer to the client's concern, nursing interventions provided, and client response as soon as possible after the occurrence. Writing scratch notes at the time of the event helps ensure accuracy in documentation. Many agencies use military time, a 24-hour system that uses digit numbers to indicate morning and afternoon and evening times (Table 1-2).

The following compares a well-organized note with a disorganized note:

Organized note	Disorganized note
7/17 0630 Client reports sharp pain 9 (scale 0-10) in left lower quadrant of abdomen, worsened by turning onto right side. Positioning on left side decreases pain to 8 (scale 0-10). Abdomen is tender to touch and rigid. Bowel sounds are absent. Dr. Phillips notified. To x-ray for CT scan of abdomen. T. Reis, R.N.	7/17 0630 Client experiencing sharp pain in lower quadrant of abdomen. MD notified. Abdomen tender to touch, rigid, with bowel sounds absent. Positioning on left side offers minimal relief of pain. CT scan ordered of the abdomen. J Adams, R.N.

CONFIDENTIALITY

Nurses are legally and ethically obligated to keep information about clients confidential. When health care professionals have reason to use records for data gathering, research, or education, there is no break in confidentiality as long as the records are used with permission and according to established guidelines.

RECORD-KEEPING FORMS

Agencies use a variety of forms to make medical record documentation easy and quick yet comprehensive. Many forms eliminate the need to duplicate repeated data in the nursing notes. The forms present special types of information in a format more accessible than the compila-

---

Medical Record Documentation Forms

NURSING HISTORY FORMS

Completed when a client is admitted to a nursing unit. Includes basic biographic data (e.g., age, method of admission, physician), admitting medical diagnosis or chief complaint, a brief medical-surgical history (e.g., previous surgeries or illnesses, allergies, medication history, client's perceptions about illness or hospitalization, physical assessment of all body systems). Encourages a systematic complete assessment and identification of relevant nursing diagnoses. Provides baseline data to compare with changes in the client's condition. The JCAHO (1993) requires a nursing assessment be completed for each client at the time of admission to a health care agency.

GRAPHIC SHEETS AND FLOW SHEETS

Include routine observations on a repeated basis using a check mark (e.g., when bath is given, client is turned). When completing a flow sheet, the nurse should review previous entries to identify changes.

COMPUTERIZED PATIENT CARE SUMMARY (see Patient Care Summary, Appendix A)

Includes pertinent information about clients and their ongoing care plans, such as the following:
1. Basic demographic data (e.g., age, physician's name, religion)
2. Primary medical diagnosis
3. Current physician's orders to be carried out routinely
4. Nursing orders or interventions
5. Scheduled tests or procedures
6. Safety precautions to be used in the client's care
7. Factors related to activities of daily living

---

tion of all progress notes. Most of the forms are self-explanatory as to the type of information required from the nurse (see box above). Sample forms are included in Appendix A.

HOME HEALTH CARE DOCUMENTATION

The current trend in health care is toward providing care in the home setting. Clients are being hospitalized primarily for acute care. More complex and technical skilled home care services are available. Medicare has specific guidelines for establishing eligibility for home care reimbursement. To fulfill Medicare guidelines, documentation by home health care nurses must clearly describe the client's health status, level of nursing care required, and the interventions needed.

Clients need home health care if they have limited mobility or are blind, senile, or otherwise unable to go out unassisted (Magliozzi, 1990). Activity restrictions after discharge also qualify clients for homebound status.

The nurse documents the extent to which clients remain homebound throughout the period that visits are made. The potential for complications after discharge can also make clients eligible for home care reimbursement for 3 weeks after discharge. The nurse documents how potential problems are linked to the primary condition (Magliozzi, 1990). When clients require skilled care, such as tasks performed or supervised by a registered nurse, Medicare will pay for home health care services. The following criteria distinguish skilled care from unskilled care:

1. The client's condition is such that significant changes may occur that would require the evaluation skills of a professional nurse.
2. The client requires direct service that employs the knowledge, skills, and judgment of a professional nurse (e.g., injections, catheter irrigations, ostomy care, bladder training, intravenous therapy, long-term airway management).
3. The client and primary care provider (spouse, family member) require teaching to perform appropriate services and observations.

In home care, good documentation is the key to reimbursement (see box below).

Guidelines for Home Care Documentation

NURSING INTERVENTIONS

Include pertinent information relating to care provided (e.g., injection, catheterization, ostomy care, intravenous therapy).

MEDICATIONS INSTRUCTION

Include action and side effects of one medication per visit. Include name of medication, action, and side effects of each medication as it is taught. Document client's or primary care giver's knowledge level after instruction. Provide written instructions (in large print if necessary).

DISEASE PROCESS INSTRUCTION

Include signs and symptoms of the primary medical diagnoses (e.g., anatomy and physiology, effect of disease on the normal body, treatment regimen). Document client's or care giver's knowledge level.

DIET INSTRUCTION

Identify menu plan taught. Indicate written material provided to client and primary care giver. Document client's or primary care giver's knowledge level.

ACTIVITY INSTRUCTION

Include activities of daily living, passive range of motion (ROM), cane ambulation, walker-assisted ambulation, non–weight bearing, ambulation with assistance. Document client's or primary care giver's knowledge level.

CHANGE-OF-SHIFT REPORT

After completing a work shift, nurses give a verbal or taped report to nurses on the next shift or conduct rounds at the client's bedside. The purpose of the report is to provide better continuity of care among nurses caring for a client. When clients see different nurses performing care in the same manner, their trust in the care givers increases.

Oral reports are given in conference rooms, with staff from both shifts participating. If an audiotape is used, it is prepared by the nurse who has completed care for the client and left for the nurse on the next shift to review. Taped reports can improve efficiency by allowing staff to report when time is available. Reports given in person or during rounds permit nurses to obtain immediate feedback when questions are raised about the client's care. Content of the report includes a detailed description of the client's progress during the shift, using a systematic approach:

1. *Background information.* Include client's name, sex, age, medical diagnosis (or reason for admission), and brief medical history.
2. *Assessment data.* Provide objective observations and measurements made by nurse during the shift. Describe client's condition and stress any recent changes. Include any relevant information reported by client.
3. *Nursing diagnoses.* Identify the nursing diagnoses appropriate for client. Clarify client's current responses to health problems. As a nursing diagnosis is resolved, it is documented as such and need not be included in subsequent reports.
4. *Interventions and evaluation.* (Steps can be combined in a report.)
   a Describe interventions, including when, where, and client response.
   b Describe instructions given in teaching plan and client's ability to demonstrate learning. This facilitates reinforcement of teaching and promotes learning.
5. *Family information.* Report on family visitation or involvement, specifically as it influenced client. Describe family members' involvement in care procedures or instruction.
6. *Discharge plan.* Client's progress in reaching discharge is reviewed on an ongoing basis. The discharge plan identifies the interventions and outcomes needed to allow the client to have a smooth transition from hospital or health care facility to home.
7. *Current priorities.* Identify the priorities to which oncoming nurse must attend. This promotes organization and continuity of care.

INCIDENT REPORTS

A client, visitor, or employee may be at risk when anything unusual occurs in a health care area. Examples of incidents include a client fall, accidental needle stick injury, medication administration error, a visitor experiencing symptoms of illness, or carelessness in performance of a procedure that leads to actual or potential client injury. When an incident occurs, the nurse involved or the nurse who witnessed the incident completes an incident report. Reporting of incidents helps in the identification of high-risk trends in nursing care or daily unit operations that warrant correction. The report is necessary even when an injury is not apparent. The information from incident reports helps nursing staff find solutions to prevent repeated incidents. The reports are an important part of a unit's quality improvement program.

When witnessing an incident, note the sequence of events involved in the incident, including time and type of incident, injuries, and factors that may have contributed to the incident. If the incident involved an injury, take steps to restore the individual's safety. A priority is to stabilize any injury to prevent worsening of the individual's condition. The report must include objective, chronological information in the event the incident leads to a lawsuit or investigation into institutional policy and procedure. The nurse who witnessed the incident or who found the client at the time of the incident files the report. (See Patient/Visitor Incident Report, Appendix A.)

CRITICAL THINKING EXERCISES

1. Mary Rodriguez, 45 years old, is admitted to the hospital with complaints of abdominal discomfort, described as a "burning, gnawing" sensation, unrelieved by food. The pain often wakes her early in the morning. Admission data include Ht 5'2", Wt 174 lb, BP 140/90, P 100 & regular, R 16. Medical history includes gastric ulcer, hypertension, and mild obesity. Mary manages a Mexican restaurant, and a nutritional history reveals Mary's diet largely consists of foods characteristic of her culture. Dietary analysis indicates Mary's diet is lacking sufficient intake of fruits and vegetables and is excessive in fat intake (e.g., cheese, red meat). She eats sporadically and is usually in a hurry. Medications include an antihypertensive drug and Zantac. Mary states she frequently does not take either drug because she "usually feels fine."

   Below are several diagnostic statements generated from the above data. Identify cues and cluster them into groups that support or validate each nursing diagnosis.
   a. Acute Pain (Abdominal) r/t unknown factors, possible gastric ulcer flare-up secondary to drug/diet noncompliance
   b. Altered Nutrition: More Than Body Requirements r/t eating habits, excessive fats
   c. High Risk for Noncompliance r/t lack of knowledge of importance of taking antihypertensive drug regardless of lack of symptoms

2. Below are a number of nursing interventions. Distinguish between interventions that clearly describe the nursing action and those that do not. If the nursing order is vague or unclear, offer an alternative description.
   a. Encourage fluid intake.
   b. Turn, cough, and deep breathe q2h while awake.
   c. Monitor weight.
   d. Implement discharge teaching.
   e. Provide written instructions for follow-up visits.
   f. Have client demonstrate changing wound dressing.
   g. Monitor vital signs.
3. Differentiate between the following pieces of documentation, deciding whether each is subjective, objective, or inference.
   a. Client c/o headache.
   b. Client is fatigued.
   c. Client states hand is numb.
   d. Client is malnourished.
   e. Respirations are 20/minute.
   f. Client reports shortness of breath.
   g. Client has low self-esteem.
   h. Skin is cool and clammy.

REFERENCES

American Hospital Association: *A patient's bill of rights,* Catalog no 157759, Chicago, 1992, The Association.

American Nurses Association: *Nursing and social policy statement,* Kansas City, Mo, 1980, The Association.

Carroll-Johnson RM: Reflections on the ninth biennial conference, *Nursing Diagnosis 1990,* 1, 1990.

CDC: Surveillance, prevention, and control of nosocomial infections, *MMWR* 41:783, 1992.

CDC: Universal precautions for prevention of human immunodeficiency virus, hepatitis B virus, and other blood-borne pathogens in health care settings, *MMWR* 37:377, 1988.

Gordon M: *Manual of nursing diagnosis,* St Louis, 1991, Mosby.

Iyer PW, Camp, NH: *Nursing documentation: a nursing process approach,* St Louis, 1991, Mosby.

Joint Commission on Accreditation of Healthcare Organizations: *Accreditation manual for hospitals,* Chicago, 1993, The Commission.

Magliozzi HM: Charting that makes it through the Medicare maze, *RN* 53:75, 1990.

McCloskey JC, Bulechek GM: *Nursing interventions classification (NIC): Iowa intervention project,* St Louis, 1992, Mosby.

ADDITIONAL READINGS

Ebersole P, Hess P: *Toward healthy aging: human needs and nursing response,* ed 4, St Louis, 1995, Mosby.

Edelstein J: A study of nursing documentation, *Nurs Manage* 21:40, 1990.

Kim MJ, McFarland GK, McLane AM: *Pocket guide to nursing diagnosis,* ed 5, St Louis, 1993, Mosby.

Lewis SM, Collier IC: *Medical surgical nursing: assessment and management of clinical problems,* ed 3, St Louis, 1992, Mosby.

Miller P, Pastorino C: Daily nursing documentation can be quick and thorough, *Nurs Manage* 20(11):47, 1990.

Naylor M: Comprehensive discharge planning for hospitalized elderly: a pilot study, *Nurs Res* 39(3):156, 1990.

Weber G: Making nursing diagnosis work for you and your client: a step by step approach, *Nurs Health Care* 12:8, 1991.

chapter 2

Facilitating Communication

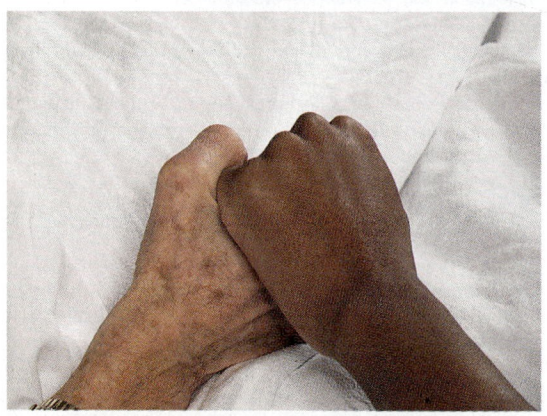

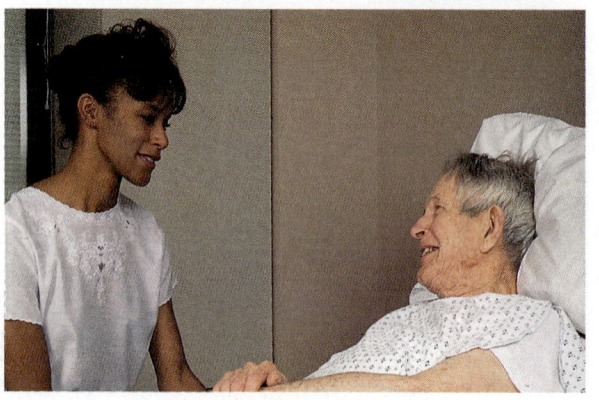

Skill 2.1
Promoting Psychological Comfort

Skill 2.2
Active Listening

Skill 2.3
Interviewing

Communication is a basic human need and the foundation for establishing a caring relationship between the nurse and the client. Each interaction is an opportunity to achieve a positive relationship and shared understanding that results in attainment of mutual goals. Nurses listen, speak, and take action to negotiate change that promotes the client's well-being.

Nurses show caring by accepting clients for who they are and respecting them as individuals. When clients feel cared for, they feel secure. Caring promotes trust and decreased anxiety, which increases the body's defenses and helps promote comfort and healing.

Therapeutic communication is not casual. It is a planned, deliberate, professional act. Nurses participate in social conversation at the beginning of an interaction to lay the foundation for developing a relationship. With practice, nurses can develop skills that limit social interactions and maintain a congenial and warm style that helps clients feel comfortable in sharing ideas and feelings.

The basic elements of communication include a message, a sender, a receiver, and feedback (Figure 2-1). The message is the information expressed, which can be motivated by experience, emotions, ideas, or actions. The message may be sent through visual, auditory, and tactile senses. Generally, the more channels used, the better the message is understood.

For communication to be effective, the receiver must be aware of the sender's message. The message received is understood as filtered through perceptions shaped from previous experiences. Feedback, verbal or nonverbal, is a response to the sender that can indicate the

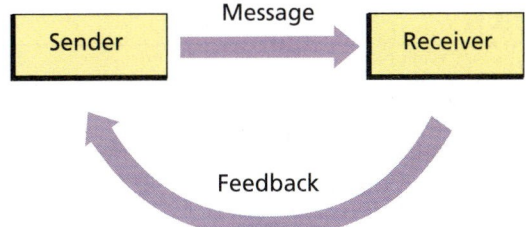

Figure 2-1 Communication is a two-way process.

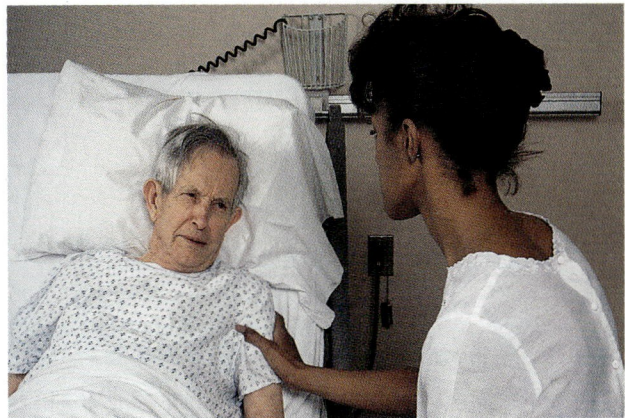

Figure 2-2 Clarify nonverbal body language.

Factors That Influence Communication

Perceptions: personal views based on past experiences

Values: beliefs a person considers important in life

Emotions: subjective feelings about a situation (e.g., anger, fear, frustration, pain, anxiety, personal appearance)

Sociocultural background: language, gestures, and attitudes common for a specific group of people relating to family origin, occupation, or lifestyle

Knowledge level: level of education and experience that influences a person's knowledge base

Roles and relationships: conversation between two nurses differs from that between nurse and client

Environment: noise, lack of privacy, and distractions influence effectiveness

Space and territoriality: distance of 18 inches to 4 feet is ideal for sitting with a client for an interaction. Clients may have different needs for personal space

meaning of the message that was received. The intent to communicate is not sufficient to ensure accurate reception of a message. Nurses need to give and seek feedback that validates understanding of messages given and received in interactions with clients.

Communication is a complex process that is influenced by many factors (see box above). Each person is unique and associates different ideas with a message and interprets it differently than any other person. For example, a facial expression may convey anger to one person and pain to another. It is essential for nurses to clarify messages so that incorrect inferences and miscommunication with the client are avoided (Figure 2-2).

Silence can be a therapeutic experience. It allows the nurse and client time to think. It is important for the nurse to notice inner feelings. It is also important to pay attention to a client's nonverbal behavior for cues that suggest what the client is feeling and to reflect the nurse's impressions to validate what the client is experiencing. If silence lasts too long or becomes uncomfortable for the client, it can be helpful to say, "You seem very quiet," or "Could you tell me what you need right now?" or "How are you feeling?"

Preoccupation with the techniques of communica-

tion can interfere rather than enhance the process; however, effective communication can be learned and requires practice, as does any other skill. An attitude of acceptance is helpful to promote open communication. To listen effectively, it helps to face clients, maintain eye contact, pay attention to what is being conveyed, and give feedback to verify accurate understanding. Even though the nurse may not agree with clients, the nurse can accept clients' rights to their opinions. It is better to avoid arguing with clients. The nurse simply reflects an understanding of what clients are communicating without agreeing or disagreeing. Ineffective communication may not halt conversation, but it tends to inhibit clients' willingness to express concerns openly. The nurse needs to find an appropriate place, allow sufficient time, and facilitate communication according to clients' circumstances and needs. Table 2-1 summarizes techniques that facilitate communication and lists factors that inhibit communication.

It is important to recognize cultural diversity and to demonstrate respect for people as unique individuals. Culture is just one factor that influences communication between two persons. Nurses need to adopt an attitude of flexibility, respect, and interest to bridge any communication barriers imposed by cultural differences.

If a client does not speak the nurse's language, a translator is needed. Often, however, the client speaks the nurse's language with limited ability or uses language with meaning different from the nurse's meaning. For example, the client may know customary greetings such as "How are you?" but not understand "pain" or "nausea." When communication fails, nurses tend to speak louder, stop talking and concentrate on the tasks, or begin doing things for, rather than with, the client. This can result in

Table 2-1 **Facilitating and Inhibiting Communication**

Technique	Examples	Rationale
INITIATING AND ENCOURAGING INTERACTION		
Giving information	"It is time for me to …" "I will be here until …"	Informs client of facts needed to understand situation. Provides a means to build trust and develop a knowledge base for client to make decisions.
Stating observations	"You are smiling." "I see you are up already."	By calling client's attention to what is observed, nurse encourages client to be aware of behavior.
Open questions/ comments	"What is your biggest concern?" "Tell me about your health."	Allows client to choose the topic of discussion according to circumstances and needs.
General leads	"And then?" "Go on …" "Say more …"	Encourages client to continue talking.
Focused questions/ comments	"Tell me about your pain." "What did your doctor say?" "How has your family reacted?" "What is your biggest fear?"	Encourages client to give more information about specific topic of concern.
HELPING CLIENT IDENTIFY AND EXPRESS FEELINGS		
Sharing observations	"You look tense." "You seem uncomfortable when …"	Promotes client's awareness of nonverbal behavior and feelings underlying the behavior. Helps clarify meaning of the behavior.
Paraphrasing	Client: "I could not sleep last night." Nurse: "You've had trouble sleeping?"	Encourages client to describe the situation more fully. Demonstrates that nurse is listening and concerned.
Reflecting feelings	"You were angry when that happened?" "You seem upset …"	Focuses client on identified feelings based on verbal or nonverbal cues.
Focused comments	"That seems worth talking about more." "Tell me more about …"	Encourages client to think about and describe a particular concern in more detail.
ENSURING MUTUAL UNDERSTANDING		
Seeking clarification	"I don't quite follow you …" "Do you mean …?" "Are you saying that …?"	Encourages client to expand on a topic that is not yet clear or that seems contradictory.
Summarizing	"So there are three things you are upset about, your family being too busy, your diet, and being in the hospital so long."	Reduces the interaction to three or four points identified by nurse as significant. Allows client to agree or add other concerns.
Validation	"Did I understand you correctly that …?"	Allows clarification of ideas that nurse may have interpreted differently than intended by client.
INHIBITING COMMUNICATION		
"Why" questions	"Why did you eat that when you know it gives you stomach pain?" "Why did you go back to bed?"	Asks client to justify reasons. Implies criticism and makes client feel defensive. Better to focus on what happened and encourage telling the whole story.
Sidestepping or changing subject	Client: "I'm having a hard time with my family." Nurse: "Do you have any grandchildren?"	This eases nurse's own discomfort. It avoids exploring topic identified by client.
False reassurance	"Everything will be okay." "Surgery is no big deal."	This is vague and simplistic and tends to belittle client's concerns. It does not invite a response.
Giving advice	"You really should exercise more." "You shouldn't eat fast food every day."	This keeps client from actively engaging in finding a solution. Often client knows what should/should not be done and needs to explore alternative ways of dealing with issue.
Stereotyped responses	"You have the best doctor in town." "All clients with cancer worry about that."	This does not invite client to respond.
Defensiveness	"The nurses here work very hard." "Your doctor is extremely busy."	Moves focus away from client's feelings without acknowledging concerns.

Special Approaches for Client Who Speaks a Different Language

Use a caring tone of voice and facial expression to help alleviate the client's fears.

Speak slowly and distinctly, but not loudly.

Use gestures, pictures, and play acting to help the client understand.

Repeat the message in different ways if necessary.

Be alert to words the client seems to understand and use them frequently.

Keep messages simple and repeat them frequently.

Avoid using medical terms that the client may not understand.

Use an appropriate language dictionary or have interpreter or family make flash cards to communicate key phrases.

Modified from Giger J, Davidhizar R: *Transcultural nursing,* St Louis, 1991, Mosby.

Communication Aids

Pad and felt-tipped pen or magic slate

Board with words, letters, or pictures denoting basic needs (e.g., water, bedpan, pain medication)

Call bells or alarms

Sign language

Use of eye blinks or movement of fingers for simple responses (e.g., "yes" or "no")

Flash cards with pictures rather than words

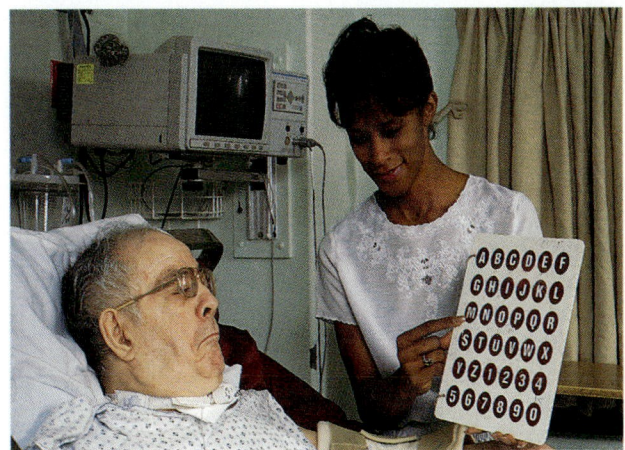

Figure 2-3 Tracheostomy interferes with speech.

painful isolation, anger, or misunderstanding and inability to cooperate. Special approaches that can help avoid these outcomes have been described (see box above).

Older adults with sensory losses require communication techniques that maximize existing sensory and motor functions (see Chapter 35). Some clients are unable to speak because of physical or neurological alterations, such as paralysis, a tube in the trachea to facilitate breathing (Figure 2-3), or a stroke resulting in aphasia. When a client experiences receptive aphasia, neither the sounds of speech nor its meaning can be distinguished, and comprehension of both written and spoken language is impaired. Expressive aphasia affects the motor function of speech so that the client has difficulty speaking and writing; however, the client can hear and understand. Communication aids can facilitate communication (see box above, right).

Nursing Diagnosis

Communication is a basic human need. **Impaired Verbal Communication** is the state in which an individual experiences a decreased or absent ability to use or understand language in human interaction (Kim, McFarland, and McLane, 1993). Difficulty communicating may be related to language barriers, altered hearing or speech, or psychological factors such as fear or anger. **Anxiety** or **Ineffective Individual Coping** may be an appropriate diagnosis when the focus is to help a client deal with a crisis. **Social Isolation** may be appropriate if the client is experiencing loneliness and inability to enjoy satisfying personal relationships.

Skill 2.1 Promoting Psychological Comfort

I t is quite common for a nurse to encounter a client who needs comfort and support while experiencing threatening situations. A newly diagnosed illness, separation from family, the discomfort of surgery or diagnostic and treatment procedures, grief, and loss are just a few examples of health-related situations that may require this skill.

Assessment

1. Observe interactions between client and others in the environment, including family or persons who provide the support system.

2. Identify medications that may alter speech. **Medications such as antidepressants, antipsychotics,**

or sedatives may cause a client to slur words or use incomplete sentences.

3. Identify body language that conveys positive or negative responses.

Planning

Expected outcomes focus on helping clients and families communicate effectively.

Implementation

EXPECTED OUTCOMES

1. Client verbalizes feelings regarding identified threat or concern.
2. Client identifies factors that provide support and comfort.
3. Client contacts one or more support systems.

Steps	Rationale
1. Provide a private, quiet, and calm environment.	Environmental factors can promote open communication.
2. Acknowledge and respond to physical discomfort by positioning, medication, or other comfort measures. Consider individual preferences and expressed needs.	Physical discomfort, difficulty breathing, or pain interferes with communication.
3. Use physical attending to convey interest by maintaining eye contact and using open, relaxed posture.	
4. Convey acceptance without judgment. Avoid facial expressions or gestures that suggest disapproval.	Acceptance is not the same as agreement but is a willingness to hear the person without conveying doubt or disagreement.
5. Provide empathy, which involves a sensitive and accurate awareness of client's feelings.	Empathy helps clients explain and explore their feelings so that problem solving might occur.
6. Remain centered on the current concern. Avoid introducing new information.	Clients may be overwhelmed by additional information. Talking about self, other people, or events shifts the focus away from clients.
7. Guide client's description of the situation to include what happened, thoughts about the experience, and feelings about the experience (e.g., "What happened then?" "How did you feel after that?").	This assists the process of clarifying the experience.
8. Communicate understanding by repeating what you understand the message to be (e.g., "I understand you . . . .," "I hear you saying . . . ," "I sense that . . .").	Communicating understanding tends to decrease the intensity of feelings.
9. Use open questions to explore possible alternatives.	Open questions cannot be answered by "yes" or "no" and encourage expression of ideas or thoughts.
10. Offer honest reassurance to the extent possible (e.g., that someone cares, that there is hope, that client is not alone) (Figure 2-4).	

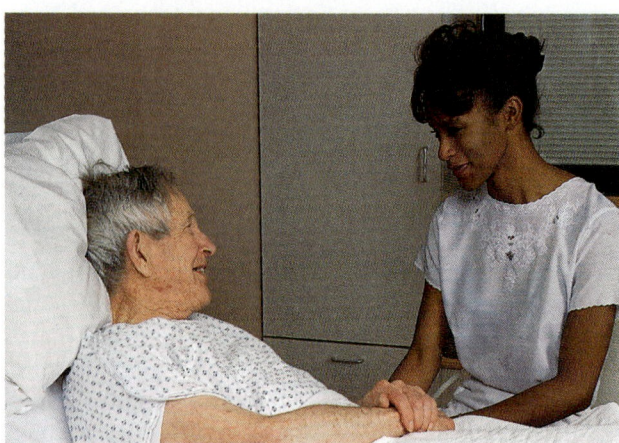

Figure 2-4

Evaluation

1. Observe client's response (body language, verbal statements) after discussion of feelings and circumstances that have been identified.
2. Ask for feedback about effectiveness of support and comfort provided.
3. Ask in what way support systems are expected to become available and helpful.

UNEXPECTED OUTCOMES AND RELATED INTERVENTIONS

1. Client is unable or unwilling to express feelings or circumstances.
   a. Consider the level of trust that has been established. If appropriate, facilitate greater level of trust in relation to other matters, such as providing for physical needs.
   b. Respect client's need, and offer opportunity to discuss the situation at another time or with another person.

2. Client expresses continued anger or discontent with alternatives available.
   a. Suggest taking more time to explore possibilities.
   b. Avoid telling client how to feel or what to think.
   c. Acknowledge and name the expressed feelings.
3. Client is unable to identify family or friends that can provide support. Family is too far away or estranged and unwilling to become involved.
   a. Identify community resources that may be helpful (e.g., church, neighbors, support groups).
   b. Facilitate a telephone support system.

SAMPLE DOCUMENTATION

1900 Client states, "The doctor said I have months, not years to live." She and her family have talked about this. Tearful when stating her son is on his way from out of state to see her today because he is worried about her. Talked about wanting to be able to finish a quilt for her daughter, but not having felt well enough to work on it lately. Requested to talk more about this later because this conversation was helpful.

Skill 2.2 | Active Listening

Active listening is one of the most effective ways to facilitate communication. It conveys interest in the client's needs, concerns, and problems and requires complete attention to understand the entire verbal and nonverbal message. A synonym for active listening is **empathy.** Empathy is the act of communicating to other persons that we have understood their feelings and what makes them feel that way. This requires acceptance of the individual in need of help. Once people know they have been understood and accepted, they do not have to struggle to explain or justify their reactions (Smith, 1992).

Listening techniques are learned behaviors. At first they seem awkward and time consuming, and as with any skill, become more comfortable with practice. It is essential that the nurse appear natural, relaxed, and at ease while listening.

Assessment

1. Assess patterns of communication with care givers:
   a. Does client initiate conversation and ask appropriate questions?
   b. Does body language support and complement the verbal message?
   c. Does client talk excessively and control the topic of conversation?
   d. Does client avoid expressing feelings or thoughts and confine conversation to necessary facts?

Awareness of communication patterns facilitates planning for the interaction.
2. Identify sensory and neurological factors that affect the client's ability to communicate. **Altered vision or hearing or expressive aphasia (in which words cannot be formed or expressed) or receptive aphasia (in which language is not understood) interferes with communication.**
3. Identify cultural influences that affect communication (Giger and Davidhizar, 1991). What language does client predominantly use in thinking? Does client need an interpreter? Is client able to read and/or write in English? What verbal or nonverbal communication shows respect (e.g., tempo, eye/body contact, topic restrictions)?

Planning

The expected outcomes focus on achieving clear understanding of client's communication.

EXPECTED OUTCOMES

1. Client demonstrates comfort and willingness to communicate, stating that the nurse is listening to identified needs.
2. Client verbalizes a sense of feeling understood.

Implementation

Steps	Rationale
1. Use physical attending to convey interest by sitting within 4 feet of client, maintaining eye contact, and using open, relaxed posture (arms and legs not crossed).	This nonverbal language conveys interest and concern.

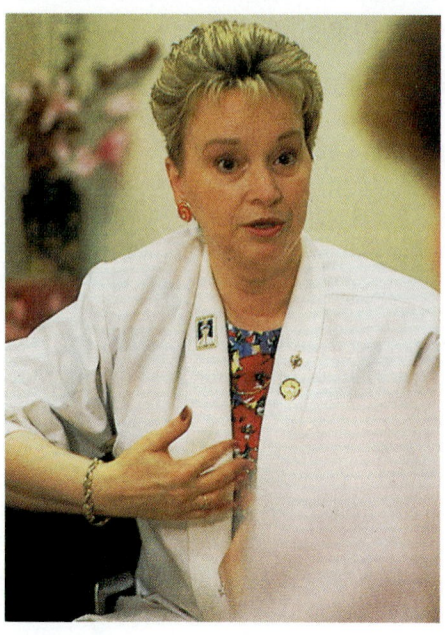

Figure 2-5 An open, relaxed posture conveys interest.

Steps	Rationale
2. Ask one related open-ended question at a time following a logical sequence that encourages client to tell the whole story.	Open questions encourage client to elaborate and provide more accurate and detailed descriptions.
3. Listen without interrupting until a natural break occurs.	This avoids interference with client's flow of thoughts.
4. Offer feedback that lets client know what you understood. **Paraphrase** by restating client's message using fewer words.	
5. If the message is unclear, back up the conversation and **clarify.** Admit confusion and ask for more information.	Without clarification, valuable information is lost.
6. **Focusing** eliminates vagueness in communication by limiting the area of discussion. Avoid numerous direct questions and "why" questions that may result in defensiveness.	When focusing, nurse asks questions that encourage full understanding of one aspect rather than allowing the focus to shift before understanding is achieved.
7. Identify incongruence, when a verbal message conflicts with nonverbal cues. **Stating observations** gives feedback that helps increase awareness of whether client communicated the intended message.	People may be unaware of the way the message was received unless the impressions created by the nonverbal cues are described.
8. Allow **silence,** which can be an effective means of allowing the organization of thoughts and processing of information. When client becomes emotionally upset or cries, a quiet period can be helpful.	Silence shows that nurse is accepting and willing to wait for client to be ready to continue.
9. At the conclusion of the interaction, **summarize** by giving a concise review of the key aspects of the main ideas.	Client is able to review information and make additions or corrections.

Evaluation

1. Ask client what facilitates or interferes with communication of needs.
2. Ask if the communication was accurately interpreted by care givers.

UNEXPECTED OUTCOMES AND RELATED INTERVENTIONS

1. Client shifts conversation back to the nurse rather than discussing own issues.
   a. Answer questions briefly if appropriate, then state your need to focus on client issues.
   b. Ask what client is most concerned about at this time.
2. Client has difficulty hearing the questions.
   a. Reduce background noise.
   b. If client has a hearing aid, be sure it is clean, inserted properly, and has a functioning battery.
   c. Adjust volume of hearing aid to a comfortable level.
   d. Speak slowly and articulate clearly.
   e. Face client to provide opportunity for lip reading.
   f. Talk toward client's best ear.
3. Client has dysarthria (difficult, poorly articulated speech from interference in control of muscles of speech) or expressive aphasia.
   a. Ask simple closed questions. Client can answer "yes" or "no" or nod or shake head in response.
   b. Allow time for understanding and a response.
   c. Use visual cues (pictures, objects, gestures).
   d. Encourage continued efforts to speak.
   e. Allow time and demonstrate an interested and patient attitude.
   f. Refer to speech therapist as needed.

SAMPLE DOCUMENTATION

1000 Client expressed concern about being able to regain ability to "do things like gardening and golf." Acknowledged being overwhelmed and discouraged. Talked at length about active lifestyle in past year. Expressed desire to work hard in physical therapy to build muscle strength as quickly as possible.

Skill 2.3 | Interviewing

The interview involves communication initiated for a specific purpose and focused on a specific content area. In nursing the interviewer obtains information about the client's health state, lifestyle, support systems, patterns of illness, patterns of adaptation, strengths and limitations, and resources. This information can be used for an admission data base or health history and provides data for identifying the client's expectations and for responding appropriately to individualized client needs.

The interview can facilitate a positive nurse-client relationship, which makes it easier for clients to ask questions about the health care environment and expectations regarding daily routines and procedures. It is important to indicate to clients that they may ask questions at any time. They also have the right *not* to answer questions. Indicating the purpose of the interview helps to establish trust and to put the client at ease.

The interview involves phases of orientation, working, and termination. The interview may be scheduled at a time when interruptions will be minimal and visitors are not present. In some cases it is possible to include family members in the interview while the focus is clearly kept with identifying the client's needs.

Orientation phase. Before beginning, the nurse tells the client the purpose for the interview and the types of data to be obtained. Then time is spent becoming acquainted with the client. Establish a time frame for the interview, and honor this commitment to the client.

Working phase. The nurse asks questions to form a data base from which a care plan can be developed (see box on p. 22). The nurse observes for evidence of discomfort and is willing to stop the interview when appropriate.

A direct-question technique is a structured format requiring one- or two-word answers and is frequently used to clarify previous information or obtain basic routine information (e.g., allergies, marital status). The open-question technique is used to promote a more complete description of identified areas of concern. Examples of open questions/comments include "What are your health concerns?" "How have you been feeling?" and "Tell me about your problem."

Termination phase. The client is given an indication that the interview is coming to an end a few minutes before conclusion is anticipated. This allows the client to ask questions and keeps the client aware of what to expect. The interview is terminated in a friendly manner, indicating specifically if there will be further contact. It is helpful to ask if anything else is needed before leaving the client's bedside.

Assessment

1. Review available information, which may include admission information such as name, address, age, marital status, employment, and reason for admission.

Interview Data Base

HEALTH-RELATED CONCERNS

Perception of health status, past health problems and therapies, effect of health status on role, influence on relationship with members of household, influence on occupation, ability to complete activities of daily living (ADLs)

EMOTIONAL CONCERNS

Support system, significant losses, major life changes or stressors (divorce, death, job change, victim of traumatic event), changes related to sexuality, sense of self-esteem or self-worth (What makes you feel good about yourself?)

KNOWLEDGE LEVEL/LEARNING NEEDS

Long-term and recent memory, intellectual abilities, education, environmental risk factors, understanding of illness, medications, treatment plans

CULTURAL AND SPIRITUAL FACTORS

Religious background, important religious practices, cultural background, values and beliefs (how this illness affects plans [goals/dreams])

2. Consider factors that may influence ability or willingness of client or significant other to respond to the questions, such as physical pain, discomfort, or anxiety. **These factors may need to be alleviated before the interview. Intellectual level affects the choice of words used in the questions.**

3. Determine if client is alert and oriented. Assess for hearing and speech difficulties (see Chapter 35). If these factors interfere with the interview, another source of information will be needed.

Planning

Expected outcomes focus on gathering information for a data base to develop an appropriate plan of care.

EXPECTED OUTCOMES

1. Client (or significant other) is able to describe health concerns.
2. Verbal and nonverbal messages are congruent.

Implementation

Steps	Rationale

Orientation phase

1. Greet client and significant others and introduce yourself by name and job title (Figure 2-6). Tell client you need to ask some questions that will require about 15 to 20 minutes. Assure client that this information will be kept confidential.

This allays anxiety about divulging information to a stranger and encourages participation.

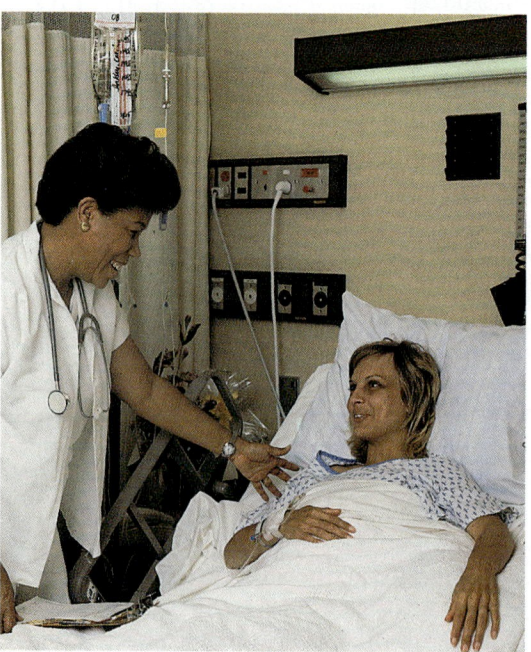

Figure 2-6 Greet client congenially.

Steps	Rationale
2. Provide privacy and eliminate distractions, unnecessary noise, and interruptions by going to a quiet unoccupied room and/or closing the door.	Controlling environmental factors is especially important when a client is anxious, angry, or depressed (Braverman, 1990).
3. Sit facing client at approximately the same eye level.	This facilitates active listening and places client more at ease.
4. If client is alert enough to state name, where he or she is, and what day it is, proceed with the interview.	If a client is disoriented or confused or information does not seem reliable, seek validation by other responsible persons (Barker and Moore, 1992).
Working phase	
5. If client is talkative, refocus the interview when client strays from the topic.	
6. Observe and clarify nonverbal behaviors.	Active listening encourages the exchange of information (see Skill 2.2). Conducting an interview by only asking questions may make client feel like a subject of interrogation.
7. Ask what led client to seek health care. Attempt to obtain a descriptive account of all the events in the order in which they occurred.	This provides a focus for collecting more specific data related to the primary areas of concern.
8. For each symptom, determine when, where, and under what circumstances it occurred. Also determine location, quality, quantity, duration, and aggravating, alleviating and associated factors (Table 2-2).	
9. Within each symptom, also clarify the absence of other symptoms that are generally associated with the problem.	
10. Identify past hospitalizations, past surgical procedures and complications, and previous major health problems.	
11. Determine whether client regularly takes medications and, if so, for what period of time. Ask the name, reason for taking, dosage, and frequency. Specifically ask about over-the-counter medications such as aspirin, acetaminophen, ibuprofen, laxatives, sleeping pills, or diet pills.	Clients may not think of over-the-counter medications, since these do not require prescriptions.
12. Also ask if client takes narcotics, insulin, digitalis, contraceptives, steroids, or hormone replacements.	Clients may not mention these if such drugs seem unrelated to the reason for admission or when they think that the physician would have previously conveyed this information.
13. Identify risk factors related to lifestyle that influence the client's health, knowledge level, and awareness of the risk.	Risk factors include smoking, alcohol use, drug abuse, lack of exercise, stress, and nutritional factors (e.g., fluids, cholesterol, carbohydrates, fiber, salt).
14. Continue with additional areas of interest or concern according to the focus of the interview (see box on p. 22).	
Termination phase	
15. Give information that tells client you are nearly finished.	This offers client a chance to ask final questions before nurse is finished.
16. Summarize your understanding of client's health concerns.	

Table 2-2 **Dimensions of a Symptom**

Dimensions	Questions to ask
Location	"Where do you feel it?" "Does it move around?" "Show me where."
Quality or character	"What is it like? Sharp, dull, stabbing, aching?"
Severity	"On a scale of 0 to 10, with 10 the worst, how would you rate what you feel right now?" "What is the worst it has been?" "In what ways does this interfere with your usual activities?"
Timing	"When did you first notice it?" "How long does it last?" "How often does it happen?"
Setting	"Does it occur in a particular place or under certain circumstances?"
Aggravating or alleviating factors	"What makes it better?" "What makes it worse?" "When does it change?" "Have you noticed other changes associated with this?"

Evaluation

1. Ask if client or significant other has had an adequate opportunity to describe health concerns.
2. Observe client's nonverbal expressions during interview. Do they match verbal statements?

UNEXPECTED OUTCOMES AND RELATED INTERVENTIONS

1. Family or significant other answers for client, even when client is capable of answering.
   a. Direct the question to client, using client's name.
   b. Avoid giving eye contact to family member.
   c. Acknowledge the answer given by a family member, then state you are interested specifically in what client has to say about it.
   d. Conclude the interview, and resume again after the family members are gone. If necessary, you may suggest that family take a break for a while, get coffee or a meal, or walk outside briefly for some fresh air.
2. Client is unable to communicate and family members are present.
   a. Interview family member as you would client.
   b. Explore the needs of family as well as of client.

SAMPLE DOCUMENTATION

Documentation involves use of a standard format for a data base (see Admission Patient Profile, Appendix A).

CRITICAL THINKING EXERCISES

1. On entering Mrs. Wilson's room, the nurse notes that she is crying. Throughout the night the nurse had difficulty controlling Mrs. Wilson's pain. Evaluate each of the following responses from the nurse now caring for Mrs. Wilson. Do the responses facilitate or block communication with Mrs. Wilson?
   a. Nurse opens the window blinds and states, "Mrs. Wilson, do you want to talk?"
   b. Nurse places her hand on Mrs. Wilson's shoulder and asks, "I'd like to help you. Mr. Tucker was just crying in the next room. This must be a good day to cry. Sometimes I feel like crying, too."
   c. Nurse leans close to Mrs. Wilson and says, "Mrs. Wilson, I know you experienced a lot of pain during the night. What can I do to help you feel better now?"
2. Various listening techniques are listed below. When would each be appropriate for the nurse to use?
   a. Using silence
   b. Speaking slowly and clearly
   c. Using visual cues
   d. Providing brief answers
   e. Paraphrasing
3. You are conducting an interview with Ted, a 22-year-old client. He is accompanied by his mother. During the interview, you note that Ted avoids eye contact and is easily distracted by noise from outside his room. Frequently, Ted's mom answers your questions to Ted. What approach should you take for the remainder of the interview?

REFERENCES

Barker E, Moore K: Neurological assessment, *RN* 55(4):28, 1992.
Braverman BG: Eliciting assessment data from the patient who is difficult to interview, *Nurs Clin North Am* 25(4):735, 1990.
Giger J, Davidhizar R: *Transcultural nursing,* St Louis, 1991, Mosby.
Kim MJ, McFarland GK, McLane AM: *Pocket guide to nursing diagnosis,* ed 5, St Louis, 1993, Mosby.
Smith S: *Communications in nursing,* ed 2, St Louis, 1992, Mosby.

ADDITIONAL READINGS

Clevenger FF: Interviewing the elderly client, *Adv Clin Care* 5(6):26, 1990.
Doenges ME, Moorehouse MF: Watch your language, *Nurs* 22(11): 1992.
Guzzetta CE et al: *Clinical assessment tools for use with nursing diagnosis,* St Louis, 1989, Mosby.
McFarland GK, McFarlane EA: *Nursing diagnosis and intervention: planning for patient care,* ed 2, St Louis, 1993, Mosby.
Vortherms RC: Clinically improving communication through touch, *J Gerontol Nurs* 17(5):6, 1991.

chapter 3

Promoting Infection Control

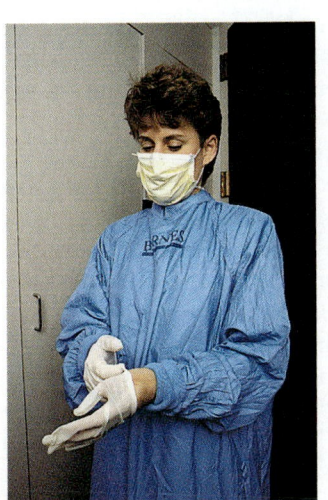

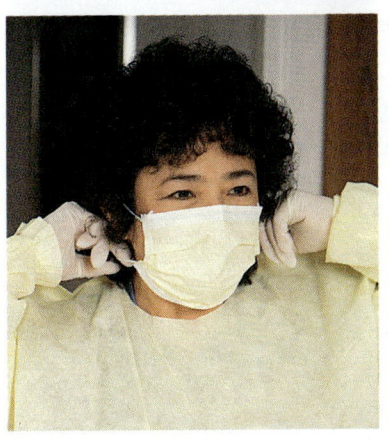

Infections present a significant hazard in all health care settings. Although protection of the client is an obvious priority, health care workers, including nurses, are at risk for contact with infectious material or exposure to a communicable disease. Knowledge of the infectious process and how a disease is transmitted, as well as the critical thinking involved in how to use and when to use aseptic technique and barrier protection, cannot be overemphasized. Today's nurse plays a vital role in the promotion of infection control.

Risk factors for acquired or nosocomial infections are greatly increased for clients in health care settings. In acute care or ambulatory care facilities, clients can be exposed to new or different microorganisms. Some of these microorganisms may be resistant to most antibiotics. In all settings, clients may have procedures or treatment modalities that lower their resistance to infections. For example, clients' immune systems may be altered if they are receiving radiation or chemotherapy treatments; therefore, they are more susceptible to infections, even from normal flora. Additionally, invasive procedures, such as the insertion of intravenous (IV) or urinary catheters, disrupt the body's natural defense barriers. In all health care settings, the nurse is responsible for teaching clients and their families about the source and transmission of infections, reason for susceptibility, and infection control principles.

Clients or health care workers do not have to develop an infection or acquire a disease with every exposure to a microorganism. This depends on the chain of infection, which is a model for the events that lead to an infection (Figure 3-1). There are six links in the chain of infection: (1) an infectious agent or pathogen, (2) the reservoir or place where the organisms reside, (3) the portal of exit from the reservoir, (4) a method or mode of transmission, (5) the portal of entrance into the host, and (6) the susceptibility of the host. Breaking any one of these links prevents an infection. For example, a nurse may prevent the client from acquiring an (IV) line infection by breaking the chain in several places. The reservoir or the microorganisms present on the skin can be altered by properly preparing the site before needle insertion. The mode of transmission can be changed by handwashing and using proper aseptic techniques.

Another example of breaking the infection chain includes alteration of a host response after a vaccination. A vaccine activates antibodies and protects the person from infection. By using infection control principles and client education, nurses can break the chain of infection.

Infections can be prevented or minimized by the use of aseptic technique. *Aseptic technique* is the purposeful prevention of the transfer of infection (Crows, 1989). Medical and surgical asepsis are the two types of techniques; both can be used in any health care setting. *Medical asepsis,* or *clean technique,* includes procedures (e.g., handwashing, disinfection of equipment) that reduce the number of microorganisms.

Medical aseptic techniques are not as rigid as surgical asepsis. *Surgical asepsis* refers to practices designed to render and maintain objects or skin maximally free from microorganisms (see Chapter 14). This also is referred to as *sterile technique.* Sterile technique must be practiced by nurses in operating rooms or during invasive procedures where sterile supplies are used. Sterile supplies have undergone a process called *sterilization,* whereby all microorganisms, including spores, have been destroyed (Rutala, 1990).

Barrier protection includes use of gowns, masks, protective eye wear, and gloves. Some form of barrier protection is indicated for all clients who potentially have an infection that can be transmitted to others. Because of the increased attention to the prevention of certain diseases, such as hepatitis B, acquired immunodeficiency syndrome (AIDS), and tuberculosis (TB), the Centers for Disease Control and Prevention (CDC) and the U.S. Occupational Safety and Health Administration (OSHA) have stressed the importance of the use of barriers and precautions.

In 1983 the CDC published guidelines for isolation precautions that encouraged decision making by the user. First, hospitals were given the choice of selecting between two systems: category-specific or disease-specific isolation. Second, personnel placing a client under precautions were encouraged to make decisions regarding need for a private room and necessity for certain types of barrier protection (Garner and Simmons, 1984). Thus, some clients were "overisolated," whereas others were "underisolated."

As new data regarding disease transmission became available, several portions of the guidelines were updated by the CDC. For example, the CDC has modified the isolation recommendation for clients with TB (CDC, 1994b) and those with suspected hemorrhagic fever (CDC, 1988b).

In 1988, the *Body Substance Isolation* (BSI) system was developed and focused personnel on selecting barrier protection whenever there was risk of contacting body substances (e.g., blood, saliva, feces, urine, and wound drainage) rather than only on the basis of isolation category or diagnosis (Jackson and Lynch, 1990).

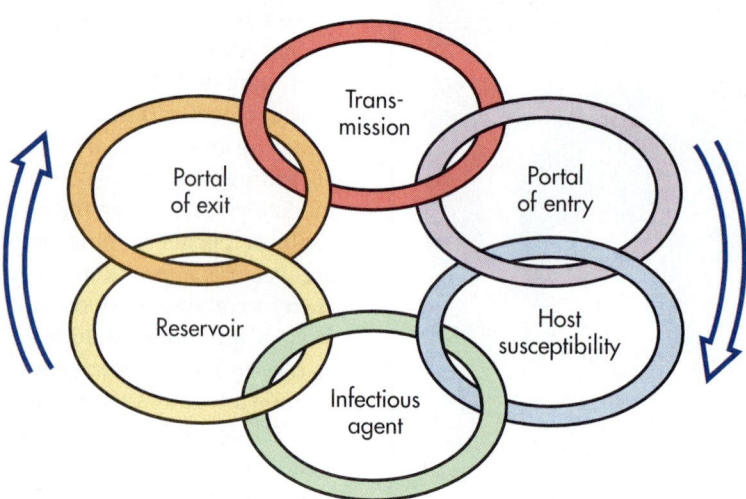

Figure 3-1   Chain of infection.

The rationale for BSI was that any client may be a source for infection. For example, nurses would wear gowns and gloves when changing the bed of an incontinent client (Jackson and Lynch, 1992).

Jackson and Lynch (1991) explain that when using BSI, workers should put on clean gloves just before contact with mucous membranes or nonintact skin of all clients. Furthermore, protective barriers should be used when it is likely that the worker will come in contact with a body substance that might soil skin or clothing. These precautions are intended to interrupt transmission of the most common source for organisms: colonized body substances.

Another system, *Universal Precautions* (UP), recommended barriers and procedures that limit an individual's exposure to infectious blood-borne agents such as the human immunodeficiency virus (HIV), which causes AIDS, and the virus that causes hepatitis (CDC, 1988a). In 1991, OSHA published regulations that required facilities to utilize UP as the minimum standard of practice (OSHA, 1991). Pugliese (1991) described UP as requiring workers to assume that all clients are potentially infected with HIV or other blood-borne agents and to use barriers to prevent exposure.

The CDC has recognized the need for a new isolation guideline that synthesizes the major features of UP and BSI and updates the previous category-specific isolation into a transmission-based precaution. The CDC's proposed new isolation guidelines containing two tiers of approach (CDC, 1994a) have not yet been approved. The first and most important tier will likely contain precautions designed to care for all clients in health care facilities regardless of their diagnosis or presumed infectiousness. This new isolation involves expanded Universal Precautions and synthesizes the major features of UP and BSI. These Precautions apply to (1) blood, (2) all body fluids regardless of whether they contain blood, (3) nonintact skin, and (4) mucous membranes. These Precautions promote handwashing and use of gloves, masks, eye protection, or gowns when appropriate for client contact (see box below, left).

The second tier will likely contain precautions for specific clients. These include highly transmissible or epidemiologically important pathogens.

The CDC further recommends the use of Universal Precautions for all immunocompromised clients. In addition, transmission-based precautions may be needed to reduce infection risks for these clients (Figure 3-2). Users

Universal Precautions*

- Standard precautions apply to blood, all body fluids, secretions, excretions, nonintact skin, and mucous membranes.
- Hands are washed if contaminated with blood or body fluid, immediately after gloves are removed, between patient contact, and when indicated to prevent transfer of microorganisms between other patients or environment.
- Gloves are worn when touching blood, body fluid, secretions, excretions, nonintact skin, mucous membranes, or contaminated items. Gloves should be removed and hands washed between patient care.
- Masks, eye protection, or face shields are worn if patient care activities may generate splashes or sprays of blood or body fluid.
- Gowns are worn if soiling of clothing is likely from blood or body fluid. Hands are washed after removing gown.
- Patient care equipment is properly cleaned and reprocessed, and single-use items are discarded.
- Contaminated linen is placed in leak-proof bag and handled so as to prevent skin and mucous membrane exposure.
- All sharp instruments and needles are discarded in a puncture-resistant container. CDC recommends that needles be disposed of uncapped or that a mechanical device for recapping be used.
- A private room is unnecessary unless the patient's hygiene is unacceptable. Check with infection control professional.

*Formerly UP and BSI.

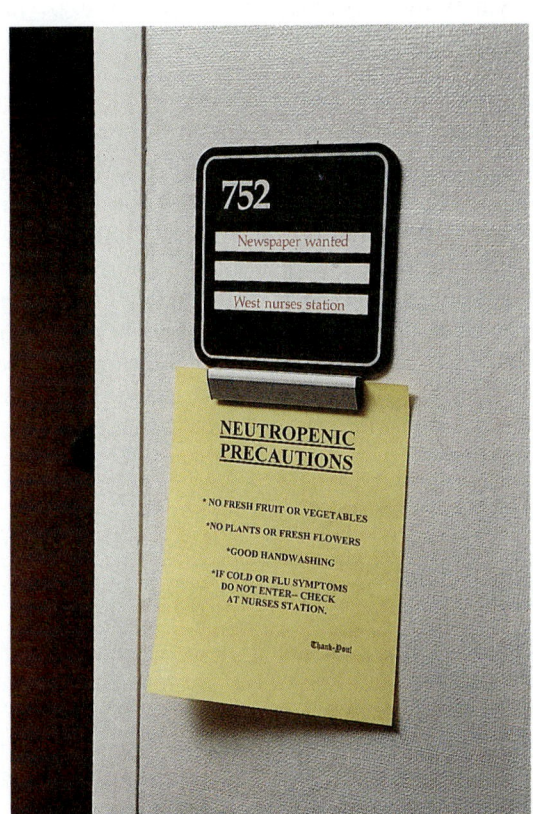

Figure 3-2 Immunosuppressed clients may be placed on nutropenic precautions (seen posted outside client's room).

of the Isolation Guidelines are referred to an additional CDC document to prevent nosocomial aspergillosis and legionnaires' disease in immunocompromised clients (CDC, 1994c).

With the increase in TB in the United States and several outbreaks of TB in clients and health care workers, the CDC (1990) published guidelines for TB control in health care facilities. These guidelines continue to be revised and challenged (CDC, 1993). In addition, OSHA has issued similar regulations. The CDC recommends workers wear a NIOSH-approved respiratory protective device when caring for potential TB clients (CDC, 1994b). The U.S. National Institute of Occupational Safety and Health (NIOSH) approved a high-efficiency particulate air (HEPA) respirator that meets or exceeds the standard, but NIOSH certification procedures are being revised. Employers are required by OSHA to establish a respiratory protection program that describes the following: standard operating procedures; medical screening; employee skin testing; training; respirator face-seal fit testing and fit checking; respirator inspections, maintenance, and storage; and evaluation process. Agencies are advised to evaluate their TB risk by analyzing numbers of confirmed cases of TB and numbers of employee skin test conversions. If risk is low, it is unlikely that stringent programs will have to be adopted. These guidelines and regulations do stress the use of TB isolation for all clients with known or suspected TB (OSHA, 1993) (see box at right).

Tuberculosis (TB) Isolation

- TB isolation should be practiced for all clients with known or suspected TB. (Suspected TB is defined by agency policy and generally means any client with a positive AFB smear, a cavitating lesion seen on chest x-ray study, or identified as high risk by a screening tool.)
- Isolation must be in a single-client room designated as negative airflow and having at least six air exchanges per hour. Room air must be vented to the outside. The door must be closed to maintain negative pressure.
- Health care workers must wear at a minimum a high-filtration mask when entering an AFB isolation room. (Check agency's policy for type of mask.)
- If HEPA mask or dust-mist-fume mask is used, workers must be fit-tested* before using a respirator for the first time. This ensures type and size of respirator appropriate for an individual.
- If HEPA mask or dust-mist-fume mask is used, workers must fit-check† the respirator's fit before each use.
- If HEPA mask or dust-mist-fume mask is used, respirator may be reused and stored according to agency policy.

AFB, Acid-fast bacillus; HEPA, high-efficiency particulate air.
*Fit test: procedure to determine adequate fit of respirator, usually by qualitative measure (wearers are exposed to a concentrated saccharin solution and asked if they can detect taste wearing respirator).
†Fit check: procedure in which worker uses negative pressure to see if mask is fitted properly.

Nursing Diagnosis

Several nursing diagnoses may be appropriate when using infection control measures. **Risk for Infection** relates to clients who may have specific risk factors that may increase their potential for acquiring an infection. These include pathological conditions (immunosuppression, chronic disease, obesity), treatments (surgery, invasive procedures, steroids), situational factors (disease exposure, inadequate immunizations, lack of handwashing by care giver), or maturation (client's age).

A diagnosis of **Knowledge Deficit** regarding infection prevention is appropriate when the nurse teaches individuals, families, or groups information about infection control measures. Clients can experience **Fear** or a feeling of **Powerlessness** when restricted to a respiratory isolation type of environment or when required to use protective barriers. **Social Isolation** may also be appropriate when use of protective barriers and environmental restrictions are required.

Skill 3.1 | Handwashing

Handwashing is the single most important means of controlling and preventing the spread of infections. The purpose of handwashing is to remove soil and transient microorganisms from the hands and to reduce total microbial count over time (Larson, 1989). The decision to wash hands depends on three factors: (1) the intensity or degree of contact with the client or infectious material, (2) the extent of contamination that may occur with the contact, and (3) the client's susceptibility to infection

(Larson, 1988). Larson further describes that for most general client care, a plain nonantimicrobial soap is acceptable in any convenient form (bar, leaflets, liquid, powder). In most health care settings, liquid or foam soap is used for handwashing. Some agencies have sinks with foot controls or an electric eye for turning the water supply on and off. This reduces the transmission of microorganisms that can occur when touching a contaminated faucet after handwashing. When performing invasive procedures, working in special care units, or dealing with immunosuppressed clients, an antimicrobial soap should be used (Garner and Favero, 1985).

Care must be taken to protect all clients from bacteria present on the nurse's hands. This is especially important if clients have an immune deficiency.

> **nurse alert**   Personnel with allergic reactions to certain antimicrobial soaps may substitute plain soap and gloving during high-risk procedures (see agency policy).

EQUIPMENT

Liquid or foam soap (antimicrobial soap under certain conditions)
Warm running water
Paper towels or air dryer

Implementation

Assessment

1. Assess client's risk for extent of infection (e.g., immunosuppressed, invasive procedure, open wound).
2. Assess client's and family's knowledge of benefits of proper handwashing.
3. Assess client's handwashing facilities in the home.

Planning

Expected outcomes focus on preventing the transmission of infection.

EXPECTED OUTCOMES

1. Client and/or family member demonstrates ability to wash hands correctly.
2. Client and/or family lists three benefits of handwashing.

Steps	Rationale
1. Wet hands with warm water.	Warm water removes less of the protective oils than hot water.
2. Apply small amount of soap on hands.	Soap decreases surface tension and facilitates removal of soil. Excess soap can dry and irritate skin.
3. Rub hands briskly using friction; keep fingertips pointed downward (Figure 3-3).	Mechanical friction helps remove microorganisms.
4. Wash hands thoroughly with soapy lather over palms, fingers, and back of hands for at least 10 to 15 seconds.	
5. Rinse thoroughly under running water, keeping fingers pointed downward (Figure 3-4).	Removes soap and microorganisms.
6. Dry hands well with paper towel or under air dryer.	
7. Turn off water supply. If faucet is used, protect hands with a paper towel.	Keep hands from contact with microorganisms on faucet handle.

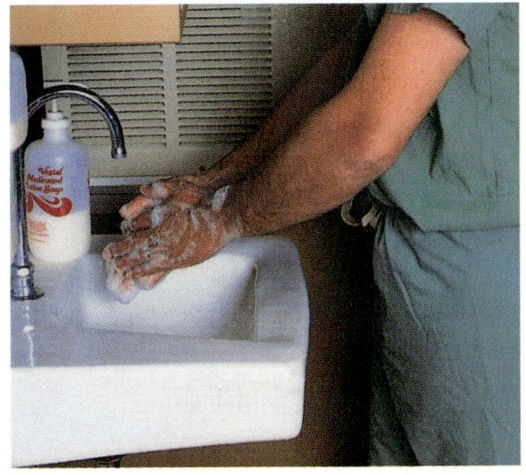

Figure 3-3

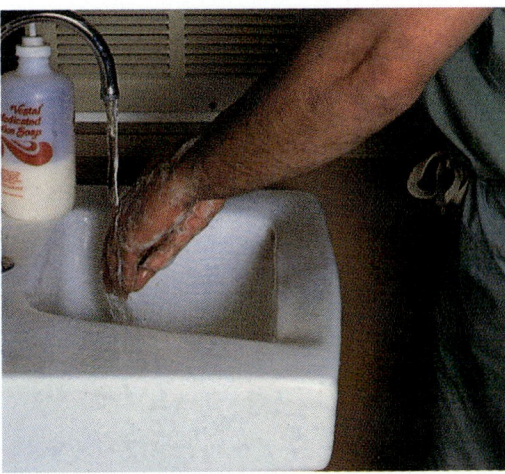

Figure 3-4

Evaluation

1. Observe client or family member wash hands. (It is best to see this performed in the home.)
2. Ask client or family to explain three benefits of hand-washing.

UNEXPECTED OUTCOMES AND RELATED INTERVENTIONS

Client or family lack motivation, equipment, or opportunity to perform handwashing.

a. Determine whether handwashing facilities can be provided or adapted in the home (e.g., proximity of facilities, running water, equipment in area).
b. Explain simply but thoroughly risks associated with failure to wash hands. Evaluate client's physical and emotional status.
c. Provide daily as much information as client and family are ready to accept.

Skill 3.2 │ Using Disposable Clean Gloves

Disposable gloves must be worn before coming in contact with mucous membranes, nonintact skin, blood, body fluids, or other infected material (Jackson and Lynch, 1991; OHSA, 1991). Additionally, gloves are indicated when there are cuts, abrasions, or oozing, draining wounds on the care giver's hands (Larson, 1989). Gloves should be inspected before use for cuts, tears, or holes. Gloves found with any of these deficiencies will not provide proper barrier protection.

EQUIPMENT

Pair of clean disposable gloves

Assessment

Inspect hands for cuts, abrasions, or wounds that indicate need for gloves.

Planning

Expected outcome focuses on preventing the transfer of microorganisms from nurse's hands to client. Additionally, nurse should be protected from infections.

EXPECTED OUTCOME

Client's signs and symptoms demonstrate lack of infection.

Implementation

Steps	Rationale
1. See Standard Protocol (Chapter 1, p. 5)	
Application	
2. Put on gloves (no special technique required). If wearing an isolation gown, pull cuffs of gloves over cuffs of gown. If not wearing a gown, pull up the gloves to cover the wrist.	Protects nurse's skin from exposure to microorganisms.
3. Interlink fingers to adjust glove fit.	Ensures proper, comfortable fit.
Removal	
4. Remove first glove by grasping outer surface of lower cuff, taking care to touch only glove to glove (Figure 3-5).	Keeps soiled part of gloves from touching skin of hand or wrist.
5. Pull glove inside out over hand, taking care to touch only inside of glove.	
6. Discard glove in receptacle.	
7. With ungloved hand, tuck finger inside cuff of remaining glove and pull it off, inside out. Discard in receptacle (Figure 3-6).	Avoids contamination of hands.

Steps	Rationale

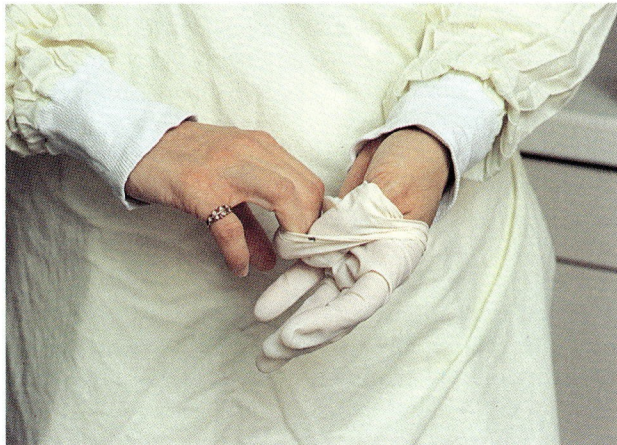

Figure 3-5   Figure 3-6

8. Wash hands thoroughly for at least 10 seconds.
9. See Completion Protocol (Chapter 1, p. 6).

---

nurse alert Gloves should be replaced as soon as practical when contaminated and after each procedure, or as soon as feasible if they are torn, punctured, or their ability to function as a barrier is compromised.

Evaluation

Evaluate client for signs of infection (e.g., temperature elevation, drainage, elevated white blood cell count, chills, malaise, nonhealing wound).

UNEXPECTED OUTCOMES AND RELATED INTERVENTIONS

Client develops signs of infection.
a. Notify physician of findings.
b. Provide appropriate therapy (e.g., wound care, hydration to reduce fluid loss, nutritional support).
c. Continue to use good handwashing.

Skill 3.3 | Caring for Clients Under Isolation Precautions

Isolation precautions and the use of barrier protection should protect the client, nurse, and others from contact with microorganisms. Gowns, gloves, eye wear, and masks are the recommended types of barrier protection. Depending on the potential for exposure, additional items such as shoe covers or hair covers may be necessary (OSHA, 1991). In assessing the type of barriers to be used, the following must be considered: the susceptibility of the client or the nurse, the potential for cross-contamination or exposure, the infectiousness of the disease or microorganism, and the facility's policies and procedures for infection control and isolation precautions.

Correct use of barrier protectors still appears to be a problem. Many nurses either overuse or underuse barrier protection. Several studies have found that nurses and other health care workers either forget or choose not to use recommended barriers (Kristensen et al., 1992; Troya et al., 1991).

Many nurses tend to use unnecessary barrier protection without exercising critical judgment about controlling transmission of infectious material or without consideration of the cost to their facilities. An example is the AIDS epidemic, which caused many health care workers to question the barrier effectiveness of gloves used in clinical settings. The fear of exposure to contaminated blood or infectious material forced some workers to wear double or even triple gloves. With this in mind, a study by Korniewicz et al. (1994) examined barrier protection with multiple vs. single gloving. They concluded that a single glove offered the same amount of protection as double gloves.

Another example of overprotection involves use of gloves, mask, eye wear, and gowns to care for a client with measles. Measles is spread by airborne droplets, so only a mask would be needed to establish the proper barrier.

When a client requires care in an isolated, private room, the nurse follows some special precautions. It is important to remember that the nurse's use of barrier precautions requires judgment. For example, a client with a respiratory infection and serious wound infection requires more precautions than one with a simple respiratory infection. Private rooms used for isolation often have negative-pressure airflow to prevent infectious particles (e.g., the particles that cause pulmonary TB) from flowing out of the closed environment. Special rooms with positive-pressure airflow are also used for highly susceptible clients such as organ transplant recipients. In this case, no organisms are able to enter a room.

When a client requires isolation in a private room, the nurse must remember that loneliness can easily develop. Isolation disrupts normal social relationships with visitors and care givers. A client who has an infectious disease may also experience self-concept or body image changes. Unless the nurse acts to minimize feelings of psychological and physical isolation, the client's emotional state can interfere with recovery.

EQUIPMENT (Figure 3-7)
Disposable gloves
Mask
Eye wear, protective goggles or glasses, face shield
Waterproof gown
Medication
Hygiene items

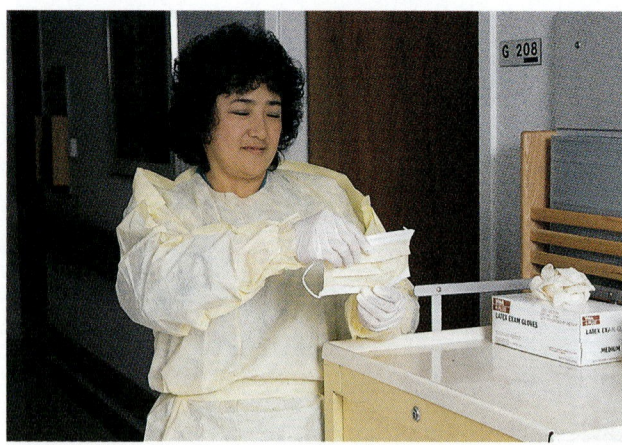

Figure 3-7

Assessment

1. Review the precautions for the specific isolation system and client's existing condition.
2. Review laboratory reports for results of culture, acid-fast bacillus (AFB) smears, and serology and for changes in white blood cell count (WBC) (see Appendix D).
3. Consider types of care measures to be performed while in client's room. **Allows nurse to organize all equipment needed in room.**
4. Determine from chart or significant other if client understands purpose of isolation and procedures to anticipate.

Planning

Expected outcomes focus on improving client's knowledge of the purpose of isolation.

EXPECTED OUTCOMES
Client and/or family verbalizes purpose of isolation.

Implementation

Steps	Rationale

1. See Standard Protocol (Chapter 1, p. 5).
2. Apply gown, mask, gloves, and goggles as appropriate.

    Reduces possibility of contamination of clothing from splashes or spatter.

   a. Apply gown, being sure it covers all outer garments; pull sleeves down to wrist. Tie securely at neck and waist (Figure 3-8).

   b. Apply disposable gloves. If worn with gown, bring cuffs over edge of gown sleeves.

    Prevents transmission of organisms from nurse to client.

   c. Apply mask around mouth and nose; tie securely. Be sure mask fits snugly.

    Reduces transfer of airborne droplet nuclei.

   d. Apply goggles to fit snugly around face and eyes (Figure 3-9).

    Goggles are worn when possibility of exposure to splashing or spattering of body fluids is likely.

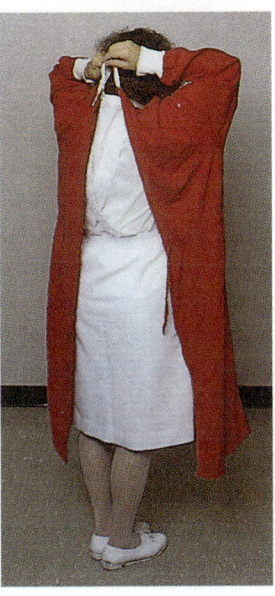

Figure 3-8

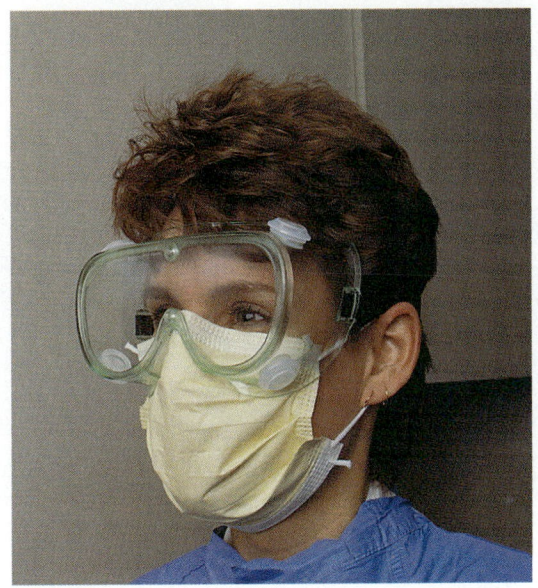

Figure 3-9

3. Enter client's room. Arrange supplies and equipment. (If equipment will be removed from room for reuse, place on clean paper towel.)

    Minimizes contamination of care items.

4. Explain purpose of isolation and precautions necessary to client, family, and visitors. Offer opportunity to participate in care and to ask questions.

    Improves client's ability to participate in care and minimizes anxiety.

5. Administer care.
6. Explain to client when you plan to return to room. Ask whether client requires any personal care items.

    Includes client in care plan.

7. Prepare to leave isolation room, removing barriers at door of room.

   a. Remove eye wear or goggles without touching hair or face.

    Gloved hands are used to remove eye wear or goggles spattered with body fluids.

   b. Untie gown at waist. Remove one glove by grasping cuff and pulling glove inside out over hand. Discard glove. With ungloved hand, tuck finger inside cuff of remaining glove and pull it off, inside out. Discard in proper receptacle.

    Gloves and gown are removed by avoiding further contamination of hands.

Steps	Rationale

c. Without touching outer surface of mask, untie mask strings; drop mask into trash receptacle.

d. Untie neck strings of gown. Allow gown to fall from shoulders. Remove hands from sleeves without touching outside of gown (Figure 3-10). Hold gown inside at shoulder seams and fold inside out (Figures 3-11 and 3-12). Discard in laundry bag.

e. Wash hands.

8. Leave room, opening door as little as possible.

9. See Completion Protocol (Chapter 1, p. 6).

Clean hands can contact clean items.

Keeping door open too long equalizes pressure in room and can allow organisms to flow out of room.

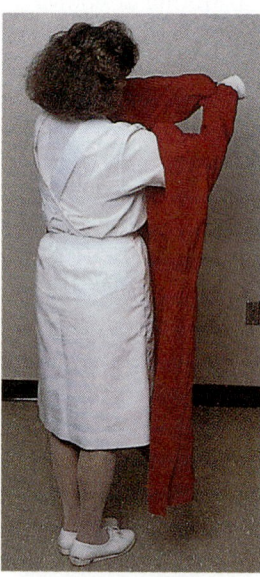   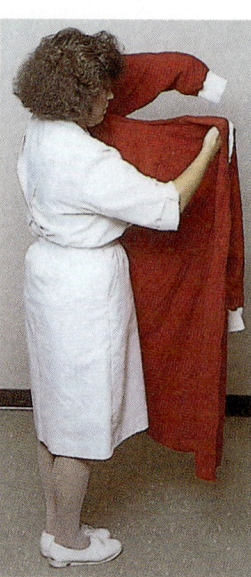   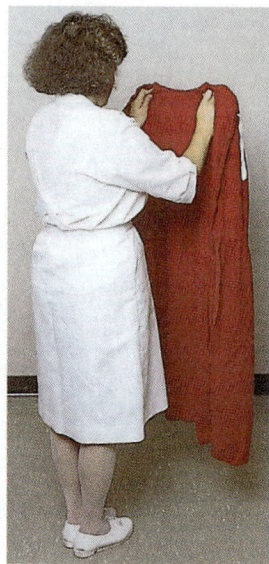

Figure 3-10   Figure 3-11   Figure 3-12

nurse alert   Needles and syringes should be disposed of uncapped in a puncture-resistant container in client's room (Figure 3-13).

Evaluation

Ask client to explain purpose of isolation in relation to diagnosed condition.

SAMPLE DOCUMENTATION

Document type of isolation and client's response.

1320 Client under respiratory precautions for TB; AFB smear shown positive. Wife present in room, wearing mask appropriately. Discussed way in which TB can be transmitted.

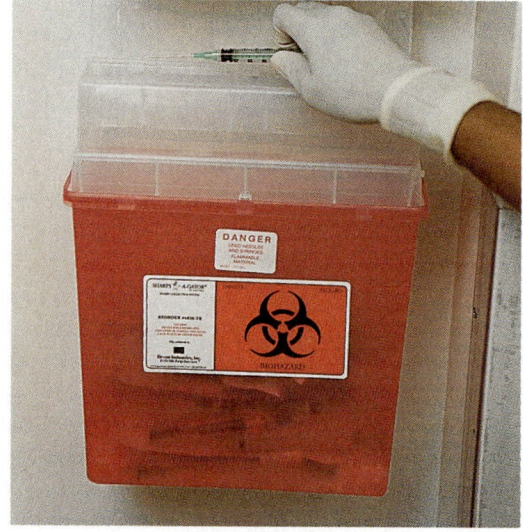

Figure 3-13

Skill 3.4 | Special Tuberculosis Precautions

The dramatic upsurge of TB cases in the United States with several outbreaks, some involving drug-resistant strains, has increased concern regarding nosocomial transfer. The CDC (1990) issued guidelines for preventing TB in health care settings, stressing the importance of early identification and treatment of persons with known or suspected TB and proper isolation in the health care setting. Again in 1994, the CDC released guidelines for even stricter adherence to infection control measures. One should suspect TB in any client with respiratory symptoms lasting longer than 3 weeks (Boutotte, 1993). Suspicious symptoms include presence of a productive cough and dyspnea, especially if accompanied by night sweats or unexplained weight loss.

Isolation for clients with known or suspected TB includes a special, private isolation room. Such rooms in existing facilities have negative pressure in relation to surrounding areas so that air is exhausted to the outside, having a minimum of six air exchanges per hour. In new construction or renovations, rooms should have at least 12 air exchanges per hour.

In 1993, OSHA issued a mandate requiring health care facilities to follow 1990 CDC guidelines for fitting health care workers potentially exposed to TB with a HEPA respirator (CDC, 1994b) (Figure 3-14). As a minimum level of protection, a 0.1-micron filter mask is used with a filter efficiency of 95% (Figure 3-15). NIOSH-approved HEPA respirators are currently the only model that meets or exceeds that standard. In agencies having major problems with drug-resistant TB, a powered air-purifier respirator (PAPR) has been used. The type of respirator protection depends on agency policy. Research has not substantiated use of any respirators or masks in preventing TB transmission.

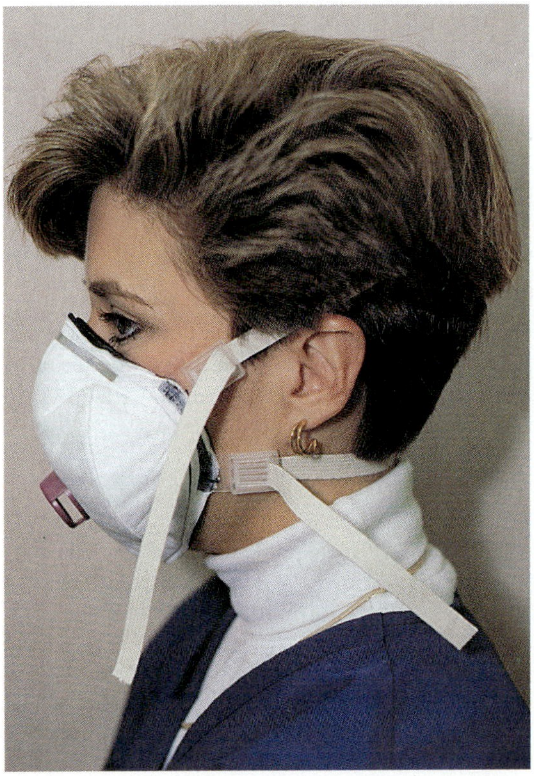

> **nurse alert** Nurses must first check their respirator protection device before entering the room. Doors to TB isolation rooms must be closed to ensure negative pressure. Sign stating proper isolation must be outside door.

OSHA also requires employers to provide training concerning transmission of TB and proven methods of prevention, especially in areas where risk of exposure is high, such as during bronchoscopy. Health care facilities must provide TB skin tests for all employees and appropriate follow-up evaluation when a previously negative skin test becomes positive (OSHA, 1993).

EQUIPMENT

TB isolation room
Respiratory protective device (check agency policy)

Assessment

1. Assess client's potential for infectious pulmonary or laryngeal TB (e.g., documentation of positive AFB smear or culture; history of fever, night sweats, or productive cough; cavitation on chest x-ray study; client

Figure 3-14 Nurse wearing HEPA respirator.

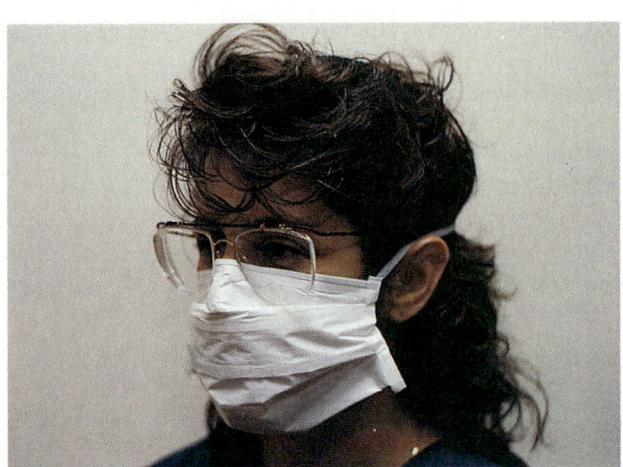

Figure 3-15 Nurse wearing 0.1-micron filter mask.

has signs or additional symptoms of TB and states a recent exposure; physician progress notes indicate plan to rule out TB).

2. Assess effectiveness of isolation room (e.g., check negative airflow using flutter strip or smoke stick, or consult with institution's plant engineering department).

Planning

Expected outcomes focus on prevention of transmission of TB and client understanding of TB transmission.

EXPECTED OUTCOMES

1. Client describes how TB may be transmitted.
2. Nosocomial transmission of TB is prevented.

Implementation

Steps	Rationale
1. See Standard Protocol (Chapter 1, p. 5).	
2. Before entering room, apply recommended mask. Be sure it fits snugly.	Reduces transmission of airborne droplet nuclei.
3. Explain purpose of AFB isolation to client, family, and others, including how TB is transmitted by inhalation of droplets that remain suspended in the air when client coughs, sneezes, speaks, or sings (Boutotte, 1993). Offer opportunity for questions.	Improves ability of client to participate in care. TB cannot be transmitted through contact with clothing, bedding, food, or eating utensils (Boutotte, 1993).
4. Instruct client to cover mouth with tissue when coughing and to wear mask when leaving the room.	Reduces spread of droplet nuclei.
5. Provide care.	
6. Leave the room and close the door.	
7. Remove respiratory protective devices such as HEPA respirator.	Most respiratory devices are reusable. The number of times depends on agency policy.
8. Place reusable device in clear plastic bag for storage, being careful not to crush device. (Check agency policy for number of times it can be reused.)	
9. See Completion Protocol (Chapter 1, p. 6).	

Evaluation

1. Assess client's laboratory data for repeated AFB smears that may be negative.
2. Ask client and/or family to identify method of transmission for TB.

UNEXPECTED OUTCOMES
AND RELATED INTERVENTIONS

Client fails to follow precautions for preventing transmission (e.g., fails to cover mouth when coughing, improperly disposes of soiled tissue).

a. Reexplain significant risk to family and friends.
b. Discuss client's concerns/feelings about the disease.

SAMPLE DOCUMENTATION

0800 AFB isolation maintained. Client instructed on TB transmission and need for isolation. Client verbalized concern about family exposure. Referred to American Lung Association and MD.

CRITICAL THINKING EXERCISES

1. You are teaching Mr. Gomez to care for his wife at home. Because she is immunosuppressed, it is important that Mr. Gomez use excellent handwashing technique. When observing Mr. Gomez, you noted that he wetted his hands with warm water, applied soap, and rubbed all areas of his hands briskly for 10 to 15 seconds. He then rinsed his hands, turned off the water, and reached for a paper towel while keeping his fingers in an upward position. How would you evaluate Mr. Gomez's demonstration? Did he follow all steps or omit steps of the procedure?

2. You are preparing to give your client an enema. You have all your supplies out, the client is positioned properly, and you have put on your disposable gloves. Just as you start the procedure, you notice that one of your gloves is torn. What should you do, and why?

3. Your friend is caring for Mrs. Jackson, a 42-year-old woman in protective isolation for diarrhea. The organism causing the diarrhea is spread by feces. Mrs. Jackson is fatigued but is able to go to the commode when she needs to have a stool. You note that your friend goes into Mrs. Jackson's room wearing a mask, protective eye gear, gown, and gloves. What advice could you give your friend that would help provide better care for Mrs. Jackson?

4. You are caring for a client with suspected tuberculosis. You have been fitted with a special mask that you wear when in the client's room. One day, a nursing student asks you why you are wearing a special mask. How would you answer the student?

REFERENCES

Boutotte J: TB: the second time around, *Nursing '93* 23(5):42, 1993.
Centers for Disease Control: Universal precautions for prevention of transmission of human immunodeficiency virus, hepatitis B virus, and other blood borne pathogens in health care settings, *MMWR* 37(24):377, 1988a.
Centers for Disease Control: Management of patients with suspected viral hemorrhagic fever, *MMWR* 37(3S):1, 1988b.
Centers for Disease Control: Guidelines for preventing the transmission of tuberculosis in the health care setting, with special focus on HIV-related issues, *MMWR* 39(RR-17):1, 1990.
Centers for Disease Control: Draft guidelines for preventing the transmission of tuberculosis in health care facilities, *DHHS* Oct 12, 1993.
Centers for Disease Control and Prevention: Draft guideline for isolation precautions in hospitals, *Federal Register* 59(214):56552, 1994a.
Centers for Disease Control and Prevention: Guidelines for preventing the transmission of tuberculosis in healthcare facilities, *Federal Register* 59(208):54242, 1994b.
Centers for Disease Control and Prevention: Recommendations for the prevention of nosocomial pneumonia, *Am J Infect Control* 22(4):267, 1994c.
Crows: Asepsis: an indispensable part of the patient's care plan, *Crit Care Nurs Q* 11(4):11, 1989.
Garner J, Favero M: *Guidelines for handwashing and environmental control,* Atlanta, 1985, Centers for Disease Control.
Garner J, Simmons B: CDC guidelines for the prevention and control of nosocomial infections: guideline for isolation precautions in hospitals, *Am J Infect Control* 12(4):103, 1984.
Jackson M, Lynch P: Implementing and evaluating a system of generic infection precautions: Body Substance Isolation, *Am J Infect Control* 18:1, 1990.
Jackson M, Lynch P: An attempt to make an issue less murky: a comparison of four systems for infection precautions, *Infect Control Hosp Epidemiol* 12:448, 1991.
Jackson M, Lynch P: Body Substance Isolation, *Infect Control Hosp Epidemiol* 13(4):191, 1992.
Korniewicz D et al: Barrier protection with examination gloves: double versus single, *Am J Infect Control* 22(1):12, 1994.
Kristensen MS, Wernberg NM, Anker-Moller E: Healthcare workers' risk of contact with body fluids in a hospital: the effect of complying with universal precautions policy (research), *Infect Control Hosp Epidemiol* 13(12):719, 1992.
Larson E: APIC guideline for use of topical antimicrobial agents, *Am J Infect Control* 16(6):253, 1988.
Larson E: Handwashing: it's essential even when you use gloves, *Am J Nurs* 89:934, 1989.
Occupational Safety and Health Administration: Blood-borne pathogens, *Federal Register* 56(235):64175, 1991.
Occupational Safety and Health Administration: *Enforcement policies on Procedures for Occupational Exposure to Tuberculosis,* Washington, DC, 1993, US Department of Labor.
Pugliese G: *Universal precautions, policies, procedures, and resources,* Chicago, 1991, American Hospital Association.
Rutala W: APIC Guidelines for selection and use of disinfectant, *Am J Infect Control* 18(2):99, 1990.
Troya S et al: A survey of nurse's knowledge, opinions, and reported uses of Body Substance Isolation Systems, *Am J Infect Control* 19(6):268, 1991.

ADDITIONAL READINGS

American Thoracic Society: Control of tuberculosis in the United States, *Am Rev Dis* 146(6):1623, 1992.
Benenson A, editor: Center of communicable diseases in man, ed 15, Washington, DC, 1990, US Government Printing Office.
DeFillippo V, Bowen R, Ingbar D: A Universal Precautions monitoring system adaptable to any health department, *Am J Infect Control* 20(3):159, 1992.
Grimes D: *Infectious diseases,* Mosby's Clinical Nursing Series, St Louis, 1991, Mosby.
Hutton M, Polder J: Guidelines for preventing tuberculosis transmission in health care settings: what's new, *Am J Infect Control* 20(1):24, 1992.
Perry A, Potter P: *Clinical nursing skills and techniques,* ed 3, St Louis, 1994, Mosby.
Pugliese G: T.B. Respirators: what's required and what isn't, *Materials Management Health Care* 3(4):30, 1994.

chapter 4

Promoting a Safe Environment

Skill 4.1
Safety Equipment

Skill 4.2
Seizure Precautions

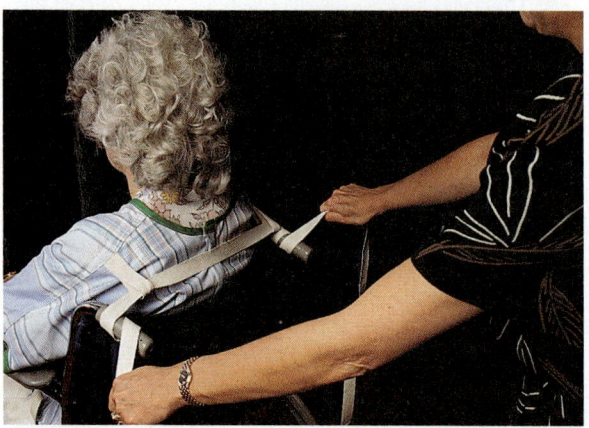

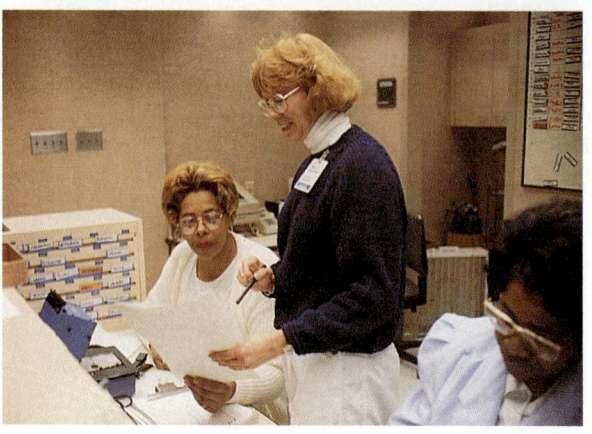

Safety, often defined as freedom from psychological and physical injury, is a basic human need that must be met. Not only is a safe environment essential for survival, but it can also decrease a client's anxiety level while increasing a sense of well-being. Feeling secure in a hospital environment allows a client to focus energies on therapeutic activities. Within the hospital setting, the nurse must assess for and eliminate many environmental hazards to ensure client safety.

Hospital units are designed and maintained with client safety in mind. Beds have wheel locks, side rails, and removable headboards for emergency care (Figure 4–1). The entire bed frame can be raised or lowered, and the entire bed can be angled up or down. The head and foot sections of the bed can also be raised or lowered. Side rails have a call button and controls to raise and lower the head and feet to change position. Clients must be informed if they are not to assume certain positions. The mattress and pillows are covered with waterproof material and are made of nonallergic materials. The mattress must be firm for client comfort and support. Many different types of mattresses have been designed to relieve pressure on a client's skin (see Chapter 24).

Call bells and/or intercom systems are available at each bedside, as well as in bathrooms and treatment rooms (Figure 4-2). Safety grips and nonskid surfaces are found in bathrooms and treatment areas. Shower chairs may be used to prevent falls (Figure 4-3). Floor surfaces are kept dry and free of clutter. Lighting, natural and artificial, must be adequate but not glaring. Proper ventilation, stable room temperature, and humidity settings provide safety as well as comfort.

Smoking is not permitted in client units because of the inherent health risks in smoking and because of the potential for starting fires. All electrical equipment must

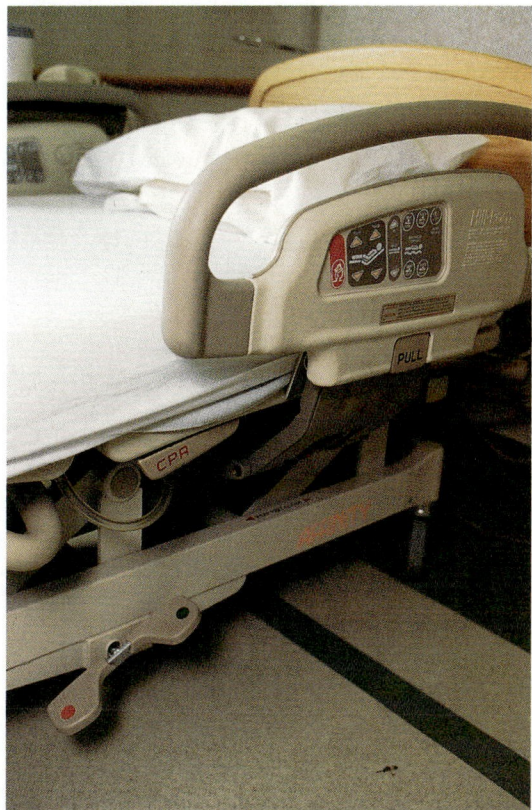

Figure 4-1 Bed should have wheels locked and be kept in a low position with side rails up. A nurse call button is on the side rail.

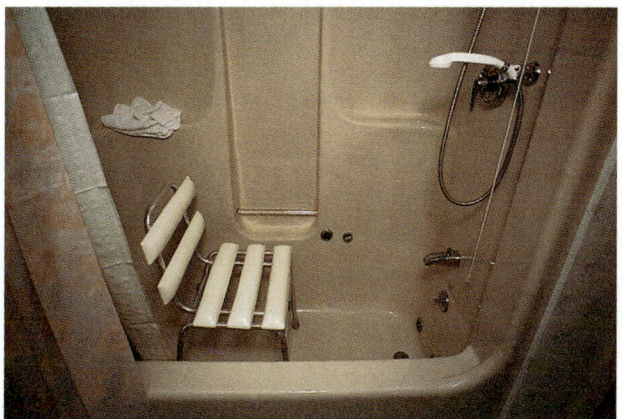

Figure 4-3 Nonslip surface in tub prevents falls. Shower chair allows clients to sit while in the shower.

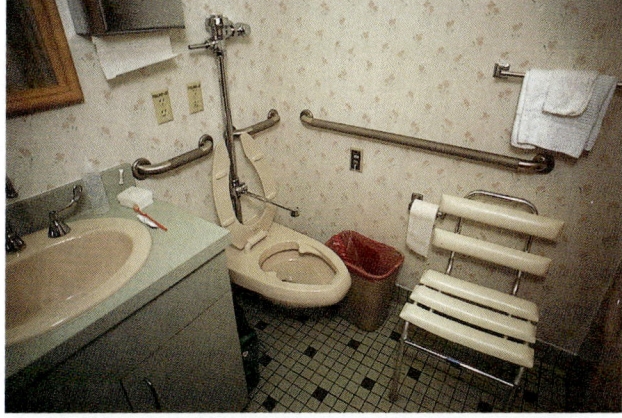

Figure 4-2 Safety features in bathrooms include safety grip bar and emergency call bell. Red bag is for disposal of hazardous waste materials, including items heavily saturated with blood.

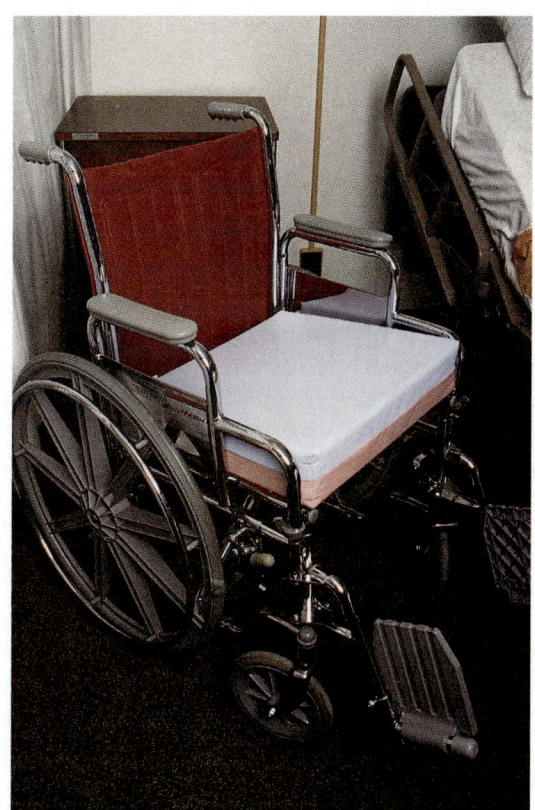

Figure 4-4 Wheelchair must have wheels locked during transfers. A wedge pillow on the seat is thicker at the front, which deters the client from getting up without assistance and eliminates the need for restraints.

Risk for Falls Assessment Tools

TOOL 1: RISK ASSESSMENT TOOL FOR FALLS

Directions: Place a check mark in front of elements that apply to your client. The decision of whether a client is at risk for falls is based on your nursing judgment. Guideline: A client who has a check mark in front of an element with an asterisk (*) or four or more of the other elements would be identified as at risk for falls.

General Data
— Age over 60
— History of falls before admission*
— Postoperative/admitted for surgery
— Smoker

Physical Condition
— Dizziness/imbalance
— Unsteady gait
— Diseases/other problems affecting weight-bearing joints
— Weakness
— Paresis
— Seizure disorder
— Impairment of vision
— Impairment of hearing
— Diarrhea
— Urinary frequency

Mental Status
— Confusion/disorientation*
— Impaired memory or judgment
— Inability to understand or follow directions

Medications
— Diuretics or diuretic effects
— Hypotensive or central nervous system suppressants (e.g., narcotic, sedative, psychotropic, hypnotic, tranquilizer, antihypertensive, antidepressant)
— Medication that increases gastrointestinal motility (e.g., laxative, enema)

Ambulatory Devices Used
— Cane
— Crutches
— Walker
— Wheelchair
— Geriatric (Geri) chair
— Braces

TOOL 2: REASSESSMENT IS SAFE "KARE" (RISK) TOOL

Directions: Place a check in front of any element that applies to your client. A client who has a check mark in front of any of the first four elements would be identified as at risk for falls. In addition, when a high-risk client has a check mark in front of the element "Use of a wheelchair," the client is considered to be at greater risk for falls.
— Unsteady gait/dizziness/imbalance
— Impaired memory or judgment
— Weakness
— History of falls
— Use of a wheelchair

Modified from Brians LK et al: *Rehabil Nurs* 16(2):67, 1991.

be periodically checked by the maintenance department and continually assessed by the nurse when in use. Three-prong adapters with grounding wires are used to avoid shocks and sparks, extension cords are avoided, and all cords are inspected for fraying.

Falls are the second leading cause of all accidental deaths for people up to age 79 years. After age 80, falls are the leading cause (*Accident facts,* 1993). Falls are a leading cause of injury of ill or physically, sensorially, or mentally impaired clients, particularly older adults (see box above). A new unfamiliar environment; inability to communicate; and impaired cognition, mobility, hearing, and sight all contribute to the risk of falling. Medications and physiological disorders, such as orthostatic hypotension and seizure disorders, are also contributing risk factors.

Clients are transported by a stretcher or wheelchair. Care must be taken to lock the wheels as the client transfers into or from the wheelchair (Figure 4-4). When the client is transported by stretcher, the side rails should

be up and the client instructed to keep hands in to prevent injury when passing through narrow doorways (Figure 4-5).

Clients at risk for self-injury or falling may need restraints for a time. Physical restraints are devices that limit a client's movement. Restraints are not a solution for a client problem, but rather a temporary means to control a client's behavior. Restraints do not necessarily prevent falls; in fact, it has been shown that clients incur less severe injuries if left unrestrained. Nurses have a responsibility to utilize all alternatives before restraining a client. These alternatives include orienting the client to the surroundings, encouraging the use of the call bell for assistance, helping the client with toileting frequently, involving the family in the client's care, and eliminating sources of disorientation. A wedge pillow, which is thicker at the front, may be used in a chair to increase the effort required to move from sitting to standing and thus deter the client from getting up without assistance and eliminate the use of restraints (Figure 4-4).

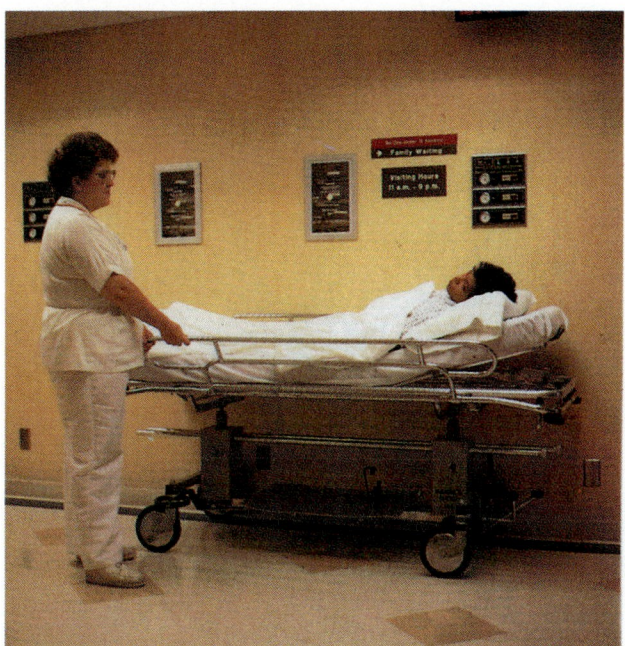

Figure 4-5 Stretcher must have side rails up during transport.

It is reported that devices such as belts, jackets, and limb or extremity restraints are used on approximately 500,000 Americans each day. This is an alarming statistic considering that restraints are associated with many complications. Almost all types of restraints have been implicated in client deaths, with most deaths associated with suffocation using the vest or jacket type (Weick, 1992). The U.S. Food and Drug Administration (FDA), which regulates restraints as medical devices and requires manufacturers to label them "prescription only," estimates that hundreds of restraint-related injuries occur each year, with at least 100 deaths taking place in nursing homes, hospitals, and private homes (Lambert, 1992).

The immobility imposed by restraining a client can lead to pressure ulcer formation, constipation, urinary and fecal incontinence, and urinary retention. Loss of self-esteem, humiliation, fear, and anger can also result (Weick, 1992). However, when applied correctly and appropriately, restraints do serve as a safety device.

Nurses caring for clients who have a seizure disorder must be familiar with "seizure precautions" if they are to protect their clients from injury during a seizure. Brief, temporary malfunctions of groups of nerve cells in the brain may produce excessive discharges from cells and result in seizures. A generalized tonic-clonic or grand mal seizure lasts 1 to 2 minutes (no longer than 5) and is characterized by a cry, loss of consciousness with falling if upright, tonicity (rigidity), and clonicity (jerking). The client may have shallow breathing, cyanosis, and possibly loss of bladder and bowel control. After the seizure, a postictal phase occurs in which the client has amnesia and confusion and may fall into a deep sleep. (*Seizure recognition and observation,* 1992). Before a convulsive episode, a few clients may report an aura, a warning or sense that a seizure is about to occur. An aura may be a bright light, a smell, or a taste (Shantz and Spitz, 1993).

Generalized tonic-clonic seizures that last longer than 5 minutes or are followed quickly by subsequent seizures are called status epilepticus. This is a medical emergency and requires intensive monitoring and treatment.

For the isolated generalized tonic-clonic seizure, it is now recommended that objects not be placed in a client's mouth. It has been found that significant injury to the client's oral cavity during a seizure is rare, even during the most violent ones (Ellis, 1993). Injury may occur from forcing an object into the mouth and from the teeth biting down on a hard object. Soft objects may break in the mouth during a seizure and be aspirated. Therefore, the Epilepsy Foundation of America, in its recommendations for seizure first aid, includes avoiding the insertion of objects into the mouth (*Seizure recognition and observation,* 1992). Clients experiencing a seizure are never restrained but need to be adequately protected from traumatic injury.

Nursing Diagnosis

Risk for Injury is appropriate when the focus involves prevention of falls related to weakness, vision changes, dizziness, incoordination, altered balance, or environmental factors. **Risk for Injury** related to insufficient knowledge of safety precautions is appropriate when teaching the client about family safety measures. It should be noted that clients with nursing diagnoses of **Impaired Physical Mobility** and/or **Sensory/Perceptual Alterations** may be predisposed to injury.

Skill 4.1 | Safety Equipment (Call Light, Side Rails, Restraints)

Every client's unit must have a call light or signaling device in good working order and accessible to the client. All hospital beds should be kept in a low position. Movable side rails prevent clients from falling out of bed. Side rails also help a client turn and position in bed. Restraints can provide for client safety if applied correctly and only when absolutely necessary. Although a nurse can apply a restraint in an emergency, a physician's order must always be obtained as soon as posible.

EQUIPMENT
Bed
Side rails
Call bell
Restraints
   Vest or jacket (Figure 4-6)
   Belt (Figure 4-7)
   Mitten (Figure 4-8)
   Extremity or limb (Figure 4-9)

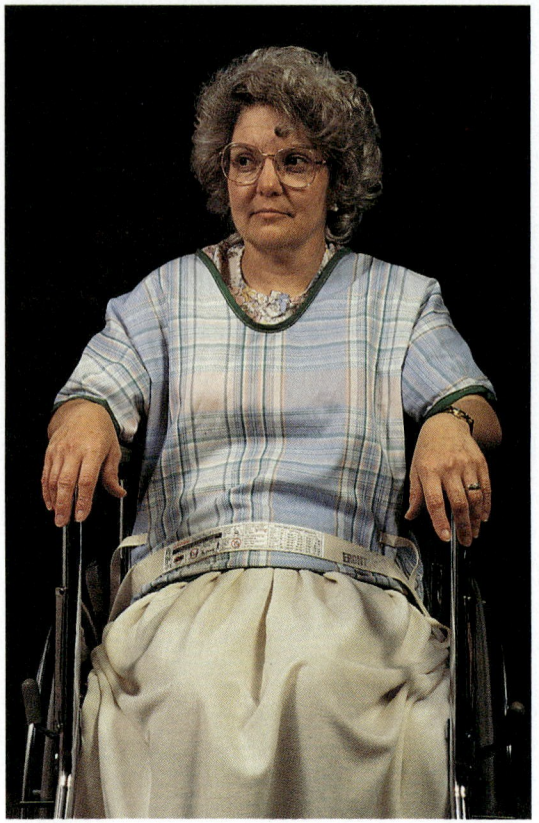

Figure 4-6 Vest or jacket restraint.

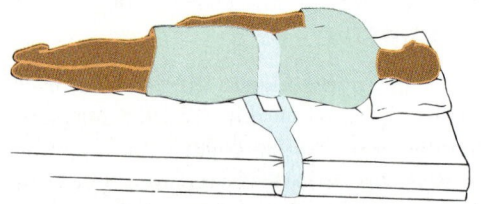

Figure 4-7 Restraint belt must be tied to bed frame rather than side rails.

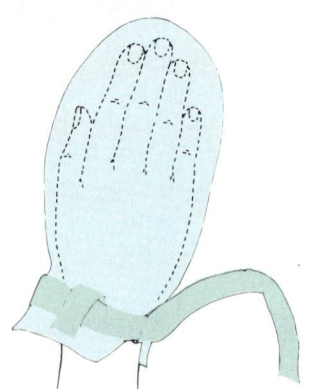

Figure 4-8 Mitten restraint.

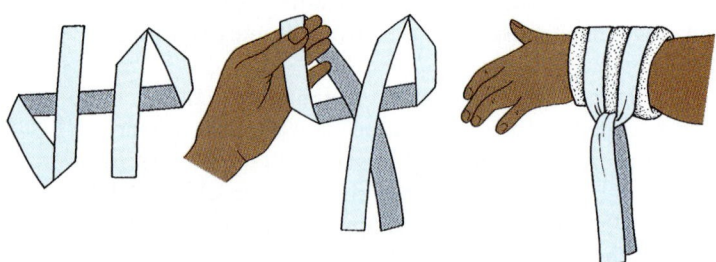

Figure 4-9 In an emergency, a clove-hitch restraint can be constructed using gauze. Make a figure 8 with the gauze and pick up loops. Place loops over a padded extremity.

Assessment

1. Assess the client's age, level of consciousness, degree of orientation, and ability to follow directions and cooperate.
2. Assess the client's mobility, hearing, and sight.
3. Assess medications and alcohol intake.
4. Assess history of hypotensive episodes and seizures.

Assessment determines the degree of assistance and type of protection a client needs to maintain safety.

Planning

Expected outcomes focus on safety, the recognition of physical hazards in the environment, the use of safety equipment, and the prevention of complications associated with the application of restraints.

EXPECTED OUTCOMES

1. Client does not fall or suffer injury or trauma while hospitalized.
2. Client demonstrates use of the call bell to obtain assistance immediately after orientation to the unit.
3. Client states two reasons side rails are used immediately after orientation to the unit.
4. Client does not experience any complication related to the use of restraints, such as impaired neurovascular integrity, impaired skin integrity, increased confusion and agitation, or any hazard of immobility during the period the restraint is in use.

Implementation

Steps	Rationale
1. See Standard Protocol (Chapter 1, p. 5).	
2. Call bell	
a. Provide client with hearing aid and glasses if used.	This facilitates client's ability to understand directions and locate and use call bell.
b. Explain and demonstrate turning call bell on and off at bedside (Figure 4-10) and in bathroom.	It is essential for client to know the locations of call bells and how to use them.

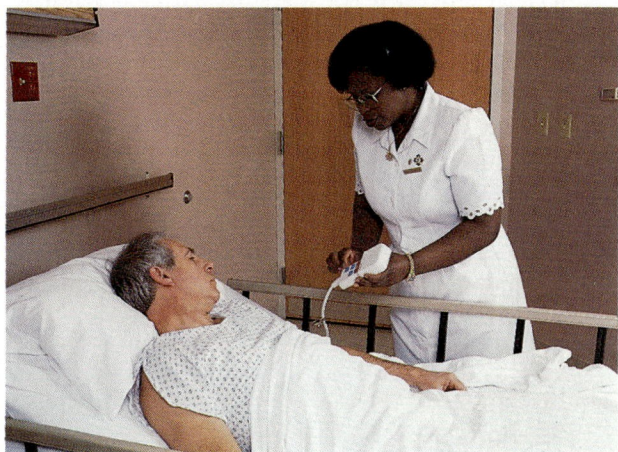

Figure 4-10

Steps	Rationale
c. Observe client return demonstration.	
d. Secure call bell to an accessible location, such as side rails or bedding. Inform client of location.	This prevents the client from overreaching and possibly falling out of bed.
3. Side rails	
a. Explain the two main reasons for using side rails: preventing falls and turning self in bed.	Client understanding promotes cooperation.
b. Check agency policies regarding age and side rail use.	Side rails often are required on all clients 65 years and older.

Steps	Rationale

c. Keep side rails in an up position and bed in a low position with locks on when client care is not being administered and the client is an older adult, weak, confused, sedated, or sleeping.

Side rails prevent older adults and confused and/or sedated clients from falling out of bed. If a client should climb over the side rails and fall, having the bed in a low position may lessen the trauma of the fall.

d. Leave one side rail up and one down on the side where the oriented and ambulatory client gets out of bed.

Client can use side rail to position self in bed.

4. Restraints

a. Assess client's need for restraint. Attempt to utilize alternatives.

Restraints are used as a last resort, since they may increase confusion and agitation and pose significant threats to a client's safety and psychological well-being.

b. Check agency policies regarding restraints. Obtain a physician's order for a particular type of restraint. Note the date and time.

A physician's order is needed. The least restrictive type of restraint should be selected. A physician's order should be time limited and should indicate specific client behaviors for which the restraint is to be used.

c. Explain to client and family the need for the restraint. Attempt to obtain consent.

d. Place client in proper body alignment.

Proper body alignment should be maintained to prevent contractures and neurovascular injury.

e. Pad bony prominences before applying restraints (Figure 4-11).

Padding protects skin from irritation.

f. Review manufacturer's instructions before applying the restraint.

Manufacturer's instructions and labeling should always be followed for client safety.

g. Apply restraint, making sure it is not over an intravenous line or other device (e.g., dialysis shunt).

Intravenous lines and other therapeutic devices may be occluded.

h. Check that two of the nurse's fingers can be inserted under the restraint (Figure 4-12).

Tight restraints may constrict circulation and ventilation and cause neurovascular injury.

   (1) Jacket/vest/posey. A vestlike garment that may cross in front or back of client. The front and back of the garment should be labeled. Apply over a gown (see Figure 4-6).

Used to prevent falls while the client is in a chair or bed. It must be applied correctly to prevent choking or suffocation.

Prevents skin irritation.

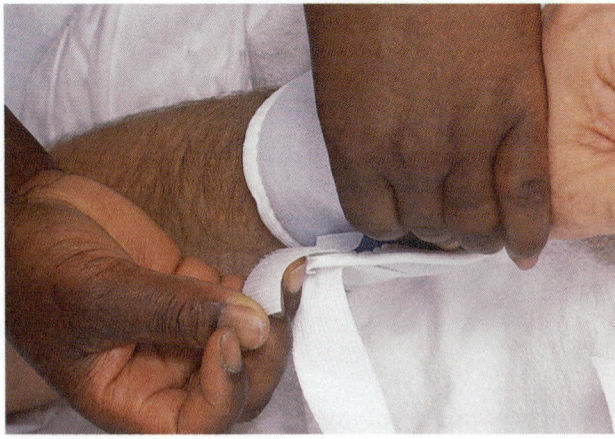

Figure 4-11

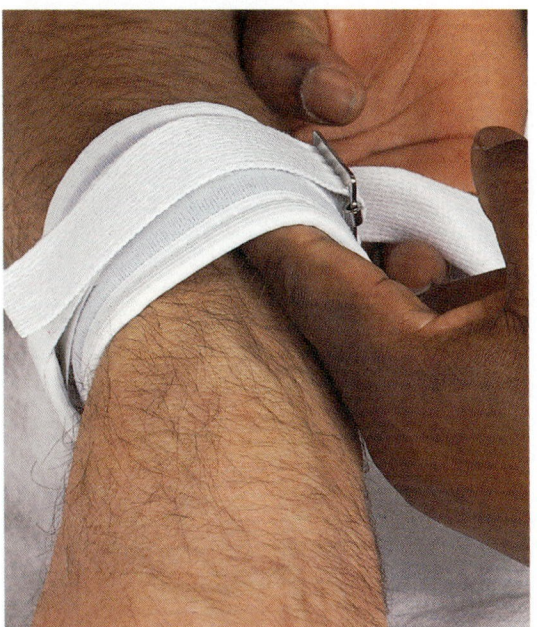

Figure 4-12

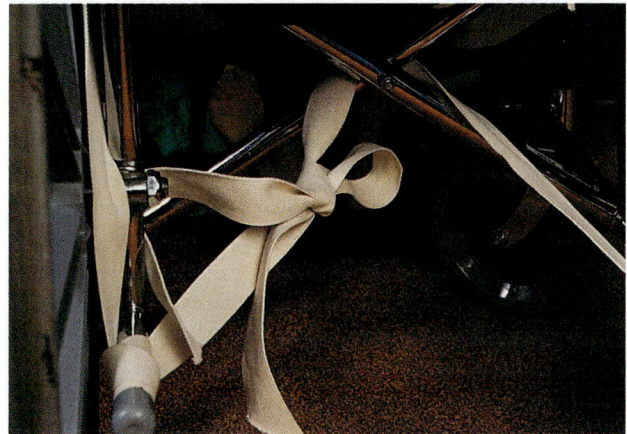

Figure 4-13 Quick-release knot.

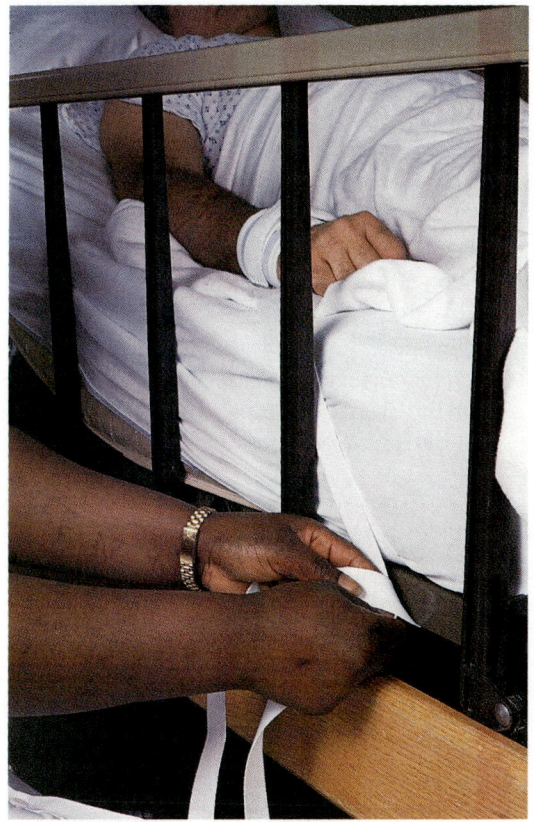

Figure 4-14 Restraint tied to bed frame.

Steps	Rationale

nurse alert Do not tie the belt in a knot. Use a quick-release tie (Figure 4-13).

Steps	Rationale
(2) Belt. Secures client to bed (Figure 4-14) or stretcher (see Figure 4-7).	Used to prevent falling off stretcher or getting out of bed.
(3) Mitten. A mitt that is applied to client's hand (see Figure 4-8).	Used to prevent dislodging of tubes and intravenous lines, scratching, and removal of dressings and other appliances.
(4) Extremity/limb. Applied to one or all four extremities.	Maintains immobility of an extremity.
(5) In an emergency, a clove-hitch restraint can be constructed using gauze. Make a figure 8 with the gauze and pick up loops. Place loops over a padded extremity (see Figure 4-9).	A clove-hitch configuration does not tighten.
i. Whenever possible, use a commercial restraint, securing according to manufacturer's directions.	Commercial restraints are designed to be secured so client cannot easily undo them and have foam padding that, when applied correctly, will not become tighter when client moves the limb.

Steps	Rationale
j. Attach restraints to the bed frame, which moves when the head of the bed is raised or lowered (see Figure 4-13). When a client is in a chair, the jacket restraint should be secured by placing ties under the arm rests and securing at the back of the chair. Attach with a bow quick-release tie (see Figure 4-14).	If restraints are secured to a side rail, client may be injured when the rail is lowered. For client in a chair, if the ties are not placed under the arm rests before securing, client may be able to stand up by sliding the restraint ties up the back of the chair. A bow quick-release tie allows for quick release in an emergency.
k. Assess client every 30 minutes while restraint is on. Check for correct application and maintenance of skin integrity; palpate pulses; and check color, temperature, and sensation in restrained body part.	Frequent observation and neurovascular assessment is essential to prevent injury to client.
l. Remove restraints for 30 minutes at least every 2 hours (q2h).	Removal allows for complete observation of the area and for full range of motion to be performed.
5. See Completion Protocol (Chapter 1, p. 6).	

Evaluation

1. Assess client for signs and symptoms of injury, and assess the environment for physical hazards continuously throughout hospitalization. Remove hazards or modify the environment as indicated.
2. Observe client using call bell.
3. Ask client to state two reasons side rails are used.
4. Observe for correct application of restraining device, observe skin, monitor pulses, and check temperature and color of restrained body part every 30 minutes. Continuously monitor for complications of immobility.

UNEXPECTED OUTCOMES AND RELATED INTERVENTIONS

1. Client experiences an injury while hospitalized. Reassess for internal risk factors and external risk factors in the environment (see Appendix A).
2. Complications occur from use of restraints.
   a. Attempt to use alternative measures to restraints.
   b. Monitor for complications continuously.
   c. Institute measures to prevent complications of immobility.

SAMPLE DOCUMENTATION

1000 Use of call bell explained and demonstrated to client. Client returned demonstration. Call bell left attached to bedding within client's reach. Use of side rails explained. Side rails left up and bed placed in low position.

1200 Client found climbing over side rails. Stated repeatedly, "I must get out of jail," despite being reoriented to surroundings frequently. Stayed with client for 20 minutes. Continuously attempted to climb out of bed.

1230 Dr. Smith notified and ordered jacket restraint. Use of restraint explained to client. Jacket restraint applied over client gown according to manufacturer's instructions and secured to bed frame.

1300 Client sitting in bed with jacket restraint on. No signs of skin impairment apparent under restraint. Depth of respirations normal. Assisted client to turn to left lateral position.

Skill 4.2 | Seizure Precautions

A sudden alteration in normal brain activity causes one of two types of seizures: generalized or partial. The most common generalized seizure is tonic-clonic, characterized by a fall to the ground and stiffening of the body (tonic phase) and subsequent jerking of the extremities (clonic phase). Partial seizures are confined to one part of the brain and can be evidenced by a variety of symptoms.

Status epilepticus is the occurrence of several seizures in succession without the client regaining consciousness between seizures. This can cause ventilation problems, hypoxia, and cardiac dysfunction and can be fatal. **This is a medical emergency.**

EQUIPMENT
Adult airway (Figure 4-15)
Padding for side rails and headboard (Figure 4-16)
Suction machine, oral suction equipment

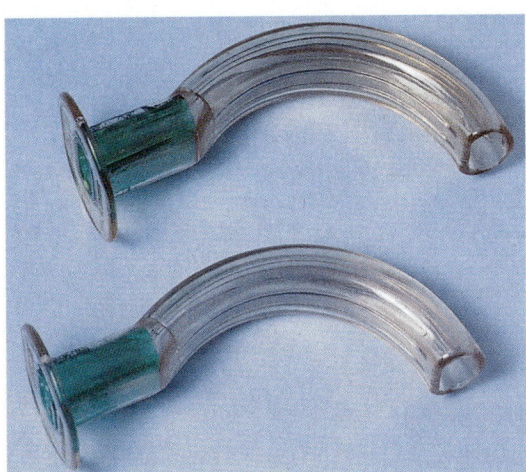

Figure 4-15 Oral airways.

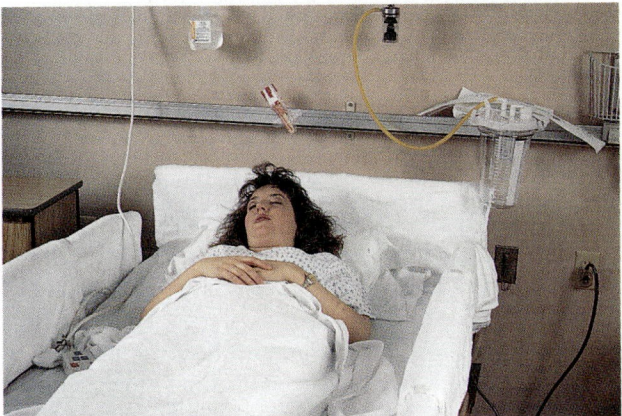

Figure 4-16 Seizure precaution: padded side rails and headboard.

Assessment

1. Assess seizure history, noting frequency of seizures, presence of aura, and sequence of events if known.
2. Assess medical and surgical conditions that may lead to seizures or exacerbate existing seizure condition.
3. Assess medication history. **Seizure medication must be taken as prescribed and not stopped suddenly. This may precipitate seizures.**

Planning

Expected outcomes should focus on safety, prevention of airway obstruction and aspiration, and maintenance of self-esteem.

EXPECTED OUTCOMES

1. Client does not suffer traumatic physical injury during a seizure episode.
2. Client's airway is maintained and secretions are not aspirated during a seizure episode.
3. Client verbalizes positive self-feelings after a seizure episode.

Implementation

Steps	Rationale
1. See Standard Protocol (Chapter 1, p. 5).	
2. Position client safely. If standing or sitting at the time of the seizure, guide client to floor and protect head by cradling in your lap or placing a pillow under head. Clear surrounding area of furniture. If client is in bed, raise side rails and put bed in low position.	These measures protect client from traumatic injury.
3. Provide privacy.	Clients may feel embarrassed after a seizure, especially if there were onlookers.
4. If possible, turn client on side, with head flexed slightly forward.	This position prevents the tongue from blocking the airway and promotes drainage of secretions, thus reducing the risk of aspiration.
5. Do not restrain client. Loosen clothing.	Restraining clients can result in musculoskeletal injury.
6. Do not force any objects into client's mouth.	Injury to the oral cavity may result from forcible insertion of a hard object. Soft objects may break or come apart and be aspirated.

Steps	Rationale
7. Observe the sequence and timing of seizure activity. Note aura (if any), level of consciousness, posture, skin color, movements of extremities, incontinence, and sleep patterns or confusion afterward. 8. Stay with client after the seizure, explaining what happened and offering support.	Accurate observation and reporting assist in the diagnosis and treatment of the seizure disorder. An *aura* is a warning clients may experience. Auras may be experienced visually, auditorily, or otherwise.
9. Status epilepticus a. Insert airway when jaw is relaxed between seizure activity (see Figure 4-15). Do not place fingers in the client's mouth. (See Chapter 30.) b. Provide oxygen and suction equipment. Prepare for intravenous insertion. (See Chapter 30.)	An open airway needs to be maintained. If seizure activity begins, the nurse could suffer from a bite injury. Status epilepticus is a medical emergency. Medications are given intravenously, the client needs to be suctioned, and oxygen is often needed.
10. Pad side rails and headboard (see Figure 4-16). 11. See Completion Protocol (Chapter 1, p. 6).	Traumatic injury is avoided.

Evaluation

1. Assess client for traumatic injury during and after the seizure episode.
2. Observe client's color and respiratory rate and pattern during the seizure.
3. Ask client to verbalize feelings after the seizure.

UNEXPECTED OUTCOMES AND RELATED INTERVENTIONS

1. Client suffers traumatic injury.
   a. Continue to protect client from further injury.
   b. Notify the physician.
2. Client verbalizes feelings of embarrassment and humiliation.
   a. Allow client to verbalize feelings.
   b. Encourage client and family to participate in decision making and planning care.

SAMPLE DOCUMENTATION

1000 Observed client sitting in chair in room. Cry heard, client observed sliding to floor, not responding to verbal stimuli. Client assisted to floor with head supported. Pillow placed under head. Tonic and clonic movements of all four extremities noted, lasting 2 minutes. Color remained good, respiratory pattern slightly irregular. No incontinence noted. At conclusion of tonic and clonic movements, client slept for 20 minutes, during which time respirations were 16 per minute and regular.

1020 Client awake and alert. Requested nurse to describe sequence of events. Stated that this was his "usual type of seizure."

CRITICAL THINKING EXERCISES

1. Critique the following sample documentation. Identify data gaps (insufficient data), unclear statements, and use of vague terminology.

   1100   Client lying in bed linens. No c/o discomfort. Unaware of time and place; knows name and birth date. Pleasant & cooperative.

   1130   Client found sitting on the floor next to the bed. Assessed for injury; no c/o pain or altered skin integrity. Stated she had to go to the bathroom. Assisted back to bed and instructed to call for assistance when getting out of bed. BP 130/80, P 88, R 14.

   1145   Client attempting to crawl out of the foot of the bed. Posey vest applied.

   1230   Client assisted with meal tray. Daughter at bedside.

2. Carla is a 26-year-old college student with a history of seizures. She is currently in the hospital for elective surgery. The morning before surgery, the nurse finds Carla unresponsive to verbal stimuli and observes jerking movements of all four extremities. The nurse lowers the side rail, positions Carla on her back, inserts a bite stick into the client's mouth, and attempts to take Carla's vital signs.

   a. Evaluate the above scenario with regard to safety precautions. What steps would you have taken to ensure safety standards were met?

   b. Distinguish between safety precautions indicated for an individual experiencing general tonic-clonic seizure activity vs. status epilepticus.

3. Analyze the following clients and judge whether each is at low (L), medium (M), or high (H) risk for injury. Use the risk assessment tool presented on p. 40 to help determine which individuals are at highest risk.

   a. Chuck is a 66-year-old client newly admitted to the hospital. He is alert and oriented to person but unable to state where he lives and is unaware of his present location. His wife states he fell at home getting out of the bathtub.

   b. Marilyn is a 78-year-old client who is alert and oriented in all spheres. She is unable to move her left leg following a stroke.

   c. Harry is a 42-year-old client with a brain tumor. He is unable to verbally express his thoughts and needs but understands and follows directions. He moves all extremities and has a slightly unsteady gait. His blood pressure medication causes orthostatic hypotension, making Harry dizzy when getting out of bed.

   d. Clarisa is a 52-year-old client admitted from a nursing home for pneumonia. She is disoriented to person, time, and place. She takes a diuretic for swelling in her legs and is weak from fever. Her own wheelchair is at the bedside.

REFERENCES

Accident facts, Itasca, Ill, 1993, National Safety Council.

Brians LK et al: *Rehabil Nurs* 16(2):67, 1991.

Ellis C: Nursing assessment and intervention for the patient experiencing seizures: a structured approach, *Clin Nurs Pract Epilepsy* 1(2):4, 1993.

Lambert V: Patient restraints, *FDA Consumer* 26(8):9, 1992.

Seizure recognition and observation, a guide for allied health professionals, ed 2, Landover, Md, 1992, Epilepsy Foundation of America.

Shantz D, Spitz M: What you need to know about seizures, *Nursing '93* 23(11):34, 1993.

Weick M: Physical restraints: an FDA update, *Am J Nurs* 92 (11):74, 1992.

ADDITIONAL READINGS

Cutchins C: Blueprint for restraint-free care, *Am J Nurs* 91(7):36, 1991.

Fletcher K: Restraints should be a last resort, *RN* 53(1):52, 1990.

Houston K, Lach H: Restraints: how do you score? *Geriatr Nurs* 11(5):231, 1990.

Leger-Krall S: When restraints become abusive, *Nursing '94* 24(3):55, 1994.

O'Brien K: Managing the seizure patient, *Nursing '91* 21(1):63, 1991.

Potter PA, Perry AG: *Fundamentals of nursing: concepts, principles, and practice,* ed 3, St Louis, 1993, Mosby.

Potter PA, Perry AG: *Clinical nursing skills and techniques,* ed 3, St Louis, 1994, Mosby.

Strumpf N, Evans L, Schwartz D: Restraint-free care: from dream to reality, *Geriatr Nurs* 11(3):122, 1990

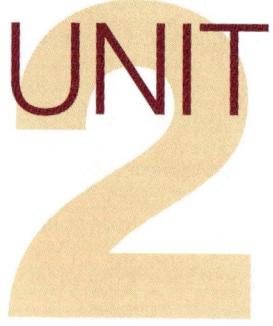

UNIT 2

Activities of Daily Living

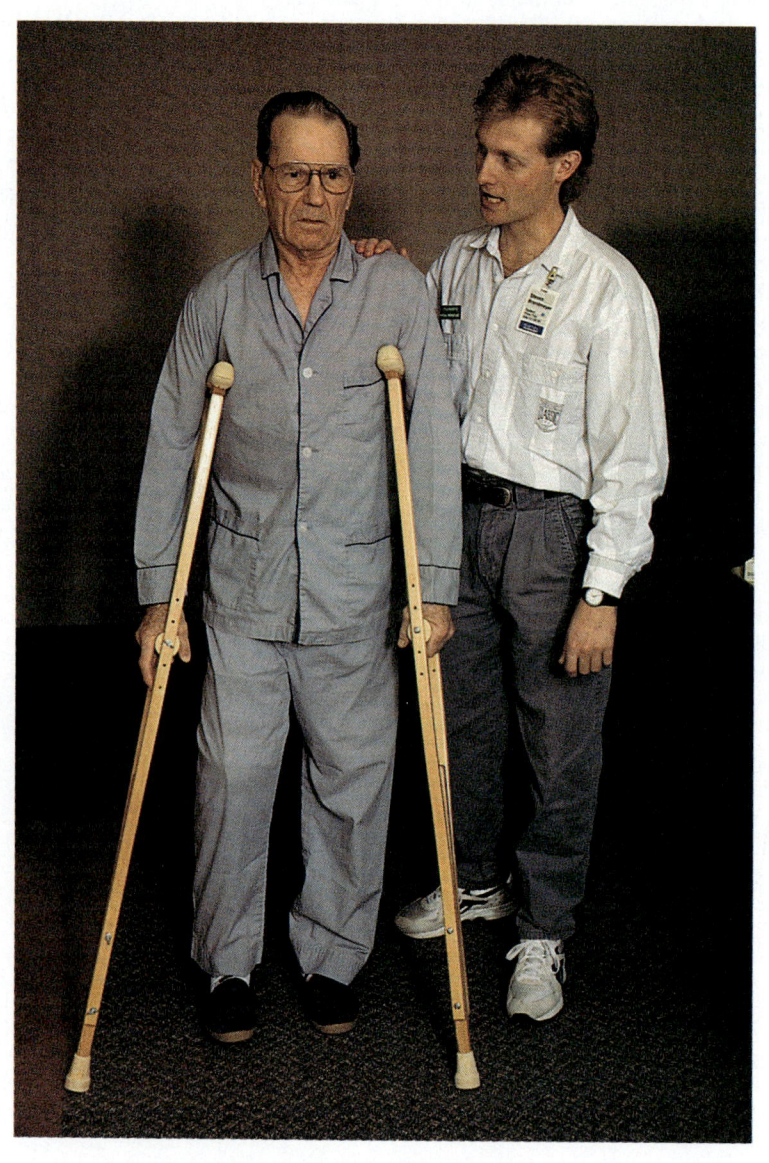

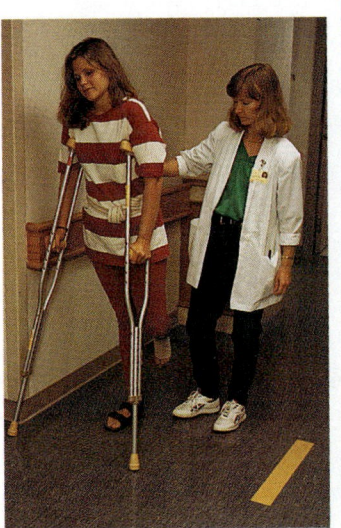

chapter 5

Promoting Activity and Mobility

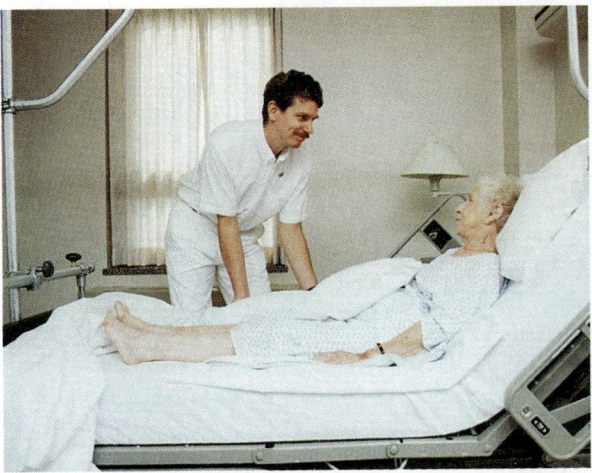

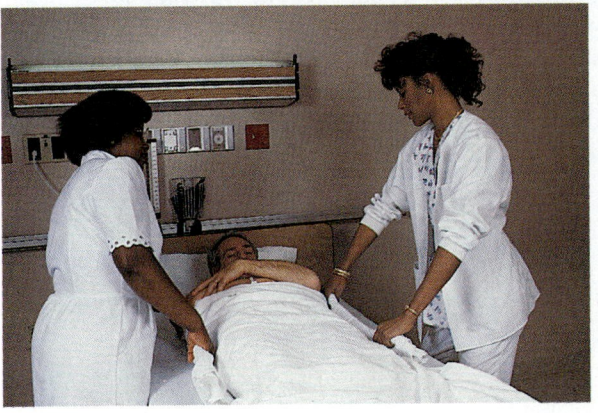

Activity is a basic human need that contributes to both physical and emotional well-being (McFarland and McFarlane, 1993). The benefits of physical activity include increased energy, improved sleep, better appetite, less pain, and improved self-esteem. It is useful to incorporate active exercises into activities of daily living (ADLs) (see box on p. 52). Every effort must be made to promote functional mobility. Physical activities that clients are able to perform indicate their physical capacity and functional ability and desires.

Three elements are essential for mobility: (1) ability to move based on adequate muscle strength, control, and coordination and range of joint motion (ROJM); (2) motivation to move; and (3) absence of restriction in the environment. To prevent injury, use of good body mechanics is essential (Table 5-1).

Immobilized older adults with chronic illnesses are at risk of developing complications that affect all body systems very quickly (Hogstel, 1992). These complications include muscle atrophy, loss of bony mass, contractures of joints and pressure ulcers, cardiovascular and respiratory problems, constipation, urinary stasis, and mental confusion.

Incorporating Exercise into Activities of Daily Living

UPPER BODY

Nodding head "yes": neck flexion
Shaking head "no": neck rotation
Reaching to bedside stand for book: shoulder extension
Scratching back: shoulder hyperextension
Brushing or combing hair: shoulder hyperextension
Eating, bathing, and shaving: elbow flexion and extension
Writing and eating: fingers and thumb flexion, extension, and opposition

LOWER BODY

Walking: hip flexion, extension, and hyperextension; knee flexion and extension; ankle dorsiflexion; plantar flexion
Moving to side-lying position: hip flexion, extension, and abduction; knee flexion and extension
Moving from side-lying position: hip extension and adduction; knee flexion and extension
While sitting, lifting knees up and straightening legs: strengthens muscles used for walking

---

Table 5-1 Body Mechanics for Health Care Workers

Action	Rationale
1. When planning to move a client, arrange for adequate help. Use mechanical aids if help is unavailable.	Two workers lifting together divide the workload by 50%.
2. Encourage client to assist as much as possible.	This promotes client's abilities and strength while minimizing workload.
3. Keep back, neck, pelvis, and feet aligned. Avoid twisting.	Twisting increases risk of injury.
4. Flex knees; keep feet wide apart.	A broad base of support increases stability.
5. Position self close to client (or object being lifted).	The force is minimized. Ten pounds at waist height close to body is equal to 100 pounds at arms' length (Patterson, 1993).
6. Use arms and legs (not back).	The leg muscles are stronger, larger muscles capable of greater work without injury.
7. Slide client toward yourself using a pull sheet.	Sliding requires less effort than lifting. Pull sheet minimizes shearing forces, which can damage client's skin.
8. Set (tighten) abdominal and gluteal muscles in preparation for move.	Preparing muscles for the load minimizes strain.
9. Person with the heaviest load coordinates efforts of team involved by counting to three.	Simultaneous lifting minimizes the load for any one lifter.

Bed rest is a medical intervention in which the client is restricted to bed for one of the following purposes: (1) decreasing oxygen requirements of the body, (2) reducing pain, and (3) allowing rest and recovery.

Nursing Diagnosis

Activity Intolerance is a situation in which clients experience altered vital signs (pulse, respiration, or blood pressure) in response to activity. **Impaired Physical Mobility** is associated with pain or discomfort resulting from trauma or surgery, decreased strength and endurance, prolonged bed rest, or restrictive external devices such as casts, splints, braces, or drainage and intravenous (IV) tubing. Psychological factors such as **Fear** relating to a history of falling also result in a client's refusal to ambulate. **Risk for Disuse Syndrome** is a diagnosis that applies when inactivity is desired or unavoidable, increasing the risk for deterioration of cardiovascular, respiratory, musculoskeletal, and psychosocial body systems (McFarland and McFarlane, 1993). In this case, maintenance of the client's present abilities is the primary focus. When a client has mental confusion, weakness, or orthostatic hypotension, **Risk for Injury** should be considered. Finally, a client with a nursing diagnosis of **Pain** is susceptible to developing impaired mobility resulting from the nature and extent of discomfort.

Skill 5.1 | Assisting with Moving and Positioning Clients in Bed

This skill includes moving dependent clients up in bed with one or two nurses and with or without a pull sheet and positioning clients in the Fowler's, supine, lateral, and semiprone (Sims') positions. The prone position is not included because it is uncomfortable, contraindicated for clients with respiratory problems, and rarely used (Bronstein, Popovich, and Stewart-Amidei, 1991). Each position offers advantages and limitations. It is important to be aware of potential pressure points (Figure 5-1). Moving a client even slightly changes the pressure points significantly.

Correct body alignment involves positioning so that no excessive strain is put on joints, tendons, ligaments, and muscles. Clients unable to move independently need to be repositioned at least every 2 hours and need a regular program of assisted range of motion (ROM) exer-

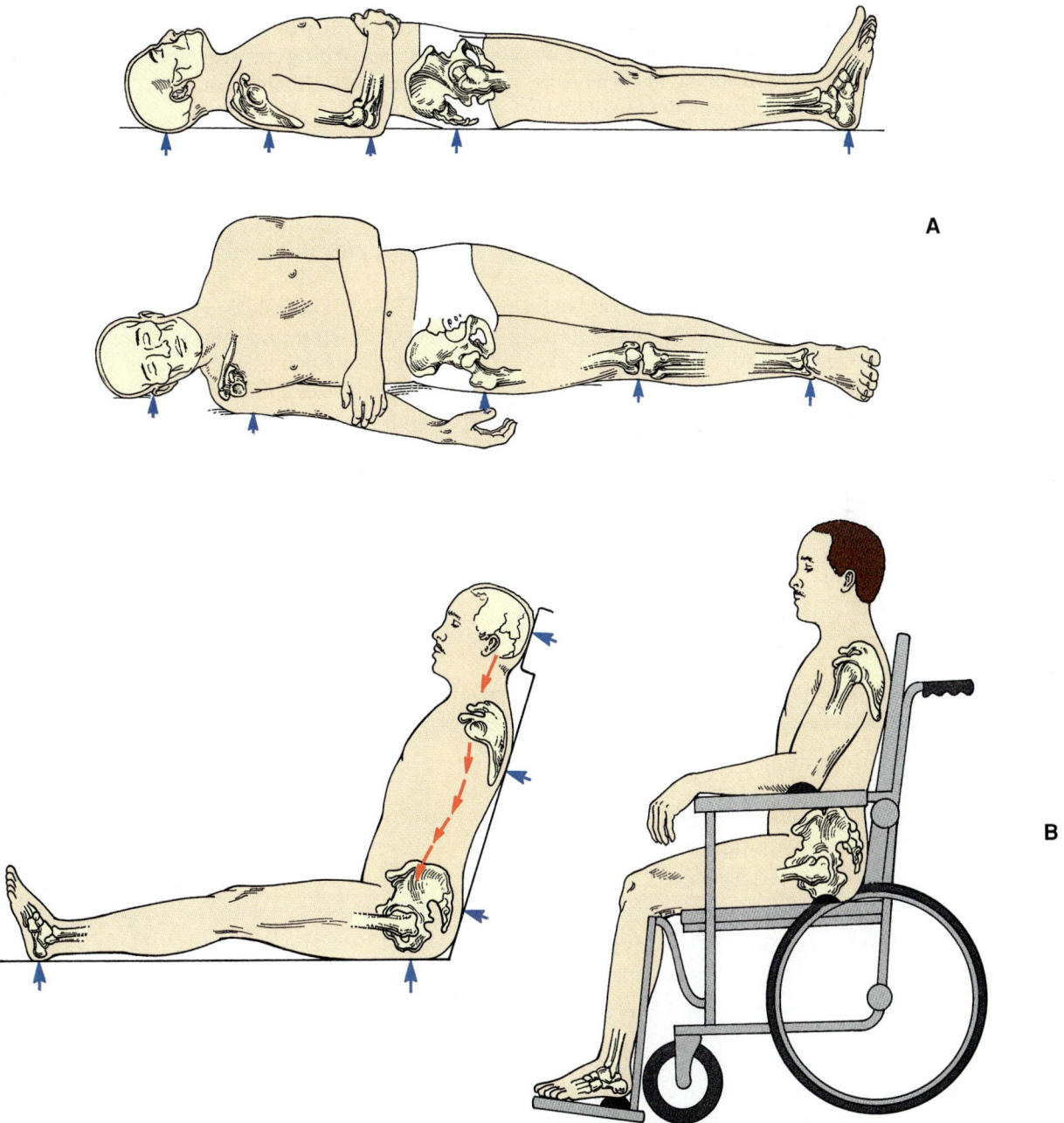

A

B

Figure 5-1 **A,** Pressure points in lying position. **B,** Pressure points in sitting position.

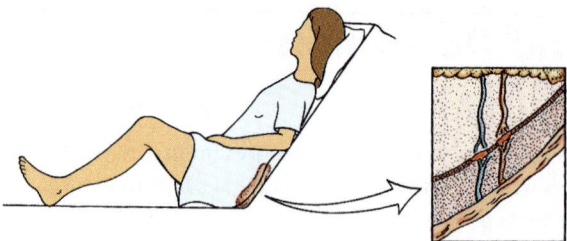

Figure 5-2 Shearing forces against sacrum cause tissue damage.

cises. Care must be taken to protect the skin from damage caused by "shearing forces" resulting from sliding the client over bed linens or rough surfaces (Figure 5-2). Shear injury occurs when the skin remains stationary and the underlying tissue shifts, resulting in tissue damage. Friction injuries may be reduced by the use of lubricants (corn starch or creams), protective films or dressings, and protective padding (USDHHS, 1992). This is especially important when the older client is thin, has fragile skin, is nutritionally compromised, or is unable to move independently.

For immobilized clients, pillows or foam wedges should be used to keep bony prominences such as heels and ankles from excessive or extended pressure. The use of air or water mattresses is also recommended (see Chapter 24).

EQUIPMENT

Pillows	Pull sheet
Hand rolls	Trapeze (optional)

Assessment

1. Assess client's weight, age, level of consciousness, and ability to cooperate. **This information determines how much assistance will be needed.**
2. Assess strength of muscles and mobility of joints to be used by observing client movement in bed and by applying gradual pressure to a muscle group (e.g., attempting to extend client's elbow). Have client resist pressure by moving against the pressure (flex elbow). Compare strength in muscle groups, including arms and legs.
3. Assess willingness to cooperate.
4. Assess need for analgesic medication 30 to 60 minutes before position changes. **Analgesics enhance client's ability to tolerate movement. Peak levels vary according to the specific analgesic and route of administration.**

Planning

Expected outcomes focus on mobility, self-care, interaction, and prevention of complications within the confines of the prescribed activity.

EXPECTED OUTCOMES

1. Normal reactive hyperemia (increased circulation) over pressure points lasts less than 1 hour.
2. Client verbalizes a sense of comfort after each repositioning.
3. Client maintains assisted changes in position in bed for at least 1 hour.
4. Client lists three benefits of position changes and good body alignment.

Implementation

Steps	Rationale
1. See Standard Protocol (Chapter 1, p. 5).	
2. Moving a dependent client up in bed with one nurse and client assistance Review principles of body mechanics (see Table 5-1). **nurse alert** This move requires that the client can assist by pushing with feet and/or lifting with trapeze. a. Adjust position of IV pole, tubes, and catheters. b. Provide client with hearing aid and glasses if used. Encourage client to assist as much as possible, discuss the steps involved, and determine ways client	 Facilitates movement without tension and disruption. Promoting client involvement motivates and speeds progress toward independence and provides a sense of control and security.

Steps	Rationale

will assist. Review each step again as move is about to be made.

c. Lower the head of the bed to the lowest position. Place the pillow near the headboard.

d. Assist client to flex knees so that soles of one or both feet are flat on the bed.

e. If there is no trapeze, slide arm nearest the head of the bed under client's shoulders, reaching under and supporting client's opposite shoulder. Place other arm under client's upper back (Figure 5-3). Have client push with feet as you lift on the count of three.

f. If there is a trapeze, assist client to grasp it. Slide both arms under the lower body (Figure 5-4).

g. Have client lift with trapeze and/or push with feet on the count of three. Repeat if needed to move up farther in the bed.

h. Ask what is needed to position client comfortably and adjust as necessary.

Minimizes effort required to move client and minimizes potential trauma from head contacting headboard. Positions client to exert effort when moving up in bed.

Coordinates client's movement with nurse's lifting action.

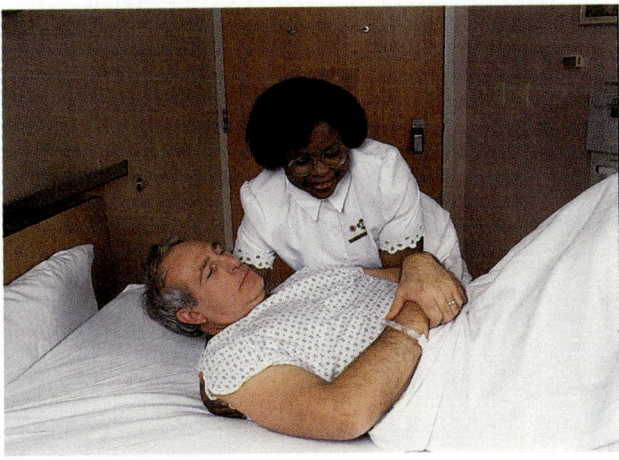

Figure 5-3

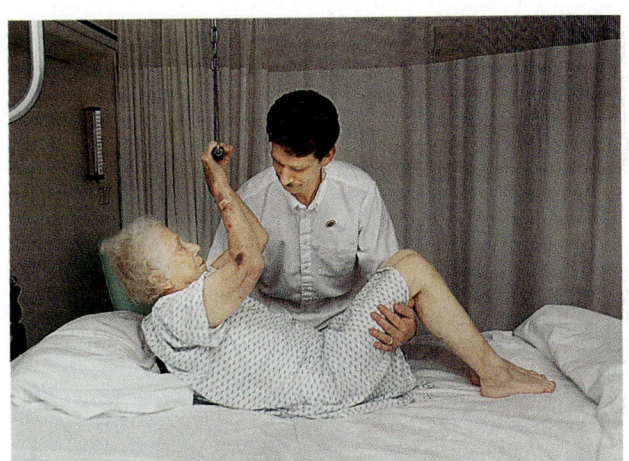

Figure 5-4

3. Assisting client to move up in bed when client cannot assist

a. Lower the head of bed to the lowest position client can tolerate and lower side rails.

b. Roll client side to side, placing a pull sheet that extends from shoulders to thighs. A pull sheet can be made using a small sheet folded in half.

c. With one nurse on each side of client, grasp pull sheet firmly with hands near client's upper arms and hips, rolling sheet material until hands are close to client.

d. Nurses' knees are flexed with body facing the direction of the move. The foot away from the bed faces forward for a broader base of support (Figure 5-5).

e. Instruct client to rest arms on body and to lift head on the count of three.

Clients with hypoxia may not tolerate lying flat.

The closer nurses are to client, the less height of lifting is required to clear the bed during the move.

nurse alert Review principles of body mechanics (see Table 5-1). This move requires at least two nurses and pull sheet when client is unable to assist. If the client is very heavy, consider the need for more assistance.

Steps	Rationale

f. Lift client toward the head of the bed on the count of three. Repeat the move if necessary.

g. Assist client as needed to shift in order to attain position of comfort.

4. Positioning in semi-Fowler's and Fowler's position

For the semi-Fowler's position, the head of the bed is raised 45 to 60 degrees. The high Fowler's position, with the head of the bed raised 90 degrees, is recommended for eating. Both positions improve breathing by decreasing pressure on the diaphragm as gravity pulls abdominal contents downward. These positions also facilitate visiting and diversional activities. Clients tend to slide toward the foot of the bed (Figure 5-6).

a. Raise the head of the bed to the appropriate level (45 to 90 degrees).

b. Use pillows to support client's arms and hands if upper body is immobilized.

c. Position a pillow under the client's head if desired, and raise the knee break of the bed slightly. Avoid pressure under the popliteal space (back of the knee).

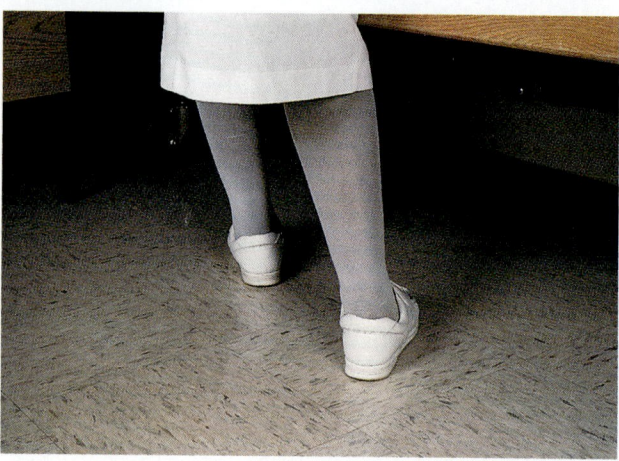

Figure 5-5

Minimizes development of dependent edema and prevents shoulder dislocation if client has upper extremity impairment.

Pressure can interfere with circulation and contribute to thromboemboli (blood clots).

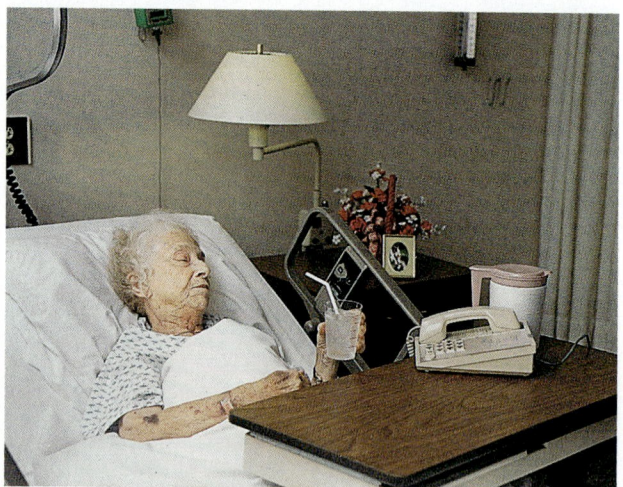

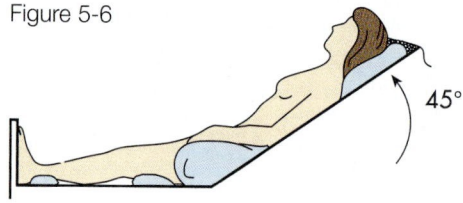

Figure 5-6

d. Change the degree of elevation of the head of bed 5 to 10 degrees frequently.

e. Identify potential pressure points, including scapulae, elbows, sacrum or coccyx, and heels (see Figure 5-1, *B*).

Alters the pressure points slightly and promotes comfort.

5. Moving dependent client to lateral (side-lying) position

This move removes pressure from bony prominences of entire back (Figure 5-7).

Steps	Rationale

a. Lower the head of bed as much as client can tolerate and lower side rail.

b. Using a pull sheet, move client to the side of the bed opposite to the one toward which the client will be turned. Raise side rail. Go to opposite side of the bed and lower side rail.
> Ensures that client will be in center of the bed when turned.

c. Assist client to raise arm nearest you above head, adjusting pillow if needed.

d. Grasp client's shoulder and hip, and assist client to roll toward you onto side.
> Turning client toward you promotes client's sense of security.
> Keeps spine in good alignment.

e. Flex client's knee that is uppermost after the turn and support leg from knee to foot.

f. Ease lower shoulder forward and check client's comfort.
> Prevents excessive pressure directly on shoulder.

g. Support upper arm with pillows so that arm is level with shoulder.
> Improves ventilation by minimizing pressure on chest.

h. Place pillow behind client's back and roll under so that it is folded lengthwise and is tucked smoothly against back.
> Provides support and prevents client from rolling onto back.

i. Make sure client's back is straight without evidence of twisting. Adjust as needed for comfort.

j. Pressure points to check include the ear, shoulder, anterior iliac spine, trochanter, lateral side of the knee, malleolus, and foot (see Figure 5-1, *A*).

nurse alert   Individuals at risk for developing pressure ulcers should not be positioned directly on the trochanter when the side-lying position is used. A 30-degree lateral position is recommended as the appropriate alternative (USDHHS, 1992).

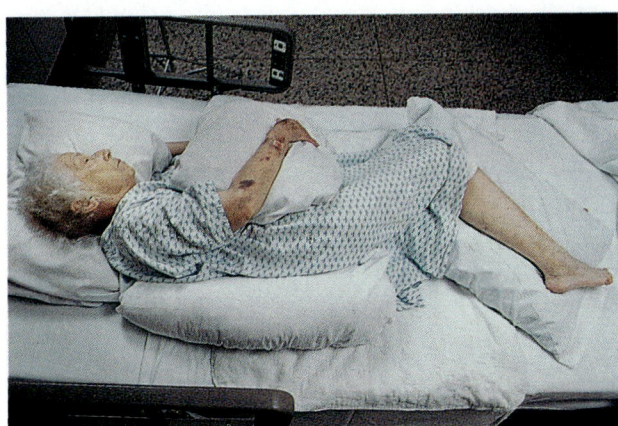

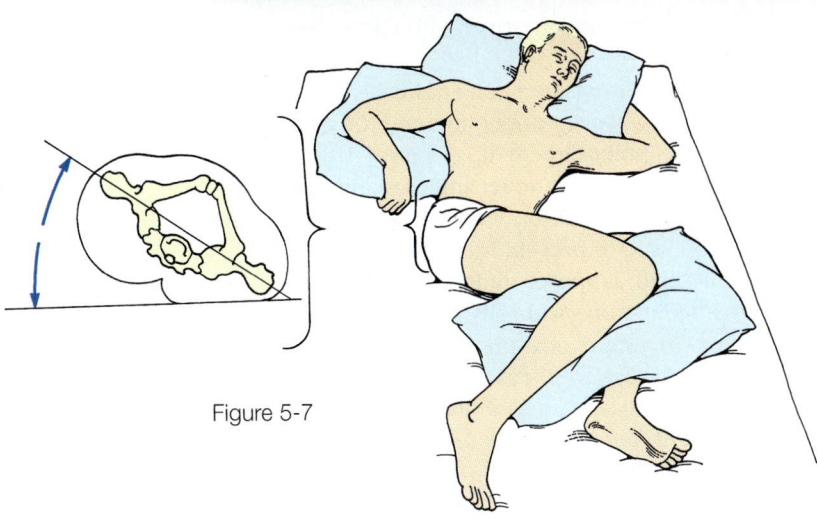

Figure 5-7

Steps	Rationale

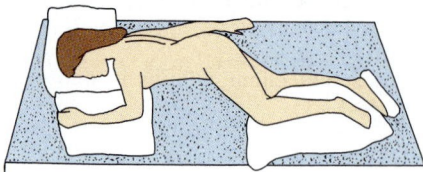

Figure 5-8

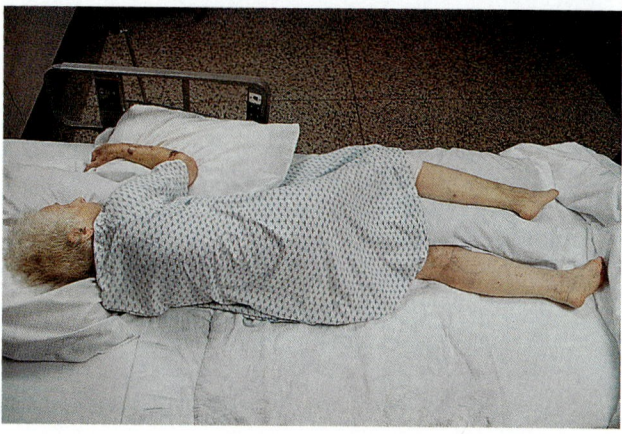

6. Moving dependent client to Sims' (semi-prone) position

For this alternative to the lateral position, client lies somewhat forward onto abdomen. This move is useful to discourage clients from rolling back to the supine position. It also minimizes pressure on the hip and shoulder (Figure 5-8).

a. With client in the lateral position, arm against mattress is externally rotated with elbow extended. Prevent internal rotation of hip and adduction of leg by extending the lowermost leg and supporting the other leg level with the hip.

b. Support client's uppermost arm in flexed position level with shoulder.

c. Pressure points include ear, front of shoulder, iliac crest, lateral knee, malleolus, and side of foot of lower leg, as well as medial knee and malleolus of upper leg.

Decreases internal rotation and adduction of shoulder and protects joint. Allows better chest expansion and improves ventilation.

7. Positioning dependent client in supine position

This alternative to the Fowler's or semi-Fowler's position decreases pressure on buttocks and minimizes client's tendency to slide to the foot of the bed (Figure 5-9).

a. Place client on back with head of bed flat.

b. Place small support (pillow) under lumbar area of back.

c. Place pillow under upper shoulders, neck, and head.

d. To position trochanter roll at client's hips, place a folded bath blanket under hips and roll ends under until toes point directly up (Figure 5-10).

e. Place small support under ankles to minimize pressure on heels. High-top tennis shoes or a footboard may be used to prevent footdrop.

f. Place small supports under forearms with hand-wrist splints or small rolls to support fingers and thumb in a functional position.

g. Pressure areas to check include the back of the head, scapulae, posterior iliac spines, sacrum or coccyx, ischium, Achilles tendons, and heels (see Figure 5-1, *A*).

8. See Completion Protocol (Chapter 1, p. 6).

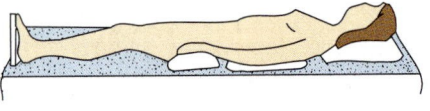

Figure 5-9

Supports normal curvature of lumbar spine.

Prevents excessive flexion of cervical spine.

Prevents external rotation of hips and may be bilateral or unilateral depending on extent and location of muscle weakness.

A functional position allows the fingers to be flexed and the thumb to touch the fingertips.

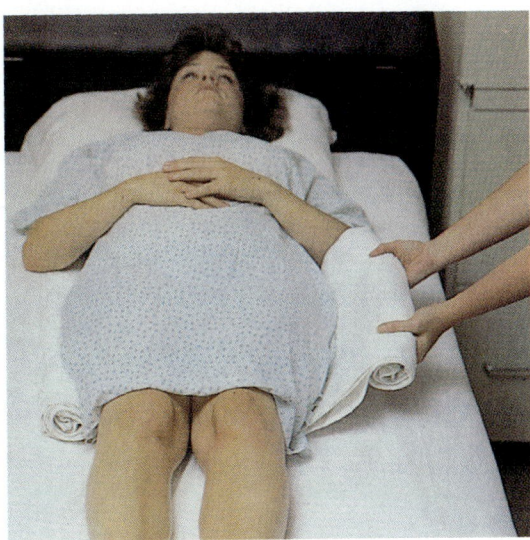

Figure 5-10

Evaluation

1. Inspect skin overlying pressure areas for erythema (redness) and blanching. Observe again in 60 minutes.
2. Ask client if position is comfortable.
3. Observe client's body alignment and position.
4. Ask client to identify three benefits of position changes and correct body alignment.

UNEXPECTED OUTCOMES AND RELATED INTERVENTIONS

1. Client develops areas of abnormal reactive hyperemia, blistering, or skin irritation.
   a. Change client's position more frequently.
   b. Avoid prolonged pressure on any one pressure area.
2. Client complains of discomfort from stretching because of altered alignment.
   a. Readjust position according to client's comfort level.
   b. Readjust supportive pillows to maintain alignment.
3. Client turns back to same position frequently and expresses discomfort with alternate positions.
   a. Reinforce the rationale for position changes.
   b. Provide diversional activities in various positions.
   c. Identify client's perception of position preference and attempt to create incentive for compliance with alternate positions.

SAMPLE DOCUMENTATION

0800 Turned from back to left lateral position. Area of erythema approximately 3 cm in diameter noted over coccyx. Blanches easily. Urged client not to lie on back.

1000 Found client lying on back. Turned to right side and supported with pillows. Coccyx remains reddened, blanches to fingertip pressure.

Skill 5.2 | Minimizing Orthostatic Hypotension

Orthostatic or postural hypotension involves a rapid drop in blood pressure of 25 mm Hg or more when changing from the supine to the sitting or standing position (Canobbio, 1990). The decreased blood pressure results in dizziness or sometimes fainting. Orthostatic hypotension may be related to bed rest, hypovolemia (decreased circulating blood volume), hypokalemia (low serum potassium level), and certain medications, including sedatives, hypnotics, analgesics, antihypertensives, antiemetics, antihistamines, diuretics, and antianxiety agents (McFarland and McFarlane, 1993).

EQUIPMENT

Blood pressure sphygmomanometer
Stethoscope

Assessment

1. Check previous blood pressure and pulse readings and assess client's activity level. **This establishes baseline criteria.**

2. Identify factors that may precipitate orthostatic hypotension, including decreased intravascular volume, hypokalemia, prolonged immobility, and medications.

Planning

Expected outcomes focus on preventing hypotension and increasing tolerance of activity with minimal risk of falls.

EXPECTED OUTCOMES

1. Client demonstrates no evidence of weakness or dizziness in response to position changes.
2. Client states three factors that influence incidents of orthostatic hypotension.
3. Client ambulates 10 feet while maintaining blood pressure within 25 mm Hg of systolic baseline.

Implementation

Steps	Rationale
1. See Standard Protocol (Chapter 1, p. 5).	
2. Explain reason for gradual position change.	
3. Raise head of bed slowly to semi-Fowler's and then to high Fowler's position and reassess blood pressure, pulse, and respirations. Instruct client to report any dizziness or lightheadedness during position change.	Raising slowly allows body to adjust to change in position. If client has a drop in blood pressure of 25 mm Hg (systolic) when upright, orthostatic hypotension is evident and risk of falls significant.

nurse alert *DO NOT attempt to ambulate if client reports dizziness or systolic blood pressure falls more than 25 mm Hg.* Lower head and allow client to rest for a few minutes and try again more gradually.

Steps	Rationale
4. If no evidence of hypotension occurs, proceed to dangle (allow feet to hang over the side of the bed). Encourage client to move shoulders in circles and flex and extend ankles and knees. Reassess blood pressure.	Movement of muscles increases venous return and stimulates circulation.
5. Proceed with planned activity.	
6. See Completion Protocol (Chapter 1, p. 6).	

Evaluation

1. Observe client for signs of weakness, dizziness.
2. Assess blood pressure, pulse, and respirations if client experiences weakness or dizziness at any point and on completion of activity. Normally, blood pressure, pulse, and respirations increase slightly in response to exercise and return to baseline within 5 minutes of resting.
3. Ask client to describe three factors pertinent to the clinical condition that may cause orthostatic hypotension.

UNEXPECTED OUTCOMES AND RELATED INTERVENTIONS

Client becomes lightheaded and dizzy when upright.
a. Return client to supine position.
b. Take blood pressure immediately.
c. After 3 to 5 minutes, attempt the same procedure. If unsuccessful, wait 1 to 2 hours before attempting again.

SAMPLE DOCUMENTATION

0900 BP with client lying down was 110/70, pulse 86, respirations 18. Was assisted to sitting position over 1 minute. Complained of dizziness. BP was 90/50, pulse 94, respirations 22. After resting in supine position for 5 minutes was assisted to upright position more slowly (over 3 minutes) without dizziness. BP 104/72, pulse 90, respirations 20. Ambulated to bathroom slowly with steady gait. Stated, "I feel weak, but not dizzy."

Skill 5.3 | Transferring from Bed to Chair

This transfer technique can be done by one nurse. Moving clients to a chair after bed rest stimulates them physically and mentally and promotes involvement in self-care activities. It is important to allow clients to proceed at their own pace, encouraging as much independence as possible. Transfers may be from bed to chair, wheelchair, or bedside commode.

EQUIPMENT

Transfer belt
Sling
Nonskid footwear
Bath blanket
Pillows

nurse alert   In general, nurses should not attempt to lift more than 35% of their own body weight. When in doubt about their ability to transfer a client safely, nurses should request assistance. It is advisable to use a transfer belt when clients have severe weakness, impaired balance, hemiparesis, or difficulty cooperating because of an altered mental state.

Wheelchair: position chair close to bed, lock brakes, and remove or fold footrests out of the way.
Bedside commode or supportive chair

Assessment

1. Assess muscle strength of legs and upper arms, comparing right with left. **Clients with hemiplegia have one-sided weakness. Clients with paraplegia may have spastic or flaccid paralysis.**
2. Assess joint mobility and limitations caused by contractures or discomfort. Assess for history of osteoporosis, which may increase risk of pathological fractures with minimal stress.
3. Assess vision, hearing, and altered sensation. **The presence of numbness or tingling of the feet or legs alters function.**

4. Assess ability to follow verbal instructions and appropriateness of response to simple commands.
5. Assess client's level of motivation. **Clients who fear falling may avoid activity or make excuses.**
6. Determine the position and functioning of IV tubing and poles, need for oxygen therapy, Foley catheter, surgical drains, and other drains or tubes.
7. Assess the need for prescribed analgesic medication minutes before transfer. Plan activity for the period in which adequate pain relief is apparent without dizziness or excessive sedation. **Analgesics enhance client's ability to tolerate movement. Peak levels vary according to the specific analgesic and route of administration.**

Planning

Expected outcomes focus on improving the client's functional abilities and strength. It is also essential to promote body alignment and safety.

EXPECTED OUTCOMES

1. Client assists with transfer to chair by standing erect, pivoting, and grasping arm of chair to sit.
2. Client feeds self while sitting in chair 30 to 40 minutes for breakfast and lunch.
3. Client participates in conversation with roommate while up in chair.

Implementation

Steps	Rationale
nurse alert Check the equipment to be used and familiarize yourself with safety factors involved, such as wheelchair brakes, removable arm, adjustable footrest or leg rest, and reclining features.	
1. See Standard Protocol (Chapter 1, p. 5).	
2. Position the chair or wheelchair so that the move will be *toward the client's stronger side.* Chair should be at an appropriate distance to allow client participation and safety. The stronger the client, the greater should be the distance.	Facilitates balance and movement.
3. Lower bed to lowest position. Lower side rails and turn client to one side with knees flexed.	
4. Raise the head of the bed to the highest position.	Minimizes orthostatic hypotension (see Skill 5.2).
5. Face the foot of the bed with feet comfortably apart and a broad base of support.	Maximizes nurse's stability and balance and prevents twisting that could result in muscle strain.
6. Assist client to the sitting position by lifting upper body as the legs swing over edge of the bed (Figure 5-11).	Client should be able to place feet flat on floor for balance and stability.
7. Encourage client to assist as much as possible as legs and feet are assisted over side of bed and client's shoulders are raised.	

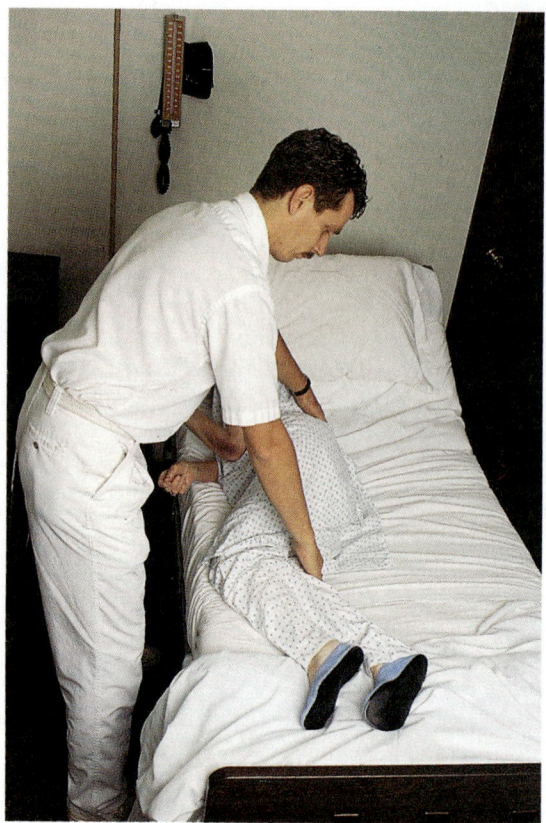

Figure 5-11

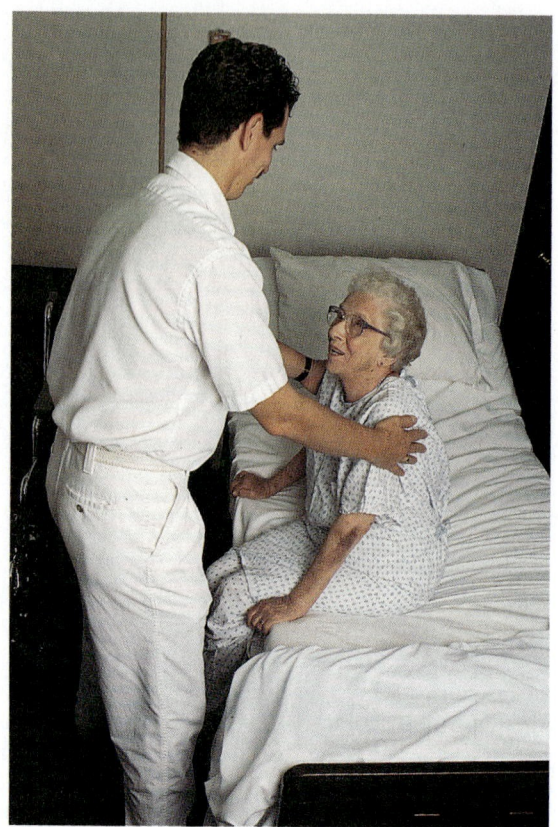

Figure 5-12

A

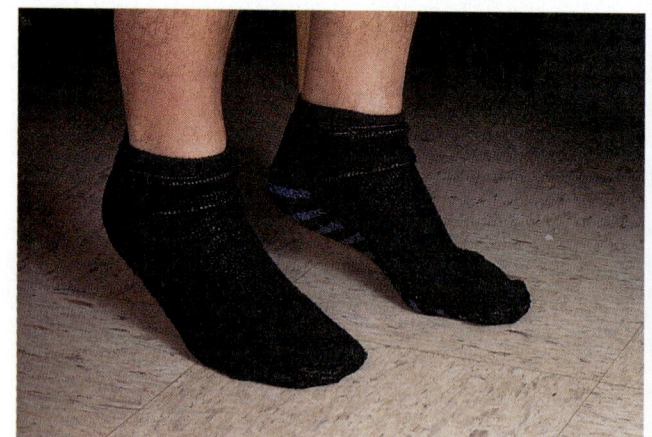

Figure 5-13

B

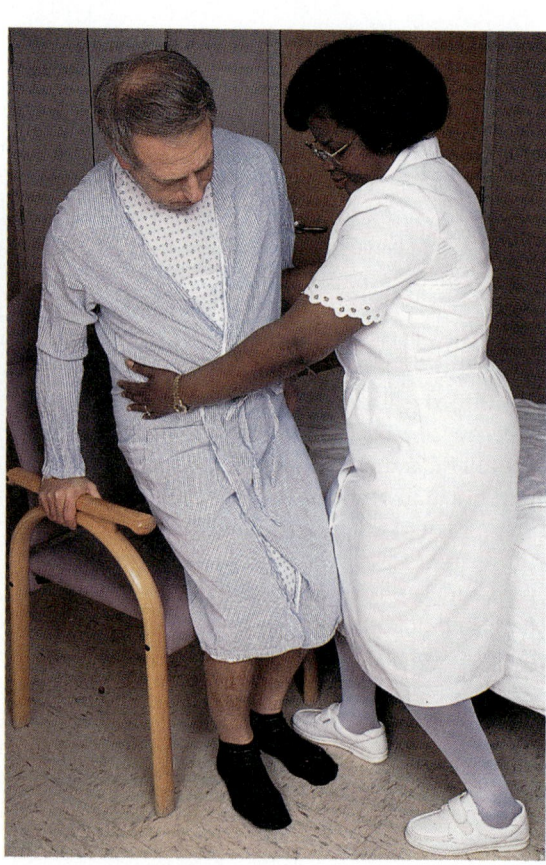

Steps	Rationale
8. Instruct client to take a deep breath and sit for 1 to 2 minutes. Encourage movement of shoulders, legs, feet, and toes (Figure 5-12).	Muscle activity promotes venous circulation and allows adjustment to the sitting position.
9. Assist client to put on nonskid slippers or shoes and place feet flat on the floor (Figure 5-13, *A*).	
10. Apply transfer belt if needed for stability.	
11. Apply a sling if client has flaccid arm.	Supports arm and prevents from stress or injury.
12. Review the steps of the transfer procedure and ways client will assist with the move.	Encourages client to participate in transfer and increases muscle strength and a sense of control.
13. Grasp the transfer belt with both hands toward the side of the client's back. Keep back straight, knees flexed with a wide base of support, and the foot farthest from the chair in a forward position. Client may place hands on your shoulders (not around neck).	Arms around neck could result in neck injury to nurse.
14. Instruct client to rock forward with each count and to stand erect on the count of three. If needed, stabilize client's affected side with pressure against the knee.	Rocking motion gives client's body momentum and reduces the effort required to lift to standing position.
15. Once standing, pivot client toward seat of chair. Client should then reach for arm of the chair and assist to ease self into chair (Figure 5-13, *B*).	
16. Observe client for proper alignment for sitting. Provide pillows to support affected (paralyzed) extremities (Figure 5-14).	
17. See Completion Protocol (Chapter 1, p. 6).	

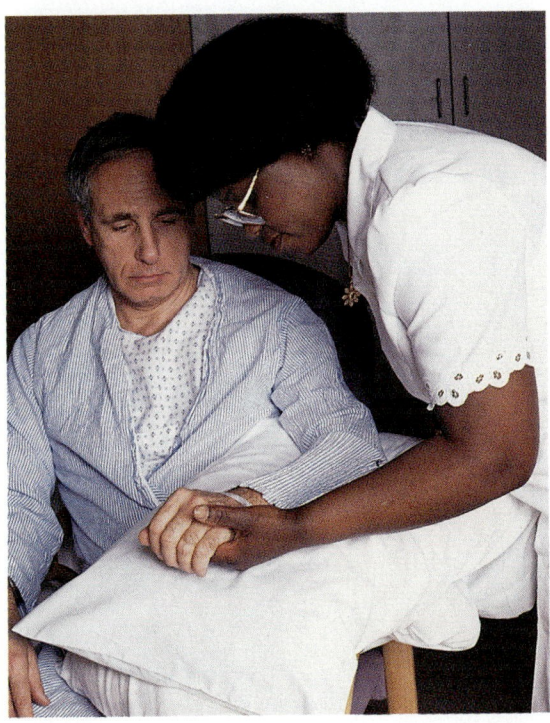

Figure 5-14

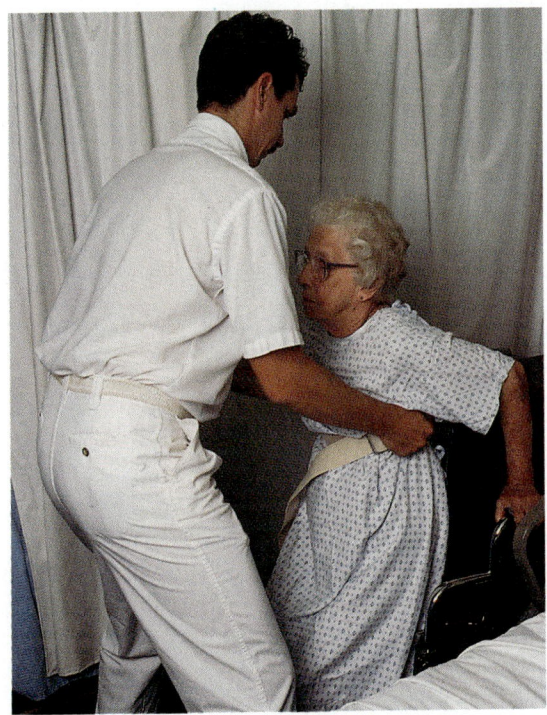

Figure 5-15

Evaluation

1. Observe client's ability to bear weight (or avoid bearing weight if prescribed), ability to pivot, and number of personnel needed. Ask client to describe level of strength and control.
2. Monitor length of time client sits in chair and observe ability to feed self while sitting in chair.
3. Observe socialization with roommate while up in chair.

UNEXPECTED OUTCOMES AND RELATED INTERVENTIONS

1. Client does not follow directions for transfer.
   a. Identify interfering factors (e.g., anxiety) and provide positive reinforcement for effort and achievement.
   b. Demonstrate the procedure for the client in a step-by-step manner.
2. Client's weakness of lower extremities does not permit active transfer.

a. Develop a plan for isotonic or isometric leg-strengthening exercises to be done while lying in bed or sitting in chair.
   b. Use a gait belt for balance and support.
3. Client tends to bear weight on non-weight-bearing leg.
   a. Have another care giver support affected leg as a reminder.
   b. Use a gait belt to facilitate balance and control (Figure 5-15).

SAMPLE DOCUMENTATION

0800 Transferred client from bed to chair with gait belt and assistance of one. Cooperative and able to stand erect with encouragement. Smiled when able to assist with self-feeding.

0815 Requested to return to bed. Stated, "I'm so tired, I just can't sit up any longer." Needed assistance of two with transfer back to bed. Knees buckled and legs were shaking during attempt to stand.

Skill 5.4 | Using a Mechanical (Hoyer) Lift for Transfer from Bed to Chair

Mechanical lifts are used for large, dependent clients who do not have spinal cord injury. Use of a lift does not require assistance from the client and should be used only when required (Baas and Ross, 1990).

EQUIPMENT

Mechanical (Hoyer) lift: hydraulic lift frame with supporting boom and attached chains, canvas sling (Figure 15-16).
Pillow

nurse alert   Before using the device, practice using controls that spread the base to provide stability, the lever that raises the sling, and the release that lowers the sling.

Assessment

1. Compare the weight limit for the lift with the client's current anticipated weight.
2. Assess muscle strength of legs and upper arms, joint mobility, and limitations from contractures or discomfort.
3. Assess vision, hearing, and altered sensation. **Decreased vision or hearing influences ability to follow verbal instructions. The presence of**

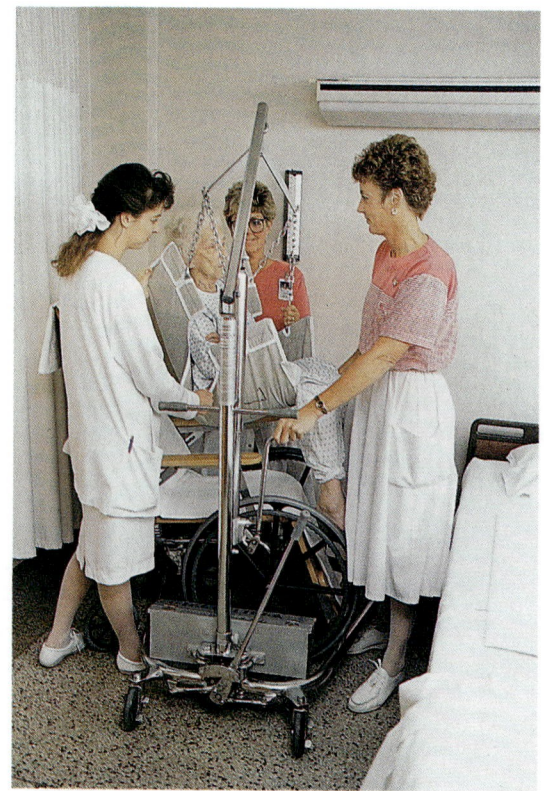

Figure 5-16

numbness or tingling of the feet or legs alters function.

4. Assess client's level of motivation. **Clients who fear falling may avoid activity or make excuses.**

Planning

Expected outcomes focus on promoting safety and comfort during the transfer.

EXPECTED OUTCOMES

1. Client verbalizes feeling secure and comfortable during transfer.
2. Client transfers safely.
3. Client maintains correct body alignment after transfer.
4. Client maintains systolic blood pressure within 25 mm Hg of baseline during transfer.

Implementation

Steps	Rationale
1. See Standard Protocol (Chapter 1, p. 5).	
2. Ask another care giver to assist. Move the lift to the bedside. Place a comfortable chair with supportive arms in a convenient location.	
3. Raise the bed to a comfortable height. Turn client to side, and place the canvas sling under the client extending from popliteal space of the knees to beneath the head. The hole is placed under the buttocks.	
4. With the client lying supine and arms crossed over the body, position the lift with the base under the bed and spread the base of the lift.	Enhances stability to prevent tipping with a broad base of support.
5. Attach the shorter chains to the section of the sling (may be narrower) that supports the upper body.	
6. Raise the boom slightly and attach the longer chains to the (wider) sling that supports the hips and thighs.	It may help if one care giver supports and flexes the client's knees as another attaches the chains to the sling.
7. Adjust the sling as necessary so that the client's weight is evenly distributed.	Promotes stability and security during the move.
8. Pump the lift to elevate it just enough to clear the bed, and guide client's legs over the side (Figure 5-17).	

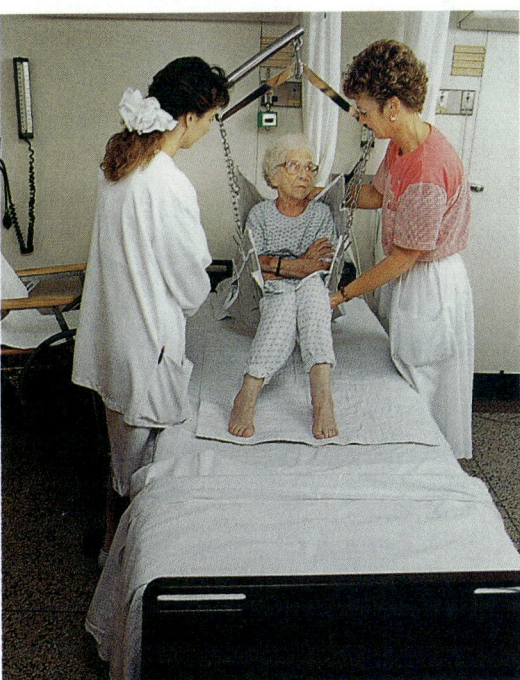

Figure 5-17

Steps	Rationale

9. Instruct the client to keep arms folded during the transfer.

Keeps the device balanced and prevents injury from bumping against objects.

10. Check the chair's position and stability before the move. While supporting the client, guide the lift toward the chair, commode, or wheelchair so that when the boom is lowered, client will be centered in the chair.

11. Release valve slowly and lower client into the chair. Protect client's head from striking the equipment. Once client is securely seated, remove the chains and store the lift nearby (Figure 5-18).

Leaving the sling under client facilitates transfer back to bed.

12. See Completion Protocol (Chapter 1, p. 6).

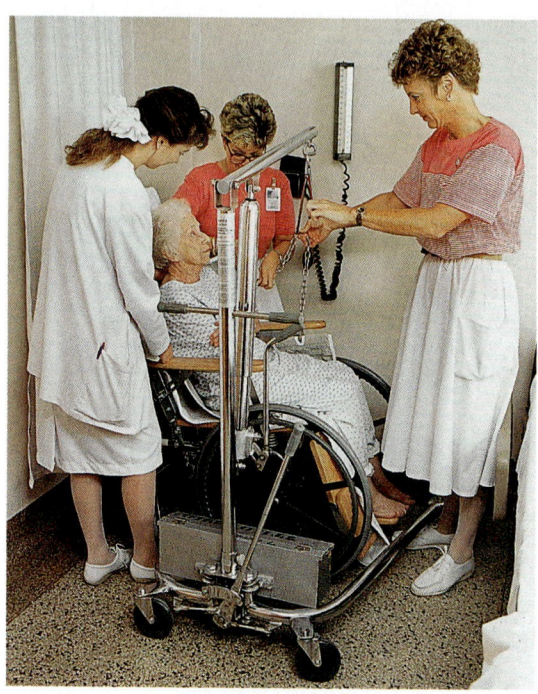

Figure 5-18

Evaluation

1. Ask client if the transfer felt safe, smooth, and comfortable.
2. Observe for correct body alignment.
3. Take blood pressure and compare with baseline.

UNEXPECTED OUTCOMES AND RELATED INTERVENTIONS

1. Client's buttocks are too far forward in the chair seat, resulting in a slouched position.
   a. Have one care giver stand in front of client to push the pelvis back into the chair.
   b. A second care giver stands behind client, placing arms under client's axillae and grasping client's wrists, which places the force on client's arms rather than at axillae and prevents injury from pressure on axillae.
   c. As care giver behind client lifts upward, second care giver pushes the knees toward back of the chair, sliding the buttocks into alignment. Avoid shearing forces.
2. Blood pressure drops more than 20 mm Hg.
   a. Have client extend and flex knees and ankles to encourage venous blood flow.
   b. If dizziness increases, lower head to position between knees and encourage deep breaths.
   c. Assess blood pressure in 5 minutes.

SAMPLE DOCUMENTATION

0900 Transferred from bed to chair using Hoyer lift. Cooperative with move. Stated "I felt very secure this time." Noted a tendency to slide down in the chair while sitting. Propped with pillows and encouraged to call for assistance when this happens. Call light is within reach.

Skill 5.5 | Transferring from Bed to Stretcher

This transfer involves movement from the bed to a stretcher for client transport from one department to another, to surgery, or for diagnostic tests when the client is too ill to tolerate sitting, client is sedated, or equipment requires a supine position.

EQUIPMENT

Stretcher with side rails or safety straps and brake locks
IV pole (if needed and not attached to stretcher)
Roller device or plastic moving device (heavy plastic to minimize shearing forces while sliding client)
Bath blanket or sheet
Pillow

nurse alert As many as five care givers may be required for a safe transfer of a heavy client who cannot assist.

Assessment

1. Assess client's level of consciousness and ability to co-operate with the move.
2. Assess client's joint mobility and limitations.
3. Assess client's pain, including location and severity. When appropriate, offer prescribed analgesic medication 30 to 60 minutes before transfer. **Analgesics enhance client's ability to tolerate movement. Peak levels vary according to the specific analgesic and route of administration.**

Planning

Expected outcomes focus on comfort and safety.

EXPECTED OUTCOMES

1. Client follows instructions for transfer to stretcher.
2. Client verbalizes feeling comfortable and secure during transfer.

Implementation

Steps	Rationale
1. See Standard Protocol (Chapter 1, p. 5). 2. Position the bed flat and raise to the same height as the stretcher. Lower side rails. 3. Cover client with a sheet or bath blanket, and remove top covers of the bed without exposing client. 4. Check for IV line, Foley catheter, tubes, or surgical drains and position them to avoid tension during the move. 5. Position the stretcher as close to the bed as possible and lock the wheels of the bed and stretcher. Side rails should be lowered (Figure 5-19).	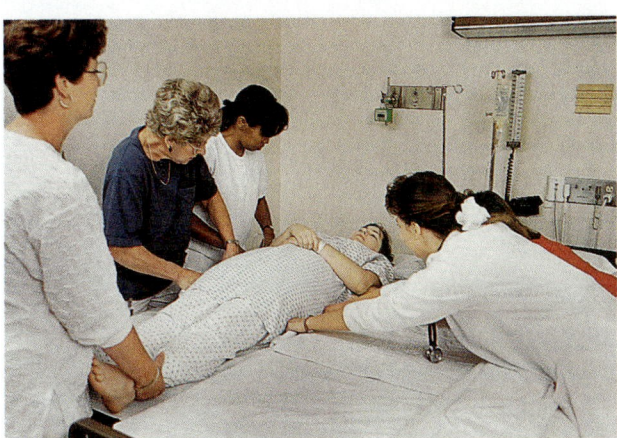 Figure 5-19
6. Transfer when client can assist a. Stand near the side of the stretcher and instruct client to move feet, then buttocks, and finally upper body to the stretcher, bringing cover along. b. After moving, check to be sure client's body is centered on the stretcher.	Promotes safety and security.
7. Client is unable to assist a. Place a folded sheet or bath blanket so that it supports client's head and extends to midthighs. b. Roll the sheet or bath blanket close to client's body. Assist client to cross arms over chest.	

Steps	Rationale
c. Two care givers reach over the bed to client, and two care givers stand as close as possible to the stretcher. A fifth care giver stands at the foot of the bed to lift the feet (Figure 5-20). d. Using a coordinating count of three, all five care givers simultaneously lift client to edge of the bed. e. With another coordinated lift, move client from edge of the bed to the stretcher.	Being closer to weight being lifted reduces risk of back injury to care giver. 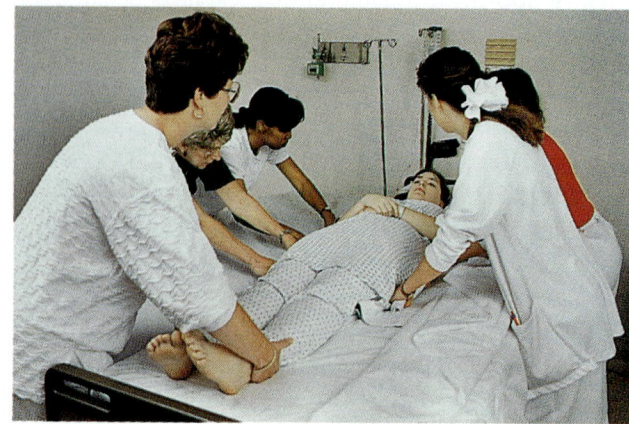 Figure 5-20
8. Raise both side rails and head of the stretcher if desired. **9.** Instruct client to keep hands inside while moving and to avoid grasping side rail, which could bump against door frames during transport. **10.** See Completion Protocol (Chapter 1, p. 6).	Improves breathing and comfort.

Evaluation

1. Observe client's ability to follow instructions and assist with transfer.
2. Ask client if the transfer felt safe, smooth, and comfortable.

UNEXPECTED OUTCOMES AND RELATED INTERVENTIONS
1. Client resists transfer and interferes with move by grasping bed or care givers.

a. Explain reason for transfer to encourage client's cooperation.
b. Reassure client that move will be made slowly and gently, according to client's level of tolerance.
c. Assess for the possibility of premedication for pain before transfer.

SAMPLE DOCUMENTATION
1030 Transferred to stretcher with assistance of 5. Client unable to assist. Reports comfortable transfer. Transported to P.T.

Skill 5.6 | **Assisting Ambulation**

In the normal walking posture, the head is erect; the cervical, thoracic, and lumbar vertebrae are aligned; the hips and knees have slight flexion; and the arms swing freely. Illness, surgery, injury and prolonged bed rest can reduce activity tolerance so that assistance is required. Clients with hemiparesis (one-sided weakness) have difficulty with balance. Temporary or permanent damage to the musculoskeletal or nervous system may necessitate use of an assistive device such as a cane, crutches, or walker (see Chapter 28). Clients with altered cardiovas-

cular or respiratory function may experience difficulty with ambulation, evidenced by chest pain, altered vital signs, dyspnea, or fatigue.

EQUIPMENT
Robe
Nonskid footwear
Portable IV pole
Gait belt (required for clients with unsteady gait or balance)

> **nurse alert** Check the availability of handrails on the walls. Consider whether the assistance of one or two care givers is required, and determine the need for an assistive device.

Assessment

1. Assess client's most recent activity experience, including distance ambulated and tolerance of activity (see Skill 5.2). **This facilitates realistic planning and identifies degree of assistance needed.**
2. Assess the best time to ambulate considering other scheduled activities such as bathing and physical therapy. **Rest is needed after activities requiring exertion and after meals. Energy is needed to digest food.**
3. Assess the environment and remove obstacles such as chairs, tables, and equipment. If client has an IV line, a rolling IV pole is needed.
4. Assess client's motivation and ability to cooperate. **Comparing this activity with activity desired by client for the home environment usually enhances motivation.**

5. Assess for medications that may alter stability including antihypertensive or narcotic medications. **These drugs may cause hypotension, dizziness, or instability.**
6. Consider the need for a place where client can sit and rest during the ambulation.

Planning

Expected outcomes focus on developing activity and rest patterns that support increased tolerance of activity. It is essential that this is tailored to each client's needs and abilities (McFarland and McFarlane, 1993).

EXPECTED OUTCOMES

1. Client ambulates to the end of the hall with assistance, stopping to rest less than three times.
2. Client maintains respirations, pulse, and blood pressure within 10% of resting values.
3. Client maintains erect posture while standing and walking.

Implementation

Steps	Rationale
1. See Standard Protocol (Chapter 1, p. 5).	
2. Assist the client to put on shoes or slippers with non-slip soles.	Provides stable walking support.
3. Assist client to stand at the bedside. Encourage to stand fully erect with shoulders back and looking ahead (not at the floor).	
4. If client is unstable, seat client and apply safety belt before proceeding. Consider the need for additional help.	If client is very heavy, unstable, or fearful, a second person is needed.
5. If client has an IV line, place the IV pole on the same side as the site of infusion, and instruct client to hold and push the pole while ambulating (Figure 5-21).	
6. If a Foley catheter is present, client or care giver carries the bag below the level of the bladder and prevents tension on the tubing.	This prevents reflux of urine from the bag back into the bladder.
7. Take a few steps supporting client with one arm around the waist and the other under the elbow of the flexed arm. Grasp safety belt in the middle of client's waist.	This provides balance and facilitates lowering client to the floor if client is unable to continue because of weakness or dizziness.
8. When ambulating in a hallway, position client between yourself and the wall. Encourage client to use handrails if available.	The wall provides stable support for clients who start to fall away from nurse.
9. See Completion Protocol (Chapter 1, p. 6).	

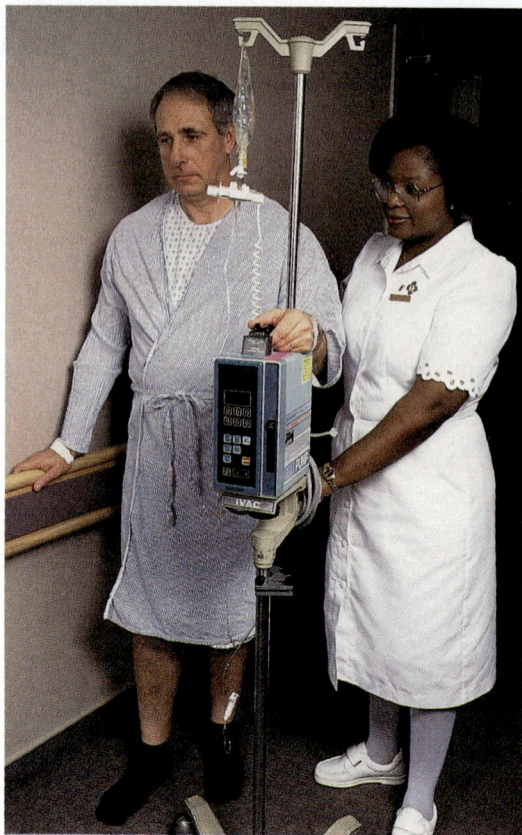

Figure 5-21

Evaluation

1. Observe tolerance of the activity by noting the frequency of rest periods.
2. Compare client's heart rate, respiratory rate, and blood pressure with baseline values immediately after ambulation and again after 5 minutes of rest.
3. Observe client's body alignment and balance while standing and walking.

UNEXPECTED OUTCOMES AND RELATED INTERVENTIONS

1. Vital signs are altered: pulse more than 20 beats over resting rate or greater than 120 beats/min, systolic blood pressure increased or decreased more than 20 mm Hg, or dyspnea, labored breathing, and wheezing present. Client reports feelings of excessive fatigue or weakness.
   a. Plan activity after adequate rest period.
   b. Pace activity to proceed more slowly, and allow time to stop and rest at regular intervals. Sitting periodically may be helpful.
   c. Provide a wheelchair to be pushed by the client to provide balance and support.
   d. Assistive devices such as a cane or walker may decrease energy required (see Chapter 28).

2. Client starts to fall.
   a. Call for help.
   b. Put both arms around client's waist from behind and spread feet apart for a broad base of support.
   c. If necessary, ease client slowly to the floor, bending knees to prevent strain on back muscles.
   d. Stay with client until assistance arrives to help lift client to wheelchair.

SAMPLE DOCUMENTATION

1300 Ambulated client 100 feet in hall with assistance of one. Vital signs stable. States, "I am not as tired as yesterday." Gait steady. Systolic blood pressure increased by 15 mm Hg and pulse increased 15 beats/min and returned to baseline within 5 minutes.

CRITICAL THINKING EXERCISES

1. Mr. Prater is acutely ill and unable to care for himself. You understand that you must keep Mr. Prater's body in proper alignment to prevent injury and maintain function.
   a. Which of the following would indicate that your outcome for preventing injury is being met?
      (1) Mr. Prater states that he frequently feels uncomfortable.
      (2) Mr. Prater is able to stay in the same position for $1\frac{1}{2}$ hours.
      (3) Mr. Prater wants to remain on his back and refuses to turn to his side.
      (4) Mr. Prater has a reddened area over his coccyx.
   b. Why are the other responses incorrect?
2. You are caring for Mrs. Vicker, a client with multiple injuries from an automobile accident. After her bath, Mrs. Vicker requests that you place a pillow behind her head, raise the head of her bed, and place two pillows under the back of her knees. How will you respond to Mrs. Vicker regarding her requests?
3. Safety is an important issue for all hospitalized clients. What important safety measure(s) was (were) overlooked in each of the following situations, and what consequence could have occurred to the clients as a result of the oversight?
   a. Sarah was transferring Martha from her bed to a stretcher. Sarah positioned the bed flat and placed a bath blanket beneath Martha from her shoulders to her hips. Sarah then moved the stretcher as close to the bed as possible and locked the wheels of the stretcher in place.
   b. Jim is in the process of transferring Mr. Blue from his bed to a chair using a mechanical lift. Jim has prepared the chair and placed it near the bed. Jim turns Mr. Blue to his side, places the sling under Mr. Blue to ensure adequate support of Mr. Blue's head, returns Mr. Blue to his back, and slowly begins to lift Mr. Blue from his bed.
   c. Tom has an order to ambulate Mrs. Rucker twice daily in her room. On entering Mrs. Rucker's room, Tom notes that she is lying in bed. He explains that she needs to take a short walk, assists her to a standing position, and encourages her to walk toward the door. Mrs. Rucker states that she is dizzy.

REFERENCES

Baas L, Ross D: Caring for patients on prolonged bedrest. In Swearingen P: *Manual of nursing therapeutics: applying nursing diagnosis to nursing disorders,* St Louis, 1990, Mosby.

Bronstein K, Popovich J, Stewart-Amidei C: *Promoting stroke recovery: a research based approach for nurses,* St Louis, 1991, Mosby.

Canobbio MM: *Cardiovascular disorders,* Mosby's clinical nursing series, St Louis, 1990, Mosby.

Hogstel MO: *Clinical manual of gerontological nursing,* St Louis, 1992, Mosby.

McFarland G, McFarlane E: *Nursing diagnoses and intervention,* ed 2, St Louis, 1993, Mosby.

Patterson DC: Minimizing back injuries in nursing home staff, *Nurs Homes* 42(4):33, 1993.

US Department of Health and Human Services, Public Health Service, Agency for Health Care Policy and Research: *Pressure ulcers in adults: prediction and prevention,* pub no 92-0047, Rockville, Md, 1992, USDHHS.

ADDITIONAL READINGS

Gulanick M et al: *Nursing care plans: nursing diagnosis and intervention,* ed 3, St Louis, 1994, Mosby.

Scopa M: Comparison of classroom instruction and independent study in body mechanics, *J Cont Educ Nurs* 24(4):170, 1993.

Tucker SM et al: *Patient care standards: nursing process, diagnosis, and outcome,* ed 5, St Louis, 1992, Mosby.

US Department of Health and Human Services, Public Health Service: *Healthy people 2000: national health promotion and disease prevention objectives,* Washington, DC, 1992, US Government Printing Office.

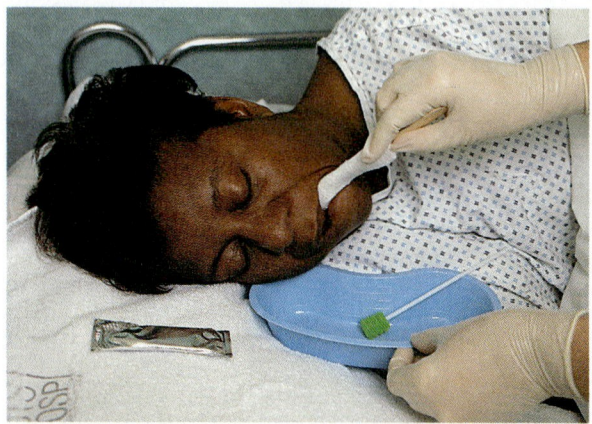

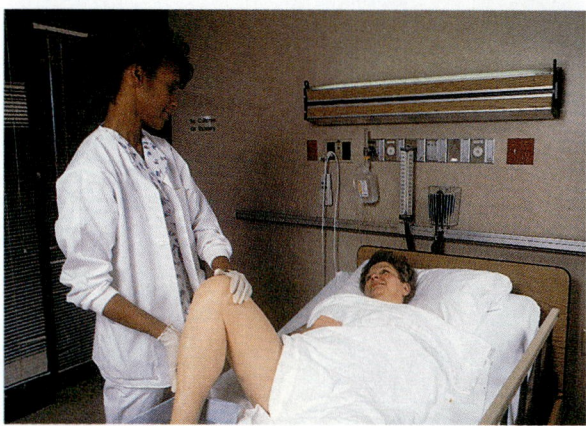

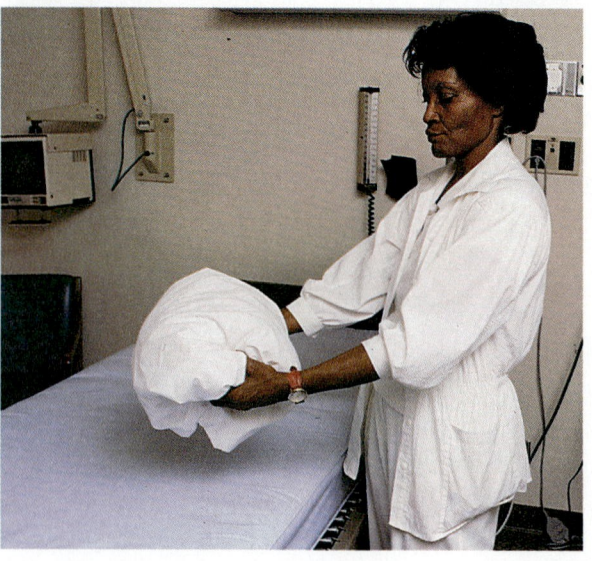

chapter 6

Promoting Hygiene

Skill 6.1
Bedmaking

Skill 6.2
Complete Bathing

Skill 6.3
Oral Care

Skill 6.4
Hair Care

Skill 6.5
Foot and Nail Care

Many clients require assistance with personal hygiene during illness or recovery. Maintenance of personal hygiene is necessary for comfort and a sense of well-being. Because personal hygiene requires close contact with the client, it provides an opportunity for interactions that focus on immediate and future emotional, social, and health-related concerns.

The nurse needs to convey sensitivity and respect for personal beliefs and habits and to ensure as much privacy as possible. Bathing should be done according to the client's usual routines and preferences. Some clients need encouragement to be independent and to participate in self-care. If the client cannot participate, the family or significant other may want to assist. Some clients lack the physical energy to perform self-care and need to be dependent in order to enhance the healing and recovery process.

Personal hygiene is essential to maintain skin integrity by promoting adequate circulation and hydration. Intact skin functions include (1) defense against infection; (2) awareness of touch, pain, heat, cold, and pressure; and (3) control of body temperature. Bathing needs to be done when any body part becomes soiled. Linen changes usually are required as well. Problems such as incontinence, wound drainage, or diaphoresis may require frequent bathing. In addition to cleansing the skin, bathing a client has several additional benefits (see box on p. 73).

Age influences the skin's condition. Normally the skin is elastic, well hydrated, firm, and smooth. With age the

<table>
<tr><td colspan="2" align="center">**Benefits of Bathing**</td></tr>
</table>

Benefits of Bathing

Cleansing the skin: removal of perspiration, some bacteria, sebum, and dead skin cells minimizes skin irritation and reduces the chance of infection.

Stimulating circulation: muscle activity, warm water, and stroking extremities enhance circulation.

Promoting range of motion (ROM): movement of extremities maintains joint function.

Reducing body odors: secretions and excretions from axillae and perineal areas result in body odors that are eliminated by bathing.

Improving self-image: promotes relaxation and feeling clean and comfortable. Care of hair and teeth enhances appearance and sense of well-being.

skin becomes thinner, dry, less vascular, more fragile, and prone to bruising and tears. Bathing is an excellent opportunity to assess the skin for common skin problems that may require special interventions (Table 6-1). Bathing older clients too frequently may contribute to dry skin and should be avoided. Three times a week may be adequate for many older clients; however, optimal frequency depends on individual needs.

Nursing Diagnosis

Bathing/Hygiene Self-Care Deficit is appropriate when the focus of care is helping the client move toward independence in bathing. The client may be unable to wash body parts, to obtain or have access to a water source, or to regulate water temperature or flow (Kim, McFarland, and McLane, 1993). Contributing factors may include impaired physical mobility in which range of motion (ROM) or muscle strength is limited. Shortness of breath with activity or excessive fatigue when bathing may also be contributing factors. **Risk for Impaired Skin Integrity** should be considered when the client has reduced sensation, immobility, impaired circulation, inadequate nutrition, or fragile skin associated with advancing age.

Altered Oral Mucous Membrane is appropriate when mucous membranes are damaged, such as by ulcerations, erythema, and irritation. Contributing factors may include sensory changes (pain, burning, numbness), decreased level of consciousness, and altered oral intake for any reason. **Dressing/Grooming Self-Care Deficit** is appropriate when the focus is to improve a client's ability to provide self-care with oral hygiene or hair care.

Body Image Disturbance is often appropriate when

Table 6-1 Common Skin Problems and Related Interventions

Problem	Interventions
Dry skin: flaky, rough texture to skin, which may crack and become infected.	Bathe less frequently; rinse away all soap or use cleansing cream rather than soap; use humidifier to add moisture to air; increase fluid intake; use moisturizing lotion.
Acne: inflammatory papulopustular skin eruption, usually involving bacterial breakdown of sebum, typically on face, neck, shoulders, and back.	Wash hair and skin daily with hot water and soap to remove oils and cosmetics (if used); cosmetics that can accumulate in pores should be used sparingly; avoid foods that aggravate condition; topical antibiotics and exposure to sunshine may minimize problems (prevent sunburn).
Hirsutism: excessive growth of body and facial hair, especially in women; may cause negative body image by giving women a male appearance.	Shaving is safest method; electrolysis permanently removes hair by destroying hair follicles; tweezing and bleaching are temporary measures; depilatories may remove unwanted hair but may cause infection, rashes, or dermatitis.
Skin rashes: skin eruption from overexposure to sun or moisture or from allergic reaction; may be flat, raised, localized, or systemic; may be associated with pruritus (itching).	Wash thoroughly; apply antiseptic spray or lotion to prevent further itching and aid in healing process; warm or cold soaks relieve inflammation.
Contact dermatitis: inflammation of skin characterized by abrupt onset with erythema, pruritus, pain, and scaly oozing lesions; usually results from contact with substance difficult to identify and eliminate.	Identify and avoid contributing agents; provide linens rinsed and sterilized to minimize irritation.
Abrasion: scraping or rubbing away of epidermis that results in localized bleeding and later weeping of serous fluid; easily infected.	Wash with mild soap and water; observe dressings for retained moisture, which can increase risk of infection.

the client loses interest in grooming or experiences hair loss. This should also be considered when the client displays a lack of interest in appearance, especially when surgery or treatment alters body appearance or function.

Altered Health Maintenance related to knowledge deficit of foot care is appropriate when client teaching is the focus of care. **Impaired Skin Integrity** is appropriate when the client has actual breaks in skin integrity, such as with pressure ulcers or vascular ulcerations from altered blood flow.

Skill 6.1 | Bedmaking

The nurse makes a client's bed with safety and comfort in mind. The sheets must always be clean, dry, and wrinkle free. Whenever a client's bed is soiled, it must be changed. The sheets should be straightened out and tightened periodically throughout the day to keep them wrinkle free.

When clients are not allowed out of bed, the nurse must make an occupied bed. Whenever a client can get out of bed, an unoccupied bed should be made and left open with the top sheets folded down. When a client is discharged and housekeeping cleans the unit, the bed is made with the top sheets left up. This is known as a *closed bed*. For clients who have gone to the operating room or a procedural area, the nurse fanfolds the top sheets lengthwise without tucking them in to facilitate the client's return to bed. This is called a *postoperative (postop)* or *surgical bed*.

EQUIPMENT

Linen bag or hamper
Bath blanket (if available)
Bottom sheet (flat or fitted)
Drawsheet
Waterproof pads (optional)
Top sheet
Blanket
Spread
Pillowcase
Disposable gloves

Assessment

1. Assess the client's ability to get out of bed, and check the activity order. **This determines whether an unoccupied or occupied bed needs to be made.**
2. Assess the client's self-toileting ability; note the presence of any wounds, drainage tubes, and so on. **This determines if waterproof pads need to be placed on the bed.**

Planning

Expected outcomes focus on the client's safety and comfort.

EXPECTED OUTCOMES

1. Client has a clean, safe environment throughout hospitalization.
2. Client verbalizes a sense of comfort while in bed.
3. Client's skin remains free of irritation throughout hospitalization.

Implementation

Steps	Rationale
1. See Standard Protocol (Chapter 1, p. 5).	
2. Unoccupied bed a. Place linen on clean overbed table or chair near bed.	Organization facilitates efficiency.
b. Raise bed to comfortable working height and lower side rail.	
c. Loosen linen from top to bottom on one side. Go to opposite side, lower rail, and loosen linen. Disconnect call bell, and check for personal items in the bed.	Gloves are worn to remove linen soiled with body secretions. Personal items may be lost in the linen.
d. Remove spread and blanket, fold in quarters, and place over bottom of bed or on back of chair if they are clean and to be reused.	

Steps	Rationale
e. Remove soiled pillowcase by grasping center of closed end with one hand and removing pillow with the other. Place pillow on client's chair or overbed table.	
f. Roll all soiled linen together, hold away from uniform, and place in linen hamper. Do not place on floor (Figure 6-1).	Reduces transmission of organisms.
g. Slide mattress, using handles on sides, to head of bed frame if necessary.	
h. Clean mattress and dry, if necessary.	
i. Place clean bottom sheet on bed with seam side down.	
(1) Most bottom sheets are fitted.	
(2) If flat, place center fold on center of bed and bottom hem at end of mattress. Fanfold sheet toward far side of bed.	Closed bed is used when no client occupies room.
j. Tuck top of sheet under top of mattress.	
k. Miter top corner of a flat bottom sheet, and tuck in side of sheet under mattress. To miter a corner: tuck sheet tightly under top of mattress, grasp edge of sheet, and bring it onto mattress at a right angle; tuck lower edge under mattress, then bring triangle fold down and tuck under mattress (Figure 6-2).	Mitered corners do not loosen easily.
l. Place folded drawsheet and/or waterproof pads on center of bed with seam side down. Fanfold toward far side of bed. Tuck drawsheet under mattress.	
m. Place waterproof pads with absorbent side up and plastic side down. Some pads go under cloth drawsheet. Newer, larger absorbent pads go on top of drawsheet or replace it. (Check agency policy.)	Waterproof absorbent pads protect bedding and keep moisture away from client's skin.
n. Move to opposite side of bed. Tuck top of bottom sheet under mattress. Miter corner (see Step k).	
o. Grasp side of flat bottom sheet tightly. Keeping it taut, place it under mattress. Proceed from head to foot.	

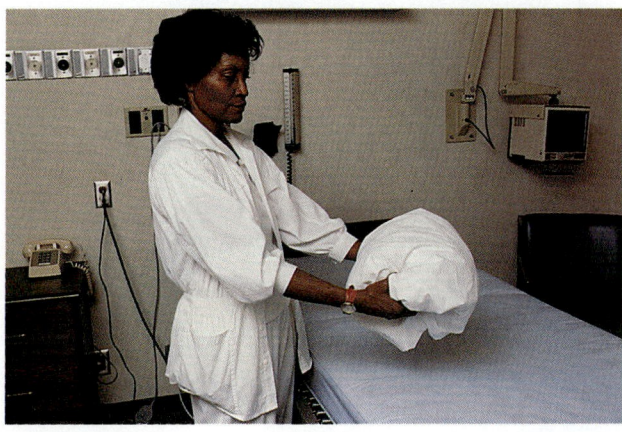

Figure 6-1

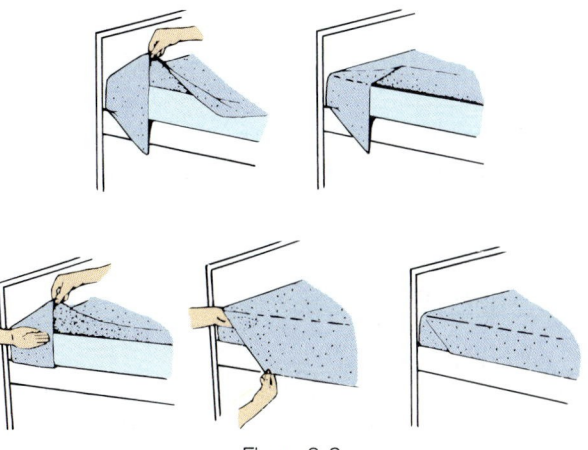

Figure 6-2

Steps	Rationale

p. Grasp drawsheet tightly at an angle. Keeping it taut, place it under mattress. Proceed from middle to top to bottom.

q. Straighten out any waterproof pads that are on top of drawsheet.

r. Place top sheet over bed with vertical fold lengthwise. Open sheet from head to foot. Leave excess sheet at bottom of bed. Make a horizontal toe pleat by fanfolding sheet 4 inches across near bottom of bed (Figure 6-3).

A toe pleat allows for movement of client's feet, prevents top linen from forcing feet into plantar flexion, and prevents pressure ulcers from developing.

s. Place blanket and spread over top sheet in same manner. Cuff top edge of top sheet over blanket and spread.

Gives a neat appearance to bed and keeps client's face off blanket and spread.

t. Make a modified mitered corner with top linens at foot of bed. Miter corner, but do not tuck in lower edge of triangle (Figure 6-4).

u. Go to other side of bed. Cuff sheet over blanket and spread. Make a modified miter corner.

v. Place clean pillowcase on pillow. Grasp center of closed end of pillowcase, and fold pillowcase inside out over closed end. Pick up pillow with hand, grasping pillowcase and pulling it over pillow. Adjust corners of pillow in case. Place pillow at head of bed.

w. Fanfold top linen down to bottom third of bed for an open bed. For a closed bed, leave top linens up.

Closed bed is used when no client occupies room.

3. Postoperative (postop) or surgical bed

Facilitates transfer of postoperative client from stretcher to bed.

a. Fold all top linen from foot of bed toward center of mattress. Linen fold should be flush with bottom edge of mattress.

b. Fold top linen that is hanging down over sides of bed toward center of mattress. Folds should be flush with side edges of mattress. Face one side of bed and fold nearest bottom corner back and over toward opposite side of bed, forming a triangle. Repeat for other side (Figure 6-5, A).

c. Grasp apex of triangle and fanfold top linen over to side of bed (Figure 6-5, B).

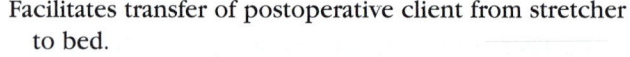
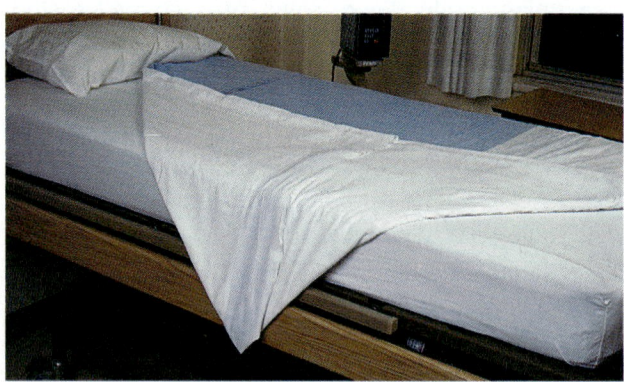

A

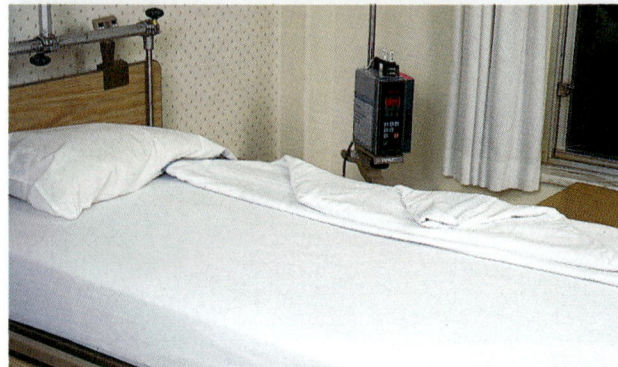

B

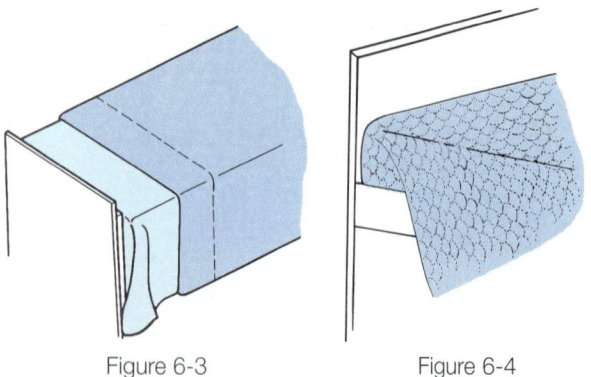

Figure 6-3   Figure 6-4

Figure 6-5

Steps	Rationale

d. Leave bed in high position with side rails down.

4. Occupied bed

a. Raise entire bed to comfortable working height. Lower head of bed, if tolerated by client. Lower side rail on nurse's side, leave far side rail up.

It is easier to apply wrinkle-free, tight linens if bed is in the flat position.

Gloves are worn to remove linen when it is soiled with body secretions.
Provides privacy.

b. Loosen all top linens. Remove spread and blanket, leaving client covered with top sheet or bath blanket. Fold spread and blanket in quarters and place over bottom of bed or on back of chair if they are clean and are to be reused.

c. Assist client to a side-lying position on far side of bed. Slide pillow over so it remains under client's head.

d. Roll bottom sheet, drawsheet, and any pads as far as possible toward client. Clean and dry mattress if necessary.

Reduces transmission of organisms and keeps new linen dry.

e. Place clean bottom sheet on bed with seam side down.
   (1) Most bottom sheets are fitted.
   (2) If flat, place center fold on center of bed and bottom hem at end of mattress. Open sheet toward client (Figure 6-6).

f. Unfold flat bottom sheet lengthwise to cover mattress. Tuck top of sheet under top of mattress.

g. Miter top corner of a flat bottom sheet, and tuck in side of sheet under mattress (Figure 6-7).

Mitered corners do not loosen easily.

h. Place folded drawsheet and/or waterproof pads on center of bed with seam side down. Fanfold toward client.

i. Cover unoccupied portion of bed with half the material, tucking drawsheet under mattress. Place remaining materials as close to client as possible.

j. Place waterproof pads with absorbent side up and plastic side down. Some pads go under cloth draw-

Waterproof absorbent pads protect bedding and keep moisture away from client's skin.

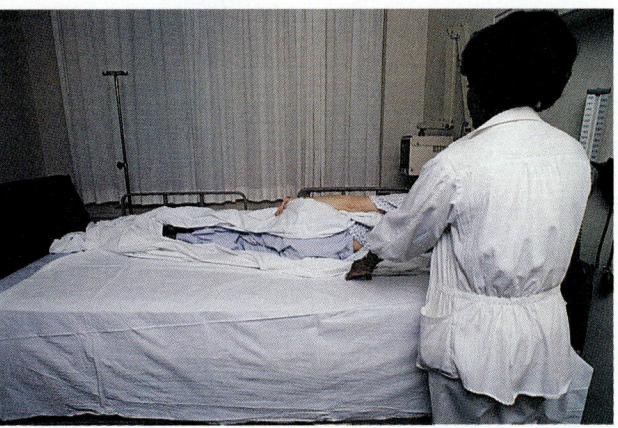

Figure 6-6

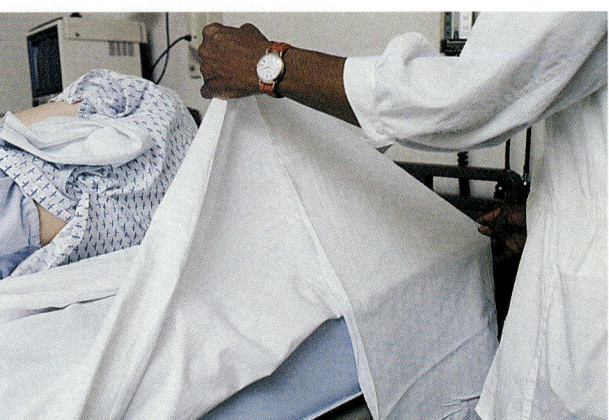

Figure 6-7

Steps	Rationale
sheet. Newer, larger absorbent pads go on top of drawsheet or replace it. (Check agency policy.)	
k. Assist client to roll over all linen and face you. Keep client covered with top sheet or bath blanket. Raise side rail on the side client is facing. Go to other side of bed and lower side rail.	
l. Remove soiled linens. Hold them away from uniform. Place on chair seat or in disposable bag or hamper if it is close by. Do not leave client with side rail down, even for a moment. Remove gloves if worn, and dispose of them properly.	Reduces transmission of microorganisms.
m. Gently slide clean linen toward you, and straighten the clean linen out.	Avoids friction of linen being pulled across it.
n. Miter the top corner of bottom sheet as before.	
o. Grasp side of flat bottom sheet tightly. Keeping it taut, tuck it under mattress. Proceed from head to foot.	
p. Repeat with a drawsheet, proceeding from middle to top to bottom.	
q. Straighten out waterproof pads that are on top of drawsheet.	
r. Assist client into a supine position; place a clean top sheet, blanket, and spread over client, leaving several inches of sheet at top to be folded down.	
s. With client grasping clean top linens, slide out used top sheet or bath blanket (Figure 6-8). Cuff top sheet over blanket and spread.	Prevents exposure of client. Gives a neat appearance to bed and keeps client's face off blanket.
t. Make a modified miter corner with top linens at foot of bed. Miter the corner as before, but do not tuck in lower edge of triangle (Figure 6-9).	
u. Loosen linen at client's feet.	Allows for movement of client's feet, prevents top linen from forcing feet into plantarflexion, and prevents pressure ulcers from developing.
v. Supporting client's head, remove pillow and change pillowcase.	

5. See Completion Protocol (Chapter 1, p. 6).

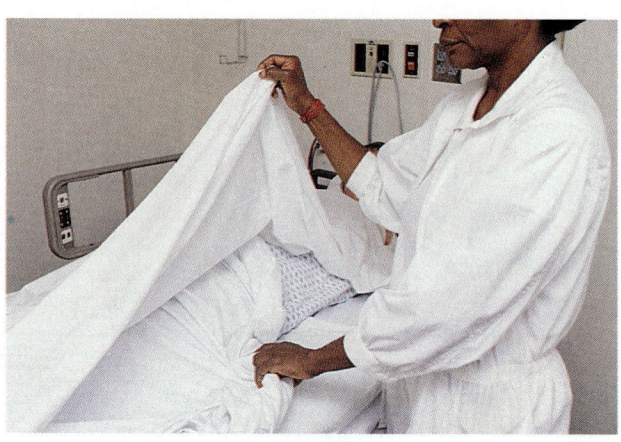

Figure 6-8

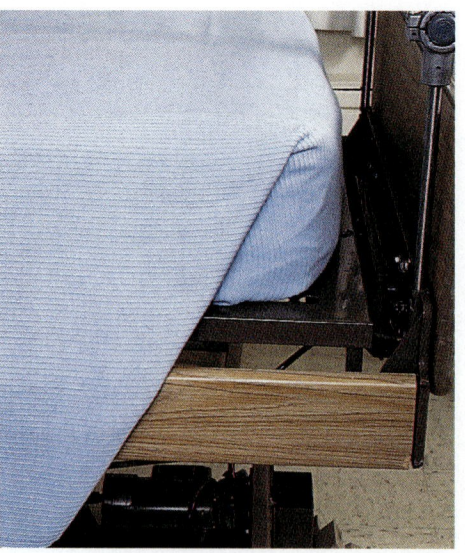

Figure 6-9

Evaluation

1. Observe client's linens for cleanliness and tightness.
2. Ask if client is comfortable after bed is made.
3. Observe client's skin for signs of irritation.

UNEXPECTED OUTCOMES AND RELATED INTERVENTIONS

1. Client is not comfortable in bed.
   a. Check that linens are clean and dry. Tighten them.
   b. Assist client to change position in bed.
2. Client's skin appears red and irritated.

   a. Gently apply lotion to intact skin.
   b. Reposition client frequently. Consider use of pressure-relieving mattress (see Chapter 24).
   c. Use nonallergenic soaps.
   d. Keep client's skin clean and dry.
   e. Notify physician if skin irritation does not subside or if a break in the skin occurs.

SAMPLE DOCUMENTATION

Bedmaking is usually not documented. Some agencies require the nurse to check off this activity on a flow sheet.

Skill 6.2 | Complete Bathing

The extent of the bath and the methods used depend on the client's ability to participate and the skin's condition. A partial bath consists of bathing only body parts that would cause discomfort or odor if left unbathed, such as hands, face, perineal area, and axillae. Clients who cannot tolerate a complete bath and self-sufficient clients unable to reach all body parts may be given a partial bed bath. A tub bath or shower can be used to give a more thorough bath. In the tub or shower, washing and rinsing all body parts is easier; however, safety is of primary concern, and clients must have adequate strength and mobility. Important guidelines need to be followed when providing a bath or shower (see box below).

EQUIPMENT

Washcloths and towels
Bath blanket
Soap and soap dish
Warm water
Toiletry items (deodorant, powder, lotion)
Clean hospital gown or pajamas
Laundry bag
Disposable gloves (for areas with potentially infected body secretions only)

Guidelines for Bath or Shower

1. Provide privacy. Close the door and/or pull curtains around the area. Expose only the areas being bathed.
2. Provide safety. If it is necessary to leave the room, be sure the call light is within reach. Provide adequate assistance.
3. Maintain warmth. The room should be comfortably warm. Use a bath blanket to minimize exposure. Rewarm bath water periodically to keep it comfortably warm throughout the bath.
4. Promote independence and participation as much as is appropriate during bathing activities.

Assessment

1. Assess degree of assistance needed for bathing. Factors may include vision, ability to sit without support, hand grasp, ROM of extremities, and cognitive ability.
2. Assess client's tolerance of activity, level of discomfort with movement, and presence of shortness of breath or chest pain with exertion.
3. Assess client's preferences for time of day, products used, and frequency of bathing.
4. Identify any problems related to condition of the skin:
   a. Excessive moisture from secretions (diaphoresis) or incontinence
   b. Drainage or excretions from lesions or body cavities
   c. External devices (catheters, drains, dressings, restraints)
   d. Rashes or skin damage related to pruritus and scratching
5. Identify any prescribed limitations of activity or positioning required by client's illness or treatment plan. This information is available from the primary care giver's report or information from a kardex or nursing care plan. (See Plan of Care, Appendix A.)

Planning

Expected outcomes focus on promoting comfort, mobility, and self-care abilities.

EXPECTED OUTCOMES

1. Client's skin is clean and free of excretions, drainage, or odor.
2. Client demonstrates functional ROM of hands and shoulders.
3. Client demonstrates ability to wash face, hands, and chest independently.
4. Client expresses comfort and relaxation.

NOTE: **This procedure assumes client is totally dependent. When client is able to assist, encourage and allow as much involvement as possible.**

Implementation

Steps	Rationale

1. See Standard Protocol (Chapter 1, p. 5).
2. With client supine, place bath blanket over client and remove top covers without exposing client. Place soiled linen in laundry bag.
3. Remove client's gown or pajamas.
    a. If an extremity is injured or has limited mobility, begin removal from unaffected side first.
    b. If client has intravenous (IV) line, remove gown from arm without IV first, then slide IV container and tubing through sleeve and rehang. Check flow rate and regulate if necessary (Figure 6-10).
    c. If IV pump is in use, turn pump off, clamp tubing, remove tubing from pump, and proceed as in Step b. Unclamp tubing and turn pump on at correct rate.

Prevents chilling and provides privacy.

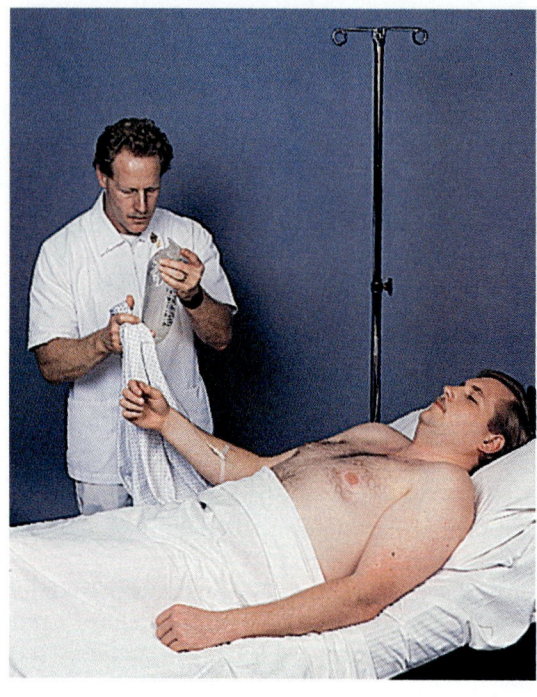

Figure 6-10

4. Remove pillow. Place one bath towel under client's head and another over chest.
5. Wash face.
    a. Form mitt with washcloth (Figure 6-11) and wash client's eyes with plain warm water using a clean area of cloth for each eye, bathing from inner to outer canthus (Figure 6-12). Dry eyes gently and thoroughly.
    b. Wash, rinse, and dry forehead, cheeks, nose, neck, and ears without using soap. Men may want to be shaved (see Skill 6.4).

Removing pillow facilitates bathing ears and neck. Towels absorb moisture.

Soap irritates eyes. Use of separate sections of cloth reduces transmission of microorganisms. Bathing inner to outer canthus prevents secretions from entering nasolacrimal duct.

Soap tends to dry face, which is exposed to air more than other body parts.

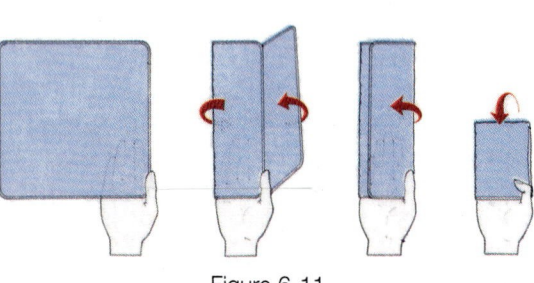

Figure 6-11

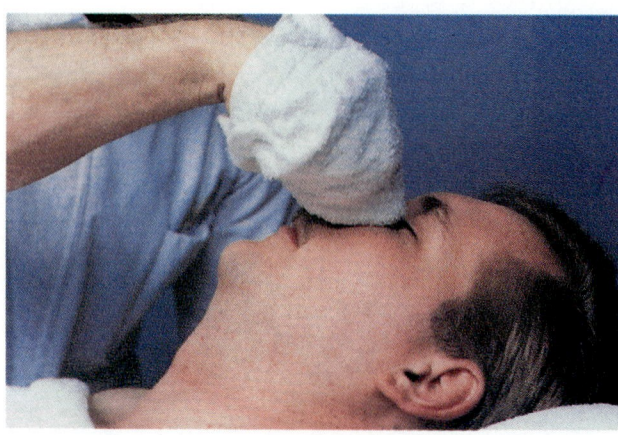

Figure 6-12

Steps	Rationale

6. Wash upper body.

a. Remove bath blanket from over client's arm farthest from nurse. Place bath towel lengthwise under arm. Bathe with minimal soap and water using long, firm strokes from distal to proximal (fingers to axilla).

Promotes circulatory return to heart.

b. Raise and support arm above head (if possible) to wash, rinse, and dry axilla thoroughly (Figure 6-13).

Raising arm promotes ROM and facilitates thorough cleansing.

c. Repeat Steps a and b with other (closer) arm. Apply deodorant or talcum powder to underarms.

d. Cover client's chest with bath towel, and fold bath blanket down to umbilicus. Bathe chest using long, firm strokes. Take special care with skin under female client's breasts, lifting breast upward if necessary. Dry well.

Skin under breasts is vulnerable to excoriation if not kept clean and dry.

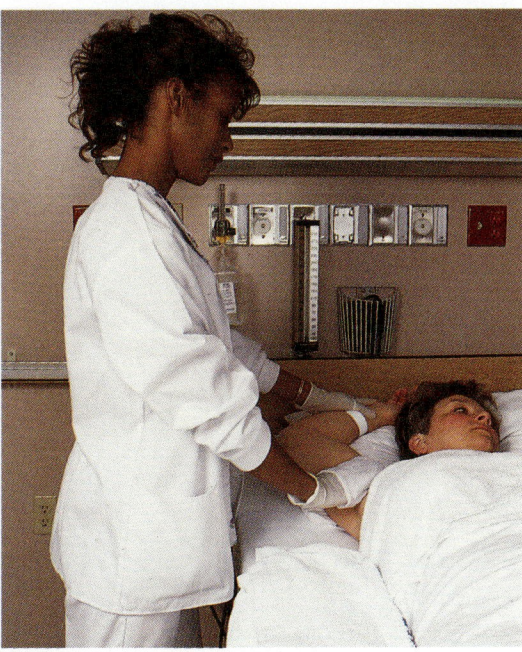

Figure 6-13

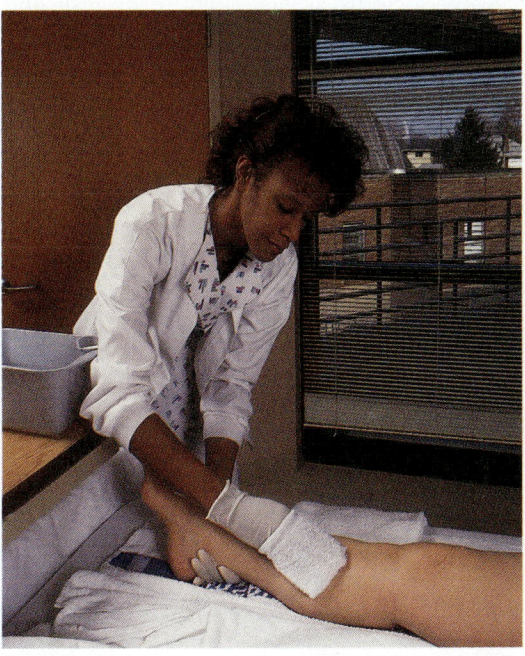

Figure 6-14

7. Wash lower body.

a. Place bath towel over chest and abdomen, and fold bath blanket down to just above pubic region. Bathe, rinse, and dry abdomen with special attention to umbilicus and skinfolds of abdomen and groin.

Keeping skinfolds clean and dry helps prevent odor and skin irritation.

b. Expose client's leg nearest to you, leaving perineum covered. Place bath towel under leg, supporting leg at knee and with foot flat on bed. If desired, place client's foot in a basin to soak while washing and rinsing. If client is unable to support leg, assistance will be needed or soaking omitted. Wash and dry leg using long, firm strokes from ankle to knee, then knee to thigh (Figure 6-14). Wash foot between toes. Dry thoroughly.

Soaking softens calluses and rough skin.

Steps	Rationale
c. Raise side rail, move to opposite side, and repeat Step b with other leg and foot. If skin is dry, apply lotion.	Promotes good body mechanics for the nurse.
d. Cover with bath blanket, and change bath water. Raise side rail.	Provides client warmth and safety.
8. Wash perineum.	
a. Assist client in assuming side-lying position, placing towel lengthwise along client's side and keeping client covered with bath blanket as much as possible.	If client is totally dependent, assistance is necessary to support client in side-lying position and to raise leg as perineum is bathed.
b. If fecal material is present, enclose it in a fold of underpad and remove as much as possible with disposable wipes first. Cleanse buttocks and anus washing from front to back or side to side. Use as many washcloths as necessary to cleanse and rinse thoroughly. Dry area completely. Remove and discard underpad and replace with a clean one.	Washing from front to back or side to side prevents transmission of microorganisms from anus to urethra or genitalia.
9. Provide female perineal care if applicable.	
a. Position waterproof pad under client's buttocks with client supine. Wash labia majora using washcloth, soap, and warm water. Then gently retract labia from thigh and wash groin from perineum toward rectum (Figure 6-15).	Washing from front to back prevents contamination of urethral meatus with fecal matter.

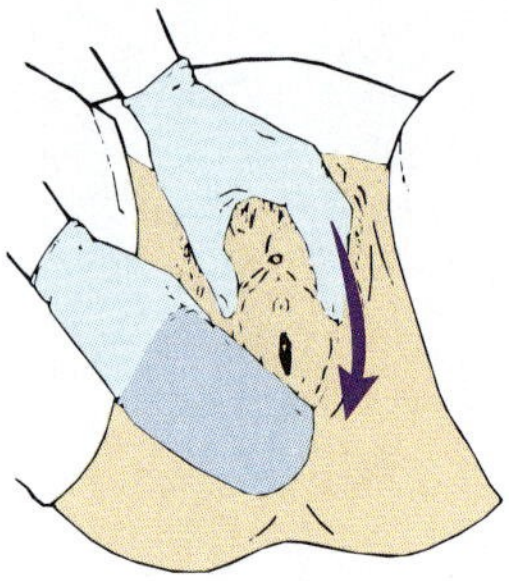

Figure 6-15

Steps	Rationale
b. Gently separate labia and expose urethra and vagina. Wash from pubic area toward rectum cleansing thoroughly. Avoid tension on indwelling catheter if present and clean area around it thoroughly.	Minimizes risk for developing infection because of presence of indwelling catheter or fecal incontinence.
c. Rinse and dry area thoroughly. Assess for redness, swelling, discharge, irritation, or skin breakdown. Make sure catheter is secured with tape to upper thigh and positioned over (not under) the thigh.	Prevents pulling of catheter on urethral canal and promotes urinary drainage.
10. Provide male perineal care if applicable.	
a. Gently grasp shaft of penis and if client is not circumcised, retract foreskin.	Gentle handling reduces risk of having an erection. Secretions and microorganisms tend to collect under foreskin.

Steps	Rationale

b. Wash tip of penis at urethral meatus first. Using circular motion, cleanse away from meatus (Figure 6-16). Replace foreskin to its natural position.

c. Gently cleanse shaft of penis, and scrotum, washing underlying skinfolds. Rinse and dry.

11. Cover client with bath blanket, and change bath water.

12. Wash back.

a. Assist client to side-lying position, and place towel lengthwise along the back. Wash, rinse, and dry back from neck to buttocks using long, firm strokes.

b. Cleanse anal area from front to back with special attention to folds of buttocks (Figure 6-17).

13. Apply body lotion to skin as needed and topical moisturizing agents to dry, flaky, or scaling areas.

14. Massage back.

Discharge may indicate presence of infection or inflammation. Replacing foreskin prevents constriction of the penis, which may result in edema.

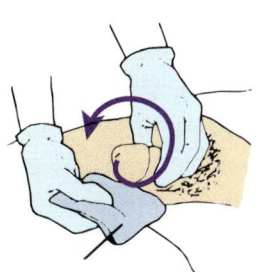 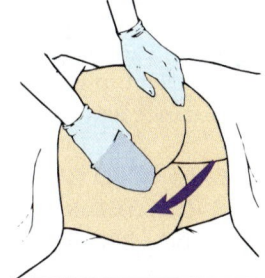

Figure 6-16   Figure 6-17

Dry skin results in reduced pliability and cracking. Moisturizers may help prevent skin breakdown (AHCPR, 1992).

nurse alert Massage over bony prominences is no longer recommended. Evidence suggests that massage may result in decreased blood flow and tissue damage in some clients (AHCPR, 1992).

a. Position client prone (on abdomen) if possible. Side-lying position is also frequently used.

b. Provide back massage using lotion to stimulate circulation (Figure 6-18). Begin at sacral area. Massaging in circular motion, stroke upward from buttocks to shoulders and upper arms and over scapulas with smooth, firm strokes (Figure 6-19). Keep hands on skin and continue massage pattern for 3 to 4 minutes.

c. Knead skin by grasping tissue between thumb and fingers. Knead upward along each side of spine and around muscles of neck, avoiding bony prominences.

d. End massage with long stroking movements, and tell client you are ending massage.

e. Observe skin for redness and skin breakdown. Remove excess lotion from back with bath towel.

f. Apply clean gown or pajamas, dressing affected side first.

13. See Completion Protocol (Chapter 1, p. 6).

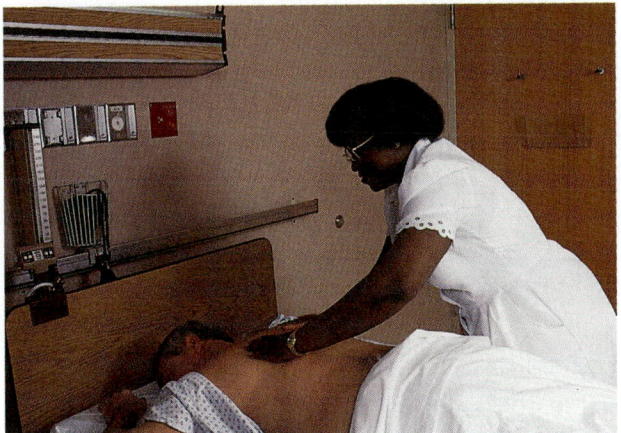

Figure 6-18

Long strokes promote comfort and relaxation.

Allows easier manipulation of gown over restricted body part.

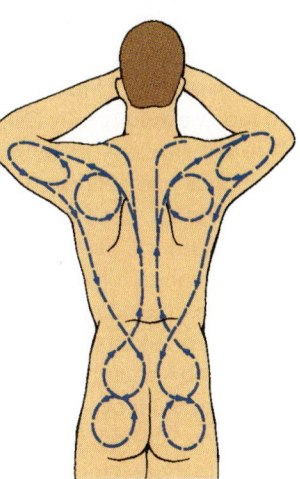

Figure 6-19

Evaluation

1. Observe areas on skin for erythema, exudate, drainage, or breakdown.
2. Measure ROM in hands, arms, and shoulders, and compare with baseline. Assess vital signs if client is experiencing distress or restlessness.
3. Observe for improved ability to assist with self-bathing and hygiene to determine progress.
4. Ask client to view self in mirror and comment on appearance and comfort.

UNEXPECTED OUTCOMES AND RELATED INTERVENTIONS

1. Client's skin on lower extremities is dry and flaky and itches.
   a. Limit the frequency of baths to every other day or less.
   b. Use a mild soap sparingly.
   c. Blot skin dry after bathing, and apply lotion to skin.
   d. Increase hydration status.
   e. Administer antipruritics as ordered to control itching.
   f. Use distraction techniques to remove focus from itching.

2. The client has evidence of rashes, redness, scaling, or cracking.
   a. Evaluate the need for a change in frequency of bathing and soap product used.
   b. Collaborate with the physician regarding application of ointments or creams to provide a protective barrier and help maintain moisture within the skin.
3. The rectum, perineum, or genital region is inflamed, is swollen, or has foul-smelling discharge.
   a. Bathe area frequently enough to keep clean and dry.
   b. Apply protective barrier or antiinflammatory cream.

SAMPLE DOCUMENTATION

Routine documentation involves a check mark on a flow sheet (see Physical Care/Activity, Appendix A). Observations made during bath are recorded on progress note.

0900 Complete bath given. Unable to assist but cooperative with turning. Skin on both legs dry and flaking, complains of severe itching. Bath oil added to bath water. Emollient lotion applied after bath. States itching is less now.

Skill 6.3 | Oral Care

Oral hygiene helps maintain healthy structures of the oral cavity and comfort of the mouth, teeth, gums, and lips. Brushing cleanses the teeth of food particles, plaque, and bacteria; massages the gums; and relieves discomfort resulting from unpleasant odors and tastes. Flossing helps remove plaque and tartar between teeth to reduce gum inflammation and infection. Many factors can influence oral hygiene (see box at right). Inadequate oral hygiene can create a general sense of discomfort and also diminish appetite.

Clients may experience altered oral mucous membranes when they are dehydrated; have inadequate nutrition, particularly vitamin B deficiency; or are unable to take food or fluids orally (NPO). Mouth breathing may result in dry mucous membranes. Trauma to oral mucous membranes may also occur from oral tubes, oxygen therapy, suctioning, hot foods, or trauma from broken teeth. Chemical injury may result from irritating substances such as alcohol, tobacco, acidic foods, or side effects of medications, including chemotherapy, antibiotics, steroids, and antidepressants. Chronic inflammatory disease may be caused by bacteria, viral or fungal infections, or ineffective oral hygiene.

Dentures should be cleaned as regularly as natural teeth to prevent gingival infection and irritation. Loose dentures can cause discomfort and make it difficult for clients to chew food and speak clearly. Loose dentures may result from weight loss.

Dentures can be easily lost or broken. They should be stored in an enclosed, labeled cup or should be soaking

Factors Influencing Oral Hygiene

Client lacks upper-extremity strength or dexterity to perform oral hygiene (e.g., is paralyzed or has limited ROM).

Client unable or unwilling to attend to personal hygiene needs (e.g., is unconscious, depressed, or confused).

Client is diabetic and prone to dryness of mouth, gingivitis, periodontal disease, and loss of teeth.

Client is prone to dehydration or has a fever. Thick secretions develop on tongue and gums. Lips become cracked and reddened.

Radiation therapy causes soreness, mild erythema, swollen mucosa, dysphagia, dryness, taste changes, and possible oral infection.

Chemotherapy causes ulcerations and inflammation of mucosa and possible oral infection.

Tissues in oral cavity become traumatized with swelling, ulcerations, inflammation, and possible bleeding.

when not worn (e.g., during surgery or a diagnostic procedure), and they should be reinserted as soon as possible. The change in appearance when they are not worn may be of major concern to the client.

Nursing Diagnosis

Altered Oral Mucous Membrane is a nursing diagnosis for clients who have damage to oral mucous membranes. This may include mild generalized erythema, small ulcerations or white patches, or hemorrhagic ulcerations. Contributing factors could include sensory changes such as numbness, chronic irritation, or decreased level of consciousness and altered oral intake. **Altered Nutrition: Less Than Body Requirements** should be considered when a client's appetite and intake are diminished because of altered mucous membranes, and the aim is to increase oral intake by improving oral hygiene. **Bathing/Hygiene Self-Care Deficit** is appropriate when the focus is to promote independence in oral hygiene and teach the use of adaptive devices. **Risk for Infection** can apply in presence of trauma or lesions in the oral cavity. **Body Image Disturbance** may be appropriate when clients are unable to wear dentures for any reason.

EQUIPMENT (Figure 6-20)

Soft-bristled toothbrush or 4 × 4 gauze (if toothbrush is contraindicated)
Antiinfective solution (diluted hydrogen peroxide) to loosen crusts
Sponge toothette
Glass of water
Padded tongue blade
Emesis basin
Portable suction machine (optional) with rubber catheter

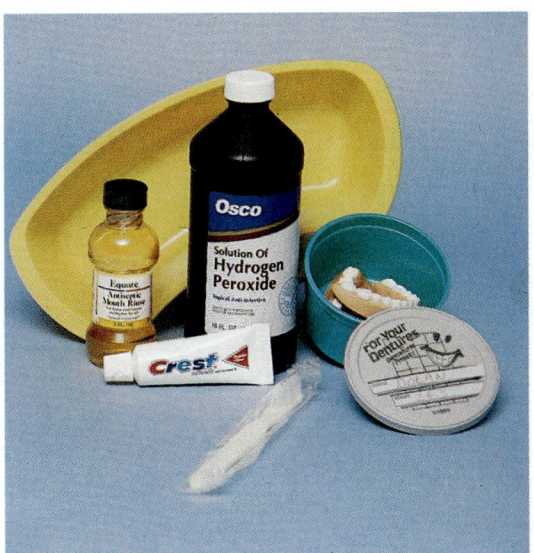

Figure 6-20

Face towel
Suction equipment (optional)
Disposable gloves
Water-soluble lubricant

Assessment

1. Determine presence or absence of gag reflex by placing tongue blade or suction tip on back of tongue. **Clients with no gag reflex are at risk for aspiration. Suction equipment must be available.**
2. Inspect lips, teeth, gums, buccal mucosa, palate, and tongue, using tongue depressor and penlight if necessary. Observe for color, texture, moisture, lesions or ulcers, and condition of teeth (or dentures). Ask if areas of tenderness exist.
3. Identify presence of oral problems.
   a. Dental caries: discoloration of tooth enamel
   b. Gingivitis: inflammation of gums
   c. Periodontitis: receding gum lines, inflammation, gaps between teeth
   d. Halitosis: bad breath
   e. Cracked lips
   f. Dry, cracked, coated tongue

FOR DENTURE CARE

1. Ask client if dentures fit and if there is any gum or mucous membrane tenderness or irritation.
2. Ask client to remove dentures and place them in basin or denture cup. Inspect oral cavity and denture surface after dentures are removed.
   If client is unable to remove dentures, grasp upper plate at front with gauze to prevent slipping. Use steady, downward pull and rotate sideways to reduce tension on lips. Gently lift lower denture from jaw and rotate to remove from mouth.
3. Ask client about preferences for denture care and products used.

Planning

Expected outcomes focus on promoting comfort, preventing aspiration, and promoting integrity of oral mucous membranes.

EXPECTED OUTCOMES

1. Client's oral mucous membranes are smooth, moist, pink, and without lesions.
2. Client maintains clean dental surfaces.
3. Client verbalizes comfort and displays no restlessness or grimace during oral care.
4. The client, spouse, or significant other demonstrates oral hygiene regimen.

Implementation

Steps	Rationale

1. See Standard Protocol (Chapter 1, p. 5).
2. Position unconscious client in side-lying position with bed flat and towel placed under chin. Have emesis basin available.

Side-lying position minimizes risk of aspiration. Debilitated client may be positioned with head of bed elevated if not in danger of aspirating.

3. Separate upper and lower teeth gently with padded tongue blade between back molars (Figure 6-21). Client needs to be relaxed. Wait until client is relaxed with mouth open, then insert blade with smooth, quick motion and without using force.

Some clients tend to bite on any object placed in mouth.

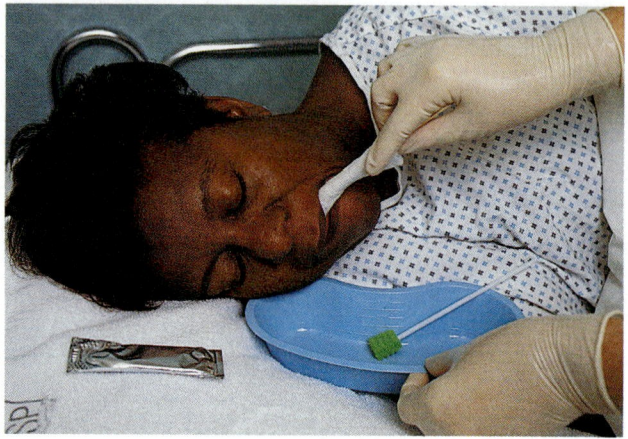

Figure 6-21

4. Suction must be on with catheter attached and ready for use if gag reflex is absent (see Skill 30.3).

Some clients who are unconscious do not have a gag reflex.

5. Clean mouth using brush or 4 × 4 gauze moistened with a 50:50 solution of peroxide and water. Clean tooth surfaces, roof of mouth, inside cheeks, and tongue. Rinse with clean toothette and water. Avoid stimulating gag reflex (if present).
6. If client cannot expectorate secretions, provide suction of oral cavity as they accumulate.

Prevents aspiration.

7. Apply water-soluble jelly to lips (Figure 6-22).

Prevents drying and cracking.

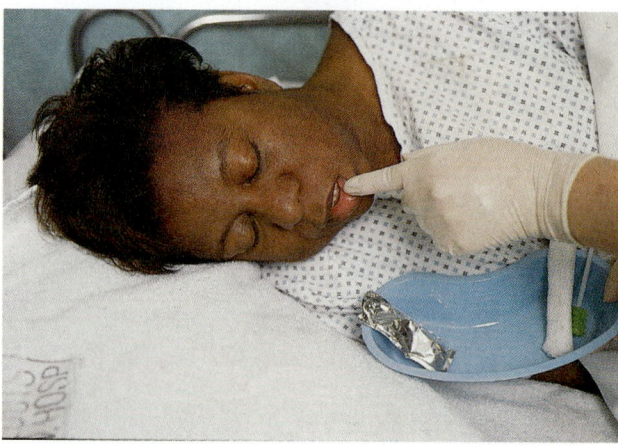

Figure 6-22

Steps	Rationale

8. For client with decreased level of consciousness or confusion, indicate that you are finished.

Provides meaningful stimulation and reality orientation.

9. Provide care of dentures.

   a. Place washcloth in sink and fill with small amount of warm water.

Cloth prevents dentures from breakage. Hot water could damage dentures.

   b. Apply cleaning agent to brush, and cleanse biting surfaces of teeth. Use short strokes from top of denture to biting surfaces to clean outer and inner tooth surfaces (Figure 6-23).

   c. Clean remaining surfaces of dentures with brush, then rinse thoroughly in tepid water.

   d. Apply toothpaste to soft toothbrush, and gently brush gums, palate, and tongue. Rinse mouth thoroughly.

Helps stimulate circulation to gums and removes residual film of debris on gums and mucosa.

   e. Some clients use an adhesive to seal dentures in place. Apply a thin layer to undersurface before inserting.

   f. If client needs assistance with insertion of dentures, moisten upper denture and press firmly to seal it in place. Then insert moistened lower denture. Ask if dentures feel comfortable.

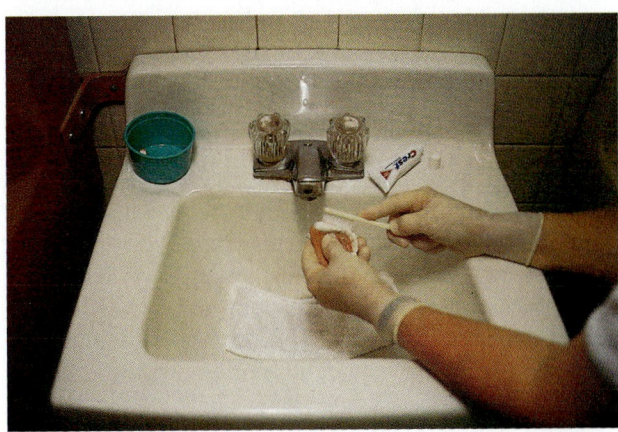

Figure 6-23

10. Store dentures.

   a. Some clients prefer to remove and store dentures in a denture cup.

Removal gives the gums a rest and prevents bacterial buildup.

   b. Label denture cup with the client's name and room number, and place in a secure place.

Keeping dentures moist prevents warping and facilitates easier insertion. Dentures are expensive to replace and can be easily misplaced.

11. See Completion Protocol (Chapter 1, p. 6).

Evaluation

1. Inspect oral mucous membranes for moistness, color, smoothness, and intact appearance.
2. Inspect dental surfaces for cleanliness.
3. Observe for restlessness or grimace during care. Ask client if mouth feels more comfortable.
4. Observe client, spouse, or significant other providing oral hygiene regimen.

UNEXPECTED OUTCOMES AND RELATED INTERVENTIONS

1. Mucosa, tongue, or gums remain coated with thick secretions.
   a. Provide mouth care more frequently.
   b. To loosen and remove thick mucus, use one part hydrogen peroxide and four parts normal saline, followed by a warm water or saline rinse (Greifzu, Radjeski, and Winnick, 1990).
2. Lips are cracked or inflamed.
   Lubricate lips more frequently.
3. Client has gurgles in back of throat from accumulation of liquid and is unable to clear throat or cough.
   Suction back of throat to clear airway and prevent aspiration.

SAMPLE DOCUMENTATION

0800 Mouth care given. Mucous membranes and lips are moist, pink, and intact. Client unresponsive. No gag reflex elicited. Oral pharynx suctioned. No grimacing or evidence of bleeding noted.

Skill 6.4 | # Hair Care

A person's appearance and feeling of well-being are influenced by how the hair looks and feels. Brushing, combing, and shampooing are basic measures for all clients unable to provide self-care. Male clients should be offered the opportunity to shave or be shaved when their condition allows. Some hospitals have a beauty shop where clients can go for professional hair care.

Fever, malnutrition, emotional stress, and depression affect the condition of hair. Diaphoresis leaves hair oily and unmanageable. Excessively dry or oily hair may be associated with hormone changes. Dry, brittle hair occurs with aging and excessive use of shampoo.

Certain chemotherapy agents and radiation therapy may cause alopecia (hair loss). Many clients choose to wear a wig; however, some choose to wear head scarves or turbans (Figure 6-24). The average growth of healthy hair is ½ inch per month. Table 6-2 describes common hair and scalp problems and nursing interventions.

When caring for clients from different cultures, it is important to learn as much as possible about the client's cultural customs and beliefs and be sensitive to the uniqueness of each client. Ask the client about preferred hair care methods or any cultural restrictions. For example, African Americans' hair is quite dry. Special lanolin conditioners may be used to maintain conditioning. The neglect of hair care may be interpreted by the client or family as rejection.

Frequency of shampooing depends on the hair's condition and the person's personal preferences. Dry hair, which often results from aging and protein deficiency, requires less frequent shampooing than oily hair or hair of people who exercise actively. Hospitalized clients who have excess perspiration or treatments that leave blood or solutions in the hair may need a shampoo.

Some clients are able to sit in a chair in front of a sink,

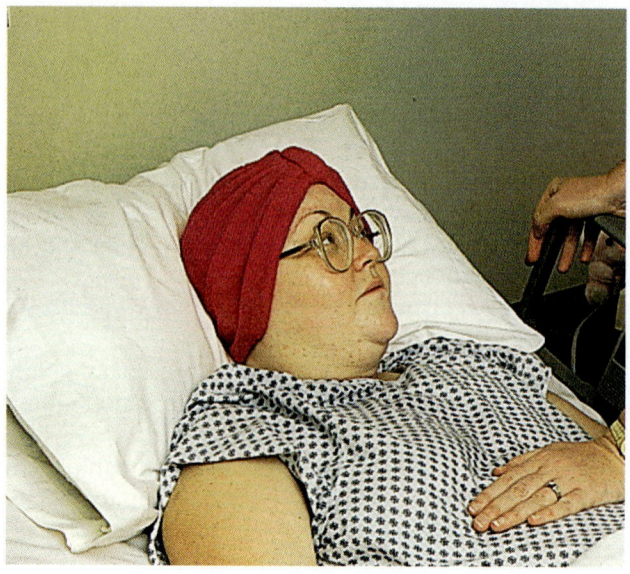

Figure 6-24

positioned facing away from the sink with the head and neck hyperextended over the sink's edge. This is contraindicated for clients who have had neck injuries or back pain.

Some clients may be placed on a stretcher with head extended over a sink. A plastic shampoo trough or board facilitates a shampoo in bed. Water is poured over the client's head and allowed to drain into a container on the side of the bed.

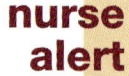 **nurse alert** Caution is needed if clients have neck pain or a neck injury.

Table 6-2 Hair and Scalp Problems and Related Interventions

Problem	Interventions
Dandruff: scaling of scalp accompanied by itching; if severe, may involve eyebrows.	Shampoo regularly with medicated shampoo.
Pediculosis	
Head lice: parasites attached to hair strands. Eggs look like oval particles. Bites or pustules may be found behind ears and at hairline. May spread to furniture and other people.	Shampoo with Kwell shampoo and repeat 12-24 hours later. Bag infested clothing and change bed linens.
Body lice: parasites tend to cling to clothing. Client itches. Hemorrhagic spots may appear on skin where lice are sucking blood. Lice may lay eggs on clothing and furniture.	For body lice, apply Kwell lotion to dry skin.
Crab lice: found in pubic hair, are grayish white with red legs, and may spread via sexual contact.	For pubic lice, notify sexual partner of proper treatment.
Alopecia (hair loss): chemotherapeutic agents kill cells that rapidly multiply, including both tumor and normal cells.	Some clients wear scarves. Some clients prefer hairpieces. Referral may be needed for professional consultation for long-term interventions.

Dependent clients with beards or mustaches need to have assistance keeping the facial hair clean, especially after eating. A brush or comb may be used. Shaving of facial hair is a task most men prefer to do for themselves. Men without beards usually shave daily. A beard or mustache should be combed or washed as needed. Food particles easily collect in the hair. Some religions and cultures forbid cutting or shaving any body hair (Galanti, 1991); therefore, nurses should not shave a client without consent.

EQUIPMENT

Brush
Comb
Shampoo board
Shampoo
Towels (two or more)
Razor
Shaving cream
Basin of very warm water
Hydrogen peroxide (optional)

Assessment

1. Determine any restrictions that may be necessary. Often a physician's order is required. If exposure to moisture is contraindicated, dry shampoo may be used. **Shampoo may be contraindicated if client has increased intracranial pressure; cerebrospinal fluid leaks; open incisions of face, head, or neck; cervical neck injuries; tracheostomy; facial edema; or respiratory distress.**

2. Assess condition of hair and scalp. Note distribution of hair, oiliness, and texture. Inspect scalp for abrasions, lacerations, lesions, inflammation, and infestation. **This determines the need for further interventions, such as conditioner or medicated shampoo.**

3. Before shaving client, assess for bleeding tendency. Review medical history and check laboratory values, including platelet count, prothrombin time (PT), and activated partial thromboplastin time (aPTT). **Clients with leukemia, hemophilia, or disseminated intravascular coagulation and clients receiving anticoagulant therapy (heparin or coumadin) or taking high doses of aspirin may have abnormally long clotting times. An electric razor is generally recommended for these clients. Electric razors may be a safety hazard in the presence of oxygen therapy.**

4. If client wants to shave himself, assess ability to manipulate razor to determine how much assistance will be needed.

Planning

Expected outcomes should focus on comfort and promoting self-concept.

EXPECTED OUTCOMES

1. Client expresses increased sense of comfort.
2. Client verbalizes improved self-image.
3. Skin remains free of cuts.

Implementation

Steps	Rationale

1. See Standard Protocol (Chapter 1, p. 5).

2. Shampoo
   a. Place a towel under head. Brush and comb client's hair by separating hair into small sections, releasing tangles with fingers.
   b. Place a waterproof pad under client's shoulders, neck, and head. Position client supine with plastic trough under head and spout extending beyond edge of mattress. Position container under spout to collect water (Figure 6-25).
   c. Pour warm water over hair until it is completely wet. The client or another care giver should protect client's face with towel or washcloth over eyes.

   d. If hair is matted with blood, apply hydrogen peroxide to dissolve it and rinse with saline.

Moistening with water or mineral oil may help free tangles. Anchoring tangled hair at scalp prevents painful pulling of scalp.

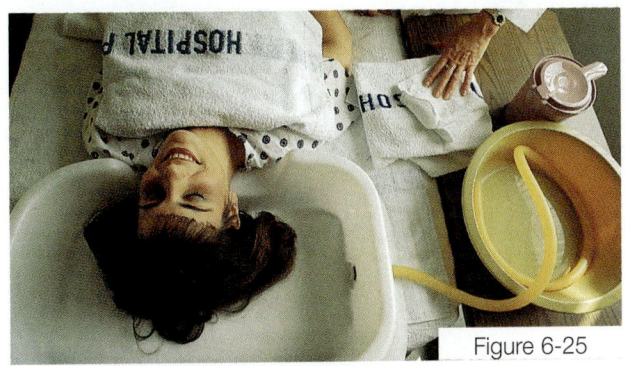

Figure 6-25

Steps	Rationale

e. Apply small amount of shampoo and work up a lather with both hands. Start at hairline and work toward back of neck. Lift head slightly to wash back of head. Massage scalp gently. Rinse thoroughly and repeat if necessary. Dry using a second towel if needed.

f. Assist client to a comfortable position and complete styling of hair. Braids may be helpful for clients with very long hair (Figure 6-26).

3. Shave beard

a. Assist client to sitting position if possible, and place towel over chest and shoulders.

b. Place a warm, moist washcloth over client's face for several seconds. Apply shaving cream.   Softens beard.

c. With the razor at a 45-degree angle, shave in direction of hair growth using short strokes. Hold skin taut to avoid pulling. Ask client to direct you with his usual technique and tell you if it becomes uncomfortable (Figure 6-27).

d. Rinse and dry face. Apply aftershave if desired.   Provides a positive effect for comfort and self-esteem.

4. See Completion Protocol (Chapter 1, p. 6).

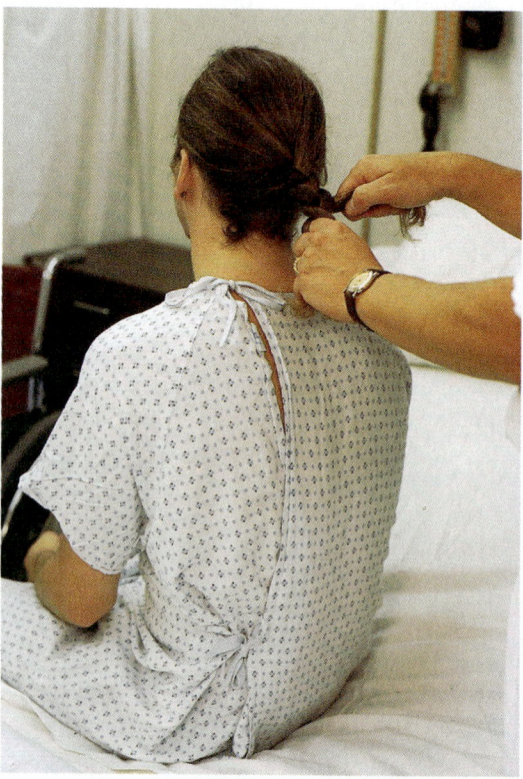

Figure 6-26

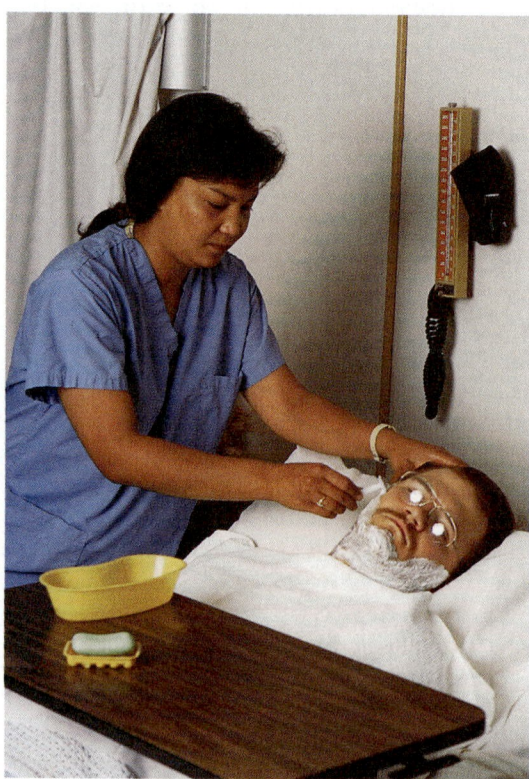

Figure 6-27

Evaluation

1. Ask if client feels more comfortable.
2. Offer a mirror and ask how client feels and looks.
3. Inspect condition of shaved area of skin for nicks.

UNEXPECTED OUTCOME
AND RELATED INTERVENTION

Client has small nicks or cuts on skin.

    Apply pressure and if necessary a small dressing or Band–Aid.

SAMPLE DOCUMENTATION

1000 Shampoo and shave completed without difficulty. Verbalized increased comfort and expressed satisfaction with appearance.

Skill 6.5 | Foot and Nail Care

Most people are required to walk or stand to perform their jobs, and foot pain can cause strain on muscle groups. Often, people are unaware of foot or nail problems until pain occurs. Various skin problems involving the feet are the result of improperly fitted shoes. Tight shoes, socks, garters, or knee-high hose may interfere with circulation. Foot pain may cause a person to change gait, resulting in strain on different muscle groups. If job performance requires a person to walk or stand comfortably, a foot disorder can become a serious problem.

    Nail and foot care should be included in a client's daily hygiene; the best time is during the client's bath. Feet and nails often require special care to prevent infection, odors, and injury to soft tissues. Problems often result from abuse or poor care of the feet and hands, such as biting nails or trimming them improperly, exposure to harsh chemicals, or wearing poorly fitting shoes. Changes also occur in the shape, color, and texture of nails that may result from various nutritional, infectious, and circulatory disorders (Table 6-3).

    Many older clients may have poor vision, hand tremors, obesity, or limited joint mobility that contributes to difficulties with foot and nail care. Older clients may also have excessive dryness of the skin and poor circulation.

    Circulation is assessed by palpation of the pedal and posterior tibial pulses. The nurse also palpates the skin for edema, texture, and coolness. Changes in skin color may be noted. Clients with peripheral vascular disease, such as diabetes, may have inadequate arterial or venous circulation or both. These clients are at high risk for neuropathy, a degeneration of peripheral nerves with loss of sensation. Sensation can be checked by light touch, use of a pinprick, or asking client to discriminate hot and cold temperatures. These clients need to inspect their feet daily, since injuries may not be felt. These injuries are easily infected and heal slowly because of inadequate circulation.

EQUIPMENT

Basin (appropriate size for soaking)
Washcloth
Bath or face towel
Nail clippers
Orange stick (optional)
Emery board or nail file

Assessment

1. Identify client's risk for foot or nail problems.
   a. Poor vision, lack of coordination, and inability to bend over contribute to older adults' difficulty in performing foot and nail care. Normal physiological changes of aging also result in nail and foot problems.
   b. Vascular changes associated with diabetes reduce blood flow to peripheral tissues. Break in skin integrity places diabetic clients at high risk for skin infection.
   c. Edema associated with cardiac or renal conditions can have symptoms of increased tissue edema, particularly in dependent areas (e.g., feet). Edema reduces blood flow to neighboring tissues.
   d. Presence of muscle weakness or paralysis of one lower extremity after a stroke may result in altered walking patterns, which increases friction and pressure on feet.
2. Inspect all surfaces of toes, feet, and nails. Pay particular attention to areas of dryness, inflammation, or cracking. Also inspect areas between toes, heels, and soles of feet. **Changes in skin associated with aging include thinning of epidermis and dryness. The nails may become opaque, tough, scaly, brittle, and hypertrophied.**
3. Assess color and warmth of toes and feet. Assess capillary refill of nails. Palpate the dorsalis pedis pulse of both feet simultaneously, comparing the strength of

Table 6-3 **Common Foot and Nail Problems**

Problem	Interventions
Callus: thickened epidermis, usually flat, painless, and on underside of foot or palm; caused by friction or pressure.	Avoid friction or protect skin with gloves or fabric and well-fitted shoes. Soak callus in warm water and Epsom salts to soften; use pumice stone to remove while soft. Apply cream or lotion.
Corns: caused by friction and pressure from shoes, mainly on toes, over bony prominence; usually cone shaped, round, raised, and tender; may affect gait.	Avoid corn pads, which increase pressure and reduce circulation. Surgical removal may be necessary.
Plantar warts: lesions on sole of foot caused by virus; may be contagious, are painful, and make walking difficult.	Treatment ordered by physician may include applications of acid, burning, or freezing for removal.
Athlete's foot: fungal infection of foot; scaling and cracking of skin occur between toes and on soles of feet; may have small blisters containing fluid. Apparently induced by tight footwear. May spread to other body parts, especially hands; is contagious; and frequently recurs.	Feet should be well ventilated. Dry well after bathing; apply powder. Wear clean socks. May be treated with medicated powder or cream.
Ingrown nails: toenail or fingernail grows inward into soft tissue around nail, often from improper nail trimming; may be painful with pressure.	Frequent hot soaks in antiseptic solution and surgical removal of portion of nail that has grown into skin. Teach client to trim nails straight across.
Ram's horn nails: long curved nails; attempts to cut may damage nail bed and risk infection.	Refer to podiatrist.
Fungus infection: thick, discolored nails with yellow streaks.	Refer to podiatrist.

pulses. **Circulatory alterations may change integrity of nails and increase client's chance of localized infection when a break in skin integrity occurs.**

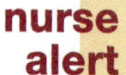 **nurse alert**   Some agencies require a physician's order for trimming nails when circulatory compromise is apparent.

4. Determine client's ability to perform self-care. **Limited vision, lack of coordination, and inability to reach feet influence degree of assistance required.**
5. Assess client's knowledge of foot and nail care practices and type of home remedies client uses for existing foot problems.
   a. Over-the-counter liquid preparations to remove corns may cause burns and ulcerations.
   b. Cutting of corns or calluses with razor blade or scissors may result in infections.
   c. Use of oval corn pads may exert pressure on toes, thereby decreasing circulation to surrounding tissues.
   d. Application of adhesive tape may tear thin and delicate skin of older adults when removed.
6. Assess type of footwear worn by clients.
   a. Type and cleanliness of socks worn?
   b. Type and fit of shoes?
   c. Restrictive garters or knee-high nylons worn?

Planning

Expected outcomes focus on self-care practices that maintain healthy nails and feet and promote circulation and comfort.

EXPECTED OUTCOMES
1. Client maintains nail integrity and cleanliness.
2. Client correctly demonstrates nail care.
3. Client walks steadily in appropriate footwear.
4. Client identifies ways to minimize sources of pressure or irritation when walking.

Implementation

Steps	Rationale

1. See Standard Protocol (Chapter 1, p. 5).

2. Soak feet

  a. Explain that soaking requires 10 to 20 minutes.

  b. Assist ambulatory client to sit in chair with disposable bath mat under feet. If confined to bed, assist to a semi-Fowler's position with a waterproof pad and bath towel under feet (Figure 6-28).

  c. Fill wash basin with warm water. Test temperature of water with back of hand.

> Warm water softens nails and thickened epidermal cells, reduces inflammation of skin, and promotes local circulation. Clients with decreased sensation to feet are unable to detect temperature of hot water.

  d. Place basin on bath mat or towel and help client place feet in basin. Place call light within client's reach and position overbed table in front of client. Offer diversional activity.

> Clients with muscular weakness or tremors may have difficulty positioning feet.

  e. If desired, allow client to soak fingers in a small basin on overbed table with arms in a comfortable position.

> Prolonged positioning can cause discomfort unless alignment is maintained.

  f. Allow client's feet and nails to soak for 10 to 20 minutes. If necessary, rewarm water after 10 minutes.

> Softening of corns, calluses, and cuticles ensures easy removal of dead cells and easy manipulation of cuticle.

  g. Using an orange stick, clean gently under nails while immersed in water. Remove basin and dry thoroughly.

> Thorough drying slows fungal growth and prevents maceration of tissues. Friction removes dead skin layers.

3. Trim nails

  a. With nail clippers, clip nails straight across and even with ends of digits. Shape nails with emery board or file (Figure 6-29).

> Cutting straight across prevents splitting of nail margins and formation of sharp nail spikes that can irritate lateral nail margins.

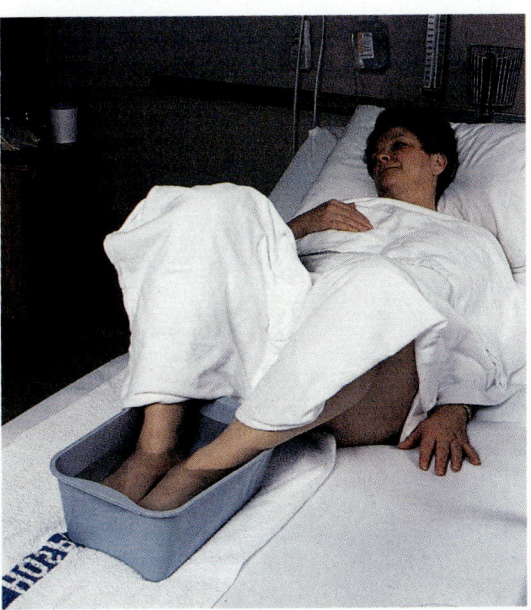

Figure 6-28

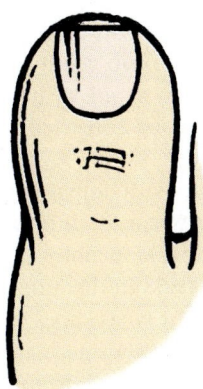

Figure 6-29

Steps	Rationale

nurse alert Clients with severe hypertrophy of nails should be referred to podiatrist for care to avoid risk of additional tissue injury.

b. If client has circulatory problems, file the nails.

Filing prevents cutting soft tissues, which could become infected and heal slowly.

c. Push cuticle back gently with orange stick and apply lotion to hands and feet.

Reduces incidence of inflamed cuticles. Lotion lubricates dry skin by helping to retain moisture.

4. Teach foot care

a. Instruct client to inspect feet daily: tops and soles, heels, and area between toes. Use a mirror to check soles and heels.

b. Instruct to wash and soak feet daily using lukewarm water and to dry thoroughly, especially between the toes.

c. Instruct to consult a physician or podiatrist rather than cutting corns or calluses or using commercial removers.

   (1) Apply moleskin to areas of feet that are under friction.

   Less likely to cause local pressure than corn pads.

   (2) Spot adhesive bandages can guard corns against friction but do not have padding to protect against pressure.

   (3) Wrap small pieces of lamb's wool around toes.

   Reduces irritation of soft corns between toes.

d. If feet tend to perspire, instruct client to use a mild foot powder.

e. Instruct client to wear clean socks or stockings daily (change twice a day if feet perspire heavily). Check for holes or roughness that might cause pressure. Wearing absorbent liners also helps reduce perspiration and foot odors.

Light-colored or white cotton socks do not contain dyes and are more absorbent (Evanski and Reinherz, 1991).

f. If dryness is noted along the feet or between the toes, instruct client to apply lanolin, baby oil, or even corn oil and rub gently into skin.

g. Instruct client to avoid wearing elastic stockings, knee high hose, or constricting garters and avoid crossing legs.

Impairs circulation to the lower extremities.

h. Instruct client with impaired sensation to wear protective footwear at all times and check inside of shoes daily for pebbles, foreign objects, and roughness or tears in the inner liners.

Reduced circulation is often accompanied by reduced sensation, allowing injuries to go untreated unless detected by inspection. Foreign objects may cause sores that go unnoticed (Osterman and Stuck, 1990).

i. Instruct client to wear shoes with flexible nonslip soles, sturdy porous uppers, and closed-in toes. Fit should not be restrictive to the feet.

j. Any minor cuts should be washed immediately and dried thoroughly. Only mild antiseptics (e.g., Neosporin ointment) should be applied to the skin. Avoid iodine or merbromin. Notify a physician.

With reduced circulation, infections are more likely and heal more slowly.

5. See Completion Protocol (Chapter 1, p. 6).

Evaluation

1. Inspect nails and surrounding skin surfaces after soaking and nail trimming. Note any remaining rough areas.
2. Ask client to explain and demonstrate nail care.
3. Observe client's walk using appropriate footwear.
4. Ask client to list ways to reduce irritation and pressure to feet when walking.

UNEXPECTED OUTCOMES AND RELATED INTERVENTIONS

1. Nails are discolored, rough, and concave or irregular in shape. Cuticles and surrounding tissues may be inflamed and tender to touch. Localized areas of tenderness are present on feet, with calluses or corns at points of friction.
   a. Repeated soakings are necessary to help relieve inflammation and remove layers of cells from calluses or corns.
   b. Change in footwear or corrective foot surgery may be needed for permanent improvement in corns or calluses.
2. Client unable to explain or perform foot care.
   a. Provide repeated opportunities for practice in controlled setting.
   b. Refer to podiatrist for regular follow-up care.
3. Client complains of pain while walking and has unsteady gait.
   a. House slippers or special footwear may be required.
   b. Muscle-strengthening exercises may promote greater stability.
   c. Clients with chronic foot pain should be seen by physician.

SAMPLE DOCUMENTATION

0900 Right great toe red, inflamed, and tender. Client states this was first noted before admission 1 week ago. Feet soaked for 10 minutes in warm water and dried thoroughly. Lotion applied. Client instructed on necessity of cutting nails straight across to avoid this problem. Stated, "This is so sore, I'll be careful how I trim my nails now."

CRITICAL THINKING EXERCISES

1. Mr. Louis, 70 years old, has a history of colon cancer. One year ago, he had a resection of the colon, and a colostomy was formed to promote passage of stool through an abdominal stoma. He is admitted for confusion and dehydration. On assessment, the nurse finds Mr. Louis incontinent of urine and diaphoretic with a fever of 101° F (38.3° C). His ankles are swollen, his skin is dry and scaly, and he is disoriented.
   Identify factors that place Mr. Louis at High Risk for Impaired Skin Integrity.
2. The nurse assesses a new client to determine the best bathing method. Mr. Nelson is 88 years old, oriented in all spheres, but somewhat forgetful regarding recent events. Mr. Nelson is unsteady and requires assistance when ambulatory. He is able to eat unassisted. The nurse decides to give Mr. Nelson a complete bed bath.
   a. What assumption did the nurse make in deciding the method of bathing?
   b. On what basis do you think the nurse made her assumption?
   c. How could you determine whether the assumption was accurate?
   d. Discuss possible consequences of making inappropriate or false assumptions when planning methods for promoting hygiene.
3. Mr. Richards, 38 years old, sustained a closed head injury 2 weeks ago. He is unresponsive, has an artificial airway (tracheostomy tube), and is flaccid on the right side. His hair and mustache are long, oily, and matted together. He is coughing up copious amount of thick, yellow sputum from the tracheostomy tube and is diaphoretic because of a low-grade fever and respiratory infection. Mr. Richards has a Foley catheter and is incontinent of feces.
   a. Discuss hygiene measures appropriate for Mr. Richards.
   b. Are there any specific hygiene measures that would be contraindicated?
4. You are assigned to two clients who both require a complete bed bath. Joseph, 30 years old, has a left leg cast, and Clarissa, 75 years old, has a red rash over her entire body.
   Discuss how the bed bath should be individualized for each of these clients.
5. As a community health nurse, you are caring for an elderly client who has severe arthritis, bilateral cataracts, and diabetes. Discuss potential difficulties the client might experience in performing foot care.

REFERENCES

AHCPR: *Pressure ulcers in adults: prediction and prevention (clinical practice guidelines),* Rockville, Md, 1992, US Dept of Health and Human Services.

Avalon Industries: Personal communication, Antoinette Taylor, Education Coordinator, PO Box 388080, Chicago, Ill, 63063, 1994.

Evanski PM, Reinherz RP: Easing the pain of common foot problems, *Patient Care* 25:38, 1991.

Galanti G: *Caring for patients from different cultures,* Philadelphia, 1991, University of Pennsylvania Press.

Greifzu S, Radjeski D, Winnick B: Oral care is part of cancer care, *RN* 53:43, 1990.

Kim MJ, McFarland GK McLane AM: *Pocket guide to nursing diagnoses,* ed 5, St Louis, 1993, Mosby.

Osterman HM, Stuck RM: The aging foot, *Orthop Nurs* 9:43, 1990.

ADDITIONAL READINGS

Beck S: Impact of systematic oral care protocol on stomatitis after chemotherapy, *Cancer Nurse* 2:185, 1979.

Belcher AE: *Cancer nursing,* St Louis, 1992, Mosby.

Ebersole P, Hess P: *Toward health aging: Human needs and nursing response,* ed 3, St Louis, 1990, Mosby.

Hogstel MO: *Clinical manual of gerontologic nursing,* St Louis, 1992, Mosby.

McFarland GK, McFarlane EA: *Nursing diagnosis and interventions: planning for patient care,* ed 2, St Louis, 1993, Mosby.

Patient information from your doctor: preventing common foot problems, *Patient Care* 25:54, 1991.

chapter 7 | Promoting Nutrition

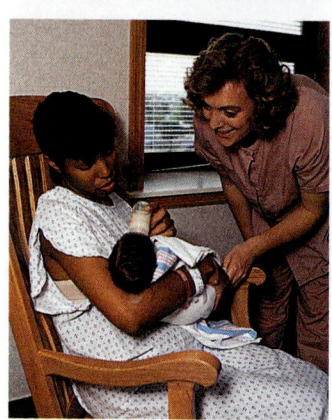

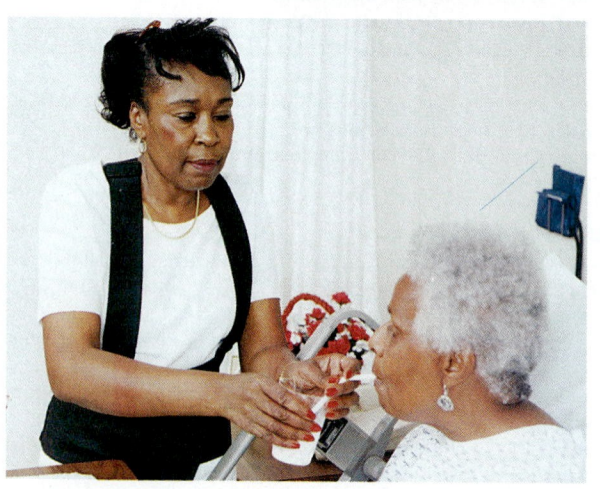

Nutrition is considered one of the foundations for life and health. It involves the process of ingesting food and using it to maintain body tissue and provide energy. The basic energy sources include carbohydrates, fats, proteins, vitamins, minerals, and fatty acids. The body needs these sources in various combinations to continue daily activities, provide energy, heal, resist infection, grow, and survive. The U.S. Department of Agriculture has recommended the Food Guide Pyramid (Figure 7-1) to emphasize the grain and cereal group as the basic food in the diet, with less desired foods in smaller quantities at the top.

Assessment of a client's nutritional status is essential for determining what dietary needs are present. Nurses are in an ideal position to perform this because of their close, bedside observation of the client throughout the day. Registered dietitians also are highly skilled at assessing client's nutritional needs. Nurses and dietitians working together are able to develop a detailed plan of care to meet nutritional needs based on a sound nutritional assessment, the client's food preferences, and any cultural or religious requirements.

A nutritional assessment has four components: (1) a diet history, (2) physical assessment of the body, (3) laboratory data, and (4) anthropometric measurements to determine the size, frame, and fat and tissue content of the body (see box on p. 97). This can be performed by a dietitian or nurse.

Clients at risk for malnutrition include those with conditions that increase metabolism (e.g., hyperthyroidism, pregnancy, burns, sepsis); diseases that impair absorption (e.g., diabetes, liver disease, gastric surgery, Crohn's dis-

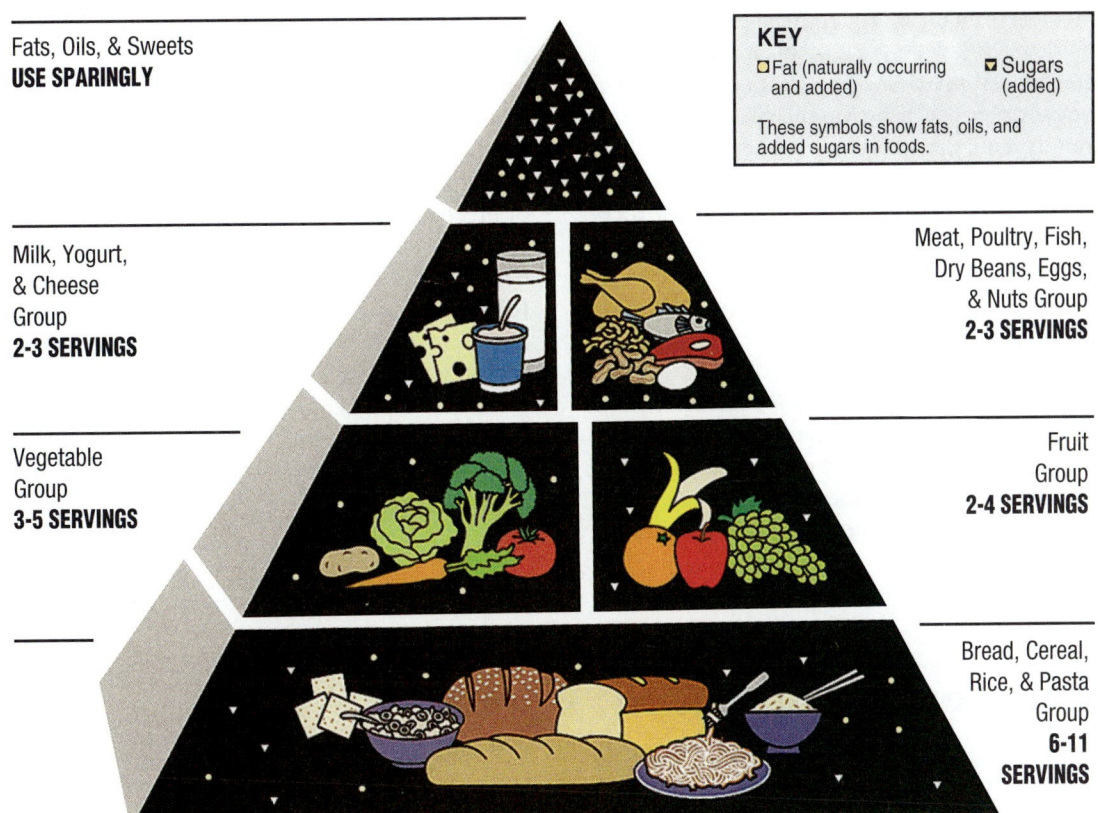

KEY
☐ Fat (naturally occurring and added) ☑ Sugars (added)

These symbols show fats, oils, and added sugars in foods.

Fats, Oils, & Sweets
USE SPARINGLY

Milk, Yogurt, & Cheese Group
2-3 SERVINGS

Meat, Poultry, Fish, Dry Beans, Eggs, & Nuts Group
2-3 SERVINGS

Vegetable Group
3-5 SERVINGS

Fruit Group
2-4 SERVINGS

Bread, Cereal, Rice, & Pasta Group
6-11 SERVINGS

Figure 7-1 Food Guide Pyramid. (From US Department of Agriculture: *USDA's food guide pyramid,* USDA Human Nutrition Information pub no 249, Washington, DC, 1992, US Government Printing Office.)

Components of a Nutritional Assessment

DIET HISTORY
Appetite (current/changing)
Weight
Food preferences
Meal patterns
Bowel problems
Existing diseases

PHYSICAL ASSESSMENT
Skin
Hair
Muscles
Teeth
Gums
Eyes
Gastrointestinal function
Abdomen
General appearance

LABORATORY DATA
Protein
Albumin
Lymphocyte
Hemoglobin
Blood urea nitrogen (BUN)
Creatinine clearance

BODY MEASUREMENTS
Size
Frame
Height
Weight
Fat content
Tissue content

ease, diverticulosis); medical procedures (e.g., abdominal surgery, mouth/neck/jaw surgery, medications, radiation therapy); mechanical problems (e.g., difficulty chewing, paraplegia, quadriplegia, cerebrovascular accident [CVA], upper extremity injury, neuromuscular diseases such as poliomyelitis or muscular distrophy); and psychosocial problems (e.g., altered level of consciousness, alcoholism, depression, anorexia, loneliness, fear of choking, stress).

Nursing Diagnosis

Altered Nutrition, Less Than Body Requirements is the general nursing diagnosis for clients when the focus is increasing the quantity or quality of nutritional intake. **Feeding Self-Care Deficit** is more appropriate when clients are unable to prepare food or feed themselves be-

cause of mobility or coordination problems, such as with paralysis, casts, or missing limbs; visual problems, such as blindness or altered depth perception; or mental problems, such as confusion or dementia. **Impaired Swallowing** is appropriate if clients have an altered gag reflex or inability to cough, weakened muscles of chewing, or mechanical alterations such as cancer of the upper airway, an obstructing tumor, or a fistula (abnormal opening between the esophagus and adjacent body cavity). **Risk for Aspiration** may also be appropriate for clients who need assistance because of inability to position themselves or who are learning to swallow after neurological damage or surgery. **Altered Nutrition, More Than Body Requirements** is appropriate when clients are more than 10% to 20% over the desired weight range for their height.

Skill 7.1 | Feeding Dependent Clients

Many hospitalized clients are unable to feed themselves adequately because of the severity of their illness or the fatigue and debilitation associated with their disease. Others are limited by loss of arm or hand movement, by impaired vision, by brain injury, or by the need to remain in a flat or prone position. When assisting the client with feeding, the nurse must ensure the client ingests an adequate volume of food and must facilitate independence when possible with the use of adaptive devices or finger foods and with comfortable and safe positioning for swallowing. Since mealtime is often viewed as a social time for clients, nurse-client communication is important.

EQUIPMENT

Meal tray
Overbed table
Adaptive utensils if appropriate (Figure 7-2)
    Utensils with padded or enlarged handles
    Cups with lids and/or handles
    Plate guard to fit around plate
    Suction device to hold plate to tray
    Hand splints to help hold utensil in hand
Damp washcloth (optional)
Oral hygiene supplies (optional)

Assessment

1. Assess client's level of consciousness, ability to cooperate, mobility/activity orders, and physical limitations to determine appropriate positioning for meals.
2. Assess client's need for toileting, handwashing, and oral care before feeding. **This reduces interruptions and improves appetite during the meal.**
3. Assess client's food preferences to determine if special foods will improve appetite and desire to feed independently.

Planning

Expected outcomes focus on increased independence with eating, improved nutritional intake, and safe intake of food.

EXPECTED OUTCOMES

1. Client's body weight remains stable or trends toward the normal level.

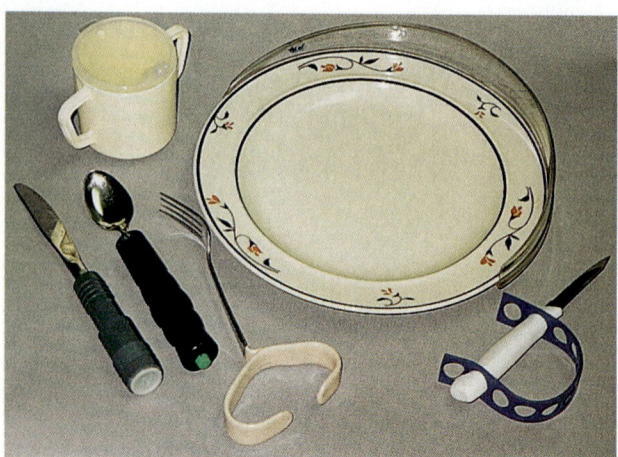

Figure 7-2

2. Client's nutrition-related laboratory values trend toward normal. (Note serum protein, albumin, and hemoglobin.)
3. Client demonstrates increased ability to feed self or open items on tray.

4. Client coughs appropriately when eating with no new signs of respiratory compromise.
5. Client demonstrates use of adaptive utensils as appropriate.

Implementation

Steps	Rationale
1. See Standard Protocol (Chapter 1, p. 5).	
2. Offer toileting and handwashing before meal.	
3. Offer toothbrush or mouthwash before meal.	May improve appetite in client with stomatitis or other oral hygiene problems.
4. Position client appropriately for safe eating within limitations of ability. a. Up in chair b. High-Fowler's position in bed (Figure 7-3) c. Side-lying position if flat in bed	Positioning helps to improve swallowing and digestion and to avoid aspiration.
5. Assist client with setting up meal tray if he or she is able: open packages, cut up food, apply seasonings/condiments, butter bread, place napkin.	
6. Place adaptive utensils on tray if indicated, and instruct in their use.	
7. If client is visually impaired, identify food location on plate as if it were a clock (Figure 7-4).	Visually impaired client may feed self if given adequate information about tray.

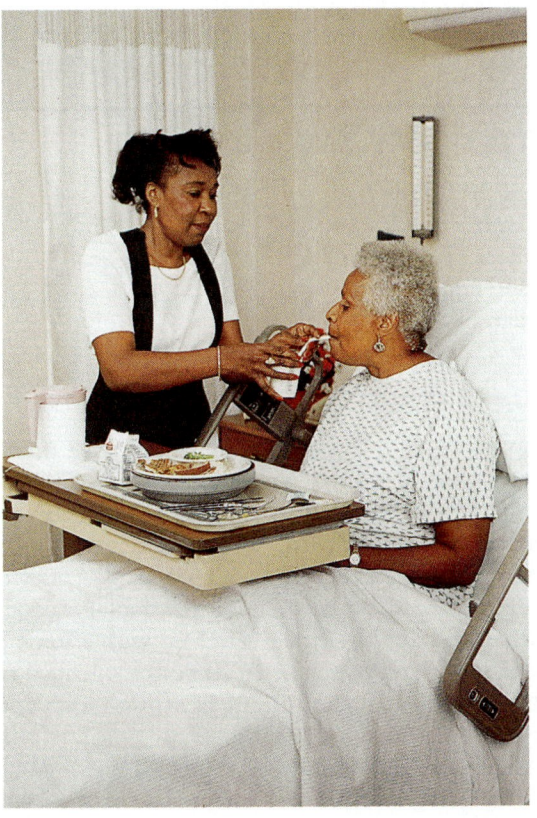

Figure 7-3

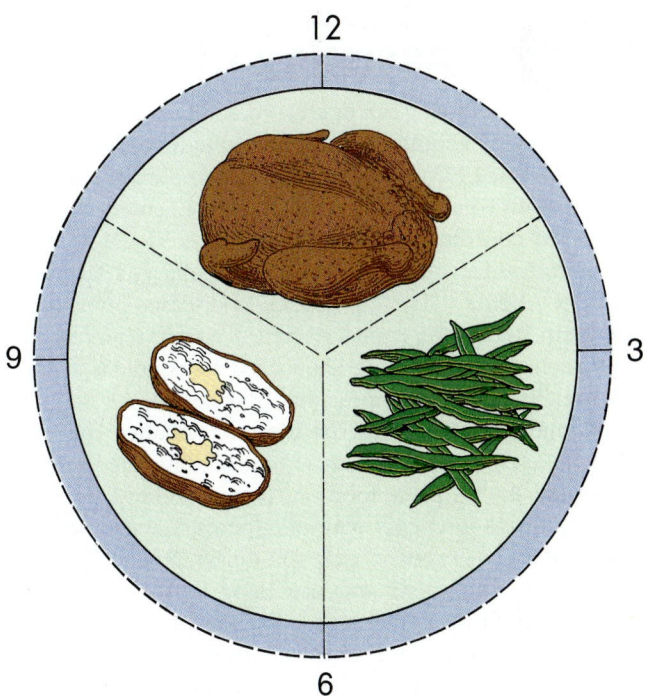

Figure 7-4 For the visually impaired client: "The potatoes are at 9 o'clock."

Steps	Rationale
8. Pace feeding to avoid client fatigue. Ask client the order in which he or she wishes to eat food. Interact with client during mealtime.	Gives client some control of situation and avoids embarrassment of limitations. Social interaction may improve appetite.
9. Assist client with washing hands and repositioning as desired.	
10. Monitor intake and output (see Skill 7.4) and calorie count.	These values help measure improvement in nutrition.
11. See Completion Protocol (Chapter 1, p. 6).	

Evaluation

1. Monitor body weight and laboratory values.
2. Observe amount of food on tray after meal.
3. Observe client's technique for self-feeding: certain items, part or all of meal.
4. Observe client during eating for choking, coughing, gagging, or food left in the mouth.
5. Observe use of adaptive utensils.

UNEXPECTED OUTCOMES AND RELATED INTERVENTIONS

1. Client refuses to eat food offered.
   a. Determine if client has other food preferences.
   b. Determine if different times of the day are better.
   c. Determine if pain or anxiety should be treated before eating.
   d. Determine if client is mentally incapable of cooperating.
2. Client chokes on food or does not choke but food sits on side or back of mouth (see Skill 7.2).
   a. Use suction equipment if necessary to clear food from airway.
   b. If choking occurs repeatedly, stop feeding and notify physician.

SAMPLE DOCUMENTATION

0800 Assisted client to high Fowler's position. Client able to feed self 5 bites with padded spoon and plate guard. Became fatigued, rest of breakfast fed to client. No coughing or aspiration noted.

Skill 7.2 | Assisting Clients with Impaired Swallowing

Impaired swallowing is a decreased ability to pass fluids and/or solids voluntarily from the mouth to the stomach (NANDA, 1993). Swallowing is a complex event, requiring both voluntary and involuntary movements. It requires the coordination of cranial nerves V, VII, IX, X, and XII, as well as the muscles of the tongue, pharynx, larynx, and jaw. Clients with neuromuscular diseases involving the brain, brainstem, cranial nerves, myoneural junction, or muscles of swallowing should be assessed for swallowing difficulties before feeding (Baker, 1993).

Maintaining an upright position to enhance the effects of gravity is important. When feeding the client, the nurse should place food on the **unaffected** side of the mouth (as in clients with hemiparesis) and observe the swallowing event closely for delays. Reducing distractions in the room and providing verbal coaching throughout the swallowing process can also greatly help the client swallow more effectively. In some cases, thickeners may be added to food or fluids to increase the consistency and thus allow the client more control of the volume in the mouth (Emmick-Herring and Wood, 1990).

EQUIPMENT

Meal tray
Thickener (if ordered)
Suction equipment
Oxygen

Assessment

1. Assess client's level of alertness; drooling; problems with speech; and wet, gurgly voice. **These factors indicate poor oral control and may put the client at risk for aspiration.**
2. Assess client's ability to cough on request, as well as the presence of gagging or involuntary coughing when back of the throat is tickled with a tongue depressor or wet cotton swab. **Absence of these functions indicates that client is at high risk for aspiration with swallowing.**
3. Assess client's swallowing reflex before feeding by placing fingers on client's throat at level of the larynx, then asking client to swallow saliva. Movement of the larynx should be palpated (Figure 7-5).

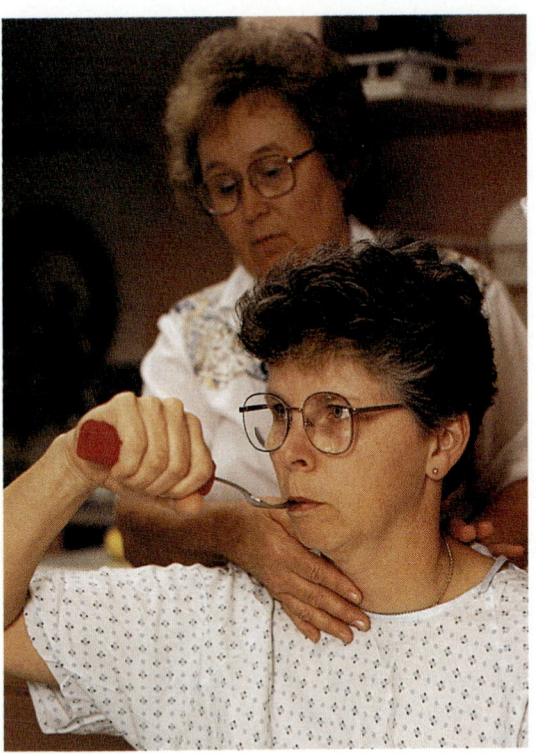

Figure 7-5

Planning

Expected outcomes focus on adequate food and fluid intake to prevent malnutrition and dehydration while avoiding aspiration.

EXPECTED OUTCOMES
1. Client swallows without retaining food in mouth.
2. Client demonstrates a complete swallowing event.
3. Client exhibits no symptoms of aspiration or respiratory distress after meals.
4. Client's body weight, thirst, skin turgor, and nutrition-related laboratory values all trend toward normal.

Implementation

Steps	Rationale
1. See Standard Protocol (Chapter 1, p. 5).	
2. Position client upright in bed or chair with head slightly flexed forward.	This position reduces risk of aspiration (Price and DiIorio, 1990).
3. Reduce distractions in the room to keep client focused on swallowing.	
4. Add thickener to thin liquids or begin serving client pureed foods.	Thin liquids such as water and fruit juice are difficult to control in the mouth and easily aspirated.
5. Place ½ to 1 tsp of food on unaffected side of the mouth, allowing utensil to touch the mouth or tongue.	
6. Provide verbal coaching while feeding client.	Verbal cueing keeps client focused on swallowing (Donahue, 1990).
a. Open your mouth.	
b. Feel the food in your mouth.	
c. Chew and taste the food.	
d. Raise your tongue to roof of your mouth.	
e. Think about swallowing.	
f. Close your mouth and swallow.	
g. Swallow again.	Swallowing twice is often necessary to clear the pharynx (see Figure 7-5).
h. Cough to clear airway.	
7. Provide positive reinforcement to client.	Enhances client's confidence in skill.
8. Observe for coughing, choking, gagging, and drooling of food; suction airway as necessary.	
9. Provide rest periods as necessary during meal to avoid fatigue.	

Steps	Rationale
10. Maintain upright position for 15 to 30 minutes after eating.	Helps avoid aspiration or regurgitation.
11. Provide mouth care after meals.	This dislodges any food or fluids that may have accumulated inside client's cheeks.
12. Advance diet to thicker foods that require more chewing and finally to thin liquids as tolerated.	Dietitian and/or speech pathologist can direct safest advancement of diet.
13. See Completion Protocol (Chapter 1, p. 6).	

Evaluation

1. Observe contents of client's mouth during meal for food pocketing.
2. Observe client for a continuous (not prolonged or delayed) swallowing event.
3. Observe client for coughing or choking during meal.
4. Monitor intake and output (Skill 7.4), calorie count, food eaten from tray, weight (Skill 7.3), and nutrition-related laboratory values.

UNEXPECTED OUTCOMES AND RELATED INTERVENTIONS

1. Client begins coughing, choking, or turning blue.
   a. Stop feeding client.
   b. Position client in high Fowler's position or, if unable, position on side.
   c. Suction airway until clear.
   d. Provide oxygen if color has not returned to normal.
2. Food and/or fluids drain out of client's nose during the meal.
   a. Stop feeding client.
   b. Suction nasopharyngeal area.
   c. Resume feeding with increased head flexion.
3. On inspection, food is found pocketed in client's cheeks.
   Teach client to use the tongue or to massage the cheek externally to move food to a more functional area of the mouth.

SAMPLE DOCUMENTATION

1200 Client fed $\frac{1}{2}$ of pureed diet and juice with thickener added. Stopped meal due to fatigue. No coughing or aspiration noted.

Skill 7.3 | Obtaining Body Weights

This skill involves obtaining an accurate body weight for the client. Care must be taken in using the same scale at or near the same time of the day, weighing the same amount of clothing or linen, and avoiding weighing client drainage bags (e.g., full colostomy or catheter bag). The client's safety is extremely important, so a bed scale or chair scale may be used if the client is unable to safely stand independently.

Some of the newer models of beds have scales built into their structures. Obtaining a client's weight on this type of scale requires following the manufacturer's instructions.

Although obtaining a body weight is a fairly simple task, it must be done accurately because it is one of the more important parameters used to evaluate and treat many diseases, including congestive heart failure, fluid overload, and renal failure. The Joint Commission for the Accreditation of Healthcare Organizations (JCAHO) requires all hospitalized clients to have height-weight mea-

surement. Height is measured using a device attached to the standing scale (Figure 7-6, *A*). A height and weight chart is used to identify the appropriate weight (see Appendix E).

EQUIPMENT
Standing platform scale
   or
Stretcher scale or bed scale
   or
Seated chair scale

Assessment

1. Assess client's weight-bearing status by asking client or by reviewing client's record to determine ability to stand independently and the previously recorded weight.

2. Assess client's level of consciousness. Alert, stable clients who have been on bed rest may require the assistance of two personnel to stand and be weighed safely or be transferred to a chair scale. If the client is not alert or is critically ill, a bed scale is the safest means to obtain a weight.

Planning

Expected outcomes focus on accuracy of the weight obtained and client's safety during the process.

EXPECTED OUTCOMES
1. Client's correct weight is determined.
2. Client does not slip or fall during the weighing process.

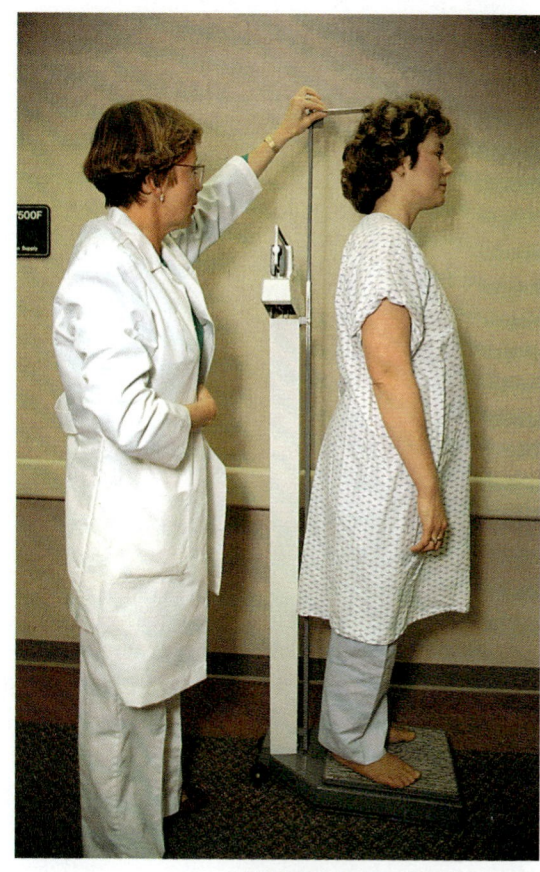

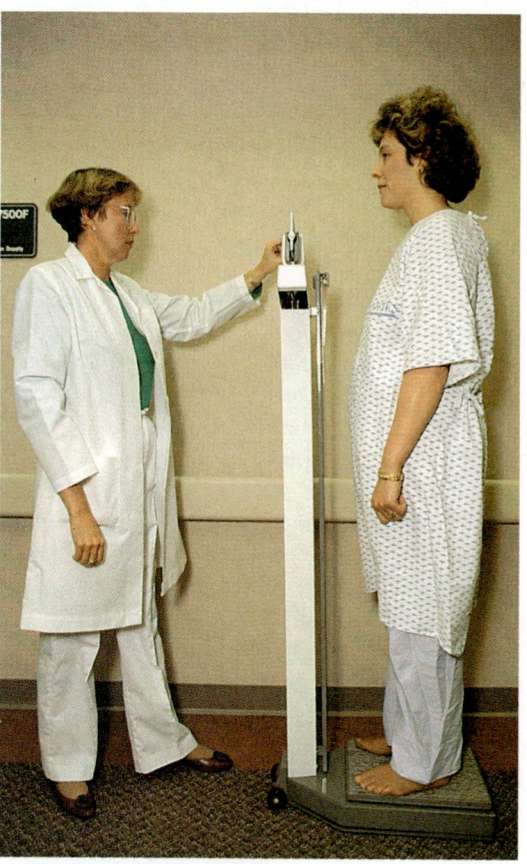

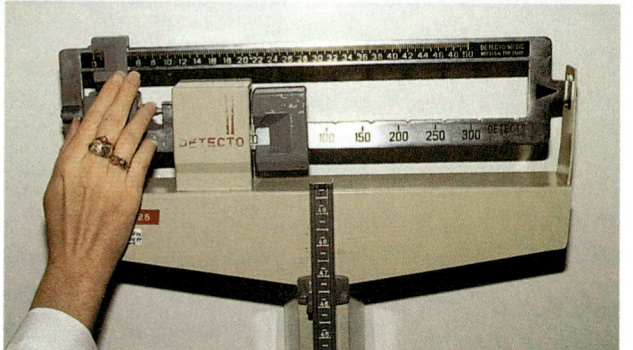

Figure 7-6 **A,** Measuring client's height. **B,** Client standing independently on platform scale. **C,** Adjust calibrating knob on scale.

Implementation

Steps	Rationale
1. See Standard Protocol (Chapter 1, p. 5).	
2. Empty any pouches attached to client that contain drainage.	Weight of drainage alters body weight.
3. Place appropriate scale at client's bedside.	Chair scale should be used if client cannot stand independently. Bed scale should be used if client is non–weight bearing.
4. Weigh client on platform scale.	Used when clients can bear weight.
a. Balance and calibrate scale to "0" pounds (or kilograms). Balance beam should be in middle of mark; digital scale should read "0."	
b. Ask client to step up onto platform scale and stand still (Figure 7-6, *B*).	
c. Adjust balance on scale until it is in middle of mark or until digital scale displays a reading (Figure 7-6, *C*).	
5. Weigh client on chair scale.	Used when clients may be out of bed but are unable to stand independently.
a. Balance and calibrate scale to "0" pounds (or kilograms). Balance beam should be in middle of mark; digital scale should read "0."	
b. Assist client onto chair scale.	
c. Adjust balance on scale until it is in middle of mark or until digital scale displays a reading.	
6. Weigh client on bed scale.	Used when clients are unable to bear weight.
a. Place sling with same type and amount of linen and a client gown on arms of scale.	
b. Calibrate scale to "0" with linens and gown.	Calibrating with linen and gown allows these to be kept on client but not included in weight.
c. With nurse on side of bed, roll client onto side. Place sling under client (Figure 7-7) using good body mechanics (see Chapter 5). Two nurses may be required for clients who are unable to assist with procedure.	Using two nurses protects client from rolling out of bed.

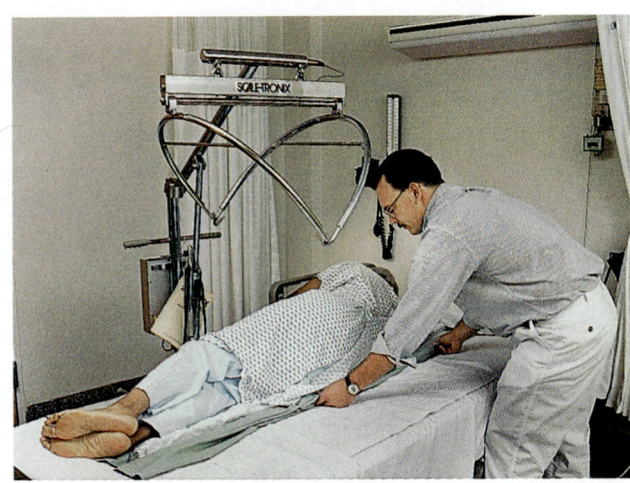

Figure 7-7

Steps	Rationale

    d. Attach scale and elevate until clear of bed (Figure 7-8).

    e. Instruct client to remain still, if possible.   Movement can cause inaccurate readings.

    f. Obtain weight from scale (Figure 7-9).

    g. Lower client onto bed, roll over stretcher, then re-move stretcher and scale from client's bed.

7. See Completion Protocol (Chapter 1, p. 6).

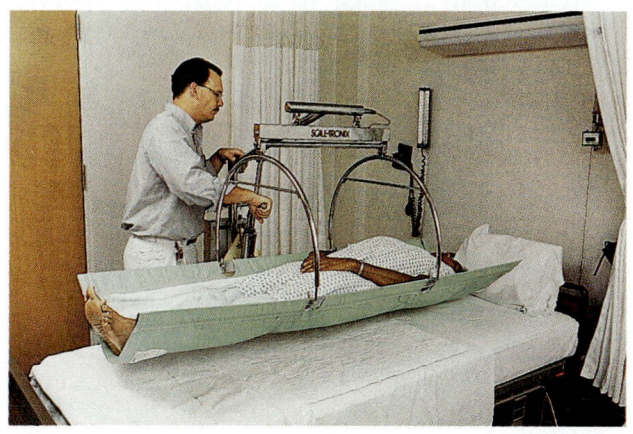

Figure 7-8

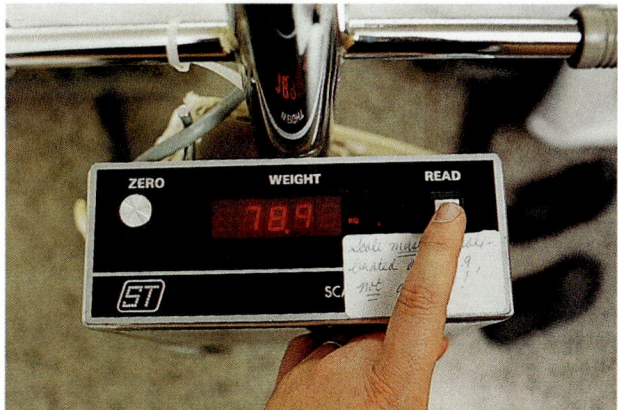

Figure 7-9

Evaluation

1. Determine how weight obtained compares with last weight obtained and current plan of treatment (e.g., diuretics, fluid bolus).

2. Observe for instability with type of scale used.

UNEXPECTED OUTCOMES AND RELATED INTERVENTIONS

1. Weight obtained varies by greater than 5 pounds from previous reading.
   a. Recheck weight with another scale.
   b. Be sure that client is not touching scale and that no one is supporting him or her during procedure.
   c. Recalibrate scale to be certain it is balanced at "0."

2. Client falls during transfer or is injured during bed scale weighing.
   a. Assist client immediately back to bed or out of in-jured position.
   b. Assess for physical injury.
   c. Contact physician as agency protocol dictates.

DOCUMENTATION

Usual documentation is simply the weight obtained recorded in the appropriate box on a flow sheet, for example, "72 kg/bed scale."

Skill 7.4 | Monitoring Intake and Output

Measuring and recording all liquid intake and output (I&O) may be an independent nursing intervention or may be ordered by the physician. The recording of I&O over a 24-hour period is appropriate if a client has a fever, has edema, is receiving intravenous or diuretic therapy, or is placed on restricted fluids. It is also important when a client has excessive fluid or electrolyte loss, as associated with vomiting, diarrhea, or gastrointestinal drainage. At specified times, usually every 8 hours, I&O is totaled and evaluated. Significant alterations are apparent by comparing 24-hour totals over several days.

Intake includes all liquids taken orally, by feeding tube, and parenterally. Oral liquids include semiliquids, such as gelatin and ice cream, and liquid medications. Liquid output includes urine, diarrhea, vomitus, gastric suction, and contents of drainage devices. When possible, assistance from the alert and cooperative client or family facilitates accuracy and independence.

EQUIPMENT

Graduated measuring container
Bedpan, urinal, or bedside commode
Specipan or "hat" (a receptacle that fits inside the commode)
Disposable gloves

Assessment

1. Identify medications that may alter urine output. For example, **diuretics cause water, sodium, and potassium excretion, and steroids (e.g., prednisone, cortisone) cause sodium and water retention and potassium excretion.**

2. Monitor hematocrit, which is part of a complete blood count (CBC). **A high hematocrit suggests a large percentage of red blood cells (RBCs) in the total blood volume and is characteristic of dehydration** (Pagana and Pagana, 1992).

3. Monitor weight changes greater than 2% within 24 to 48 hours in adult clients. One liter of water weighs 1 kg (2.2 pounds) (see Chapter 36). **Weight loss greater than 2% suggests dehydration, whereas sudden weight gain greater than 2% may indicate edema and fluid overload.**

4. Assess client's knowledge of the purpose for I&O measurement and ability to participate actively in measurement. **Severely ill or disoriented clients may be unable to participate actively in measuring or recording.**

Planning

Expected outcomes focus on maintaining fluid balance, encouraging adequate fluid intake, and achieving normal laboratory values and body weight.

EXPECTED OUTCOMES

1. Client's urine is neither concentrated nor dilute, with specific gravity WNL (1.010 to 1.025).
2. Client maintains fluid balance, as evidenced by intake approximately 600 ml greater than output, with total 24-hour output at least 1500 ml.
3. Client's hematocrit is within a range of 40% to 54% for males or 38% to 47% for females.
4. Client's weight remains within 2% of normal.

Implementation

Steps	Rationale
1. See Standard Protocol (Chapter 1, p. 5).	
2. Explain to client and family that accurate I&O measurements are important to identify potential fluid overload or excessive losses.	Alert, cooperative ambulatory clients can be active participants with recording I&O.
3. Measure and record all fluid intake.	
a. Liquids with meals may include gelatin, custards, ice cream, popsicles, and sherbets. Ice chips are recorded as 50% of measured volume (e.g., 100 ml ice equals 50 ml water).	
b. Liquid medicines such as antacids are counted as fluid intake.	
c. Enteral nutrition (tube feedings) (see Chapter 32).	
d. Intravenous fluids (see Chapter 29).	

Steps	Rationale

4. Instruct client and family to call nurse to empty urinal, drainage bag, bedpan, commode, or "hat" each time it is used (Figure 7-10). Alert, cooperative clients may keep own tally using scratch paper or a copy of facility's I&O chart.

Promotes accurate method for recording output. Report any urine output less than 30 ml/hr, which may indicate decreased renal perfusion.

5. Empty and record urine output from Foley catheter into clean, graduated container at end of each shift (Figure 7-11). Cleanse the drainage port before recapping.

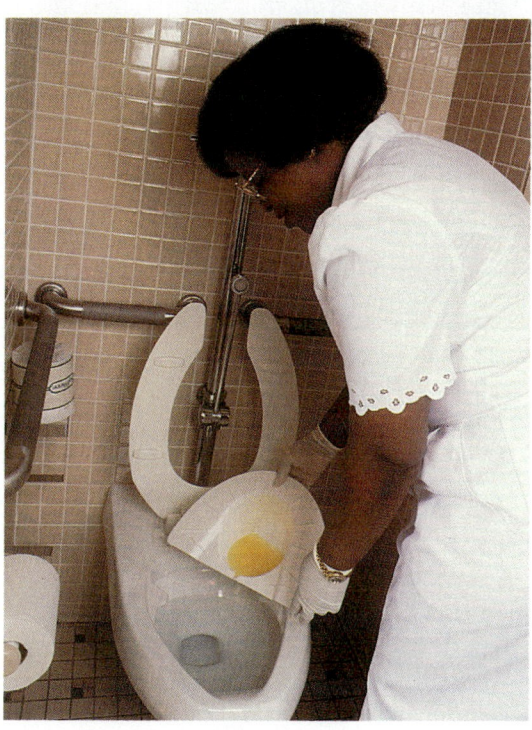

Figure 7-10

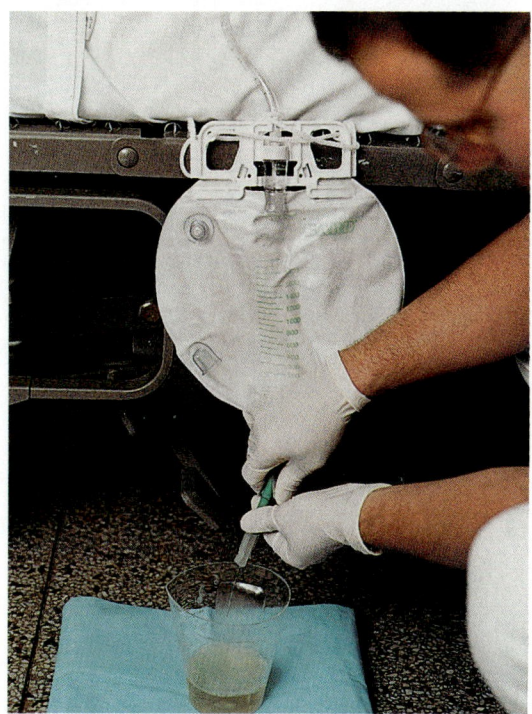

Figure 7-11

6. Observe color and characteristics of urine in Foley bag. Some clients may have a special device that is emptied into the larger container hourly. Urine output less than 30 ml/hr can indicate decreased renal perfusion and should be reported.

Dark, concentrated urine suggests dehydration.

7. Measure and record all drainage from all other sources, including nasogastric suction (see Chapter 31) and all measurable wound drainage (Figure 7-12, *A*), or measure chest tube drainage by marking and recording the time on the collection chamber (Figure 7-12, *B*). (See Chapter 20.)

8. Weigh client with the same scale, at the same time of day, and with comparable articles of clothing, including bed linen if bed weights are necessary (see Skill 7.3)

9. See Completion Protocol (Chapter 1, p. 6).

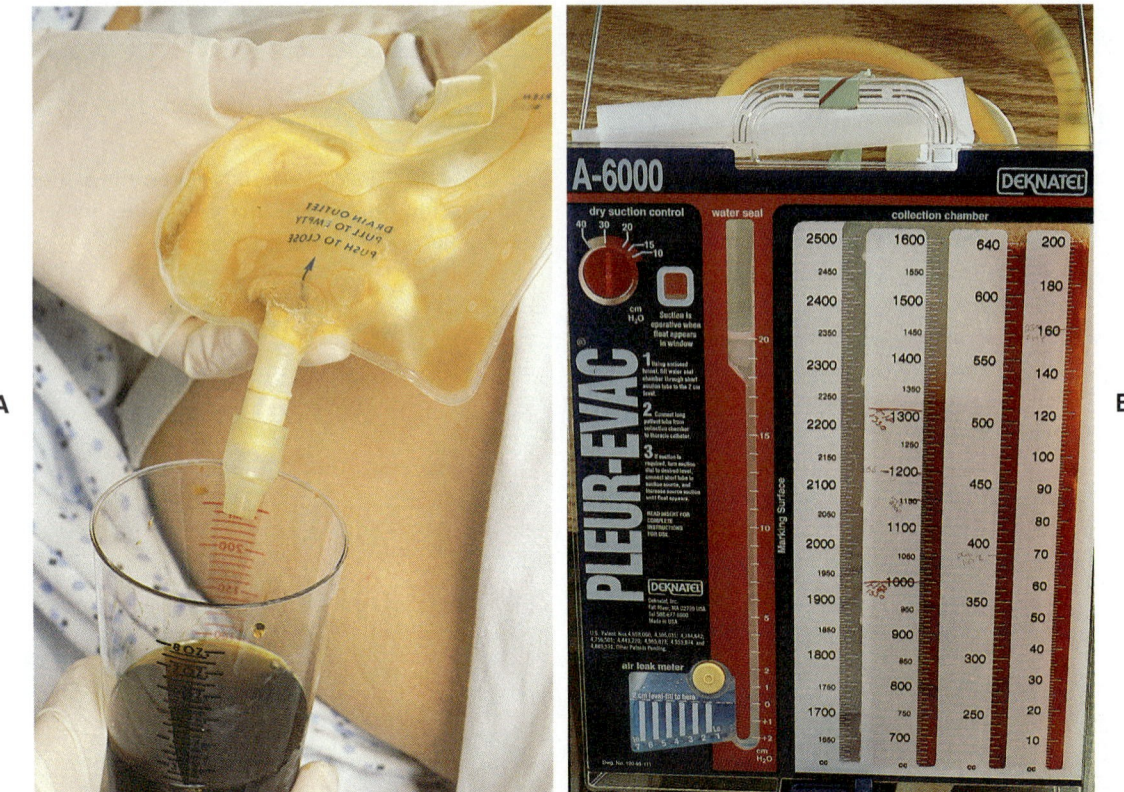

Figure 7-12 **A,** T-Tube drainage; **B,** chest-tube drainage (for I&O).

Evaluation

1. Observe amount and characteristics of urine, including color and specific gravity (normal, 1.010 to 1.025). Specific gravity can be measured using a reagent test strip with a color chart. **Diluted, watery urine results in low specific gravity readings, and dark-yellow, concentrated urine results in high specific gravity readings.**
2. Calculate total I&O at the end of each shift and for 24 hours.
3. Monitor serum hematocrit values.
4. Compare daily weights, noting increase or decrease greater than 2% within 48 hours.

UNEXPECTED OUTCOMES AND RELATED INTERVENTIONS

1. Client develops fluid volume excess or fluid overload (see Chapter 36), as evidenced by intake greater than output and weight gain greater than 2% over 24 to 48 hours and a low hematocrit.
2. Client develops fluid volume deficit (see Chapter 36), as evidenced by output greater than intake and weight loss greater than 2% in 24 to 48 hours and a high hematocrit.

SAMPLE DOCUMENTATION (see Figure 7-13)

1500 Very little p.o. fluid intake today (total of 300 ml in 8 hours). Client has complained of nausea, refused to eat or drink. Temperature 38.5° C. Urine output 350 ml per Foley, dark and concentrated. Physician notified. IV fluids started as ordered.

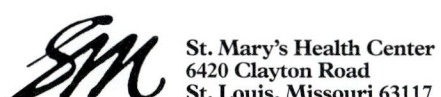

St. Mary's Health Center
6420 Clayton Road
St. Louis, Missouri 63117

John Martinez

PATIENT LABEL

INTAKE AND OUTPUT SUMMARY

	DATE 6-10-XX	2200 – 0600	0600 – 1400	1400 – 2200	24 Hr.	
INTAKE	P.O. Intake	120	800	650	1570	TOTAL INTAKE
	Tube Feedings					
	Hyperalimentation					
	I.V. Primary					
	I.V.P.B.	50		50	100	1670
	Blood/Blood Products					
OUTPUT	Urine	325	700	500	1525	TOTAL OUTPUT
	Emesis					
	G.I. Suction					
	Drainage	50	75	30	155	1855
	Chest tube	75	50	50	175	

	DATE	2200 – 0600	0600 – 1400	1400 – 2200	24 Hr.	
INTAKE	P.O. Intake					TOTAL INTAKE
	Tube Feedings					
	Hyperalimentation					
	I.V. Primary					
	I.V.P.B.					
	Blood/Blood Products					
OUTPUT	Urine					TOTAL OUTPUT
	Emesis					
	G.I. Suction					
	Drainage					

	DATE	2200 – 0600	0600 – 1400	1400 – 2200	24 Hr.	
INTAKE	P.O. Intake					TOTAL INTAKE
	Tube Feedings					
	Hyperalimentation					
	I.V. Primary					
	I.V.P.B.					
	Blood/Blood Products					
OUTPUT	Urine					TOTAL OUTPUT
	Emesis					
	G.I. Suction					
	Drainage					

	DATE	2200 – 0600	0600 – 1400	1400 – 2200	24 Hr.	
INTAKE	P.O. Intake					TOTAL INTAKE
	Tube Feedings					
	Hyperalimentation					
	I.V. Primary					
	I.V.P.B.					
	Blood/Blood Products					
OUTPUT	Urine					TOTAL OUTPUT
	Emesis					
	G.I. Suction					
	Drainage					

Figure 7-13 (Courtesy St. Mary's Health Center, St. Louis, Mo.)

CRITICAL THINKING EXERCISES

1. Mrs. Cupp had jaw surgery yesterday. Mr. Russ had a stroke 2 days ago.

   a. What primary problem will the nurse need to monitor for in both these clients that relates to their nutritional status?

   b. What measures will be necessary when feeding Mr. Russ that will not be required for Mrs. Cupp? For both Mr. Russ and Mrs. Cupp?

2. As the nurse obtains weights on each of the following clients, what scale should be used and what precautions should be taken to ensure accurate measurements?

   a. Ethel is 76 years old, has a colostomy, and is unable to stand without assistance.

   b. Mark is a 52-year-old male who recently had a heart attack. He has no activity restrictions and is being discharged in the morning.

   c. Elmer is 68 years old and receives diuretics for fluid retention. After weighing Elmer today, you noted that he has lost 7 pounds. He can ambulate to the bathroom with assistance.

3. Mr. Carl is a 70-year-old client who is on accurate intake and output recordings.

   a. From the following data, calculate Mr. Carl's intake and output for the past 8 hours.

	Diet		**Medications**
0800	1 cup coffee	0900	1 oz Milk of Magnesia
	1 egg		
	1 piece toast		
	½ cup cereal		
	½ cup skimmed milk		**Urine output**
1000	1 cup ice chips	1000	450 ml urine
1230	½ tuna sandwich	1400	250 ml urine
	½ cup custard		
	½ cup jello		
	6 oz iced tea		
1400	4 oz popsicle		

   b. What conclusions can be drawn from Mr. Carl's intake and output?

REFERENCES

Baker DM: Assessment and management of impairments in swallowing, *Nurs Clin North Am* 28(4):793, 1993.

Donahue PA: When it's hard to swallow: feeding techniques for dysphagia management, *J Gerontol Nurs* 16(4):6, 1990.

Emmick-Herring B, Wood P: A team approach to neurologically based swallowing disorders, *Rehabil Nurs* 15(3):132, 1990.

Pagana DK, Pagana TJ: *Mosby's diagnostic and laboratory test reference,* St Louis, 1992, Mosby.

Price ME, DiIorio C: Swallowing: a practice guide, *Am J Nurs* 90(7):42, 1990.

ADDITIONAL READINGS

DiIorio C, Price ME: Swallowing: an assessment guide, *Am J Nurs* 90(7):39, 1990.

LaBlance GR, Kraus K, Steckol KF: Rehabilitation of swallowing and communication following glossectomy, *Rehabil Nurs* 16(5):266, 1991.

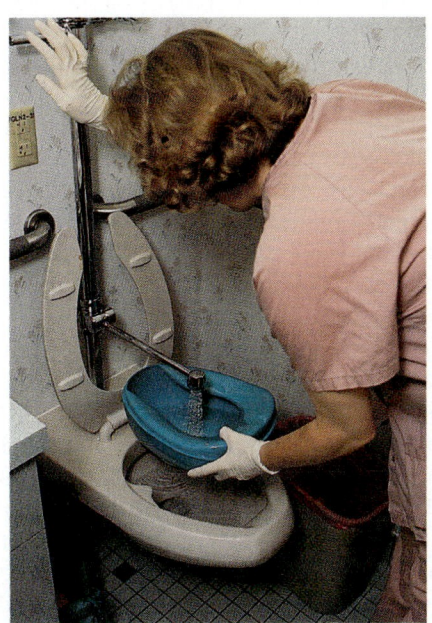

chapter 8 | Assisting with Elimination

Skill 8.1
Providing a Bedpan and Urinal

Skill 8.2
Caring for Incontinent Clients

Skill 8.3
Applying an External Catheter

Skill 8.4
Administering an Enema

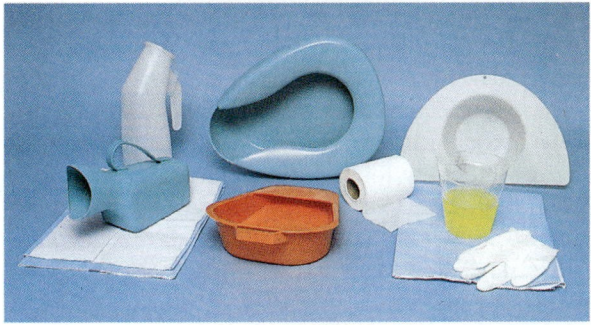

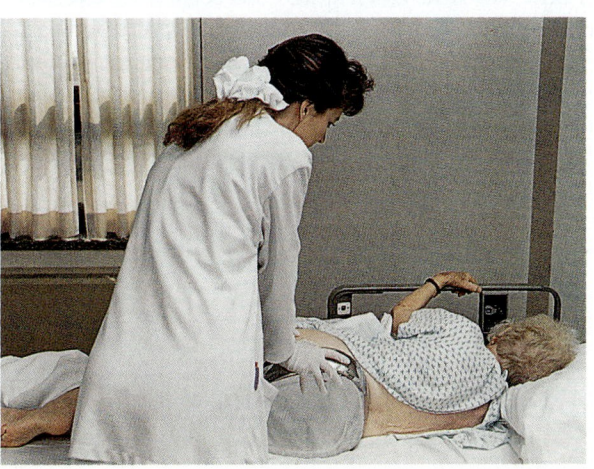

Clients' normal elimination patterns are often disturbed by physiological or psychological factors during illness. To promote normal elimination, nurses determine a client's normal pattern of elimination and attempt to accommodate that pattern. Maintaining privacy during elimination is difficult in the hospital, where bathroom facilities are often shared with a roommate. Clients who have difficulty ambulating or rising from a sitting position may need an elevated toilet seat, a bedside commode, bedpan, or urinal. The sights, sounds, and odors associated with elimination may be embarrassing. Embarrassment may prompt the client to decrease fluid intake to minimize the need to void or to ignore the urge to eliminate for as long as possible.

Emotional stressors are likely to affect bowel and urinary elimination. When an individual is anxious, afraid, or angry, the stress response may accelerate peristalsis, resulting in diarrhea and gaseous distention. When a person is depressed, peristalsis can decrease, resulting in reabsorption of water from the stool and constipation. Anxiety may also result in urinary frequency and urgency or inability to empty the bladder completely.

Urinary incontinence is the loss of control over voiding. Leakage of urine may be continuous or intermittent and is a very common problem among older clients. The U.S. Public Health Service's Agency for Health Care Policy and Research has concluded that approximately 80% of clients with urinary incontinence can be treated or cured (USDHHS, 1992). Most can be helped by bladder training and pelvic muscle exercises. Others can benefit from medication or surgery (Mondoux, 1994).

Older adults may have special problems with incontinence because of restricted mobility and urgency or frequency related to sphincter muscle control or diuretics. Prolonged immobility and damage to muscles from surgery or trauma may influence urinary continence. Continuous drainage of urine through an indwelling catheter often causes loss of bladder tone or damage to urethral sphincters. While the catheter is in place, the bladder is kept empty and is not stretched to capacity, altering bladder control.

Immobility also tends to slow peristalsis, resulting in increased absorption of fluid and hardening of feces. Decreased fluid intake or excessive fluid loss may result in dry, hard stools. *Fecal incontinence* is the involuntary passage of stool and can vary in severity and duration. *Transient incontinence* is most frequently associated with severe diarrhea. *Chronic incontinence* is typically associated with loss of sphincter control, decreased sensory awareness, or chronic changes in mental status (Doughty and Jackson, 1993).

Nursing Diagnosis

Several different nursing diagnoses pertain to clients with difficulties associated with bladder or bowel elimination. **Self-Toileting Deficit** is appropriate for clients with impaired ability to complete toileting activities independently and is used when the focus is to promote self-care.

For nursing diagnoses associated with urinary incontinence, the focus involves preventing episodes of uncontrolled voiding. Five nursing diagnoses are related to urinary incontinence: **Functional, Stress, Reflex, Urge,** and **Total. Functional Incontinence** refers to involuntary, unpredictable passage of urine because of a nonurinary problem, such as immobility. **Stress Incontinence** involves urine loss of less than 50 ml with increased abdominal pressure, as with coughing or sneezing. **Reflex Incontinence** is involuntary loss of urine at somewhat predictable intervals when a specific bladder volume is reached, often related to lack of awareness of bladder filling or absence of feelings of bladder fullness. This may be associated with spinal cord injury or impairment. **Urge Incontinence** is involuntary passage of urine soon after a strong sense of urgency to void and is related to bladder spasms, decreased bladder capacity, increased fluids, or concentrated urine. **Total Incontinence** is continuous and unpredictable loss of urine without distention or bladder contractions. Clients are unaware of this type of incontinence. **Urinary Retention** may be associated with overflow incontinence, in which the individual is unable to empty the bladder, has a sensation of bladder fullness, and experiences dribbling with a distended bladder.

Colonic Constipation refers to decreased frequency in the passage of stool and/or passage of hard, dry stool. This may be related to low roughage in the diet, low fluid intake, decreased activity level, altered routines (time), or chronic use of laxatives or enemas. Clients with **Perceived Constipation** have the expectation of a daily bowel movement at the same time every day, resulting in habitual use or abuse of laxatives, enemas, or suppositories.

Diarrhea is characterized by the frequent passage of loose, liquid, and unformed stools associated with abdominal pain, cramping, and urgency or loss of control. **Bowel Incontinence** involves the inability to retain a bowel movement because of weakness of the rectal sphincter or inability to know when a bowel movement occurs. Loss of sensation in the anal area from dysfunction of the defecation reflex may be associated with previous anal surgery, cerebrovascular accident (CVA), dementia, spinal cord injury, or ulcerative colitis.

When bowel or bladder continence is not realistic, **Risk for Impaired Skin Integrity** or **Impaired Skin Integrity** related to bowel or urinary incontinence may be appropriate. **Care Giver Role Strain** may also be appropriate when urinary or bowel incontinence results in prolonged difficulty for family members providing care (Gordon, 1993). **Self-Esteem Disturbance** related to incontinence or **Social Isolation** related to the fear of being incontinent suggests a focus that promotes emotional well-being.

Fluid Volume Deficit may be related to excessive fluid loss from diarrhea. In addition, severe diarrhea results in losses of serum electrolytes, including sodium, potassium, chloride, and bicarbonate, and contributes to fluid and electrolyte imbalance (see Chapter 36).

Skill 8.1 | Providing a Bedpan and Urinal

Squatting is the normal position during defecation and urination for females. Standing to void is customary for males. For the client confined to bed, it may be difficult to assume the normal position, but the upright position should be facilitated to the extent possible.

Clients restricted to bed who have control of elimination must use bedpans for defecation. Women use bedpans for both urine and feces, whereas men use bedpans for defecation and urinals for urination.

nurse alert
Check physicians' orders for prescribed bed rest. When determining the need for a bedpan or urinal, consider factors that limit mobility (e.g., fractures, pain, surgery, postcardiac catheterization, arteriogram with potential for bleeding). Unless contraindicated, it is generally beneficial for clients to get up from bed to use the bathroom.

EQUIPMENT

Bedpan (regular or fracture)
Urinal (male and female)
Specipan
Toilet paper
Underpads
Disposable gloves

Assessment

1. Discuss client's elimination needs in a professional, open manner using common language familiar to client. **Language and facial expressions that indicate disapproval or revulsion contribute to embarrassment and create communication barriers.**

2. Assess elimination pattern. When does client normally defecate (e.g., after breakfast)? Are laxatives or stool softeners routinely used? **The normal defecation pattern varies widely. However, reports indicate a frequency of two to seven stools per week, with one stool per day the most common bowel elimination pattern** (Sandler, Jordan, and Shelton, 1990). **Clients normally void five or more times per day on awakening, after meals, and before bedtime.**

3. Assess the length and extent of immobility. **Physical activity promotes peristalsis, increases circulation to the bowel, and promotes digestion.**

4. Assess client's ability to assist, including ability to lift hips or turn. **Determines the type of assistance needed to assist client on and off bedpan.**

5. Determine if a urine or stool specimen is to be collected.

6. Assess patterns of fluid intake. Adequate hydration (1200 to 1500 ml water daily) facilitates normal bowel elimination by keeping stools soft. Hot fluids are especially effective in softening stool and increasing peristalsis. **Decreased fluid intake slows the passage of food through the intestines, peristalsis slows, and there is increased absorption of fluid and hardening of feces.**

7. Assess dietary intake, including high-fiber foods such as raw fruit, whole grains, bran, and green leafy vegetables. **High-fiber foods increase bulk, which helps increase fluid content in stool, normalize consistency, and decrease transit time in the colon.**

8. Assess extent and location of pain that may influence ability to void, defecate, or position on a bedpan. It may be advisable to administer a prescribed analgesic about a half hour before the normal time of elimination.

9. Assess bowel sounds and palpate abdomen for distention. Ask client if flatus is being passed. **Normal bowel sounds are heard as clicks and gurgles that occur irregularly at the rate of about 5 to 35 per minute** (Doughty and Jackson, 1993). **A feces-filled colon can be palpated as a soft, rounded mass. A distended bladder can be palpated as a smooth, round mass above the symphysis pubis** (Barkauskas et al., 1994).

Planning

Expected outcomes focus on the client regaining a management of elimination rather than on dealing with the effects of the soiling (McFarland and McFarlane, 1993).

EXPECTED OUTCOMES

1. Client assists with movement onto bedpan and self-cleaning.
2. Client successfully defecates soft stool on the bedpan.
3. Client uses the bedpan or urinal to void more than 300 ml two times by 1300 today.
4. Client's skin remains intact without redness or irritation.

Implementation

Steps	Rationale

1. See Standard Protocol (Chapter, 1 p. 5).
2. Lower head of the bed so that it is nearly flat, and assist client to roll toward you.
3. Raise side rail and have client grasp it if necessary to maintain the side-lying position.

Facilitates placement of the bedpan.

4. Go to opposite side of the bed and place the powdered bedpan under the buttocks with the lower end just under the upper thighs.

Powder keeps pan from sticking to the skin. Many agencies have plastic bedpans. Warming a metal pan under running water promotes comfort and the relaxation necessary for elimination.

5. Press the bedpan firmly down into the mattress and against the buttocks (Figure 8-1). Keeping one hand against the bedpan, place the other on client's hip and assist client to roll back onto the pan.
6. If client is able to lift buttocks, place the pan under the buttocks as they are lifted. Use of a fracture pan requires less lifting (Figure 8-2). Check position of the pan by looking between client's legs. Front of the pan should be centered and visible.

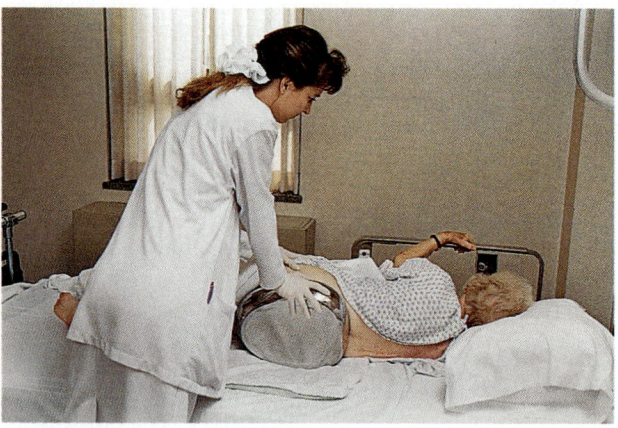

Figure 8-1

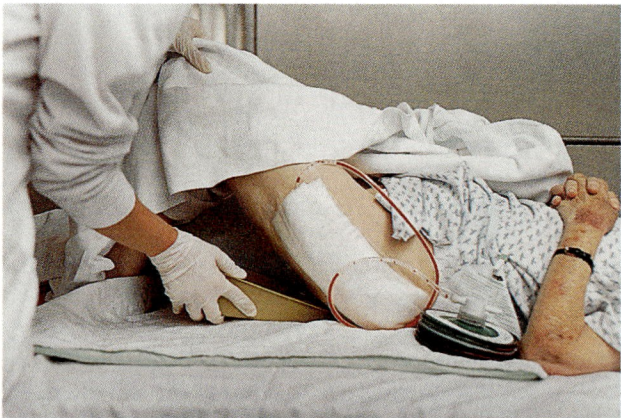

Figure 8-2

7. If not contraindicated, raise head of the bed at least 30 to 45 degrees. Have client bend knees to assume a squatting position.

This approximates the normal position for defecation as much as possible.

8. Raise the side rail and place the call light and toilet paper within easy reach. Provide privacy.

Privacy is essential for some clients to empty bowel and bladder successfully.

9. When client is finished, lower side rail and assist client to roll away from you onto one side as you hold the bedpan securely in place.

Prevents spilling contents on the bedding.

10. Assist client with wiping as needed. If necessary, clean perineum from front to back using a washcloth and warm soapy water.

Cleaning front to back prevents transmission of microorganisms from anus to urethra, which may contribute to a urinary tract infection.

11. Provide opportunity for client to wash hands.

Steps	Rationale

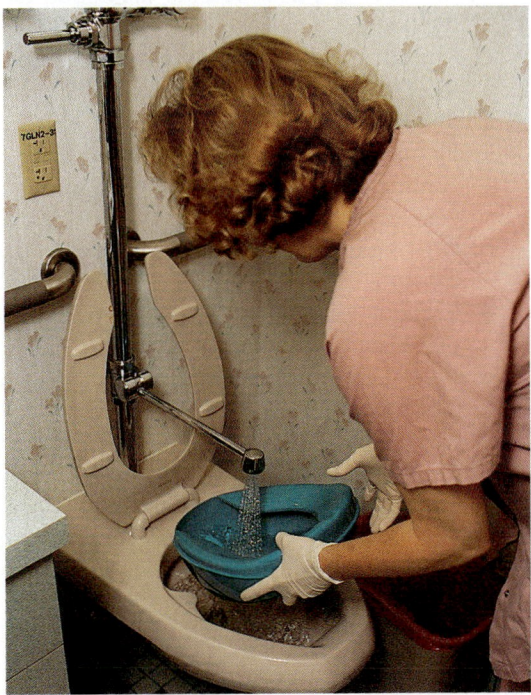

Figure 8-3

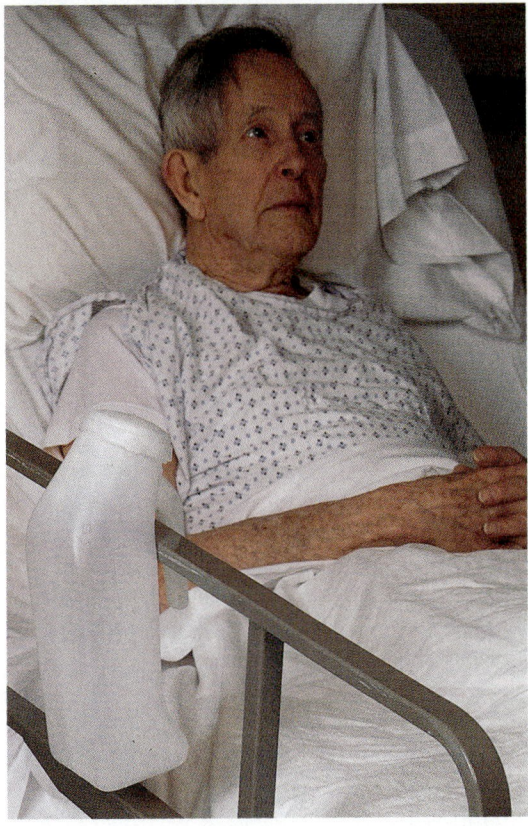

Figure 8-4

nurse alert   Before emptying the bedpan, note the color and appearance of urine and stool. Measure the amount if intake and output (I&O) are being recorded, and check for whether a specimen is needed (see Chapter 13).

12. Empty the contents into the toilet and rinse thoroughly with spray faucet attached to the toilet (Figure 8-3).

13. Store bedpan and urinal in appropriate location, normally in the bathroom. Some clients need or want to have the bedpan within easy reach. If so, bedpan may be placed on a chair seat and covered with a disposable cover.

Promotes rapid accessibility when there is urgency or frequency of bowel or bladder elimination.

14. **Providing a urinal for a male client**
    a. Position on side, back, or sitting with head of the bed elevated, or assist to a standing position.
    b. If lying in bed, client should hold urinal with base flat on the bed between the thighs, and if possible, client places penis into neck of the urinal. Assist as needed.
    c. Instruct client to notify care giver so that the urinal can be emptied each time it is used. If needed, measure and record urine output.
    d. Urinals may be attached to the side rail for easy access (Figure 8-4).

15. See Completion Protocol (Chapter 1, p. 6).

Men find it easier to void and empty the bladder while standing.
Minimizes spilling.

Avoids overfilling; minimizes odors and growth of microorganisms. Provides accuracy in recording amount of each voiding.

Evaluation

1. Observe client's ability to assist with movement onto and off the bedpan and participate in self-cleaning.
2. Observe and record the appearance and characteristics of stool, including color, odor, consistency, frequency, amount, shape, and constituents. Observe and record the appearance and amount of urine.
3. Observe skin integrity in the perineal area.

UNEXPECTED OUTCOMES AND RELATED INTERVENTIONS

1. Client is unable to void using a bedpan or urinal.
   a. Provide sensory stimulation that promotes voiding, such as running water in the sink or pouring warm water over perineum, stroking the inner thigh, placing hand in warm water, or providing a drink (if not contraindicated).
   b. Male clients may need to stand in order to void. Obtain adequate assistance if client is at risk of falling.
2. Client is unable to defecate using a bedpan.
   a. Assist to as normal a position as possible. Encourage client to massage upper abdomen from right to left to promote peristalsis.

   b. Provide reading materials and allow ample time and privacy for the process.
   c. Consider use of a bedside commode rather than the bedpan if client is able to be up in a chair.
   d. Consider collaborating with the physician for stool softener or laxative orders.
3. Client is incontinent (see Skill 8.2).
   a. Identify detailed information about episodes of incontinence, including how often, amount, and circumstances involved.
   b. Offer bedpan or urinal more frequently (e.g., every 2 hours).
   c. If client experiences the urge but cannot wait, place urinal within client's reach.
   d. Male clients may benefit from an external catheter. (See Skill 8.3.)

SAMPLE DOCUMENTATION

0800 Client had difficulty voiding on bedpan. Voided 200 ml dark-amber urine after drinking 240 ml water. Encouraged to drink more fluids (see I&O sheet, Appendix A).

Skill 8.2 | Caring for Incontinent Clients

Incontinence is a very common problem, especially among older adults. Regardless of the cause, incontinence is psychologically distressing and a socially disruptive problem.

Urinary incontinence occurs because pressure in the bladder is too great or because the sphincters are too weak. Incontinence may only involve a small leakage of urine when the person laughs, coughs, or lifts something or may reflect total lack of bladder control. Pelvic floor exercises (Kegel's exercises) involve tightening of the ring of muscle around the vagina and anus and holding them for several seconds. This is done at least 10 times, three times a day. Alert clients need a product that is discreet and promotes self-care. Some incontinence products are designed for small amounts of leakage. Persistent urge, stress, or overflow incontinence may need referral for urological evaluation.

When urinary incontinence results from decreased perception of bladder fullness or impaired voluntary motor control, bladder training can be helpful. Bladder training provides cooperative clients with opportunity to void at regular intervals (every $1\frac{1}{2}$ to 2 hours) to achieve continence. On such a schedule, clients need to be asked if they are wet or dry, checked for wetness, reminded or assisted to the toilet, and praised for appropriate toileting. Limiting fluids after the evening meal minimizes the need for voiding during the night.

When paralyzed clients have overflow incontinence, Crede's method may be used. This involves manual pressure over the lower abdomen to express urine from the bladder at regular intervals.

Total incontinence characterized by urine flow at unpredictable times without distention or bladder spasms requires the use of disposable adult undergarments or underpads as the primary means of management. Urine is very irritating to the skin. Skin that is continuously exposed to urine quickly becomes inflamed and irritated. Cleansing the skin thoroughly after each episode of incontinence with warm soapy water and drying it thoroughly help prevent skin breakdown.

Assessment

1. Assess the frequency of episodes of incontinence. Determine if there is a pattern.
2. Assess the amount of leakage experienced. Determine if it is frequent dribbling of small amounts or unpredictable loss of large amounts of urine and stool. **Helps determine type of incontinence and appropriate choice of therapies.**

3. Assess episodes related to specific events such as coughing, sneezing, or exercise.
4. Assess the condition of client's skin in the perineal area. **Identifies the need for special skin care products, barrier films, or creams.**
5. Assess fluid intake and the color, odor, and appearance of urine. **Some clients drink less to minimize incontinence, resulting in dark, concentrated urine and increased risk for infection.**

Planning

The expected outcomes focus on promoting continence.

EXPECTED OUTCOMES

1. Client achieves continence 75% of the time.
2. Client remains clean and dry 90% of the time.
3. Client maintains skin integrity without redness or irritation of the perineum.

Implementation

Steps	Rationale
1. See Standard Protocol (Chapter 1, p. 5).	
2. Provide client with opportunity to use the bathroom, bedpan, or commode to void and defecate at appropriate regular times.	Promotes episodes of continence.
3. Keep a record of episodes of continence and incontinence events for 48 hours.	Record allows identification of patterns of elimination.
4. Cleanse the perineum in a professional, caring, and matter-of-fact manner. Avoid all negative verbal and nonverbal expressions.	This approach minimizes embarrassment. Under no circumstances should client be reprimanded or humiliated for having "accidents."
5. Turn client to the supine position with legs abducted (see Skill 5.1).	
a. **Female.** Wash labia using a washcloth, soap, and warm water. Then gently retract labia from thigh and wash groin from perineum toward rectum (front to back).	Cleansing from front to back prevents transmission of microorganisms from anus to urethra.
b. **Male.** Wash the penis beginning with the urinary meatus, retracting the foreskin if client is uncircumcised. Gently cleanse shaft of penis and scrotum, taking care to thoroughly reach all skinfolds. Return foreskin to its natural position.	
6. Turn client to side and continue cleansing, using as many washcloths as necessary and drying thoroughly.	
7. Place absorbent underpad from waist to knees with absorbent side toward client.	Use of incontinence products should be limited to severely impaired clients. Use of one product only promotes client dignity.
8. If skin is red or irritated, exposure to air whenever possible is beneficial. A vitamin-enriched cream may promote healing. Apply a skin barrier or sealant to protect the skin from moisture (see Chapter 23).	
9. Ambulatory clients may wear briefs with pads to absorb urine (see box on p. 118).	Sanitary pads can hold small amounts of urinary leakage but are not intended for this purpose.
10. See Completion Protocol (Chapter 1, p. 6).	

Containment Devices

Diapers can hold large amounts of urinary leakage. They are large and bulky and best used for clients with total incontinence and confined to bed or wheelchair.

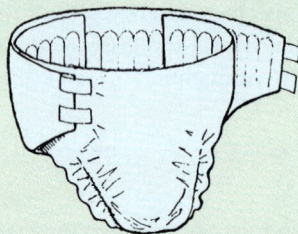

Adult undergarments can hold relatively large amounts of urinary leakage and are best for ambulatory clients.

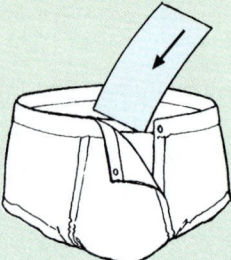

Underpants with absorbent pads can hold relatively large amounts of urinary leakage.

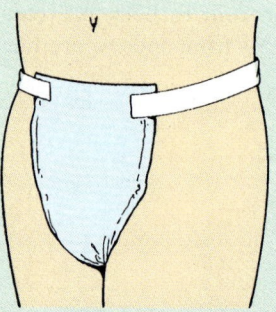

Sanitary pads can hold small amounts of urinary leakage. They are constructed for menstrual flow and are not as absorbent as incontinent pads.

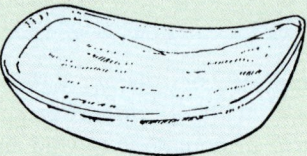

Male drip collectors can absorb small amounts of urine and fit comfortably over the penis.

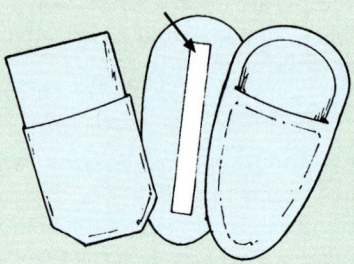

Modified from Gray M: *Genitourinary disorders,* Mosby's Clinical Nursing Series, St. Louis, 1992, Mosby.

Evaluation

1. Determine percentage of continent episodes in relation to total number of events of elimination in specified time.
2. Observe effectiveness of absorbent pads or garments used to contain incontinent episodes.
3. Observe the perineum for evidence of redness or irritation.

UNEXPECTED OUTCOMES AND RELATED INTERVENTIONS

1. Client describes episodes of incontinence as urgency, associated with frequency and burning with voiding.
   a. Increase fluid intake and encourage cranberry juice.
   b. Consider the possibility of urinary tract infection. Report to physician for evaluation and treatment.
2. Client experiences overflow incontinence associated with urinary retention and bladder distention.

a. Teach and encourage voiding according to a planned schedule.

b. Notify physician if prescribed drugs may be contributing to urinary retention (e.g., anticholinergics, antispasmodics, antidepressants, seizure medications). Dosage or schedule of administration may be adjusted.

c. Intermittent catheterization may be necessary (see Chapter 34).

SAMPLE DOCUMENTATION
0800 Complains of urgency and frequency of urination that started yesterday. Voiding 50 to 100 ml concentrated urine every 1 to 2 hours. States burning and some pain are associated. Increased fluid intake encouraged. Perineum red around urinary meatus and labia, cleansed with warm soapy water and dried thoroughly.

Skill 8.3 | Applying an External (Condom or Texas) Catheter

The external application of a urinary drainage device is a convenient, safe method of draining urine in male clients. The external catheter is suitable for incontinent or comatose clients who still have complete and spontaneous bladder emptying. The external catheter is a soft, pliable rubber sheath that slips over the penis. A self-adhesive device may be available at some agencies. External catheters have elastic adhesive provided to secure them in place. The catheter may be attached to a leg drainage bag or a standard urinary drainage bag.

An external catheter should be assessed every 4 hours to detect potential problems and changed once every 24 hours. With each catheter change, the nurse cleanses the urethral meatus and penis thoroughly and looks for signs of skin irritation.

EQUIPMENT
Urinary external catheter (appropriate size) with elastic or Velcro adhesive (if not using self-adhesive device) (Figure 8-5)
Urinary collection bag with drainage tubing or leg bag and straps
Skin preparation (tincture of benzoin)
Towels and washcloths
Bath blanket
Clean disposable gloves
Scissors

Assessment

1. Assess urinary elimination patterns, ability to urinate voluntarily, and continence. **External catheter is suitable for incontinent or comatose male clients with complete and spontaneous bladder emptying.**

2. Assess mental status of client so appropriate teaching related to external catheter can be implemented. Teaching can include self-application. Assess client's knowledge of the purpose of an external catheter.

3. Assess condition of penis. **Provides a baseline to compare changes in condition of skin after application of the external catheter.**

Planning

Expected outcomes focus on promoting dryness and preventing continual exposure of skin to urine.

EXPECTED OUTCOMES
1. Client voids five or more times daily.
2. Penile shaft remains free from skin irritation or breakdown.
3. Catheter remains secure with adequate penile circulation 1 hour after application and every 4 hours thereafter.

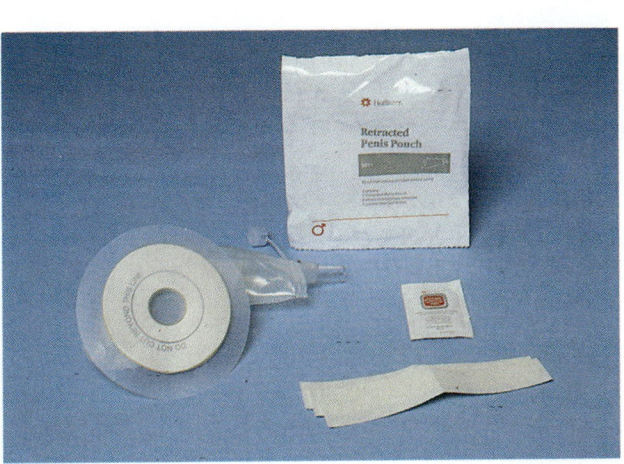

Figure 8-5

Implementation

Steps	Rationale
1. See Standard Protocol (Chapter 1, p. 5).	
2. Assist client into supine position with a bath blanket over upper torso and lower extremities covered; only genitalia should be exposed.	Promotes comfort and prevents unnecessary exposure of body parts.
3. Prepare urinary drainage collection bag and tubing. Clamp off drainage exit ports. Secure collection bag to bed frame; bring drainage tubing up between side rails and bed frame. Be sure tubing is not pulled when side rails are raised. Prepare leg bag for connection to external catheter, if necessary.	Provides easy access to drainage equipment.
4. Using warm soapy water remove all secretions from the penis and dry thoroughly.	Prevents skin breakdown from exposure to secretions. Rubber sheath rolls onto clean, dry skin more easily.
5. Clip hair at base of penis if necessary.	Hair adheres to adhesive and pulls during external catheter removal.
6. Apply skin preparation to penis and allow to dry. A thin layer of plasticized skin spray protects skin from irritation. If client is uncircumcised, return foreskin to normal position.	Skin preparation has an alcohol base. Evaporation prevents irritation. Returning foreskin prevents foreskin from tightening around penile shaft, which impedes circulation to penis, and causes trauma to tissue.

7. With self-adhesive external catheter

Application:

a. A plastic collar positions the inner flap for application (Figure 8-6).

b. Pinch catheter closed (Figure 8-7). Place against glans as shown so tip, not entire glans, protrudes approximately 0.6 cm (¼ inch) into opening (Figure 8-8). Foreskin should remain in natural position so tip of glans and foreskin protrude 0.6 cm (¼ inch) into opening.

    Allows free flow of urine into collecting tubing when client voids.

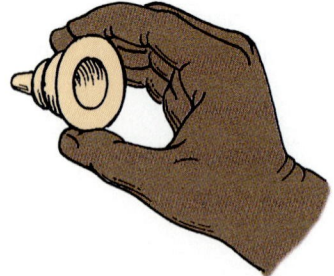

Figure 8-6

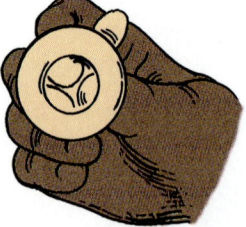

Figure 8-7

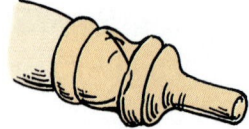

Figure 8-8

c. With nondominant hand, grasp penis along shaft. With the other hand, unroll catheter up the shaft of the penis with as little wrinkling as possible. Discard plastic collar.	Plastic collar is for application of external catheter. *Do not* push it onto the penis.
d. Gently squeeze catheter to adhere sheath to skin. Once applied, do not attempt to reposition catheter. Pinch wrinkles to seal openings.	Condom must be snug, but not tight enough to cause constriction of blood flow.

Steps	Rationale

8. For external catheter without adhesive (Figure 8-9)

Application:

a. Apply sheath to penis as in Step 7c.

b. Allow 2.5 to 5 cm (1 to 2 inches) of space between tip of glans penis and end of external catheter.

c. Encircle penile shaft with strip of elastic adhesive only in contact with sheath. Apply snugly, but not tightly.

Allows free passage of urine into collecting tubing when client voids.

Constriction of blood flow may occur if applied too tightly.

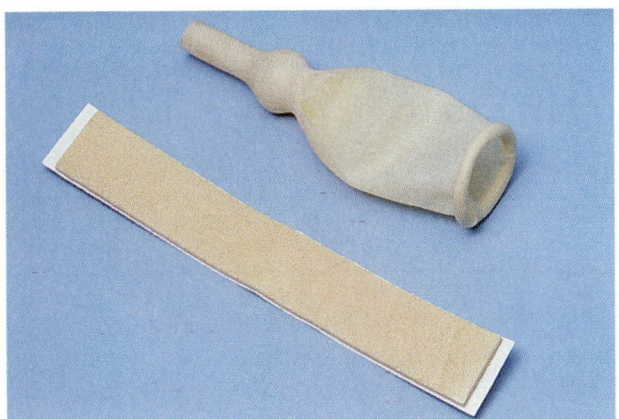

Figure 8-9

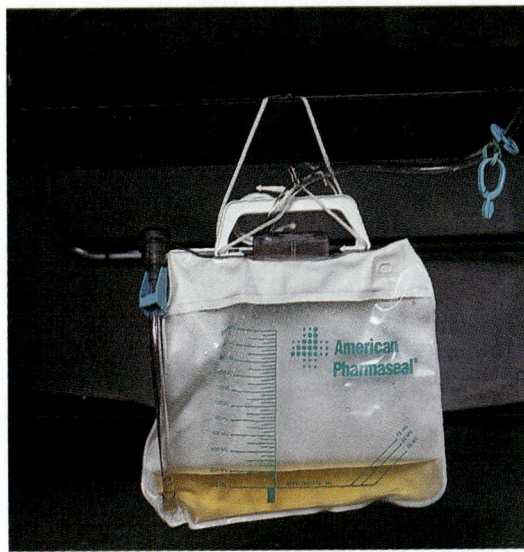

Figure 8-10

9. Connect drainage tubing to end of external catheter. A urine drainage bag (Figure 8-10) or leg bag attached above or below the knee may be used (Figure 8-11, *A*). Be sure sheath is not twisted.

10. Secure so that tubing is not looped and promotes free drainage of urine (Figure 8-11, *B*).

Allows urine to be collected and measured. Keeps client dry. Twisted sheath obstructs urine flow.

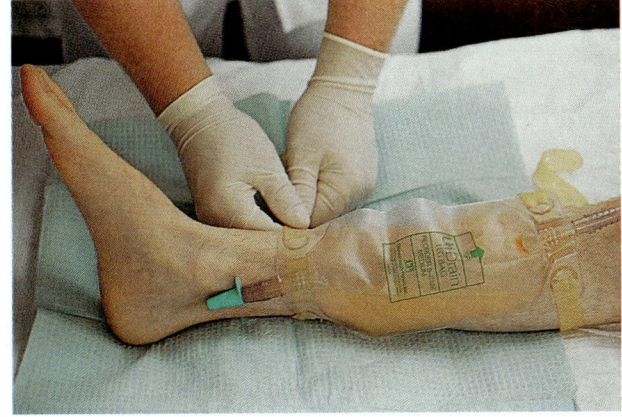

A

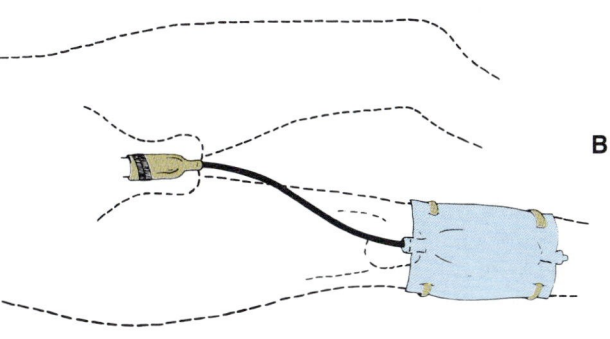

B

Figure 8-11

11. Remove sheath for 30 minutes every 24 hours to allow assessment and cleansing of skin.

12. See Completion Protocol (Chapter 1, p. 6).

Evaluation

1. Observe frequency and amount of urine output in drainage container every 4 hours.
2. Remove sheath and inspect skin on penile shaft for signs of breakdown or irritation at least daily during hygiene and when external catheter is reapplied.
3. Observe circulation of glans penis 1 hour after application and every 4 hours thereafter to determine that sheath has not been applied too tightly.

UNEXPECTED OUTCOMES AND RELATED INTERVENTIONS

1. Urination is reduced or infrequent, indicating possible urinary retention.
   a. Check for urinary retention and bladder distention.
   b. Monitor urine output.
2. Skin irritation is noted. Client may have allergy to adhesive product or irritation from contact with urine.
   a. Increase frequency of skin cleansing and remove external catheter for 30 minutes each shift to promote healing.
   b. Make sure urine drains readily rather than sitting in contact with penis.
3. Urine leaks from tubing.
   Remove catheter and reapply more snugly.
4. Penile swelling occurs.
   a. Remove catheter and allow swelling to decrease.
   b. Reapply more loosely.

SAMPLE DOCUMENTATION

0900 Self-adhesive external urinary catheter applied and connected to drainage bag. No swelling or redness noted on skin. Client voided 350 ml clear amber urine without discomfort or difficulty.

1000 Circulation to penis intact under external urinary catheter. Denies discomfort from pressure on penis.

Skill 8.4 | Administering an Enema

The primary reason for an enema is promotion of defecation. The volume and type of fluid instilled can lubricate or break up the fecal mass, stretch the rectal wall, and initiate the defecation reflex. Clients should not rely on enemas to maintain bowel regularity because they do not treat the cause of irregularity or constipation. Frequent enemas disrupt normal defecation reflexes, resulting in dependence on enemas for elimination (Clarke, 1989).

An enema is the instillation of a solution into the rectum and sigmoid colon. Cleansing enemas promote complete evacuation of feces from the colon by stimulating peristalsis through infusion of large volumes of solution.

An impaction involves presence of a fecal mass too large or hard to be passed voluntarily. Either constipation or diarrhea can suggest the presence of an impaction. An oil-retention enema lubricates the rectum and colon, softens the feces, and facilitates defecation. An oil-retention enema can be used alone or as adjunct therapy to manual removal of a fecal impaction.

Medicated enemas contain pharmacological therapeutic agents and are used to reduce dangerously high serum potassium levels, as with a sodium polystyrene sulfonate (Kayexalate) enema, or to reduce bacteria in the colon before bowel surgery, as with a neomycin enema.

EQUIPMENT

Enema bag (disposable or reusable)
Disposable gloves
Waterproof absorbent underpads
Adult: 750 to 1000 ml warm water or prepackaged disposable enema with prelubricated tip
Water-soluble lubricant
Bath blanket
Toilet tissue
Bedpan, bedside commode, or access to toilet
Wash basin, washcloths, towel, and soap
Intravenous (IV) pole

Assessment

1. Assess last bowel movement and presence or absence of bowel sounds. **This determines the need for enema administration.**
2. Assess ability to control external sphincter. **Client with paralysis and no sphincter control must be placed on bedpan because enema solution cannot be retained.**
3. Assess presence or absence of hemorrhoids, which may obscure the rectal opening and cause discomfort or bleeding with evacuation.
4. Assess for abdominal pain. May affect client's ability to tolerate the enema.
5. Determine client's level of understanding and previous experience with enemas in order to provide appropriate teaching measures.

Planning

Expected outcomes focus on establishing a normal pattern of bowel elimination and normal consistency of stools.

EXPECTED OUTCOMES

1. Client verbalizes relief of abdominal discomfort.
2. Client expels gas and feces from the colon.
3. Client empties rectum and lower colon of stool.

Implementation

Steps	Rationale
1. See Standard Protocol (Chapter 1, p. 5).	
2. If using an enema bag, fill it with 750 to 1000 ml warm tap water as it flows from faucet. Check temperature of solution by pouring small amount over inner wrist. Remove air from tubing by allowing solution to fill tubing. Clamp tubing.	Hot water can burn intestinal mucosa. Cold water can cause abdominal cramping and is difficult to retain.
3. Add soap solution if ordered.	
4. Assist client into left side-lying (Sims') position with right knee flexed.	Allows enema solution to flow downward by gravity along natural curve of sigmoid colon and rectum, thus improving retention of solution.

nurse alert Clients with minimal sphincter control may not be able to retain all of enema solution and require placement of a bedpan under the buttocks. Administering enema with client sitting on toilet is ineffective because solution will not effectively infuse against gravity into bowel.

Steps	Rationale
5. Place waterproof pad absorbent side up under hips and buttocks to prevent soiling of linen.	
6. Cover client with bath blanket, exposing only rectal area, and clearly visualize anus.	Provides warmth, reduces exposure of body parts, allows client to feel more relaxed and comfortable. Presence of hemorrhoids obscures anal opening and increases discomfort with bowel elimination.
7. If client will be expelling contents in toilet, ensure that toilet is available and place client's slippers and bathrobe in easily accessible location. If client is unable to get out of bed, place bedpan in easily accessible position.	
8. Prepackaged disposable container	
a. Remove plastic cap from rectal tip. Tip may be already lubricated. More lubricant can be applied if needed.	Lubrication provides for smooth insertion of rectal tube without rectal irritation or trauma.
b. Gently separate buttocks and locate rectum. Instruct client to relax by breathing out slowly through mouth.	Breathing out promotes relaxation of external rectal sphincter. Presence of hemorrhoids obscures location of rectum. Probe gently with gloved finger to locate rectal opening if necessary.
c. Insert lubricated tip of bottle gently into rectum approximately 7.5 to 10 cm (3 to 4 inches) for an adult.	

Steps	Rationale

d. Squeeze bottle continuously until all of solution has entered rectum and colon. (Most bottles contain approximately 250 ml solution.)

Hypertonic solutions require only small volumes to stimulate defecation. Intermittent squeezing results in return of solution to the bottle.

9. Enema bag

a. Lubricate 7.5 to 10 cm (3 to 4 inches) of tip of rectal tube with lubricating jelly.

b. Gently separate buttocks and locate anus. Instruct client to relax by breathing out slowly through mouth.

Breathing out promotes relaxation of external anal sphincter.

c. Insert tip of rectal tube slowly by pointing tip in direction of client's umbilicus. *Adult:* 7.5 to 10 cm (3 to 4 inches) past the internal sphincter.

Careful insertion prevents trauma to rectal mucosa from accidental lodging of tube against rectal wall. Forceful insertion beyond 10 cm (4 inches) could cause bowel perforation.

d. Hold tubing in rectum constantly until end of fluid instillation.

Bowel contraction can cause expulsion of rectal tube.

e. With container at client's hip level, open regulating clamp and allow solution to enter slowly.

Rapid infusion can stimulate evacuation and cause cramping.

f. Raise height of enema container slowly to 30 to 45 cm (12 to 18 inches) above the anus. Infusion time varies with volume of solution administered (e.g., 1 L may take 7 to 10 minutes). Hang container on IV pole (Figure 8-12).

Raising container too high causes rapid infusion and possible painful distention of colon.

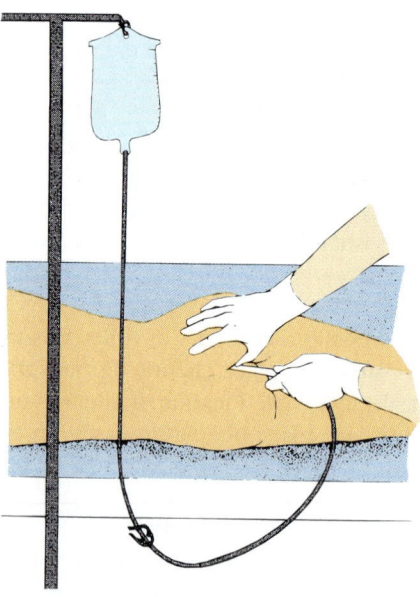

Figure 8-12

g. Lower container or clamp tubing if client complains of cramping or if fluid escapes around rectal tube.

Temporary cessation of infusion minimizes cramping and promotes ability to retain all the solution.

h. Clamp tubing after all the solution is infused. Tell client that the procedure is completed and that you will be removing rectal tube. Then gently withdraw tube.

Clients may misinterpret the sensation of removing the tube as loss of control.

Steps	Rationale
10. Explain to client that feeling of distention is normal. Ask client to retain solution as long as possible (5 to 10 minutes) while lying quietly in bed.	Solution distends bowel. Length of retention varies with type of enema and client's ability to contract rectal sphincter. Longer retention promotes more effective stimulation of peristalsis and defecation.
11. Discard enema container and tubing in proper receptacle, or rinse out thoroughly with warm soap and water if container is to be reused.	
12. Assist client to bathroom or commode if possible. If necessary to use the bedpan, assist to as near the normal position for evacuation as possible.	Normal squatting position promotes defecation.
13. Instruct clients with a history of cardiovascular disease to exhale while expelling enema to avoid the Valsalva maneuver (forced effort against a closed airway), especially if client is dehydrated.	The Valsalva maneuver in strenuously trying to move a constipated stool may result in cardiac arrest (Anderson, Anderson, and Glanze, 1994).
14. Instruct client to call for nurse to inspect results before flushing the toilet. Observe character of feces and solution.	When enemas are ordered "until clear," enemas are repeated until client passes fluid that is clear and contains no formed fecal matter. Usually three consecutive enemas are adequate.
15. Assist client as needed to wash anal area with warm soap and water.	Fecal contents can irritate skin. Hygiene promotes client's comfort.
16. See Completion Protocol (Chapter 1, p. 6).	

Evaluation

1. Ask client if abdominal discomfort has been relieved. Palpate abdomen to determine if distention is relieved. An impaction may be palpated as a hard mass. Client may experience rectal fullness. Frequent, small, liquid or loose stools may occur around the stool (Barkauskas et al., 1994).
2. Inspect color, consistency, and amount of stool and fluid passed. Note abnormalities such as presence of blood or mucus.
3. When "enemas until clear" is ordered in preparation for surgery or diagnostic testing, the water expelled is colorless and contains no particles of feces.

UNEXPECTED OUTCOMES AND RELATED INTERVENTIONS

1. Client is unable to hold enema solution.
   a. Pinch the buttocks together to assist retention.
   b. Position on bedpan while administering the solution.
2. Severe cramping, bleeding, or sudden severe abdominal pain occurs and is unrelieved by temporarily stopping or slowing flow of solution.
   a. Stop enema.
   b. Notify physician.
3. With an order for "enemas until clear," after three enemas the water is highly colored or contains solid fecal material.
   a. Notify the physician before continuing.
   b. Excessive loss of electrolytes is a dangerous possibility.

SAMPLE DOCUMENTATION

2000 Retained 900 ml tap water enema for 10 minutes with return of large, formed, hard, dark-brown stool and large amounts of colored water. Complained of "mild" cramping during administration. Comfortable after evacuation of enema. Distention relieved. Abdomen is soft.

CRITICAL THINKING EXERCISES

1. Consider the following client situations. Distinguish between the types of urinary elimination problems each presents by selecting the appropriate nursing diagnosis from the following list: (A) Stress Incontinence; (B) Reflex Incontinence; (C) Urge Incontinence; (D) Urinary Retention; and (E) Functional Incontinence.
   a. Charles is a 77-year-old client who had a stroke 3 years ago. He is immobile because of paralysis of the left side. He has no evidence of renal or bladder disease, but he is unable to control urination.
   b. Conrad is a 35-year-old male who sustained a traumatic spinal cord injury 6 months ago after falling from a 10-foot scaffold. He is paralyzed from the nipple line down and cannot sense when his bladder is full. Approximately every 4 hours, Conrad is incontinent of urine.
   c. Gladys is a 55-year-old mother of five children. She is seeing her gynecologist and complains of dribbling urine every time she laughs or coughs.
2. For each of the clients in Exercise 1, identify a specific approach to bladder management.
3. Of the following individuals, determine who is at highest risk for developing colonic constipation. Rank the four examples in order from highest to lowest risk (1 = highest risk, 4 = lowest risk).
   a. Joseph, an active 66-year-old male, walks for 20 minutes three times a week and enjoys eating at fast-food restaurants.
   b. Twila is 72 years old and resides in a long-term care facility. She is confused and bedridden, requires assistance with feeding, and has a history of chronic laxative abuse.
   c. Elton is 97 years old and cares for himself at home. He ambulates with a cane and enjoys going with his long-time buddies to the American Legion for his noon meal.
   d. Marsha is a 45-year-old client admitted to the hospital after a car accident in which she sustained multiple fractures and a broken jaw. She is currently receiving IV normal saline and is unable to eat or drink.
4. You are in the process of administering a tap water enema to a 51-year-old female client. She begins complaining of abdominal cramping, and fluid starts to leak from the rectum. What should you do?

REFERENCES

Anderson KN, Anderson LE, Glanze, WD: *Mosby's medical, nursing, and allied health dictionary,* ed 4, St Louis, 1994, Mosby.

Barkauskas VH et al: *Health and physical assessment,* St Louis, 1994, Mosby.

Clarke B: Making sense of enemas, *Nurs Times* 84(30):40, 1989.

Doughty DB, Jackson DB: *Gastrointestinal disorders,* Mosby's Clinical Nursing Series, St Louis, 1993, Mosby.

Gordon M: *Manual of nursing diagnosis, 1993-1994,* St Louis, 1993, Mosby.

Gray M: *Genitourinary disorders,* Mosby's Clinical Nursing Series, St Louis, 1993, Mosby.

McFarland GK, McFarlane EA: *Nursing diagnosis and intervention: planning for patient care,* ed 2, 1993, Mosby.

Mondoux LC: Patients won't ask, *RN* 57(2):35, 1994.

Sandler RS, Jordan MC, Shelton BJ: Demographic and dietary determinants of constipation in the U.S. population, *Am J Public Health* 80:185, 1990.

US Department of Health and Human Services: *Clinical practice guidelines: urinary incontinence in adults,* Pub no 92-0038 Rockville, Md, 1992, Public Health Service, Agency for Health Care Policy and Research.

ADDITIONAL READINGS

Carlson-Catalano J: Bedpans and blood—changing perceptions about nursing, *RN* 56(8):80, 1993.

Fox B: Recurring urinary tract infections: incidence and risk factors, *Am J Public Health* 80(3):331, 1990.

Gulanick M et al: *Nursing care plans: nursing diagnosis and intervention,* ed 3, St Louis, 1994, Mosby.

Lange J: Today's rules for using incontinence products, *Nurs Homes* 43(3):45, 1994.

Pagana DK, Pagana TJ: *Mosby's diagnostic and laboratory test reference,* St Louis, 1992, Mosby.

chapter 9

Promoting Comfort, Sleep, and Relaxation

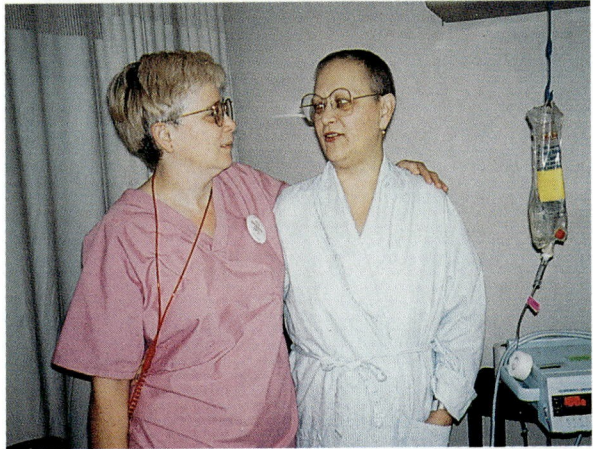

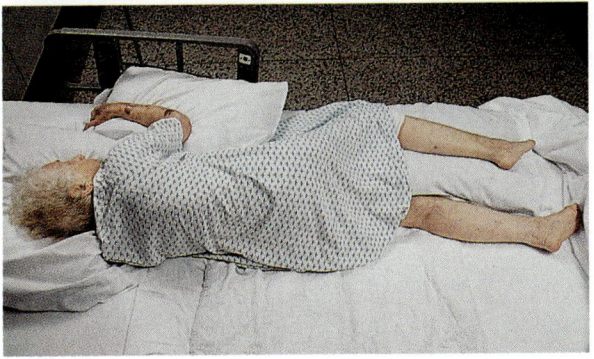

Skill 9.1
Comfort Measures that Promote Sleep

Skill 9.2
Progressive Relaxation

Skill 9.3
Guided Imagery

The theory that sleep is associated with healing suggests that achieving optimum sleep quality is important for the recovery of health care clients. Identifying sleep disturbances and promoting sleep, comfort, and relaxation are basic aspects of the nursing role.

The major complaint in sleep disturbances is insufficient quantity and quality of sleep and is usually associated with some underlying physical (e.g., pain) or psychological (e.g., anxiety) disorder. The benefits of sleep often go unnoticed until a person develops problems resulting from sleep deprivation, which lead to changes in reflexes, memory, equilibrium, pain tolerance, and attention span. Severity of symptoms is highly variable and relates to the duration of the sleep deprivation (see box on p. 128). Research has shown that older adults have a tendency to experience changes in sleep patterns that can result in impaired judgment and concentration. The use of sedatives or hypnotics tends to create troublesome side effects (Johnson, 1993).

Sleep studies have revealed the phases and stages of sleep. Sleep involves two phases: non–rapid eye movement (NREM) and rapid eye movement (REM) sleep. During NREM a sleeper progresses through four stages in a typical sleep cycle. The cycles do not occur once but cycle back and forth several times during the course of sleep. At the end of each NREM phase, REM sleep occurs. REM sleep is the deepest level of sleep and is associated with changes in cerebral blood flow and vivid

---

Sleep Deprivation Symptoms

PHYSIOLOGICAL
Hand tremors
Decreased reflexes
Slowed response time
Reduction in word memory
Decreased reasoning and judgment
Cardiac irregularities
Decreased alertness

PSYCHOLOGICAL
Moods
Disorientation
Irritability
Decreased motivation
Fatigue and sleepiness
Hyperactivity
Agitation

---

dreams. REM sleep assists learning, emotional adaptation, and problem solving. People progress in various ways through cycles depending on the amount of time spent sleeping. The 24-hour sleep-wake cycle is a circadian rhythm that influences physiological function and behavior.

Pain and discomfort are subjective and highly individualized sensations and are greatly influenced by psychosocial and cultural factors. The gate control theory suggests that pain impulses can be regulated or blocked by "closing gates" that transmit pain sensations to the spinal cord. A bombardment of sensory impulses, such as from a backrub, closes the gates to pain stimuli. This theory also suggests that gating mechanisms can be altered by thoughts, feelings, and memories. (For additional information on pain management, refer to Chapter 21.) The focus of this chapter is the nurse's role in providing basic comfort measures.

Pain has been shown to stimulate the autonomic nervous system as part of the stress response. This response involves physiological changes, including increased heart rate, respirations, blood pressure, oxygen consumption, metabolism, and muscle tension. Clients may lose the ability to concentrate and may become less aware of environmental stimuli (Peddicord, 1991). Nurses need to be able to use and teach stress management techniques and comfort measures that can promote falling and remaining asleep.

Life-threatening illness, changes in family structure, job stress, depression, and grief increase the anxiety of clients and their families. Anxiety can increase a client's level of pain and discomfort, interfere with learning, lower resistance to disease, and delay the recovery process (McFarland and McFarlane, 1993). Stress-related conditions frequently bring clients into the health care system. Recent studies support the effectiveness of progressive relaxation and guided imagery in managing pain and stress-related conditions. Although these techniques alone will not cure a disease, they do have a positive effect on stress-related symptoms, pain, and disease processes accelerated by stress, when used in addition to prescribed medical treatment (Benson and McKee, 1993).

Nursing Diagnosis

Sleep Pattern Disturbance is the state in which disruption of sleep causes discomfort or interferes with a person's desired activities (Gordon, 1993). Related factors may include physical discomfort, personal or family stress, depression, environmental or habit changes, inactivity, or fear. The focus of care involves reducing factors that interfere with sleep. **Fatigue** is an overwhelming sense of exhaustion and decreased capacity for physical and mental work, even after sleeping. The focus for clients with fatigue becomes conservation of energy and providing rest periods. **Anxiety** is a feeling of apprehension and tension with a nonspecific or unknown cause and frequently is associated with insomnia and depression. The nursing focus with anxiety is promoting relaxation and stress management. **Fear** is a feeling of dread related to a specific threat or danger. The nursing focus with fear is elimination of the potential, actual, or imagined threat.

Skill 9.1 | Comfort Measures that Promote Sleep

The hospital environment is likely to influence clients' ability to fall and remain asleep. Acutely ill clients require frequent assessment and are exposed to unavoidable environmental stimulation to the point of having difficulty differentiating night and day. Disruptive sounds include paging systems, alarms, monitors, telephones, flushing toilets, suctioning equipment, and nursing activities. This is especially problematic for clients in intensive care units (ICUs). In this environment, normal sleep-wake cycles are frequently disrupted.

In addition, any illness that causes pain, difficulty breathing or swallowing, itching, nausea, or nocturia (urination at night) results in discomfort. Discomfort, emotional stress, anxiety, and depression may interfere with

Table 9-1 Common Sedative and Hypnotic Medications

Drug Class/ Specific Agents	Comments
BENZODIAZEPINES Dalmane (flurazepam) Ativan (lorazepam) Restoril (temazepam) Halcion (triazolam)	May remain in body for longer than 24 hours Onset: 30-60 minutes Duration: 7-8 hours Elderly and debilitated clients need smaller doses.
BARBITURATES Phenobarbital (long acting) Seconal (short acting) Nembutal (short acting)	Begin with lowest dose and increase as needed based on client response. Effect as sedative or hypnotic is dose related. Clients may develop dependence and abrupt withdrawal is contraindicated.
MISCELLANEOUS Noctec (chloral hydrate) Placidyl (ethchlorvynol) Doriden (glutethimide)	Onset: 30-60 minutes Duration: 4-8 hours

Modified from Edmunds MW: *Introduction to clinical pharmacology,* St. Louis, 1991, Mosby.

Table 9-2 Effects of Some Medications on Sleep

Drug Class	Effects
Hypnotics	Interfere with reaching deeper sleep stages Provide only temporary (1 week) increase in quantity of sleep Eventually cause "hangover" during day: excess drowsiness, confusion, decreased energy May worsen sleep apnea in adults
Beta blockers	Cause nightmares, insomnia, awakening from sleep
Antianxiety agent (Valium)	Decreases stage 2, stage 4, and REM sleep; decreases awakenings
Narcotic analgesics (morphine, meperidine [Demerol])	Suppress REM sleep If discontinued quickly, can increase risk of cardiac dysrhythmias because of rebound Cause increased awakenings and drowsiness
Antidepressants and stimulants	Suppress REM sleep

falling asleep or may cause frequent awakening or early awakening.

When comfort measures are inadequate, short-term use of prescribed sedatives or hypnotics may be necessary. A *sedative* is medication that relaxes the client and promotes rest. A *hypnotic* actually produces sleep. A medication may act as a sedative with a smaller dose and a hypnotic with larger doses (Edmunds, 1991). Table 9-1 lists drugs frequently used as sedatives and hypnotics.

EQUIPMENT
Night light
Side rails
Alarm system (optional) for clients at risk for falls
Television monitoring system (optional) for clients at risk for falls

Assessment

1. Ask client to describe location of any discomfort, as well as onset, precipitating factors, quality, duration, and severity.
2. To identify client's normal sleep pattern, ask:
   a. What time do you usually go to sleep?
   b. How quickly do you fall asleep?
   c. What is the average number of hours you sleep?
   d. How many times do you awaken during that time?
   e. When do you typically awaken?
   f. Do you rise once you awaken, or do you stay in bed?
3. When a problem is identified, use open questions to help client describe the problem more fully.
   a. What interferes with your sleep?
   b. What type of sleep problem do you experience?
   c. When did you notice the problem? How long has it lasted?
   d. How often do you have trouble sleeping?
   e. Compare your sleep now with your normal sleep.
   f. What do you do just before going to bed?
   g. What do you think about as you fall asleep?
   h. Have you had any recent changes at work or at home?
   i. How has the loss of sleep affected you?
   j. Have you or your partner noted any changes in behavior since the sleep problem started? Irritability, fatigue, trouble concentrating, others?
4. Identify medications that may influence sleep patterns (Table 9-2).
5. Identify indications of sleep apnea. **Sleep apnea is the temporary cessation of airflow through the nose and mouth for 10 seconds or more during sleep** (Barkauskas et al., 1994). The sleeping partner may be a better source of information than the client.
   a. Snores loudly and irregularly?

b. Stops breathing for a while and then starts up again?
c. Has headaches after awakening?
d. Awakens coughing or choking?
e. Makes grunting or gurgling noises during sleep?

Planning

Expected outcomes focus on providing comfort and assisting client in identifying and adopting sleep-promoting measures.

Implementation

EXPECTED OUTCOMES
1. Client describes discomfort as less than 4 (scale of 0 to 10).
2. Client falls asleep within 30 minutes of preparing for sleep.
3. Client tries two new methods or techniques that promote sleep.
4. Client reports 4 or more hours of restful sleep on awakening.

Steps	Rationale
1. See Standard Protocol (Chapter 1, p. 5).	
2. Promote usual bedtime routines (reading, eating a snack, watching TV). Encourage client to empty bladder. Provide opportunity to wash face and hands, brush teeth or dentures, and cleanse mouth.	
3. Suggest avoiding caffeine at bedtime. Schedule diuretics early in the day to minimize nocturia.	Caffeine in coffee, tea, colas, and chocolate is a stimulant and can interfere with sleep. It also acts as a diuretic and may cause the need to void during the night.
4. Make sure client gown and linens are clean and dry. Tighten and smooth wrinkled bed linen. Provide adequate warmth, especially feet and shoulders.	
5. Provide cutaneous stimulation such as a massage (see Skill 6.2). A warm bath or a warm or cold compress may promote comfort.	Massage promotes muscle relaxation. The gate control theory suggests that stimulation of certain nerve fibers closes gates to transmission of discomfort.
6. Assist client to a comfortable position, providing support to body parts to minimize muscle tension. If sleep disturbance is related to sleep apnea, place a pillow at the client's back to support in lateral position (Figure 9-1). Continuous positive airway pressure (CPAP) may also control symptoms (see Skill 30.2).	CPAP helps keep airway open.

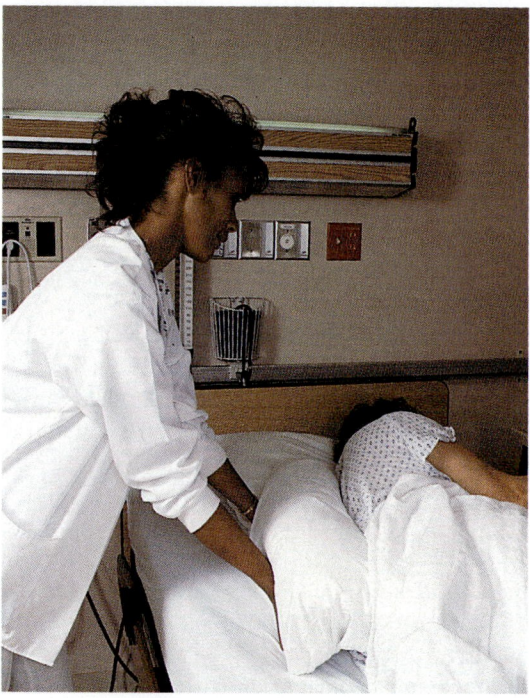

Figure 9-1 Client position for sleep.

Steps	Rationale

7. Raise side rails and place call light within reach. Remind client to call for help if getting up for any reason is necessary. Assure client you will respond to calls as quickly as possible.

Clients who have urinary urgency may attempt to go to the bathroom alone rather than experience soiling the bed.

8. Identify need for safety system. Some beds have alarm systems that alert nurses to client getting out of bed. Some rooms can be monitored by a television screen for safety (Figure 9-2).

Many clients become disoriented when in an unfamiliar environment, which increases risk for falls (see agency policy).

9. Eliminate environmental noise as much as possible. Closing door to the hallway may minimize disturbing sounds. Some clients are accustomed to music or the sound of radio or television (see box at right).

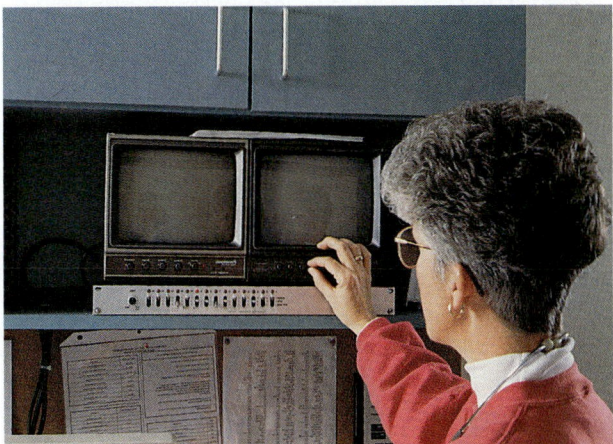

Figure 9-2 T.V. monitor at nurses' station allows observation of clients while they sleep.

Control of Noise in the Hospital

Close doors to client's room.
Provide a sign on the door requesting avoidance of interruptions.
Reduce volume of nearby telephone and paging equipment.
Wear rubber-soled shoes.
Turn off equipment if possible (e.g., oxygen, suction).
Drain humidified oxygen tubing of water accumulation periodically.
Avoid flushing a toilet or moving beds if possible.
Keep talking at low levels, especially at night.
Conduct nursing reports and discussions in areas away from client rooms.
Turn off television or radio or provide soft music.

10. Provide an acceptable level of indirect light. Use of a night light may be beneficial.

May reduce confusion if client awakens at night.

11. Schedule necessary assessments, medications, and treatments to minimize the number of times client must be awakened and assure client of this plan.

Increases the opportunity for quality sleep and REM/NREM sleep cycling.

12. See Completion Protocol (Chapter 1, p. 6).

Evaluation

1. Ask client to rate discomfort level on a scale of 0 to 10 (10 is the worst).
2. Observe client for evidence of sleep 30 minutes after preparing for sleep and every hour thereafter.
3. Ask client if methods tried to help promote sleep seemed to help.
4. Assess client's perception of feeling rested on awakening.

UNEXPECTED OUTCOME AND RELATED INTERVENTIONS

Client reports frequent awakenings during the night or not feeling rested on awakening.

a. Have client keep a sleep-wake log. Each morning, record evening and bedtime rituals, the time attempting to begin sleep, number and length of awakenings, and time of morning awakening.
b. Monitor for signs of sleep deprivation (see box on p. 128).
c. Offer hypnotics or antianxiety agents (if ordered) 30 to 40 minutes before usual bedtime (see Table 9-1). Sedative-hypnotics should be used short term only (less than 1 week).
d. Clients should avoid alcohol, smoking, and drinking caffeine while taking hypnotics. **Alcohol can increase the sedation produced by these drugs and can dangerously depress brain**

function. Smoking and drinking caffeine interfere with effectiveness.

nurse alert Hypnotics do not have pain-relieving qualities. If client has pain, an analgesic is more appropriate. More than one type of medication may be needed.

SAMPLE DOCUMENTATION

0700 Client states he kept waking up when turning, when anyone entered the room, or when roommate moved. Very tired and wants to sleep without interruption. Discussed using soft music for distraction and getting pillow from home to enhance comfort.

Skill 9.2 | Progressive Relaxation

Clients can alter the ability to relax physically and mentally, resulting in many beneficial physical and psychological benefits. Relaxation can promote rest and sleep as well as significantly relieve tension headaches and acute and chronic pain. Basic to relaxation therapy is alteration of breathing patterns. The client should learn deep, relaxed diaphragmatic breathing, which requires less energy. Evidence suggests that it stimulates the vagus nerve, resulting in parasympathetic dominance (Peddicord, 1991), the opposite of the sympathetic nervous system response.

For effective relaxation, the client's participation and cooperation are needed. The technique requires practice and is best taught when the client is not experiencing acute pain. The nurse guides the client slowly through the steps of the exercise. Relaxation training may take 5 to 10 training sessions before clients can use it effectively. It can be practiced indefinitely and usually has no side effects.

EQUIPMENT

Cassette tape player
Taped instructions for relaxation, nature sounds, or music

Assessment

1. Assess facial expressions and verbal indications of discomfort. Clients may cry, moan, grimace, clench jaws, or tightly close or widely open mouth or eyes.

2. Observe body movement indicating physical or psychological distress. This may include restlessness, muscle tension, hand and finger movements, pacing, rhythmical or rubbing motions, or immobilization.
3. Observe social interactions that suggest physical or psychological distress. Clients may avoid conversation, have reduced attention span, avoid eye contact, or display irritability, anger, or withdrawal.
4. Assess for physiological signs of anxiety or stress, which may include tachycardia (increased heart rate), increased respirations or hyperventilation, elevated blood pressure, sweaty palms, trembling, and dry mouth.

Planning

Expected outcomes focus on reducing discomfort and distress as well as increasing client's sense of control.

EXPECTED OUTCOMES

1. Client identifies two factors that minimize discomfort.
2. Client expresses feelings of well-being and relaxation.

Implementation

Steps	Rationale
1. See Standard Protocol (Chapter 1, p. 5). **2.** Assist client to assume position of comfort with entire body well supported. Encourage to settle in comfortably. Instruct client to notice areas of tension. a. **Sitting:** entire back rests against back of chair and head supported in line with spine, feet flat on	Adequate support enhances relaxation.

Steps	Rationale

floor, legs apart, and arms resting comfortably on arms of chair or lap (Figure 9-3).

b. **Lying:** keep head aligned with spine, a thin small pillow under head, arms resting at sides without touching sides of body, legs separated, and toes slightly outward (Figure 9-4).

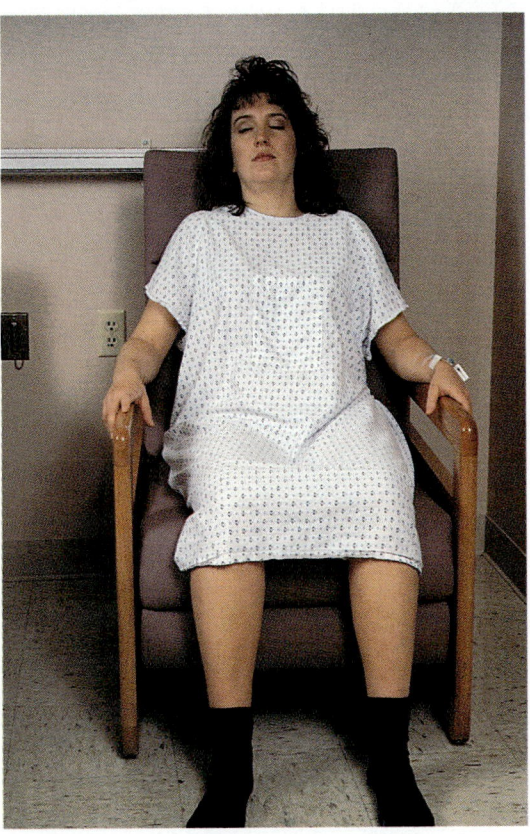

Figure 9-3

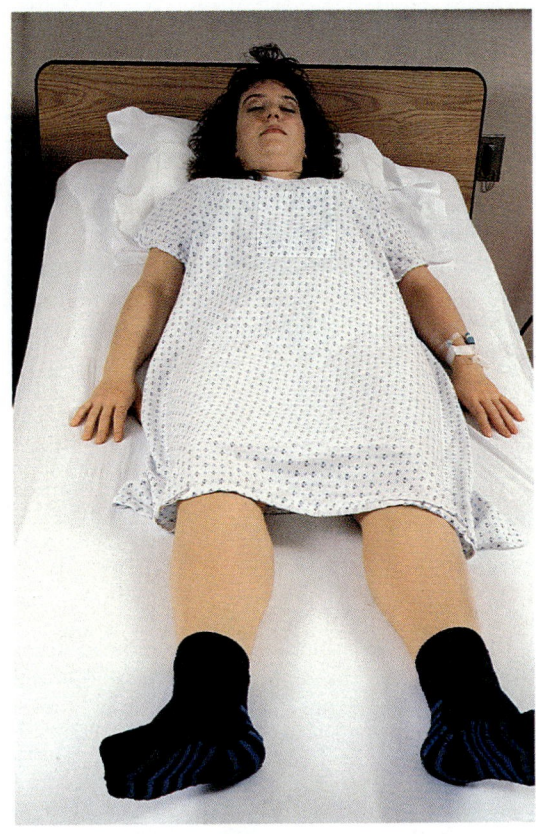

Figure 9-4

3. Tell client to close eyes, relax, and breathe slowly and deeply, allowing the abdomen to rise and fall with each breath.

Deep, regular breathing pattern creates a sensation of removing all discomfort and stress.

4. Coach client to locate an area of muscle tension, think about how it feels, tense muscles, and hold the tension, then completely relax.

Focusing on muscle tension provides awareness of need for relaxation.

5. Concentrate on each of the following groups of muscles, beginning by holding tension and then relaxing: face, jaw, neck, shoulders, arms, hands, fingers, chest, abdomen, back, hips, thighs, legs, and feet.

Systematic practice facilitates a conditioned response and provides a sense of control.

6. When full relaxation is achieved, allow client to continue in this state for 30 minutes without interruption. Soft music may facilitate continued relaxation.

Full relaxation lowers anxiety and tension, and pain perception is diminished.

7. See Completion Protocol (Chapter 1, p. 6).

Evaluation

1. Ask client to identify factors that improved comfort.
2. Ask the client to describe perception of well-being and level of relaxation.

UNEXPECTED OUTCOMES AND RELATED INTERVENTIONS

1. Client becomes agitated or verbalizes inability to follow instructions.
   a. Stop the exercise.
   b. Discuss and use alternative measures for relief.
   c. Encourage practicing at another time when discomfort is less.

2. Client has difficulty relaxing one part of the body.
   a. Slow the progression.
   b. Add suggestion of a sensation of warmth or heaviness or lightness of that body part.
   c. Repeat relaxation of body part several times.

SAMPLE DOCUMENTATION

2200 Client reported restlessness and severe headache (10 on scale 0-10). States she can't go to sleep. Participated in progressive relaxation exercise. States headache is relieved (<4 on scale 0-10). Resting in bed with eyes closed.

Skill 9.3 | Guided Imagery

In guided imagery the client creates an image in the mind, concentrates on that image, and gradually becomes less aware of discomfort. The nurse coaches the client in forming the image and enhancing the sensory experience. The nurse uses information from the client and does not make changes in the client's image.

EQUIPMENT
Tape recorder (optional)
Tape with verbal description of image or nature sounds (optional)

Assessment

1. Assess the onset and duration of the most bothersome symptoms of discomfort. Encourage full description of the symptoms.
2. Identify what client has tried previously for pain control and degree of success.
3. Assess previous experience with relaxation training.
4. Assess sleep pattern, exercise, and use of medication.
5. Assess sources of physical and psychological stress.

Helps determine when guided imagery can be used.
6. Assess willingness to learn and continue to practice the technique. **Guided imagery requires concentration.**

Planning

Expected outcomes focus on promoting comfort and independent management of symptoms.

EXPECTED OUTCOMES

1. Client reports feeling completely relaxed.
2. Client states decreased intensity (less than 4 on scale of 0 to 10) or elimination of symptoms of discomfort or anxiety.
3. Client demonstrates ability to complete self-guided imagery exercise independently.

Implementation

Steps	Rationale
1. See Standard Protocol (Chapter 1, p. 5).	
2. Assist client to assume position of comfort with entire body well supported (see Skill 9.2, Step 2).	The ability to relax physically promotes mental relaxation.
3. Ask client to think of a pleasant scene or experience that promotes use of many senses—vision, hearing, smell, taste, and touch.	
4. Sit close to client and speak in a soft, calm voice.	The experience of discomfort can be altered by concentrating on a serene, tranquil voice.
5. Begin by helping client breathe in a slow, rhythmical fashion as you count, and suggest inhaling on 1 and 2, exhaling on 3 and 4.	

Steps	Rationale
6. Suggest relaxation with a phrase such as, "Your body is beginning to relax . . . think relax . . . continue to breathe slowly and relax."	Focusing on the sensation of relaxation enhances the ability to relax.
7. Describe the scene identified by client as pleasurable and relaxing; for example, "Imagine yourself lying on a cool bed of grass with the sounds of rushing water from a nearby stream. It's a sunny day, and there is a gentle cool breeze." Have client travel mentally to the scene.	
8. Ask questions to help client experience the scene: "How does this look? Sound? Smell? Feel? Taste?"	
9. Encourage client to practice the imagery. It may be helpful to tape-record the imagined experience for repeated practice opportunities.	
10. End the experience: "Experience the comfort and relaxation. When you open your eyes, you will feel alert and renewed. Breathe deeply. Be aware of where you are now, stretch gently, and when you are ready, open your eyes."	
11. See Completion Protocol (Chapter 1, p. 6).	

Evaluation

1. Ask client if muscles feel completely relaxed.
2. Ask client to state level of discomfort using a scale (0 to 10), with 10 being the worst.
3. Observe client perform self-guided imagery.

UNEXPECTED OUTCOMES AND RELATED INTERVENTIONS

1. Client expresses fear of loss of control.
   a. Reassure that client is always in control and can choose to stop the exercise at any time by opening eyes.
   b. Tell client to raise a finger when you instruct to do so. This confirms ability to remain in control.
2. Client completes guided imagery exercise only when assisted by another person.
   a. Identify a family member or friend who is willing to participate regularly for a time.
   b. Suggest that with practice, client will be able to use the technique mentally at will.
   c. A shorter version of the exercise may be helpful.

SAMPLE DOCUMENTATION

2100 Guided imagery practiced for 5 minutes in preparation for sleep. Client states feeling "much more relaxed and comfortable now." Plans to practice this regularly using "favorite fishing spot" as setting.

CRITICAL THINKING EXERCISES

1. Ruth is scheduled for abdominal surgery in the morning. She is very anxious. Explain how her anxiety can affect each of the following if not addressed by the nurse.
   a. Her comfort level
   b. Her ability to understand her preoperative teaching
   c. Her ability to sleep tonight
2. Yesterday the nurse taught Mattie progressive relaxation techniques to help her deal with her chronic pain. Today Mattie complains that the relaxation techniques are not helping. How would you respond to Mattie's statement?
3. How do the concepts of relaxation and guided imagery differ? What is the primary benefit of both?

REFERENCES

Barkauskas VH et al: *Health and physical assessment,* ed 4, St Louis, 1994, Mosby.

Benson H, McKee MG: Relaxation and other alternative therapies, *Patient Care* 27(20):75, 1993.

Edmunds MW: *Introduction to clinical pharmacology,* St Louis, 1991, Mosby.

Gordon M: *Manual of nursing diagnosis,* 1993-1994, St Louis, 1993, Mosby.

Johnson JE: Progressive relaxation and the sleep of older men and women, *J Community Health Nurs* 10(1):31, 1993.

McFarland GK, McFarlane EA: *Nursing diagnosis and intervention: planning for patient care,* ed 2, St Louis, 1993, Mosby.

Peddicord K: Strategies for promoting stress reduction and relaxation, *Nurs Clin North Am* 26(4), 1991.

ADDITIONAL READINGS

Berman TM: Sleep disorders: take them seriously, *Patient Care* 24:85, 1990.

Durham E, Frost-Hartzer P: Relaxation therapy works, *RN* 54(8):40, 1991.

Feierman JR: Disordered sleep, *Emerg Med* 17:160, 1985.

Metzler DJ, Finesilver CA: When to worry if your patient can't sleep, *RN* 53:52, 1990.

Paice JA: Unraveling the mystery of pain, *Oncol Nurs Forum* 18(5):843, 1991.

Wilkie DJ: Cancer pain management: state-of-the-art nursing care, *Nurs Clin North Am* 25(2):331, 1990.

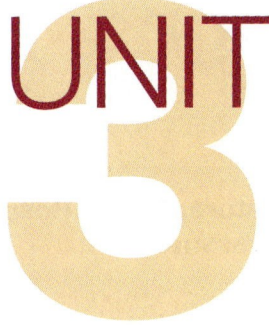

UNIT 3

Assessment Skills

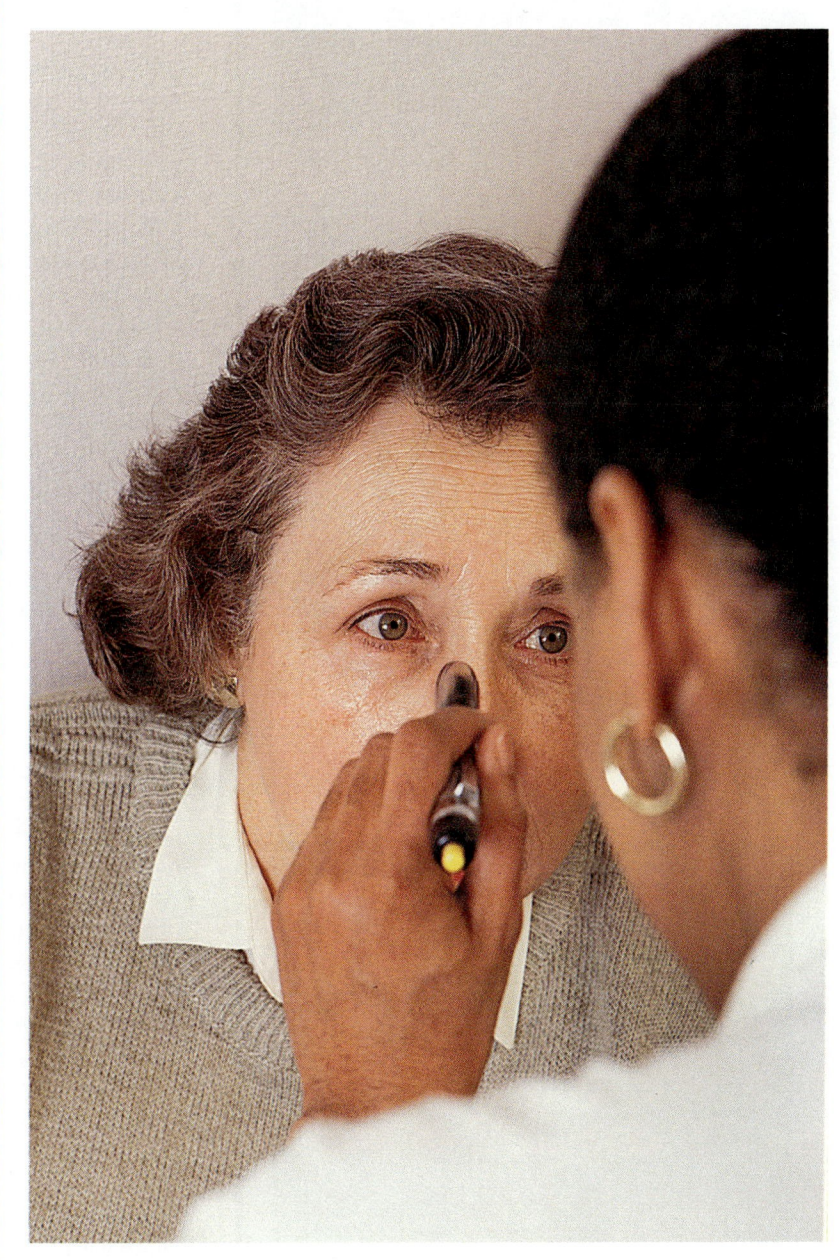

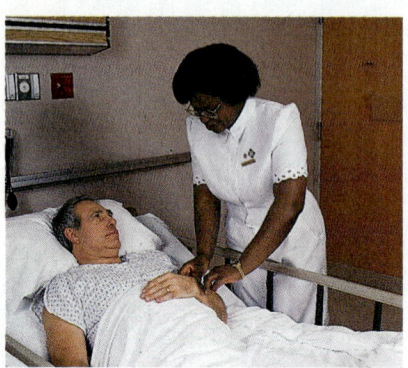

chapter 10

Vital Signs

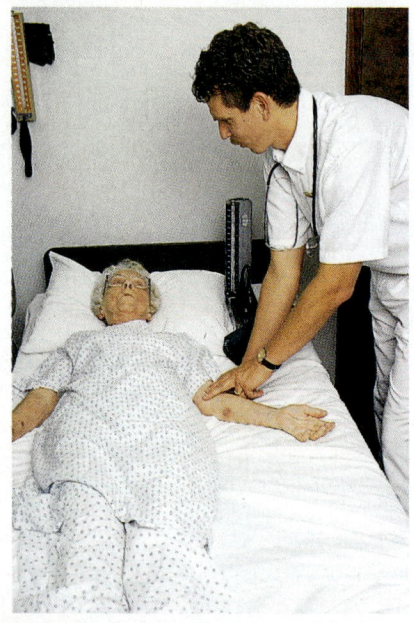

Skill 10.1
Assessing Temperature, Pulse, Respirations, and Blood Pressure

Skill 10.2
Measuring Oxygen Saturation

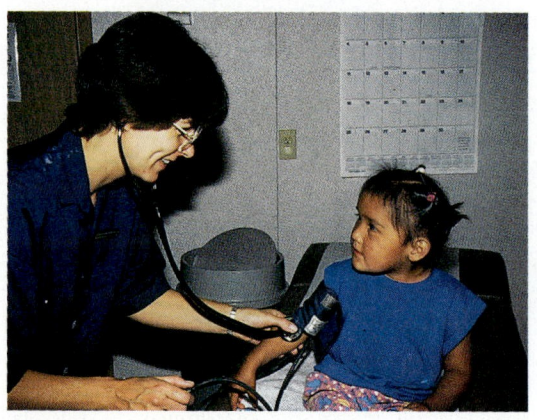

Temperature, pulse, respirations, and blood pressure (BP) are the vital signs, which indicate the body's ability to regulate body temperature, maintain blood flow, and oxygenate body tissues. Vital signs indicate clients' responses to physical, environmental, and psychological stressors. Any difference between a client's normal baseline and current vital signs is an indication for the nurse to further evaluate the client's condition (Table 10-1). Alterations in one of the vital signs (e.g., body temperature) are accompanied by changes in pulse and respirations as well. The nurse must be able to measure vital signs correctly, understand and interpret the values, begin interventions as needed, and report findings appropriately.

The frequency of vital signs assessment is individualized to the client's needs and condition (see box on p. 139). Vital signs may reveal sudden changes in a client's condition, as well as changes that occur progressively over a long time.

TEMPERATURE

The body functions best within a relatively narrow temperature range, the average being 37° C (98.6° F). No single temperature is normal for all people, and fluctuations normally occur throughout the day and night; temperature is lowest between 1 and 4 AM, rises steadily throughout the day, and peaks at about 6 PM. Temperature can be measured using several sites (Table 10-2) and using different types of thermometers. Body temperature is physiologically regulated by vasodilation, vasoconstriction, and sweating and behaviorally by avoidance of temperature extremes. Clients may experience hyperthermia with flushed, warm skin and increased pulse and respiratory rates or hypothermia with cool pale skin, slow capillary refill, cyanotic nail beds, and shivering. Nursing interventions to promote temperature control may include warming or cooling the environment, removing or adding covers, and administering antipyretic medication.

Table 10-1 **Vital Signs: Normal Ranges for Adults**

Vital sign	Range
TEMPERATURE	
Oral/tympanic	37.0° C; 98.6° F (range, +/−1° F)
Rectal	37.6° C; 99.6° F (range, +/−1° F)
Axillary	36.4° C; 97.6° F (range, +/−1° F)
PULSE	60-100 beats/min, strong and regular
RESPIRATIONS	12-20 breaths/min, deep and regular
BLOOD PRESSURE*	Systolic: 90-140 mm Hg (average, 120)
	Diastolic: less than 90 mm Hg

*In some clients, BP is consecutively measured lying, sitting, and standing or in both arms. In normal individuals, the change from lying to standing causes a decrease in systolic blood pressure of less than 15 mm Hg (Barkauskas et al., 1994). Record the position and extremity, and compare the measurements for significant differences.

When to Take Vital Signs

1. On client's admission to a health care facility and during visits to a clinic or physician's office.
2. According to routine established hospital policy or as specified by physician's order; may be twice a day (b.i.d) or once per shift (every 8 hours).
3. Before and after surgical procedure or invasive diagnostic procedures. Monitoring during recovery may be every 5 to 15 minutes initially, then every 30 minutes, every hour, and every 4 hours as condition stabilizes.
4. Before and after administration of medications that affect cardiovascular or respiratory function and before and after temperature regulation.
5. When general physical condition changes (e.g., loss of consciousness, increased restlessness, or intensity of pain).
6. Before and after nursing interventions (e.g., ambulating a client who has dyspnea on exertion).
7. Whenever client reports nonspecific symptoms of distress (e.g., "feeling funny" or "different").

Table 10-2 **Sites for Temperature Measurement**

Tympanic (Figure 10-1)	Oral (Figure 10-2)	Rectal (Figure 10-3)	Axillary (Figure 10-4)
Check ear for presence of ear wax or drainage.		Position in Sims' position. Lubricate tip of thermometer.	
Contraindicated in presence of ear drainage (blood or spinal fluid)	Contraindications: infants, small children, confused clients, clients with shaking chills or recent seizure activity, which could risk glass breakage and tissue damage. Limitations: mouth breathing, hot or cold fluids, and smoking affect accuracy.	Contraindicated after rectal surgery or recent myocardial infarction (heart attack). Placement risks tissue damage in presence of hemorrhoids or rectal tumors or with clients unable to assume lateral position for sufficient visualization of anus.	Requires longer time for accurate readings
2 seconds	2 minutes	2 minutes	5 minutes
Place into external ear canal with gentle firm pressure. Pressure is required for accurate reading.	Place under tongue in posterolateral subinguinal pocket.	Insert lubricated tip into anus toward umbilicus to a depth of 1.5 cm (½ inch).	Place bulb or tip into center of axilla and firmly hold arm against client's side.
37° C +/−1° C	37° C +/−1° C	37.6° C +/−1° C	36.4° C +/−1° C

Keeping clients informed of their body temperature changes promotes understanding of their health status.

TYPES OF THERMOMETERS

Electronic thermometers with battery-powered units

The tympanic thermometer has a temperature-sensitive probe with a disposable plastic cover placed in contact with the opening of the external ear canal (Figure 10-5). Within seconds the probe registers the temperature of the blood flowing near the tympanic membrane, which shares blood supply with the hypothalamus. Accuracy is very good; and since it does not contact body fluids, infection control is enhanced.

An electronic thermometer for measuring oral, rectal, or axillary temperatures has a cord to a temperature-

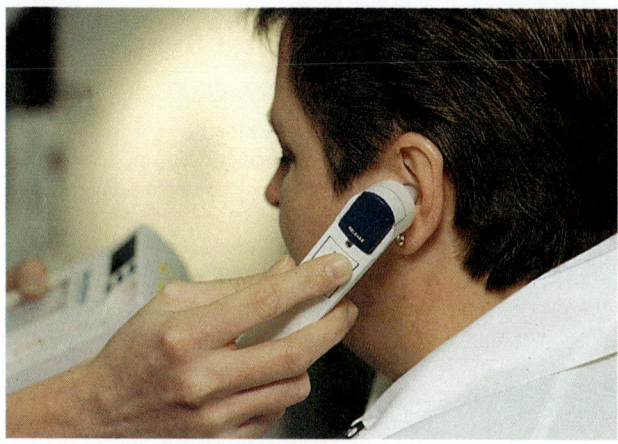

Figure 10-1 Electronic tympanic thermometer placement.

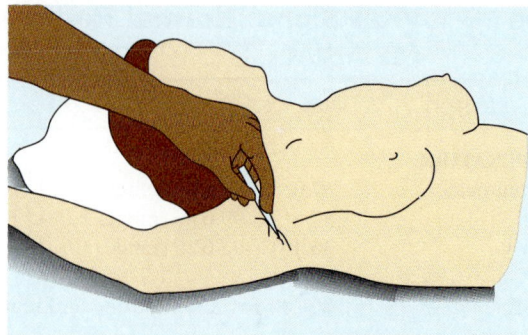

Figure 10-4 Placement of glass thermometer for axillary temperature.

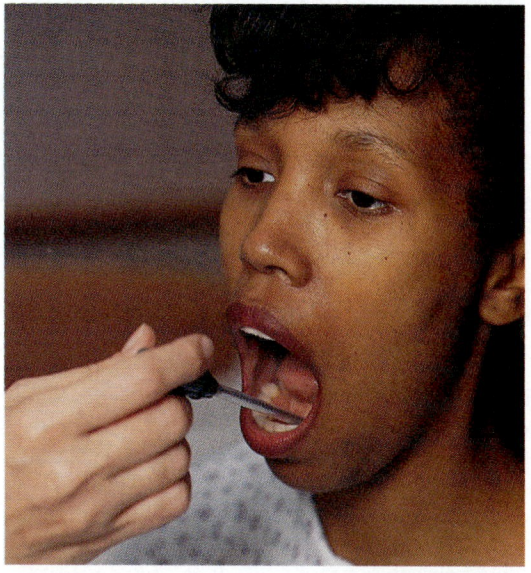

Figure 10-2 Electronic oral thermometer placement.

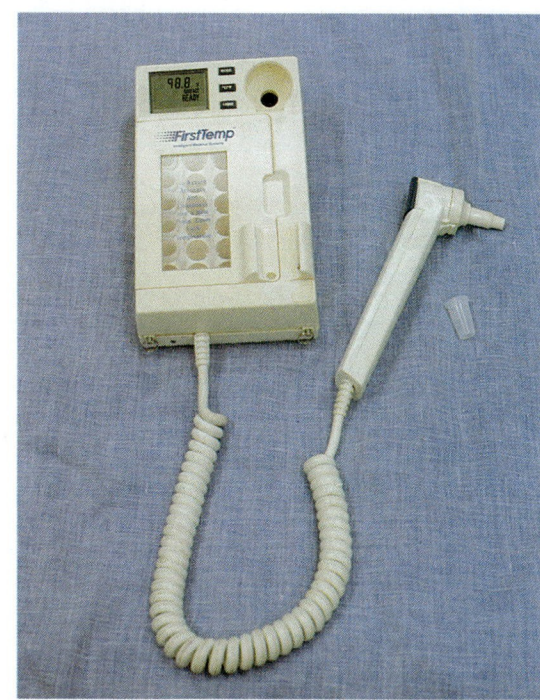

Figure 10-5 Electronic tympanic thermometer.

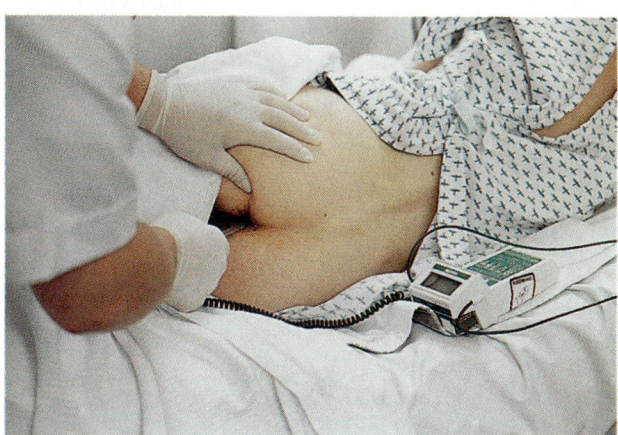

Figure 10-3 Electronic rectal thermometer placement.

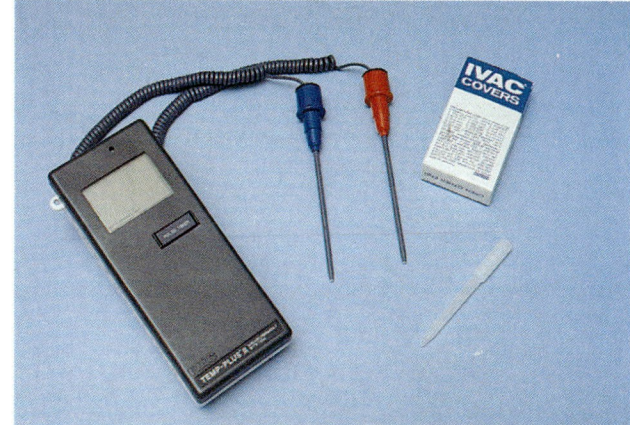

Figure 10-6 Electronic thermometer. Blue probe for oral or axillary use. Red probe for rectal use.

sensitive probe covered by a disposable plastic sheath. Separate probes are available for different sites: oral (with a blue tip) and rectal (with a red tip). Digital readings are displayed in less than a minute (Figure 10-6).

Glass (mercury) Thermometer

Glass thermometers are inexpensive and readily available. To reduce the risk of cross-contamination, each client has a personal thermometer that is stored at the bedside in a dry container and sent home when the client is discharged. Glass thermometers are held at the end opposite the bulb, which may be elongated or stubby (Figure 10-7). Glass thermometers may have either a Celsius or a Fahrenheit scale (Figure 10-8). Conversion charts are available to convert from one system to the other.

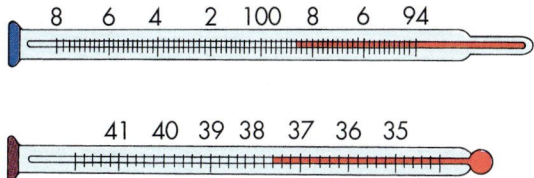

Figure 10-7 Comparison of oral and rectal glass thermometers. Elongated bulb is for oral or axillary use. Stubby bulb may be used for any site. Typically, the red bulb indicates rectal use.

PULSE

The pulse is a pressure wave transmitted from the left ventricle to the aorta, larger arteries, and peripheral arteries, and provides an indication of heart rate and tissue perfusion (circulation). The radial pulse is the site for routine pulse assessment. If abnormalities are noted, an apical pulse is assessed using a stethoscope to listen to the heart through the chest wall. The pulse of a healthy adult is regular with the normal rate ranging between 60 and 100 beats/min. The normal pulse is easily palpable,

does not fade in and out, and is not easily obliterated. Changes in the pulse can reflect the client's metabolic rate and physiological responses to stress, exercise, blood loss, and pain.

Cardiac output can be altered by bradycardia (pulse less than 60 beats/min), tachycardia (pulse greater than 100 beats/min) or dysrhythmia (irregular pulse). Weak, feeble, and thready are descriptive words for a pulse of low volume that is difficult to palpate. *Bounding* is the term used to describe a pulse that is easy to palpate. Strength (amplitude) of pulses may be rated by the following scale: 4+ bounding, 3+ full, 2+ normal, 1+ weak, 0+ absent (Canobbio, 1990).

If the radial pulse is not accessible, an apical pulse may be assessed (Figure 10-9). If pulse irregularities are noted, the apical pulse should be assessed for a full minute. The apical pulse is the most accurate measure of the rate and rhythm of the heart (see Chapter 11). It is auscultated (heard with a stethoscope) by placing the diaphragm over the point of maximum impulse (PMI) at the fifth intercostal space on the midclavicular line (Figure 10-10).

The construction of a stethoscope magnifies the sounds as they are transmitted through tubing to the listener. The use of a stethoscope should be practiced before use with a client (see box on p. 143).

RESPIRATIONS

Movement of air between the environment and the lungs involves three interrelated processes: *ventilation,* which is mechanical movement of air in and out of the lungs; *diffusion,* which involves movement of respiratory gases (oxygen and carbon dioxide) between the alveoli and red blood cells (RBCs); and *perfusion,* which involves distribution of blood through the pulmonary capillaries. Assessment of respirations involves observing the rate, depth, and rhythm of respiratory movements. *Rate* refers to the number of times the person breathes in and out in 1 minute. *Depth* of respirations is estimated by observing

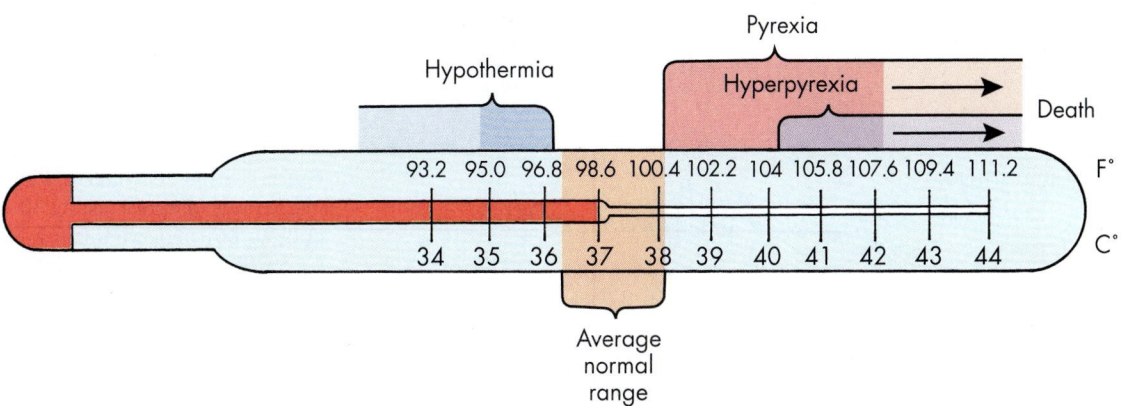

Figure 10-8 Celsius and Fahrenheit temperatures related to temperature ranges.

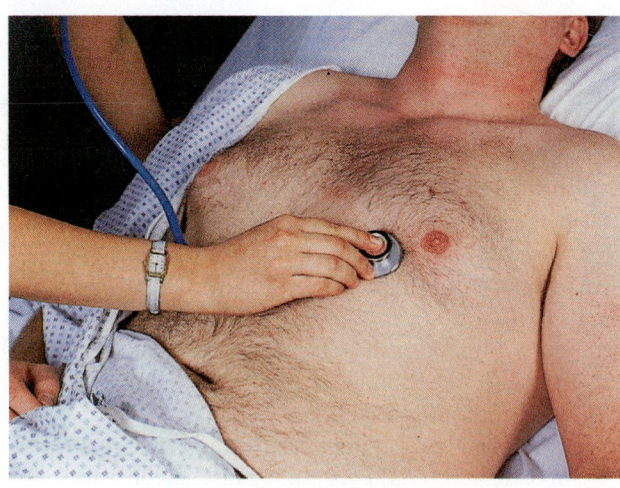

Figure 10-9 Assessing apical pulse.

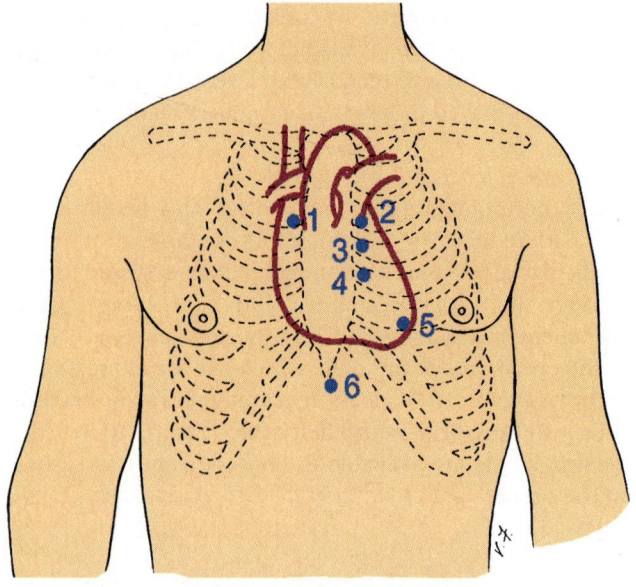

Figure 10-10 Point of maximum impulse is at *5*. Other heart sounds are auscultated at points 1 to 4.

Table 10-3 **Alterations in Respiration**

Type	Diagram	Description
Normal		12-20 breaths/min; regular in rhythm and symmetrical.
Bradypnea		Breathing is slow and regular.
Tachypnea		Breathing is rapid and regular.
Apnea		Respirations cease for several seconds. If persistent, referred to as respiratory arrest.
Hyperventilation		Increase in both rate and depth; associated with CO_2 loss and dizziness.
Cheyne-Stokes respirations		Irregular rhythm characterized by alternating periods of apnea lasting 10-20 seconds and by hyperventilation.
Kussmaul's respirations		Deep rapid respirations associated with diabetic ketoacidosis.

Learning to Use a Stethoscope

1. Place earpieces in both ears with tips of earpieces turned toward the face. *Lightly* blow against the diaphragm (flat side of chestpiece). Now place the earpieces in both ears with the tips turned toward the back of the head and again blow against the diaphragm. Compare comfort in the ears and amplification of sounds with earpieces in both directions. Most people find pointing earpieces toward the face more comfortable and effective.

2. If the stethoscope has both a diaphragm (flat side) and a bell (bowl shaped with a rubber ring) (Figure 10-11, *A*), put earpieces in ears and lightly blow against the diaphragm. If sound is faint, lightly blow into the bell. Then turn the head and blow again against both the diaphragm and the bell. NOTE: The chestpiece can be turned to allow sound to be carried through either side (bell or diaphragm) of the chestpiece. The diaphragm is used for higher-pitched heart sounds, bowel sounds, and lung

sounds (Figure 10-11, *B*). The bell is used for lower-pitched heart sounds and vascular sounds (Figure 10-11, *C*).

3. With earpieces in place and amplification set for the diaphragm, move the diaphragm lightly over the hair on your arm. The bristling sound mimics a sound heard in the lungs. When listening for significant sounds, the diaphragm should be held firmly and still, eliminating extraneous sounds.

4. Place the diaphragm over the front of your chest and listen to your own breathing comparing the bell and the diaphragm. Repeat the process while listening to heartbeat. Ask someone to speak in a conversational tone and note how the speech detracts from hearing clearly. When using a stethoscope, both the client and the examiner should remain quiet.

5. With the earpieces in your ears, gently tap tubing. Note that this also generates extraneous sounds. When listening to a client, maintain a position that allows tubing to hang free. Movement may allow tubing to rub or bump objects, creating extraneous sounds.

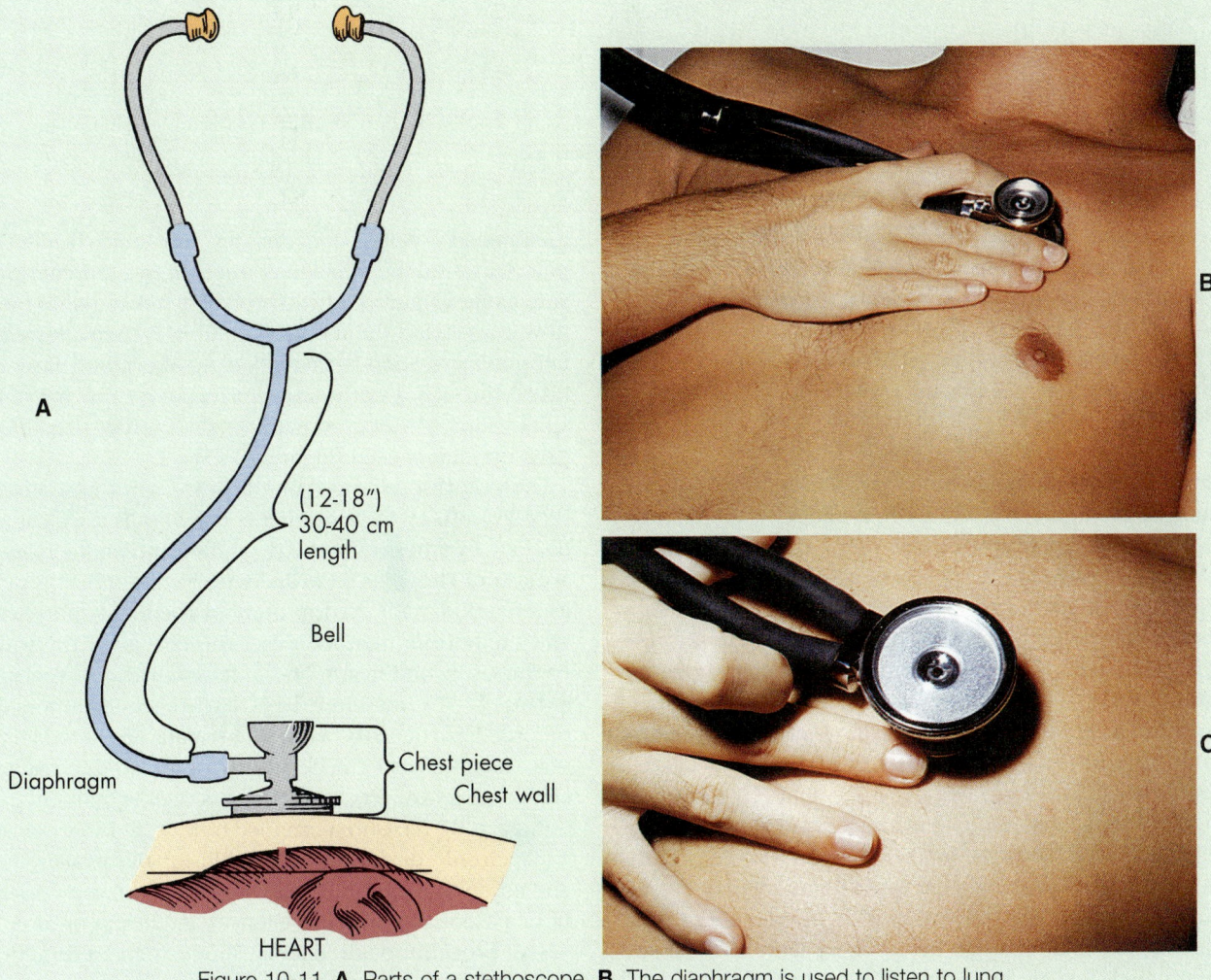

Figure 10-11 **A,** Parts of a stethoscope. **B,** The diaphragm is used to listen to lung and bowel sounds. **C,** The bell must be placed lightly on the skin to hear low-pitched vascular and heart sounds.

the movement of the chest during inspiration and can be described as deep or shallow. *Rhythm* of respirations is normally regular; however, irregular respiration patterns may occur (Table 10-3).

Normally, men and children have diaphragmatic breathing, which is most visible in the abdomen, and women breathe more with the thorax, most apparent in the upper chest. Labored respirations usually involve use of the accessory muscles of respiration in the neck. When something interferes with airflow, the intercostal spaces usually retract during inspiration. A longer expiration phase is evident when outflow is obstructed. If a client is experiencing *dyspnea,* a subjective experience of inadequate or difficult breathing, lung sounds should be assessed with a stethoscope. In some clients, abnormal sounds, such as wheezing, can be heard even without a stethoscope. Dyspnea may be associated with increased effort to inhale and exhale and active use of intercostal and accessory muscles. *Orthopnea* is difficulty breathing while lying flat and is relieved by sitting or standing.

BLOOD PRESSURE

Blood pressure (BP) is the force exerted by the blood against the vessel walls. The unit for measuring BP is millimeters of mercury (mm Hg). The *systolic* pressure is determined by the amount of blood being forced into the aorta and arteries and the force of contraction of the heart ventricles. The aortic valve closes as the pressure in the aorta and large blood vessels falls. The level of the pressure before the next ventricular compression is the *diastolic* pressure (Jolly, 1991).

BP reflects a relationship between cardiac output (CO) and peripheral vascular resistance (R):

$$BP = CO \times R$$

Normally, the volume of blood circulating remains constant: approximately 5000 ml in an adult. If circulating blood volume increases, such as after a rapid intravenous (IV) infusion, BP may temporarily rise. If blood volume falls with hemorrhage or dehydration, BP falls. BP can also be affected by blood viscosity and elasticity of vessel walls. Arteriosclerosis involves a loss of elasticity of arterial walls from the presence of fibrous tissue that does not stretch easily resulting in rising BP. Hypertension (high BP) is a major contributing factor for death, heart attack, and cerebrovascular accident (CVA, stroke) in the United States and Canada. Risk factors include obesity, increased sodium intake, increased cholesterol, smoking, and lack of exercise. One BP recording does not qualify as a diagnosis of hypertension; however, repeated measurements should be made on at least two subsequent visits to a clinic or physician.

Measurement of BP requires the use of a sphygmomanometer and stethoscope. The cuff of the sphygmo-

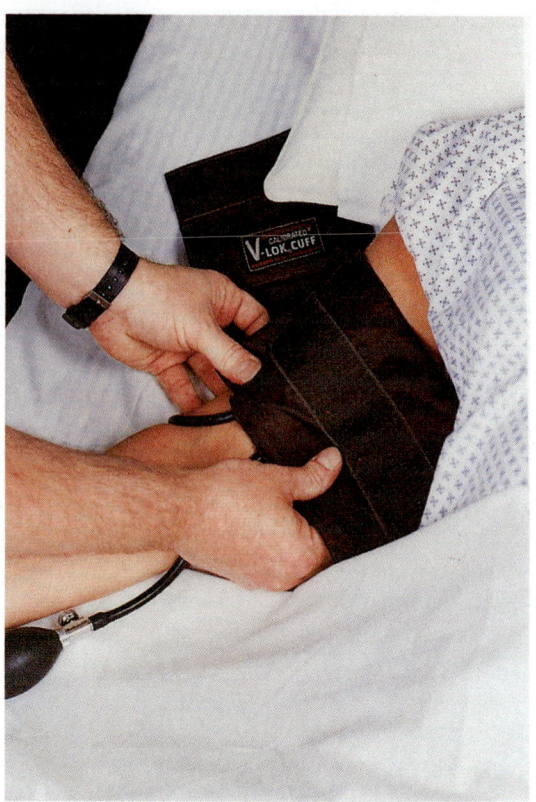

Figure 10-12 Placement of blood pressure cuff.

manometer, which contains an inflatable bladder, is placed around the arm and connected to a mercury pressure gauge (Figure 10-12). The cuff is inflated until blood flow ceases, and the mercury column is then allowed to fall gradually. Sounds that relate to the blood flow are heard through a stethoscope placed over the artery. Results will not be accurate unless the correct-sized blood pressure cuff is used (Figure 10-13).

Korotkoff sounds are sounds heard when auscultating BP (Table 10-4). In some clients the sounds are clear and distinct. In others only the beginning and ending sounds are heard. The BP is recorded with two numbers written as a fraction, with the top number the first sound heard and the bottom number either the change of the sound or the last sound heard. The American Heart Association (AHA, 1987) recommends that three numbers be recorded, particularly when the sounds are heard all the way down to zero. Check agency policy so that readings are consistently recorded. Various factors influence accuracy in BP measurement (see box on p. 145).

Electronic devices are available for BP measurement and are used for frequent BP monitoring in the critically ill or potentially unstable client (e.g., during or after invasive procedures, circulatory shock, increased intracranial pressure). Electronic equipment monitors and displays systolic and diastolic BP, mean arterial pressure (MAP), and pulse rate (Figure 10-14). Alarm parameters

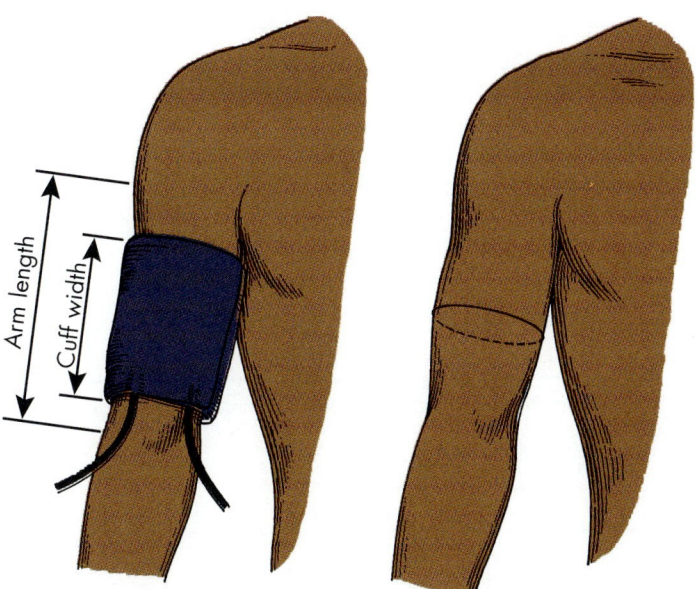

Figure 10-13 Guidelines for proper cuff size. Cuff width = 20% more than upper arm diameter, or 40% of circumference and ⅔ of arm length.

Table 10-4 **Korotkoff Sounds**

Phase	Sounds
I	Pressure level at which the first faint, clear tapping sounds are heard (systolic blood pressure). Sounds gradually increase in intensity.
II	Sounds soften or become swishing.
III	Sounds are sharper and more crisp and increase in intensity.
IV	Distinct, abrupt muffling of sounds, more soft and blowing, occurs.
V	All sounds cease. Artery remains open during entire cardiac cycle.

Modified from Anderson DA et al: *Am J Crit Care* 4(2):269, 1993.

can be set to alert care givers to significant changes. In some cases the monitor can generate printouts. Monitors can be attached to an IV pole and batteries used for transfers, but they should be plugged in whenever possible to keep the battery charged.

Table 10-5 in the box on p. 146 lists proper cuff sizes, and the box on p. 146 describes electronic BP monitoring.

Nursing Diagnosis

Risk for Altered Body Temperature is an appropriate nursing diagnosis for a client unable to maintain a normal body temperature 36° to 37.5° C (97° to 99.5° F). Clients at risk include those with dehydration, infection, major surgery, compromised neurological status, or en-

Common Errors in Blood Pressure Measurement

CAUSES OF FALSE-HIGH MEASUREMENTS
Physical activity within 5 minutes before measurement
Client talking during measurement
Arm not supported during measurement
Pain, anxiety, discomfort

CAUSES OF FALSE-LOW MEASUREMENTS
Extremity lower than heart
Mercury column below eye level
Failure to identify auscultatory gap (period of silence below actual systolic pressure)
Faint or inaudible volume of sounds

NOTE: Incorrect cuff size will cause a **false-low** reading if too large and a **false-high** reading if too small. The AHA has recommended that the bladder of the blood pressure cuff, when turned lengthwise, should encircle 40% of the circumference of the extremity (Frohlich et al., 1987).

Faulty equipment, including problems with inflation or deflation and leaking, may result in inaccurate measurement. Equipment should be repaired or replaced.

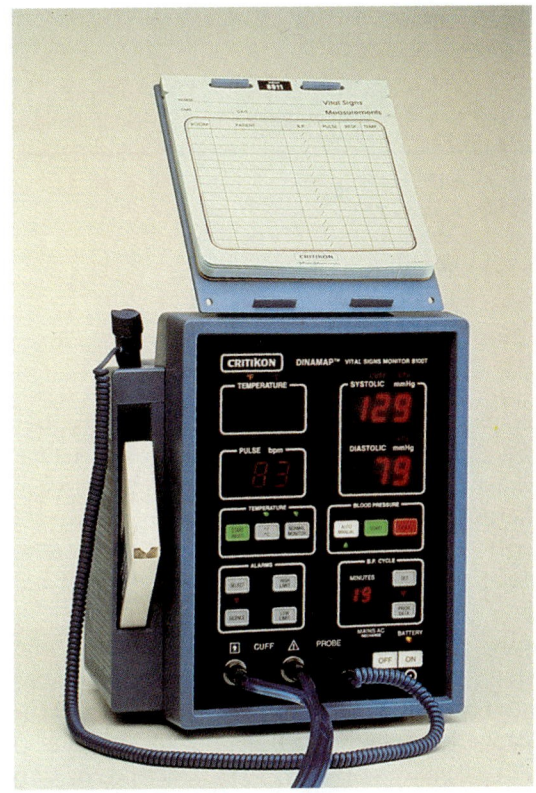

Figure 10-14 Automatic blood pressure monitor. (Dinamap* Vital Signs Monitor is a trademark of Critikon, Inc. Photo courtesy Critikon, Inc., Tampa, Fla.)

Electronic Blood Pressure Monitoring

1. Determine best site for BP monitoring. Upper arm, forearm, or lower leg is appropriate as long as circulation is adequate and cuff is the correct size (see Table 10-5 and Figure 10-15).
2. Determine baseline BP with sphygmomanometer using the same site as will be used with the electronic monitor. **Allows comparison with electronic monitor to check accuracy.**
3. Explain the alarm system, which sounds audible tones with the first reading and when certain factors interfere with monitoring at the established intervals. **Clients become anxious when alarms are not understood.**

Table 10-5 Proper Cuff Size for Electronic Monitor* (Figure 10-15)

Cuff type	Limb circumference (cm)
Small adult	17-25
Adult	23-33
Large adult	31-40
Thigh	38-50

*It is mandatory for the 12- to 24-foot cord to be used for adult monitoring.

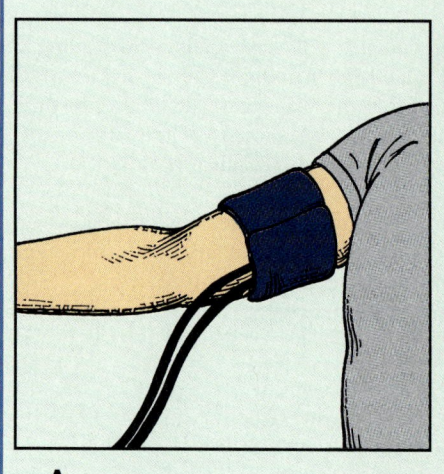 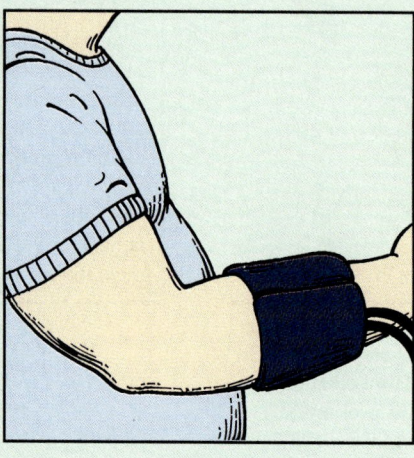 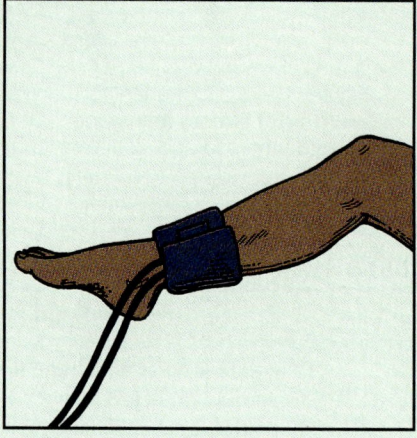

A B C

Figure 10-15 Placement of blood pressure cuff for electronic monitoring.

vironmental exposure. **Ineffective Thermoregulation** is an appropriate nursing diagnosis when an individual's body temperature fluctuates between hyperthermia (above normal) and hypothermia (below normal). This may be related to ineffective temperature-regulating mechanisms (McFarland and McFarlane, 1993).

Activity Intolerance should be considered when an individual has insufficient energy to endure or complete required or desired daily activities. This is often related to imbalance between oxygen supply and demand (Kim, McFarland, and McLane, 1993). **Decreased Cardiac Output** may be appropriate when the client has hemorrhage or dehydration or when the heart muscle is too weak to pump effectively, as manifested by decreased BP,

decreased or irregular peripheral pulses, and difficulty breathing.

Ineffective Airway Clearance is appropriate for clients who are unable to maintain airway patency (clear secretions or obstructions). **Ineffective Breathing Pattern** is appropriate when an individual's breathing does not enable adequate mechanical movement of air into and out of the lungs. The client's breathing may include hypoventilation or hyperventilation and dyspnea. Clients with **Impaired Gas Exchange** have altered vital signs and require frequent assessment for critical changes. Impaired gas exchange refers to altered oxygen or carbon dioxide exchange in the lungs or at the cellular level with hypoxia manifested by cyanosis, tachycardia, dizziness, and mental confusion.

4. Connect the cuff to the pneumatic hoses. Squeeze all air from the cuff.
5. Place the monitor cuff on the selected site making sure the "artery" arrow is correctly placed. Secure the cuff for a snug fit (Figure 10-15). **Excessive tightness may cause venous congestion and discoloration of the limb. Too loose a cuff may result in no readings and/or inaccurate readings.**

nurse alert Do not place the cuff on an extremity being used for IV infusion or any area where circulation is compromised.

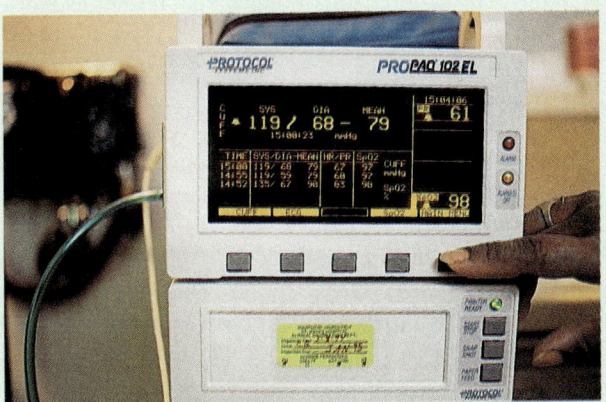

Figure 10-16 Controls on electronic blood pressure monitor.

6. Support the extremity at heart level, and instruct the client to remain still while the pressure determination is being made. **Cuff motion results in inaccurate readings.**
7. Set the control for automatic or manual, then press the start button (Figure 10-16). The first BP measurement sequence initially pumps the cuff to a pressure of about 178 mm Hg. After the initial pressure is reached, the monitor begins a deflation sequence that determines BP.
8. Set alarm parameters using the "high" and "low" limit buttons for systolic pressure, MAP, pulse rate, and diastolic pressure. **Limits depend on client's condition and baseline readings.**
9. Set the frequency of BP determination by pressing the "set" button until the display reads the desired time interval in minutes. Additional readings may be determined at any time by pressing the "start" button. Pressing the "cancel" button immediately deflates the cuff. Intervals may be set from 1 to 90 minutes. The monitor displays the most recent reading and flashes the time in minutes that has elapsed since that reading. Previous data are retrieved by pressing the "prior data" button.
10. If BP determinations are frequent, the cuff may be left in place and rotated to alternate sites at least every 2 hours. **Frequent BP readings become uncomfortable.**
11. A digital display of previous data can be retrieved by pressing the "prior data" control. With some monitors, a printout option is available.

Skill 10.1   Assessing Temperature, Pulse, Respirations, and Blood Pressure

The nurse routinely obtains a baseline measurement of vital signs at initial contact with a client to provide a means for comparison with subsequent vital sign values. The nurse's findings aid in determining whether it is necessary to assess specific body systems more thoroughly. For example, after assessing an abnormal respiratory rate, the nurse also auscultates lung sounds. In certain situations, vital sign assessment may be limited to measurement of a single vital sign for the purpose of reviewing a specific aspect of a client's condition. For example, after administering an antihypertensive medication, the nurse measures the client's BP to evaluate the drug's effects. Part of the nurse's clinical judgment involves deciding which vital signs to measure, when measurements should be made, and the frequency of assessment.

This skill includes temperature measurement with an electronic thermometer using the oral site, palpating the radial pulse, and auscultating blood pressure.

EQUIPMENT
Electronic thermometer with disposable probe
Stethoscope
Sphygmomanometer

BP cuff of appropriate size
Alcohol swab
Watch (sweep second hand or digital watch that displays seconds)

Assessment

1. Consider normal daily fluctuations: body temperature is lowest in the early morning, peaks in late afternoon, and falls gradually at night (Figure 10-17). **BPs follow a similar circadian rhythm.**

2. Identify factors likely to interfere with accuracy of temperature reading, including oral intake of hot or cold fluids, caffeine, or smoking. To avoid inaccuracy, wait 20 to 30 minutes.

3. Identify medications that may influence vital signs (e.g., antiarrhythmics, cardiotonics, bronchodilators, antihypertensives).

4. Identify factors that influence vital signs. **Exercise increases metabolism and heat production, resulting in increased temperature, pulse, respirations, and BP. Anxiety and pain also tend to increase vital signs through hormonal and neural stimulation.**

5. Identify conditions that precipitate fever, including infections. Monitor white blood cell count (WBC). **A WBC greater than 12,000 suggests presence of infection. A WBC less than 5000 suggests immunosuppression, which increases risk of infection.**

6. Identify factors that influence BP. **High BP is associated with pain, rapid IV infusion of fluids or blood products, increased intracranial pressure, cardiovascular disease, and renal disease. Low BP is associated with rapid vasodilation, shock, hemorrhage, and dehydration.**

7. Assess pertinent laboratory values, including complete blood count (CBC), which includes hemoglobin, hematocrit, and RBC count; oxygen saturation; and arterial blood gases (ABGs). **A low hemoglobin, hematocrit, and RBC count are associated with decreased oxygen transport to tissues and hypoxia. ABGs reflects adequacy of oxygenation and ventilation** (see Appendix D).

8. Determine previous baseline vital signs from client's record. **Baseline information provides basis for comparison and assists in assessment of current status.**

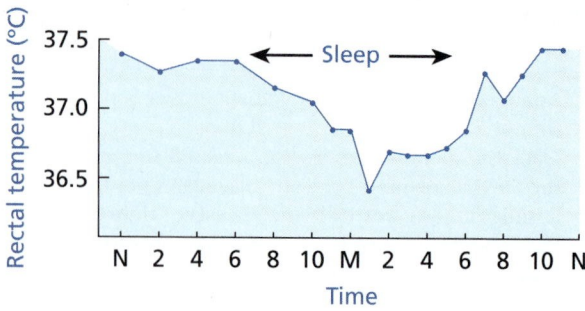

Figure 10-17 Temperature cycle for 24 hours. (From Mountcastle VB: *Medical physiology,* vol 2, ed 14, St. Louis, 1980, Mosby.)

Planning

Expected outcomes focus on identifying abnormalities and restoring homeostasis.

EXPECTED OUTCOMES

1. Client's vital signs are within normal range.
2. Client identifies factors that influence vital signs.
3. Baseline is established for clients with chronic diseases that alter vital signs such as chronic obstructive pulmonary disease (COPD).
4. Client describes alterations in vital signs related to

Implementation

Steps	Rationale
1. See Standard Protocol (Chapter 1, p. 5).	
2. Assist client to comfortable position either lying or sitting. Avoid injured arm or one with IV infusion, previous breast or axilla surgery, cast, or arteriovenous shunt for renal dialysis.	Good circulation facilitates accuracy in BP measurement. BP measurement temporarily disrupts circulation.
3. Temperature a. Attach oral probe (blue tip) to thermometer unit. Grasp top of stem, avoiding pressure on the ejection button. Slide disposable plastic probe cover over thermometer probe until it snaps in place.	

Steps	Rationale

b. Ask client to open mouth, and gently place probe under tongue in posterior sublingual pocket lateral to center of lower jaw (Figure 10-18). Ask client to hold thermometer with lips closed.

Facilitates contact with blood vessels for accurate reading.

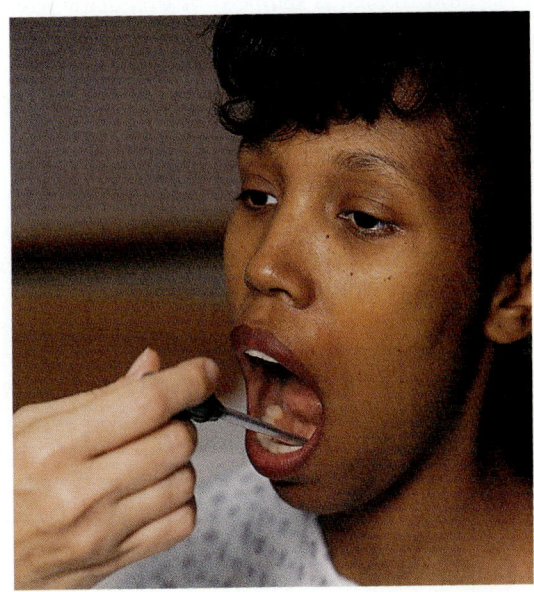

Figure 10-18

c. When the audible signal indicates completion, note and record the reading. Remove probe from under tongue, and inform client of temperature reading.

d. Push ejection button on thermometer probe to discard cover into proper receptacle, and return to storage position.

Digital reading automatically disappears when the probe is replaced.

4. Pulse

a. Locate radial pulse by placing two fingers on inner aspect of client's wrist, which should rest on the upper abdomen or chest. Assess regularity of the pulse (Figure 10-19).

   (1) If the pulse is regular, count the rate for 30 seconds and multiply total by 2.

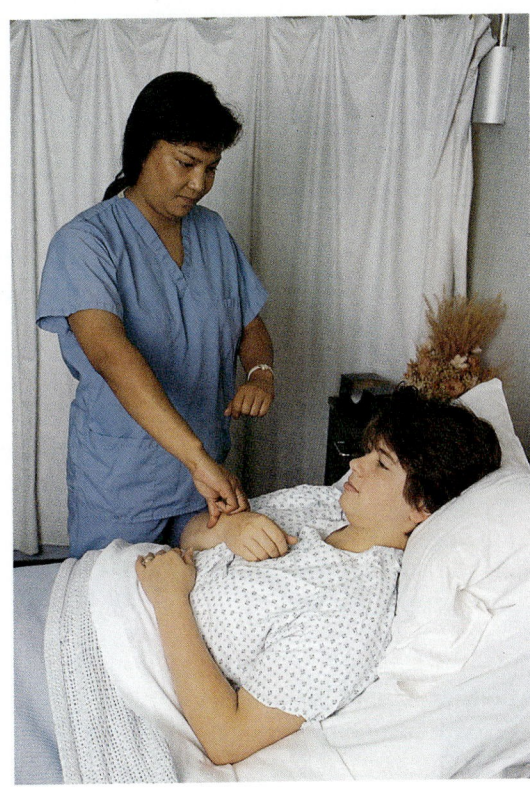

Figure 10-19

Steps	Rationale
(2) If pulse is irregular, count for a full minute. Note if it is regularly irregular (e.g., every fourth beat is skipped) or irregularly irregular (i.e., no pattern to irregularity).	A longer period increases accuracy of count in the presence of irregularity. Irregularity may indicate abnormal electrical cardiac function or heart contractions too weak to generate a pulse wave. An apical pulse is the standard in some agencies (see agency policy).
b. Determine quality of the pulse as weak, strong, or bounding.	Quality reflects volume of blood ejected against arterial wall with each heart contraction.

5. Respirations

Steps	Rationale
a. Without changing the position of your hand on the pulse, observe and count each respiratory cycle (one inspiration and one expiration).	Maintaining the same position keeps client from being aware that you are counting respirations. Awareness can result in altered respirations.
(1) If the rhythm is regular, count for 30 seconds and multiply by 2.	
(2) If respirations are irregular or very slow or fast, count for a full minute.	Assessment with irregularities requires at least 1 minute (see Table 10-3).
b. Observe amount of movement of the chest, and describe quality as shallow, normal, or deep.	Depth of respirations reveals volume of air moving into and from the lungs.
c. Observe for evidence of increased effort to inhale and exhale. Ask client to describe subjective experience of shortness of breath compared with usual breathing pattern.	Clients with chronic lung disease may experience difficulty breathing all the time and can best describe their own discomfort from shortness of breath.

6. Blood Pressure

> **nurse alert** Eliminate extraneous noise, such as television and conversation. Noise interferes with accuracy.

Steps	Rationale
a. Verify appropriateness of cuff size.	Improper cuff size results in inaccurate readings. If cuff is too small, it tends to come loose as it is inflated (see Figure 10-13).
b. Remove restrictive clothing.	BP is altered by tight clothing, causing congestion of blood.
c. Support forearm at heart level and position palm of the hand upward.	Blood pressure is altered by contraction of muscles.
d. Palpate the brachial artery over the antecubital fossa at the midline toward the medial side (Figure 10-20).	Permits proper placement of the cuff and stethoscope so that the BP can be heard accurately.
e. Verify center of the bladder by folding it in half with center over the brachial artery and lower edge of the cuff at 2.5 to 5 cm (1 to 2 inches) above the antecubital space (inner aspect of the elbow). Wrap the cuff snugly and smoothly in place.	Bladder of cuff should be evenly distributed over the artery as it inflates. Avoids extraneous sounds from movement of the cuff against stethoscope.
f. If you do not know client's usual BP, estimate systolic pressure by palpating the pulse while inflating the cuff until the pulse disappears. Note pressure on sphygmomanometer; this is the estimated systolic pressure.	Estimating prevents false-low readings, which may result from the presence of an auscultatory gap (inaudible sounds below the actual systolic pressure). This phenomenon occurs in about 5% of adults and is prevalent in individuals with hypertension (Barkauskas et al., 1994).
g. Deflate the cuff completely and wait at least 60 seconds before measuring the BP.	Sudden pressure changes alter the accuracy of BP measurement.

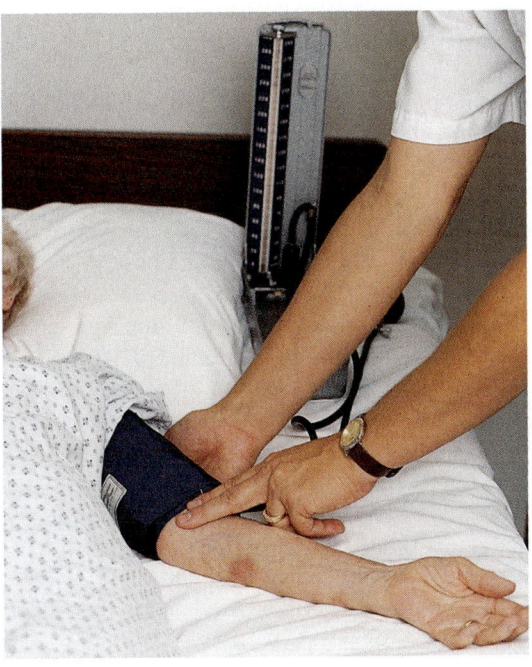
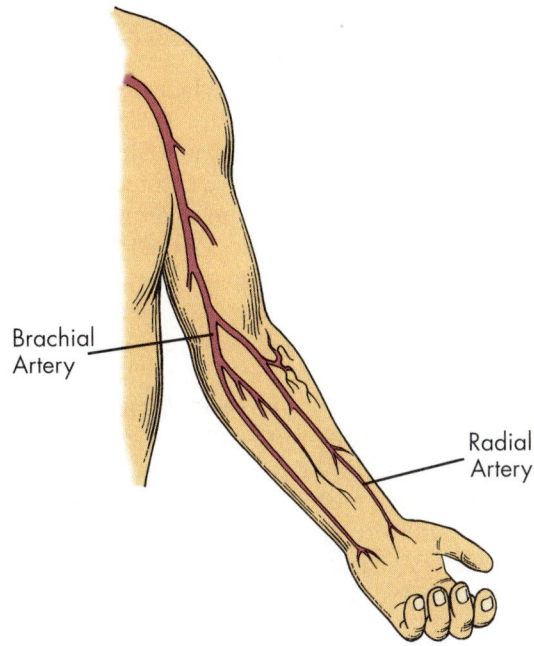

Brachial Artery

Radial Artery

Figure 10-20

Steps	Rationale

h. Place bell or diaphragm of the stethoscope gently and firmly over the artery where the pulse was palpated.

Too much pressure against the artery may alter the point at which blood would make the first sound. If the stethoscope has a bell, use it for auscultation. Low-frequency sounds are heard best with the bell.

i. Position yourself so that you can see the manometer easily and at eye level.

j. Ask the client not to talk, and avoid bumping stethoscope.

Extraneous sounds interfere with precise hearing of Korotkoff sounds.

k. Rapidly and steadily inflate the cuff to approximately 30 mm Hg above the estimated or baseline BP. Make sure there are no sounds at this point.

Silence interrupted by the first Korotkoff sound substantiates accurate perception of systolic reading.

nurse alert If you hear sounds immediately, release the pressure, wait 60 seconds, and estimate systolic pressure at a higher reading. Reinflation of a partially deflated cuff is uncomfortable for client and may render an inaccurate reading.

l. Open valve on the manometer and allow the mercury to drop 2 to 3 mm per heartbeat (Figure 10-21).

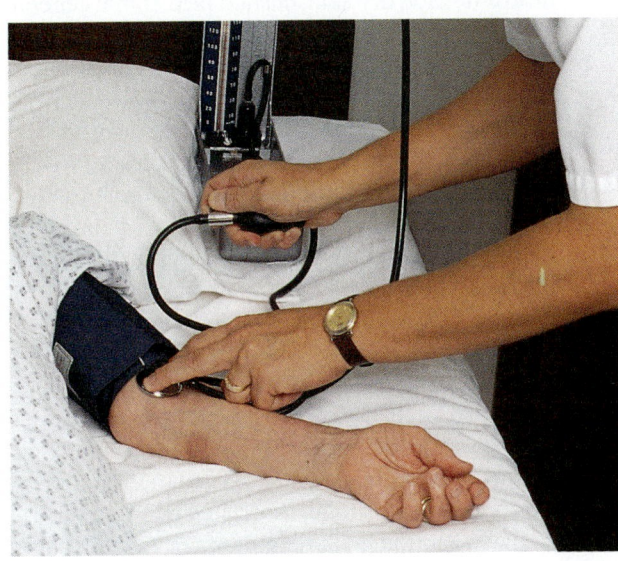

Figure 10-21

Steps	Rationale
m. Note point on the manometer when the first clear sound is heard, which is phase I of Korotkoff sounds (see Table 10-4) and the systolic pressure. The sounds will slowly increase in intensity.	Systolic pressure is the point at which blood in the artery is first able to force its way through the vessel.
n. As the cuff continues to deflate, note the point at which the sound first becomes muffled (phase IV) and the point at which the sound completely disappears (phase V). Listen for 10 to 20 mm Hg after the last sound, and then allow remaining air to escape quickly.	The diastolic pressure is the force produced during ventricular relaxation and filling. Phase IV (when sounds first becomes muffled) and phase V of Korotkoff sounds may occur at the same time or separately and should be recorded (Canobbio, 1990).
o. Inform client of the BP. If possible, discuss risk factors for high BP. If BP is elevated and client takes antihypertensive medications, assess whether any doses have been missed.	
p. Remove and store BP cuff and return thermometer to battery charger promptly.	Maintains thermometer battery charge.
7. See Completion Protocol (Chapter 1, p. 6).	

Evaluation

1. Compare vital signs with client's baseline and normal expected ranges.
2. Ask client to identify factors that influence vital signs.
3. Identify a baseline for clients with chronic diseases that alter vital signs.
4. Ask client to describe changes in vital signs related to therapies (e.g., ambulation, medications).

UNEXPECTED OUTCOMES AND RELATED INTERVENTIONS

1. Client has a fever 1° C or more above normal.
   a. Assess for additional related data suggesting systemic infection, including loss of appetite, headache, hot, dry skin, flushed face, thirst, general malaise, or chills.
   b. Further assess for possible site of localized infection.
   c. Report fever if indicated to facilitate appropriate treatment, which may include blood tests (WBC), cultures, antibiotics, or antipyretics (fever-reducing medications).
   d. Increase fluid intake to at least 3 L daily unless contraindicated.
   e. Remove excess blankets. Keep bed linens dry.
2. Client has tachycardia (pulse greater than 100 beats/min) or pulse is weak and difficult to palpate.
   a. Identify related data, including pain, fear or anxiety, recent exercise, low BP, blood loss, elevated temperature, or inadequate oxygenation.
   b. Observe for symptoms associated with abnormal cardiac function, including dyspnea, fatigue, chest pain, orthopnea, syncope, palpitations (unpleasant awareness of pulse), jugular vein distention, edema of dependent body parts, cyanosis, or pallor of skin.
3. Client has bradycardia (pulse less than 60 beats/min) or dysrhythmias (pattern that may be regularly irregular or irregularly irregular).
   a. Auscultate the apical pulse by listening with a stethoscope over apex of the heart located at fifth intercostal space left of the midclavicular line. Normal heart sounds are identified as "lub-dub." Count for a full minute and report rate and regularity.
   b. Observe for factors that may alter heart rate and regularity, including medications such as digoxin and antiarrhythmics. It may be necessary to withhold prescribed medications until the physician can evaluate the need to alter the dosage.
4. Client has abnormal respiratory rate, depth, or pattern of dyspnea with complaints of feeling short of breath.
   a. Observe for related factors, including obstructed airway; noisy respirations; cyanosis of nail beds, lips, mucous membranes, and skin; restlessness; irritability; confusion; dyspnea (labored breathing); shortness of breath; productive cough; and abnormal breath sounds.
   b. Consider possible effects of anesthesia or medications such as narcotic analgesics (pain relievers).
   c. Assist client to a supported sitting position, which improves ability to take a deep breath.
   d. Encourage client to cough to clear the airway of secretions and consider the need for suctioning or oxygen therapy.

5. Client has elevated BP, as evidenced by diastolic pressure greater than 90 mm Hg or moderate to severe elevation, as evidenced by diastolic pressure greater than 105 mm Hg.

   NOTE: **A diagnosis of hypertension involves three or more elevated readings on separate occasions.**

   a. Observe for related symptoms. Often, none is apparent unless extremely high. Client may have a headache (usually occipital), flushing of face, or nosebleed; older adult client may notice fatigue.

   b. Be certain size of cuff is appropriate. A cuff that is too small gives false-high readings. Recheck or have another nurse recheck readings.

   c. Administer antihypertensive medication as ordered. If none is ordered, report blood pressure to initiate appropriate evaluation and treatment.

6. Client is hypotensive when blood pressure is not sufficient for adequate perfusion and oxygenation of tissues.

   a. Compare to baseline. A systolic reading of 90 may be normal for some persons and cause no ill effects.

   b. Observe for symptoms associated with hypotension related to decreased cardiac output, which include tachycardia; weak thready pulse; weakness, dizziness, or confusion; pale, dusky, or cyanotic skin; or cool mottled skin over extremities.

   c. Position in supine position to enhance circulation.

   d. Increase rate of IV infusion or administer vasoconstricting drugs if ordered.

7. It is difficult to hear sounds when checking the BP. Raising the arm over the head helps relieve congestion, increases pressure differences, and makes sounds louder and more distinct as blood enters the lower arm.

   a. Raise client's arm above the head for 15 seconds.

   b. Inflate cuff with the arm elevated and gently lower the arm while continuing to support it.

   c. Position the stethoscope and proceed as before.

8. If unable to auscultate BP, the palpation method or a Doppler instrument may be used. This method provides systolic reading only.

   a. Palpate brachial or radial artery with fingertips of one hand. Inflate cuff to a pressure 30 mm Hg above point at which pulse disappears.

   b. Slowly deflate cuff, allowing mercury to fall 2 mm Hg/sec.

   c. When pulse is again palpable or audible with the Doppler, note manometer reading. This represents the systolic blood pressure.

   d. Deflate cuff rapidly and completely. Remove from client's arm unless frequent reassessment is necessary.

SAMPLE DOCUMENTATION

0700 Client has nosebleed. Ice and pressure applied to bridge of nose. BP 230/110, pulse 88, respirations 22, temperature 37.2° C. Denies headache. Physician notified. (See Vital Signs Record, Appendix A.)

Skill 10.2 | Measuring Oxygen Saturation (Pulse Oximetry)

Pulse oximetry is a noninvasive measurement of arterial oxygen saturation (Sao_2) to detect the presence of hypoxemia. The Sao_2 is the ratio of oxygenated hemoglobin to the total amount of hemoglobin and is expressed as a percentage; for example, an Sao_2 of 96% indicates that 96% of the total available hemoglobin have oxygen molecules attached to them (Pagana and Pagana, 1992). The normal Sao_2 is greater than 95%. An Sao_2 less than 70% is life-threatening (Sonnesso, 1991). The more hemoglobin saturated by oxygen, the higher is the Sao_2.

NOTE: When hemoglobin levels are low, the client may not have adequate tissue oxygenation even if the Sao_2 shows an acceptable level on the monitor.

The pulse oximeter sensor can be placed on the client's finger, toe, nose, or earlobe. The sensor emits two wavelengths of light, one red and one infrared, which are transmitted through the tissues and blood vessels. Blood that is well oxygenated (red) absorbs light differently than blood that is deoxygenated (blue). Values obtained by oximetry become less accurate if the Sao_2 is less than 80%. At this level, oxygenated blood is darker, making it more difficult for the oximeter to distinguish between oxygenated and deoxygenated blood (Lewis and Collier, 1992).

EQUIPMENT

Pulse oximeter (Figure 10-22)
Cutaneous sensor probe
Acetone

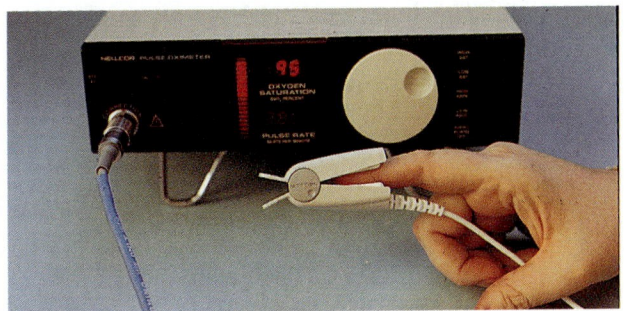

Figure 10-22

Assessment

1. Identify clients at risk for unstable oxygen status. **This includes clients in critical condition or who require a ventilator and clients with chest pain or activity intolerance; also done after anesthesia or sedation for surgery or procedures such as endoscopy, bronchoscopy, cardiac catheterization, or sleep testing.**
2. Assess type and level of supplemental oxygen required and hemoglobin level. **Any abnormalities in the type or amount of hemoglobin affect the amount of oxygen available.**
3. Assess capillary refill at site for sensor probe placement (finger, toe, nose, earlobe). Site should be clean and dry and nails free of polish.

Planning

Expected outcomes focus on monitoring and maintaining adequate oxygenation when client is at risk for hypoxemia.

EXPECTED OUTCOMES

1. Sao_2 level greater than 90% is maintained during sleep, after removal of secretions with suctioning, and with exertion of ambulating in the hall for 5 minutes. (NOTE: Acceptable level must be individualized for each client.)
2. Client maintains good skin color and is not restless; pulse and respirations are within normal limits.

Implementation

Steps	Rationale
1. See Standard Protocol (Chapter 1, p. 5). **2.** Select site, which may include ear, nail bed, or bridge of nose. If finger is used, remove fingernail polish and acrylic nails (if worn).	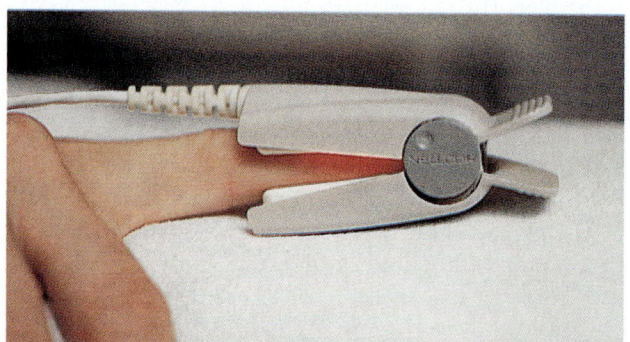 Figure 10-23 Application of sensor to finger.
3. Check capillary refill at the site. **4.** Apply sensor to site (Figure 10-23), making sure photodetectors are aligned opposite each other. If finger is used, support lower arm and instruct client to keep extremity still.	Decreased circulation could alter readings. Movement interferes with measurement.
5. Determine that client's radial pulse correlates with the pulse on the oximeter. **6.** Read digital display of Sao_2 level. **7.** Check alarm limits, which are usually preset at a high Sao_2 of 100% and low Sao_2 of 85%. High and low pulse rates can also be set. Limits can be changed as indicated by condition.	Ensures accuracy of oximeter and checks pulse against machine.
8. Move the sensor periodically.	Minimizes tissue irritation from adhesive sensor and pressure from spring tension sensor.
9. Periodic ABGs may be needed (physician's order required). **10.** Compare Sao_2 when awake and asleep or before, during, and after planned activity. **11.** See Completion Protocol (Chapter 1, p. 6).	Validates accuracy. Oxygen desaturation may occur during sleep or activity.

Evaluation

1. Compare Sao₂ levels before and during sleep, after removal of secretions with suctioning, and before, during, and after activity.
2. Observe for indications of hypoxemia, which include the presence of cyanosis, restlessness, apnea, and tachycardia.

UNEXPECTED OUTCOMES AND RELATED INTERVENTIONS

1. Client's Sao₂ is less than 90%.
   a. Observe for and minimize factors that alter Sao₂, such as secretions in the lungs, increased activity, and decreased hemoglobin levels.
   b. Administer oxygen according to physician's orders (see Chapter 30).
2. Pulse rate indicated on oximeter is inaccurate. Compare with ABG measurements.
   a. Client may have inadequate perfusion. Assess apical and radial pulses to evaluate. Make sure sensor is not applied so as to constrict blood flow.
   b. Clients who have cold hands may have inaccurate readings. Use a different site for measurement.
   c. Clients who smoke cigarettes or use nicotine gum may have reduced peripheral circulation, which reduces accuracy of readings.
   d. Protect sensor from strong light (sunlight, lamp for procedures), which may interfere with accuracy.

SAMPLE DOCUMENTATION

1330 Pulse ox at rest 92%. Up to ambulate. C/O shortness of breath after 5 min at slow, steady gait. Pulse ox 82%, P 96, R 24. Rested sitting for 5 min; pulse ox back up to 90%. Back to bed. Plans to repeat ambulation during evening to increase endurance.

CRITICAL THINKING EXERCISES

1. Consider each of the following clients. For each, what system is involved, and what is the correct term for the problem(s) the client is experiencing?
   a. Mr. Peck is being treated for pneumonia. He is sitting in his chair, leaning over and breathing heavily. You recognize that he is having difficulty breathing. When you ask him if he would like assistance getting back into bed, he states that he can't breathe well when in bed.
   b. Mrs. Reed is a 67-year-old client being treated for fluid retention. Her ankles and legs are very swollen. When you take her pulse, you note that it is fast (104 beats/minute) and very strong.
2. Mr. Smith is an elderly male who has an open leg ulcer. He complains of being tired and has a temperature of 101.4° F (38.5° C) and irregular peripheral pulses.
   a. Write two or three appropriate nursing diagnoses addressing Mr. Smith's problems.
   b. The nurse is monitoring Mr. Smith's fever pattern, vital signs, oral intake, urine output, and lung and abdominal status. What other assessments should the nurse perform?
   c. When monitoring Mr. Smith's temperature, why would the nurse select a tympanic thermometer rather than an oral thermometer for Mr. Smith?
3. You are to place a pulse oximeter on Mrs. Perkins. When you take the monitor into her room, she states that she doesn't want to have it on because it hurts and she doesn't have a fever that needs to be monitored.
   a. How would you respond to Mrs. Perkins' statement?
   b. If Mrs. Perkins continues to appear reluctant, what else can you do to help alleviate her anxiety?

REFERENCES

American Heart Association: *Recommendations for human blood pressure determination by sphygmomanometers,* Dallas, 1987, The Association.

Anderson DA, Cunningham SG, Maloney JP: Indirect blood pressure measurement: a need to reassess, *Am J Crit Care* 4(2):269, 1993.

Barkauskas VH et al: *Health and physical assessment,* ed 4, St Louis, 1994, Mosby.

Canobbio MM: *Cardiovascular disorders,* Mosby's Clinical Nursing Series, St Louis, 1990, Mosby.

Frohlich ED et al: *Recommendations for human blood pressure determination by sphygmomanometers,* AHA pub no 70-1005, Dallas, 1987, American Heart Association.

Jolly A: Taking blood pressure, *Nurs Times* 87(15):40, 1991.

Kim MJ, McFarland GK, McLane AM: *Pocket guide to nursing diagnoses,* ed 5, St Louis, 1993, Mosby.

Lewis SM, Collier IC: *Medical-surgical nursing,* ed 3, St Louis, 1992, Mosby.

McFarland GK, McFarlane, EA: *Nursing diagnosis and intervention: planning for patient care,* ed 2, St Louis, 1993, Mosby.

Pagana KD, Pagana TJ: *Diagnostic and laboratory test reference,* St Louis, 1992, Mosby.

Sonnesso G: Are you ready to use pulse oximetry? *Nursing '91* 21(8):60, 1991.

ADDITIONAL READINGS

Ebersole P, Hess P: *Toward healthy aging: human needs and nursing response,* ed 5, St Louis, 1995, Mosby.

Flynn JM, Bruce NP: *Introduction to critical care nursing skills,* St Louis, 1993, Mosby.

Hill MN, Grim CM: How to take a precise blood pressure, *Am J Nurs* 91:38, 1991.

Hollerbach AD et al: Accuracy of radial pulse assessment by length of counting interval, *Heart Lung* 19:258 May 1990.

Matthews JP: How to use an automated vital signs monitor, *Nursing '91* 21(2):60, 1991.

Perry AG, Potter PA: *Clinical nursing skills and techniques,* ed 3, St Louis, 1994, Mosby.

Schnapp LM, Cohen NH: Pulse oximetry: uses and abuses, *Chest* 98:1244, 1990.

Spyr J, Preach MA: Pulse oximetry: understanding the concept, knowing the limits, *RN* 53(5):38, 1990.

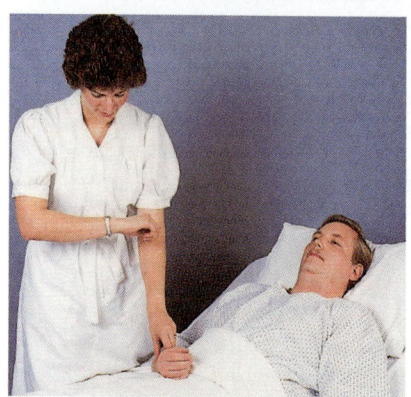

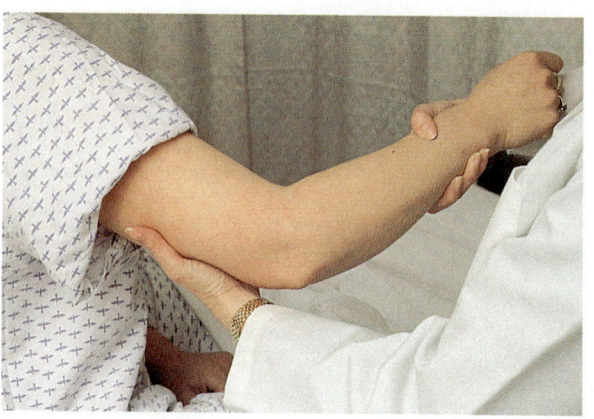

chapter 11

Shift Assessment

Skill 11.1
General Survey and Inspection of Integument

Skill 11.2
Auscultating Lung Sounds

Skill 11.3
Auscultating Apical Pulse

Skill 11.4
Assessing the Abdomen

Skill 11.5
Assessing Extremities and Peripheral Circulation

The shift assessment involves a brief systematic review of a client's condition at the beginning of each shift, with the nurse collecting subjective and objective data to identify changes in the client's status compared with the previous assessment. This routine brief assessment takes 10 to 15 minutes and reveals information that supplements the data base for the client. Once data are gathered, the nurse groups significant findings into patterns of data that confirm or reveal actual or high-risk nursing diagnoses. Information gathered provides the information about a client's functional abilities and serves as a comparison for future assessment findings. In addition, the information helps the nurse select appropriate nursing measures to manage the client's health.

A shift assessment is usually performed using a consistent, organized sequence that improves accuracy of findings. Sometimes, priorities for assessment are based on a client's presenting signs and symptoms or health care needs. For example, a client who develops sudden shortness of breath should first undergo an assessment of the lungs.

Clients are often knowledgeable about their physical condition and can verify whether certain findings are normal for them and when actual changes have occurred. A client's sensory or physical limitations can affect how quickly the nurse is able to complete the assessment. If a client becomes fatigued, a brief rest period may be necessary.

Inspection, palpation, auscultation, olfaction (smell), and percussion are techniques used in physical examination. All, except percussion, are used for a shift assessment. *Percussion* is a more advanced technique used in comprehensive examinations (see Chapter 12).

Inspection involves visual examination of body parts. It is helpful to recognize normal physical characteristics of clients before trying to distinguish abnormal findings. Experience is needed to recognize normal variations among clients and ranges of normal in an individual. Good lighting and adequate exposure of body parts are essential for inspection. When necessary, use additional light (e.g., penlight).

Palpation involves use of the sense of touch to detect characteristics of body parts such as texture, temperature, perception of vibration or movement, and consistency. The nurse uses the back of the hand to determine temperature variations. The pads of the fingertips detect changes in texture, shape, size, consistency, and pulsation. Asking the client to take slow, deep breaths enhances muscle relaxation, which improves the ability to palpate effectively. Tender areas are palpated last. Clients appreciate warm hands, short fingernails, and a gentle approach.

Auscultation is listening with a stethoscope for sounds created in body organs to detect variations from normal. Most sounds can be heard only with a stethoscope. The nurse learns the normal type of sounds arising from body structures (e.g., passage of blood through an artery) before learning to recognize abnormal sounds. Likewise, the nurse learns the areas that normally do not emit sounds. To auscultate, the nurse needs to hear well, have a good stethoscope and know how to use the stethoscope properly.

The final skill a nurse may use during assessment is *olfaction* (smell). Certain changes in body functions create characteristic body odors (Table 11-1). The sense of smell can detect abnormalities that go unrecognized by any other means.

Performing a shift assessment efficiently requires skill and practice. The nurse may need to integrate additional assessment into routine nursing care, such as bathing, administration of medications, or other therapies, or while conversing with a client. In addition, health education can be integrated with assessment activities. The nurse can teach clients about their health problems during assessments. This is an ideal time to discuss changes in symptoms, the implications for changes, and approaches the client may use for self-assessment. More comprehensive assessment skills are described in Chapter 12.

Nursing Diagnosis

Ineffective Airway Clearance is appropriate when the client is unable to clear secretions or obstructions from the respiratory tract. **Ineffective Breathing Pattern** involves altered inhalation or exhalation and may include either hypoventilation or hyperventilation. Influencing factors may include decreased muscle strength or energy, pain, and anxiety.

Activity Intolerance applies when physiological energy is inadequate for the completion of desired activities because of altered cardiac function. **Decreased Cardiac Output** is appropriate when there is need to reduce cardiac workload or improve cardiac performance.

Pain related to unknown etiology may be appropriate when the focus of nursing care involves identifying factors that contribute to pain.

Table 11-1 **Assessment of Characteristic Odors**

Odor	Site or source	Potential causes
Alcohol	Oral cavity	Ingestion of alcohol
Ammonia	Urine	Urinary tract infection
Body odor	Skin, particularly in areas where body parts rub together (e.g., under arms, beneath breasts)	Poor hygiene, excess perspiration (hyperhidrosis), foul-smelling perspiration (bromidrosis)
Feces	Wound site	Wound abscess
	Vomitus	Bowel obstruction
	Rectal area	Fecal incontinence
Foul-smelling stools in infant	Stool	Malabsorption syndrome
Halitosis	Oral cavity	Poor dental and oral hygiene, gum disease
Sweet, fruity ketones	Oral cavity	Diabetes acidosis
Stale urine	Skin	Uremic acidosis
Sweet, heavy, thick odor	Draining wound	*Pseudomonas* (bacterial) infection
Musty odor	Casted body part	Infection inside cast
Fetid, sweet odor	Tracheostomy or mucous secretions	Infection of bronchial tree (*Pseudomonas* bacteria)

Constipation or **Diarrhea** may be associated with abdominal pain or cramping and altered peristalsis resulting in either infrequent hard stools or frequent unformed stools and fluid loss.

Altered Peripheral Tissue Perfusion involves a chronic deficit in blood supply to the extremities and is appropriate when findings reveal alteration in arterial or venous circulation. **Activity Intolerance** related to pain secondary to ischemia may be an appropriate diagnosis when clients require improved circulation to increase endurance of activity. Activity intolerance may also be related to prolonged immobility, weakness, and muscle atrophy.

Impaired Skin Integrity or **Risk for Impaired Skin Integrity** related to impaired circulation is appropriate when changes have caused or may cause skin ulcerations. Related factors need to be individualized to arterial or venous factors based on the client's condition if possible (Gordon, 1993; McFarland and McFarlane, 1993).

Skill 11.1 | General Survey and Inspection of Integument

The general survey is the preliminary portion of the assessment during which the client's vital signs, general behavior, and appearance are identified. If abnormalities or signs of problems are revealed during the assessment, the nurse can direct attention to specific concerns. This information influences how the nurse communicates instructions to the client and conducts remaining portions of the assessment.

Clients develop skin lesions from trauma to the skin, exposure to pressure while immobilized, continued exposure to moisture and irritating fluids, or reaction to medications used in therapy. This is a particular concern for debilitated or older adults. Nurses routinely assess the skin each shift using inspection, palpation, and olfaction.

EQUIPMENT
Stethoscope
Sphygmomanometer and cuff
Wristwatch with second hand
Tape measure (optional)
Penlight
Thermometer

Assessment

1. Obtain previous vital signs from client records. Often this information is kept on a clipboard just outside the door. **Previous data provide means to compare nurse's assessment findings to detect change. Compare current data with previous data to detect alterations.**
2. Consider factors or conditions that may normally alter vital sign readings (see Chapter 10).
3. Review client's recent fluid intake and output (I&O) records. Intake includes all liquids taken orally, by feeding tube, and parenterally. Liquid output includes urine, diarrhea, vomitus, gastric suction, and drainage from postsurgical tubes, such as chest tubes or Jackson-Pratt drains.
4. Assess client's general perceptions about personal health. Nurse's assessment of client's general appearance coupled with client's own perceptions may reveal problem areas.

Planning

Expected outcomes focus on accuracy in collection of assessment data.

EXPECTED OUTCOMES
1. Client demonstrates alert, cooperative behaviors without evidence of physical or emotional distress during assessment.
2. Client's skin is smooth, soft, dry, and warm.
3. Client provides appropriate subjective data related to physical condition.

Implementation

Steps	Rationale
1. See Standard Protocol (Chapter 1, p. 5).	
2. Take temperature, pulse, respiration, and blood pressure (BP) unless gathered within last 3 hours (see Chapter 10). During examination, inform client about vital signs compared with previous data.	Data used to compare with client's baseline.

Steps	Rationale

3. Assess the following aspects of behavior and appearance.

   a. Signs of distress (e.g., shortness of breath, acute pain, anxiety).

   b. Race, gender, and age.

Such distress requires immediate attention and helps establish priorities.

These are important variables that influence assessment findings and techniques to use.

4. Determine the level of consciousness and orientation by talking to client (Figure 11-1).

May reveal subtle or obvious change in client's condition. Level of consciousness influences ability to cooperate with examination.

   a. Is client alert, confused or lethargic?

   b. Eyes open spontaneously, to speech, to pain, or not at all.

   c. Verbal response may be oriented, confused, inappropriate, or incomprehensible.

   d. Motor response may be appropriate in relation to commands, withdraw in response to pain only, or no response apparent.

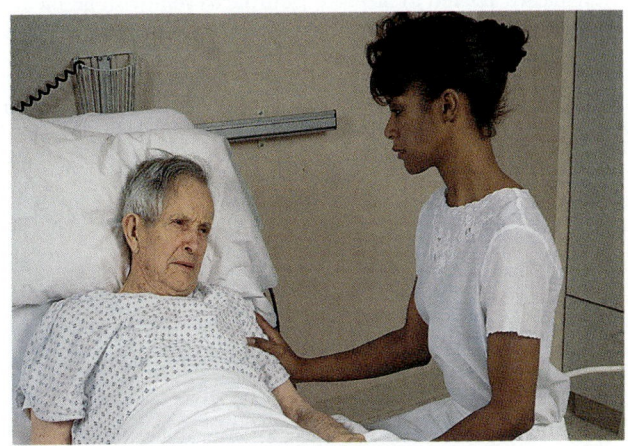

Figure 11-1

5. Assess affect and mood: note if verbal expressions match nonverbal behavior. Note appropriateness to situation.

Reflects client's feelings and emotional status.

6. Assess if speech is understandable and properly paced. Is there an association with client's behavior?

Alterations reflect neurological impairment, injury or impairment of mouth, or differences in dialect and language.

7. Note body type (trim and muscular, obese, excessively thin).

Reflects level of health, risk factors and lifestyle.

8. Assess position and posture: note alignment of shoulders and hips. Reposition for comfort if needed.

Reveals musculoskeletal problem, mood, or presence of pain.

9. Assess body movements: are they purposeful? Are there tremors of the extremities?

Indicates neurological problem or emotional stress.

10. Assess hygiene and grooming: observe for presence or absence of makeup, type of clothes (hospital or personal), and general state of cleanliness.

May reflect client's mood, sociocultural preferences, economic status, self-care habits, culture, and lifestyle.

11. Assess for presence or absence of body odor.

Results from physical exercise, inadequate hygiene, or certain conditions, including infections or tissue necrosis.

12. Inspect color of skin surfaces. Compare color of symmetrical body parts, including areas unexposed to sun.

Changes in color can indicate pathological alterations (Table 11-2).

13. Inspect oral mucosa, tongue, teeth, and gums of oral cavity for hydration and obvious lesions (Figure 11-2).

Reveals need for oral hygiene. Identifies sources of irritation that can affect ability to chew or swallow.

Table 11-2 **Pathological Color Changes**

Color changes	Light skin	Dark skin
Cyanosis: related to hypoxia (decreased oxygen)	Blue tinge, especially in conjunctiva, nail beds earlobes, oral membranes, soles, and palms	Ashen-gray lips and tongue
Pallor: related to decreased perfusion (blood flow)	Loss of rosy glow in skin, especially face	Ashen-gray appearance in black skin
Erythema: related to increased blood flow (fever, irritation)	Redness easily seen anywhere on body	Difficult to assess; rely on palpation for warmth or edema
Jaundice: related to deposits of bilirubin in tissue, liver disease	Yellow staining in sclera of eyes, skin, fingernails, soles, palms, and oral mucosa	Most reliably assessed in sclera, hard palate, palms, and soles
Ecchymoses: related to bleeding into skin, often trauma	Purple to yellowish green areas resulting from bleeding into skin, usually related to trauma	Difficult to see except in mouth or conjunctiva
Petechiae: minute hemorrhages into skin	Purple pinpoints most easily seen on buttocks, abdomen, and inner surfaces of arms or legs	Usually invisible except in oral mucosa, conjunctiva, or eyelids and covering eyeballs

Modified from Whaley LF, Wong DL: *Nursing care of infants and children,* ed 5, St Louis, 1995, Mosby.

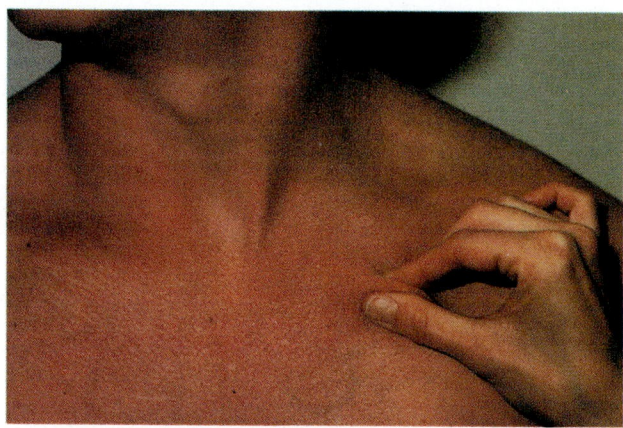

Figure 11-3 (From Seidel HM et al: *Mosby's guide to physical examination,* ed 3, St. Louis, 1995, Mosby.)

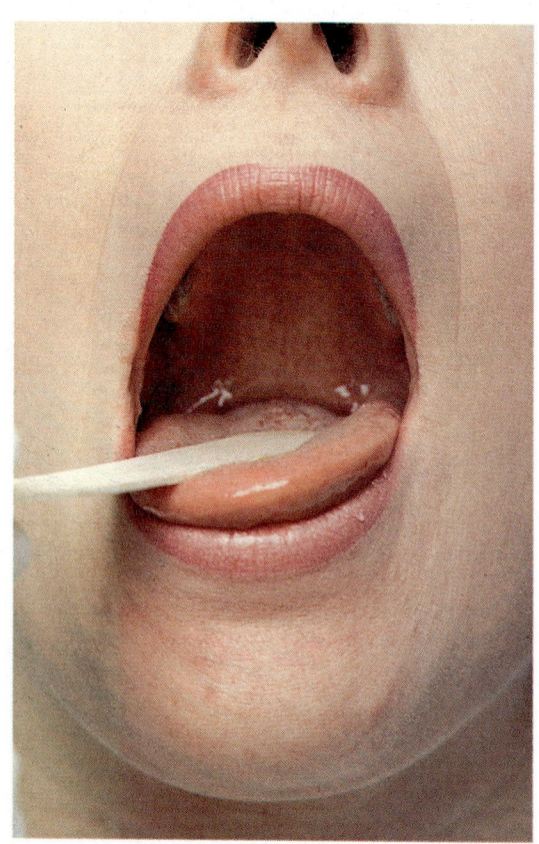

Figure 11-2

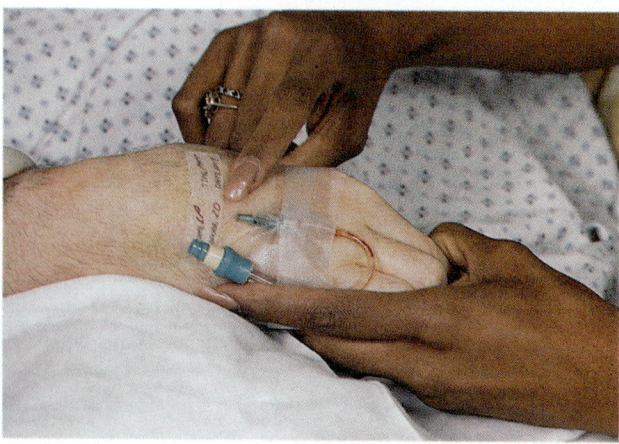

Figure 11-4

Steps	Rationale
14. Inspect color of oral mucosa, nail beds, lips, palms of hands, sclerae, and conjunctivae.	Nurse can more readily identify abnormalities in areas of body where melanin production is least. Reveals oxygen and status of circulation.
15. Palpate skin surfaces with fingertips.	Changes in skin texture may be the only indication of skin rashes in dark-skinned clients.
a. Feel moisture of the skin using fingertips. 	Skin moisture is affected by environment and body temperature regulation. Description of secretions helps to indicate type of lesion.
b. If secretions or drainage are noted, describe color, odor, amount, and consistency (e.g., thin and watery or thick and oily).	
c. Use dorsum (back) of hand to palpate temperature of skin surfaces (nurse may remove a glove temporarily if worn). Compare symmetrical body parts and upper to lower body parts. Note distinct temperature differences. Note localized areas of warm or cool skin.	Cool skin temperature reflects decreased blood flow. A stage I pressure ulcer may cause warmth and erythema of an area (see Chapter 23).
d. Stroke skin surfaces lightly with fingertips to detect texture (smooth or rough) and if there are localized areas of hardness or lesions.	Changes may result from dehydration and localized trauma or skin lesions.
e. Assess skin turgor by first grasping fold of skin over client's sternum, forearm, or abdomen. Release skinfold and note ease and speed with which skin returns to place (Figure 11-3).	Turgor is measure of skin's elasticity and hydration status. Skin may remain suspended or "tented" for few seconds before slowly returning to place, indicating dehydration, inadequate nutrition, and effects of aging. Do not test over back of hand, due to looseness of skin (Seidel, 1995).
f. Assess condition of skin, paying particular attention to regions of pressure. If areas of redness are noted, place fingertip over area and apply gentle pressure, then release.	Normal reactive hyperemia (redness) is visible effect of localized vasodilation, the body's normal response to lack of blood flow to underlying tissue. Affected area of skin will blanch with fingertip pressure.
g. If lesions are detected, inspect color, location, size, type, grouping (e.g., clustered or linear), and distribution (localized or generalized). Be sure skin is well illuminated.	Certain skin lesions can be identified by a characteristic pattern of features (see box on p. 162).
h. Gently palpate any lesion to determine mobility, shape, contour (flat, raised, or depressed), and consistency (soft or hard).	Gentle palpation prevents accidental rupture of underlying cysts.
i. Ask if client has tenderness during palpation.	Tenderness may be indicative of inflammation or pressure on body part.
j. Palpate intravenous (IV) site (Figure 11-4) if present for evidence of inflammation (redness, heat, swelling, or tenderness) or infiltration (puffiness, pallor and coolness) (see Chapter 29).	Report or correct identified problems with infusion immediately. Presence of phlebitis on infiltration requires relocation of IV catheter or needle.
16. Check IV fluids and medications, including rate and type. Note the expiration date of fluids and tubing.	Too rapid or too slow infusion rate can cause fluid excess or deficit. Tubing is changed every 48 to 72 hours (check agency policy).
17. Observe drainage (color, amount, consistency) and function of any drainage systems (see Chapter 20).	Character and amount of drainage to expect will vary with excessive bleeding or the type of drainage system.
18. Examine dressings to determine if they are clean, dry, and intact.	Drainage or moisture may indicate need for dressings to be changed (see Chapter 20).
19. See Completion Protocol (Chapter 1, p. 6).	

Types of Skin Lesions

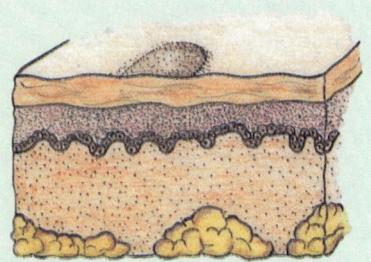

Macule: flat, nonpalpable, change in skin color, smaller than 1 cm (e.g., freckle or petechia)

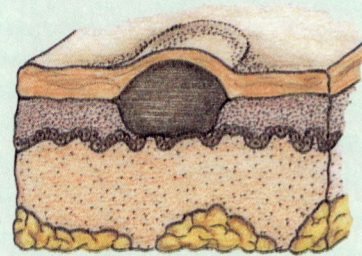

Papule: palpable, circumscribed, solid elevation in skin, smaller than 0.5 cm (e.g., elevated nevus)

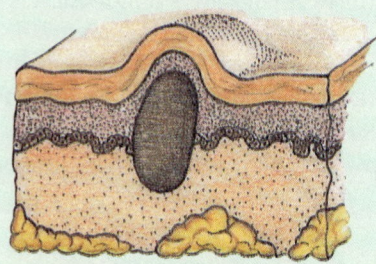

Nodule: elevated solid mass, deeper and firmer than papule, 0.5 to 2.0 cm (e.g., wart)

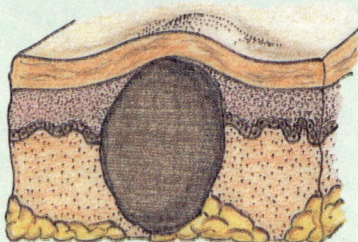

Tumor: solid mass that may extend deep through subcutaneous tissue, larger than 1 to 2 cm (e.g., epithelioma)

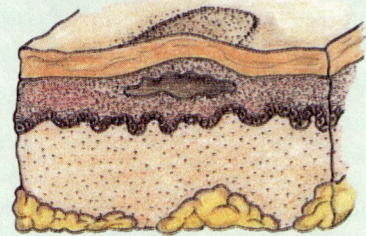

Wheal: irregularly shaped, elevated area or superficial localized edema, varies in size (e.g., hive or mosquito bite)

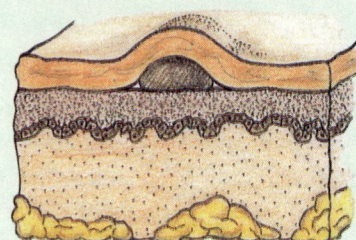

Vesicle: circumscribed elevation of skin filled with serous fluid, smaller than 0.5 cm (e.g., herpes simplex or chicken-pox)

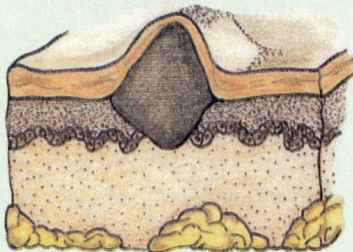

Pustule: circumscribed elevation of skin similar to vesicle but filled with pus, varies in size (e.g., acne or staphylococcal infection)

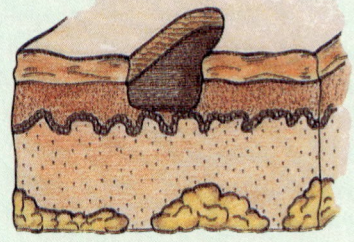

Ulcer: deep loss of skin surface that may extend to dermis and frequently bleeds and scars, varies in size (e.g., venous stasis ulcer)

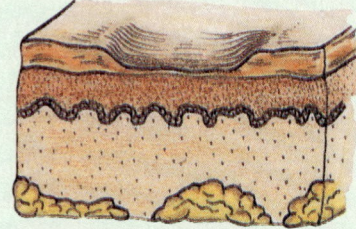

Atrophy: thinning of skin with loss of normal skin furrow with skin appearing shiny and translucent, varies in size (e.g., arterial insufficiency)

Evaluation

1. Observe throughout the assessment for evidence of physical or emotional distress.
2. Compare assessment findings with previous observations of skin.
3. Ask the client if there is information about physical condition that has not been discussed.

UNEXPECTED OUTCOMES AND RELATED INTERVENTIONS

1. Client displays signs of distress, such as shortness of breath, acute pain, or anxiety.

   a. Respond immediately to identified need (reposition, administer oxygen or medication as appropriate).

   b. Notify charge nurse or physician if orders are needed for relief of acute symptoms.

2. Client's skin has abnormal coloring, dry texture, reduced turgor, lesion, or erythema.

   a. Identify contributing factors (see Chapter 23).

   b. Prevent continued irritation and damage as appropriate (e.g., loosen constricting or pressure-causing devices, turn, provide hygiene).

3. Client is unwilling or unable to provide subjective information relating to identified concerns.
   a. Seek information from family members if present.
   b. Review client's record for baseline data.

SAMPLE DOCUMENTATION

Documentation involves the use of an assessment flow sheet (see Routine Nursing Assessment, Appendix A). Significant changes or deviations may need additional description in the nurse's progress notes.

Skill 11.2 | Auscultating Lung Sounds

Assessment of respiratory function is one of the most critical assessment skills, since alterations can be life-threatening. Routine shift assessment is essential because changes in respirations can occur quickly as a result of a variety of factors, including immobility, infection, and fluid overload. Shift assessment includes auscultation, which assesses the movement of air through the tracheobronchial tree. Normally, air flows through the airways unobstructed. Recognizing the sounds created by normal airflow allows the nurse to detect sounds

Table 11-3 Adventitious Sounds

Sound	Site auscultated	Cause	Character
Crackles (also called *rales*)	Are most commonly heard in dependent lobes: right and left lung bases	Random, sudden reinflation of groups of alveoli*	Are fine, short, interrupted crackling sounds heard during inspiration, expiration, or both; vary in pitch: high or low; may or may not change with coughing*
Gurgles (also called *rhonchi*)	Are primarily heard over trachea and bronchi; if loud enough, can be heard over most lung fields	Fluid or mucus in larger airways, causing turbulence	Are low-pitched, continuous musical sounds heard more during expiration; may be cleared by coughing
Wheezes	Can be heard over all lung fields	Severely narrowed bronchus	Are high-pitched, continuous musical sounds heard during inspiration or expiration; do not clear with coughing†
Pleural friction rub	Is heard best over anterior lateral lung field (if client is sitting upright)	Inflamed pleura, parietal pleura rubbing against visceral pleura	Has grating quality heard best during inspiration; does not clear with coughing

*Data from Forgacs P: *Chest* 73:399, 1978.
†Data from Wilkins RL, Hodgkin JE, Lopez B: *Lung sounds: a practical guide,* St. Louis, 1988, Mosby.

caused by obstruction of the airways. Auscultation of the lungs requires familiarity with landmarks of the chest. During the assessment, the nurse should keep a mental image of the location of the lung lobes.

Adventitious sounds are abnormal sounds resulting from air passing through moisture, mucus, or narrowed airways; alveoli suddenly reinflating; or an inflammation between the pleural linings. The four types of adventitious sounds include *crackles* (also referred to as *rales*), *gurgles* (also referred to as *rhonchi*), *wheezes,* and *pleural friction rub* (Table 11-3). The location and characteristics of the sounds should be noted, as well as diminished breath sounds or the absence of breath sounds (found with collapsed or surgically removed lobes). Since palpation and percussion are not included in a routine shift assessment, they are not described in this skill.

EQUIPMENT
Stethoscope

Assessment

1. Check client record to determine if client has smoking history: length of time has smoked, number of cigarettes per day, cigar or pipe smoking, or length of time since smoking stopped. (To calculate pack years, multiply the number of packs smoked per day times

the number of years a smoker; for example, ½ pack per day times 4 years equals 2 pack years.) **Smoking predisposes client to lung disease and affects secretion of mucus in airways.**

2. Ask if client is experiencing any of the following: persistent cough (productive or nonproductive), sputum production, shortness of breath (at rest or with exertion), chest pain, or orthopnea. If cough is productive, obtain a description of sputum.

3. Check for history of allergies to pollens, dust, or other airborne irritants, as well as to any foods, drugs, or chemical substances. **Allergies are associated with wheezes on auscultation, dyspnea, cyanosis, and diaphoresis.**

4. Determine the rate, rhythm, and depth of breathing (see Chapter 10). **Used to compare with baseline to assess change in client condition.**

Planning

Expected outcomes focus on identifying alterations in respiratory function.

EXPECTED OUTCOME
Client's breath sounds are clear to auscultation in all lung fields.

Implementation

Steps	Rationale

1. See Standard Protocol (Chapter 1, p. 5).
2. Position for auscultation of lungs.
  a. Have client sit upright or elevate head of bed 45 to 90 degrees for bedridden client.
  b. If client cannot tolerate sitting, supine position is allowed for anterior chest and side-lying position is used for posterior chest.
3. Remove or raise gown, avoiding unnecessary exposure and providing full visibility of thorax (Figure 11-5).
	Promotes full lung expansion during examination.

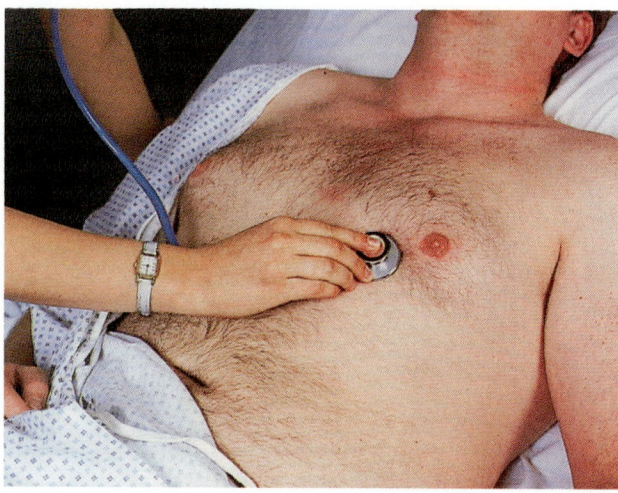

Figure 11-5

Steps	Rationale

4. Instruct client to relax and breathe deeply but normally through the mouth.

Anxiety may increase client's respiratory rate, thus interfering with analysis of findings.

5. Auscultate breath sounds. For adult, place diaphragm of stethoscope on chest wall over intercostal spaces). Move stethoscope systematically from apex of lung down to lower lobes. Ask client to take slow, deep breaths through the mouth each time you place the stethoscope on the chest.

Easy, passive movement indicates no respiratory distress.

6. Listen to entire inspiration and expiration at each stethoscope position. Systematically compare breath sounds over right and left sides. If sounds are faint, ask client temporarily to breathe harder and faster. Figures 11-6 and 11-7 identify correct posterior and anterior pattern for assessment of lungs.

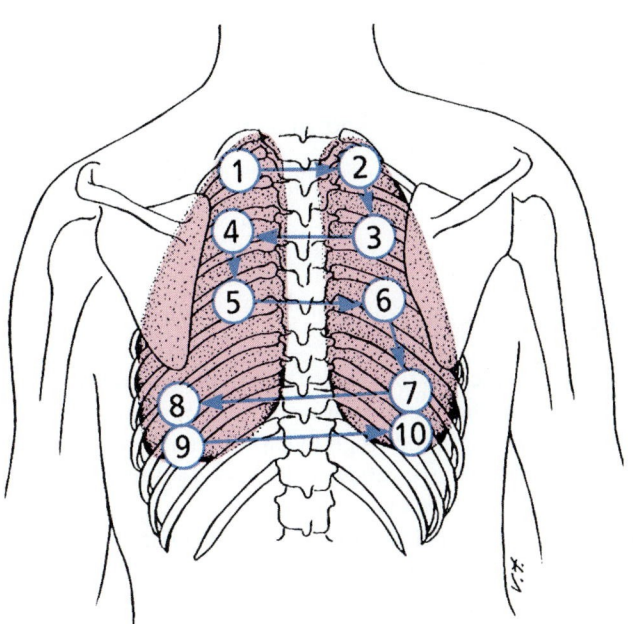

Figure 11-6   Posterior chest.

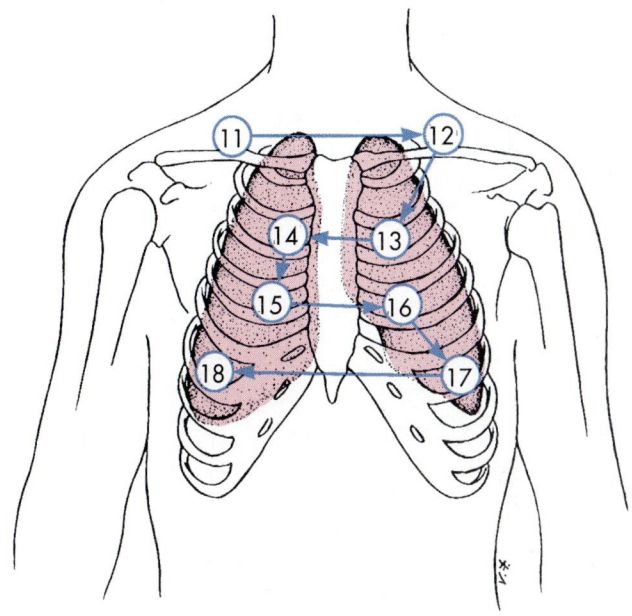

Figure 11-7   Anterior chest.

7. Assess client's respiratory character, observing symmetry and degree of chest wall and abdominal movement.

Assesses client's effort to ventilate.

8. If adventitious sounds are auscultated, have client cough. Listen again with stethoscope to determine if sound has cleared with coughing (see Table 11-3).

Gurgles caused by fluid or mucus in larger airways can be diminished or eliminated by effective coughing. Crackles may or may not change with coughing.

9. If client has a productive cough, and mucus is purulent, record amount, color, and odor of mucus. Obtaining a specimen may be indicated (see Chapter 13).

10. See Completion Protocol (Chapter 1, p. 6).

Evaluation

Compare respirations (depth, regularity, rate) and breath sounds with findings of previous shift.

UNEXPECTED OUTCOMES AND RELATED INTERVENTIONS

Client is unable to clear secretions from airway, and adventitious sounds are auscultated over one or both lungs.
a. Encourage increased fluid intake if not contraindicated.

b. Position with head of bed elevated, turning side-to-side every 2 hours.
c. If client is experiencing respiratory distress, suction and/or oxygen administration may be indicated (see Chapter 30).

SAMPLE DOCUMENTATION
0730 Wheezes noted on anterior upper lobes bilaterally. Respiratory rate 26. C/O shortness of breath even at rest. M.D. notified. HOB raised to 90 degrees.

Skill 11.3 | Auscultating Apical Pulse

The apical pulse provides information about the heart rate and rhythm. Changes in the client's pulse may result from responses to many factors, including stress, exercise, fatigue, blood loss, and pain. Responses to medications and medical treatment can also be monitored by changes in the pulse.

Auscultation of the apical pulse is done as part of the routine shift assessment after auscultation of the lungs,

since the client is already in a suitable position with the chest exposed. The nurse forms a mental image of the heart's location in the center of the chest to the left of the sternum. The apex of the heart is the bottom tip (Figure 11-8) and actually touches the anterior chest wall at approximately the fourth to fifth intercostal space along the midclavicular line, known as the point of maximal impulse (PMI).

EQUIPMENT
Stethoscope

Assessment

1. Review records for history of smoking, alcohol ingestion, cocaine use, absent or reduced regular exercise, and intake of foods high in carbohydrates and cholesterol. **These are important risk factors for cardiovascular disease.**
2. Determine medications the client is taking related to cardiovascular function (e.g., digoxin, antidysrhythmics, antihypertensives). Determine if client knows their purpose, dosage, and side effects.

Planning

Expected outcomes focus on identification of alterations in cardiovascular function.

EXPECTED OUTCOME
Client's heart rhythm is regular at a rate between 60 and 100 beats/min.

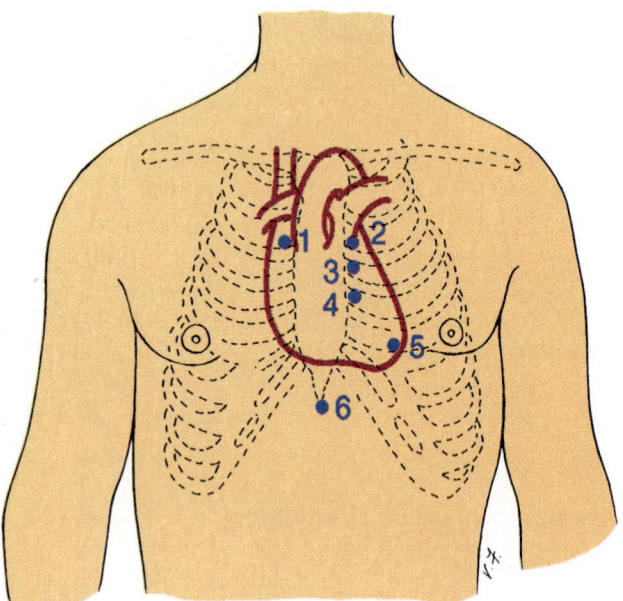

Figure 11-8

Implementation

Steps	Rationale

1. See Standard Protocol (Chapter 1, p. 5).
2. Prepare client: have client assume semi-Fowler's or supine position.

   Provides adequate visibility and access to left thorax and mediastinum. Client with heart disease may experience shortness of breath while lying flat.

3. Explain procedure and be sure client is relaxed and comfortable.

   Client with previously normal cardiac history may become anxious if nurse shows concern.

4. Locate anatomical landmarks used to assess cardiac function.

   Familiarity with landmarks allows nurse to describe findings more clearly and ultimately may improve assessment.

5. Locate PMI by palpating with fingertips along fifth intercostal space in midclavicular line (Figure 11-9). Note a light tap in an area 1 to 2 cm ($\frac{1}{2}$ to 1 inch) in diameter at the apex.

   NOTE: In the presence of cardiac enlargement associated with left-sided heart disease, PMI is located to the left of the midclavicular line. If associated with right-sided heart failure, PMI is moved toward the sternum.

6. If palpating PMI is difficult, turn client onto left side.

   Maneuver moves the heart closer to the chest wall.

7. Ask client not to speak. Using the stethoscope's diaphragm, place lightly against chest wall over the PMI (Figure 11-10).

   Pressing too firmly may decrease transmission of sounds. Cardiovascular sounds may be difficult to hear, so a quiet room and focused attention are essential (Barkauskas et al., 1994).

   a. Listen for "lub-dub" sounds (S_1 and S_2).
   b. After both sounds are heard clearly as "lub-dub," count each combination of S_1 and S_2 as one heartbeat. Count the number of beats for 1 minute to determine the apical pulse rate.

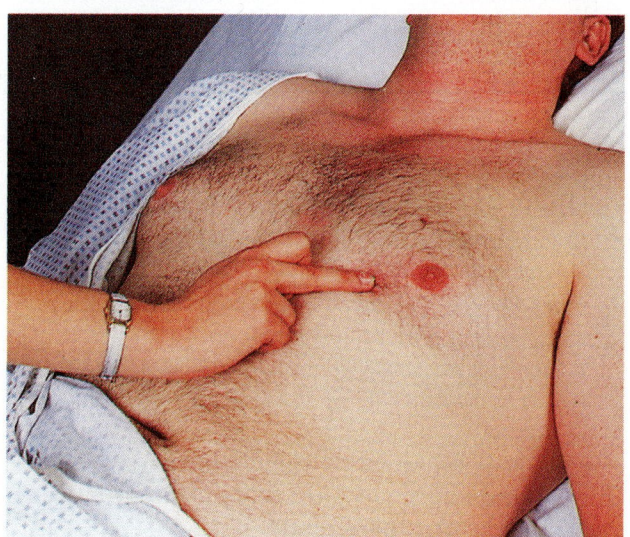

Figure 11-9

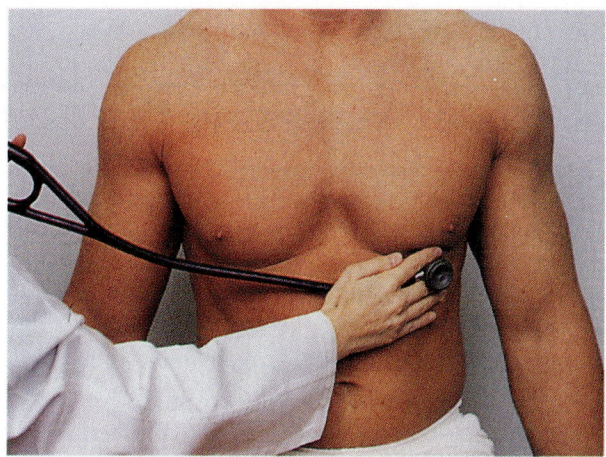

A

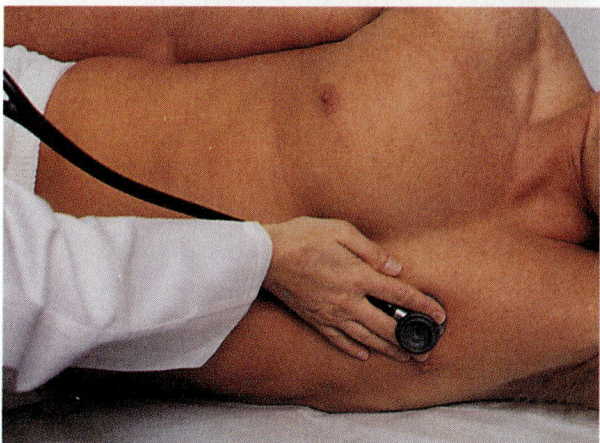

B

Figure 11-10 **A,** Sitting; **B,** lying on left side. (From Seidel HM et al: *Mosby's guide to physical examination,* ed 3, St. Louis, 1995, Mosby.)

Steps	Rationale
8. Identify if the rhythm is regular or irregular. This may be further identified as regularly irregular or irregularly irregular.	An irregular heartbeat is a dysrhythmia, which interferes with heart's ability to pump effectively and may result in decreased cardiac output.
9. When heart rate is irregular, compare apical and radial pulses. This is best done with a colleague, who can count the radial pulse simultaneously while the apical pulse rate is counted (see Chapter 12). NOTE: Additional information about cardiac assessment is included in Chapter 12.	If a pulse deficit exists (radial pulse is slower than apical), this indicates that ineffective contractions of the heart fail to send pulse waves to the periphery.
10. See Completion Protocol (Chapter 1, p. 6).	

Evaluation

Compare heart rate and rhythm with previous shift assessment.

UNEXPECTED OUTCOME AND RELATED INTERVENTIONS

Client's heart rate is irregular; rate is less than 60 or greater than 100 beats/min.

a. Respond immediately to acute distress (oxygen or medication if ordered).

b. Identify and alleviate contributing factors if possible.

c. Notify charge nurse or physician if orders are needed for relief of acute symptoms.

SAMPLE DOCUMENTATION

0730 Pulse rate 104 and irregularly irregular. Blood pressure 120/70. Client denies discomfort. Resting quietly in bed without complaints of distress. (See Routine Nursing Assessment: Cardiovascular, Appendix A.)

Skill 11.4 | Assessing the Abdomen

Routine abdominal assessment may identify changes resulting from dietary changes, procedures that interfere with peristalsis, or prolonged bed rest. Abdominal pain can be caused by many different problems relating not only to the gastrointestinal (GI) system, but also the urinary system, reproductive system, or spinal or muscular injury. When performing abdominal assessment, the nurse should maintain a mental image of the anatomical location of each of the organs, including the kidneys, which are toward the back.

Abdominal shift assessment includes inspection, auscultation, and palpation. The order of an abdominal assessment differs from previous assessments in that auscultation precedes palpation. Otherwise, palpation may alter the frequency and character of bowel sounds.

EQUIPMENT
Stethoscope
Tape measure

Assessment

1. If client has abdominal or low back pain, assess the character of pain in detail (location, onset, frequency, precipitating factors, aggravating or relieving factors, type of pain, severity). Compare findings with baseline. **Knowing characteristics of pain helps determine its source.**
2. Carefully observe client's movement and position.
    a. Lying still with knees drawn up.
    b. Moving restlessly to find a comfortable position.
    c. Lying on one side or sitting with knees drawn up to chest.
    Positions assumed by the client may reveal nature and source of pain (e.g., peritonitis, renal [kidney] stone, pancreatitis).
3. Assess when client last had a stool, character of stool, and any recent changes in character of stools.
4. Identify measures usually used to promote elimination (e.g., laxatives, enemas, dietary intake, eating and drinking habits). **This may help to identify cause and nature of elimination problems.**
5. Determine if client has had abdominal surgery or trauma. **Surgery or trauma influences approach to assessment of the abdomen and can be associated with pain.**
6. Assess if client has had any recent changes in weight or intolerance to diet (e.g., nausea, vomiting, cramp-

ing), especially in last 24 hours. **Changes may indicate stomach, gallbladder, or lower intestinal tract alterations.**

7. Assess for difficulty in swallowing, belching, flatulence, bloody emesis (hematemesis), black or tarry stools (melena), heartburn, diarrhea, or constipation.

Planning

Expected outcomes should focus on identifying alterations in function relating to organs located within the abdomen (stomach, gallbladder, intestines, kidneys).

EXPECTED OUTCOMES

1. Abdomen is soft and symmetrical with even contour. No mass, distention, or tenderness is palpable.
2. Bowel sounds are active and audible in all four quadrants.

Implementation

Steps	Rationale
1. See Standard Protocol (Chapter 1, p. 5).	
2. Prepare client.	
a. Ask if client needs to empty bladder.	Palpation of full bladder can cause discomfort and feeling of urgency and can make it difficult for client to relax.
b. Keep upper chest and legs covered.	Maintains client's warmth during examination, promoting relaxation.
c. Have client lie supine with arms down at sides. Knees may be flexed.	Position promotes optimal relaxation of abdominal muscles. Tightening of muscles prevents adequate palpation of underlying muscles.
d. Maintain conversation during assessment except during auscultation. Explain steps calmly and slowly.	

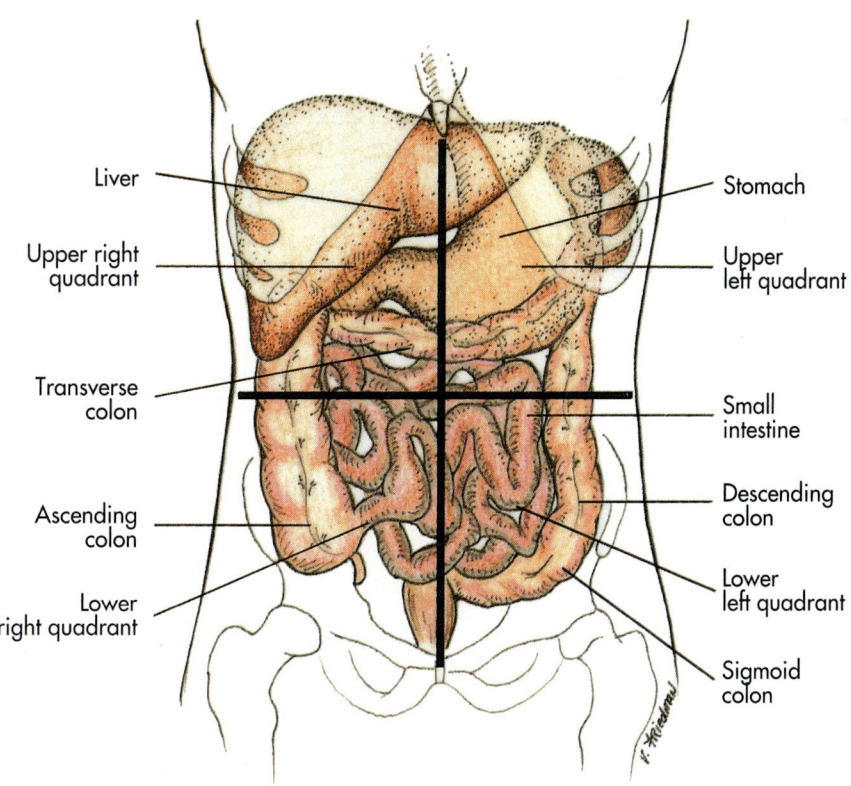

Figure 11-11

Steps	Rationale
e. Ask client to locate tender areas and assess painful areas last.	Manipulation of body part can increase pain and client's anxiety and make remainder of assessment difficult to complete.
3. Describe observations or findings in relation to quadrants. A line extending from tip of xiphoid process to symphysis pubis crossed by a line intersecting umbilicus divides abdomen into four equal sections (Figure 11-11).	Provides consistent reference points.
4. Inspect skin of abdomen's surface for scars, venous patterns, rashes, lesions, silvery white striae (stretch marks), and stomas or ostomies.	Scars reveal evidence client has had past trauma or surgery. Striae indicate stretching of tissue by growth, obesity, pregnancy, ascites, or edema. Venous patterns may reflect liver disease (portal hypertension). Artificial openings indicate bowel or urinary diversion (see Chapters 33 and 34).
5. Observe for visible pulsations and movement as client inhales and exhales.	Normal ventilation involves rhythmical movement of abdomen as diaphragm descends and rises. Normally, the aorta pulsates slightly with each beat of systole.
6. To assess bowel sounds, provide a quiet environment. Ask client not to talk. If nasogastric (NG) or intestinal tube is connected to suction, turn off momentarily.	Sound obscures bowel sounds.
7. Place the stethoscope's diaphragm lightly over each of the four abdominal quadrants. Listen until repeated gurgling or bubbling sounds are heard at each location (Figure 11-12).	

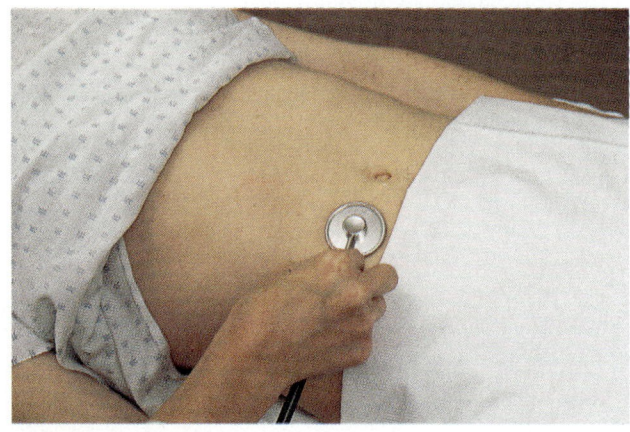

Figure 11-12 (From Doughty DB, Jackson DB: *Gastrointestinal disorders,* Mosby's Clinical Nursing Series, St. Louis, 1993, Mosby.)

Steps	Rationale
8. Describe sounds as normal or audible, absent, and hyperactive or hypoactive.	Normal bowel sounds occur irregularly every 5 to 15 seconds. Hyperactive sounds occur almost continuously. This is normal after meals. Hypoactive bowel sounds occur less than once every 15 to 20 seconds.
9. Listen 3 to 5 minutes before reporting bowel sounds are absent.	Suggests absence of peristalsis, which may require medical or surgical intervention.
10. Ask client if abdomen feels unusually tight. Observe skin for a taut, stretched, shiny appearance.	Continued sensation of fullness helps to detect distention. Feeling of fullness after a heavy meal causes only temporary distention. Tightness is not felt with obesity.
11. If distention is suspected, place tape measure around abdomen at level of umbilicus and note measurement. Compare with previous measurements if available (Figure 11-13).	Assesses changes in abdominal size. All measurements of abdominal girth should be done at the umbilicus.

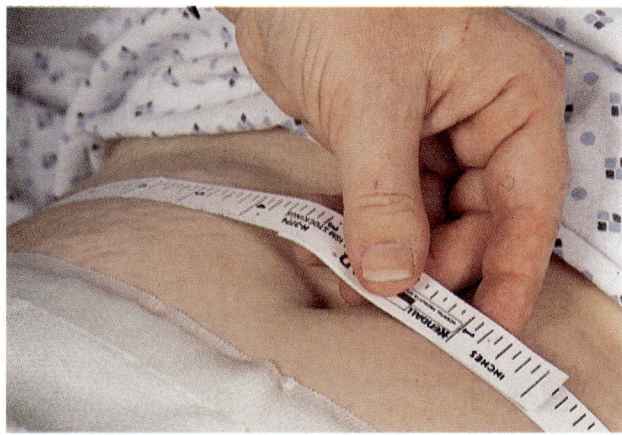

Figure 11-13

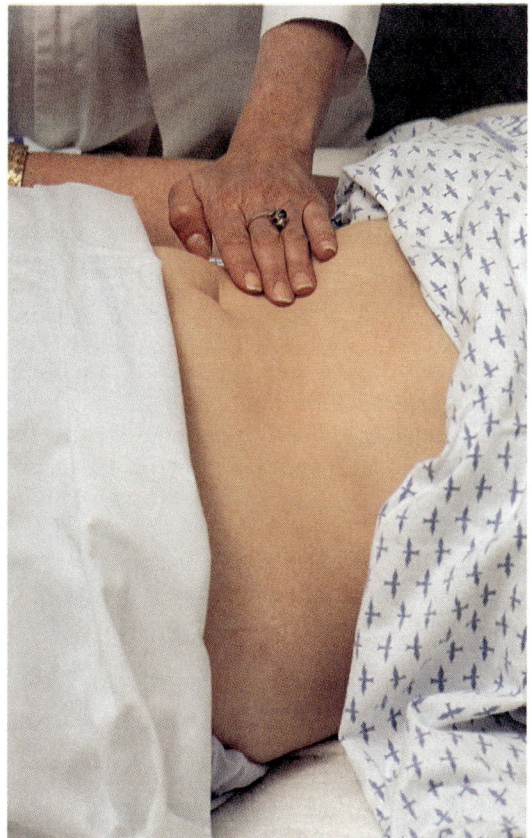

Figure 11-14

Steps	Rationale
12. Have client roll onto side. If distention is present, entire abdomen protrudes.	Distention results from accumulation of intestinal gas, a tumor, or fluid in abdominal cavity. If gas causes distention, flanks do not bulge. If fluid is source of distention, flanks bulge and protuberance forms on dependent side.
13. Lightly palpate over each abdominal quadrant, using palm and pads of fingertips in smooth, coordinated movement. Depress skin approximately 1 cm ($\frac{1}{2}$ inch). Note if abdomen is firm or soft to touch. Palpate painful areas last, avoiding quick jabs (Figure 11-14).	Detects areas of localized tenderness, degree of tenderness, and presence and character of underlying masses. Palpation of sensitive areas last minimizes guarding, which is voluntary tightening of underlying abdominal muscles.
14. Observe client's verbal and nonverbal cues, which may indicate discomfort from tenderness.	Firm abdomen may indicate accumulation of fluid or gas.
15. Palpate for a full bladder just above symphysis pubis, felt as a smooth, rounded mass.	Detects presence of a distended bladder.
16. If masses are palpated, note size, location, shape, consistency, tenderness, mobility, and texture.	Characteristics help to reveal type of mass.
17. If tenderness is present, press one hand slowly and deeply into the involved area and then let go quickly. Note if pain is aggravated.	Tests for rebound tenderness. Results are positive if pain increases. Additional assessment may include increased pain with coughing or dropping onto heels from a tiptoe position. Rebound abdominal tenderness, if found, can result from peritoneal irritation (e.g., appendicitis, pancreatitis).
18. See Completion Protocol (Chapter 1, p. 6).	

Evaluation

1. Observe throughout the assessment for evidence of discomfort.
2. Compare assessment findings with previous shift assessment.

UNEXPECTED OUTCOMES AND RELATED INTERVENTIONS

1. Client has a firm, protruding, symmetrical abdomen with taut skin. Client complains of tightness and is not passing flatus resulting in gaseous distention.
   a. Encourage ambulation (if permitted).
   b. Encourage hot liquids (if permitted).
   c. NG intubation may be required if bowel sounds are absent and client has nausea and vomiting (see Chapter 31).
2. Client has an increased abdominal girth with ascites (a buildup of fluid within peritoneal cavity).
   a. Determine the extent of the pressure, which can press against the diaphragm, causing difficulty breathing.
   b. Position with head of bed elevated to minimize discomfort.
3. Client has a distended urinary bladder palpable over the symphysis pubis.

a. If a Foley catheter is in place, check that it is properly secured and that tubing and bag are positioned to promote drainage.
   b. Ask if there has been a change in voiding pattern (ability to urinate) or pain when urinating.
   c. If unable to urinate, see Chapter 34.
4. Hyperactive bowel sounds are evident, which results from an increase in GI motility.
   a. Assess for anxiety, diarrhea, and use of laxatives, which stimulate peristalsis.
   b. Caution clients about dangers of excessive regular use of laxatives or enemas, which can result in dependence.
   c. Bowel sounds normally tend to be increased after meals.

SAMPLE DOCUMENTATION

1030 Client complains of feeling "bloated." Denies nausea. Abdomen firm and nontender. Abdominal girth increased from 38" to 41" since yesterday. Bowel sounds hypoactive. Denies passing flatus. Encouraged to drink hot tea and ambulate more frequently. (See Routine Nursing Assessment: Gastrointestinal and Abdomen, Appendix A.)

| Skill 11.5 | **Assessing Extremities and Peripheral Circulation** |

Prolonged illness or immobility may result in muscle weakness and atrophy. Hospitalized clients may experience altered peripheral circulation as a result of high or low BP, immobility, prolonged bed rest, altered fluid balance, or pressure and constriction of the extremities with dressings or a cast.

Inadequate tissue perfusion results in an inadequate delivery of oxygen and nutrients to cells, a condition called *ischemia*. This can be caused by constriction of the vessels or by occlusion (blockage) from clot formation. The effects of the ischemia depend on the duration of the problem and the metabolic needs of the tissues. Ischemia results in pain. If lack of oxygen to tissues is unrelieved, tissue necrosis (death) occurs. An embolus is a blood clot that breaks loose and travels through the circulation. If the clot obstructs circulation to the lungs or the brain, it can be life-threatening.

Assessment of extremities and circulation routinely includes inspection and palpation.

EQUIPMENT
Stethoscope

Assessment

1. Determine if client is taking medications for cardiovascular function (e.g., antidysrhythmics, antihypertensives) and if client knows their purpose, dosage, and side effects. **This allows nurse to assess client's compliance with and understanding of drug therapies. Medications for cardiovascular function cannot be taken intermittently.**
2. Ask if client experiences dyspnea, chest pain or discomfort, palpitations, excess fatigue, fainting, cyanosis, orthopnea, or edema of the feet. Ask if symptoms occur at rest or during exercise. **These are the cardinal symptoms of heart disease. Cardiovascular function may be adequate during rest but not during exercise.**
3. Ask if client experiences leg cramps, numbness or tingling in extremities, or sensation of cold appendages. Also determine if client has noted swelling of feet, ankles, or hands. **These are common signs and symptoms of peripheral vascular disease.**
4. If client experiences pain or cramping in the lower

extremities, ask if it is relieved or aggravated by walking. **Relationship of symptoms to exercise can clarify whether problem is vascular or musculoskeletal. Pain caused by vascular conditions tends to increase with activity.**

Planning

Expected outcomes focus on identifying alterations in muscle strength and altered peripheral circulation.

EXPECTED OUTCOMES

1. Client demonstrates strong grasp and leg strength that is equal bilaterally.
2. Client's peripheral pulses are normal (3+) and equal; extremities are warm and pink, with capillary refill less than 3 seconds.
3. Client has no dependent edema.

Implementation

Steps	Rationale
1. See Standard Protocol (Chapter 1, p. 5).	
2. Observe ability to use arms and hands for grasping objects (Figure 11-15).	
3. Assess muscle strength of upper extremities by asking client to grasp your hands and squeeze as hard as possible. Note weakness, and compare right with left.	Muscle weakness may be generalized or confined to certain muscle groups. Dominant side is often slightly stronger.
4. Inspect the knees, ankles, and feet for redness or swelling. Note abnormal positioning or alignment.	
5. Assess strength of lower extremities by having client move legs. Then ask client to push and pull feet against your hands. Note weakness, and compare right with left.	
6. Inspect lower extremities for changes in color and condition of the skin (Table 11-4). Note skin and nail texture, hair distribution, venous patterns, edema, and scars or ulcers.	Determines if venous or arterial insufficiency is present.

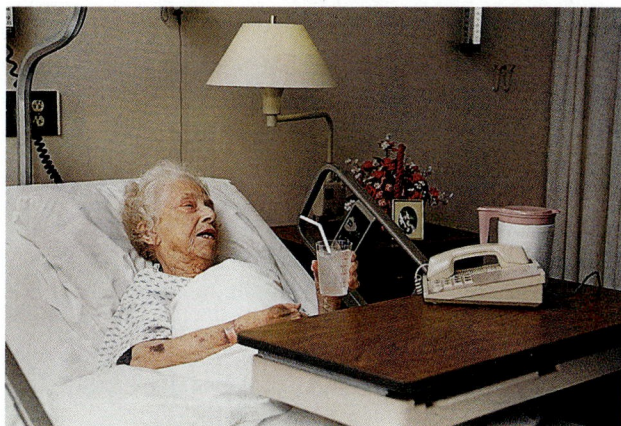

Figure 11-15

Table 11-4 **Comparison of Venous and Arterial Insufficiency**

Assessment	Arterial	Venous
Pain	Burning, throbbing, cramping, increases with exercise	Aching, increases in evening and with dependent position
Paresthesia	Numbness, tingling, decreased sensation	None
Temperature/color	Cool to touch, pale when elevated	Warm, flushed, cyanotic, brown discolorations on ankles
Capillary refill	>3 seconds	Not applicable
Pulses	Diminished or absent	Present
Ulcerations	Deep, well defined at site of trauma or tips of toes	Shallow ulcers around ankles (chronic venous stasis); edema apparent

Steps	Rationale

7. Inspect areas of skin for edema, paying particular attention to dependent body parts such as feet and ankles, sacrum, and scapular areas. Note color, location, and shape of area.

Edema results from fluid in tissues. Inadequate venous return causes edema in the sacrum if client confined to bed, in the feet and ankles if sitting. Direct trauma causes localized edema.

   a. Palpate edematous areas, noting mobility, consistency, and tenderness.

Assists in determining extent of edema.

   b. Assess for pitting edema by pressing area firmly for 5 seconds, then releasing. Depth of edema determines severity (Figure 11-16).

      2 mm indentation: +1 edema
      4 mm indentation: +2 edema
      6 mm indentation: +3 edema
      8 mm indentation: +4 edema

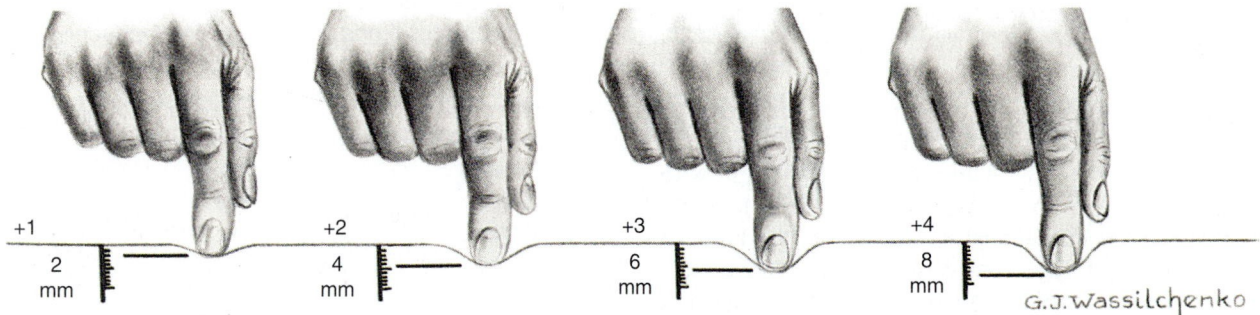

Figure 11-16 (From Canobbio MM: *Cardiovascular disorders,* Mosby's Clinical Nursing Series, St. Louis, 1990, Mosby.)

8. Check capillary refill by grasping client's fingernail, and note color of nail bed. Next, apply gentle, firm pressure with the thumb to the nail bed. Release thumb quickly. Watch for color change. On release of pressure, circulation is restored and normally returns to pink color in less than 3 seconds.

Cold temperature with vasoconstriction and vascular disease may impair refill. Local pressure from cast or bandage may also impair refill.

9. If client complains of tenderness or pain in legs, test for Homans' sign.

Homans' test for thrombophlebitis.

   a. Support the leg while flexing the foot in dorsiflexion.

   b. Note if client complains of pain.

10. Note tenderness or firmness of leg muscle and gently palpate calf muscles.

Signs of phlebitis include inflammation of veins and reddened or swollen areas over vein sites.

11. Palpate temperature of extremities with dorsum (back) of hand.

Temperature measures degree of blood flow to body part.

12. Assess each peripheral artery for following characteristics.

Palpation of peripheral arteries determines adequacy of blood flow to extremities.

   a. Elasticity of vessel wall: depress and release artery, noting ease with which it springs back to shape.

Determines integrity of vessel. Artery should be easily palpable and should return to shape after pressure is released.

   b. Rate and rhythm of pulse: measure rate for 1 minute.

Radial pulse is chosen to assess heart rate. Other peripheral pulses are assessed only to determine condition of local blood flow.

   c. Strength of pulse indicates force of blood against arterial wall.

Steps	Rationale

Rating scale for strength (Seidel, 1995):

    0: No pulse is palpable.

   1+: Pulse is difficult to palpate, weak and thready in character, and easy to obliterate.

   2+: Pulse located with light pressure, and touch senses it is stronger than 1+.

   3+: Normal pulse, easy to palpate, and not easily obliterated.

   4+: Strong pulse, easily palpated, bounds against fingertips, and cannot be obliterated.

  d. Equality of pulses: comparison of both sites allows nurse to determine any localized obstruction or disturbance in blood flow.

13. Palpate dorsalis pedis (pedal pulses). Have client lie supine with feet relaxed. Gently place fingertips between great and first toe and slowly move along groove between extensor tendons of great and first toe until pulse is palpable (Figure 11-17).

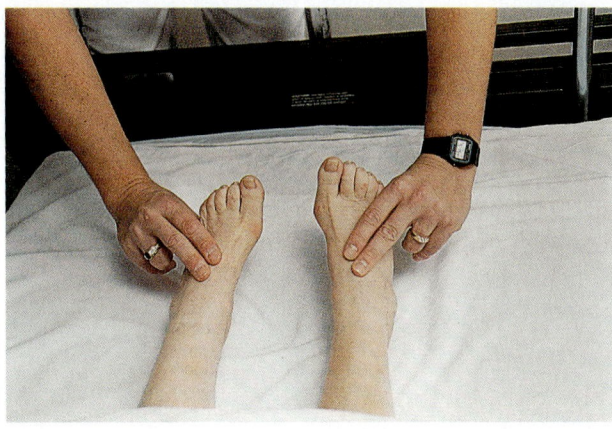

Figure 11-17

Artery lies superficially and does not require deep palpation. Too much pressure can obliterate pulse. Pulse is absent from birth in some healthy individuals.

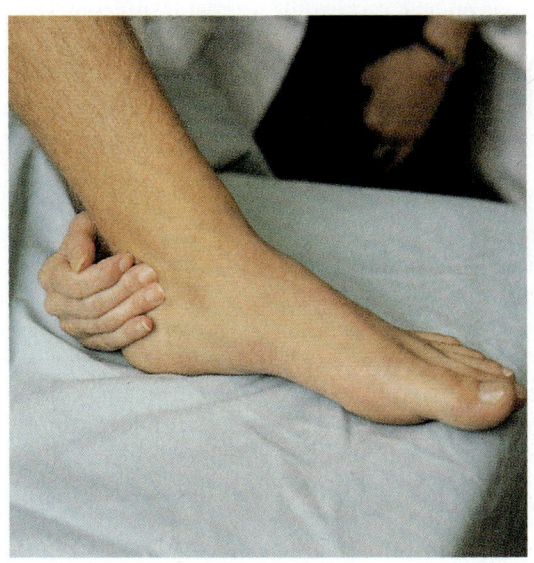

Figure 11-18

14. Palpate posterior tibial pulse. Have client relax and slightly extend feet. Place fingertips behind and below medial malleolus (ankle bone) (Figure 11-18).

Artery is easily palpable with foot relaxed.

15. If it is difficult to palpate a pulse or the pulse is not palpable, use a Doppler instrument over the pulse site (see Chapter 12).

Doppler amplifies sounds, allowing nurse to hear low-velocity blood flow through peripheral arteries.

16. See Completion Protocol (Chapter 1, p. 6).

Evaluation

1. Compare muscle strength and range of motion with previous shift assessment.
2. Compare pulses and capillary refill with previous shift assessment.
3. Compare absence or presence and extent of edema with previous shift assessment.

UNEXPECTED OUTCOMES AND RELATED INTERVENTIONS

1. Previously palpable pedal pulses are diminished or absent.

> **nurse alert** If pulses were previously palpable and cannot be located, ask another nurse to assess client's pulses. Loss of peripheral pulse must be reported to the physician immediately for appropriate medical intervention.

2. Client's lower extremities have pale, cool, thin, and shiny skin, with reduced hair growth and nail thickening, indicating chronic arterial insufficiency.
   a. Client may benefit from having legs in dependent position (hanging down) to promote circulation.
   b. Assess strength of pedal pulses. Absent pulses or pulses less than 2+ help to determine the extent of the problem.
3. Client has warm but cyanotic skin with dependent edema present in ankles; brown pigmentation is noted, indicating venous stasis (decreased venous circulation).

   Keep legs elevated to promote venous circulation.
4. Client demonstrates a positive Homans' sign, which indicates risk for clot in client's deep leg veins.
   a. Assess for redness, tenderness, and warmth.
   b. Measure circumference of both legs at the same distance from the knee to determine presence of swelling.
   c. Do not massage extremity, which could dislodge clot, resulting in an embolus.
   d. Report condition promptly to nurse in charge or physician.

SAMPLE DOCUMENTATION

1530 Client's right lower leg is red, warm, and tender to touch. Circumference of right leg is 16″ and left leg 14″. Client was instructed to remain in bed. Findings reported to Dr. H. (See Routine Nursing Assessment: Cardiovascular, Appendix A.)

CRITICAL THINKING EXERCISES

1. Josephine is a 70-year-old client admitted to the hospital for pneumonia. During shift report, the nurse notes the following findings: alert, oriented female; skin warm, dry with slight tenting; 1+ edema of the lower extremities; T 100, P 82 irregularly irregular, BP 140/82, R 22 with c/o shortness of breath; color pink; 33-pack-year smoking history; diminished breath sounds in the bases; productive cough; AP 120; client states she is "on some heart pills" but does not know dosage or exact purpose.
   a. Based on this report, differentiate normal from abnormal findings.
   b. Identify three or four diagnostic categories that would be priority problems. In parentheses, note the data that support each diagnosis.
   c. Later in the shift, you note that Josephine has rhonchi bilaterally in the upper lung fields and rales in the bases. Her respirations are 24 and labored. Compare these findings with those of the previous nurse, and offer priorities for further assessment.
2. During the 3 to 11 PM shift, Gerald, a 52-year-old male with a diagnosis of nausea and vomiting and possible bowel obstruction, is admitted to your unit. Gerald has a nasogastric (NG) tube to low suction.
   a. To assess this client's abdominal status adequately, discuss how you would proceed with your shift assessment.
   b. You determine that Gerald has four bowel sounds within a 5-minute period. Discuss the significance of this finding.
   c. On palpation, Gerald's abdomen feels firm and distended. How would you distinguish between gas and fluid as potential causes?
3. Jack is a 50-year-old black male who has come to the hospital with a complaint of cramping in the lower extremities. During shift assessment, Ed, the nurse assigned to Jack, gathers the following data:
   Cardiovascular: no c/o chest pain, shortness of breath; c/o mild fatigue
   Peripheral circulation: lower extremities cool; pedal pulses 1+ bilaterally; no dependent edema noted; sparse hair growth and thick nails on the great toes; states leg cramping is aggravated by walking; capillary refill 4 seconds; Homans' sign negative; color improved when legs dangling from edge of bed
   Musculoskeletal: hand grasp and leg strength equal bilaterally
   a. What data lead Ed to believe Jack's problem is vascular vs. musculoskeletal?
   b. Ed identifies the problem as Altered Peripheral Tissue Perfusion: Arterial. Discuss how he was able to differentiate between an arterial vs. a venous cause.

REFERENCES

Barkauskas VH et al: *Health and physical assessment,* ed 4, St Louis, 1994, Mosby.

Canobbio MM: *Cardiovascular disorders,* Mosby's Clinical Nursing Series, St Louis, 1990, Mosby.

Doughty DB, Jackson DB: *Gastrointestinal disorders,* Mosby's Clinical Nursing Series, St Louis, 1993, Mosby.

Gordon M: *Manual of Nursing Diagnosis, 1993-1994,* St Louis, 1993, Mosby.

McFarland GK, McFarlane EA: *Nursing diagnosis and intervention: planning for patient care, ed 2,* St Louis, 1993, Mosby.

Seidel HM et al: *Mosby's guide to physical examination,* ed 3, St Louis, 1995, Mosby.

ADDITIONAL READINGS

Brown M: How do you spell assessment? *Am J Nurs* 91(9):55, 1991.

Fellows E, Joez A: Getting the upper hand on lower extremity arterial disease, *Nursing* 21(8):34, 1991.

Finesilver C: Respiratory assessment, perfecting the art, *RN* 55(2):22, 1992.

Gehring P: Vascular assessment, perfecting the art, *RN* 55(1):40, 1992.

Holmgren C: Abdominal assessment, perfecting the art, *RN* 55(3):28, 1992.

McConnell EA: Clinical do's and don't's, assessing the skin: *Nursing* 22(4):86, 1992.

McGovern M, Kuhn JK: Skin assessment of the elderly client, *J Gerontol Nurs* 18(4):39, 1992.

Seidel HM et al: *Mosby's guide to physical examination,* ed 2, St Louis, 1991, Mosby.

Yacone-Norton LA: Cardiac assessment, perfecting the art, *RN* 54(12):28, 1991.

chapter 12 | Comprehensive Health Assessment

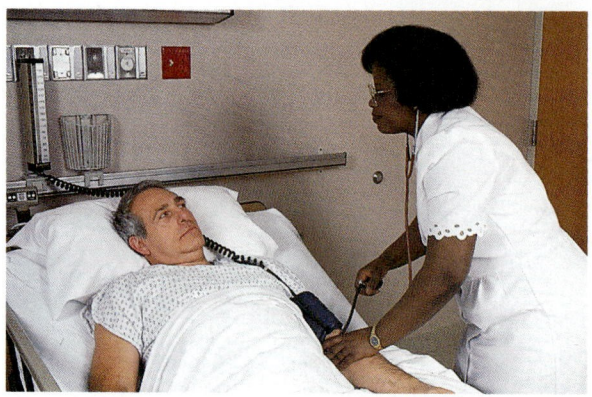

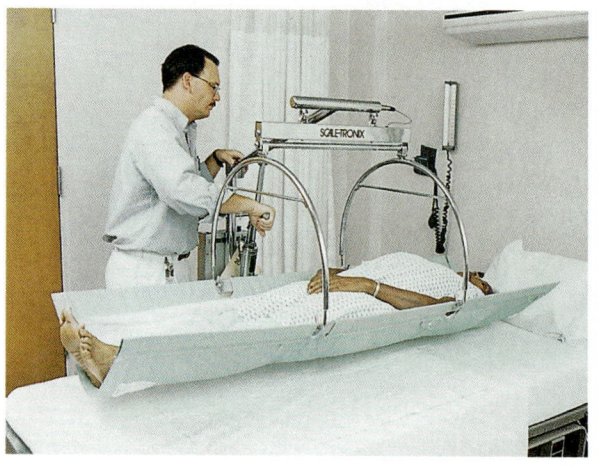

Health assessment involves a detailed review of a client's condition, with the nurse collecting a nursing history to provide a complete picture of a client's health status. The physical examination reveals information that refutes, confirms, or supplements the data base for the client. With the gathered data, the nurse groups significant findings into patterns of data that reveal nursing diagnoses. Abnormal findings require the nurse to gather additional data. Results of a health assessment and physical examination allow the nurse and the physician to collaborate on an appropriate plan of care. The information provides a baseline for the client's functional abilities and helps in the nurse's selection of nursing measures to facilitate management of the client's health problems or health promotion.

For priorities for health assessment and basics of assessment techniques, refer to Chapter 11.

SKILLS OF PHYSICAL EXAMINATION

Inspection, palpation, percussion, auscultation, and olfaction are examination techniques that enable the nurse to collect a broad range of physical data about clients. Inspection, palpation, and auscultation are skills used in the shift assessment (see Chapter 11) as well as in a comprehensive examination.

Percussion is a specialized technique that denotes location, size, and density of underlying structures. When the body's surface is struck with a finger, a vibration travels through body tissues. The sound from the vibration depends on the density of underlying tissues. Direct percussion involves striking the body surface directly with one or two fingers. Indirect percussion involves placing the middle finger of the examiner's nondominant hand firmly against the body surface. With palm and fingers remaining off the skin, the tip of the middle finger of the dominant hand strikes the other using a quick, sharp stroke (Figure 12-1). The wrist must remain relaxed to deliver the proper blow. Accurate use of percussion takes time and practice.

There are five different percussion sounds. *Tympany* is a drumlike sound that indicates an air-containing space (e.g., gastric air bubble, puffed-out cheek). *Resonance* is a hollow sound heard over a normal lung. *Hyperresonance* is a louder booming sound heard over a hyperin-

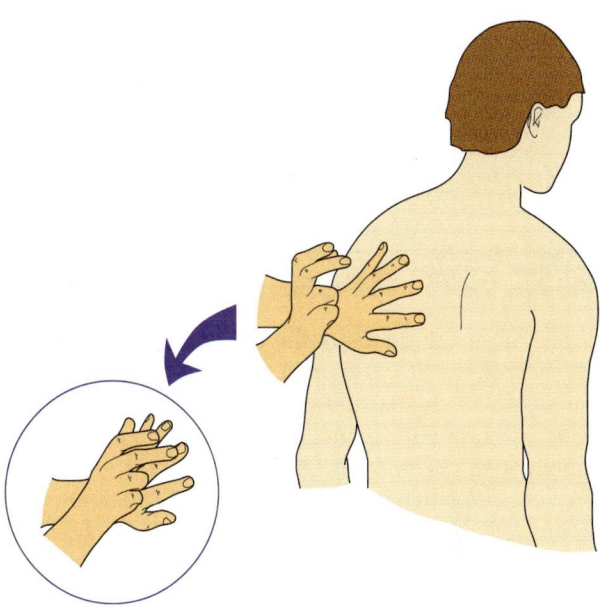

Figure 12-1 Percussing the chest.

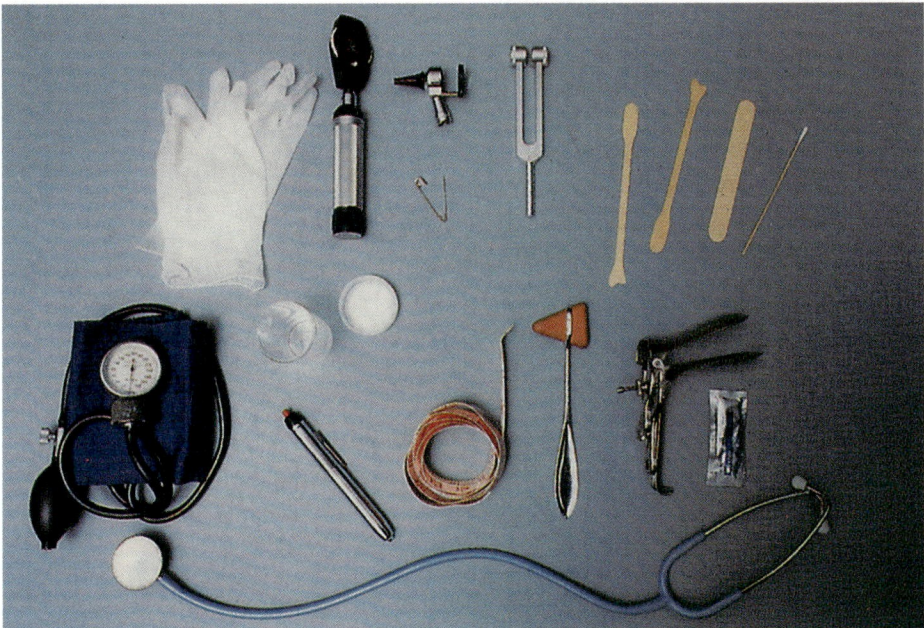

Figure 12-2 Standard equipment for physical assessment. Equipment shown includes: *(top, left to right)* disposable gloves, ophthalmoscope with battery handle, otoscope attachment, safety pin, tuning fork, cervical spatulas, tongue depressor, cotton-tip swab; *(middle, left to right)* sphygmomanometer, specimen cup, penlight, tape measure, reflex hammer, vaginal speculum, lubricant; *(bottom)* stethoscope.

flated lung, as with emphysema. *Dullness* is a soft or moderate thud, as heard over the liver. *Flatness* is a soft sound heard over muscle. Each sound allows an examiner to locate anatomical landmarks as well as underlying abnormalities.

A variety of instruments are used for physical examination. Instruments should be clean or sterile and in good working order. An ophthalmoscope has a light and system of lenses and mirrors that is used to examine the interior structures of the eyes. An otoscope illuminates the inner ear canal and tympanic membrane (eardrum). It can also be used for examination of the nose. A percussion (reflex) hammer is used to test deep tendon reflexes. A vaginal speculum is used to examine the vaginal canal and cervix. A tuning fork can be used to test hearing and vibratory perception. (See Figure 12-2.) All equipment should be ready for use when an examination begins. This prevents delays, thus ensuring a smooth, organized approach.

Skill 12.1 | Assessing Mental Health Status

Mental health status is the initial step in a comprehensive health assessment. Mental health status encompasses six mental and emotional components: orientation, attention and concentration, judgment, memory, thought content and processes, and mood and affect. The level of consciousness is a priority concern. The client's level of consciousness influences the ability to follow directions and participate in a complete health assessment and examination.

Nonverbal observation findings such as crying, frowning, or a masklike face give the nurse clues for further questioning of a client's mental health. Mental health status can be impacted by situational and maturational crises. The client's race, culture, gender, and age also need to be considered. These important variables influence assessment findings and techniques used.

Nursing Diagnosis

Altered Thought Processes is appropriate when the client lacks orientation to time, place, person, and/or event or demonstrates an abnormality in any of the six components of the mental health examination.

EQUIPMENT
None

Assessment

1. Assess if the client is pain free and comfortable without recent pain medication.
2. Assess if the client has a history of deviations in mental status and if these are recent or longstanding.
3. Determine if the client is taking medications such as analgesics, sedatives, hypnotics, antipsychotics, antidepressants, or nerve stimulants. **Medications can depress mental status or cause agitation.**

Planning

EXPECTED OUTCOMES
1. Client is alert, oriented, and responds appropriately to all questions.
2. Client demonstrates immediate recall of recent and past events.
3. Client is able to interpret abstract ideas and make associations of related concepts.

Table 12-1 **Glasgow Coma Scale**

Action	Response	Score
Eyes open	Spontaneously	④
	To speech	3
	To pain	2
	None	1
Best verbal response	Oriented	⑤
	Confused	4
	Inappropriate words	3
	Incomprehensible sounds	2
	None	1
Best motor response	Obeys commands	⑥
	Localized pain	5
	Flexion withdrawal	4
	Abnormal flexion	3
	Abnormal extension	2
	Flaccid	1
	Total Score	⑮

From Potter PA, Perry AG: *Basic nursing,* ed 3, St. Louis, 1995, Mosby.

Implementation

Steps	Rationale
1. See Standard Protocol (Chapter 1, p. 5). **2.** Assess mental and emotional status. a. Assess level of consciousness (LOC), directing questions and giving instructions that require response. Be sure client is as fully awake as possible before testing alertness.	Alteration in mental status may result from brain disorders, drug effects, or electrolyte and metabolic changes. Nurse can assess client's optimal level of alertness only by being assured client is fully responsive.
b. Use Glasgow Coma Scale (GCS) to measure consciousness objectively (Table 12-1).	GCS is used to evaluate neurological status over time. The higher the score, the more normal the level of function.

c. Note appropriateness of emotions, responses, and ideas expressed.
  d. Rephrase or ask similar questions if it is uncertain whether client understands.
  e. If client has inappropriate responses, ask questions such as, "Tell me your name," "Tell me where you live," "Tell me what day this is," and "Tell me the name of this place."
	Measures client's orientation to person, place, and time within environment.

f. If client is unable to respond to questions of orientation, offer simple commands: "Squeeze my fingers" or "Move your toes."
  g. When client fails to respond to verbal command, test painful stimuli response.
    (1) Apply firm pressure with thumb on root of client's fingernail. Client's inappropriate response may be caused by a communication or language problem rather than deterioration of mental status.
    (2) Avoid pinching skin to elicit response.
	LOC exists along a continuum from fully alert and responsive, to inability to initiate meaningful behaviors consciously, to unresponsiveness to external stimuli.
	The more reduced the level of consciousness, the greater the impairment of cerebral function.
	Client should withdraw from pain.
	
	Causes bruising.

3. Assess behavior and appearance.
  a. Observe client's mannerisms and actions. Note response to directions and what mood client displays. Does client participate with examination?
  b. Observe manner of speech.
 	
  c. Observe appearance: hygiene, cleanliness, appropriateness of makeup, clothes (state of repair, appropriateness to weather and setting).
	Mood and behavioral responses may indicate a specific disease process. Client is normally concerned and anxious about findings. Euphoria or lack of concern is inappropriate.
	Tone, pitch of voice, and speed of spoken word may reveal mood and behavior status.
	Appearance can reflect numerous conditions. An unkempt appearance may reflect poor self–image, inability to groom, an emergency, inability to keep clothing clean or a lack of finances or resources.

4. Assess language function. If unclear client communication, assess the following, asking client to:
  a. Name a familiar object to which you point.
  b. Respond to a simple verbal or written command such as, "Sit up."
  c. Read simple sentences out loud.
	Assesses client's ability to understand spoken or written English words.

5. Assess intellectual function. a. Ask client to repeat a short series of numbers forward, then backward (e.g., 7, 3, 1, 4). Gradually increase number of digits until client fails to repeat digits correctly.	Assesses immediate recall. Normally a person can recite a series of five to eight digits forward and four to six backward.

Steps	Rationale
b. Ask client to recall what was eaten for breakfast or the form of transportation used to arrive at the clinic or hospital. Validate accuracy with family member.	Assesses recent memory.
c. Ask client to recall birthday and previous medical history or family history.	Assesses past memory.
d. Ask what client knows about illness or reason for examination or hospitalization.	Assesses knowledge level and ability to learn.
e. Have client explain meaning of simple proverb such as, "Don't count your chickens before they hatch." Note if explanation is literal or abstract.	Determines ability for higher level of intellectual functioning for abstract thinking. Client with altered mentation interprets phrase literally or merely rephrases words.
f. Ask client to identify similarities or associations between terms or simple concepts, for example, "A dog is to a beagle as a cat is to a ___ " or "What do a tree and a rose have in common?"	Association is a higher intellectual function.
6. See Completion Protocol (Chapter 1, p. 6).	

Evaluation

1. Observe client responses: relates history in clear, sequential, and logical manner; answers questions directly without drifting from the subject; accurately recalls history and facts; and indicates ability to manage various aspects of life.
2. Observe client to exhibit subtle, sustained mood with mild anxiety during assessment and appropriate fluctuations of affect according to subject being discussed.
3. Observe that client regarded examiner appropriately during interaction.
4. Ask client if any information about mental state has not been discussed.

UNEXPECTED OUTCOMES
AND RELATED INTERVENTIONS

1. Client is confused and at times difficult to arouse by verbal stimulus.
   Stop examination and investigate reasons for confusion.
2. Client is not consistently oriented to person, place, time, or events.
   Provide reality orientation as needed.

3. Speech is slow and slurred.
   Provide more time for examination. If this represents a change, notify M.D.
4. Client is able to recall past events but unable to repeat a series of five numbers.
   Be sure to note age of client; older adults may normally have this problem.
5. Client is unable to interpret proverbs or associate related concepts.
   Reassess client's cultural and educational background. Nurse may need to rephrase concepts in terms with which client is familiar.

SAMPLE DOCUMENTATION

0800 Client exhibits orientation to person, place, time, and events. Past and recent memory intact. Higher level of intellect demonstrated by interpretation of proverb and association of related concepts. Responded to questioning quickly and with cooperation. Denies mood swings.

Skill 12.2 | Assessing the Head, Face, and Neck

Although many structures are located in the head, neck, and face, this skill focuses on the skull, face, thyroid gland, trachea, and lymph node chains. Assessment of the carotid and jugular veins is usually deferred until the cardiovascular assessment (Skill 12.6). Facial muscles are innervated by cranial nerve (CN) V (trigeminal) and CN VII (facial). The function of these nerves is also tested as part of the neurological examination (Skill 12.9) but is usually carried out at this time. The assessment techniques are normally painless and involve inspection, palpation, and auscultation.

Nursing Diagnosis

Risk for Infection is appropriate when the assessment findings reveal enlarged lymph nodes with accompanying signs and symptoms. An enlarged node alone does not indicate infection. **Impaired Skin Integrity** is appropriate when lesions are found on the scalp, face, or neck.

EQUIPMENT
Stethoscope
Transparent pocket ruler
Cup of water

Assessment

1. Assess client for a history of recent cold or infection.
2. Determine if client has history of thyroid problem or takes thyroid medicine.
3. Ask if client has history of neck pain or has noted any enlargements or nodules.
4. Determine if medical condition indicates pneumothorax, hemothorax, pleural effusion, or bronchial tumor.

Planning

EXPECTED OUTCOMES
1. Client has no deviations from normal:
   a. Lymph nodes are nonpalpable, small, mobile, and nontender.
   b. Trachea is at midline.
   c. Facial nerves are intact.
   d. Scalp is clean and intact.
2. Client responds appropriately to instructions.

Implementation

Steps	Rationale
1. See Standard Protocol (Chapter 1, p. 5).	
2. Have client sit upright. Ask client to remove wigs, hairpieces, or toupees. Nurse examines posterior, lateral, and anterior skull and scalp.	Provides easy access.
3. Inspect and palpate the following:	
a. Skull for size, shape, contour, and position.	Note size in proportion to overall body size; ovoid shape; long diameter on anteroposterior axis; symmetrical and smooth with prominent occipital and frontal areas. Assess lesions in same manner as for skin lesions (see Skill 11.1). Use ruler to size lesions.
b. Scalp for color, texture, lesions, hygiene, and tenderness. Part hair in several areas to inspect fully.	
c. Face for color, proportions, expressions, and movement.	May reveal facial nerve involvement.
4. Assess trigeminal and facial nerves.	Determines presence of bilateral equal muscle strength.
a. CN V: Instruct client to clench teeth while examiner palpates muscles over jaw (Figure 12-3).	
b. CN VII: Instruct client to raise eyebrows, close eyes tightly, frown, smile, show teeth, and puff out cheeks (Figure 12-4).	Reveals symmetrical facial movement.
5. Palpate temporal artery bilaterally for rhythm and tenderness.	

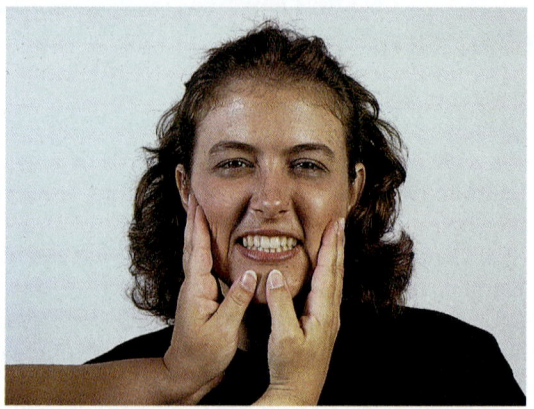

Figure 12-3 (From Chipps E et al: *Neurologic disorders,* Mosby's Clinical Nursing Series, St. Louis, 1992, Mosby.)

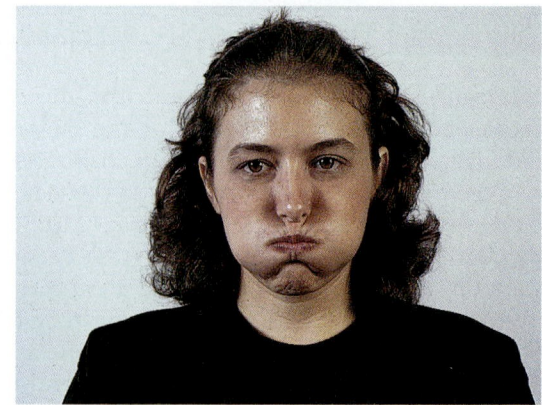

Figure 12-4 (From Chipps E et al: *Neurologic disorders,* Mosby's Clinical Nursing Series, St. Louis, 1992, Mosby.)

Steps	Rationale
6. Assess CN XI (spinal accessory). Instruct client to shrug shoulders against resistance of examiner's hands and then to turn head to one side against resistance of examiner's hand.	Maneuver shows ability to oppose resistance or presence of pain, weakness, or discomfort.
7. Inspect neck for symmetry, masses, scars, movement, and range of motion (ROM).	When evaluating ROM, proceed slowly and judge each movement separately.
a. Have client flex neck with chin toward sternum.	Observe for reduced flexion less than 70 degrees.
b. Have client extend neck with chin pointing toward the ceiling without tensing neck muscles. Palpate any apparent masses to determine size, shape, tenderness, consistency, and mobility. Use pads of fingers.	Neck extension provides for exposure of underlying structures. Observe for reduced extension less than 30 degrees. Tensing muscles prevents access to lymph nodes for palpation.
c. Have client bend neck laterally with ear toward shoulder, then rotate neck, with chin toward shoulder, right and left.	Observe for reduced lateral bending less than 35 degrees from midline and rotation with chin less than 70 degrees.
8. Inspect and palpate trachea for location. Place the thumbs on each side of the trachea, just above the suprasternal notch (Figure 12-5). Note space between thumb and sternocleidomastoid muscle. Trachea is normally in midline above suprasternal notch. Avoid forceful pressure.	Gentle palpation prevents eliciting cough reflex.

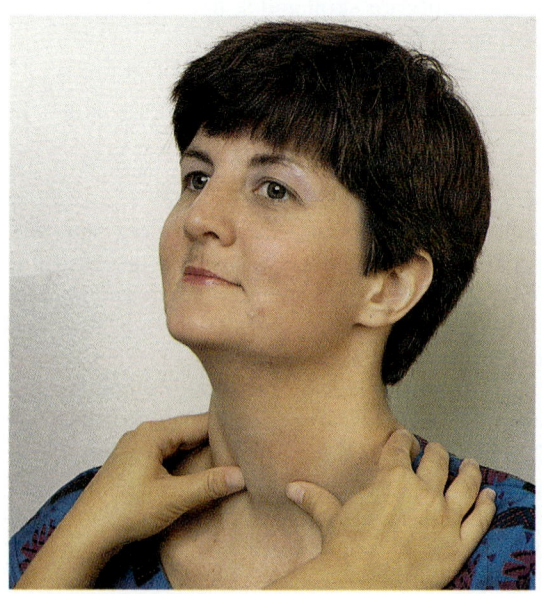

Figure 12-5 (From Belcher AE: *Cancer nursing,* Mosby's Clinical Nursing Series, St. Louis, 1992, Mosby.)

Steps	Rationale

9. Assess lymph nodes.
   a. Inspect both sides of neck as client relaxes with neck slightly flexed forward.

   b. Stand either in front of or to the side of client and palpate each lymph node chain systematically. Use pads of fingers and gently palpate in rotary fashion over region where nodes are normally found. Be sure to press underlying tissue. Note size, shape, location, mobility, symmetry, and surface characteristics (Figure 12-6).

   c. Ask client to bend head forward and relax shoulders. Palpate supraclavicular nodes. It may be necessary to hook the index and third fingers over the clavicle, lateral to the sternocleidomastoid muscle, to palpate these nodes.

10. See Completion Protocol (Chapter 1, p. 6).

Allows for clear view of all lymph node chains.

Improves access for node palpation. Methodical palpation over each lymph chain prevents omission of any nodes. Vigorous palpation may obliterate small nodes and cause stimulation of carotid sinus with a slowing of the heart rate.

Position relaxes the muscles to ease palpation of nodes.

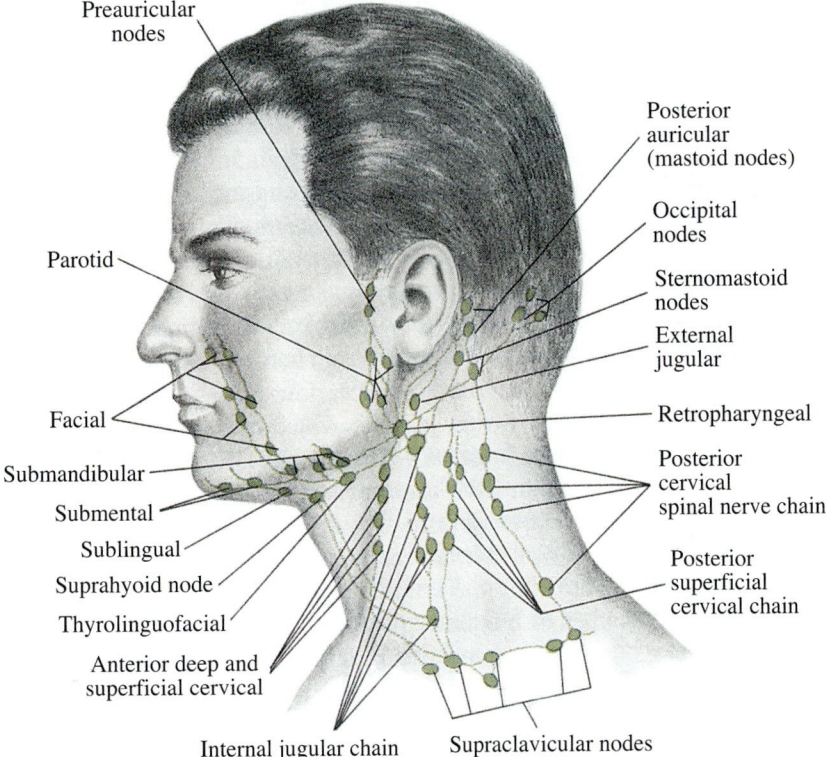

Figure 12-6 (From Seidel HM et al: *Mosby's guide to physical examination,* ed 3, St. Louis, 1995, Mosby.)

Labels: Preauricular nodes, Parotid, Facial, Submandibular, Submental, Sublingual, Suprahyoid node, Thyrolinguofacial, Anterior deep and superficial cervical, Internal jugular chain, Posterior auricular (mastoid nodes), Occipital nodes, Sternomastoid nodes, External jugular, Retropharyngeal, Posterior cervical spinal nerve chain, Posterior superficial cervical chain, Supraclavicular nodes

Evaluation

1. Compare findings with client's baseline and normal expected findings.
2. Ask for feedback on whatever instruction was given to the client.

UNEXPECTED OUTCOMES AND RELATED INTERVENTIONS

1. Lymph nodes are palpable, nontender, fixed, and hard.
   Refer to physician; fixed, hard, nontender nodule may indicate malignant lesion.

2. Lymph nodes are large, tender, and mobile.
   a. Ask more questions about infection, since findings indicate inflammation or infection.
   b. Check temperature.
3. Trachea is deviated to right or left.
   Assess for lung problems, including degree of respiratory distress (Skill 12.5).

SAMPLE DOCUMENTATION

1000 Head, face, and neck negative for any lesions and lymph node enlargement.

Skill 12.3 | Assessing the Nose, Sinuses, and Mouth

Assessment of the client's nose and sinuses takes little time, and procedures are relatively simple using inspection and palpation. If clients have nasogastric (NG) or nasotracheal tubes (NT) inserted, however, the nurse should take care to inspect the nasal mucosa thoroughly. Presence of the tubes can cause mucosal irritation and even erosion. Nasal flaring, especially in children, may indicate respiratory difficulty. Discharge from one nostril may be caused by a foreign body in the nares.

Condition of the oral cavity can reveal significant information about a client's health, such as state of hydration, nutritional status, hygiene practices, and specific pathological conditions. The procedure is to be done thoroughly so as not to miss a lesion or local area of inflammation under or around the tongue and along the mucosal surfaces. A convenient time to perform this assessment is during administration of oral hygiene.

Nursing Diagnosis

Ineffective Breathing Pattern is appropriate when a client's inhalation or exhalation pattern is inadequate. **Pain** is appropriate when open lesions or inflammation occur. **Altered Oral Mucous Membrane** is appropriate when observation reveals a break in the oral mucosa. **Bathing/Hygiene Self-Care Deficit** is appropriate if the client exhibits inability to use upper extremities or lacks availability of a care giver.

EQUIPMENT

Tongue depressor
Penlight
Disposable gloves
Gauze square

Assessment

1. Determine if client has experienced any trauma to the nose or mouth.
2. Assess if client has history of allergies, nasal discharge, epistaxis, postnasal drip, smoking, chewing tobacco, alcohol consumption, recent change in appetite, dentures (comfort and fit), and dental hygiene practices.
3. Ask if client uses nasal sprays, drops, or sniffs toxic substances.
4. Ask if client snores at night or has difficulty breathing through the nose.

Planning

EXPECTED OUTCOMES

1. Client has no deviations from normal:
   a. Nose is aligned, symmetrical, without obvious lesions, and nontender.
   b. Nasal mucosa is pink, clear, and dry; septum is midline.
   c. Sinuses are nontender and glow when illuminated.
   d. Mouth mucosa is glistening pink or red, soft, moist, and smooth.
   e. Teeth, if present, are white, smooth, and shiny.
   f. Gums are pink, moist, smooth, and firm.
   g. Tongue is midline, moist, and mobile, with smooth lateral margins.
   h. Client is able to explain recommended hygiene schedule, proper use of nasal spray, and signs of oral cancer.
2. Client is able to describe appropriate hygiene measures, use of nasal spray, and signs of oral cancer.

Implementation

Steps	Rationale
1. See Standard Protocol (Chapter 1, p. 5).	
2. Examine nose and sinuses.	
a. Inspect nose externally for placement, alignment, and symmetry. If swelling or deformities exist, palpate more gently for tenderness, swelling, or deviations.	Asymmetry may indicate trauma and may affect patency.
b. Use penlight to illuminate anterior nares and inspect nasal mucosa and position of septum at anterior end of nose.	Reveals any nasal obstruction interfering with breathing. Character of discharge and inflammation reveals allergy (clear or whitish color) or infection (yellowish color).
c. If nasogastric or nasotracheal tubes are present, inspect nares for excoriation, inflammation, or sloughing of skin.	Swallowing or coughing reflex causes movement of tubes against nares. Failure to anchor tube properly results in pressure against mucosa.

Steps	Rationale

d. Ask client to tip head back slightly. Inspect septum for deviation, lesions, or superficial blood vessels.

Position provides clear view of septum and turbinate.

e. Palpate frontal sinus by placing thumb over ridge of upper orbit of each eye and pressing gently upward (Figure 12-7).

Pressure elicits tenderness if sinus is swollen or inflamed.

f. Palpate maxillary sinuses by placing thumbs over maxillary sinus, just to each side of nose, and applying gentle upward pressure (Figure 12–8).

Elicits tenderness in presence of inflammation.

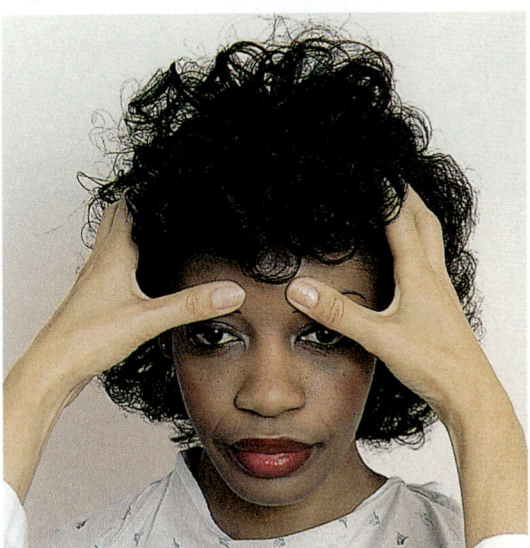

Figure 12-7 (From Wilson SF, Thompson JM: *Respiratory disorders,* Mosby's Clinical Nursing Series, St. Louis, 1990, Mosby.)

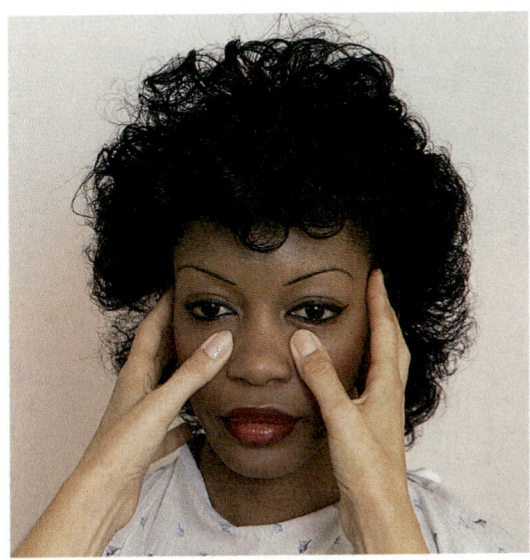

Figure 12-8 (From Wilson SF, Thompson JM: *Respiratory disorders,* Mosby's Clinical Nursing Series, St. Louis, 1990, Mosby.)

g. Shine penlight against the inner aspect of the supraorbital ridge of the frontal bone. Darken room for better visualization.

Light passes through bone to illuminate frontal sinuses. Normally the light outlines the sinuses.

h. Place penlight below each orbital ridge while inspecting the hard palate through the client's open mouth. Look for areas of darker color.

3. **Examine mouth.**

a. Have client open mouth halfway and inspect lips for color, texture, hydration, contour symmetry, and lesions.

Provides full view of lips. Asymmetry may be caused by paralysis.

b. Inspect inner mucosa by gently pulling lower then upper lip from teeth (Figure 12–9). Note color, texture, hydration, and any ulcers, abrasions, or cysts.

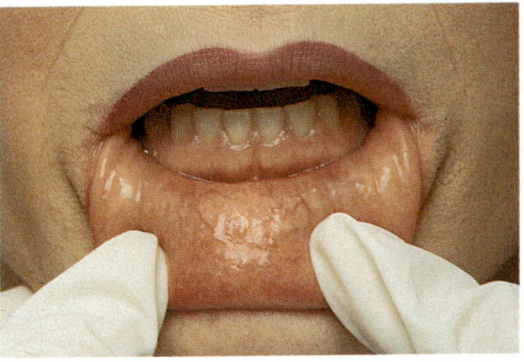

Figure 12-9

Steps	Rationale

c. If lesions present, palpate with fingers for tenderness, size, and consistency.

d. Ask client to open mouth; inspect lining of cheeks by gently retracting lips and cheeks with tongue depressor. View surface of mucosa right to left and top to bottom (Figure 12–10).

e. Palpate cheek with one finger along the inner mucosa and the thumb along the outside cheek.

f. While retracting cheeks, inspect gums for color, edema, retraction, bleeding, and lesions. Ask if client has any tenderness. If client wears dentures, be sure they are removed.

Allows discrimination between cancerous lesion, ulceration, and cyst.

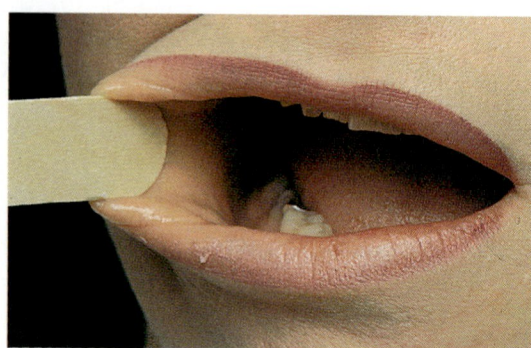

Figure 12-10

g. Palpate gums gently with tongue blade and note resistance.

h. To examine teeth, ask client to open lips and clench teeth. Note position of teeth. Ask to open mouth wide and note caries or missing teeth.

i. To assess tongue, ask client to relax mouth and protrude tongue halfway. Note color, size, position, and texture. Ask client to elevate it, then move it side to side. Illuminate with penlight.

j. Inspect undersurface of tongue by asking client to lift tongue toward roof of mouth (Figure 12-11).

Client may fear sensation of inability to swallow. Detects areas of hardening.

May reveal hygiene or chewing problems.

Tongue should move freely.

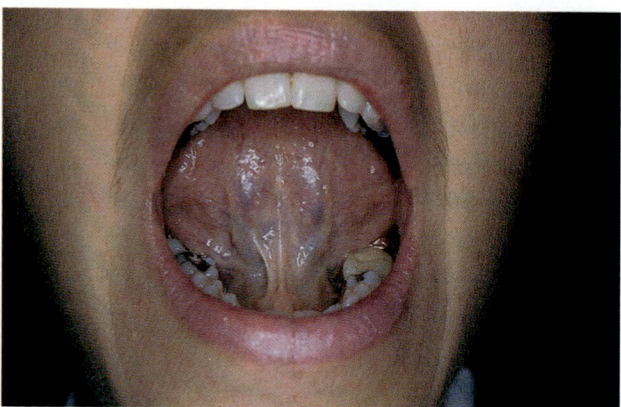

Figure 12-11

k. To palpate tongue, first explain procedure. Then, as client protrudes tongue, grab tip with gauze and gently retract to side. Palpate full length of tongue, base, and any lesions of floor of the mouth. Release tongue.

l. With client extending head backward and holding mouth open, inspect hard and soft palates using penlight for illumination.

Undersurface of tongue and floor of mouth are common sites for cancerous lesions.

Hard palate is anterior; soft palate extends toward pharynx.

Steps	Rationale
m. Ask client to say "ah." Place tongue blade on middle third of tongue (Figure 12-12).	Tongue depressor placed anteriorly may cause posterior tongue to mound up and obstruct view; placed posteriorly may elicit gag reflex. Assesses CN X (vagus). Uvula and soft palate should rise without deviation to either side.
n. With penlight, inspect posterior pharynx, including anterior and posterior tonsillar pillars. Observe color, hydration, drainage, and any lesions. Note the tonsils in cavity between the pillars. 4. See Completion Protocol (Chapter 1, p. 6).	Common sites for infection. 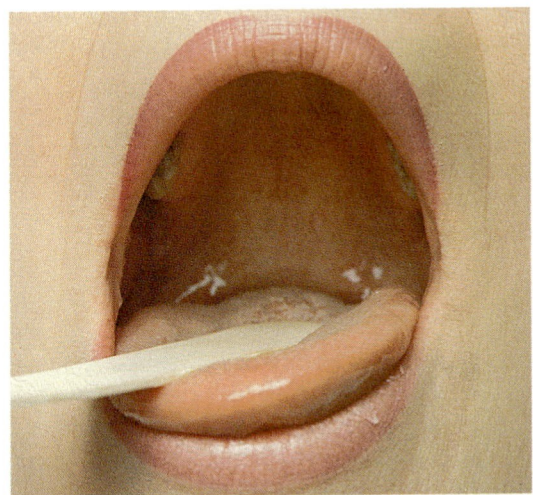 Figure 12-12

Evaluation

1. Compare findings with client's baseline and normal expected findings.
2. Ask client to describe recommended hygiene schedule, indications for use of nasal spray, or signs of oral cancer.

UNEXPECTED OUTCOMES AND RELATED INTERVENTIONS

Client has evidence of asymmetry, inflammation, drainage, lesions, tenderness, dry mucosa, or inadequate oral hygiene. Tongue is edematous and coated. Sinuses are tender or obstructed. Illuminated areas are dark in color.

a. Ask client more details about history as related to findings.
b. Group significant findings into patterns of data that reveal actual or high-risk diagnoses.
c. Identify functional abilities and concerns.
d. Communicate pertinent findings to appropriate health care team member.

SAMPLE DOCUMENTATION

0900 Nasal passages patent without deviation, lesions, or abnormal drainage. Oral mucous membranes and palates clear and moist without lesions, redness, or tenderness. Full dentition without cavities. Intact cranial nerve X.

Skill 12.4 | Assessing the Eyes and Ears

Vision is vital to performing activities of daily living (ADLs), communicating effectively with others, and analyzing and learning about events. Clients often have preexisting visual alterations or may be undergoing diagnostic or therapeutic procedures that can impair vision.

A hearing disorder is caused by one of four types of problems: (1) mechanical dysfunction—blockage of external ear by cerumen or a foreign body; (2) trauma impact, blows, falls, and motor vehicle accidents—foreign bodies or excess noise exposure; (3) neurological disorders—auditory nerve damage (e.g., after use of medications); and (4) acute illnesses after inner ear infection. Conduction deafness results from sound waves failing to pass through external or middle ear structures; it is often curable. Nerve deafness, which involves the internal ear, is more serious.

Examination of the eyes include skills for assessing visual acuity, visual fields, extraocular movements, and external eye structures. Assessment of the ear includes inspection of the external ear and the test for gross hearing.

Nursing Diagnosis

Risk for Injury is appropriate when the deficit impairs the client's ability to be functional or perform ADLs. **Sensory/Perceptual Alterations: Visual or Auditory** are appropriate when the client has a deficit in vision or hearing. **Pain** is appropriate for clients with eye or ear infection.

EQUIPMENT
Newspaper or magazine
Penlight
Cotton–tipped applicator

Assessment

1. Question if client has history of eye disease, trauma, itching, discharge, diabetes, or hypertension; also ask about blurred vision, diplopia, spotters, floaters, flashes of light, or halos around lights. **These warning signs may indicate visual problems.**

2. Question if client has history of ear disease or trauma; ask if there is itching, discharge, or tinnitus (ringing) of the ears.

3. Determine occupational history and use of glasses, contacts, hearing aid, and medications (e.g., antibiotics, large doses of aspirin).

Planning

EXPECTED OUTCOMES
1. Client has no deviations from normal:
   a. Normal visual acuity with or without correction.
   b. Full visual fields and parallel eye movement in each cardinal gaze.
   c. Normal position of eyes, lids, and eyebrows; clarity of sclera with clear, pink conjunctiva; equal, round, briskly reactive pupils; and equal corneal light reflex.
   d. Clear and smooth ear canal, translucent eardrum, normal hearing acuity, and cerumen in ear canal.
2. Client is able to explain early signs and symptoms of visual and hearing loss.

Implementation

Steps	Rationale
1. See Standard Protocol (Chapter 1, p. 5). 2. Test visual acuity: CN II. a. If client wears glasses or contact lenses, ask to read print from newspaper while wearing glasses. Note distance from the eyes that client holds the newspaper (Figure 12-13).	Be sure client is able to read and can read English. It may help to have client read aloud if illiteracy is suspected.

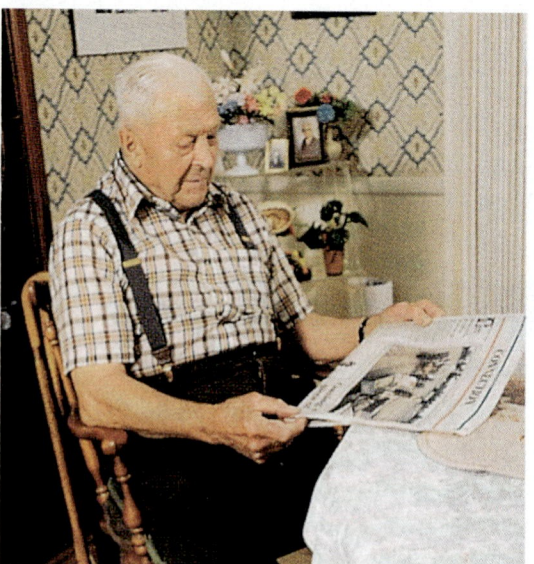

Figure 12-13 (From Barkauskas VH et al: *Health and physical assessment*, St. Louis, 1994, Mosby.)

Steps	Rationale

b. If client is unable to see print clearly, test each eye separately by placing index card over one eye at a time. (A more detailed examination involves use of a Snellen eye chart.)

Determines extent of involvement of each eye.

3. Test visual fields.

a. Have client sit or stand 60 cm (2 feet) away and face you. Your eyes should be at eye level of client (Figure 12-14).

b. Ask client to gently close or cover one eye and to look at your eye directly opposite. Close or cover other eye on side of client's closed eye.

Nurse's field of vision is superimposed on client's.

c. Move finger or object equidistant from you and client outside of own field of vision. Slowly bring it back into field, asking client to state when it is first seen. Repeat procedure for all visual fields and for both eyes.

The point at which finger can first be viewed indicates farthest limit of visual field for that direction.

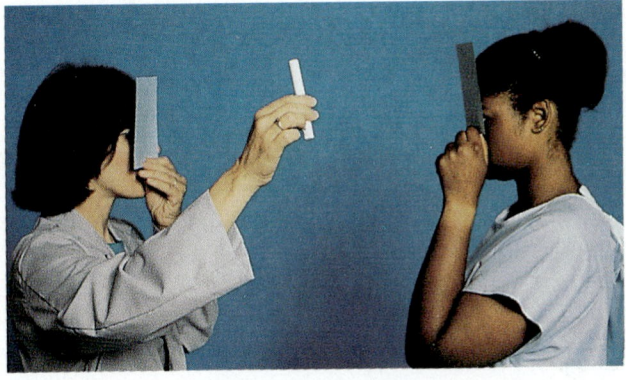

Figure 12-14 (From Barkauskas VH et al: *Health and physical assessment*, St. Louis, 1994, Mosby.)

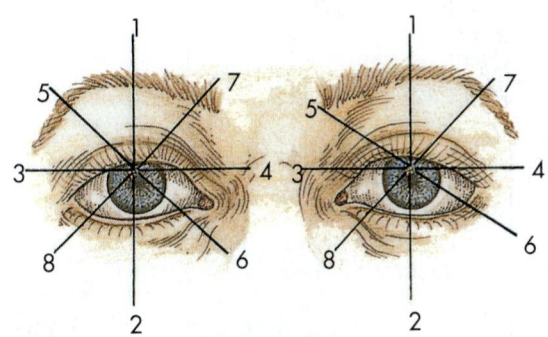

Figure 12-15

4. Test extraocular movements: CNs III, IV, and VI.

a. Instruct client to look straight ahead toward nurse, keeping head motionless throughout examination.

b. Hold finger 15 to 30 cm (6 to 12 inches) in front of client's eyes.

Comfortable distance prevents nystagmus.

c. Ask client to follow movement of finger with eyes, keeping head still. Move finger slowly through each of eight cardinal gazes (Figure 12-15).

The point at which finger can first be viewed indicates farthest limit of visual field for that direction.

d. Nurse keeps finger within normal field of vision.

Forcing client to look beyond visual field may cause nystagmus (rhythmical oscillation of eyes).

e. Nurse observes parallel eye movement, position of upper lid in relation to iris, and presence of nystagmus.

Eyes move together in parallel. Upper eyelid should cover iris only slightly. Eyelid does not cover pupil.

5. Test pupillary reflexes: CN III. Dim room lights so you can still see pupils. As client looks straight ahead, move penlight from side of client's face and direct light on pupil (Figure 12-16). Observe pupillary response of both eyes (Figure 12-17). Normal pupils are round, clear, and equal in size. Defects

Darkened room normally ensures brisk response of pupils to light. Pupil that is illuminated constricts; pupil in other eye should constrict equally (consensual light reaction).

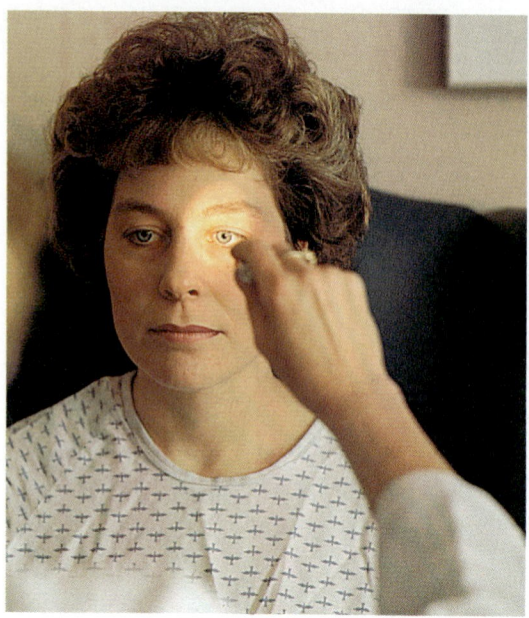

Figure 12-16

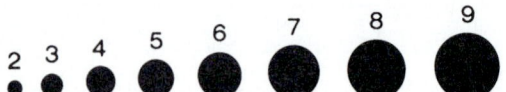

Figure 12-17 Chart showing pupil sizes in millimeters.

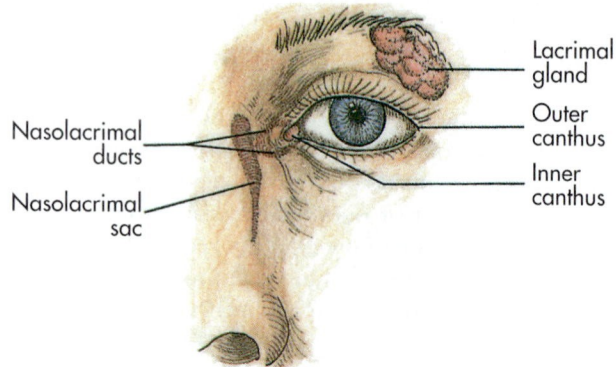

Figure 12-18

Steps	Rationale
along inner margins of iris may be from surgical correction for glaucoma.	
6. Test accommodation. Ask client to look at wall in distance. Then quickly bring finger within 10 to 15 cm (4 to 6 inches) of client's nose and ask client to look at finger. Finally, move finger smoothly toward nasal bridge; watch for pupil movement.	When focusing on near object, pupils in both eyes should constrict when gaze comes in from a distance. Pupils normally converge.
7. Assess external eye.	
a. Inspect eye position with eyes open. Note if any portion of lower conjunctiva is visible.	Normally, eyelids do not cover pupil, and sclera cannot be seen above iris.
b. Ask client to close both eyes; inspect lid position. Raise eyebrows and inspect upper eyelids for color, edema, and presence of lesions. Have client open eyes, and note blink reflex.	Eyelids should close completely. Persons blink as many as 20 times per minute.
c. Inspect lacrimal apparatus (Figure 12-18) and note edema or inflammation. Palpate to detect tenderness. (NOTE: Apply gloves if drainage present.) Inspect for excess tearing or edema of inner canthus.	Normally, lacrimal gland cannot be seen or palpated.
d. Inspect conjunctiva for color, edema, or lesions by gently depressing lower lid with thumb pressed against bony orbit. Ask client to look up (Figure 12-19).	Prevents pressure from being exerted on eye.

Figure 12-19 (From Barkauskas VH et al: *Health and physical assessment,* St. Louis, 1994, Mosby.)

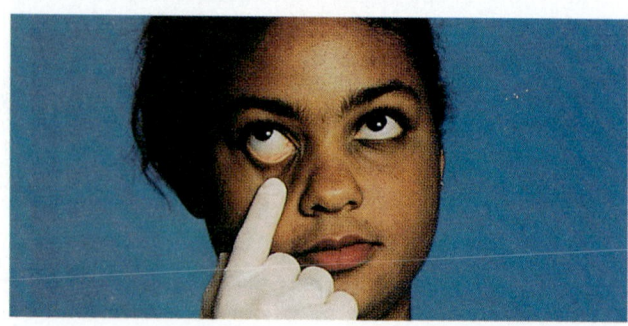

Steps	Rationale
e. Inspect cornea for opacities by shining light at an angle toward the cornea. Check pupils for size, shape, and equality. Inspect iris for symmetry.	Illumination should show a clear and transparent cornea. Normal pupils are round, clear, and equal in size. Defects along inner margins of iris may be from surgical correction for glaucoma.
8. Examine external ear.	
a. Inspect auricle for placement, size, symmetry, and color.	Normally, ears are level with each other, and upper point of attachment to head is in straight line with lateral outer canthus or corner of eye.
b. Palpate auricle for texture, tenderness, and presence of lesions. If client complains of pain, gently pull auricle and press on tragus and behind ear over mastoid bone.	If palpation of external ear increases the pain, external ear infection is likely. If palpation does not increase pain, infection may involve middle ear. Palpate any lesions gently.
c. Observe opening of ear canal for lesions, discharge, swelling, foreign bodies, or inflammation. Illumination should show a clear and translucent cornea.	
d. Inspect canal for buildup of cerumen. If canal is clear, ask how often client usually cleans ears.	Small amounts of cerumen normally should be in ears. Cotton-tipped swabs or other objects should not be used to clean ear canals. Cerumen can cause conduction deafness.
9. Assess hearing acuity.	
a. Ask client to close eyes. Test one ear at a time while occluding the other. Stand 15 to 60 cm (6 inches to 2 feet) away, exhale fully, and softly whisper a sequence of numbers with two equally accented syllables (e.g., "nine four").	Determines if client can hear voice tones.
b. Ask client to repeat. Repeat in conversational or loud tones if needed.	Reflects hearing deficit.
10. See Completion Protocol (Chapter 1, p. 6).	

Evaluation

1. Compare findings with client's baseline and normal expected findings.
2. Ask client to describe early symptoms of visual deficits and hearing loss.

UNEXPECTED OUTCOMES AND RELATED INTERVENTIONS

1. Client has evidence of decreased visual acuity or visual fields, inflammation, change in color of sclera from white, ptosis of eyelids, or crusty yellow or white drainage on lid margins.
   a. Gently cleanse eyes, taking care not to facilitate transmission of microorganisms (see Skill 6.2).
   b. Consider need for referal to ophthalmologist.
2. Nurse detects auricle or ear canal that is swollen, inflamed, or tender to palpation; drainage or lesions; or decreased hearing acuity.
   a. Gently cleanse auricle.
   b. Consider possibility of ear irrigations (see Skill 35.5).
   c. Consider referral for hearing evaluation.
3. Client exhibits a lack of awareness for early symptoms of hearing loss or visual defects.
   a. Offer appropriate teaching and follow-up for early detection.
   b. Consider adaptations to facilitate safety and communication (see Chapter 2).

SAMPLE DOCUMENTATION

1000 Client exhibits no dysfunction in accommodation, visual fields, hearing, and visual acuity. Extraocular muscle function intact without nystagmus. Pupils equal, react briskly to light bilaterally, and constrict from 4 to 2 mm.

Skill 12.5 | Assessing the Thorax, Lungs, and Breasts

Any alteration in pulmonary function usually affects other body systems. Care must be taken to assess findings from all body systems when determining the nature of pulmonary problems. For example, if a client's ventilation is impaired, the nurse should also assess the client's level of orientation, skin color, and capillary refill to determine if oxygenation to tissues is adequate.

The optimal time to complete the thorax and chest assessment is when the client is dangling or sitting in a chair. To perform an assessment accurately, the nurse should be familiar with the anatomical landmarks of the chest (Figure 12-20).

Assessment of male and female breasts are alike, even though the female examination is more detailed. Breast cancer affects one of every nine women in the United States (ACS, 1995). The disease is the second leading cause of death in women with cancer. Early detection is the key to cure.

Nursing Diagnosis

Anxiety is appropriate when a client has a history of air hunger, cancer, or high-risk factors related to cancer. **Ineffective Airway Clearance** might be indicated with reduced chest excursion or inability to elicit a cough. **Impaired Gas Exchange** might occur when trauma, congestion, or infection is present in the lungs unilaterally or bilaterally. **Knowledge Deficit** regarding breast self-examination (BSE) is appropriate for clients who are inexperienced or not using the proper technique.

EQUIPMENT

Gloves
Stethoscope

Assessment

1. Review family history for cancer, tuberculosis, allergies, asthma, and chronic obstructive pulmonary disease (COPD).
2. Ask if client experiences any of the following: persistent cough (productive or nonproductive), shortness of breath at rest or with activity, chest pain, orthopnea, or frequent respiratory infections.
3. **Assess Risk Factors for Lung Cancer**
   a. Determine if client works in environment or participates in hobbies that contain pollutants (e.g., asbestos, coal dust, chemical irritants).
   b. Ask if client has smoking history or exposure to smoke: length of time; number of cigarettes per day, cigar, pipe, or marijuana smoking; or length of time since exposure or smoking stopped.

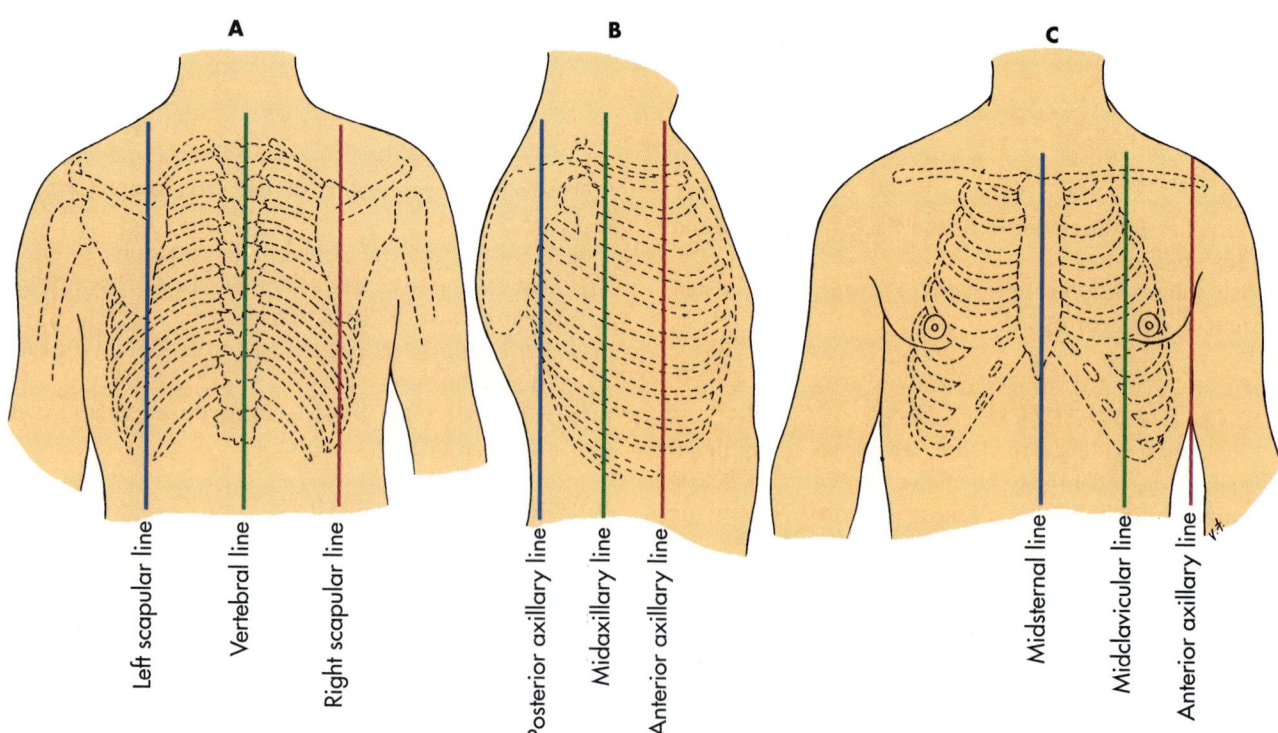

Figure 12-20 **A,** Posterior thorax; **B,** lateral thorax; **C,** anterior thorax.

4. **Assess Risk Factors for Breast Cancer**
   a. Determine if female client has family history of breast cancer, previous breast cancer, history of fibrocystic disease, never had children, or had first child after age 30 or did not breast-feed.
   b. Ask if client (either sex), has noticed pain, lump, thickening, or tenderness in breast; discharge, distortion, retraction, or scaling of nipple; or changes in size of breast. Have client point out any lumps.
   c. Determine if client is taking oral contraceptives, digitalis, diuretics, steroids, or estrogen hormones.
5. Determine if female client performs monthly breast self-exams (BSEs) and when in relation to menstrual cycle. Have client demonstrate or describe method.

Planning

EXPECTED OUTCOMES

1. Client has no deviations from normal:
   a. Chest excursion is symmetric; regular, passive, and diaphragmatic or costal respirations; clear, equal breath sounds.
   b. Young to middle-aged breasts—smooth, symmetrical without retraction or flattening; firm, elastic tissue with presence of soft lobular underlying tissue; smooth symmetrical nipples and areolas; no drainage from nipples.
   c. Older adult breasts—smaller, shrunken, wrinkled, and sagging; stringy, nodular tissue; nipples may point downward.
   d. Nonpalpable lymph nodes.
2. Client describes findings of breast cancer and factors that predispose to lung disease and cancer.
3. Client correctly demonstrates BSE.

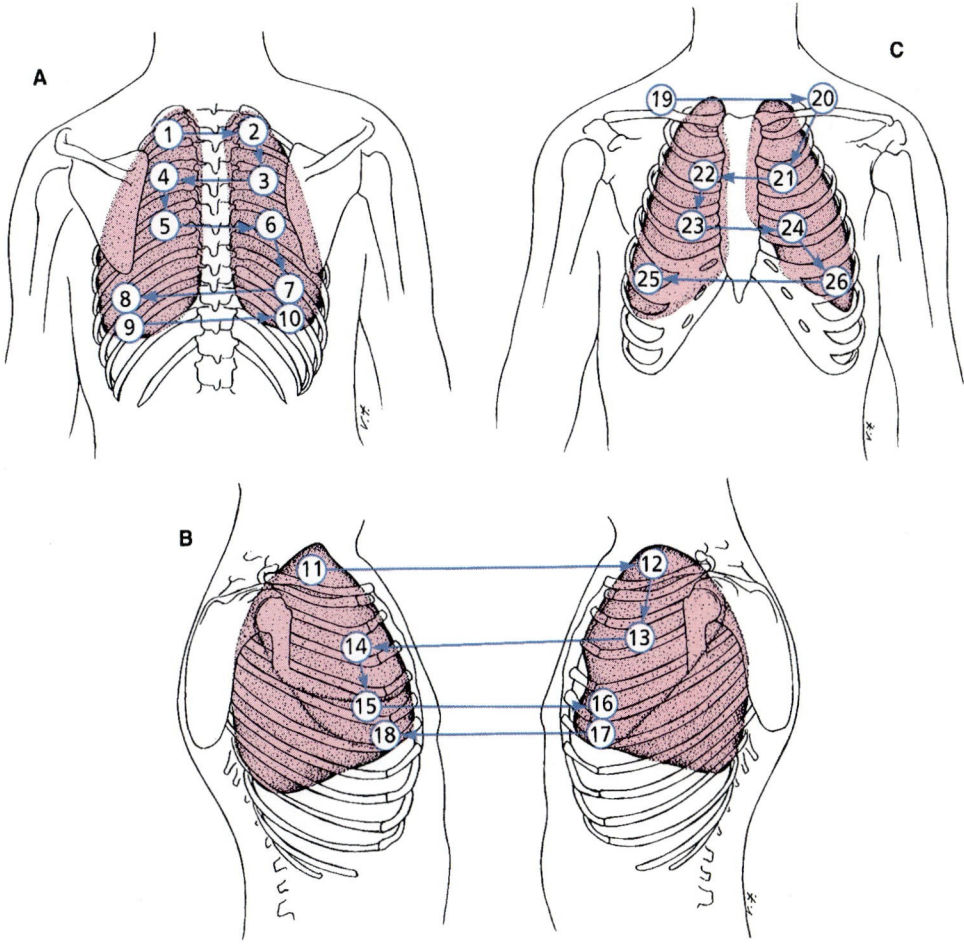

Figure 12-21

Implementation

Steps	Rationale
1. See Standard Protocol (Chapter 1, p. 5). **2.** Sequence of assessment moves from posterior to lateral, then to anterior thorax, and then to breast assessment. Describe findings made during the examination in relation to the imaginary lines formed from anatomical landmarks: sternum, intercostal spaces, clavicle, spine, scapulae, and axilla (Figure 12-21). **3.** Assess posterior thorax. a. Standing at midline position behind the client, inspect thorax for shape, deformities, retractions or bulging of intercostal spaces, slope of ribs, and alignment of scapulae. Note client's posture.	
	Allows for identification of any factors that may impair chest expansion and any symptoms of respiratory distress. COPD results in 1:1 anterior/posterior diameter ratio. A client with breathing problem often leans forward with hands on knees for support.
b. Determine rate, depth, and rhythm of breathing (see Skill 10.1). c. Palpate posterior chest wall, costal spaces and intercostal spaces, for masses or localized areas of tenderness. If suspicious mass or swollen area is detected, palpate for size, shape, and typical qualities of lesion. If painful, do not palpate deeply.	Fractured rib can be painful and should not have pressure applied.
d. Palpate for chest excursion. Place hand on lower third of each rib cage, with hands parallel and thumbs approximately 5 cm (2 inches) apart, pointing to spine. Fingers point out laterally. Press hands toward client's spine to form small skinfolds between thumbs (Figure 12-22). After exhalation, client takes deep breath. Note movement of thumbs, which normally separate 3 to 5 cm ($1\frac{1}{2}$ to 2 inches) during chest excursion (Figure 12-23).	Assesses client's ability to breathe deeply. 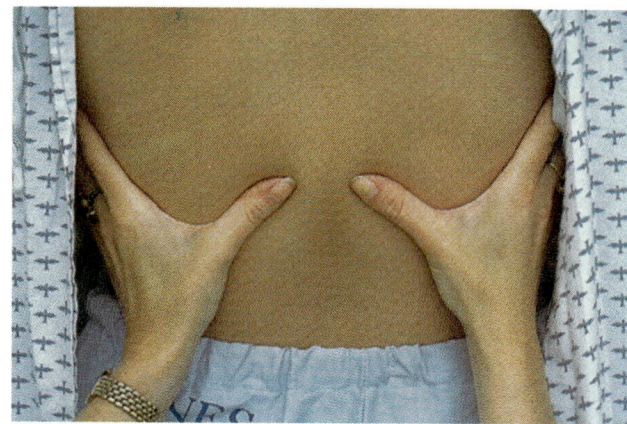 Figure 12-22 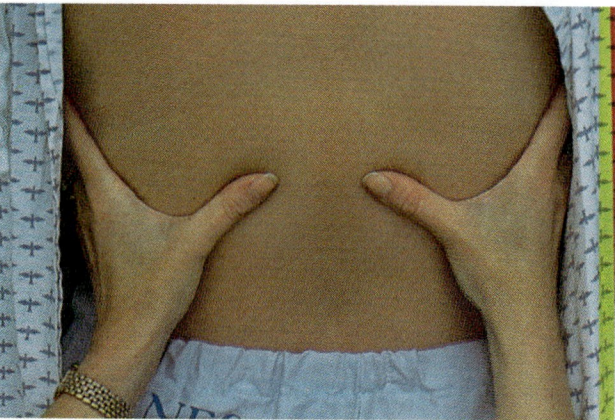 Figure 12-23

Steps	Rationale

e. Palpate for vocal or tactile fremitus by first placing ball or lower palm of hands on area of thorax over intercostal space. Then ask client to say "99" in voice of uniform intensity. Place hand over symmetrical areas of thorax (Figure 12-24). Feel faint vibration.

Vibration created by movement of vocal cords travels through lung tissue to chest wall. Failure to palpate vibration indicates airway obstruction. Palm of hand is most sensitive to vibrations.

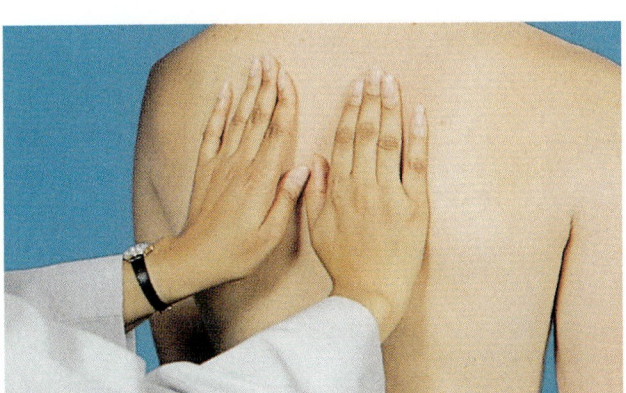

Figure 12-24 (From Barkauskas VH et al: *Health and physical assessment,* St. Louis, 1994, Mosby.)

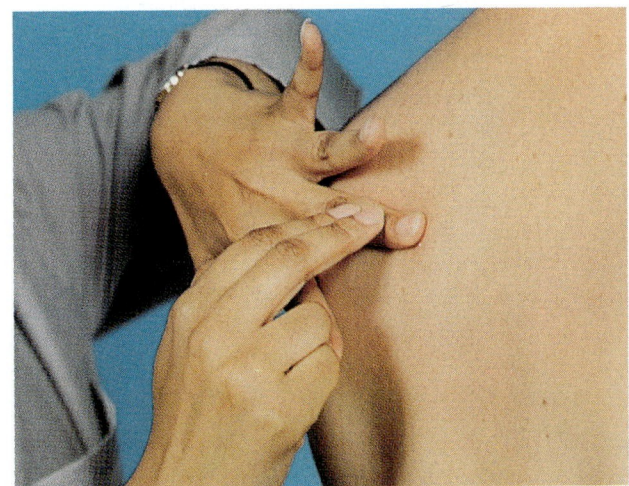

Figure 12-25 (From Barkauskas VH et al: *Health and physical assessment,* St. Louis, 1994, Mosby.)

f. Ask client to fold arms forward across chest. Follow same pattern as with palpation; using indirect percussion, percuss intercostal spaces (Figure 12-25) for comparison of posterior lobes.

g. Auscultate lung sounds (see Skill 11.2).

h. If any abnormalities, place stethoscope over intercostal spaces systematically. Ask client to say "e" and "99" in a normal tone of voice.

Position separates scapulae to expose more lung tissue. Percussion determines underlying lung tissue density. Normal is resonant. Dull or flat sounds reflect fluid-filled tissue.

Tests for spoken voice sounds. Normally, expect "e" to sound like "e" and "99" to sound muffled. Abnormal if "e" sounds like "a" and "99" is clear and distinct, reflecting fluid or consolidation of lung tissue.

4. Assess lateral thorax.

a. Instruct client to raise arms straight into air and inspect, palpate, percuss, and auscultate chest wall. Omit excursion maneuver.

b. Give particular attention during auscultation to the right lateral wall at the fourth to fifth intercostal spaces, since this is the location of the right middle lobe.

The right middle lobe is the most common site for aspiration.

5. Assess anterior thorax.

a. Inspect the width or spread of angle made by costal margins and tip of sternum; it is usually greater than 90 degrees between margins.

b. Measure client's respiratory character, observing for symmetry and degree of chest wall and abdominal movement.

Assesses client's effort to ventilate.

c. Palpate for areas of swelling, tenderness, and tactile fremitus. In female, retract breast tissue and lift breasts gently for chest wall palpation.

Steps	Rationale

d. Percuss thorax between intercostal spaces by using same sequence as in palpation.

Percussion over anterior thorax enables nurse to locate position of the heart, liver, and stomach. Location of findings by common reference points helps successive examiners to confirm findings and locate abnormalities.

e. For auscultation, see Skill 11.2.
6. Inspect breasts.
a. Describe findings made during examination in relation to imaginary lines that divide breasts into four quadrants and tail (Figure 12-26).

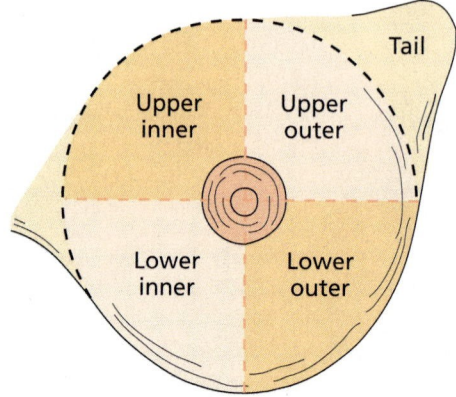

Figure 12-26 Left breast divided into four quadrants and an axillary tail.

b. Inspect both breasts for size symmetry, position of breasts, and position of the nipples in relation to underlying intercostal space.

Changes in size or shape may indicate underlying mass or presence of inflammation.

c. Observe contour or shape of breast and note any masses, retraction of tissue, or flattening. If retraction is suspected, ask client to raise arms above head or press hands against hips (Figure 12-27).

Underlying mass, swelling, or inflammation may cause bulging or retraction of breast tissue. Maneuver causes contraction of pectoral muscles, which accentuates presence of retraction.

d. Inspect underlying skin for color and venous pattern. If breasts are large, carefully lift breasts to inspect underlying surfaces. Normal breasts are color of surrounding skin surfaces.

Vascular changes, edema, and inflammation cause skin color changes. Breast undersurface is a common site for redness and excoriation caused by rubbing against chest wall.

e. Inspect areolas and nipples for color, size, and shape. Note direction in which nipples point and presence of rashes or ulcerations. If nipple discharge present, apply gloves. Note color and amount of discharge.

Hormonal changes cause differences in color and size of areolas and nipples throughout the life span.

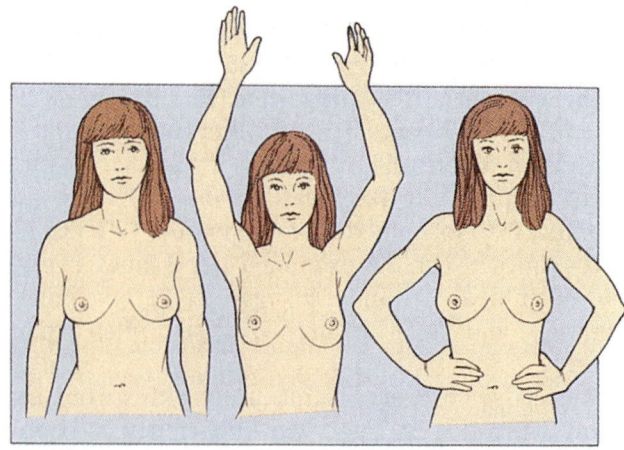

Figure 12-27 (From Payne WA, Hahn DB: *Understanding your health,* ed 2, St. Louis, 1989, Mosby.)

Steps	Rationale

7. Palpate lymph nodes.

  a. Client position: arms at side and muscles relaxed. Face client, stand on the side being examined, and support this arm while abducting arm from chest wall.

Position allows for easy palpation of axillary nodes.

  b. Place hand against client's chest wall and high in the axillae. Palpate axillary nodes with fingertips, pressing gently down over the surface of the ribs and muscles (Figure 12-28).

  c. Palpate the following areas: edge of the pectoralis major muscle along anterior axillary line; chest wall in midaxilla; upper part of humerus; and anterior edge of latissimus dorsi muscle along posterior axillary line (Figure 12-29).

Breast cancer can metastasize to lymph nodes.

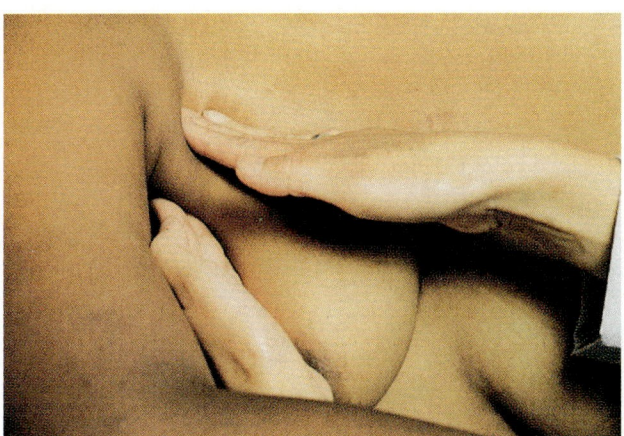

Figure 12-28 (From Barkauskas VH et al: *Health and physical assessment,* St. Louis, 1994, Mosby.)

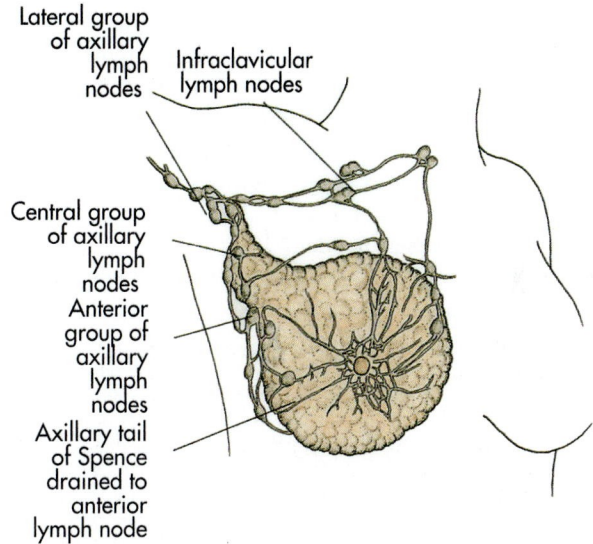

Figure 12-29 Anatomical position of axillary and clavicular lymph nodes.

  d. Palpate along upper and lower clavicular ridges.

  e. Note number, location, consistency, mobility, and size of nodes. If enlarged node is present, ask if tender.

Location of supraclavicular and infraclavicular nodes.
Characteristics of node help to determine cause of enlargement.

8. Palpate breasts.

  a. If client has lump or mass, examine opposite breast first.

Ensures objective comparison between normal and abnormal tissue.

  b. Client position: lying with right arm abducted and hand placed above head (Figure 12-30, *A*). A small towel can be placed under right shoulder blade. During this portion, nurse can ask client to demonstrate BSE, or nurse can perform and teach to client.

Position allows breast tissue to flatten evenly against client's chest wall.

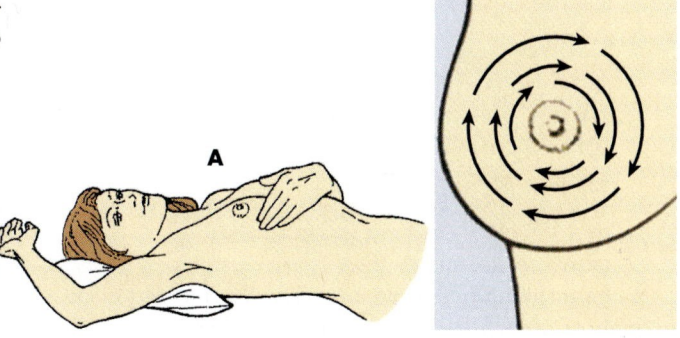

Figure 12-30 (From Payne WA, Hahn DB: *Understanding your health,* ed 2, St. Louis, 1989, Mosby.)

Steps	Rationale

c. Stand at client's right side. Using systematic approach, gently palpate breast tissue with palmar surface of first three fingers of right hand moving in rotary fashion and compressing breast tissue against chest wall. Begin in one quadrant and thoroughly examine all surfaces before moving to other three quadrants and tail. Each quadrant may be examined by moving from nipple outward (Figure 12-30, *B*).

d. Note consistency of breast tissue.

e. If mass is found, palpate for location in relation to quadrants, size in centimeters, shape (round or discoid), consistency (soft, firm, hard), tenderness, mobility, and discreetness (are boundaries of mass easily detected?).

f. Use finger to compress areola gently. Then, with thumb and index finger, gently compress nipple while observing for a discharge (Figure 12-31). (Apply gloves as needed.)

g. Repeat procedure in opposite breast after repositioning client.

h. For large breasts, bimanual palpation may be needed; support inferior portion of breast in one hand while palpating breast tissue against supporting hand (Figure 12-32).

i. In male clients, conduct same technique and note any breast swelling.

9. See Completion Protocol (Chapter 1, p. 6).

Entire breast must be thoroughly palpated to rule out presence of a mass. Young women: breast normally firm and elastic; older women: normally often feels stringy and nodular. Note time of examination vs. time of menstrual cycle. If done during the week before or within the first few days of the menstrual cycle, examination may not reveal true findings. Menstrual cycle may cause breast to be tender and engorged.

Consistency of underlying tissue changes with age, pathological conditions, and hormonal variations.

Lower edge of breast, inframammary ridge, may normally feel firm and hard.

Involvement of glandular tissue may cause discharge from nipple.

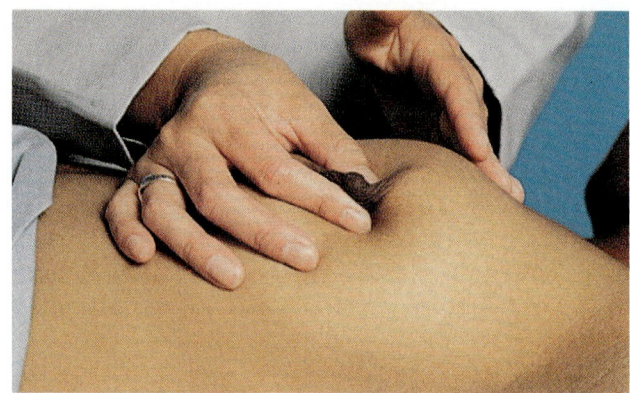

Figure 12-31 (From Barkauskas VH et al: *Health and physical assessment,* St. Louis, 1994, Mosby.)

Signs of breast cancer are same as for female client.

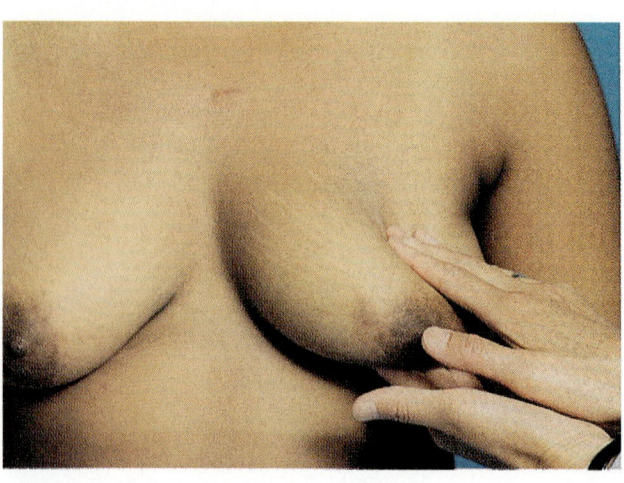

Figure 12-32 (From Barkauskas VH et al: *Health and physical assessment,* St. Louis, 1994, Mosby.)

Evaluation

1. Compare findings with client's baseline and normal expected findings.
2. Ask client to explain risk factors predisposing to lung disease.
3. Ask client to describe signs and symptoms of breast cancer.
4. Ask client to demonstrate BSE.

UNEXPECTED OUTCOMES AND RELATED INTERVENTIONS

1. Client has evidence of anterior/posterior diameter in ratio of 1:1, limited chest excursion, and abnormal chest auscultation, percussion, and palpation.
   a. Compare to baseline for client, consider presence of pain, and consider recent use of medication (e.g., sedatives).
   b. Monitor frequently for changes back to normal or deterioration of respiratory condition.
   c. Communicate new changes in condition to appropriate health care team member.

2. Client has evidence of localized hard, fixed, non-tender, and irregularly shaped mass; dimpling or retraction unilaterally; palpable lymph nodes; or serous, bloody nipple drainage.
   a. These are signs of breast cancer.
   b. Refer to client's physician.
3. Client has evidence of lumpy, painful breasts, occasional nipple discharge; and lumps that are soft, well differentiated, and movable.
   a. These are common signs of fibrocystic disease.
   b. Encourage client to become familiar with own breast tissue and to notify physician if abnormalities present.

SAMPLE DOCUMENTATION

1000 Client exhibits no respiratory distress or abnormalities. Breast exam negative for tenderness, lumps, drainage, or abnormal contour. Client unable to perform BSE independently. Follow-up instructions scheduled tomorrow.

Skill 12.6 | Assessing the Heart and Circulation

An alteration in cardiac function frequently results in changes in the vascular system. A client who presents with findings of cardiac problems such as chest pain may have a life-threatening condition. The nurse must be able to prioritize essential assessments.

Assessment of the heart follows examination of the thorax, with the client in a semirecumbent position. Assessment then proceeds to the vascular system. All four examination techniques are used.

Central cyanosis is evident from bluish discoloration of the mucosa at base of the tongue or inside the mouth. This indicates poor oxygenation. Peripheral cyanosis is evident from bluish discoloration of lips, extremities, and nail beds. This condition results from low cardiac output or local vasoconstriction. Older adults should be routinely assessed for carotid bruits. In addition, varicosities are common in the elderly population and in people who must stand for prolonged periods.

Nursing Diagnosis

Altered Peripheral Tissue Perfusion is appropriate when the client has cyanotic extremities, diminished peripheral pulses, cold clammy skin, and a change in LOC. **Pain** is appropriate when diminished peripheral arterial flow or stagnant venous flow presents in acute or chronic fashion or when compromised cardiac circulation produces cardiac pain. **Decreased Cardiac Output** is indicated when the client has diminished cardiac contractility or a damaged heart. **Activity Intolerance** is appropriate when the client has insufficient physiological energy (e.g., from a low blood count) to endure or complete daily activities.

EQUIPMENT
Stethoscope
Doppler stethoscope with conducting gel (optional)

Assessment

1. Assess client for risk factors for heart/vascular disease, including history of smoking; alcohol ingestion; high-fat, low-fiber diet; cocaine use; absent or irregular exercise; stressful lifestyle; diabetes; hypertension; family history of heart disease; obesity; excessive caffeine intake; history of phlebitis or varicose veins; or wearing tight-fitting clothing about the legs.
2. Ask if client has experienced leg cramps; edema of hands, ankles, or feet; numbness; or tingling in extremities or a sensation of cold extremities. **Reveals circulatory alterations.**
3. If client experiences pain or cramping in the lower extremities, ask if it is relieved or aggravated by walking. **Differentiates vascular from musculoskeletal pain.**

Planning

EXPECTED OUTCOMES

1. Client has no deviations from normal:
   a. Normal rhythm and heart rate, normal heart sounds, and a point of maximal impulse (PMI) at the fifth intercostal space, midclavicular line.
   b. Blood pressure (BP) within normal parameters for client; equal, strong, bilateral pulses; no jugular vein distention; and warm, pink extremities with normal hair growth and nails.
2. Client describes behavior aimed at improving cardiovascular function and decreasing risk factors for cardiovascular disease.

Implementation

Steps	Rationale
1. See Standard Protocol (Chapter 1, p. 5).	
2. Heart assessment	
a. Stand on client's right side and view chest at an angle to the side. Locate anatomical landmarks used to assess cardiac function (Figure 12-33). Inspect and palpate simultaneously over the six landmarks. Look for visible pulsations. Palpate each site, alternating with the fingertips and ball of the hand (Figure 12-34).	Familiarity with landmarks allows nurse to describe findings more clearly and ultimately may improve assessment. The fingertips best sense pulsations; the ball of the hand detects vibrations.
b. If pulsations or vibrations are palpated, time their occurrence in relation to systole or diastole by feeling the carotid pulse simultaneously.	
c. Locate the PMI by palpating with fingertips at apex at fifth intercostal space in an area 1 to 2 cm in diameter (about the size of a quarter). Normally at the PMI, the apical pulse is felt as a light tap.	The PMI (apical impulse) may be located to the left of the midclavicular line in clients with enlarged hearts.
d. Inspect the epigastric area; palpate the abdominal aorta. Note a localized strong beat.	Rule out reduced blood flow or diffuse aortic pulse.

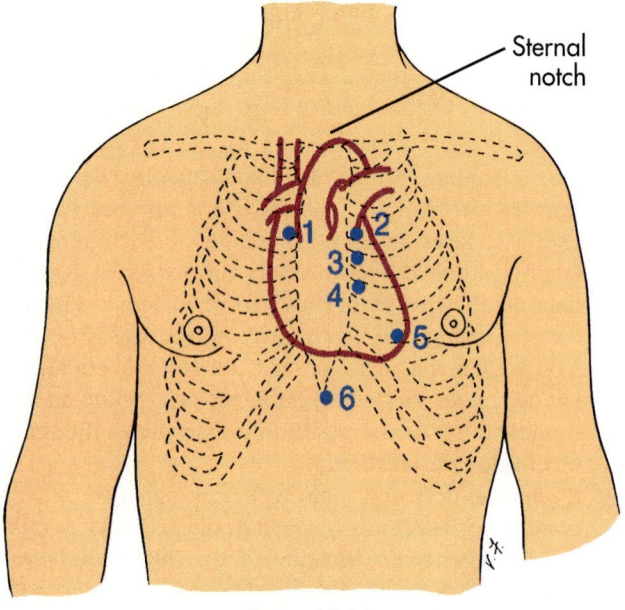

Figure 12-33

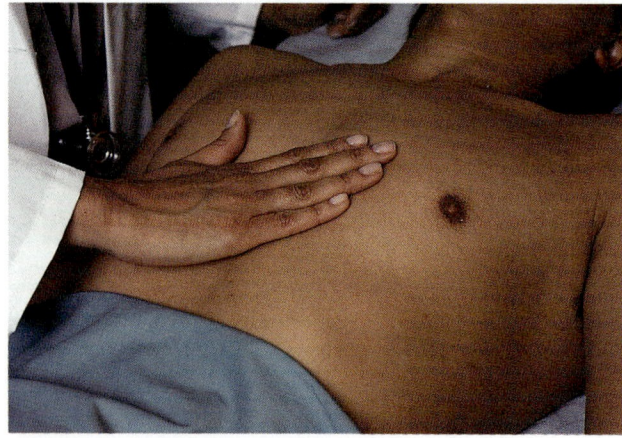

Figure 12-34 (From Canobbio MM: *Cardiovascular disorders,* Mosby's Clinical Nursing Series, St. Louis, 1990, Mosby.)

Steps	Rationale

e. Auscultate heart sounds (Figure 12-35).

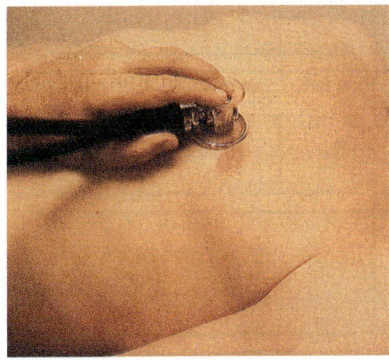

Figure 12-35 (From Seidel HM et al: *Mosby's guide to physical examination,* ed 3, St. Louis, 1995, Mosby.)

(1) With client supine and head of bed elevated 45 degrees, locate the anatomical sites for auscultation of cardiac function.

    (a) Angle of Louis is felt as a ridge in the sternum approximately 5 cm (2 inches) below the sternal notch (see Figure 12-33).

    (b) Intercostal spaces are just below each rib. The second intercostal space on the right is the aortic area *(dot 1)* and on the left is the pulmonic area *(dot 2).*

    (c) Erb's point is at the third intercostal space *(dot 3).*

    (d) Tricuspid area *(dot 4)* is at the fourth intercostal space.

    (e) Apical area is located at the fifth intercostal space at the left midclavicular line *(dot 5).*

    (f) Epigastric area is at tip of the sternum *(dot 6).*

NOTE: In clients with serious heart disease, the PMI is located to the left of the midclavicular line.

(2) If locating PMI is difficult, turn client onto left side (Figure 12-36).

Maneuver moves the heart closer to the chest wall.

(3) Ask client not to speak. Place stethoscope's diaphragm lightly against chest wall.

Pressing too firmly may decrease transmission of sounds.

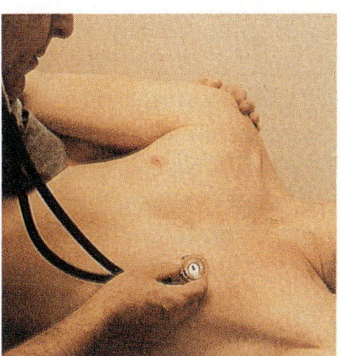

Figure 12-36 (From Seidel HM et al: *Mosby's guide to physical examination,* ed 3, St. Louis, 1995, Mosby.)

(4) Listen at the apex. Normal first and second heart sounds (S_1, S_2) are high pitched, are best heard with diaphragm, and sound like "lub-dub."

(5) After both sounds are heard clearly as "lub-dub," count each combination of S_1 and S_2 as one heartbeat. Count the number of beats for 1 minute to determine the apical pulse rate.

f. Identify if heart rhythm is regular or irregular. This may be further identified as regularly irregular or irregularly irregular.

An irregular heartbeat is a dysrhythmia, which interferes with the heart's ability to pump effectively.

g. When heart rate is irregular, compare apical and radial pulses. This is best done with a colleague, who can assess the radial pulse while the nurse simultaneously assesses the apical pulse.

If a pulse deficit exists (radial pulse slower than apical), ineffective heart contractions are failing to send pulse waves to the periphery.

h. Listen for clicks as short, high-pitched extra sounds.

Clicks are caused by abnormalities such as mitral valve prolapse or prosthetic valves.

i. Listen for pericardial friction rubs as "squeaky" or rubbing sounds.

Rubs result from inflamed visceral and parietal layers of the pericardium rubbing against one another.

j. Auscultate for heart murmurs. Murmurs are swishing or blowing sounds caused by altered blood flow.

Sounds may be caused by increased flow through a normal valve, forward flow through a stenotic (narrowed) valve or into a dilated vessel or chamber, or backward flow through a valve that fails to close.

Steps	Rationale

3. Vascular assessment

The sequence of vascular assessment is blood pressure, carotid arteries, jugular neck vein distention, and then peripheral pulses.

    a. Compare lying and standing blood pressures.

        Abnormalities may suggest atherosclerosis or diseases of aorta. Comparing pressure readings with client in different positions rules out orthostatic hypotension and volume depletion.

    b. Assess carotid arteries with client in sitting position. Inspect neck bilaterally for obvious pulsations, then palpate each artery separately (Figure 12-37). Note if pulsation changes with inspiration or expiration.

        Simultaneous occlusion of both arteries could cause loss of consciousness from inadequate circulation.

    c. Place bell of stethoscope over each carotid artery, auscultating for blowing sound or bruit (Figure 12-38).

        Narrowing of lumen results in turbulence with a harsh blowing sound.

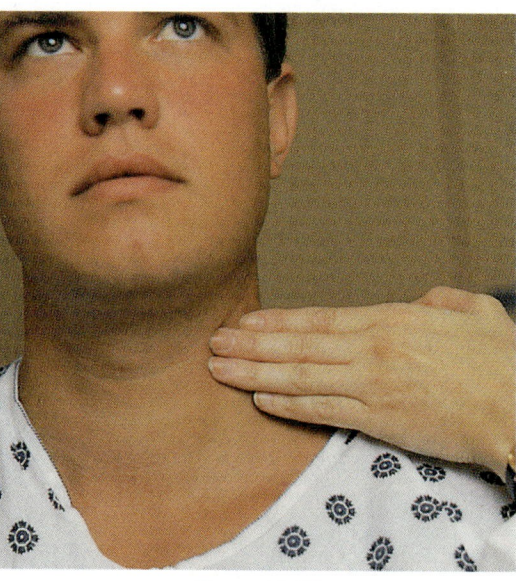

Figure 12-37

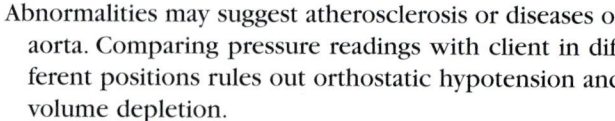

Figure 12-38 (From Barkauskas VH et al: *Health and physical assessment,* St. Louis, 1994, Mosby.)

    d. Assess jugular veins in supine position, where normally distention occurs. Reposition client with head elevated to at least a 30- to 45-degree angle. Look for the usual position of the internal jugular vein, just visible 2.5 cm (1 inch) above the sternal angle or suprasternal notch (Figure 12-39). Repeat measurement on other side. Note any elevations greater than about 1 inch.

        Higher than 1 inch indicates volume overload with a venous pressure increase and *NVD,* neck vein distention.

    e. Assess integrity of vascular system.

        (1) Inspect skin, mucous membranes, nail beds (Figure 12-40) and lower extremities for changes in color, texture, edema, ulcers, or hair distribution (Table 12-2).

        (2) If veins in calves reddened or swollen, palpate gently for tenderness or firmness of muscle.

45° angle

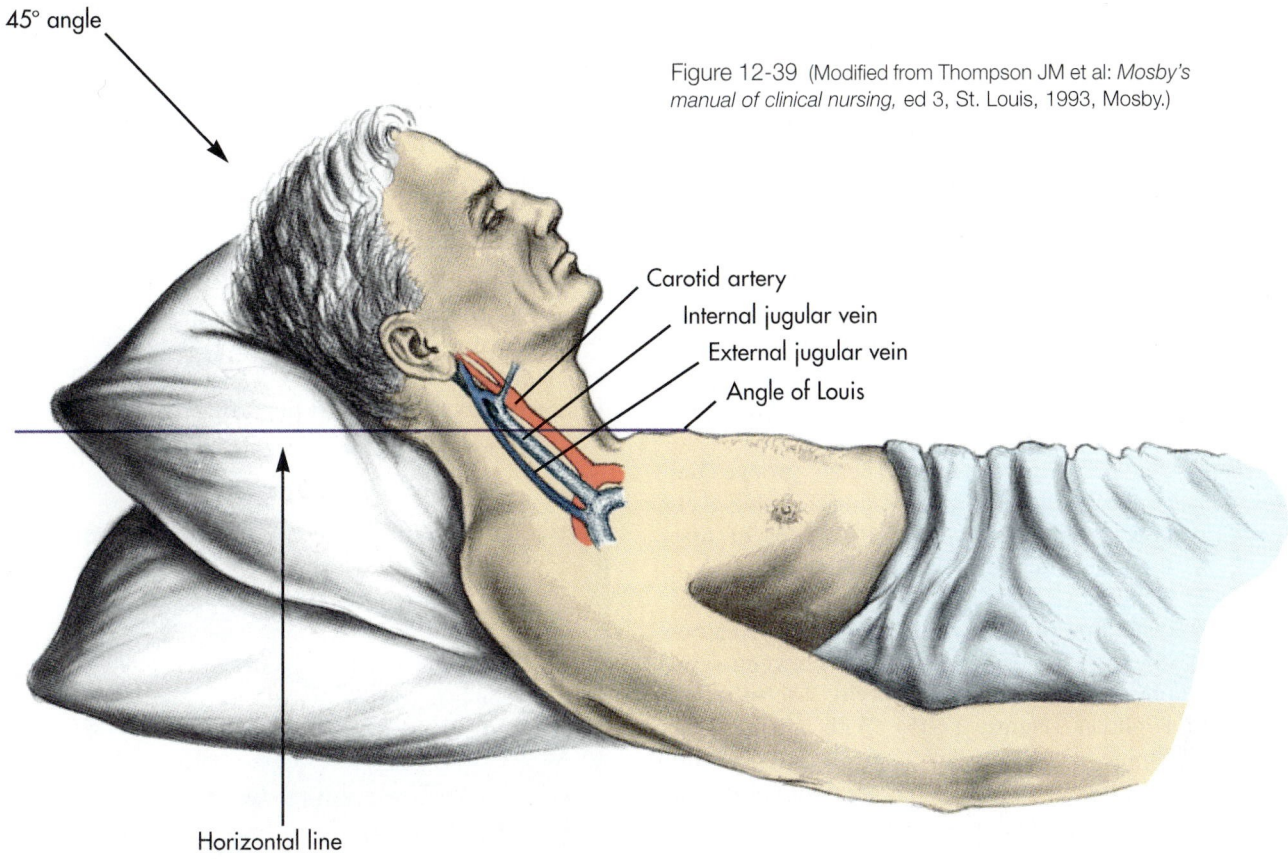

Figure 12-39 (Modified from Thompson JM et al: *Mosby's manual of clinical nursing,* ed 3, St. Louis, 1993, Mosby.)

Carotid artery
Internal jugular vein
External jugular vein
Angle of Louis

Horizontal line

Table 12-2 **Skin Color Variations**

Color	Cause	Assessment location
Blue (cyanosis)	Heart or lung disease, cold environment	Nail beds, lips, mouth, skin (severe cases)
Pallor (decrease in color)	Anemia, shock	Face, skin, nail beds, conjunctivae, lips
Yellow-orange (jaundice)	Liver disease, destruction of red blood cells	Sclerae, mucous membranes, skin
Red (erythema)	Fever, direct trauma, blushing, alcohol intake	Face, area of trauma
Tan-brown	Suntan, pregnancy, endocrine disorder	Areas exposed to sun, face, areolas, nipples

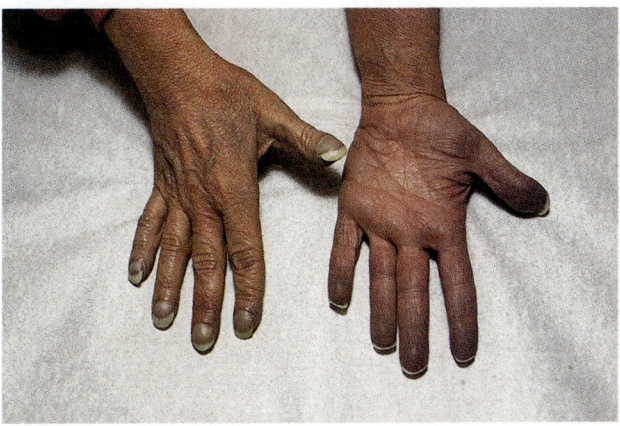

Figure 12-40 Cyanosis of hands and clubbing of nails. (From Canobbio MM: *Cardiovascular disorders,* Mosby's Clinical Nursing Series, St. Louis, 1990, Mosby.)

Steps	Rationale

With tenderness, support the leg while client dorsiflexes foot. Note if client complains of sharp pain.

   (3) If edema present, assess for pitting (see Skill 11.1). Palpate and note temperature.

  f. Palpate peripheral arteries.

   (1) Radial (Figure 12-41). Lightly place tips of first and second fingers in groove formed along radial side of forearm, lateral to flexor tendon of wrist.

   (2) Ulnar (Figure 12-42). Place fingertips along ulnar side of forearm.

   (3) Brachial (Figure 12-43). Locate groove between biceps and triceps muscles above elbow at antecubital fossa. Place tips of first three fingers in muscle groove.

   (4) Femoral (Figure 12-44). With client supine, place first three fingers over inguinal area below inguinal ligament, midway between symphysis pubis and anterosuperior iliac spine.

   (5) Popliteal (Figure 12-45). With client lying supine or prone, flex knee slightly. Palpate with fingers of both hands deep into popliteal fossa, just lateral to midline.

   (6) Dorsalis pedis (Figure 12-46). With client supine and feet relaxed, gently place fingertips between great and first toe and slowly move along groove between extensor tendons of these toes until pulse is palpated.

   (7) Posterior tibial (Figure 12-47). Have client relax and slightly extend feet. Place fingertips behind and below medial malleolus (ankle bone).

    Assess each site for rate and rhythm, strength, and elasticity. (Depress and release artery, noting ease with which it springs back.)

  g. If pulses are difficult to palpate, use an ultrasound stethoscope over the pulse site. Apply conductance gel over site; then apply probe at a 45- to 90-degree angle on skin (Figure 12-48). Turn up volume as needed.

4. See Completion Protocol (Chapter 1, p. 6).

Rationale

Homans' test for thrombophlebitis.

The higher degree of pitting, the more severe the edema.

Rating scale for strength of pulses (Seidel et al., 1995):
0,   No pulse
1+, Weak, thready, barely palpable
2+, Normal pulse
3+, Full, increased
4+, Strong, bounds against fingertips

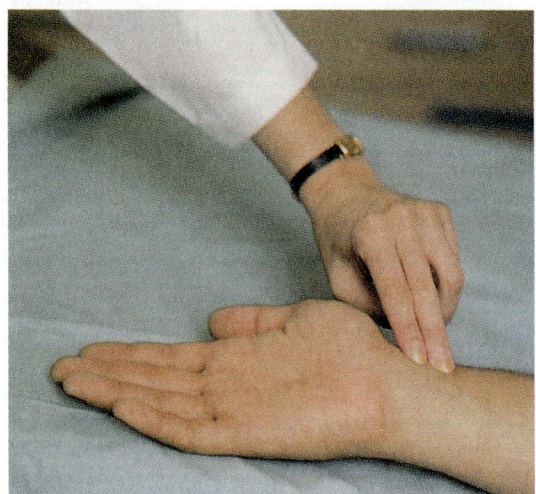

Figure 12-41

Excess pressure can obliterate pulse.

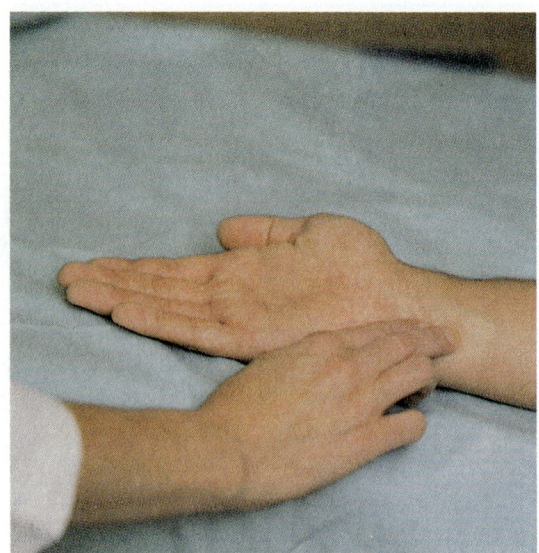

Figure 12-42

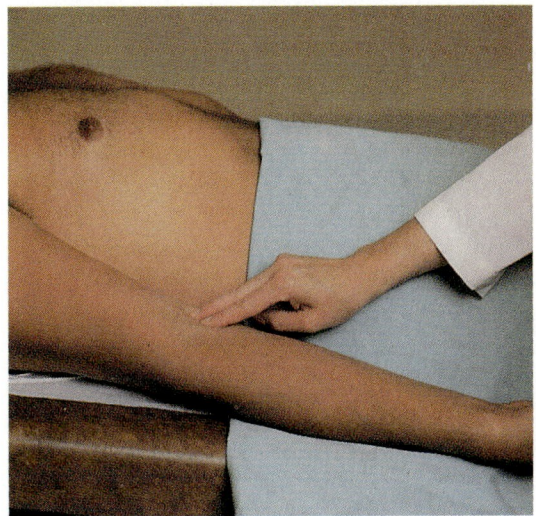

Figure 12-43

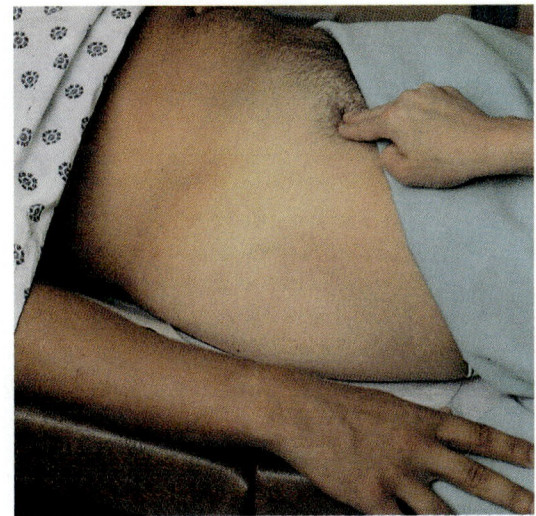

Figure 12-44

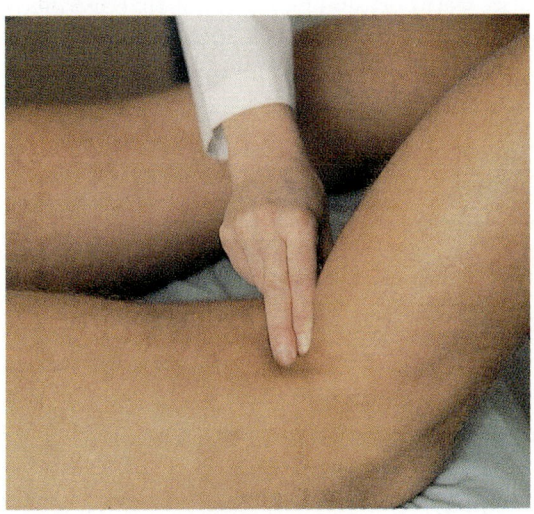

Figure 12-45

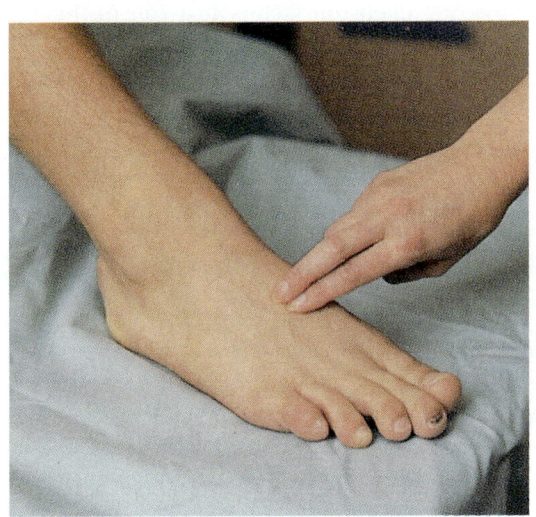

Figure 12-46

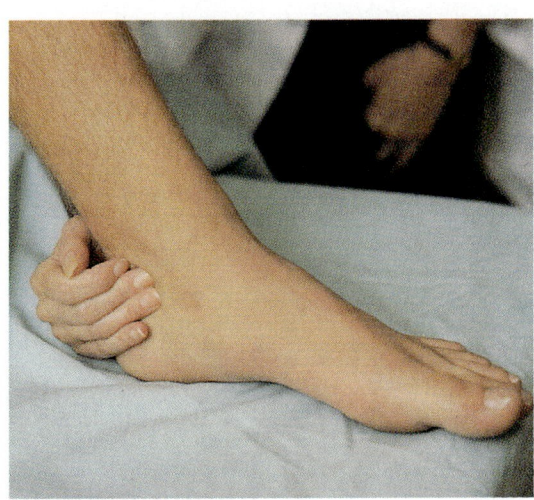

Figure 12-47

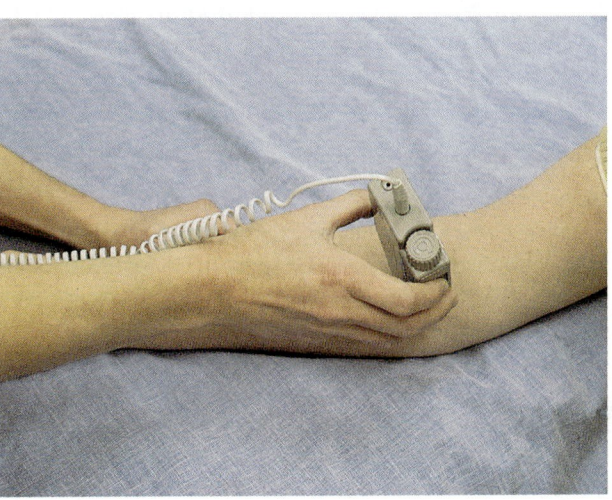

Figure 12-48

Evaluation

1. Compare findings with client's baseline and normal expected findings.
2. Ask client to describe risk factors of cardiovascular disease.
3. Have client explain exercise routine to follow for improvement of cardiovascular function.

UNEXPECTED OUTCOMES AND RELATED INTERVENTIONS

1. Client has evidence of hypertension, hypotension or elevated neck vein distention.
   a. Monitor closely for changes in vital signs.
   b. Notify physician of findings.
   c. If client is unstable, be sure resuscitation equipment is nearby (see Chapter 37).
2. Evidence of edema of extremities, diminished arterial circulation, or stasis of venous circulation.
   a. Instruct client on factors that can further impair circulation.
   b. Determine client's knowledge of foot care practices.

3. Positive Homans' sign is detected.
   a. Evaluate for additional evidence of thrombophlebitis (i.e., redness, swelling, and inflammation).
   b. Instruct client to remain in bed.
   c. Notify physician.
4. Heart sounds are abnormal with gallops or rubs.
   a. Refer to past history. Compare with previous findings.
   b. If findings differ, refer client to physician for follow-up.
5. Client is unable to offer interventions to improve cardiovascular function.
   Review with client means to improve cardiovascular function, exercise, elimination of risk factors.

SAMPLE DOCUMENTATION

1100 Pulses 3+ at radial, femoral, and posterior tibial. Extremities warm, dry, and pink in color. Hair distribution of lower legs adequate. NVD at 30 degrees absent. Heart rate regular, S_1 and S_2 present without abnormal sounds.

Skill 12.7 | Assessing the Abdomen

Within the abdominal cavity are multiple organs: stomach, intestines, pancreas, gallbladder, liver, kidneys, and bladder. When performing the assessment, the nurse should maintain a mental image of the anatomical location of each organ (Table 12-3; Figure 12-49). Specific historical data are essential to pinpoint findings to localize organ involvement.

The abdominal assessment should be completed in depth for any client reporting gastrointestinal (GI) and urinary complaints. The sequence differs for the abdominal area in that inspection is followed by auscultation. Percussion and palpation are done last because these maneuvers stimulate an increase in bowel sounds.

Nursing Diagnosis

Pain or **Chronic Pain** is appropriate if the client reports discomfort of the anterior or posterior trunk. Altered elimination, such as **Diarrhea, Constipation,** or **Urinary Retention,** is indicated when assessment data confirm abnormal peristalsis of the intestines, resulting in loose or constipated stools or bladder dysfunction with abnormal urination patterns. **Altered Nutrition: More** or **Less than Body Requirements** is appropriate if the client reports factors of indigestion, cramping, or emesis after eating and if the client's weight is 20% over or under ideal body weight.

Table 12-3 **Location of Abdominal Organs**

Right upper quadrant	Left upper quadrant
Liver and gallbladder	Left lobe of liver
Pylorus	Spleen
Duodenum	Stomach
Head of pancreas	Body of pancreas
Right adrenal gland	Left adrenal gland
Portion of right kidney	Portion of left kidney
Hepatic flexure of colon	Splenic flexure of colon
Portions of ascending and transverse colon	Portions of transverse and descending colon

Right lower quadrant	Left lower quadrant
Lower pole of right kidney	Lower pole of left kidney
Cecum and appendix	Sigmoid colon
Portion of ascending colon	Portion of descending colon
Bladder (if distended)	Bladder (if distended)
Ovary and salpinx	Ovary and salpinx
Uterus (if enlarged)	Uterus (if enlarged)
Right spermatic cord	Left spermatic cord
Right ureter	Left ureter

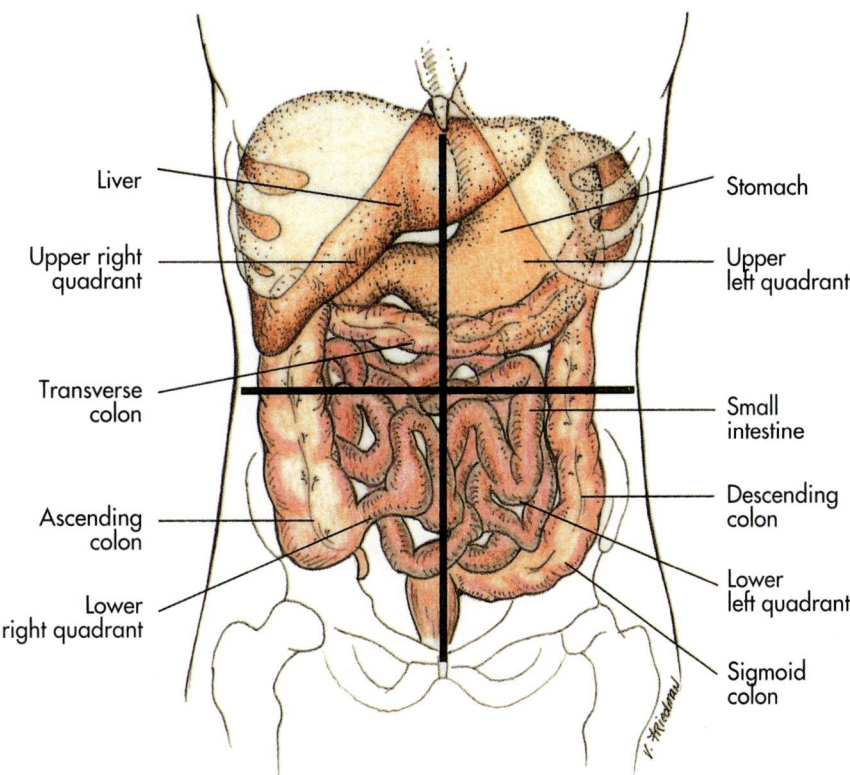

Figure 12-49 Abdominal quadrants.

Liver

Upper right quadrant

Transverse colon

Ascending colon

Lower right quadrant

Stomach

Upper left quadrant

Small intestine

Descending colon

Lower left quadrant

Sigmoid colon

EQUIPMENT
Stethoscope
Tape measure
Marking pen

Assessment

1. Elicit details of abdominal or low back pain: location, onset, frequency, precipitating factors, aggravating factors, type of pain, and severity. For female clients, determine if they are pregnant.
2. Note position and movement of client. Usually leans into, splints or positions toward the pain? Moves more slowly? **Positioning may reveal nature of pain.**
3. Obtain detailed data about elimination patterns for bowel and bladder along with measures used to promote elimination: laxatives, enemas, and eating and drinking habits vs. patterns of weight gain or loss.

4. Inquire about history of surgeries of the trunk and family history of cancer, kidney disease, alcoholism, drug use, and hypertension.

Planning

EXPECTED OUTCOMES

1. Client has no deviations from normal:
   a. Soft, symmetrical abdomen with even contour and no masses or tenderness; active bowel sounds in all four quadrants; percussion reveals tympanic sounds.
   b. Normal borders of liver without any enlargement or tenderness.
   c. No costovertebral angle or suprapubic tenderness.
2. Client states warning signs of colon cancer.

Implementation

Steps	Rationale
1. See Standard Protocol (Chapter 1, p. 5).	
2. After emptying bladder, have client assume a recumbent position with knees slightly flexed or a small pillow under knees. Ask client to point with one fin-	Full bladder can cause discomfort and feeling of urgency, preventing ability to relax. Position promotes optimal relaxation of abdominal muscles.

Steps	Rationale

ger to any painful areas and to show how pain moves or radiates.

Painful areas are assessed last.

3. Inspect abdominal surface.

Keep in mind the landmarks mapped out by quadrants.

   a. For skin alterations: scars, venous patterns, and openings.

   b. For contour and symmetry.

   c. For position, shape, and color of umbilicus and visible pulsations.

An everted, pouched-out umbilicus usually indicates distention or hernia.

   d. For distention, ask client if abdomen feels tight. If distention suspected, measure size of abdominal girth by placing tape measure around abdomen at level of umbilicus and note measurement. Mark site with marker pen.

Assesses increases in abdominal size caused by distention.

4. Repeat inspection with client taking a deep breath and holding it, then raising head up. At this time, observe for bulges.

Position causes superficial abdominal wall masses and hernias to become apparent.

5. Auscultate bowel by placing diaphragm of stethoscope lightly over each of the four quadrants (Figure 12-50). Ask client not to speak. If NG tube present, disconnect it from suction or turn suction off during auscultation. If client has no history of bowel problems, only the left lower quadrant needs to be auscultated for bowel sounds. If sounds are abnormal here, assess all quadrants.

Determines presence or absence of peristalsis. Absent sounds indicate cessation of gastric motility in the large bowel.

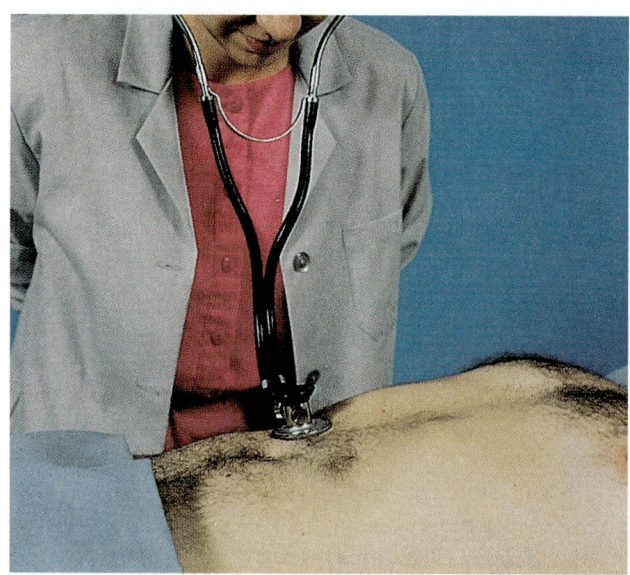

Figure 12-50 (From Barkauskas VH et al: *Health and physical assessment,* St. Louis, 1994, Mosby.)

6. Listen 2 to 5 minutes for succession of clicks or gurgles in each quadrant before deciding bowel sounds are absent. Describe sounds as audible or normal, absent, hyperactive (prolonged, loud, multiple gurgles), hypoactive (paralytic ileus with absent or infrequent sounds), or borborygmi (exaggerated waves of peristalsis that indicate attempt to push fluid and air against an obstruction).

Normal sounds range from 8 to 20 per minute.

7. Percuss abdomen. Gently percuss each of the four quadrants systematically to note areas of tympany and dullness (Figure 12-51).

Normal percussion sounds are tympanic sounds.

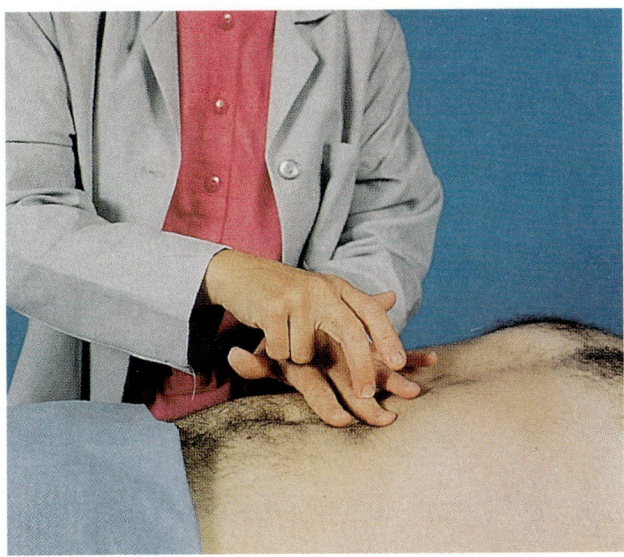

Figure 12-51 (From Barkauskas VH et al: *Health and physical assessment,* St. Louis, 1994, Mosby.)

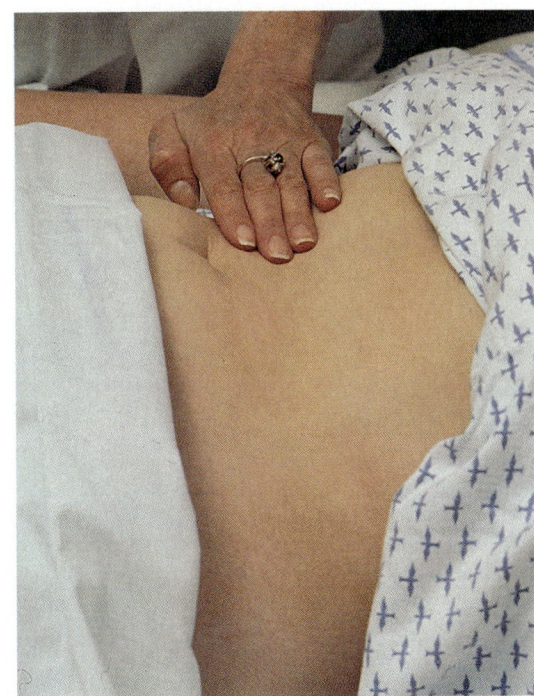

Figure 12-52

Steps	Rationale
8. Palpate abdomen. Lightly palpate over abdominal quadrants by using palm and pads of fingertips in smooth, coordinated movement. Depress skin approximately 1.25 cm (½ inch) and note muscle tone, abdominal stiffness, presence of masses, and tenderness. Observe client's face for grimacing, which may indicate tenderness or pain. Note if abdomen is firm or soft to touch (Figure 12-52). Remember to palpate painful areas last and to avoid quick jabs.	Detects areas of localized tenderness, degree of tenderness, and presence and character of underlying masses.
9. Just below umbilicus and above symphysis pubis, palpate for smooth, rounded mass.	Detects the top of a distended bladder.
10. If abdominal masses are palpated, note size, location, shape, consistency, tenderness, mobility, and texture.	
11. If tenderness is present, press one hand slowly and deeply into the involved area, then let go quickly.	Tests for rebound tenderness. Results are positive if pain increases with maneuver. Note if pain is aggravated.
12. Assess liver. Locate the liver's lower border by placing left hand under client's right posterior thorax, just under small of the back. Apply gentle pressure with left hand. With fingers pointing toward right costal margin, place right hand on right upper quadrant below costal margin. Ask client to take a deep breath, and gently palpate right hand in and up. As client inhales, liver's edge may be felt (Figure 12-53) as it descends.	Liver's edge cannot usually be palpated in normal adults. If liver is enlarged, pressure in this area causes pain; be sure to observe client's face during this maneuver.
13. Place bell of stethoscope over midline of abdomen and auscultate for vascular sounds. If aortic bruit is heard, stop assessment and notify physician.	Determines presence of turbulent blood flow (bruits) through thoracic or abdominal aorta.

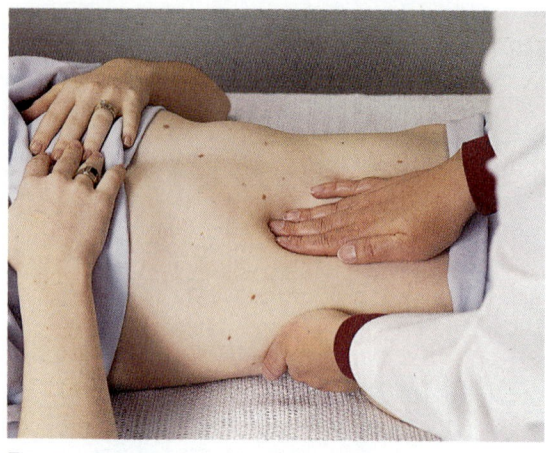

Figure 12-53 (From Seidel HM et al: *Mosby's guide to physical examination,* ed 3, St. Louis, 1995, Mosby.)

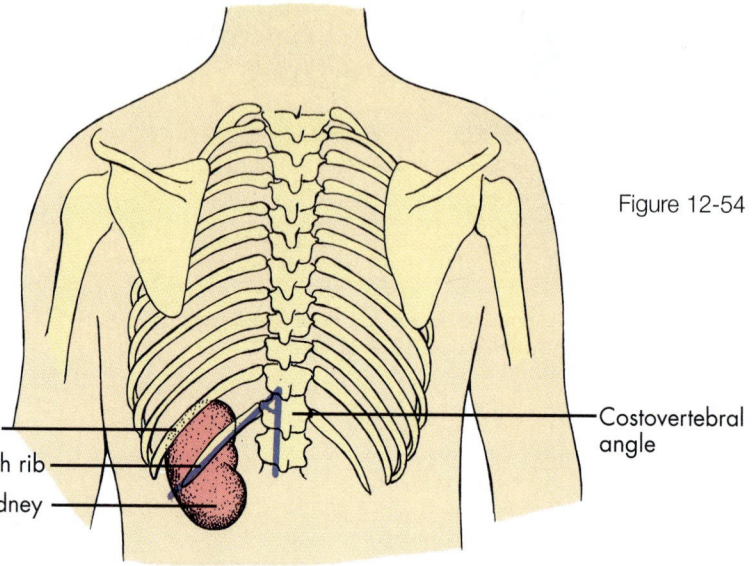

Eleventh rib

Twelfth rib

Kidney

Costovertebral angle

Figure 12-54

Steps	Rationale
14. Assess posterior trunk. Have client sit upright. Place bell of stethoscope posteriorly over costovertebral angle (CVA) (Figure 12-54) and listen for bruits. If found, stop and notify physician. Next, firmly percuss over each CVA along scapular lines. Use ulnar surface of fist to percuss directly or indirectly. Note if client has pain.	Pain may indicate presence of kidney inflammation.
15. See Completion Protocol (Chapter 1, p. 6).	

Evaluation

1. Compare findings with client's baseline and normal expected findings.
2. Ask client to describe signs of colon cancer.

UNEXPECTED OUTCOMES
AND RELATED INTERVENTIONS

1. Client has abnormal bowels sounds; abdominal pain; asymmetrical abdomen with palpable masses; dullness to percussion; rebound abdominal tenderness; or findings of enlarged liver.
   a. Compare established baseline with new findings.
   b. Report to physician any new findings.
   c. Position to reduce abdominal discomfort.

2. Client has bladder that is palpable over the symphysis pubis or has a tender kidney area.
   a. Report findings to appropriate health care personnel, charge nurse, or physician.
   b. Implement actions to facilitate bladder emptying, or insert urinary catheter as ordered (see Chapter 34).
3. Client is unable to describe signs of colon cancer.
   Review with client appropriate signs of colon cancer.

SAMPLE DOCUMENTATION

1300 Bowel sounds active in LLQ; abdomen soft, flat, and without tenderness on palpation. Percussion notes normal. Negative for bladder distention or kidney tenderness.

Skill 12.8   Assessing the Genitalia and Rectum

The nurse should complete the assessment of the external genitalia and rectum after obtaining a sexual activity health history. This is especially important to screen for sexually transmitted disease (STD). These data will guide the nurse in what to inspect in more detail or defer to another health care team member.

Typically, the client feels anxious during the examination. To avoid embarrassing the client, the nurse uses a calm, reassuring, and attentive approach. Comfort is established through correct positioning and draping. Each portion of the examination is explained so that the client can anticipate the nurse's action.

Nursing Diagnosis

Impaired Skin Integrity is appropriate when lesions, rashes, or drainage are evident. **Knowledge Deficit** is indicated if the client has inadequate perineal care or verbalizes minimal knowledge in the prevention of sexually transmitted diseases (STDs) or cancer risk factors. **Risk for Infection** is appropriate if the client reports multiple sex partners. **Sexual Dysfunction** or **Altered Sexuality Patterns** is indicated if reported by the client.

EQUIPMENT
Gloves
Examination light

Assessment

1. Assess client's sexual history for use of safer sex behaviors; reproductive history; pain during intercourse; and history of any lesions or drainage in the perineal area.

2. Assess client for elimination problems such as change in bowel habits; melena; hemorrhoids; use of laxatives, iron, or codeine; rectal pain; and history of genitourinary problems.
3. Determine if client has had previous illness or surgery involving reproductive organs or rectal area.
4. For males, determine if client has had prior feelings of heaviness or painless enlargement of the testes.
5. Assess dietary history for intake of fat and fiber.
6. Determine family history for cancer of the reproductive organs or colon.

Planning

EXPECTED OUTCOMES
1. Client exhibits normal genitalia.
   a. Female: symmetrical labia majora, triangular pattern of hair growth, pink clitoris and labia minora, symmetrical vaginal orifice without tissue prolapse, nonpalpable Bartholin's and Skene's glands, and absence of lesions, inflammation, edema, or foul-smelling drainage.
   b. Male: pink, smooth glans with meatus at tip; freely hanging scrotum with both testes descended; loose scrotal skin; smooth, ovoid, and nontender testes; shaft without swelling; and no bulging or protrusion in scrotal or inguinal area.
   c. Client exhibits anal area without redness, lesions, or hemorrhoids.
2. Client describes symptoms of STD.
3. Client describes the findings of reproductive organ cancers and methods for screening.

Implementation

Steps	Rationale
1. See Standard Protocol (Chapter 1, p. 5). 	
2. For female client a. After client empties bladder, position in lithotomy position: supine, knees flexed perpendicular to the bed, thighs relaxed with legs abducted to the side, and arms to the side or over chest. b. Place rectangular sheet with corner draping over sternum, adjacent corners falling over each knee, and fourth corner covering perineum (Figure 12-55).	Provides for privacy.

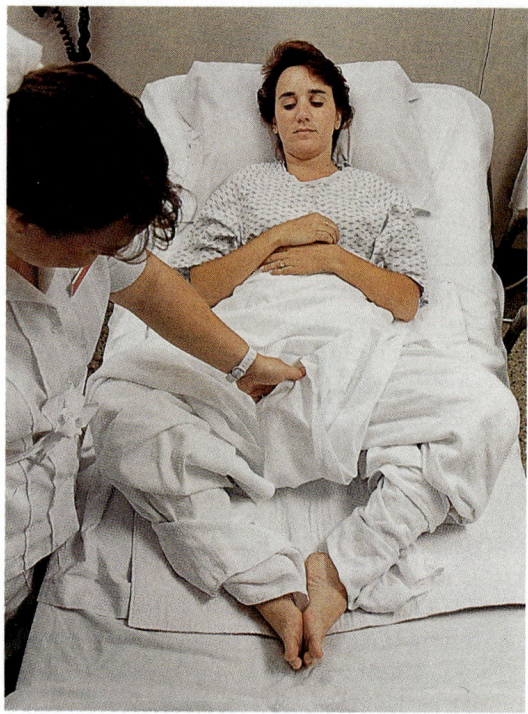

Figure 12-55

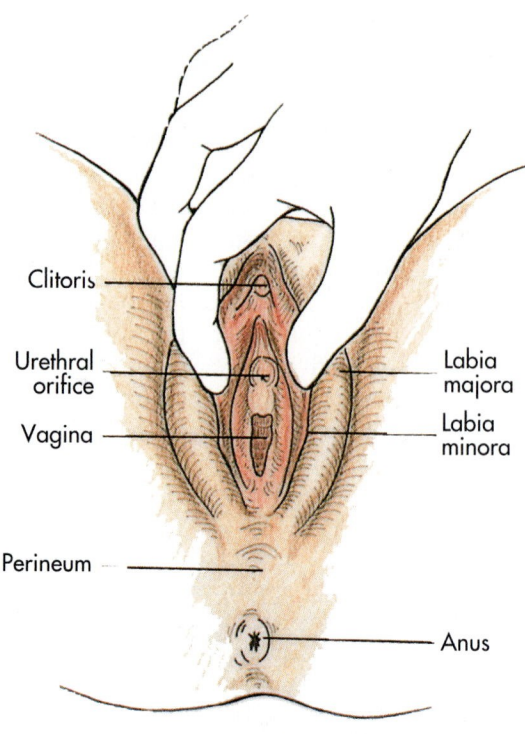

Clitoris

Urethral orifice

Vagina

Labia majora

Labia minora

Perineum

Anus

Figure 12-56

Steps	Rationale
c. With perineum well illuminated, inspect quantity and distribution of hair growth, color of skin, and size and contour of labia. Note any areas of inflammation, edema, lacerations, lesions, or discharge. Inspect skin and hair of pubic area for lice. If structures appear distorted or if vaginal orifice is asymmetrical, palpate tissues later in examination.	
d. Before touching perineum, touch neighboring thigh. Explain that it is necessary to inspect deeper perineal structures.	
e. With nondominant hand, gently place thumb and index finger inside labia minora and retract tissues outward (Figure 12-56). Be sure to have firm hold during retraction.	Ensures clear view for inspection.
f. Inspect clitoris, labia minora, vaginal opening, and urethral orifice (a small slit or pinhole opening just above vaginal canal) for size, color, drainage, edema, inflammation, or lesions.	
g. Nurse may also examine rectal area at this time. Use nondominant hand and retract buttocks. Inspect condition of perianal tissues, noting color of skin, closure of anal sphincter, and presence of lesions, hemorrhoids, ulcers, inflammation, rashes, or discoloration.	Perianal area is more pigmented and more coarse than skin overlying buttocks.
h. Ask client to bear down as though having a bowel movement.	Maneuver causes any hemorrhoids or fissures within anal canal to appear.

Steps	Rationale

i. Clean any moisture or drainage from perineal area. Assist client to sitting position while draping protects privacy.

Restores comfort.

3. For male client

a. After client empties bladder, have him lie supine with chest, abdomen, and lower legs draped. Throughout the examination, manipulate genitalia gently.

b. Expose area, then observe size and shape of the penis and testes, color of the scrotal skin, and character and distribution of pubic hair.

Scrotal skin is darker than surrounding skin and is wrinkled. Adult client has pubic hair extending from base of penis over the symphysis pubis; hair is coarse and curly.

c. Inspect skin over genitalia for lice, rashes, excoriations, or lesions.

d. Inspect structures of penis.

(1) In uncircumcised males, retract foreskin to reveal glans and urethral meatus. Note position of meatus and observe for discharge, edema, inflammation, and lesions of glans. Be sure to check entire circumference (Figure 12-57).

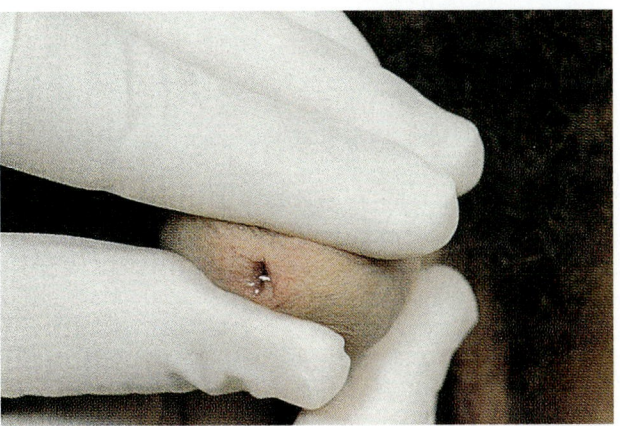

Figure 12-57 (From Barkauskas VH et al: *Health and physical assessment,* St. Louis, 1994, Mosby.)

(2) Carefully inspect area between foreskin and glans.

Common site for venereal lesions. Small amount of thick, white secretion between glans and foreskin is normal. Be sure to replace foreskin over glans if it was retracted, since edema will result if it is not replaced properly.

(3) Inspect scrotum's size, shape, and symmetry and for presence of lesions.

Normally, left testis is lower than right. Scrotum should hang freely from perineum behind penis.

(4) Gently lift scrotal sac to view posterior surface. Gently palpate each testis and epididymis using thumb and first two fingers. Palpate for size, shape, and consistency. Ask if client has sensation of tenderness (Figure 12-58).

Teach or reinforce principles and technique of testicular self-examination at this time.

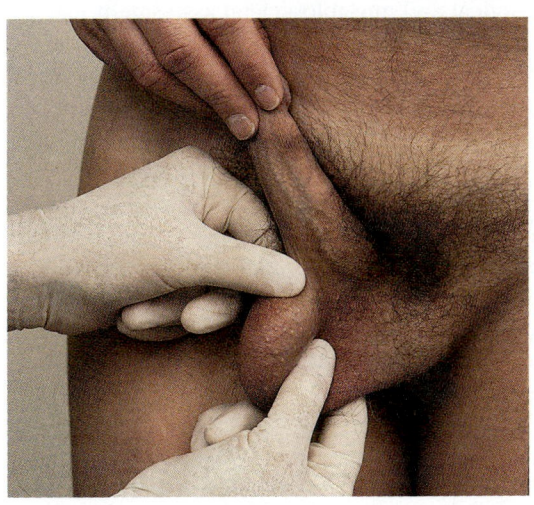

Figure 12-58 (From Seidel HM et al: *Mosby's guide to physical examination,* ed 3, St. Louis, 1995, Mosby.)

Steps	Rationale
e. Explain technique of testicular self exam (to be performed monthly after age 15). Have client perform exam after warm bath or shower, when scrotum is relaxed. Client should stand naked in front of mirror and look for swelling of or lumps in skin. Using both hands, he should place the index and middle fingers under testicles and place thumbs on top, then gently roll testicle, feeling for lumps, thickening, or hardening.	Testicular cancer is common solid tumor among young men age 18 to 34.
f. Ask client to assume a side-lying position. Examine the rectal area. Refer to Steps 2g and 2h to complete examination.	
4. See Completion Protocol (Chapter 1, p. 6).	

Evaluation

1. Compare findings with client's baseline and normal expected findings.
2. Ask client to describe the findings of STDs.
3. Ask client to demonstrate/describe screening for reproductive organ cancers.

UNEXPECTED OUTCOMES AND RELATED INTERVENTIONS

1. Client has evidence of inflammation, foul-smelling discharge, lesions, or edema in genitalia area or tender, reddened anal area with or without hemorrhoids.
   a. Obtain further details of history as indicated.
   b. Culture any vaginal or urethral discharge.
   c. Refer to appropriate agency for follow-up and treatment.
2. Client is unable to describe the risk factors for colorectal cancer or STDs or when to monitor for reproductive organ cancers.
   a. Review selected risks that are pertinent to client.
   b. Provide supplementary reading materials.

SAMPLE DOCUMENTATION

1400 Normally developed genitalia without lesions, discharge, or lice. Rectum without hemorrhoids, lesions, or discharge. Normal bowel patterns without use of laxatives or cathartics.

Skill 12.9 | Assessing Neurological Function

Neurological and musculoskeletal assessment may be conducted simultaneously. Information gathered from both examinations is valuable in determining a client's ability to perform ADLs or to tolerate exercise.

The extensiveness of the neurological assessment may be limited if the client's LOC is diminished. A client's chief complaint often determines whether a neurological assessment is necessary. For example, if a client has headaches, this assessment is mandatory. However, if a client complains of oral pain or skin rash, a neurological assessment is not as urgent.

Nursing Diagnosis

Risk for Injury is appropriate when the client has muscle weakness or altered LOC. **Impaired Physical Mobility** involves findings of cerebellar disease, which causes a wide-based shuffling gait; parkinsonian slow shuffle with increased rapidity and propulsive nature; paresis; diminished sensation of extremities; and any type of "plegia"—paraplegia: paralysis of lower extremities; quadriplegia: paralysis of upper and lower extremities; or hemiplegia: paralysis of one half of body. **Risk for Impaired Skin Integrity** is appropriate if client is unconscious or has impaired voluntary movement. **Unilateral Neglect** applies when a client who has suffered a stroke is perceptually unaware of and inattentive to one side of the body.

EQUIPMENT

Cotton applicator or cotton ball
Safety pin (sterile)

Two test tubes, one filled with hot water and one with cold water
Reflex hammer
Vials containing coffee or vanilla extract

Assessment

1. Determine if the client is taking medications, such as analgesics, sedatives, hypnotics, antipsychotics, antidepressants, or nerve stimulants.
2. Screen client for headaches, seizures, dizziness, vertigo, numbness or tingling of body part, visual changes, weakness, pain, or changes in speech.
3. Discuss with significant other any recent changes in client's behavior, such as increased irritability, mood swings, or memory loss.

4. Assess client for history of changes in any of the senses: vision, hearing, smell, taste, or touch.

Planning

EXPECTED OUTCOMES

1. Client exhibits normal function:
   a. Client is alert, oriented, carries on appropriate discussion.
   b. Sensation is intact for pain, temperature, light touch, and position.
   c. Cranial nerves are intact.
   d. Muscle strength is normal and symmetrical; gait is even and balanced; reflexes are symmetric and 2+.
2. Client/family identifies safety factors related to neurological deficits.

Implementation

Steps	Rationale
1. See Standard Protocol (Chapter 1, p. 5).	
2. Assess mental and emotional status, behavior, appearance, language function, and intellectual function. (See Skill 12.1.)	
3. Assess function of each cranial nerve if not completed (Table 12-4; see Skill 12.2).	Detects presence of motor and sensory impairment of nerves extending from intracranial sites.
a. CN I: Ask client to identify different aromas, such as coffee, vanilla, and alcohol swab (Figure 12-59). Have client close eyes if test aroma has labeled container.)	
b. CNs II, III, IV, and VI: Refer to Skill 12.4.	Tests sensory and motor function.
c. CNs V and VII: Ask client to close eyes and lightly measure sensation of light pain and soft touch across skin of face (Figure 12-60). With client's eyes open, lightly touch cornea with wisp of sterile cotton. As client smiles, frowns, puffs out cheeks, and raises and lowers eyebrows, look for symmetry. Have client identify salty or sweet taste on front of tongue.	Tests sensory and motor function.

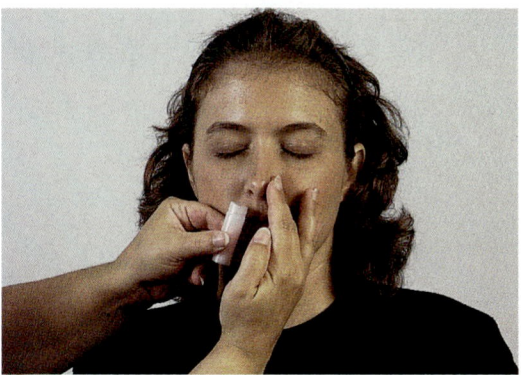

Figure 12-59 (From Chipps E et al: *Neurologic disorders,* Mosby's Clinical Nursing Series, St. Louis, 1992, Mosby.)

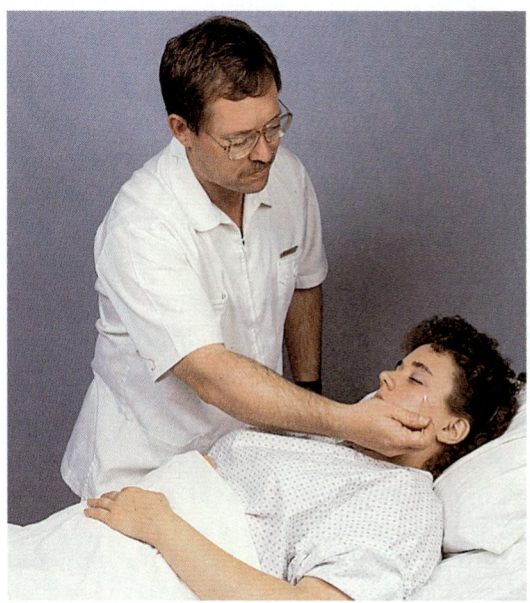

Figure 12-60

Table 12-4 **Cranial Nerve Function and Assessment**

Number	Name	Type	Function	Method
I	Olfactory	Sensory	Sense of smell	Ask client to identify different nonirritating aromas such as coffee and vanilla.
II	Optic	Sensory	Visual acuity	Use Snellen chart or ask client to read printed material while wearing glasses.
III	Oculomotor	Motor	Extraocular eye movement	Assess directions of gaze.
			Pupil constriction and dilation	Measure pupil reaction to light reflex and accommodation.
IV	Trochlear	Motor	Upward and downward movement of eyeball	Assess directions of gaze.
V	Trigeminal	Sensory and motor	Sensory nerve to skin of face	Lightly touch cornea with wisp of cotton. Assess corneal reflex. Measure sensation of light pain and touch across skin of face.
			Motor nerve to muscles of jaw	Palpate temples as client clenches teeth.
VI	Abducens	Motor	Lateral movement of eyeballs	Assess directions of gaze.
VII	Facial	Sensory and motor	Facial expression	As client smiles, frowns, puffs out cheeks, and raises and lowers eyebrows, look for symmetry.
			Taste	Have client identify salty or sweet taste on front of tongue.
VIII	Auditory	Sensory	Hearing	Assess ability to hear spoken word.
IX	Glossopharyngeal	Sensory and motor	Taste	Ask client to identify sour or sweet taste on back of tongue.
			Ability to swallow	Use tongue blade to elicit gag reflex.
X	Vagus	Sensory and motor	Sensation of pharynx	Ask client to say "ah." Observe palate and pharynx movement.
			Ability to swallow	Use tongue blade to elicit gag reflex.
			Movement of vocal cords	Assess speech for hoarseness.
XI	Spinal accessory	Motor	Movement of head and shoulders	Ask client to shrug shoulders and turn head against passive resistance.
XII	Hypoglossal	Motor	Position of tongue	Ask client to stick out tongue to midline and move it from side to side.

Steps	Rationale
d. CN VIII: Assess client's ability to hear the spoken word at normal and whispered levels of voice.	Tests auditory sensory function.
e. CNs IX, X, and XII: Ask client to identify sour, salty, or sweet taste on back of tongue. Use a tongue blade to elicit gag reflex. Ask client to say "ah" while you observe movement of palate, pharynx, signs of hoarseness, and ability to stick out tongue to midline and move side to side.	Tests sensory and motor function.
f. CN XI: Have client shrug shoulders and turn head against examiner's passive resistance. (See Skill 12.2.)	Tests motor function.

Table 12-5 **Assessment of Sensory Nerve Function**

Function	Equipment	Method	Precautions
Pain	Safety pin	Ask client to voice when dull or sharp sensation is felt. Alternately apply pointed and blunt ends of pin to skin's surface. Note areas of numbness or increased sensitivity.	Remember that areas where skin is thickened, such as heel or sole of foot, may be less sensitive to pain.

Figure 12-61

Function	Equipment	Method	Precautions
Temperature	Two test tubes, one filled with hot water and other with cold	Touch skin with tube. Ask client to identify hot or cold sensation.	Omit test if pain sensation is normal.
Light Touch	Cotton ball or cotton-tip applicator	Apply light wisp of cotton to different points along skin's surface. Ask client to voice when sensation is felt.	Apply at areas where skin is thin or more sensitive (e.g., face, neck, inner aspect of arms, top of feet and hands).
Vibration	Tuning fork	Apply vibrating fork to distal interphalangeal joint of fingers and interphalangeal joint of great toe. Have client voice when the vibration stops.	Be sure client feels vibration and not merely pressure.
Position		Grasp finger, holding it by its sides with thumb and index finger. Alternate moving finger up and down. Ask client to state when finger is up or down. Repeat with toes.	Avoid rubbing adjacent appendages as finger or toe is moved.
Two-point discrimination	Two safety pins	Lightly apply points of two safety pins simultaneously to skin's surface. Ask client if one or two pinpricks are felt.	Apply pins to same anatomical site (e.g., fingertips, palm of hand, or upper arms). Minimum distance at which client can discriminate two points varies (2-3 mm on fingertips).

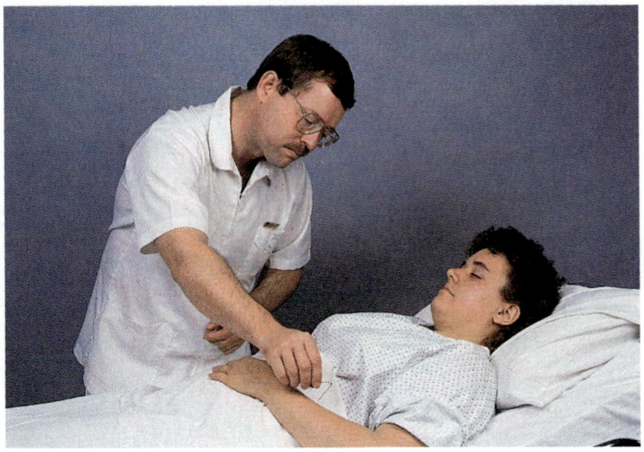

Steps	Rationale

4. Assess sensory function.
   a. Perform all sensory testing with client's eyes closed. Sensory can be integrated into site-specific assessments.
   b. Assess sensation to pain (Figure 12-61), temperature, light touch, vibration, position, and two–point discrimination (Table 12-5).
   c. Apply sensory stimuli in random, unpredictable order. Note anatomical area where sensation is reduced.
   d. Compare symmetrical areas of body while applying stimuli to face, arms, legs, and trunk.
   e. Ask client to say when particular stimulus is perceived.

5. Assess motor function.
   a. Assess gait, stance, and muscle strength and tone.

   b. Have client stand with feet close together and eyes closed (Figure 12-62). Then ask client to stand on one foot, then the other (Figure 12-63).
   c. Ask client to sit. Demonstrate method for rapidly striking thigh with palm of hand evenly and without hesitation. Have client repeat.

Client should not be able to see when or where stimulus strikes skin.

Changes may reflect lesions in peripheral nerves, spinal cord, or cerebral cortex.
Note swaying. Romberg's test assesses balance. Cerebellar disease causes imbalance even with eyes open.

Note smoothness of movement. Assesses upper extremity coordination.

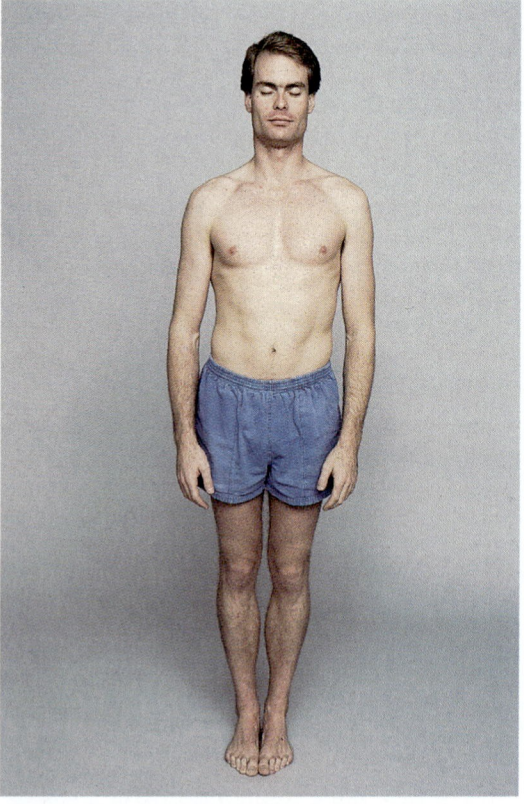

Figure 12-62 (From Chipps E et al: *Neurologic disorders,* Mosby's Clinical Nursing Series, St. Louis, 1992, Mosby.)

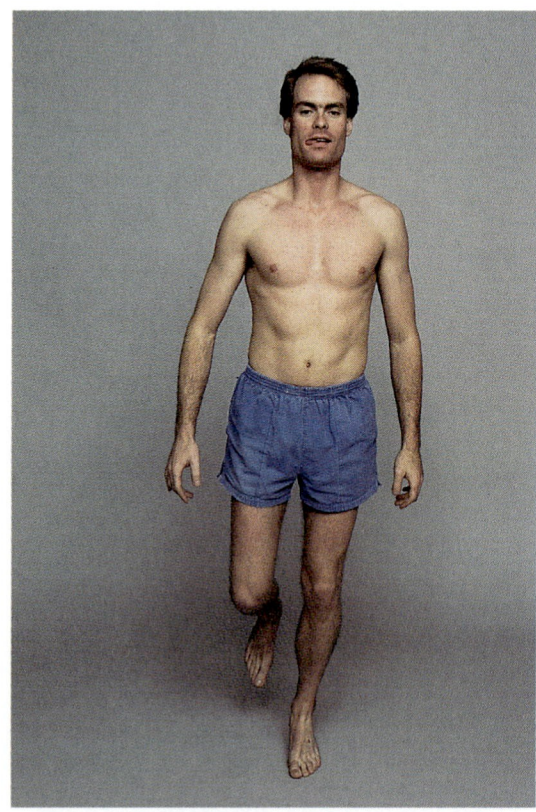

Figure 12-63 (From Chipps E et al: *Neurologic disorders,* Mosby's Clinical Nursing Series, St. Louis, 1992, Mosby.)

Steps	Rationale

d. Have client alternately strike thigh with hand supinated and then pronated.

e. Stand in front of client; hold index finger 60 cm (2 feet) stationary in front of client's face. Ask client to touch your index finger with his or her index finger (Figure 12-64, *A*) and then to touch the nose alternately (Figure 12-64, *B*).

Speed and symmetry of movement are disturbed in cerebellar dysfunction. Note tremors of hand or awkward movement.

Point-to-point test assesses upper extremity coordination.

A 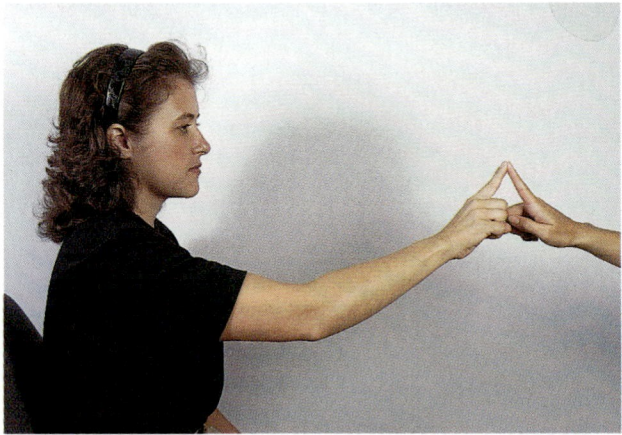 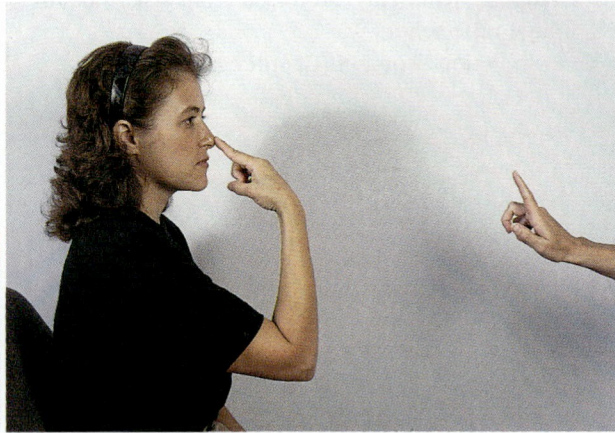 B

Figure 12-64 (From Chipps E et al: *Neurologic disorders,* Mosby's Clinical Nursing Series, St. Louis, 1992, Mosby.)

f. Ask client to close eyes and place heel of one foot just below knee of opposite leg and then slide heel down to shin toward foot. Repeat for other leg (Figure 12-65).

Presence of involuntary movements or difficulty in controlling heel may indicate cerebellar problem.

g. With client supine, place hand at ball of client's foot. Ask client to tap hand with foot as quickly as possible.

Note speed and smoothness of movement. Assesses lower extremity coordination.

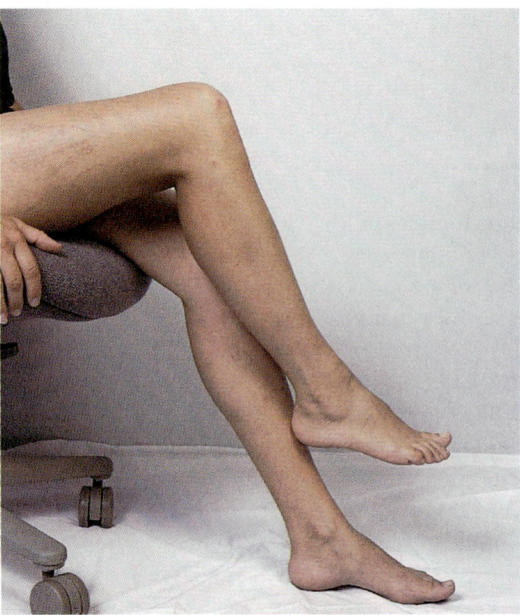

Figure 12-65 (From Chipps E et al: *Neurologic disorders,* Mosby's Clinical Nursing Series, St. Louis, 1992, Mosby.)

Steps	Rationale
6. Assess reflexes. a. Assess deep tendon reflexes (Table 12-6). Reflexes should be symmetrical on both sides of body. b. Ask client to relax extremity. c. Position limb to slightly stretch muscle being tested. d. Hold reflex hammer loosely between thumb and fingers. e. Tap tendon briskly (Figure 12-66). f. Compare symmetry of reflex from one side of body to the other. **7.** See Completion Protocol (Chapter 1, p. 6).	The more common tested reflexes are *plantar* and *patellar*. Reflexes are graded on scale: 0, No response 1+, Low-normal slight muscle contraction 2+, Normal visible muscle twitch 3+, Brisker than normal 4+, Hyperactive, very brisk; spinal cord disorder suspected Asymmetry of reflex response indicates alteration in reflex pathway. 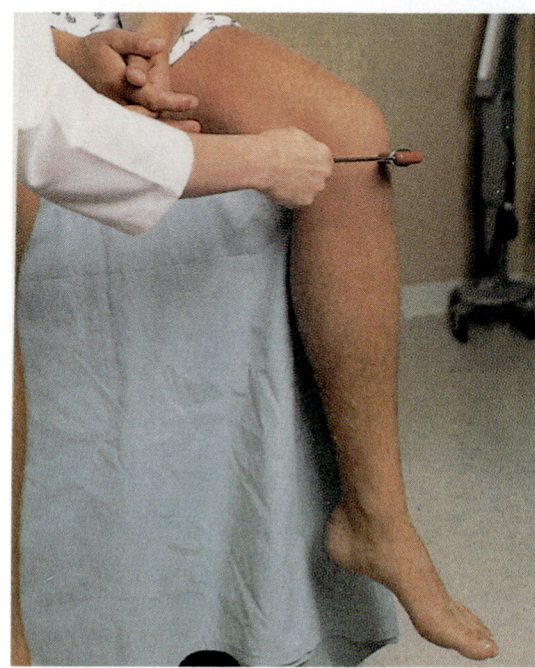 Figure 12-66

Evaluation

1. Compare findings with client's baseline and normal expected findings.
2. Ask what safety measures are being taken to adapt to motor/sensory deficits.

UNEXPECTED OUTCOMES AND RELATED INTERVENTIONS

Client demonstrates evidence of confusion; intact sensory and motor function but slow response to instructions; reduced sensation to temperature, touch, and painful stimuli; unsteady gait or dragging foot; reflexes of 0 to 1+ or 3+ to 4+; or abnormal cranial nerve function.

 a. Provide for client's safety (e.g., remove barriers to mobility in the home; provide appropriate assistive devices; supervise ambulation).
 b. Compare findings to prior history to identify if they are new.
 c. If new findings, refer client and significant other to appropriate health care professional or agency.

SAMPLE DOCUMENTATION

0800 Client appropriate and oriented × 3 without deficits in mobility, coordination, or motor and sensory functioning of upper and lower extremities. Deep tendon reflexes 2+ for plantar and patellar and bilaterally equal.

Table 12-6 **Assessment of Common Reflexes**

Type	Procedure	Normal reflex
DEEP TENDON REFLEXES		
Biceps	Flex client's arm at elbow with palms down. Place your thumb in antecubital fossa at base of biceps tendon. Strike thumb with reflex hammer.	Flexion of arm at elbow
Triceps	Flex client's elbow, holding arm across chest, or hold upper arm horizontally and allow lower arm to go limp. Strike triceps tendon just above elbow.	Extension at elbow
Patellar	Have client sit with legs hanging freely over side of bed or chair or have client lie supine and support knee in flexed position. Briskly tap patellar tendon just below patella.	Extension of lower leg at knee
Achilles	Have client assume same position as for patellar reflex. Slightly dorsiflex client's ankle by grasping toes in palm of your hand. Strike Achilles tendon just above heel.	Plantar flexion of foot
Plantar (Babinski's)	Have client lie supine with legs straight and feet relaxed. Take handle end of reflex hammer and stroke lateral aspect of sole from heel to ball of foot, curving across ball of foot toward big toe.	Bending of toes downward
CUTANEOUS REFLEXES		
Gluteal	Have client assume side-lying position. Spread buttocks apart and lightly stimulate perineal area with cotton applicator.	Contraction of anal sphincter
Abdominal	Have client stand or lie supine. Stroke abdominal skin with base of cotton applicator over lateral borders of rectus abdominis muscle toward midline. Repeat test in each abdominal quadrant.	Contraction of rectus abdominis muscle with pulling of umbilicus toward stimulated side

Skill 12.10 | Assessing Musculoskeletal Function

Musculoskeletal assessment includes a general inspection of gait, posture, and body position as well as thorough assessment of specific muscle, bone, and joint groups. This assessment is easily integrated into routine activities of care or when assessing other body systems.

With aging, abilities decrease for response to multiple stimuli, and ROM decreases in all joints because of reduction in muscle fiber size and tightening of joints. Allow more time for older adults because they are slower to complete tasks.

Nursing Diagnosis

Risk for Injury is appropriate when the client is not immobilized and has a deficit in musculoskeletal functioning. **Body Image Disturbance** is indicated when the client expresses concern or negative comments about lack of abilities for locomotion. **Impaired Physical Mobility** is appropriate when findings of muscle weakness, loss of strength, or skeletal abnormalities are present. **Pain** is indicated with a report of injury or misalignment of the skeletal frame.

EQUIPMENT
Tape measure

Assessment

1. Ask client to describe history of problems in bone, muscle, or joint function (e.g., recent falls, trauma, lifting heavy objects) and history of bone or joint disease with sudden or gradual onset.
2. Assess nature and extent of client's pain: type, location, severity, predisposing and aggravating factors, and relieving factors.
3. Determine how alterations influence client's ability to perform ADLs, household chores, work, and social functions.
4. Assess height loss of women older than age 50 by subtracting current height from recall of maximum adult height (Reed and Birge, 1988). May be indicator for osteoporosis.

Planning

EXPECTED OUTCOMES

Client exhibits normal function:
a. Gait is even and balanced with arms swinging freely at side, and posture is erect.
b. Full active ROM in all joints, joints without deformities or crepitus, and normal thoracic and lumbar curves.
c. Strong muscle groups without deformity.

Implementation

Steps	Rationale
1. See Standard Protocol (Chapter 1, p. 5).	
2. Inspect gait as client walks into examination room and stands. Observe for foot dragging, shuffling, or limping; balance; and presence of obvious deformity in lower extremities.	Gait is more natural if client is unaware of observation. Nature of gait may indicate type of alteration. Ambulation can accentuate presence of deformity.
3. Stand behind client and observe postural alignment: position of hips relative to shoulders. Look sideways at cervical, thoracic, and lumbar curves (Figure 12-67). Note abnormalities.	

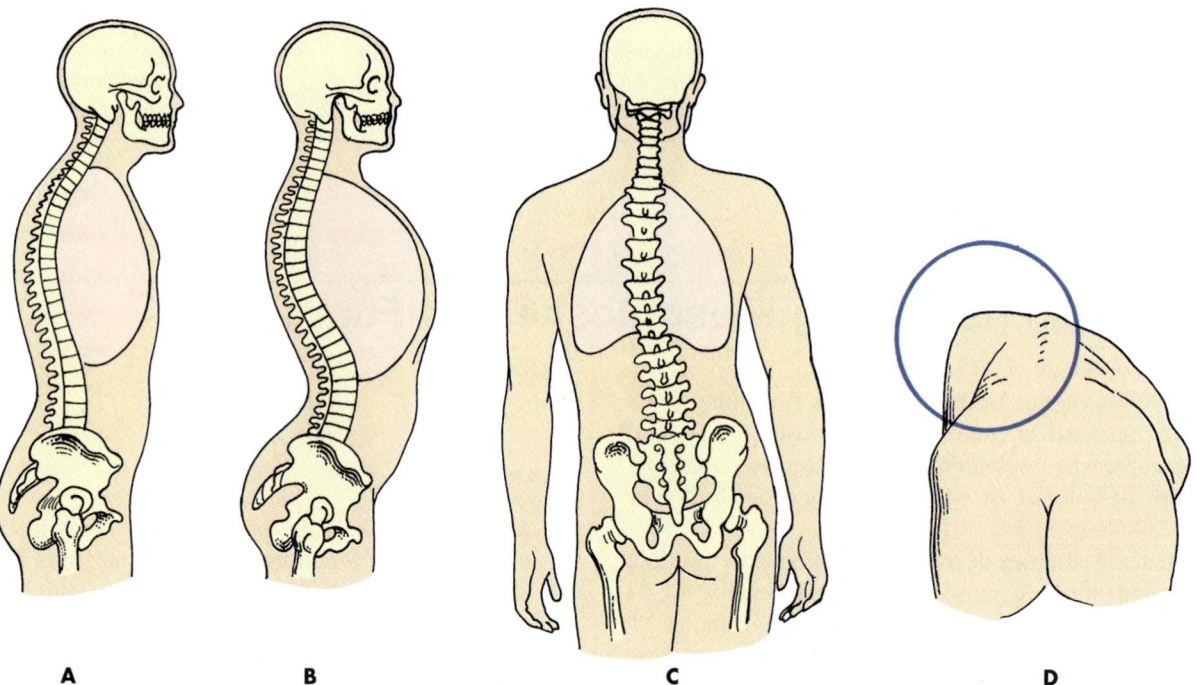

Figure 12-67 Spinal deformities: **A,** kyphosis; **B,** lordosis; **C,** scoliosis; **D,** scoliosis with client bending forward.

Steps	Rationale
4. Make a general observation of symmetry of joints, muscles, and extremity length. Look for obvious deformities.	General review helps to pinpoint areas requiring in-depth assessment.
5. Assist client in putting each joint through its full ROM (Figure 12-68). Observe for equality of motion in same body parts.	Assessment of client's normal ROM provides baseline for assessing later changes after surgery or procedures.
a. Active motion: Client needs no support or assistance and is able to move joint independently.	

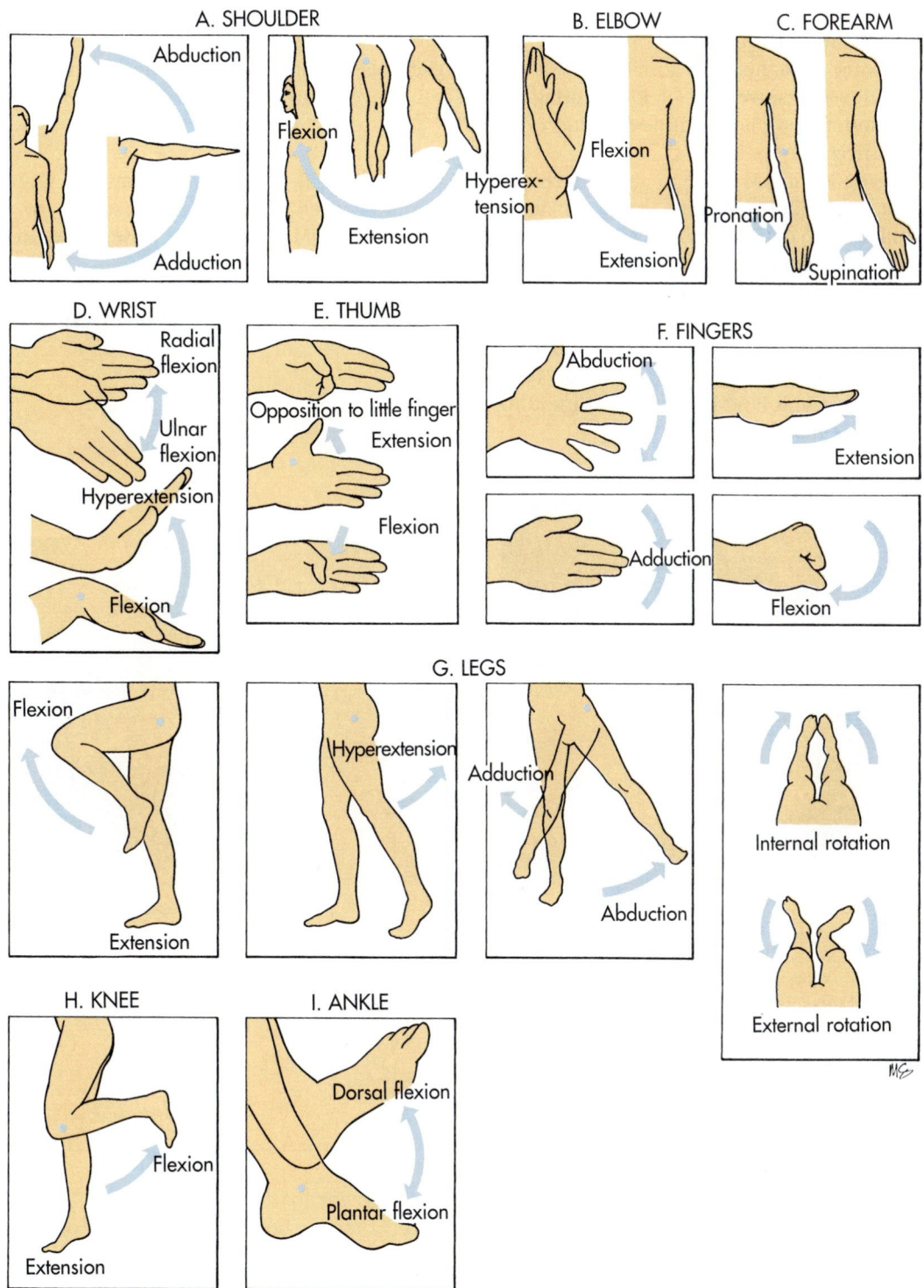

Figure 12-68 Range of motion, standards for mobility. **A** to **F,** Upper extremities. **G** to **I,** Lower extremities. (Modified from Beare PG, Myers JL: *Principles and practice of adult health nursing,* ed 2, St. Louis, 1994, Mosby.)

Steps	Rationale

b. Passive motion: Nurse supports extremity and moves joints through full ROM.

6. While observing ROM, note any instability of joint. Palpate for unusual movement of joint during its movement and for swelling, stiffness, tenderness, redness, and heat.

7. While assessing ROM, ask client to allow extremity to relax or hang limp. Support extremity, move through full ROM to detect muscular resistance. Observe position changes (standing, sitting, lying) for coordination, strength, and flexibility.

8. Assess muscle strength by having client resist pressure applied to the muscle group by the nurse to move against resistance (e.g., push with foot) (Figure 12-69). Have client hold resistance until told to stop. Compare symmetrical groups.

Crepitus is crunching or grating that occurs when joint is moved; it indicates a pathological condition.

Detects muscle tone in major muscle groups. Normal tone causes mild, even resistance to movement through ROM. If tone is increased (hypertonicity), any sudden movement of joint is met with considerable resistance.

Hypotonic muscle moves without resistance and feels flabby.

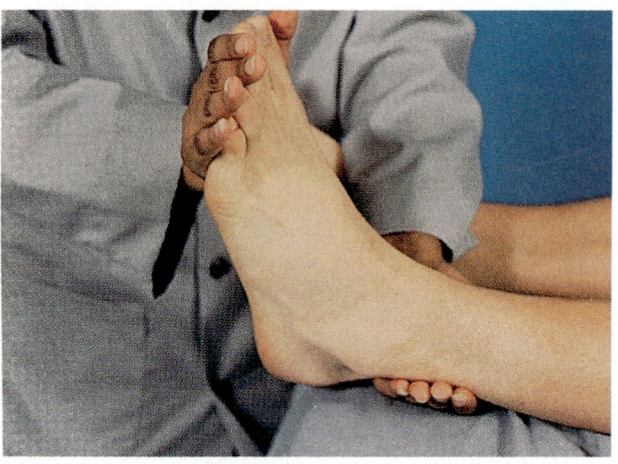

Figure 12-69 (From Barkauskas VH et al: *Health and physical assessment,* St. Louis, 1994, Mosby.)

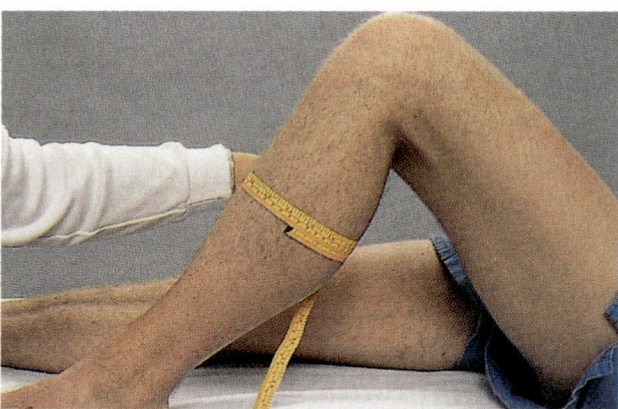

Figure 12-70 (From Seidel HM et al: *Mosby's guide to physical examination,* ed 3, St. Louis, 1995, Mosby.)

9. If muscle weakness is identified, measure muscle size with tape measure placed around body of muscle (Figure 12-70). Compare with same muscle on opposite side of body.
10. See Completion Protocol (Chapter 1, p. 6).

Evaluation

Compare findings with client's baseline and normal expected findings.

UNEXPECTED OUTCOMES AND RELATED INTERVENTIONS

Client demonstrates evidence of reduced ROM in one or more major joints, weakness in one or more muscle groups, or postural abnormalities with poor balance and shuffling or stumbling feet.

a. Provide for client's safety.
b. Compare findings to prior history to identify if these are new findings.
c. Refer to the appropriate health care agency or physician.
d. See Skill 25.1.

SAMPLE DOCUMENTATION

1400 ROM without restrictions for all joints. Strength equal and without weakness in all muscle groups. Gait steady and smooth.

CRITICAL THINKING EXERCISES

1. Label the parts of the following mental status assessment using the following letters: (A) orientation, (B) attention/concentration, (C) judgment, (D) memory, (E) thought content/processes, and (F) mood/affect.

   Sarah is a 69-year-old female of German heritage. She is visiting her daughter in the United States and has developed severe headaches. After a mental status assessment, the nurse practitioner records the following data:

   Client alert and aware that she is at the health clinic.

   Client gives a reliable health history and correct sequence of the day's events, as confirmed by her daughter.

   Client is unable to read the newspaper because of a language barrier, but she is able to follow commands and responds appropriately to general questions.

   Client appears neat in appearance.

   Client's nonverbal behavior (grimacing, rubbing forehead) is congruent with the complaint of headache.

   Client is mildly distracted because of the headache.

   Client has difficulty interpreting the proverb "a bird in the hand is worth two in the bush."

   Client is able to associate related concepts.

2. Ronald is a 42-year-old male visiting the community health clinic for a routine health assessment. The nurse practitioner records the following findings:

   Head, face, and neck: skull normal contour without notable lesions; jaw muscle strength equal bilaterally, symmetrical facial movement; discomfort noted on neck flexion at 40 degrees; trachea in midline; neck negative for lymph node palpation

   Nose, sinuses, and mouth: no septal deviation or nasal drainage noted; oral mucous membranes red with white patch noted on left cheek; denies tenderness; central cyanosis noted; intact CN X

   Eyes and ears: normal visual acuity with glasses; extraocular muscle function intact without nystagmus; right pupil sluggish to light; mildly diminished hearing acuity in left ear

   Thorax, lungs, and breasts: anterior/posterior diameter ratio 1:1; limited chest excursion; hyperresonant lung fields on percussion; wheezing noted on expiration

   Heart and circulation: apical rate 82/min, regular; normal S_1 and S_2 at the apex without abnormal sounds; BP lying 138/78, standing 124/68; posterior tibial and pedal pulses 2+ bilaterally; no NVD noted

   a. From the above assessment, determine which data would prompt you to gather additional data. Offer suggestions for additional assessment in relation to the data you identify as abnormal.

   b. Based on the above assessment, evaluate whether the listed expected outcomes have been met (M), not met (N), or insufficient data to evaluate (I).

   Client has intact facial nerves.

   Client's nasal mucosa is pink and dry; septum is in midline.

   Client's oral mucosa is pink/red and smooth without lesions.

   Client has normal visual acuity with glasses.

   Client demonstrates full visual fields.

   Client has normal hearing acuity.

   Client has clear, equal breath sounds.

   Client demonstrates symmetrical chest excursion.

   Client has smooth, symmetrical breasts.

   Client has normal heart rate, rhythm, and heart sounds.

   Client's blood pressure is within normal limits.

   Client has equal, strong, bilateral pulses.

   Client's extremities are warm and pink with normal hair and nail growth.

3. Discuss possible positive and/or negative consequences of each of the following assessment methods and approaches.

   a. Assessing S_1 and S_2 with the bell of the stethoscope

   b. Palpating and percussing the thorax before auscultation

   c. Auscultating the thorax, moving from anterior to posterior with each position change of the stethoscope

   d. Retracting the penile foreskin during a genital assessment

   e. Assessing breast tissue during the menstrual cycle

   f. Performing sensory function techniques with client watching application of each stimulus

4. Discuss the logic of conducting neurological and musculoskeletal assessments together.

REFERENCES

American Cancer Society: *1995 Cancer facts and figures,* New York, 1995, The Society.

Barkauskas VH et al: *Health and physical assessment,* St Louis, 1994, Mosby.

Beare PG, Myers JL: *Principles and practice of adult health nursing,* ed 2, St Louis, 1994, Mosby.

Belcher AE: *Cancer nursing,* Mosby's Clinical Nursing Series, St Louis, 1992, Mosby.

Burggraf V, Donlon B: Assessing the elderly, *Am J Nurs* 85(9):974, 1985.

Canobbio MM: *Cardiovascular disorders,* Mosby's Clinical Nursing Series, St Louis, 1990, Mosby.

Chipps E et al: *Neurologic disorders,* Mosby's Clinical Nursing Series, St Louis, 1992, Mosby.

Kaufman J: Assessing the 12 cranial nerves, *Nursing '90* 20:56, 1990.

Lower J: Rapid neuro assessment, *Am J Nurs* 92(6):38, 1992.

McConnell E: Auscultating bowel sounds, *Nursing '90* 20:106, 1990.

Merkley K: Assessing chest pain, RN 57(6):58, 1994.

Payne WA, Hahn DB: *Understanding your health,* ed 2, St Louis, 1989, Mosby.

Potter PA, Perry AG: *Basic nursing,* ed 3, St Louis, 1995, Mosby.

Seidel HM et al: *Mosby's guide to physical examination,* ed 3, St Louis, 1995, Mosby.

Reed AT, Birge SJ: Screening for osteoporosis, *J Gerontol Nurs* 14(7):18, 1988.

Thompson JM et al: *Mosby's manual of clinical nursing,* ed 3, St Louis, 1993, Mosby.

Wilson SF, Thompson JM: *Respiratory disorders,* Mosby's Clinical Nursing Series, St Louis, 1990, Mosby.

Yacone-Morton LA: Cardiac assessment, *RN* 54(12):28, 1991.

ADDITIONAL READINGS

DeWitt S: Nursing assessment of the skin and dermatologic lesions, *Nurs Clin North Am* 25(1):235, 1990.

Ebersole P, Hess P: *Toward healthy aging: human needs and nursing response,* ed 4, St Louis, 1994, Mosby.

McHugh J, McHugh W: How to assess deep tendon reflexes, *Nursing '90* 20:62, 1990.

Phipps W et al: *Medical-surgical nursing: concepts and clinical practice,* ed 5, St Louis, 1995, Mosby.

chapter 13

Laboratory and Diagnostic Tests

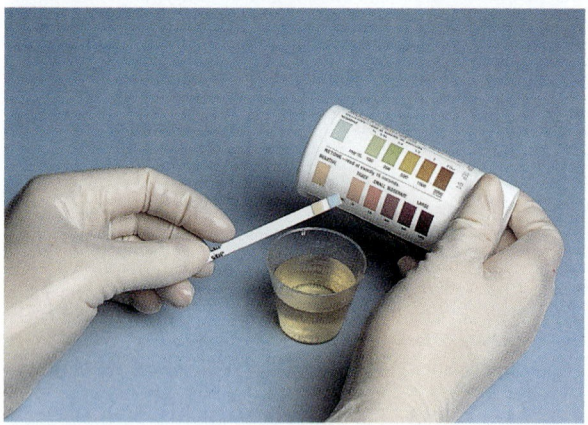

Skill 13.1
Specimen Collection

Skill 13.2
Unit Specimen Testing

Skill 13.3
Assisting with Aspirations

Skill 13.4
Assisting with Diagnostic Procedures

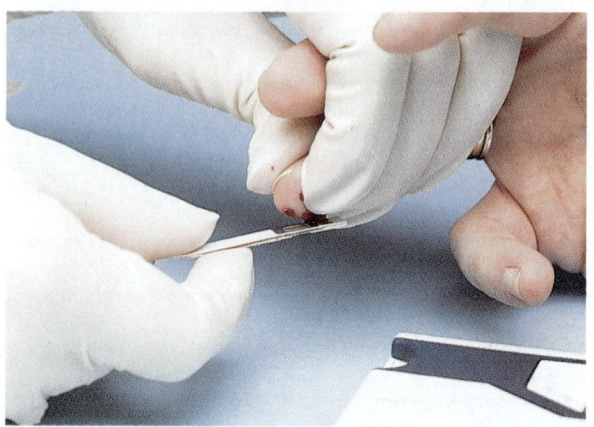

Results of laboratory and diagnostic tests provide valuable information about body functioning and contribute to the assessment of a client's health status. Analysis of test results can facilitate the diagnosis of health care problems, provide information about the stage and activity of a disease process, and measure the client's response to therapy.

Nurses often assume the responsibility for collection of specimens of body secretions and excretions (Table 13-1). Most persons believe secretions and body excretions should be handled discreetly; therefore, it is important to provide the client with as much comfort and privacy as possible. With proper instruction, many clients are able to obtain their own specimens of urine and stool, thus avoiding embarrassment.

Diagnostic tests may be performed by a physician at the client's bedside or in a room equipped specifically for therapeutic or diagnostic purposes. The nurse is responsible for assessing the client's knowledge of the procedure, preparing the client, and caring for the client after tests are completed. The nurse's knowledge of each test and the application of the nursing process ensure the safe performance of the procedure. The nurse also anticipates the physician's needs to have supplies ready and keeps the client adequately informed of procedural details that could cause discomfort.

Table 13-1 **Specimen Collection**

Source	Type of specimen	Assessment
Urine specimens	Routine urinalysis Culture/sensitivity Clean-voided (midstream) From indwelling catheter	Urinary tract infection: frequency, urgency, dysuria, hematuria, back pain, cloudy urine with sediment, foul odor, fever
Stool specimens	Hemoccult Culture	Possibility of blood in stool, visible or not visible (occult) Diarrhea
Nose and throat Sputum Wound drainage	Culture Culture Culture	Sore throat, upper respiratory or sinus infection Productive cough Fever; increased tenderness/deep pain at wound site; drainage, especially purulent, foul smelling, green, yellow, or brown

The nurse must consider legal implications when dealing with diagnostic procedures. Most invasive diagnostic tests require a signed informed consent. The physician is ultimately responsible for disclosure, but the nurse must be aware of institutional policies regarding consent forms and ensure that informed consent is signed before the procedure. The nurse must also record and report the client's status before and after the procedure.

Nursing Diagnosis

Anxiety is often caused by the manner in which a specimen is obtained or a procedure is performed. Fear of the unknown test results can also cause anxiety. Clients often experience a **Knowledge Deficit** regarding the purpose of the specimen collection or diagnostic test and the manner in which the specimen is collected or the diagnostic test performed. **Risk for Infection** exists when a client's skin and/or tissue integrity is broken during a diagnostic procedure. **Pain** is often associated with diagnostic tests when some type of instrument is inserted into a part of the body.

Skill 13.1 | Specimen Collection (Urine, Stool, Cultures)

The laboratory examination of collection specimens provides valuable clues about the human body's function. A urinalysis can provide information about the status of kidney function, nutrition, metabolic function, and certain systemic diseases. Another common test performed on urine is a culture and sensitivity measurement, which is collected during the middle portion of voiding (midstream or clean-voided specimen). Urine may also be collected from an indwelling catheter; this urine is considered sterile.

Analysis of stool provides useful information about pathological conditions such as tumors, infection, and malabsorption problems. A nasal or throat culture specimen is a simple diagnostic tool for determining the nature of a client's problem when signs and symptoms of upper respiratory or sinus infections are present. A specimen of wound drainage is analyzed to determine the type and number of pathogenic microorganisms present.

Clients can often assist the nurse in obtaining specimens. Clients should receive careful instructions about the purpose and technique of urine and stool collection

to ensure specimens are not accidentally contaminated. For cultures of the nose, throat, or wound, the specimen is collected by the nurse with client's cooperation.

EQUIPMENT
Random urine specimen
Disposable gloves
Washcloth, towel, soap, and water
Clean collection container (e.g., specimen "hat") to place under toilet seat (Figure 13-1), bedpan, or urinal
Wide-mouth specimen container with lid
Midstream (clean-voided) urine specimen
Disposable gloves
Commercial kit for clean-voided urine (Figure 13-2) containing:
    Antiseptic towelettes
    Sterile specimen container
Soap, water, washcloth, and towel
Bedpan (for nonambulatory client) or specimen "hat" (for ambulatory client)
Sterile urine specimen from an indwelling catheter

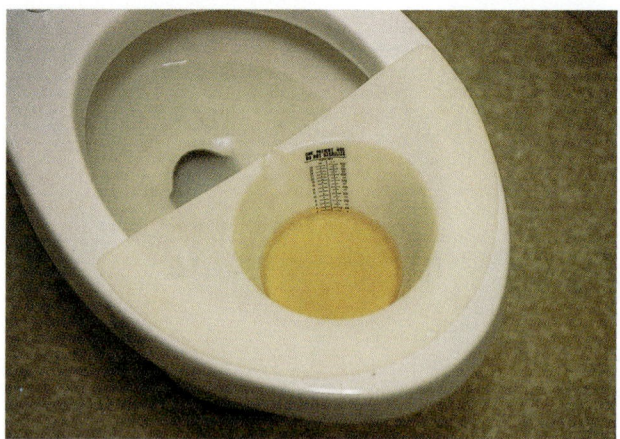

Figure 13-1

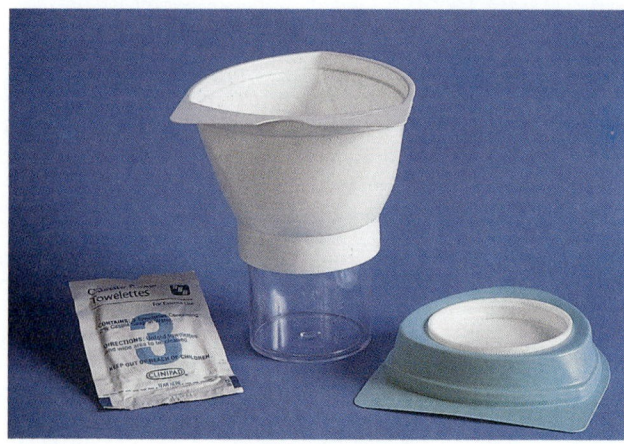

Figure 13-2

Disposable gloves

3 ml syringe with 1-inch needle (21 to 25 gauge) for culture

or

20 ml syringe with 1-inch needle (21 to 25 gauge) for routine analysis

Metal clamp or rubber band

Alcohol, povidone-iodine, or other disinfectant swab

Specimen container (nonsterile for routine urinalysis, sterile for culture)

Stool specimen

Disposable gloves

Plastic container with lid

Two tongue blades

Paper towel

Bedpan, specimen "hat," or bedside commode

"Save Stool" signs

Nasal and throat specimen

Disposable gloves

Two sterile swabs in sterile culture tubes (Flexible wire swab with cotton tip may be used for nose cultures.)

Nasal speculum (optional)

Emesis basin or clean container (optional)

Tongue blades

Penlight

Facial tissues

Wound drainage specimen

Culture tube with swab and transport medium for aerobic culture

Anaerobic culture tube with swab (Tubes contain carbon dioxide or nitrogen gas.)

5 to 10 ml syringe and 21-gauge needle

Sterile gloves

Protective eye wear

Antiseptic swab

Sterile dressing materials (determined by type of dressing)

Paper or plastic disposable bag

Assessment

1. Assess client's ability to assist with urine and stool specimen collection: able to position self and hold container. **This determines ability to cooperate and level of assistance required.**
2. Assess client's understanding of need for the specimen. **This determines the need for health teaching. Client's understanding of purpose promotes cooperation.**
3. Assess for signs and symptoms of urinary tract infection (frequency, urgency, dysuria, hematuria, flank pain, cloudy urine with sediment, foul odor, fever), upper respiratory infection (increased cough, increased sputum production, changes in sputum color), sinus infection (sinus headache or tenderness, nasal congestion, sore throat, inflammation or purulent drainage of posterior pharynx), and wound infection (fever, increasing tenderness and deep pain at the wound site, change in color or amount of drainage, elevated white blood cell count [WBC] in conjunction with erythematous wound). Signs and symptoms help reveal nature of problem.
4. Assess stool or urinary elimination pattern to allow for more effective planning.

Planning

Expected outcomes focus on the collection of an uncontaminated specimen by nurse or client with client knowledgeable of the purpose of the specimen examination.

EXPECTED OUTCOMES

1. Client's specimen is free of contaminants, such as urine or toilet tissue in stool or stool or toilet tissue in urine.
2. Client explains procedure for specimen collection before collection is attempted.
3. Client explains purpose of specimen analysis before collection is attempted.

Implementation

Steps	Rationale

1. See Standard Protocol (Chapter 1, p. 5)

2. Perform random urine collection.

   a. Explain procedure to client and/or family member. Discuss reason for specimen collection, how client/family member can assist, and how to obtain specimen free of feces and tissue.

       Promotes cooperation. Client may be able to obtain the specimen independently. Prevents accidental disposal of urine.

   b. Give client or family member towel, washcloth, and soap to cleanse perineal area, or assist client to cleanse perineum.

       Cleansing prevents contamination of specimen as urine passes from urethra.

   c. Give male client specimen container and direct to bathroom; give female client specimen "hat" and direct to bathroom. Assist client as needed to void into bedpan or urinal.

       Maintains as much independence in client as possible.

   d. If client did not void directly into specimen container, transfer 4 oz of urine into it.

       Avoids contamination of specimen and ensures collection of correct volume.

   e. Place lid tightly on container without touching inside of lid.

       Prevents contamination of specimen by other substances and loss from spillage.

   f. If urine has been splashed on outside of container, wash it off.

       Prevents spread of bacteria.

3. Collect midstream (clean-voided) urine specimen.

   a. Explain procedure to client and/or family member. Discuss reason midstream specimen is needed, how client/family member can assist, and how to obtain specimen free of feces and tissue.

       Promotes cooperation and participation. Client may be able to obtain specimen independently. Prevents accidental disposal of specimen. Feces and tissue alter chemical composition of specimen.

   b. Give client or family member towel, washcloth, and soap to cleanse perineum, or assist client to cleanse perineum.

       Prevents contamination of specimen after urine passes from urethra.

   c. Assist bedridden client onto bedpan.

       Provides easy access to perineal area to collect specimen.

   d. Using sterile technique, open commercial specimen kit (Figure 13-2), maintaining sterility of inside of specimen container.

   e. Open specimen container, and place cap with sterile inside surface up. Do not touch inside of container.

       Contaminated specimen is most frequent reason for inaccurate reporting on urine cultures and sensitivities.

   f. Assist or allow client to cleanse perineum and collect specimen independently.

    Male

    (1) Hold penis with one hand; using circular motion and antiseptic towelette, cleanse end, moving from center to outside (Figure 13-3).

       Decreases bacterial levels at urinary meatus.

    (2) If agency procedure indicates, rinse area with sterile water and dry with cotton balls or gauze pad.

       Prevents contamination of specimen with antiseptic solution.

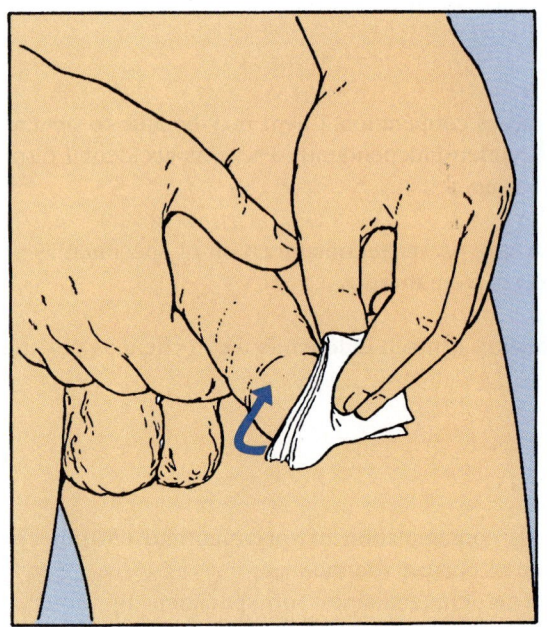

Figure 13-3 (Modified from Grimes D: *Infectious diseases,* Mosby's Clinical Nursing Series, St. Louis, 1991, Mosby.)

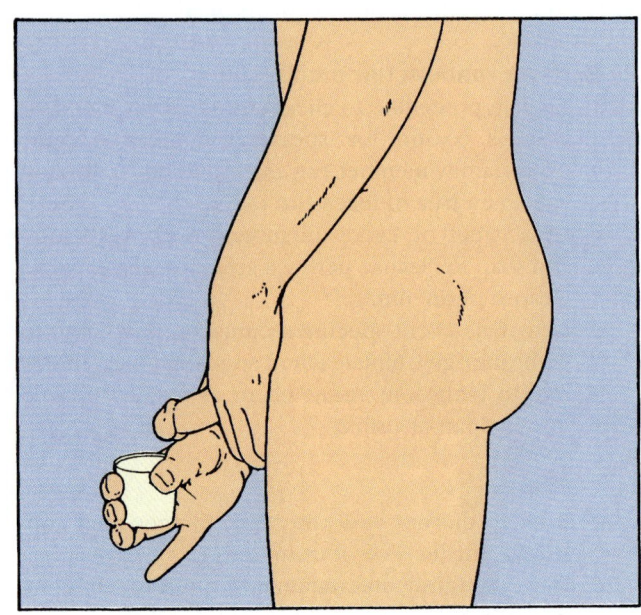

Figure 13-4 (Modified from Grimes D: *Infectious diseases,* Mosby's Clinical Nursing Series, St. Louis, 1991, Mosby.)

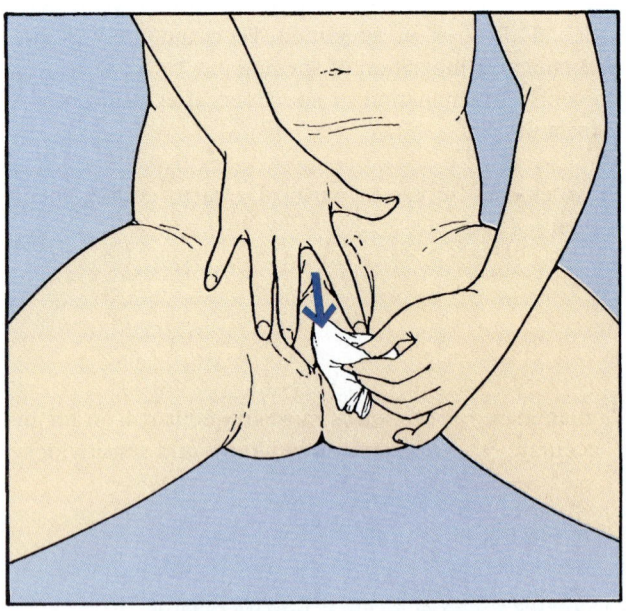

Figure 13-5 (Modified from Grimes D: *Infectious diseases,* Mosby's Clinical Nursing Series, St. Louis, 1991, Mosby.)

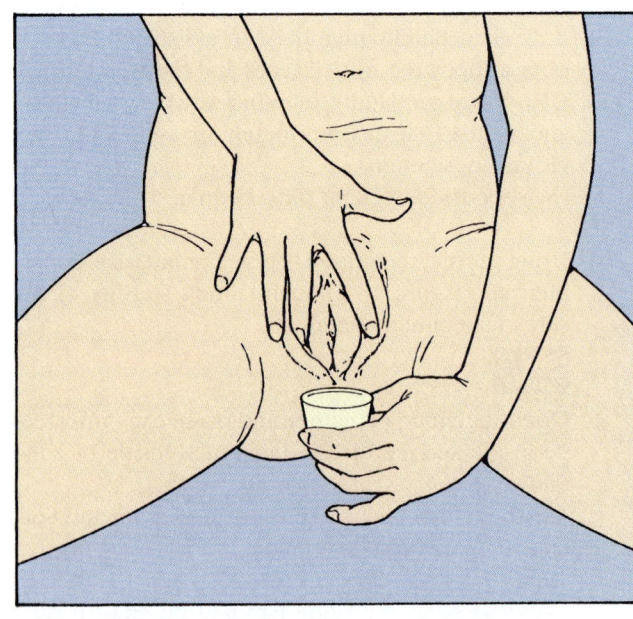

Figure 13-6 (Modified from Grimes D: *Infectious diseases,* Mosby's Clinical Nursing Series, St. Louis, 1991, Mosby.)

Steps	Rationale

(3) After client has initiated urine stream, pass urine specimen container into stream and collect 30 to 60 ml (Figure 13-4).

Initial urine stream flushes out microorganisms that normally accumulate at urinary meatus and prevents collection of these microorganisms in specimen.

Female

(1) Spread labia minora with fingers of nondominant hand.

Provides access to urethral meatus.

(2) Use dominant hand to cleanse area with antiseptic towelette, moving from front (above urethral orifice) to back (toward anus) (Figure 13-5).

Prevents contamination of urinary meatus with fecal material.

(3) If agency procedure indicates, rinse area with sterile water and dry with cotton.

Prevents contamination of specimen with antiseptic solution.

(4) While continuing to hold labia apart, client should initiate urine stream. After stream achieved, pass specimen container into stream and collect 30 to 60 ml (Figure 13-6).

Initial urine stream flushes out microorganisms that normally accumulate at urethral meatus.

g. Remove specimen container before flow of urine stops and before releasing labia or penis. Client finishes voiding into bedpan or toilet.

Prevents contamination of specimen with skin flora.

h. Replace cap securely on specimen container (touch only outside).

Maintains sterility of inside of container and prevents spillage of urine.

i. Cleanse urine from exterior surface of container.

Reduces transmission of microorganisms.

4. Collect sterile urine specimen from an indwelling catheter.

a. Explain procedure to client and/or family member. Emphasize that although a syringe with a needle is used to remove the urine from the catheter, client will not experience any discomfort.

Prevents anxiety when nurse manipulates catheter and aspirates urine with syringe and needle. Promotes client cooperation.

b. Explain why catheter will need to be clamped for 30 minutes before obtaining a urine specimen and why it is not obtained from drainage bag.

Prevents development of anxiety over clamping and promotes understanding of need for urine to collect within bladder.

c. Clamp drainage tubing with clamp or rubber band for up to 30 minutes (Figure 13-7) below the site chosen for withdrawal.

Permits collection of fresh, sterile urine in catheter tubing.

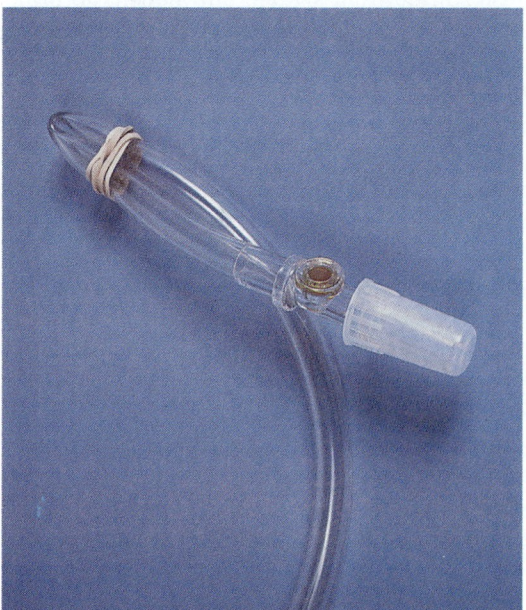

Figure 13-7

Steps	Rationale

d. Return to room and inform client that the procedure to collect a specimen from a catheter will begin.

Allows client to anticipate manipulation of urinary catheter and cope more effectively with discomfort that may occur when catheter is moved.

e. Position client so catheter is easily accessible.

f. Cleanse entry port for needle with disinfectant swab.

Prevents entry of microorganisms into catheter.

g. Insert needle at 30-degree angle just above where catheter is attached to drainage tube or at 90-degree angle from a collection port in the drainage tube of an indwelling catheter (Figure 13-8).

Ensures entrance of needle into catheter lumen and prevents accidental puncture of lumen leading to balloon that holds catheter in place in bladder. Aspiration of water from lumen can result in catheter falling out of bladder.

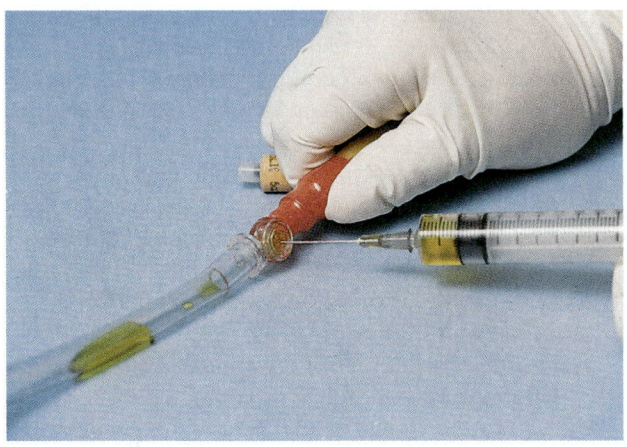

Figure 13-8

h. Draw urine into 3 ml syringe for culture, or draw urine into 20 ml syringe for routine urinalysis.

Allows collection of urine without contamination. Proper volume is needed to perform test.

i. Transfer urine from syringe into nonsterile urine container for routine urinalysis, or transfer urine from syringe into sterile urine container for culture.

Prevents contamination of urine during transfer procedure.

j. Place lid tightly on container.

Prevents contamination of specimen by air and loss by spillage.

k. Unclamp catheter and allow urine to flow into drainage bag.

Allows urine to drain by gravity and prevents stasis of urine in bladder.

5. Collect stool specimen.

a. Explain procedure to client and/or family member. Discuss reason stool specimen is needed, how client/family member can assist, and how to obtain specimen free of urine and tissue.

Promotes cooperation.

b. Assist client as needed into bathroom or onto commode or bedpan.

Client's physical mobility and level of fatigue influence amount of assistance needed.

c. Instruct client to void into toilet before defecating (discard urine before collecting specimen in bedpan).

Feces should not be mixed with urine or toilet tissue. Urine inhibits fecal bacterial growth. Toilet tissue contains bismuth, which interferes with test results.

d. Provide client with clean, dry bedpan and specimen "hat" in which to defecate.

Feces should not be mixed with urine or water.

Steps	Rationale
e. If needed, assist client in washing after toileting and leave in safe, comfortable position after defecation.	Promotes comfort and sense of well-being.
f. Take covered bedpan or container with stool to bathroom or utility room.	Covering bedpan and removing it from client's room reduces odor and client's embarrassment.
g. Obtain specimen. (1) *For culture.* Remove swab from sterile test tube, gather bean-sized piece of stool, and return swab to tube. If stool is liquid, soak cotton swab in it and return to tube.	Stool is touched only by sterile swab to prevent introduction of bacteria.
(2) *For other tests.* Obtain specimen by using tongue blades to transfer portion of stool to container (2.5 cm [1 inch] of formed stool or 15 ml of liquid stool).	Use of tongue blades prevents transfer of bacteria to hands or other objects.
(3) *For timed stool specimen.* All of each stool is placed in waxed cardboard containers for specific time ordered and kept in specimen refrigerator.	Tests for dietary products and digestive enzymes such as fat content or bile require analysis of all feces over time.
h. For timed tests, place signs that read "Save all stool (with appropriate dates)" over client's bed, on bathroom door, and above toilet.	Helps prevent accidental disposal of stool.
i. Immediately place lid on container tightly.	Prevents spread of microorganisms by air or contact with other articles.
6. Collect throat, nasal, and wound drainage cultures.	
a. Explain procedure to client and/or family member.	Decreases anxiety and promotes cooperation.
b. Explain that client may have tickling sensation or gag during swabbing of throat, urge to sneeze during nasal swabbing, and tickling or painful sensation during swabbing of wound. State that procedure takes only a few seconds.	Clients who have been made aware of sensations to expect are able to cooperate with uncomfortable experiences (Beare and Myers, 1994).
c. Ask client to sit erect in bed or chair facing you for nose or throat culture. Acutely ill client may lie back against bed with head of bed raised to 45-degree angle.	Provides easy access to nasal or oral structures.
d. Have swab in tube ready for use. You may want to loosen top so swab can easily be removed.	Nurse should be able to grasp swab easily without danger of contaminating it. Most commercially prepared tubes have a top that fits securely over end of swab, which allows nurse to touch outer top without contaminating swab stick.
e. Collect culture. **Throat culture** (1) Instruct client to tilt head backward. For clients in bed, place pillow behind shoulders.	Facilitates visualization of pharynx.
(2) Ask client to open mouth and say "ah."	Permits exposure of pharynx, relaxes throat muscles, and minimizes gag reflex.
(3) If pharynx not visualized, depress tongue with tongue blade and note inflamed areas of pharynx or tonsils. Depress anterior third of tongue only. (Illuminate with penlight as needed.)	Area to be swabbed should be visualized. Placement of tongue blade along back of tongue more likely initiates gag reflex.

Steps	Rationale

(4) Insert swab without touching lips, teeth, tongue, or cheeks (Figure 13-9).

(5) Gently but quickly swab tonsillar area side to side, making contact with inflamed or purulent sites.

Touching lips or oral mucosal structures can contaminate swab with resident bacteria.

These areas contain the most microorganisms.

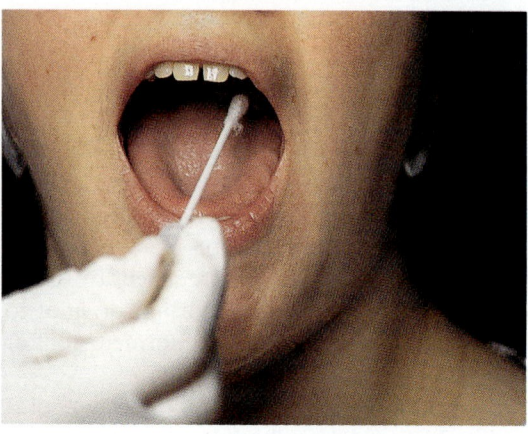

Figure 13-9

(6) Carefully withdraw swab without striking oral structures. Immediately place swab in culture tube, and crush ampule at bottom of tube. Push tip of swab into liquid medium.

Retains microorganisms within culture tube. Mixing swab tip with culture medium ensures life of bacteria for testing.

Nasal culture

(1) Encourage client to blow nose, and check nostrils for patency with penlight.

(2) Ask client to occlude each nostril alternately and exhale.

(3) Ask client to tilt head back. Clients in bed should have pillow behind shoulders.

(4) Gently insert nasal speculum in one nostril (optional). Carefully pass swab through center of speculum (if used) into nostril until it reaches that portion of mucosa that is inflamed or containing exudate.

(5) Rotate swab quickly.

(6) Remove swab without touching sides of speculum.

(7) Carefully remove nasal speculum (if used) and place in basin. Offer client facial tissue.

(8) Insert swab into culture tube. Crush ampule at bottom of tube, and push tip of swab into liquid medium.

Clears nasal passage of mucus that contains resident bacteria.

Determines nostril with greater patency, from which specimen will be collected.

Facilitates visualization of nasal septum and sinuses.

Allows retraction of mucosa for easier swab insertion. Swab should remain sterile until it reaches area to be cultured. Rotating swab covers all surfaces with exudate.

Prevents contamination of swab by resident bacteria.

Retains microorganisms within culture tube. Mixing swab tip with culture medium ensures life of bacteria for testing.

Nasopharyngeal culture

Follow steps for nasal culture *except* use a special swab on a flexible wire that can be flexed downward to reach the nasopharynx via the nose.

Sputum culture

(1) Position client on side of bed or in high semi-Fowler's position.

(2) Provide opportunity to cleanse or rinse mouth with water.

Reduces oral contamination that can alter results.

Steps	Rationale

(3) Provide sputum cup and instruct client not to touch inside.

(4) After several deep breaths tell client to inhale deeply and cough forcefully, expectorating sputum directly into specimen container (Figure 13-10).

Full inhalation provides enough force to move sputum out of deeper airways.

(5) Repeat until 5 to 10 ml (1 to 2 tsp) of sputum (not saliva) has been collected.

Wound drainage culture

(1) Remove old dressing. Observe drainage. Fold soiled sides of dressing together and then dispose of in bag.

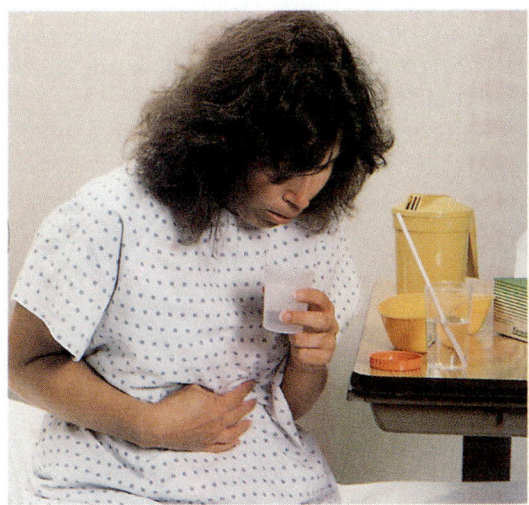

Figure 13-10 (From Grimes D: *Infectious diseases*, Mosby's Clinical Nursing Series, St. Louis, 1991, Mosby.)

(2) Cleanse area around wound edges with antiseptic swab. Remove old exudate.

Removes skin flora, preventing possible contamination of specimen.

(3) Discard swab and dispose of soiled gloves in bag.

Reduces spread of infection.

(4) Open package containing sterile culture tube and dressing supplies.

Provides sterile field from which nurse can pick up and handle sterile supplies.

(5) Apply sterile gloves.

Allows nurse to maintain sterility of items while collecting specimen.

(6) Aerobic culture

Take swab from culture tube, insert tip into wound near area of drainage, and rotate swab gently. Remove swab and return to culture tube (Figure 13-11, *A*). Crush ampule of medium and push swab into fluid (Figure 13-11, *B*).

Swab should be coated with fresh secretions (not drainage) from within wound. Medium keeps bacteria alive until analysis is complete.

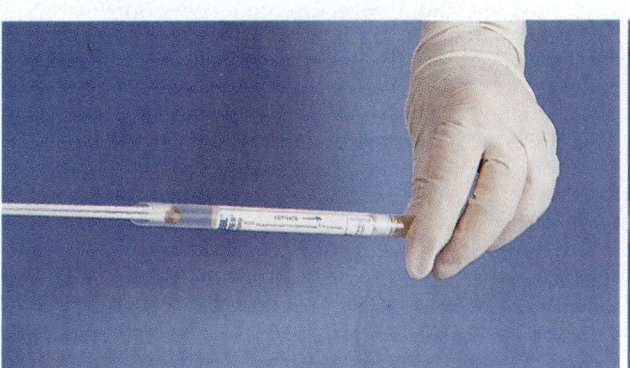
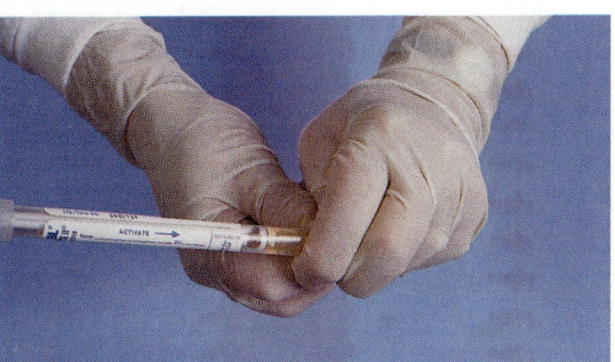

A   B

Figure 13-11

Steps	Rationale

(7) Anaerobic culture
Take swab from special anaerobic culture tube, swab deeply into body cavity, and rotate gently. Remove swab and return to culture tube.

or

Insert tip of syringe (without needle) into wound and aspirate 5 to 10 ml of exudate. Attach 21-gauge needle, expel *all* air, and inject drainage into special culture tube.

(8) Clean wound as ordered and apply new sterile dressing.

Specimen is taken from deep cavity where oxygen is not present. Carbon dioxide or nitrogen gas keeps organisms alive until analysis is complete.

Air injected into tube would cause organisms to die.

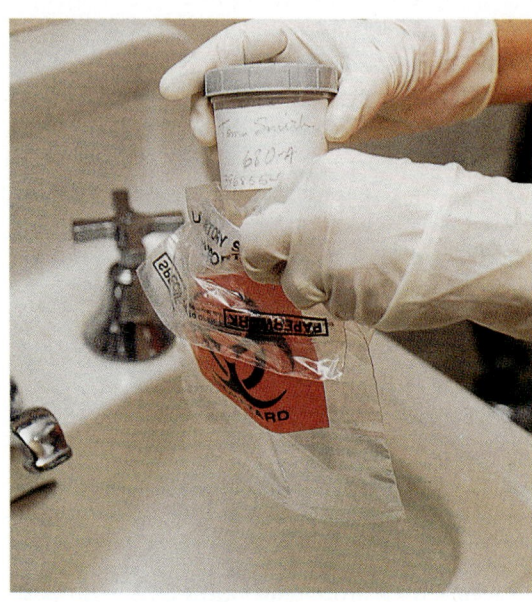

Figure 13-12

f. Place top on tube securely.

7. Securely attach properly completed identification label and laboratory requisition to side of specimen container (not lid). Enclose in a plastic bag (Figure 13-12).

8. Send specimen immediately to laboratory or refrigerate.

9. See Completion Protocol (Chapter 1, p. 6).

Prevents contamination from microorganisms.
Incorrect identification of specimen could result in diagnostic or therapeutic errors.

Specimen left at room temperature may increase bacterial content.

Evaluation

1. Inspect specimen for contaminants, such as urine or tissue in stool or stool or tissue in urine.
2. Ask client to identify steps in specimen collection procedure.
3. Ask client to state purpose of specimen analysis.

UNEXPECTED OUTCOMES AND RELATED INTERVENTIONS

1. Client is unable to produce a urine or stool specimen.
   a. Offer fluids (if permitted) to enhance ability to void.
   b. Administer a suppository or enema as ordered to promote passage of stool.

2. Client's urine specimen is contaminated with stool and tissue.
   a. Reinforce importance of obtaining specimen free of contaminants.
   b. Assist client with specimen collection: place specimen "hat" as close to front of commode as possible.

3. Client experiences minor nasal bleeding.
   a. Apply mild pressure over bridge of nose.
   b. Apply ice pack over bridge of nose.

SAMPLE DOCUMENTATION

0900 Abdominal dressing removed with a moderate amount of yellow drainage. Wound edges are not approximated, are erythematous, and are warm to touch. Aerobic wound culture obtained. Wound packed with iodoform gauze and covered with sterile 4 × 4 dressing.

Skill 13.2 | Unit Specimen Testing (Glucose, Hemoccult, Gastroccult)

This skill includes tests done on the nursing unit (Table 13-2). When the screening test for the presence of substances in the urine is positive, other tests are used to determine the diagnosis or measure the effectiveness of treatment. The capillary blood glucose test is used to measure blood glucose for monitoring the control of diabetes mellitus. Test results are used to direct diet, amount and type of medication, and exercise prescription. The Hemoccult test measures microscopic amounts of blood in the stool. It is a useful diagnostic tool for conditions such as colon cancer, upper gastrointestinal (GI) ulcers, and localized gastric or intestinal irritation. Measuring gastric occult blood via the Gastroccult test reveals bleeding in the esophagus, stomach, or duodenum and is similar to measuring stool for occult blood. The Gastroccult test also measures pH level of (GI) secretions.

The nurse can easily perform these tests at the bedside with minimal discomfort to the client. Clients should receive instructions about the purpose of the tests and if any discomfort is to be anticipated, such as during skin puncture for a capillary blood sample for glucose measurement and during insertion of a nasogastric (NG) tube if needed for the Gastroccult test.

EQUIPMENT

Urine glucose
Disposable gloves
Reagent test strip
Test strip color chart
Glucose monitoring (Figure 13-13)
Disposable gloves
Antiseptic swab
Cotton ball
Sterile blood-letting device
Paper towel
Glucose testing meter
Blood glucose reagent strips (brand determined by meter used)
Hemoccult
Disposable gloves
Paper towel
Wooden applicator
Hemoccult test (Figure 13-14)
   Cardboard Hemoccult slide
   Hemoccult developing solution
Gastroccult
Disposable gloves
Facial tissues
Emesis basin
Wooden applicator or 1 ml syringe
Gastroccult test (Figure 13-15)
   Cardboard Gastroccult slide
   Gastroccult developing solution
60 ml bulb or catheter-tip syringe
NG tube and supplies for insertion (if indicated)

Table 13-2 Tests Done by Nurses on the Unit

Test	Assessment
Accu-Chek (capillary glucose)	Hyperglycemia (high blood glucose): thirst, polyuria, polyphagia, weakness, fatigue, headache, blurred vision, nausea, vomiting, abdominal cramps
	Hypoglycemia (low blood glucose): sweating, tachycardia, palpitations, nervousness, tremors, weakness, headache, mental confusion, fatigue
Multistix (urine screening test for pH, protein, glucose, ketones, and/or blood)	Protein or blood: abnormal kidney function or urinary tract infection
	pH: concentration
	Glucose: inadequate glucose metabolism
	Ketones: abnormal metabolism of proteins associated with inadequate food intake or excessive vomiting
Hemoccult (stool)	Gastrointestinal alterations: abdominal cramping, pain, vomiting, diarrhea, appearance of blood or suspected presence of unseen (occult) blood in stool, vomitus, or gastric aspirate
Gastroccult (gastric contents or drainage from NG tube)	

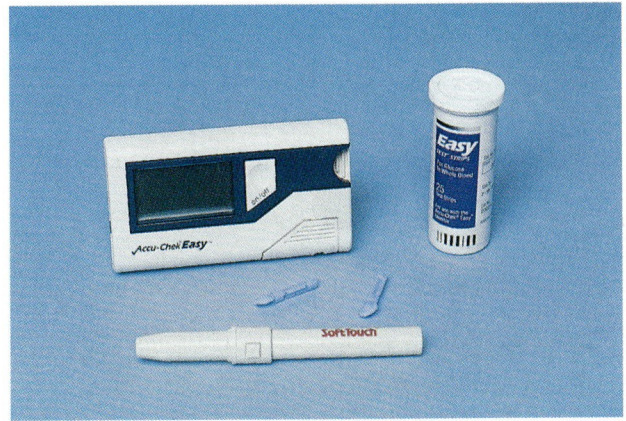

Figure 13-13

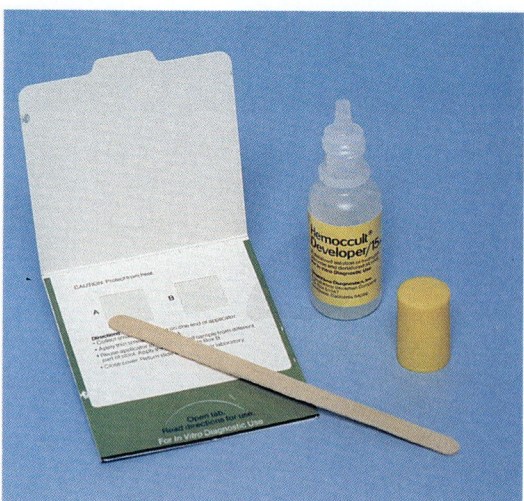

Figure 13-14

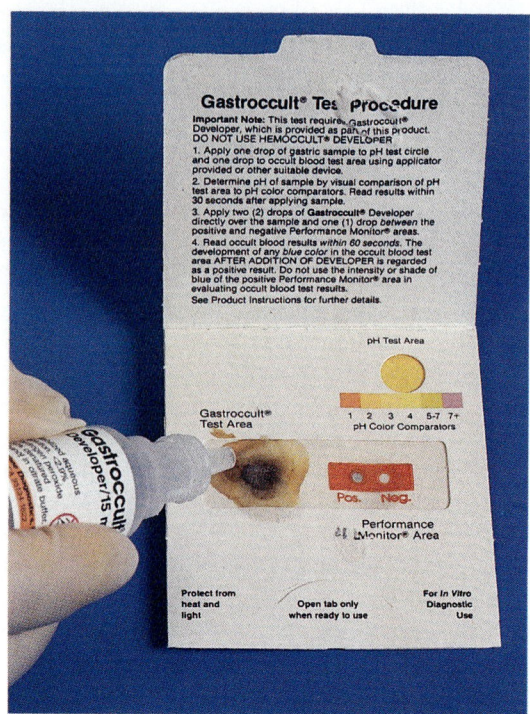

Figure 13-15

Assessment

1. Assess client's understanding of need for the specimen. **This provides nurse with a data base on which to provide necessary teaching.**
2. Assess client for types of medications received and foods eaten. **Drugs such as cortisone preparations, diuretics, and anesthetics increase blood glucose levels. Anticoagulants increase risk of bleeding in the GI tract, and long-term use of steroids and acetylsalicylic acid can irritate the gastric mucosa.**
3. Assess client for related signs and symptoms (Table 13-2), which help reveal nature of the problem.

Planning

Expected outcomes focus on collecting an appropriate specimen, with client knowledgeable of the purpose of specimen examination, and decreasing client's anxiety when these types of specimens are collected.

Implementation

EXPECTED OUTCOMES

1. Client explains purpose of the unit test ordered before specimen collection is attempted.
2. Client explains basic steps of the procedure for the unit test ordered before specimen collection is attempted.
3. Client's specimen is appropriate for the unit test analysis.
4. Client verbalizes lack of fear of specimen collection and unit test results after nurse reviews the procedure.

Steps	Rationale
1. See Standard Protocol (Chapter 1, p. 5).	
2. Explain procedure to client and/or family member.	Promotes cooperation.
3. Perform urine glucose screening test for pH, protein, ketones, and blood.	
a. Obtain double-voided specimen when testing urine for glucose.	Stagnant urine stored in bladder overnight or for long periods does not reveal amount of glucose excreted by kidney at time of testing.
(1) Ask client to collect random urine specimen and discard.	
(2) Have client drink at least 8 oz water or preferred liquid.	Facilitates ability to void again within short period.

Steps	Rationale

(3) 30 to 45 minutes later, have client collect another random specimen.

b. Use Multistix reagent test strip to assess for glucose, pH, protein, ketones, and/or blood simultaneously (Figure 13-16).

Fresh specimen provides accurate test measurements. If client is catheterized, a single, fresh specimen from catheter is adequate.

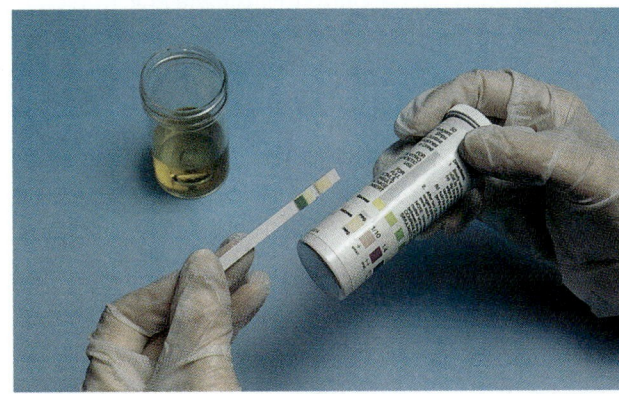

Figure 13-16

(1) Immerse end of chemically impregnated test strip into urine.

Exposes reagent to urine.

(2) Remove strip immediately from container and tap it gently against container's side.

Excess urine can dilute reagents.

(3) Hold strip in horizontal position.

Prevents possible mixing of chemical reagents.

(4) Time for number of seconds specified on container, and compare color of strip with color chart on container.

Accurate interpretation of results depends on precise timing.

c. Discuss test results with client.

Participation in care improves understanding and compliance.

4. Perform blood glucose measurement (Accu-Chek used as example).

a. Instruct client to wash hands with soap and warm water, if able.

Reduces presence of microorganisms. Promotes vasodilation at selected puncture site. Establishes practice for client when test is performed at home.

b. Position client comfortably in chair or semi-Fowler's position in bed.

Ensures easy accessibility to puncture site.

c. Remove reagent strip from container and tightly seal cap.

Protects strips from accidental discoloration.

d. Turn on glucose meter.

Activates meter.

e. Insert strip into glucose meter (see manufacturer's directions) and make necessary adjustments.

Some machines must be calibrated; others require zeroing of timer. Each meter is adjusted differently.

f. Remove unused reagent strip from meter and place on paper towel or clean, dry surface with test pad facing up.

Moisture on strip can change its color, altering reading of final test results.

g. Choose puncture site.

Puncture site should be vascular. Side of finger is less sensitive to pain.

h. Hold finger to be punctured in dependent position while gently massaging finger toward puncture site.

Increases blood flow to area before puncture.

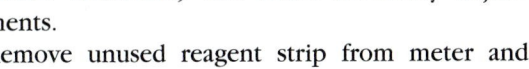

Steps	Rationale

i. Clean site with antiseptic swab and *allow to dry completely.*

Alcohol can alter accuracy of test.

j. Remove cover of blood-letting device.

Cover keeps tip of needle sterile.

k. Place blood-letting device firmly against finger and push release button, causing needle to pierce skin (Figure 13-17).

Pierces skin to appropriate depth, ensuring adequate blood flow.

l. Wipe away first droplet of blood with cotton ball. (See manufacturer's directions for meter used.)

First droplet of blood generally contains large portions of serous fluid, which can dilute specimen and cause false results.

m. Lightly squeeze (but do not touch) puncture site until large droplet of blood has formed.

Ensures proper coverage of test pad on reagent strip.

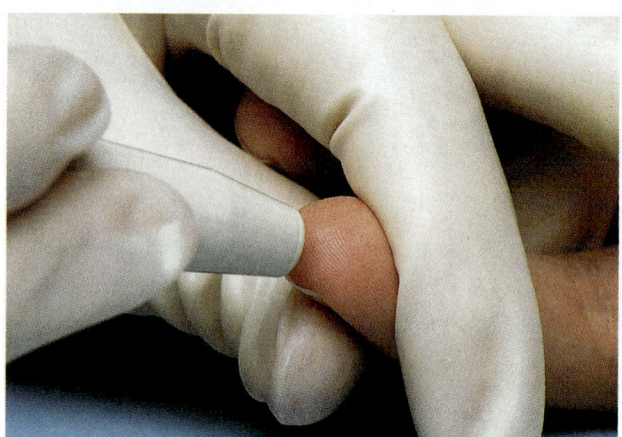

Figure 13-17

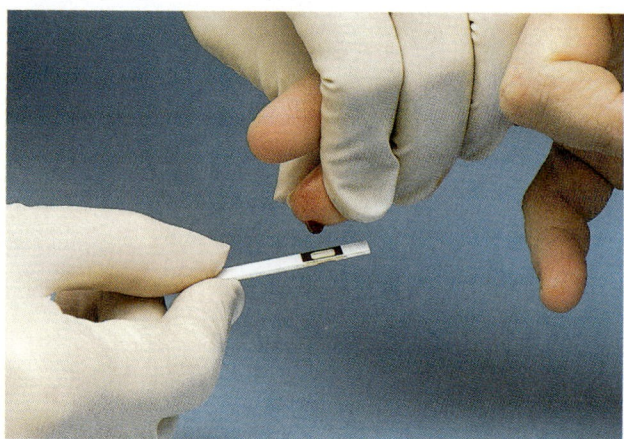

Figure 13-18

n. Hold reagent strip test pad close to drop of blood, and lightly transfer droplet to test pad (Figure 13-18). Do not smear blood.

Ensures proper chemical reaction. Smearing causes inaccurate test results.

o. Immediately press timer on glucose meter, and place reagent strip on paper towel or on side of timer. (See manufacturer's directions for meter used.)

Accurate timing ensures correct results. Strip should lie flat so blood does not pool on only one part of pad. Some meters (e.g., One Touch) require blood sample to be applied to test strip already in meter.

p. Apply pressure to skin puncture site.

Promotes hemostasis.

q. When timer displays 60 seconds (for Accu-Chek III model), use moderate pressure to wipe blood from test pad with cotton ball. No blood should remain on test pad for some meters. (See manufacturer's directions for meter used.)

For meter to read glucose levels, some strips must be dry. Refer to product directions for timing used with each type of meter.

r. While timer continues to count, place reagent strip into meter (Figure 13-19).

Strip must be inserted correctly to obtain accurate reading.

s. Read meter, noting reading on display (Figure 13-20).

t. Turn meter off. Dispose of test strip, cotton balls, and blood-letting device in proper receptacles.

Meter is battery powered. Proper disposal reduces spread of microorganisms.

u. Share results with client.

Promotes participation and compliance with therapy.

5. Perform Hemoccult test.

a. Obtain uncontaminated stool specimen (see Skill 13.1) in clean, dry container. Avoid contamination with urine, water, or toilet tissue.

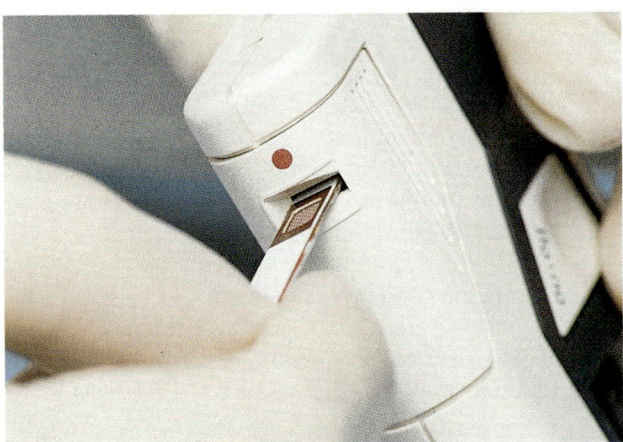
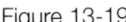

Figure 13-19

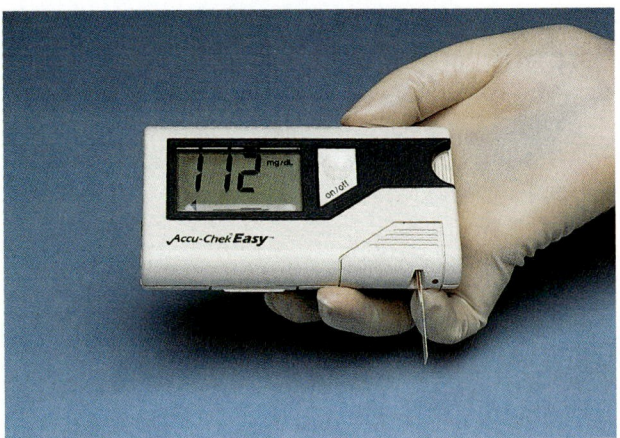

Figure 13-20

Steps	Rationale
b. Use tip of wooden applicator to obtain small portion of feces.	Small specimen is sufficient for measuring blood content.
c. Open flap of Hemoccult slide and apply thin smear of stool on paper in first box.	Guaiac paper inside box is sensitive to fecal blood content. Occult blood from upper GI tract is not always equally dispersed through stool.
d. Obtain second fecal specimen from different portion of stool and apply thinly to slide's second box (Figure 13-21).	Findings of occult blood are more conclusive when entire specimen is found to contain blood.
e. Close slide cover and turn slide over to reverse side. Open cardboard flap and apply two drops of Hemoccult developing solution on each box of guaiac paper (Figure 13-22).	Developing solution penetrates underlying fecal specimen. Blood is indicated by change in color of guaiac paper.
f. Read results of test after 30 to 60 seconds. Note color changes.	Bluish discoloration indicates occult blood (guaiac positive). No change in color of guaiac paper indicates negative results.

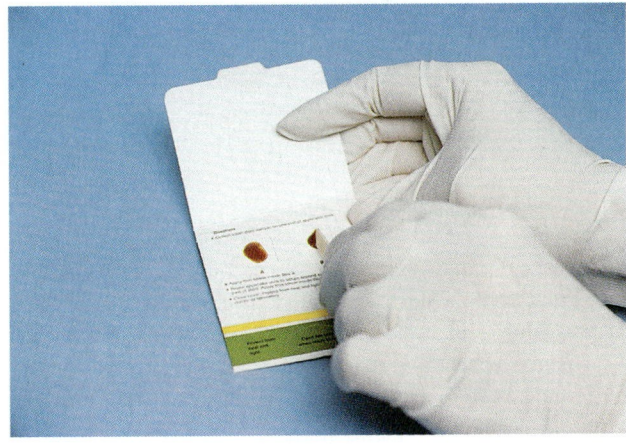

Figure 13-21

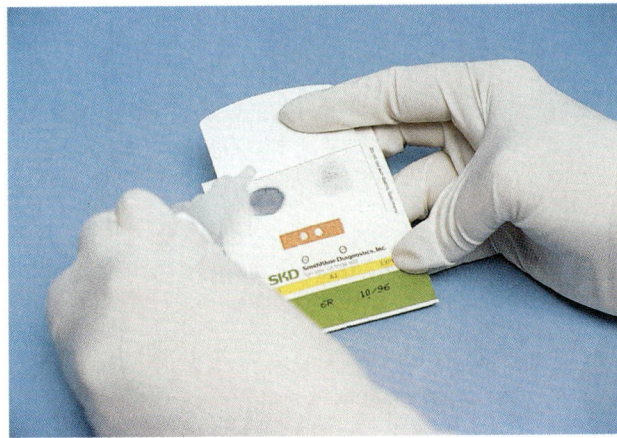

Figure 13-22

Steps	Rationale

6. Perform Gastroccult test.

a. To obtain specimen of gastric contents using NG tube, position client in high Fowler's position in bed or chair.

Minimizes aspiration of gastric contents. Position relieves pressure on abdominal organs. If client is nauseated, flat position in bed or one in which client cannot sit straight may cause abdominal discomfort.

b. Insert NG tube as indicated, if not already placed (see Skill 31.1).

Allows aspiration of gastric contents.

c. Obtain specimen of gastric contents by attaching bulb syringe to NG tube and aspirating 5 to 10 ml. Obtain sample of emesis with 1 ml syringe or wooden applicator.

Only small amount of specimen is needed for pH and occult blood testing.

d. Apply 1 drop of gastric sample to Gastroccult blood test paper.

Sample must cover guaiac paper for test reaction to occur.

e. Apply 2 drops of commercial developer solution over sample and 1 drop between positive and negative performance monitors (Figure 13-23).

Developer initiates chemical reaction of solution with guaiac paper.

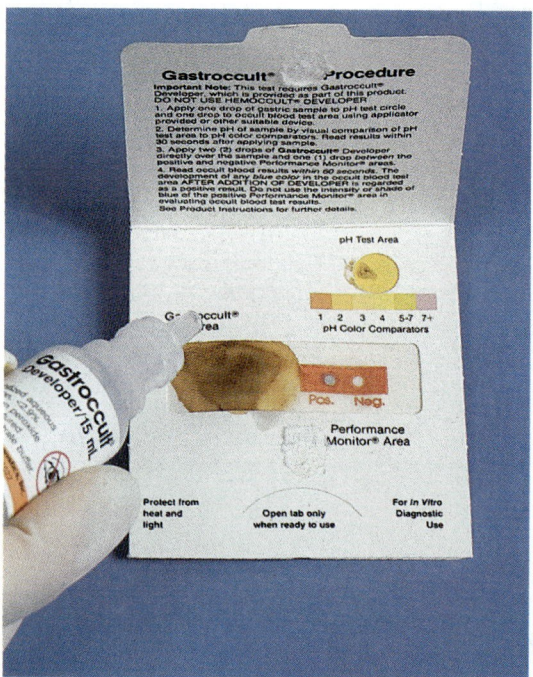

Figure 13-23

f. After 60 seconds, compare color of gastric sample with that of performance monitors.

Positive performance monitor turns blue in 30 seconds, and negative monitor remains white or beige. If sample turns blue, test is positive for occult blood. If sample turns green, test is negative.

g. Explain results to client.

Immediate results are obtained. Allows client to participate in care.

7. See Completion Protocol (Chapter 1, p. 6).

Evaluation

1. Ask client to state purpose of the specific unit test ordered.
2. Ask client to state the specimen collection procedure required.
3. Inspect client's specimen for appropriateness.
4. Ask if client has questions or concerns about the unit test procedure before specimen collection and later about unit test results. Assess nonverbal behaviors of anxiety before, during, and after procedure.

UNEXPECTED OUTCOMES AND RELATED INTERVENTIONS

1. Puncture site from Accu-Chek is bruised or continues to bleed.
   a. Apply pressure to site for at least 1 minute.
   b. Apply pressure to site for at least 5 minutes if client is taking anticoagulants or acetylsalicylic acid.

2. Hemoccult test results are positive.
   a. Assess client for hemorrhoids that can cause bleeding. (Bleeding could be misinterpreted as upper GI bleeding.)
   b. Assess client for intake of medications that may increase risk of GI bleeding (e.g., anticoagulants, steroids, acetylsalicylic acid) (Pagana and Pagana, 1992).
   c. Repeat Hemoccult at least three times while client is on a meat-free, high-residue diet. (Red meats cause false-positive results.)

SAMPLE DOCUMENTATION

0730 Blood glucose 110. No sliding-scale insulin administered. (See Diabetic Management Record, Appendix A.)

1200 Blood glucose 240. Regular insulin (4 units) administered subcutaneously as ordered per sliding scale.

1000 Nasogastric tube draining 100 ml of light-brown fluid with dark flecks. Gastroccult test is positive for occult blood. Physician notified of results.

1030 Infusion of Zantac 250 mg in 250 ml 5% dextrose initiated via IV at 10 ml per hour.

| Skill 13.3 | Assisting with Aspirations (Bone Marrow Aspiration, Lumbar Puncture, Paracentesis, Thoracentesis, Liver Biopsy) |

These procedures are performed at the client's bedside or in a treatment room by a physician assisted by a nurse. A consent form is signed by the client. The nurse assists the client throughout a procedure. Most of these procedures cause moderate discomfort, and the client may tolerate the procedure better if a well-informed nurse stays at the bedside and explains each step (Table 13-3).

EQUIPMENT

Most institutions purchase trays with contents appropriate for the specific aspiration, or the trays are compiled by the institution's central supply department. Contents of trays may differ from one institution to another. Equipment needed but not found in aspiration trays includes:

Two pair sterile gloves of appropriate size for physician

Laboratory requisitions and labels

Mask, goggles, and gowns for physician and nurse

Standard aspiration trays may contain:

Antiseptic solution (e.g., povidone-iodine)

Gauze sponges (4 × 4)

Sterile towels

Anesthetic agent (e.g., lidocaine 1%)

Two 3 ml sterile syringes with 23- to 25-gauge needles

2-inch adhesive tape

Bandaids

The box on p. 246 lists equipment usually found in specific aspiration trays.

Assessment

1. Assess client's knowledge of procedure to determine level of health teaching required.
2. Observe verbal and nonverbal behaviors to determine client's anxiety.
3. Assess client's ability to understand and follow directions. **Procedure requires client to follow directions closely and assume proper position.**
4. Assess client's ability to assume position required for procedure and ability to remain still. **Client must maintain position without moving to avoid complications during needle or trocar insertion.**
5. Determine whether client is allergic to antiseptic or anesthetic solutions to decrease risk of complications. **Common allergic reactions to anesthetic agents are central nervous system depression, respiratory difficulties, and hypotension. Aller-**

gic reactions to antiseptic solutions are usually skin irritations.

6. Assess vital signs to provide baseline data for comparison with postprocedural vital signs.

7. Assess client's coagulation status (use of anticoagulants, platelet count, prothrombin time) to determine factors that can increase risk of bleeding.

8. Assess according to aspiration being performed (see Table 13-3).

9. Assess need for preprocedural pain medication. **Procedure may be painful, and client must remain still throughout procedure because of potential complications.**

Table 13-3 **Aspirations**

Test	Purpose	Assessment specific to test
Bone marrow aspiration	Removal of cells from bone marrow for diagnosis of leukemias and other malignancies, anemias, and thrombocytopenia	Assess complete blood count for abnormalities.
Lumbar puncture	Aspiration of spinal fluid for testing and/or measurement of pressure for diagnosis of meningitis, encephalitis, brain or spinal cord tumors, and cerebral hemorrhage	Assess neurological status, including movement, sensation, and muscle strength of legs, to provide baseline for comparison after procedure.
Paracentesis	Removal of fluid from peritoneal cavity to determine presence of blood, bile, bacteria, or protein; also to decrease intraabdominal pressure in presence of ascites (accumulation of fluid in peritoneal cavity)	Assess bladder for distention and determine last voiding. Bladder should be empty to minimize risk of puncture. Weigh client, assess abdomen, and measure abdominal girth at largest point. Mark location.
Thoracentesis	Aspiration of fluid to evaluate cell types for the presence of a tumor. May also be used to remove excess fluid in pleural cavity to minimize difficulty breathing	Establish baseline by assessing respiratory rate and depth, symmetry of chest on inspiration and expiration, type of cough, and sputum.
Liver biopsy	Aspiration of cells from liver for diagnosis of cancer, effects of hepatotoxic drugs, or assessment of treatment for chronic liver disease such as hepatitis	Bladder should be empty.

Contents of Aspiration Trays

BONE MARROW ASPIRATION TRAY
Sterile syringes: two 10 ml and two 50 ml for marrow aspiration
Two bone marrow needles with inner stylus
Test tubes and/or glass slides

LUMBAR PUNCTURE TRAY
Three spinal needles (various sizes) with inner obturators (5 to 12.5 cm [2 to 5 inches] long)
Glass or plastic manometer with three-way stopcock
Four test tubes

PARACENTESIS TRAY
Four 10 to 60 ml syringes with 19- to 20-gauge needles
Small, sterile knife blade
Two sterile cannula needles, sizes 10 or 12, with inner trochar or catheter
Sterile specimen cups and receptacle

(2 to 3 L IV fluids and macrodrip-size (10 gtt/ml) IV tubing [as ordered by physician] are not included in tray.)

THORACENTESIS TRAY
Two 50 ml syringes with 14- to 17-gauge needles, 5 to 7 cm (2 to 3 inches) long, for drainage of pleural fluid
Receptacle for fluid
Three-way stopcock
Two-way stopcock with extension tubing
Test tubes

LIVER BIOPSY TRAY
Scalpel
Two True-Cut disposable needles (4½-inch straight and 6-inch straight)
One bottle 30 ml sterile 0.9% normal saline
Formalin solution

Planning

Expected outcomes focus on client's knowledge of the procedure, including the need to remain still to prevent complications; client's anxiety regarding procedure and results; and control of discomfort during and after the procedure.

EXPECTED OUTCOMES

1. Client explains purpose and basic steps of the procedure before it is begun.
2. Client assumes the correct position and remains still throughout the entire procedure.
3. Client does not verbalize fear of procedure and its results after nurse reviews procedure.
4. Client verbalizes minimal pain, which requires no analgesics after procedure.
5. Client has nonlabored respirations within normal range after abdominal paracentesis and thoracentesis.
6. Client has few changes in heart rate and blood pressure during and after aspiration.
7. Puncture site dressing remains clean, dry, and intact.
8. Client is able to explain position and activity restrictions after aspirations.

Implementation

Steps	Rationale
1. See Standard Protocol (Chapter 1, p. 5).	
2. Assist with bone marrow aspiration.	
a. Explain steps of skin preparation, anesthetic injection, needle insertion, and position required.	Anticipation of expected sensation reduces anxiety.
b. Set up sterile tray or open supplies to make accessible for physician.	Reduces risk of contamination of sterile field and promotes prompt completion of procedure.
c. Assist client in maintaining correct position. (Position required depends on bone marrow aspiration site. Iliac crest is most common site, but sternum or tibia may also be used.) Reassure client while explaining procedure.	Decreases chance of complications during procedure. Explanations increase client comfort and relaxation.

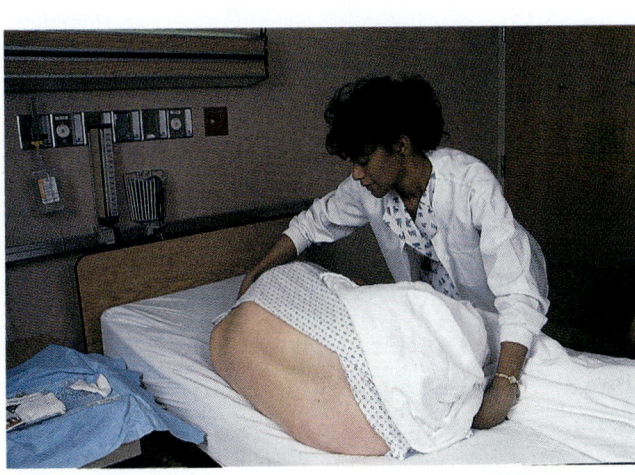

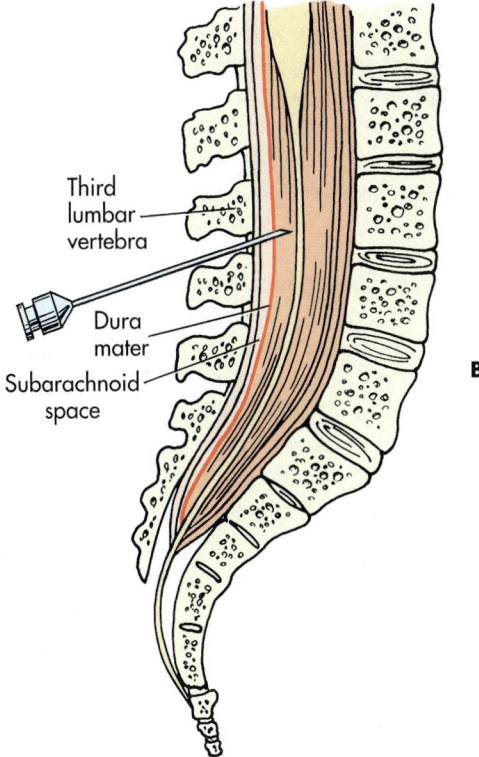

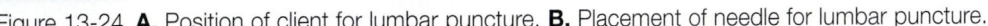

Figure 13-24 **A,** Position of client for lumbar puncture. **B,** Placement of needle for lumbar puncture.

Steps	Rationale
d. Assess client's condition during procedure: comfort, respiratory status, and vital signs if indicated.	Identifies any changes that may indicate a complication.
e. Note characteristics of bone marrow aspirate (e.g., amount, color).	Characteristics are used for observation, reporting, and recording.

3. Assist with lumbar puncture.

Steps	Rationale
a. Explain steps of procedure, and assist client in assuming flexed side-lying position for entire procedure (Figure 13-24, *A*).	Ensures no movement of spinal needle within spinal column and canal. Spinal needle is inserted into spinal canal anywhere between third lumbar (L3) and first sacral (S1) vertebrae (Figure 13-24, *B*).
b. Set up sterile tray or open supplies to make accessible for physician.	
c. Gently but firmly hold client's arms and legs in flexed position.	Prevents sudden movement by client.
d. Caution client not to cough and to breathe slowly and deeply.	Coughing or changes in breathing increase cerebrospinal fluid (CSF) pressure and give false reading.
e. Explain each step that may cause discomfort.	Client should know exactly what is occurring so that discomfort can be anticipated and surprises eliminated.
f. Properly label tubes with client information and name of test desired.	Nurse is responsible for labeling tubes with client's name and tests desired. Test tubes are numbered in sequence of collection (e.g., nos. 1 through 4).
g. Assist with placement of direct pressure and gauze dressing over puncture site.	Pressure helps minimize CSF loss and bleeding.
h. Ask client to maintain dorsal recumbent position (flat), usually for 4 to 12 hours after procedure. Client may turn from side to side.	Dorsal recumbent position reduces risk of spinal headache, which may result if client sits upright.
i. Provide for client's comfort with medication as ordered.	Procedure is usually described as painful by client. Postprocedural headache may require that client be medicated.
j. During and after procedure, observe client for: (1) Changes in level of consciousness (LOC) and pupil size/reaction. (2) Respiratory status and vital signs. (3) Numbness, tingling, or pain radiating down legs.	Changes in LOC, pupil size/reaction, respiratory status, and vital signs indicate increasing intracranial pressure. May result from spinal nerve irritation.
k. Encourage client to force fluids by mouth if not contraindicated.	Needed to replace CSF lost and resume hemodynamics.

4. Assist with paracentesis.

Steps	Rationale
a. Explain steps of procedure and position required (either semi-Fowler's in bed or sitting upright on side of bed or in chair with feet supported) (Figure 13-25).	
b. Set up sterile tray or open sterile supplies and make accessible for physician.	
c. Describe steps of procedure as they are implemented by physician.	Allows client opportunity to ask questions and helps to decrease anxiety.
d. Assess vital signs every 15 minutes during procedure.	Identifies possible complications of procedure, such as shock.
e. After physician attaches intravenous (IV) tubing to cannula, administer physician-ordered amount of fluid at prescribed rate.	Promotes infusion of prescribed fluid into peritoneum.
f. Clamp IV tubing after fluid is instilled, and place drainage tubing below client's abdominal level.	Promotes gravitational drainage of fluid from peritoneal cavity.

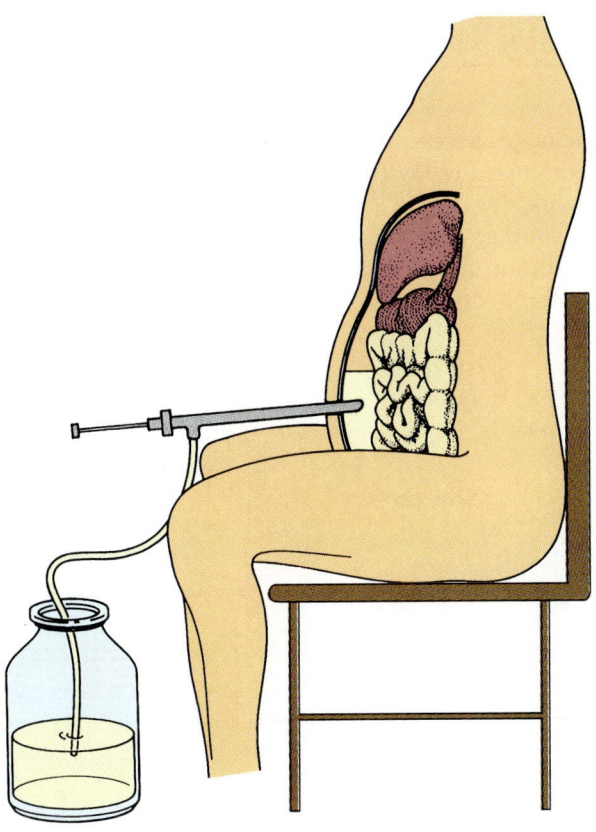

Figure 13-25 (Modified from Beare PG, Myers JL: *Principles and practice of adult health nursing,* ed 2, St. Louis, 1994, Mosby.)

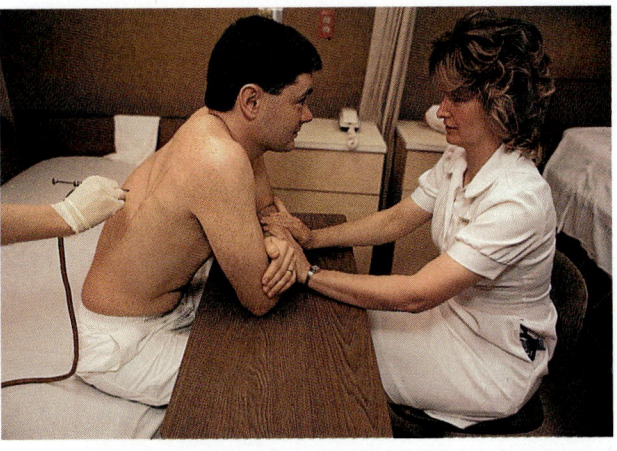

Figure 13-26 (From Wilson SF, Thompson JM: *Respiratory disorders,* St. Louis, 1990, Mosby.)

Steps	Rationale
g. Open tubing clamp to allow drainage of ascitic or peritoneal lavage fluid. Maximum amount of ascitic fluid usually allowed to drain is 1500 ml.	Permits gravitational flow of fluid or solution from abdomen. Maximum of 1500 ml drainage prevents hypovolemic shock.
h. Collect any necessary laboratory specimens in sterile containers.	
5. Assist with thoracentesis.	
a. Explain steps of procedure and position required.	
b. Set up sterile tray or open supplies to make them accessible to physician.	
c. Assist client in assuming correct position: leaning over a bedside table padded with pillows (Figure 13-26).	Positions client appropriately for procedure and prevents sudden movement by client.
d. Assist client through procedure by holding shoulders or sides and reassuring in coaching manner.	Procedure is usually uncomfortable.
e. Assess client's respiratory status during procedure: rate, difficulty, and color of mucous membranes and nail beds.	Enables nurse to detect tolerance to procedure and possible complications.
f. Assist client in assuming comfortable position in bed after procedure.	If leakage into pleural space is suspected, client is positioned recumbent with punctured chest side up.
6. Assist with liver biopsy.	
a. Explain steps of procedure and position required.	
b. Set up sterile tray or open sterile supplies and make them accessible for physician.	

Steps	Rationale

c. Ask client to empty bladder.

d. Assist client to correct position: supine at far right edge of bed with head turned left and right arm extended above head (Figure 13-27, *A*).

Facilitates access to liver biopsy site. Needle is inserted through the lower chest, between the sixth and seventh ribs (Figure 13-27, *B*).

e. Teach client breathing used during procedure: take deep breath in, blow all air out, and hold breath. After physician removes needle, client can breathe normally.

This brings the liver and diaphragm to their uppermost position and immobilizes them (Wilkinson, 1990).

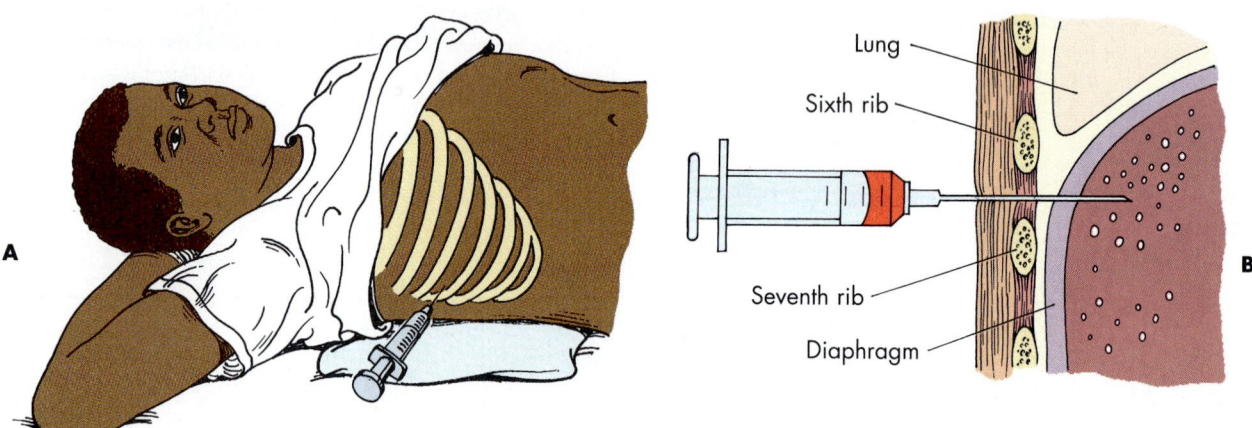

Figure 13-27

f. Assist client in changing position after the procedure: move to center of bed and roll onto right side. Instruct to maintain position for 2 hours.

Liver capsule is compressed against the chest wall at the site of needle insertion, which prevents blood from leaking (Wilkinson, 1990).

g. Advise client to remain in bed for 6 hours.

h. Assess pulse, blood pressure, and respirations every 15 minutes for 1 hour, every 30 minutes for 2 hours, every 1 hour for 4 hours, then every 4 hours.

Enables nurse to identify possible complications of procedure, such as shock.

7. Securely attach properly completed identification label and laboratory requisition to specimen(s).

Incorrect identification of specimen could result in diagnostic or therapeutic errors.

8. Send specimen immediately to laboratory.

9. See Completion Protocol (Chapter 1, p. 6).

Evaluation

1. Ask client to state purpose and explain steps of the procedure before it is started.

2. Ask client to demonstrate body position required for procedure. Assess client's body position throughout procedure and assist to maintain position as necessary.

3. Ask if client has questions or concerns about the procedure before it begins and later about test results. Assess nonverbal behaviors of anxiety before, during, and after procedure.

4. Observe client's level of comfort during and after procedure.

5. Assess client's respiratory status (rate, rhythm, and depth of respirations; symmetry of chest movement) during and after abdominal paracentesis and thoracentesis.

6. Assess client's heart rate and blood pressure during and after procedure. (Check hospital policy; may be as often as every 15 minutes for 2 hours.)

7. Inspect dressing over puncture site for drainage every hour after the procedure until client's condition is stable.

8. Ask client to describe postprocedural positioning and activity restriction for lumbar puncture, liver biopsy, and thoracentesis.

UNEXPECTED OUTCOMES AND RELATED INTERVENTIONS

1. Client develops a suboccipital headache after lumbar puncture.
   a. Instruct client to lie flat in bed.
   b. Encourage fluid intake of at least one glass per hour if not contraindicated.
   c. Administer analgesics as prescribed.
   d. Apply ice pack to area of discomfort.
2. Client found ambulating to bathroom while on strict bed rest after liver biopsy.
   a. Instruct client to remain in bed, positioned on right side. Reinforce that this position prevents blood or bile from leaking from puncture site.
   b. Inspect dressing for blood or bile leakage.
   c. Place call light within client's reach and reinforce when to use it.
   d. Check blood pressure, pulse, and respirations.
3. Client complains of lightheadedness while sitting at side of bed after abdominal paracentesis.
   a. Assist client to supine position.
   b. Check blood pressure and pulse.
   c. Inspect abdominal dressing for bleeding or peritoneal fluid.

SAMPLE DOCUMENTATION

0930 Abdominal paracentesis completed with 1100 ml cloudy liquid aspirated. Respirations 18 with moderate depth, pulse 98, and blood pressure 138/86. Rates pain at 6 on scale of 1-10. 2 × 2 gauze dressing applied to puncture site; remains dry and intact. 0940 Demerol 50 mg given in right dorsal gluteal for abdominal pain.

1010 States pain has decreased to 2, which is tolerable. Abdominal girth measures 34 inches at umbilicus. Weight decreased to 168 pounds.

Skill 13.4 | Assisting with Diagnostic Procedures (Angiography [Arteriography], Bronchoscopy, Endoscopy, CT, MRI, ECG)

The diagnostic procedures addressed in this skill may be performed by a variety of health care personnel. Roles of the nurse include assisting with the preparation of the client before the procedure, providing support during the procedure if indicated, and providing appropriate nursing care after the procedure (Table 13-4).

EQUIPMENT

Angiogram (arteriogram)
Special packs are usually available from central supply. The packs contain various sizes and types of catheters for performing the procedures, as well as the necessary specialized equipment.
Sterile gown
Sterile gloves
Mask
Goggles
Bronchoscopy
Bronchoscopy tray, if available from central supply, may include:
   Flexible fiberoptic bronchoscope
   Gauze sponges (4 × 4)
   Local anesthetic spray (lidocaine)
   Sterile tracheal suction catheters
   Sterile gloves
   Sterile water-soluble lubricating jelly
Mask, goggles, and gown
Emesis basin
Oxygen equipment

Endoscopy
Endoscopy tray may include:
   Fiberoptic endoscope
   Camera
   Solutions for biopsied specimens
Local anesthetic spray
Tracheal suction equipment
Blood pressure equipment
Sterile water-soluble jelly
Mask, goggles, and gown
CT scanning
None
MRI
Contrast medium: gadolinium (Magnevist) (optional and must be ordered by physician)
ECG
ECG machine
Electrode paste (gel)
ECG leads or electrodes
Alcohol wipes
Razor

Assessment

1. Assess client's knowledge of the procedure to determine level of understanding and what education may be necessary.
2. Observe verbal and nonverbal behaviors to determine level of client's anxiety.

Table 13-4 **Selected Diagnostic Procedures**

Procedure	Description	Assessment
Angiography (arteriography)	Injection of radiopaque material through catheter threaded into femoral, brachial, or carotid artery and viewed with x-ray study to show vasculature of heart and arterial system	Assess peripheral pulses to establish baseline. Auscultate heart and lung sounds to establish baseline. Assess complete blood count, platelets, prothrombin time, electrolytes, blood urea nitrogen, and creatinine levels to evaluate possible contraindications (Schroeder et al, 1992).
Bronchoscopy	Examination of tracheobronchial tree with flexible fiberoptic bronchoscope. Sputum or mucus plugs may be aspirated or tissues can be examined or biopsied for abnormalities.	Assess heart and lung sounds, type of cough, and sputum to establish baseline. Assess for allergy to local anesthetic used to spray throat, which could cause laryngeal edema or laryngospasm.
Endoscopy	Visualization of gastrointestinal (GI) tract using a long, flexible fiberoptic scope with a light source attached	Assess for upper GI bleeding, which may obscure viewing lens with blood, preventing visualization.
Esophagogastroduodenoscopy (EGD)	Visualize upper GI tract	
Proctoscopy, colonoscopy, or sigmoidoscopy	Visualize lower GI tract	
Computed tomography (CT or CAT scan)	Multiple x-ray studies of specific body organs and tissues to provide three-dimensional view	Assess for claustrophobia, which indicates need for sedation or alternative diagnostic test.
Magnetic resonance imaging (MRI)	Noninvasive scanning to visualize internal organs and structures by use of magnetic forces rather than radiation	Assess for cardiac pacemaker, aneurysm clips, or history of valve replacement, which are contraindications because magnet may move metal or electronic objects (Pagana and Pagana, 1992).
Electrocardiogram (ECG or EKG)	Graphic representation of electrical impulses generated by heart during a cardiac cycle; identifies abnormalities that interfere with electrical conduction through cardiac tissue	Assess for chest pain, dyspnea, and heart rate and rhythm. Assess blood pressure, pulse, and respirations.

3. Assess if client is allergic to iodine dye (for clients undergoing angiography, CT scanning, and MRI). If so, notify cardiologist or radiologist. **In angiography and CT scanning, a hypoallergenic contrast medium can be used.**

4. Assess vital signs to provide baseline data for comparison with findings during and after procedure.

5. Assess peripheral pulses (for clients undergoing angiography) to provide baseline data for comparison with findings during and after procedure.

6. Auscultate heart and lung sounds (for clients undergoing angiography and bronchoscopy) to provide baseline data for comparison with findings during and after procedure.

7. Assess respiratory status—lung sounds, type of cough, and sputum produced (for clients undergoing bronchoscopy)—to provide baseline data for comparison with respiratory status during and after procedure.

8. Assess whether client has signed consent form (check institution's policy). **Angiography, bronchoscopy, CT (if dye used), MRI (if dye used), and endoscopy usually require a signed consent form to reduce legal risk to institution.**

9. Assess time of last ingested fluid or food (for clients undergoing angiography, bronchoscopy, CT, and upper GI endoscopy). Clients should receive nothing by mouth (NPO) 6 to 8 hours before angiography, 8 hours before endoscopy and bronchscopy, and 4 hours before CT to prevent possible aspiration. **Excessive hydration causes dilution of contrast medium, making structures more difficult to visualize. Iodine dye may cause nausea.**

10. Assess client's ability to remain still and cooperate throughout the procedure.

11. Assess according to procedure being performed (see Table 13-4).

Planning

Expected outcomes focus on client's knowledge of the procedure, client's level of anxiety, prevention of complications, and control of discomfort during and after the procedure.

EXPECTED OUTCOMES

1. Client explains the purpose and basic steps of the procedure before it is begun.
2. Client assumes the correct position and remains still throughout the entire procedure.
3. Client verbalizes fear of procedure and results, even after the procedure is reviewed by nurse.
4. Client has little pain, which requires no analgesia after the procedure.

5. Client does not experience postprocedural complications, such as:
   a. Hypotension and tachycardia, which may signify hemorrhage or allergic reaction to dye.
   b. Diminished or absent peripheral pulses, which may signify thrombosis or embolism.
   c. Flushing, itching, and urticaria, which signify possible allergic reaction to dye.
   d. Sudden, severe shortness of breath, which signifies laryngospasm and bronchospasm in response to irritation from bronchoscope or topical anesthetic.
   e. Abdominal pain, fever, and bleeding, which occur with perforation of abdominal structures.
   f. Respiratory depression, decreased cardiovascular function, confusion, and diminished reflexes, which are side effects of drugs used for IV sedation (client conscious).

Implementation

Steps	Rationale
1. See Standard Protocol (Chapter 1, p. 5).	
2. Explain purpose and steps of procedure.	Reduces anxiety and increases cooperation.
3. Assist client to empty bladder before procedure.	Ensures that client will not need to void during procedure.
4. Assist with angiography (arteriography). (Figure 13-28 shows an example of abdominal angiography.)	
a. Establish IV access using large-bore cannula (see Chapter 29).	Provides access for delivery of IV fluids and/or drugs.
b. Assist client in assuming comfortable position on x-ray table.	Position may need to be maintained for 1 to 3 hours.
c. Structures can be visualized as dye circulates.	

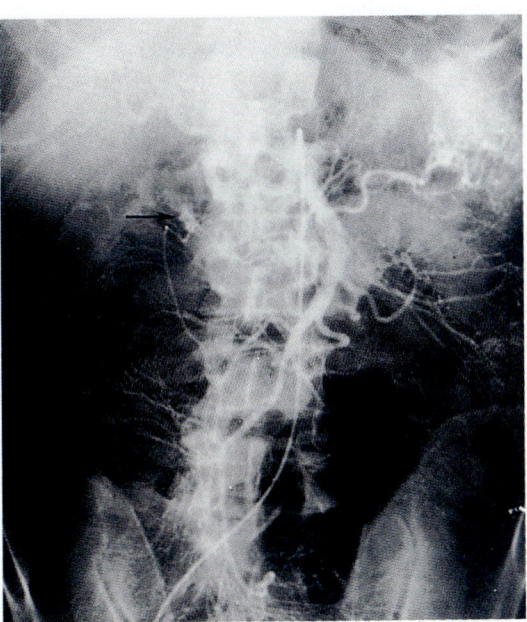

Figure 13-28 (From Doughty DB, Jackson DB: *Gastrointestinal disorders,* Mosby's Clinical Nursing Series, St. Louis, 1993, Mosby.)

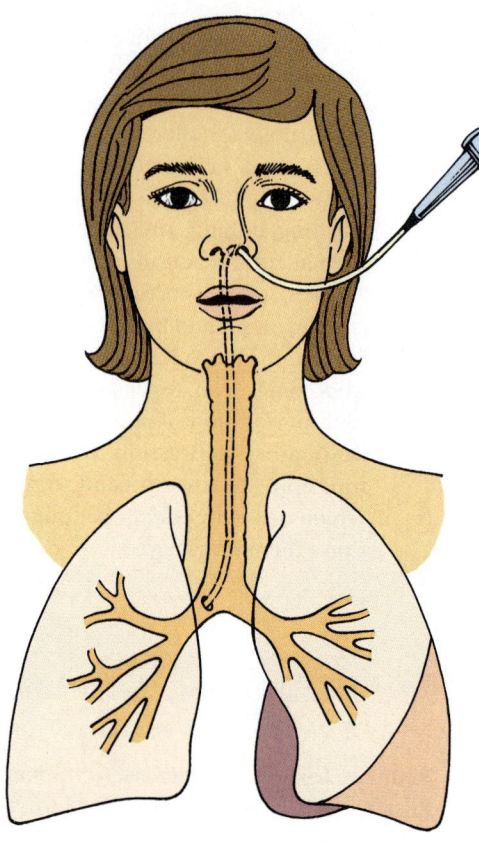

Figure 13-29 Bronchoscope inserted through the client's nose, into the trachea, and to the bronchus.

Steps	Rationale

5. Assist with bronchoscopy (Figure 13-29).

a. Remove and safely store client's dentures and eyeglasses (if applicable).

b. Establish IV access using large-bore cannula (see Chapter 29).

    Provides access for delivery of IV fluids and/or drugs.

c. Assist client in maintaining position desired by physician: semi-Fowler's or supine (Pagana and Pagana, 1992).

    Provides maximal visualization of lower airways and adequate lung expansion.

d. Instruct client not to swallow local anesthetic; provide emesis basin.

    Anesthetic may be absorbed systemically and cause severe central nervous system and cardiovascular reactions.

e. Assist client through procedure by explanations.

    Although premedicated and drowsy, clients need to be reminded not to change position and to cooperate.

f. Monitor ECG, pulse, and blood pressure for changes every 5 minutes during procedure.

    Side effects of drugs used for IV sedation (client conscious) may include respiratory depression, decreased cardiovascular function, confusion, and diminished reflexes. Interval for assessment may be lengthened to 15 minutes if perioperative nurse determines client's condition is within normal parameters (Watson and James, 1990).

g. Assess client's respiratory status every 5 minutes during procedure: observe degree of restlessness and respiratory rate; observe capillary refill and color of nail beds; monitor pulse oximetry (oxygen saturation).

    Bronchoscope may cause feelings of suffocation; also, because airway is partially occluded, client may become hypoxic during observations. Side effects of drugs used for IV sedation (client conscious) include respiratory depression and somnolence (Watson and James, 1990).

Steps	Rationale
h. Note characteristics of suctioned material.	Information used to record and report and to make further client observations.
i. Wipe client's nose to remove lubricant after bronchoscope is removed.	Promotes hygiene and comfort.
j. Assess LOC, gag reflex, pulse oximetry, respiratory rate, blood pressure, pulse, heart rate, and capillary refill after the procedure. (Use tongue depressor to touch pharynx to test for presence of gag reflex.)	Assesses for postprocedural complications.
k. Do not allow client to eat or drink until the tracheobronchial anesthesia has worn off and gag reflex returns.	Prevents aspiration of food or fluid, which could cause pneumonia.

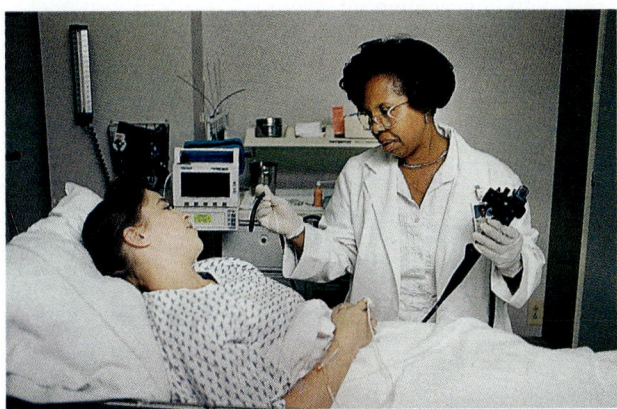

Figure 13-30 Preparing client for an esophagogastroduodenoscopy (EGD).

6. Assist with endoscopy (Figure 13-30).	
a. Remove client's dentures and partial bridges (if applicable).	Prevents dislodgment of dental structures during intubation phase.
b. Establish IV access using large-bore cannula (see Chapter 29).	
c. Assist client in maintaining left lateral position.	Unexpected change of position can cause accidental perforation of esophagus, stomach, or duodenum.
d. Assist client through procedure by anticipating needs, promoting comfort, and telling client what is happening.	Client is unable to speak after tube is passed into throat. Reassures client about procedure and how long it will last.
e. Monitor ECG, pulse, and blood pressure for changes every 5 minutes during procedure.	Side effects of drugs used for IV sedation (client conscious) may include respiratory depression, decreased cardiovascular function, confusion, and diminished reflexes. Interval for assessment may be lengthened to 15 minutes if perioperative nurse determines client's condition is within normal parameters (Watson and James, 1990).
f. Place tissue specimens in proper laboratory containers.	Ensures proper labeling and preparation of specimens for microscopic examination.
g. Suction if client begins to vomit or accumulate saliva.	Prevents aspiration of gastric contents or oral secretions.
h. Assess LOC, gag reflex, pulse oximetry, respiratory rate, blood pressure, pulse, heart rate, and capillary refill after the procedure. (Use tongue depressor to touch pharynx to test for presence of gag reflex.)	Assesses for postprocedural complications.

Steps	Rationale
i. Assist client to comfortable position, then wash hands.	Promotes rest and relaxation.
7. Assist with CT (Figure 13-31).	
a. Instruct client not to move, talk, or sigh during procedure once technician assists to desired position.	Movement causes computer-generated artifacts on image produced.
b. Observe client for signs of anaphylaxis if iodinated dye administered.	Signs include respiratory distress, palpitations, itching, and diaphoresis.
8. Assist with MRI (Figure 13-32).	
a. If possible, show client picture of MRI machine and encourage questions.	Helps to decrease anxiety by providing information.
b. Remove all metallic objects from client, such as watch, jewelry, coins, keys, hairpins, credit cards, prosthesis, and dentures containing metal (Pagana and Pagana, 1992).	Metallic objects create artifacts on the scan, and some metal objects may be damaged by the magnetic field. Also metallic objects may be moved by the magnetic field.

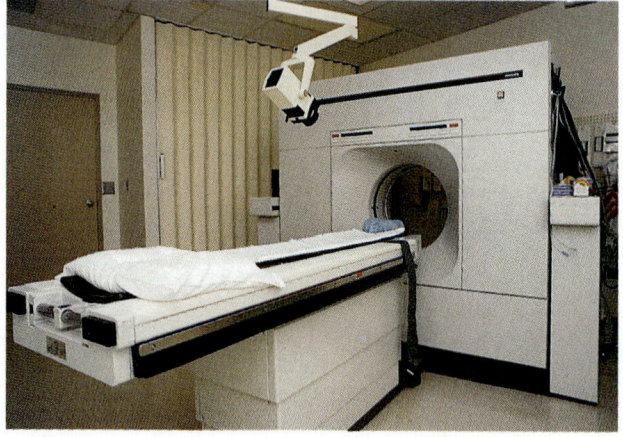

Figure 13-31 Computerized tomography can scan any part of the body, with or without contrast media. (From Brundage DJ: *Renal disorders,* St. Louis, 1992, Mosby.)

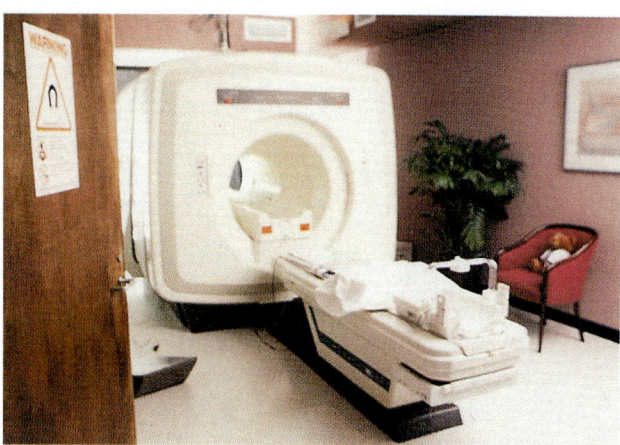

Figure 13-32 Magnetic resonance imaging is the most precise diagnostic tool available. (From Brundage DJ: *Renal disorders,* St. Louis, 1992, Mosby.)

Steps	Rationale
9. Perform ECG (Figure 13-33).	
a. Cleanse and prepare skin; wipe sites with alcohol.	Promotes adherence of leads (electrodes) to chest or extremity.
b. Apply electrode paste and attach leads. For 12-lead ECG:	Position of leads promotes proper display of ECG on paper.
(1) Chest (precordial leads)	

V_1—Fourth intercostal space (ICS) at right sternal border

V_2—Fourth ICS at left sternal border

V_3—Midway between V_2 and V_4

V_4—Fifth ICS at midclavicular line

V_5—Left anterior axillary line at level of V_4 horizontally

V_6—Left midaxillary line at level of V_4 horizontally

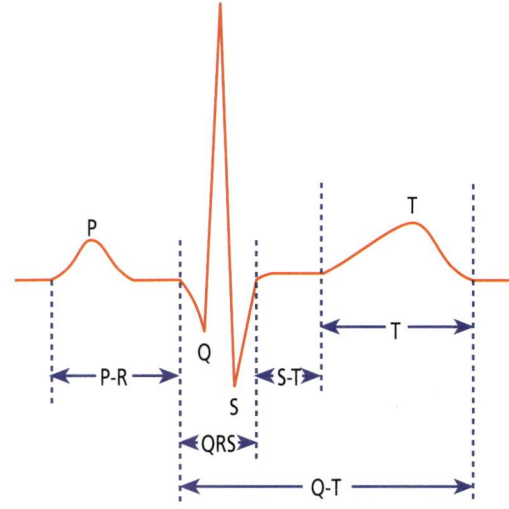

Figure 13-33 Normal ECG waveform (lead II). (From Canobbio MM: *Cardiovascular disorders,* St. Louis, 1990, Mosby.)

Steps	Rationale
(2) Extremities: one on lower portion of each extremity aVR—Right wrist aVL—Left wrist aVF—Left ankle	
c. Obtain tracing; 12-lead ECG may be obtained without removing precordial leads.	Transfers electrocardiac conduction on ECG tracing paper for subsequent analysis by cardiologist.
d. Disconnect leads, wipe excess electrode paste from chest, and wash hands.	Promotes comfort and hygiene.
e. Deliver ECG tracing to appropriate laboratory or nursing unit.	Provides for review of ECG by cardiologist.
10. See Completion Protocol (Chapter 1, p. 6).	

Evaluation

1. Ask client to explain purpose and basic steps of the procedure.
2. Ask client to demonstrate body position required for procedure. Assess client's body position during procedure.
3. Ask if client has questions or concerns about the procedure before it begins and later about test results. Assess nonverbal behaviors of anxiety before, during, and after procedure.
4. Observe client's level of comfort during and after procedure.
5. Assess client for postprocedural complications.
   a. Assess client for a decrease in blood pressure and tachycardia (could signify hemorrhage or allergic reaction to dye).
   b. Assess client's peripheral pulses. (A diminished or absent pulse could signify thrombosis or embolism.)
   c. Assess client for flushing, itching, and urticaria (could signify allergic reaction to dye).
   d. Assess client's respiratory status for sudden, severe shortness of breath (could signify laryngospasm and bronchospasm).
   e. Assess client for abdominal pain, fever, and bleeding (could signify perforation of abdominal structures).
   f. Assess client for unarousable sleep, low oxygen saturation, decreased rate and/or depth of respirations, apnea, cyanosis or mottled skin, hypotension, changes in heart rate and/or rhythm (usually bradycardia), and decreased or nonpalpable pe-

ripheral pulses (side effects of IV conscious sedation).

UNEXPECTED OUTCOMES AND RELATED INTERVENTIONS

1. Client's dorsalis pedis pulses are nonpalpable bilaterally 2 hours after an angiogram.
   a. Assess dorsalis pedis pulses with a Doppler scope.
   b. Notify physician immediately.
2. One hour after gastroscopy, client attempts to drink water furnished by a family friend.
   a. Reinforce to client and friend that liquids or solid food should not be taken orally until gag reflex returns.
   b. Teach client possible complications from eating or drinking substances before gag reflex returns (aspiration pneumonia).
   c. Check gag reflex each hour.
   d. Inform client when it is appropriate to eat and drink.
3. In the recovery room after an endoscopy, client is sleepy but responds to verbal stimulation, respirations shallow at rate of 10 per minute, oxygen saturation 85%, and ECG reading normal sinus rhythm.
   a. Instruct client to take deep breaths.
   b. Administer oxygen at 2 L per nasal cannula.
   c. Elevate head of bed 30 degrees.
   d. Notify physician.

SAMPLE DOCUMENTATION

0800 Client returned from angiogram per stretcher. Dorsalis pedis and posterior tibial pulses are +2 bilaterally. No bleeding, swelling or discoloration noted at catheter insertion site in left groin. Sandbag in place over left groin. Left leg extended. Complains of mild discomfort at left groin, but denies need for analgesics.

1000 MRI of lower extremities completed without contrast medium. Able to maintain position without moving. Client states, "It took a long time, but I got through it okay."

CRITICAL THINKING EXERCISES

1. Analyze the following client situations. Identify factor(s) that may contribute to procedural revisions and/or negatively affect the results of the test ordered.
   a. A 65-year-old client undergoes a bone marrow aspiration. Platelet count is low, and client reports no use of anticoagulants or aspirin.
   b. A 21-year-old client is scheduled for an MRI scan and is allergic to lidocaine and iodine.
   c. An 85-year-old female has rheumatoid arthritis and severe back pain. The physician has ordered a midstream urine specimen.
   d. A 54-year-old male is scheduled for a lumbar puncture. He is pacing across the room, unable to sit still during an explanation of the procedure. He currently has a respiratory infection with persistent, productive cough. History includes knee surgery with subsequent painful knee flexion.
   e. An 82-year-old male who is incontinent of stool needs a stool specimen for culture.
   f. After a finger stick, the first drop of blood is placed on the glucose strip, and the strip is positioned propped up on the reagent strip container lid during the timing process.
   g. An infant is to have a fecal specimen for occult blood testing and is having diarrheal stools.
   h. A client's first-voided AM urine specimen yields an unusually high urine glucose level.
2. For each of the following postprocedural situations, identify high-risk complications.
   a. 1700 ml ascitic fluid drained from peritoneal cavity after paracentesis
   b. Client up walking around room after a lumbar puncture
   c. Client lying on right side after liver biopsy; BP 100/62, P 110, R 20
   d. Client observed drinking a glass of water immediately after a bronchoscopy; alert and oriented; no c/o pain or discomfort
3. Walter is a 65-year-old client scheduled for an angiography. He is very anxious, stating he has heard of other people having a heart attack or dying from a blood clot during the procedure. Walter is reluctant to sign the informed consent. How would you proceed in this situation?
4. The physician has requested an aerobic culture from an open leg wound.
   a. Since you are using sterile swabs provided in the culture tube, you determine that sterile gloves are not necessary. Evaluate the logic of this decision.
   b. As you begin to place the swab near the wound drainage, you touch the client's leg. What step should you take next?
   c. How would this procedure differ if the physician had ordered an anaerobic culture?

REFERENCES

Beare PG, Myers JL: *Principles and practices of adult health nursing,* ed 2, St Louis, 1994, Mosby.

Brundage DJ: *Renal disorders,* St Louis, 1992, Mosby.

Canobbio MM: *Cardiovascular disorders,* St Louis, 1990, Mosby.

Doughty DB, Jackson DB: *Gastrointestinal disorders,* Mosby's Clinical Nursing Series, St Louis, 1993, Mosby.

Grimes D: *Infectious diseases,* Mosby's Clinical Nursing Series, St Louis, 1991, Mosby.

Pagana KD, Pagana TJ: *Mosby's diagnostic and laboratory test reference,* St Louis, 1992, Mosby.

Schroeder SA et al, editors: *Current medical diagnosis and treatment,* East Norwalk, Conn, 1992, Appleton & Lange.

Watson DS, James DS: Intravenous conscious sedation: implications of monitoring patients receiving local anesthesia, *AORN J* 51(6):1512, 1990.

Wilkinson M: Your role in needle biopsy of the liver, *RN* 53(4):62, 1990.

Wilson SF, Thompson JM: *Respiratory disorders,* St Louis, 1990, Mosby.

ADDITIONAL READINGS

Centers for Disease Control: Recommendation for prevention of human immunodeficiency virus and hepatitis B to patients during exposure-prone invasive procedures, *MMWR 40*(RR-8), July 12, 1991.

Cuzzell J: The right way to culture a wound, *Am J Nurs* 93(5):48, 1993.

Kestel F: Using blood glucose meters: what you and your patient need to know. Part 1, *Nursing '93* 23(3):34, 1993.

Kestel F: Using blood glucose meters: what you and your patient need to know. Part II, *Nursing '93* 23(4):50, 1993.

Kestel F: Using blood glucose meters: what you and your patient need to know. Part III, *Nursing '93* 23(5):51, 1993.

McConnell EA: Obtaining an aerobic wound culture specimen, *Nursing '91* 21(5):21, 1991.

Meeker MH, Rothrock JC, editors: *Alexander's care of the patient in surgery,* ed 10, St Louis, 1995, Mosby.

Perdue B: Cardiac catheterization—before and after, what the patient should understand: what the nurse needs to know! *Adv Clin Care* 5(2):16, 1990.

Perry AG, Potter PA: *Clinical nursing skills and techniques,* ed 3, St Louis, 1994, Mosby.

Potter PA, Perry AG: *Fundamentals of nursing: concepts, process, and practice,* ed 3, St Louis, 1993, Mosby.

Renkes J: GI endoscopy: managing the full scope of care, *Nursing '93* 23(6):50, 1993.

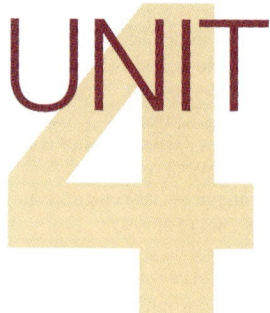

UNIT
4

Application of Surgical Asepsis

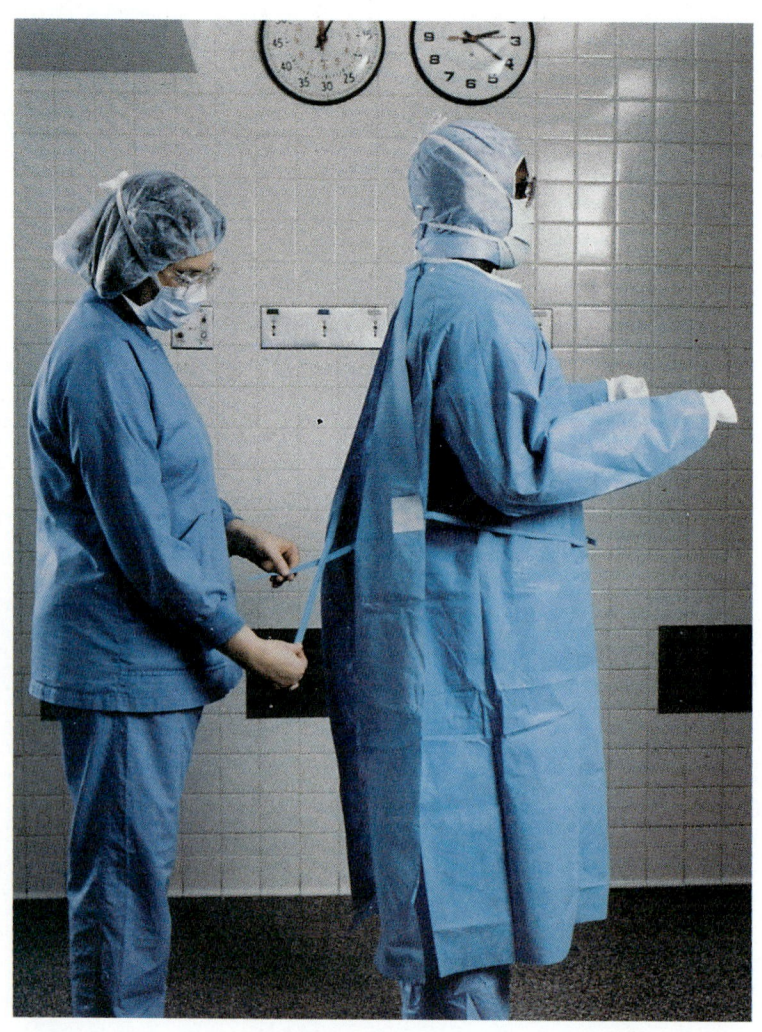

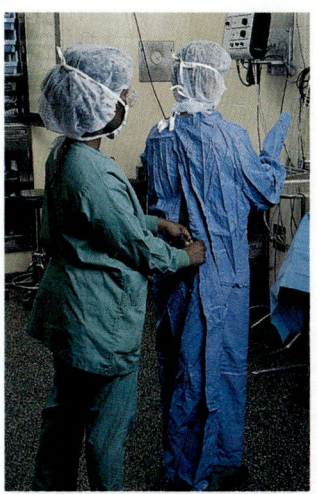

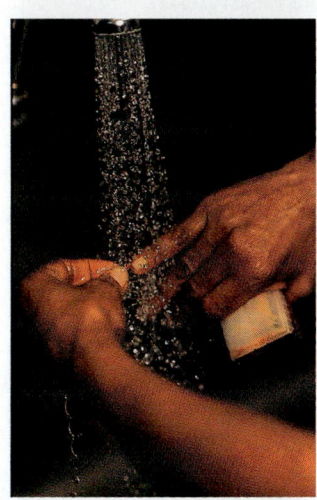

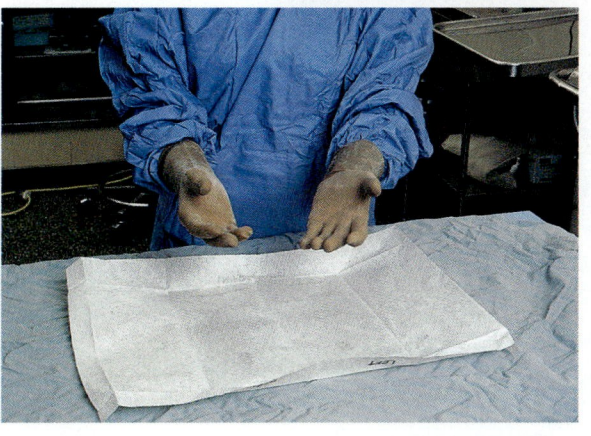

chapter 14 | Basic Sterile Techniques

Skill 14.1
Sterile Gloving

Skill 14.2
Creating and Maintaining a Sterile Field

Sterile technique or surgical asepsis is the method of creating and maintaining a controlled area free of all microorganisms, including spores and pathogens. Strict adherence to the principles of sterile (aseptic) technique limits a client's risk for infection during invasive procedures.

Asepsis is the absence of disease-causing organisms. To render an item *sterile* is to make it free of all microorganisms. Microorganisms can be *endogenous,* from within the body, or *exogenous,* from outside the body.

A *sterile field* is an area that includes surfaces and equipment draped or prepared for a sterile procedure.

A sterile field must (AORN, 1994):

- Never be covered because it is too difficult to uncover without contaminating the field
- Always be within view to avoid unobserved contamination
- Be established immediately before the procedure because of a direct relationship between the time the sterile field is created and the length of exposure to airborne contaminants

There are primarily three situations that require using surgical aseptic technique (Perry and Potter, 1994):

- During procedures requiring an incision or puncture of a client's skin
- When client's skin integrity is compromised or broken because of trauma or burns
- During procedures requiring insertion of devices or instruments into a sterile body cavity

All members of the health care team must develop a *sterile conscience* that guides them to act appropriately to maintain sterility and correct any breaks inadvertently occurring during the procedure. As the client's advocate, the nurse can set an excellent example for other members of the health care team. Physicians and other care givers may need education and direction regarding strict adherence to the principles of aseptic technique (see the box on p. 262).

Principles of Aseptic Technique

1. All items used within a sterile field must be sterile.
2. A sterile barrier that has been permeated by punctures, tears, or moisture must be considered contaminated.
3. Once a sterile package is opened, the edges are considered unsterile.
4. Gowns, once put on, are considered sterile in front from chest to waist or table level; sleeves are considered sterile from 5 cm (2 inches) above elbows to fingertips of gloved hand. (NOTE: Cuffs are not considered sterile once glove has been removed.)
5. Tables draped as part of sterile field are considered sterile only at table level.
6. If there is any question or doubt of an item's sterility, the item is considered to be unsterile.
7. Sterile persons or items contact only sterile areas; unsterile persons or items contact only unsterile areas.
8. Movement around and in the sterile field must not compromise or contaminate the sterile field.

NURSING DIAGNOSIS

The major nursing diagnosis related to clients undergoing procedures involving surgical asepsis is **Risk for Infection.** Unless strict aseptic technique is used when performing invasive procedures, clients could experience a local or systemic response, manifested by redness, pain, edema, or drainage from the procedure site as well as positive cultures, elevated temperature, or elevated white blood cell count (WBC).

Skill 14.1 | Sterile Gloving

Sterile gloves act as a barrier against the transmission of pathogenic microorganisms and should be put on before performing any sterile procedure, such as a sterile dressing change or Foley catheter insertion. The nurse must remember that sterile gloves do not replace vigorous handwashing.

The open glove method is used for most sterile procedures not requiring a sterile gown. The nurse must take care not to contaminate the gloved hands by touching unsterile items or areas. The hands should remain clasped in front of the body until ready to perform the procedure. If a glove becomes contaminated, it must be changed immediately.

EQUIPMENT
Package of correctly sized sterile gloves (Figure 14-1)

Assessment

Determine if procedure to be performed is considered a sterile procedure.

Planning

Expected outcomes focus on prevention of localized or systemic infection.

EXPECTED OUTCOMES
1. Client remains afebrile 24 to 48 hours after the procedure or throughout the course of repeated procedures.
2. Client displays no signs of localized infection (redness, tenderness, edema, drainage) at procedure site.

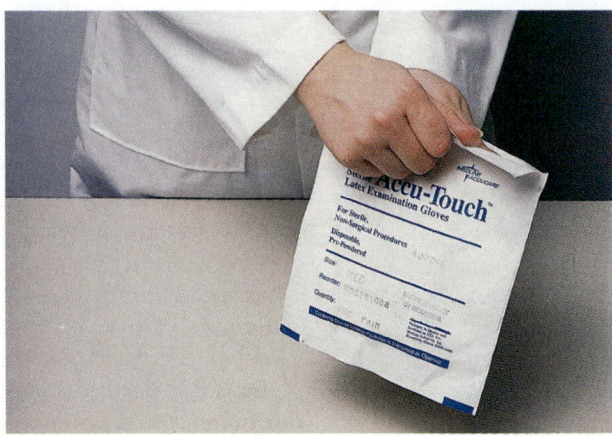

Figure 14-1

Implementation

Steps	Rationale

1. See Standard Protocol (Chapter 1, p. 5).
2. Open sterile gloves by peeling back adhered package edges (Figure 14-2).
3. Remove inner wrapper and carefully open without touching the wrapper's inner surface (Figure 14-3).
4. Select glove of dominant hand and grasp folded edge of cuff with nondominant hand. Touch only the inside surface of glove (Figure 14-4).

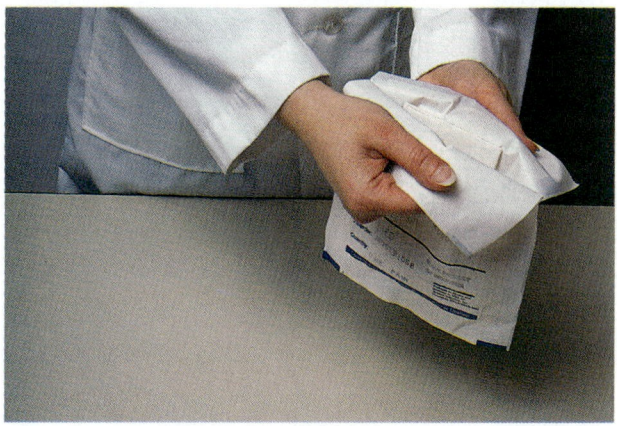

Figure 14-2

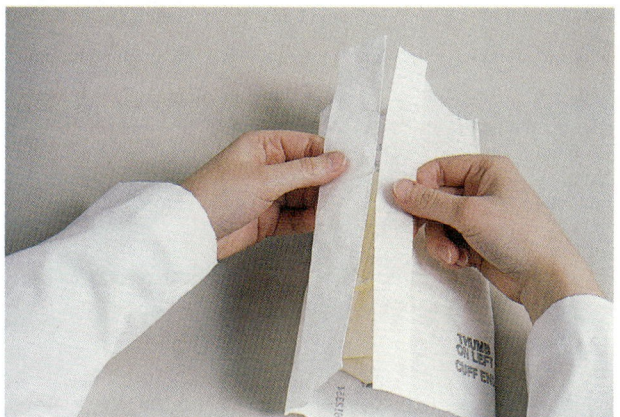

Figure 14-3

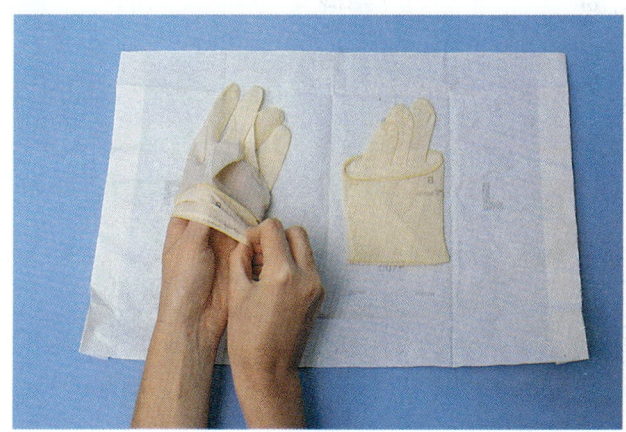

Figure 14-4

5. Pull glove over dominant hand, carefully working thumb and fingers into correct spaces. Gently let go of cuff while preventing it from rolling up wrist (Figure 14-5).

Inner edge of cuff will touch skin and is no longer considered sterile.

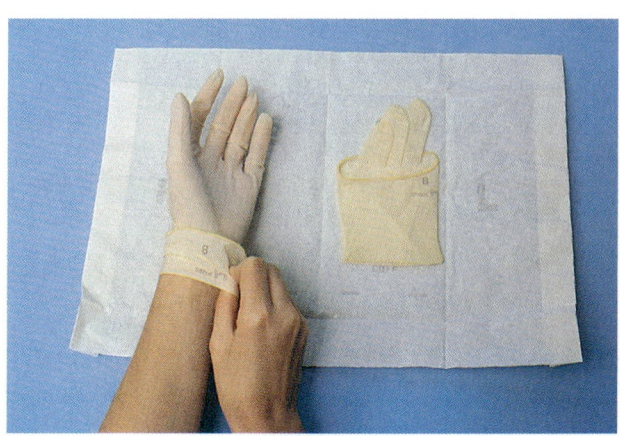

Figure 14-5

Steps	Rationale

6. Slide fingers of gloved hand underneath second glove's cuff (Figure 14-6), and pull over fingers of nondominant hand. Do not touch exposed areas with gloved hands; keep thumb of dominant hand abducted back (Figure 14-7).

Cuff protects gloved fingers; abducting thumb prevents contamination from contact with unsterile surface.

7. Interlock fingers of gloved hands and hold away from body until beginning procedure.

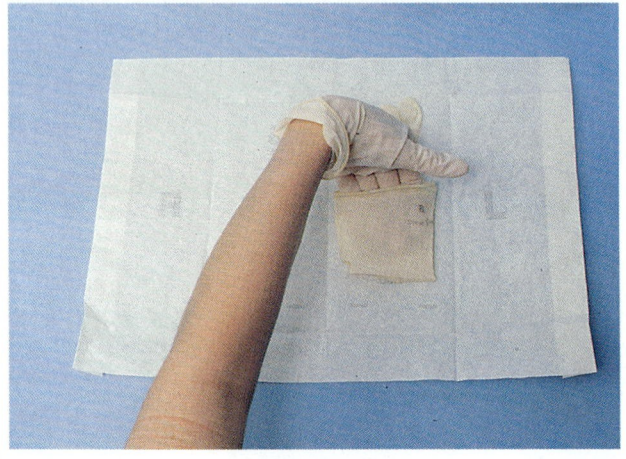

Figure 14-6

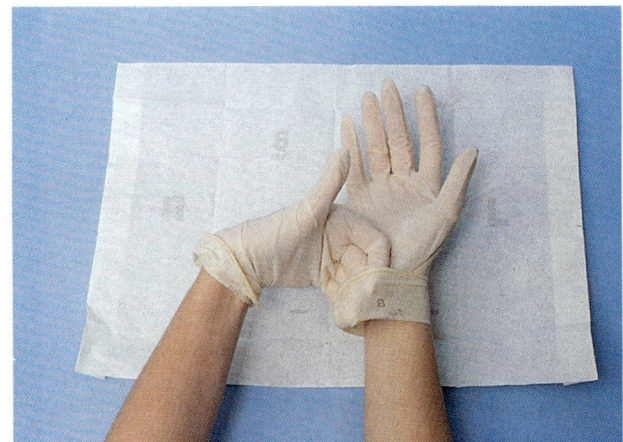

Figure 14-7

Glove disposal

8. Pull off glove of one hand, turning inside out by grasping outside of the cuff with other gloved hand. Discard in proper receptacle.

Minimizes contamination of bare hands.

9. Remove remaining glove by placing fingers of bare hand under cuff, and pull off by turning inside out. Discard in proper receptacle.

10. See Completion Protocol (Chapter 1, p. 6).

Evaluation

1. Evaluate client for fever for 48 hours after the procedure.
2. Inspect treated area for localized signs of infection (redness, swelling, odor, drainage).

UNEXPECTED OUTCOMES AND RELATED INTERVENTIONS

Client develops signs of infection.
   a. Notify physician of findings.
   b. Continue to use good handwashing.
   c. Strictly adhere to principles of aseptic technique.
   d. Monitor temperature every 4 hours.
   e. Encourage client's intake of fluids.

SAMPLE DOCUMENTATION

1000 Rt forearm dressing and packing removed and discarded. Wound gently irrigated with saline. No drainage, redness, tenderness, or swelling noted at site. Wound packed with $\frac{1}{4}$" gauze and dressed with sterile 4 × 4 sponges and silk tape. Client remains afebrile.

Skill 14.2 | **Creating and Maintaining a Sterile Field**

A sterile field provides a microorganism-free environment in which to perform a procedure. For minor procedures, a sterile kit or bundle of supplies can be opened on a clean surface and used as the sterile field (Figure 14-8). For more complicated procedures or those requiring several supplies, a table can be covered with a sterile, water-repellent drape. Sterile drapes can be linen, paper, or plastic but must be water repellent. Sterile supplies and solutions can then be delivered to the sterile field.

The inside of a sterile kit may also serve as a sterile field. Examples of sterile kits are Foley catheter insertion kits or triple-lumen catheter kits. Some institutions wrap and process their own bundles of equipment for procedures such as lumbar punctures or thoracentesis trays. Bundles packaged by the institution generally contain external and internal sterile (chemical) indicators that indicate the item has completed a sterilization process (Figure 14-9).

EQUIPMENT

Sterile gloves
Sterile, water-repellent drapes
Sterile, water-repellent gown (see institutional policy)
Disposable cap and mask (see institutional policy)
Sterile supplies/solutions specific to procedure
Waist-high table
Protective eye wear

Assessment

1. Verify that procedure requires surgical aseptic technique.
2. Check commercially packaged kits (which are usually disposable) for package integrity and expiration date or statement of sterility. If the package was processed by the agency, integrity, expiration date, and sterile indicator must be checked. Moisture, punctures, tears, and outdated or unsterile supplies entering the sterile field result in contamination.

Planning

Expected outcomes focus on prevention of localized or systemic infection.

EXPECTED OUTCOMES

1. Client remains afebrile 24 to 48 hours after the procedure or during course of repeated procedures.
2. Client displays no signs of localized infection (redness, tenderness, edema, drainage) 24 hours after the procedure.

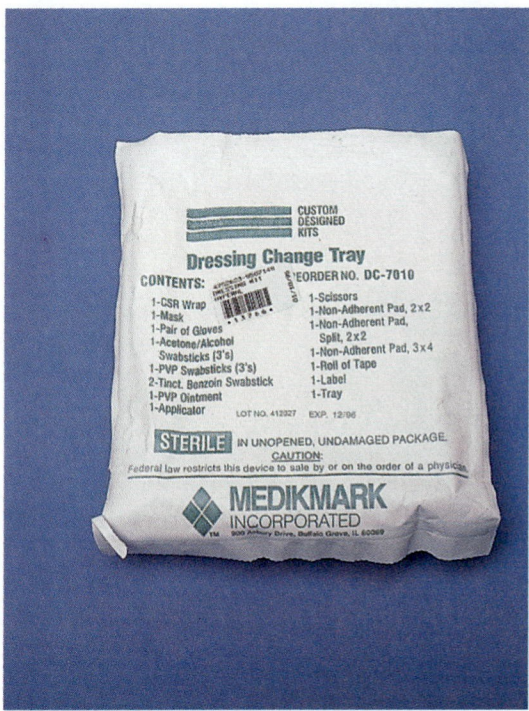

Figure 14-8 Sterile dressing change kit.

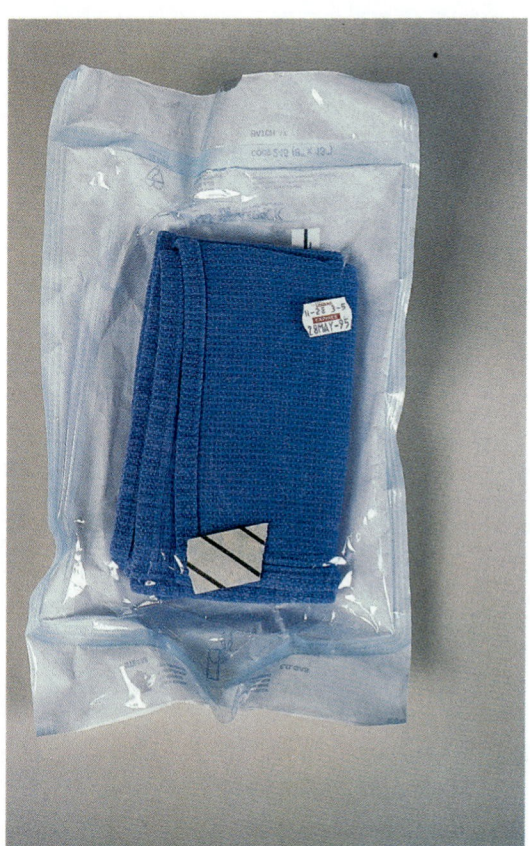

Figure 14-9 Tape with stripes changes color after sterilization.

Implementation

Steps	Rationale

1. See Standard Protocol (Chapter 1, p. 5).
2. Select a flat, clean, dry work surface at or above waist level. Instruct client not to touch work surface.
3. Put on cap and mask, if indicated (check agency policy).
4. Prepare commercially packaged kit.
  a. Remove kit from outer dust cover.
  b. Place on selected work surface.
  c. Locate and grasp tip of outermost flap and open away from yourself (Figure 14-10).
  d. Open first side flap in same manner but to the side and without reaching over sterile field (Figure 14-11).
  e. Repeat as above for flap on other side (Figure 14-12).
  f. Carefully grasp final and innermost flap corner and open toward yourself (Figure 14-13).
	Once created, sterile field is sterile only at table level.

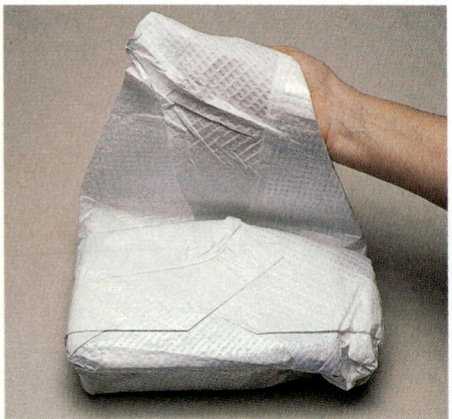

Figure 14-10

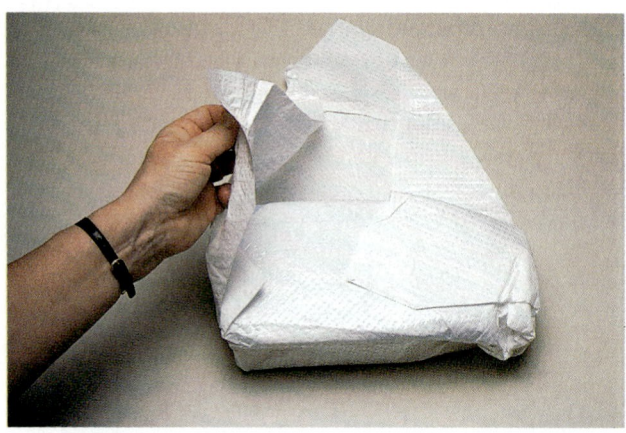

Figure 14-11

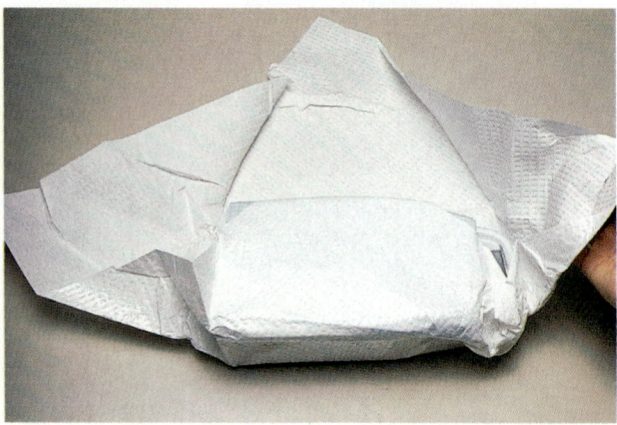

Figure 14-12

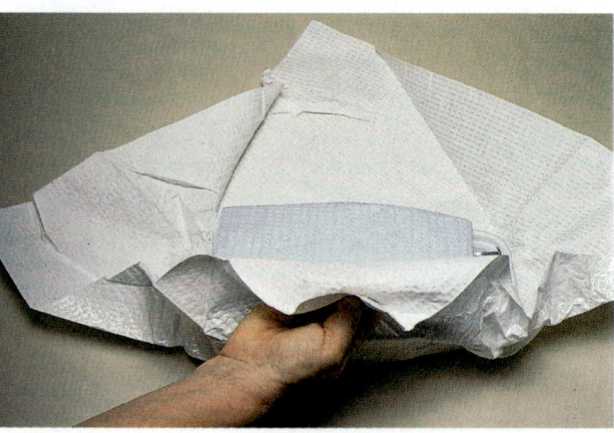

Figure 14-13

Steps	Rationale

5. Prepare linen-wrapped supply bundle (processed by agency).
  a. Place on selected work surface.
  b. Remove sterile (chemical) indicator tape from outside of package.
  c. Open both wrapper layers (one at a time) as with above kit.

Linen-wrapped items have two layers. The first is a dust cover, and the second layer must be opened to view the sterile (chemical) indicator. If dropped, linen packages are considered contaminated.

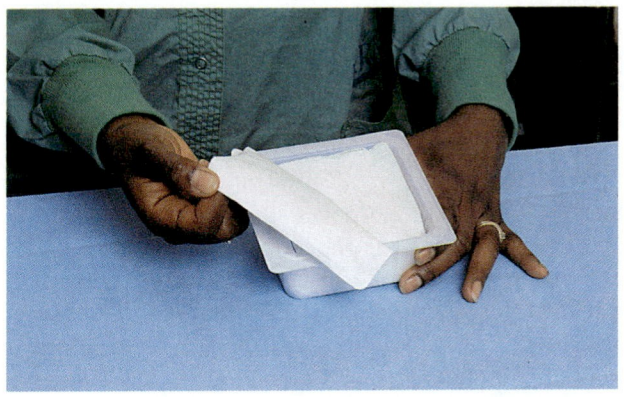

Figure 14-14

6. Delivering sterile items to the sterile field.
  a. Add packaged items to sterile field (following package directions) by carefully pulling back the edges of the outer wrapper (Figure 14-14).
  b. Gently toss item onto the sterile field while preventing wrapper from touching sterile field.
  c. Dispose of outer wrapper.

Reaching over or touching sterile field contaminates field.

7. Pouring sterile solutions.
  a. Verify contents and expiration date of solution.
  b. Remove seal and cap from bottle, keeping inside of cap sterile.
  c. Pour solution slowly into sterile container without splashing and while maintaining safe distance from the sterile field (Figure 14-15).
  d. Label container with expiration date and time (Figure 14-16).

Splashing liquids causes fluid permeation of the sterile barrier, called "strike through," resulting in contamination.

Solution is considered contaminated 24 hours after opening (check agency policy).

8. See Completion Protocol (Chapter 1, p. 6).

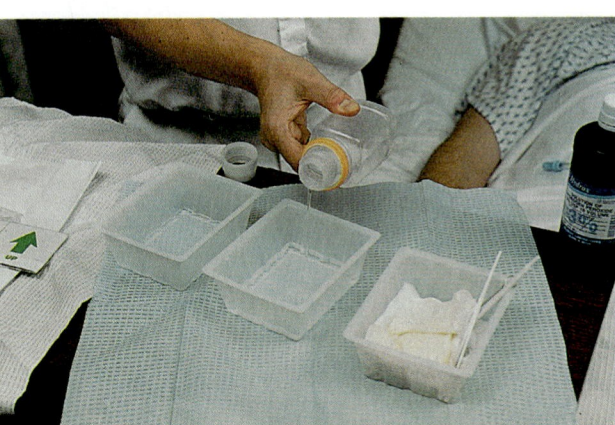

Figure 14-15

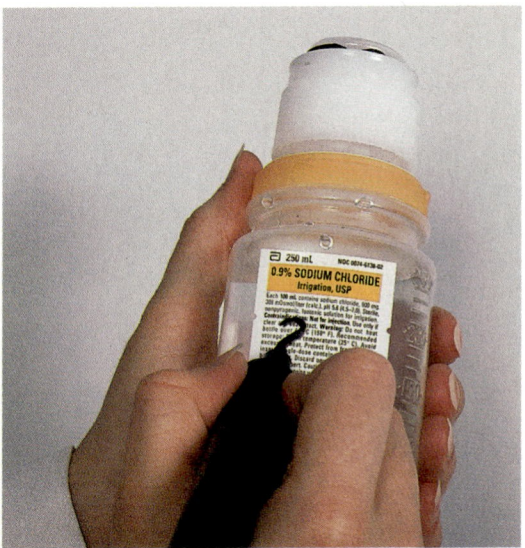

Figure 14-16

Evaluation

1. Evaluate client for fever for 48 hours.
2. Inspect treated area for localized signs of infection (redness, tenderness, edema, warmth, odor, drainage).

UNEXPECTED OUTCOMES AND RELATED INTERVENTIONS

Client develops signs of infection.
  a. Notify physician of findings.
  b. Continue strict aseptic technique and vigorous handwashing.
  c. Monitor temperature every 4 hours.
  d. Encourage client's intake of fluids.

SAMPLE DOCUMENTATION

1400 24 hr after lumbar puncture. Puncture site without redness, tenderness, or edema. Bandaid dry and intact. Client denies complaints of pain or discomfort. Remains afebrile.

CRITICAL THINKING EXERCISES

1. Critique each of the following situations involving sterile technique. Are the nurse's actions appropriate, or do corrections need to be made? Explain.
   a. After washing hands, the nurse opened the indwelling urinary catheter tray and put on sterile gloves in preparation for inserting a Foley catheter into the client's urinary bladder. Following the procedure, the nurse disposed of the used supplies, removed the gloves by turning them inside out, and disposed of them in the trash receptacle. The nurse washed hands before leaving the client's room.
   b. In report at 7:00 AM the nurse learns that Dr. Redd plans to remove a small lesion from a client's arm at 2:00 PM. The nurse decides to prepare the surgical supplies and equipment immediately after report in case activity gets busy later. Before leaving the treatment room, the nurse covers the sterile field with a sterile towel.
   c. The nurse is preparing to perform a sterile dressing change on a client with an abdominal incision. After putting on sterile gloves, the nurse realizes that the gloves are too small but proceeds with the procedure, assuming that the dressing can be changed quickly.
2. You are the nurse caring for Mr. Block. Mr. Block had abdominal surgery 2 days ago, and his incisional dressing has been changed twice.
   a. When changing Mr. Block's dressing, what steps should you take to prevent wound contamination?
   b. If encountered, what assessment findings would indicate that Mr. Block may be developing a wound infection?
3. Is it appropriate to use sterile technique or clean technique for each of the following?
   a. Taking the client's temperature
   b. Applying medication to the client's burned skin
   c. Irrigating the client's wound with normal saline
   d. Removing a dressing following foot surgery
   e. Administering a subcutaneous injection

REFERENCES

Association of Operating Room Nurses: Recommended practices for aseptic technique. In *AORN standards and recommended practices for perioperative nursing,* Denver, 1994, AORN.

Perry A, Potter P: *Clinical nursing skills and techniques,* ed 3, St Louis, 1994, Mosby.

ADDITIONAL READINGS

Atkinson L: *Berry and Kohn's operating room technique,* ed 7, St Louis, 1992, Mosby.

Meeker M, Rothrock J: *Alexander's care of the patient in surgery,* ed 10, St Louis, 1995, Mosby.

chapter 15 | Providing Wound Care

Skill 15.1
Changing Dry Sterile Dressings

Skill 15.2
Changing Moist Dressings

Skill 15.3
Changing Transparent Dressings

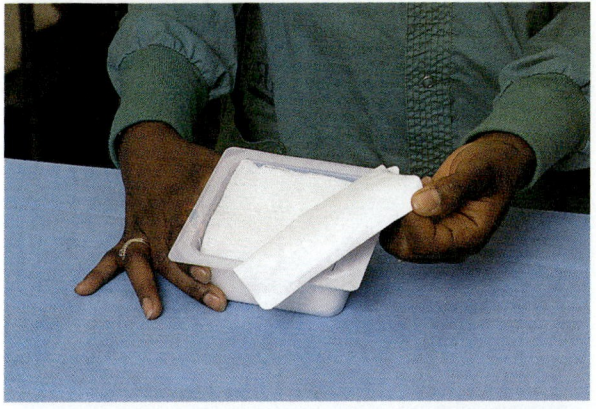

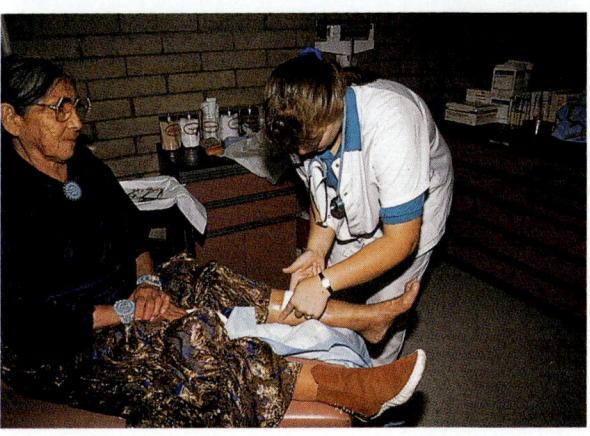

Unbroken skin is a protective barrier against disease-causing organisms and a sensory organ for pain, temperature, and touch. Injury to the skin poses risks for infection and triggers a complex healing response. Knowing the normal healing pattern helps the nurse recognize alterations that require intervention. The nurse's main responsibilities are to prevent infection and to support the body's defenses for healing. When choosing dressings, the nurse considers the type of wound, the pain associated with it, conditions that affect healing, and the client's psychological responses.

There are three components of wound healing: epithelialization, contraction, and collagen formation. Surface wounds, such as abrasions, heal by epithelialization; new skin cells replace the epithelium lost in the injured area. Full-thickness open wounds, such as a deep pressure ulcer, heal by contraction and filling of the defect with collagen (Doughty, 1992).

The first phase of healing is inflammation, which is apparent by warmth, redness, and swelling. During this phase, platelets control bleeding and substances are released that stimulate the growth of new capillaries and connective tissue cells (fibroblasts). White blood cells (WBCs) and macrophages destroy bacteria and help eliminate dead cells. New capillaries and fibroblasts appear as granulation tissue. The capillaries supply oxygen and vital nutrients; the fibroblasts produce collagen. Deposits of collagen give the wound strength, and epithelial cells cover it.

Most surgical incisions and some traumatic injuries heal by *primary intention,* since tissue is cleanly cut and the edges are well approximated. New capillary circulation bridges the wound in 3 to 4 days, and once normal tissue oxygenation is achieved, the wound is considered to be healed. Susceptibility to infection is greatest during the first 4 days.

Burns, infected wounds, and deep pressure ulcers heal by *secondary intention.* The wound is left open (not sutured). Granulation tissue and epithelialization close the defect. This healing occurs much more slowly.

Wound infection is the second most common nosocomial infection (see Chapter 3). The chances of wound infection are greater when the wound contains dead or necrotic tissue, when there are foreign bodies in or near the wound, and when blood supply and local tissue defenses are reduced. Many factors may delay healing and increase risk of infections (Table 15-1). According to the Centers for Disease Control and Prevention (CDC), a wound is infected if purulent material drains from it (Table 15-2), even if a culture has negative results or is not taken. A sample of drainage from an infected wound may not reveal bacteria in a culture because of inadequate technique or previous treatment with antibiotics (see Skill 13.1). Positive cultures may contain colonies of noninfective resident bacteria.

A contaminated or traumatic wound may show signs of infection within 2 to 3 days. A surgical wound infection usually develops on the fourth or fifth day. The client will have fever, tenderness, and increasing pain at the wound site and an elevated WBC count. The edges of the wound appear inflamed (red and swollen). Drainage, if visible, is purulent, is odorous, and has a yellow, green, or brown color, depending on the causative organism (Table 15-2).

Nursing Diagnosis

Risk for Infection is appropriate when skin integrity is broken and additional factors are present that

Table 15-1 **Factors that Delay Healing and Increase Risk for Infection**

Factor	Reason for increased risk
Older adult	Physiological changes of aging alter the immune system, resulting in decreased resistance to pathogens.
Obesity	Fatty subcutaneous tissue has diminished vascularity. Fatty tissue makes approximation of wound edges difficult and creates tension on the wound.
Diabetes	Associated vascular changes reduce blood flow to peripheral tissues; leukocyte malfunction results from hyperglycemia.
Compromised circulation	Results in inadequate supply of nutrients, blood cells, and oxygen to wound.
Malnutrition	Chronic illness or alcoholism often results in malnutrition, which impairs the normal inflammatory process and formation of new tissue.
Immunosuppressive therapy	
Chemotherapy	Decreases inflammatory response and collagen synthesis.
Steroids	Slow rate of tissue growth and development of new capillaries. Radiation in area of wound decreases blood supply to tissues.
High levels of stress	Increased cortisol levels reduce number of lymphocytes and decrease inflammatory response.

Table 15-2 **Types of Wound Drainage**

Type	Appearance
A. Serous	Clear, watery plasma

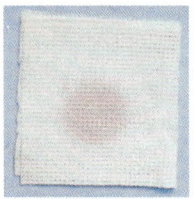

| B. Purulent (PUS) | Thick, yellow, green, tan, or brown |

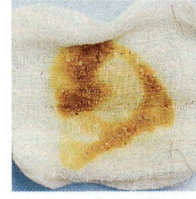

| C. Serosanguineous | Pale, red, watery: mixture of serous and sanguineous |

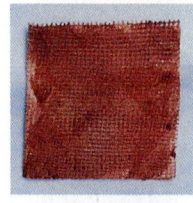

| D. Sanguineous | Bright red: indicates active bleeding |

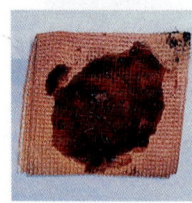

increase the client's risk for infection (see Table 15-1). When the wound is a painful surgical incision in an otherwise healthy individual, **Impaired Physical Mobility** related to incisional pain may be an appropriate nursing diagnosis, in which interventions involve immobilization of the wound to minimize pain. **Altered Health Maintenance** related to a knowledge deficit regarding the dressing change technique requires interventions focused on teaching clients home care.

Skill 15.1 | Changing Dry Sterile Dressings

Dry dressings protect the wound from injury, prevent introduction and spread of bacteria, reduce discomfort, and speed healing. Drainage from surgical or traumatic wounds may be serous, sanguineous, or serosanguineous (Table 15-2). Dressings promote hemostasis by direct pressure and absorption of drainage. Dressings also may support or immobilize a body part. The ideal dressing is easy to apply, conforms to body contours, is durable but flexible, is able to absorb or contain exudate, is easily removed without damage to the healing surface, and is acceptable in appearance (Boston and Rijswijk, 1991).

Dry dressings are most often used for abrasions and postoperative incisions when minimal drainage is anticipated. Gauze dressings come in a variety of sizes, such as 4×4 (16 inches square), 4×8 (rectangle), precut drain sponge, and rolls. Telfa gauze dressings contain a shiny, nonadherent surface on one side that does not stick to the wound. Drainage passes through the nonadherent surface to the outer gauze dressing (Figure 15-1). If a dry dressing adheres to a wound, the nurse should moisten the dressing with sterile normal saline or sterile water before removing the gauze to minimize trauma to the wound as it is removed.

Most dressings are secured with tape, which may be paper, plastic, woven, or elastic material with adhesive. Some clients are allergic to the adhesive. Frequent removal of tape for dressing changes is irritating to the skin. These dressings should be secured with Montgomery straps, which use ties that allow changing the dressing without changing the tape each time (see Skill 15.2). Dressings on an extremity may be secured with rolls of gauze (Table 15-3). The dressing is secured by several turns around the extremity (Figure 15-2, A), continuing with a figure-eight method of application (Figure 15-2, B).

EQUIPMENT
Clean and sterile gloves

A

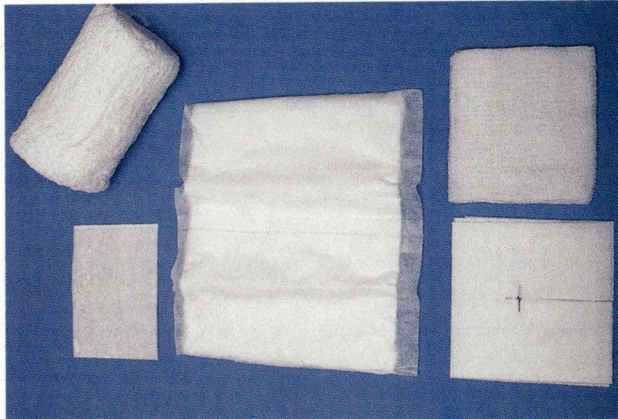

B

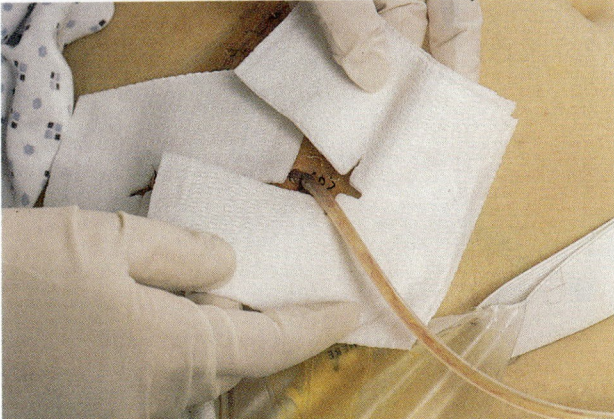

Figure 15-1 **A,** Types of dressings. *Left to right:* rolled gauze, telfa, ABD, 4 × 4, and drain dressing. **B,** Applying a drain dressing.

Table 15-3 **Principles for Wrapping an Extremity**

Action	Rationale
Position body part in comfortable position of normal alignment.	Reduces risk of deformity or injury.
Prevent friction between and against skin surfaces by placing gauze or cotton padding (e.g., between toes).	Skin surfaces that touch may cause friction or skin breakdown.
Apply securely to prevent slipping beginning at distal end and moving toward trunk.	Promotes venous return and minimizes edema or circulatory impairment.
Observe areas distal to bandage for signs of circulatory impairment (cool, pale, swollen, numbness, tingling, slow capillary refill).	Prompt attention to circulatory impairment prevents serious complications.

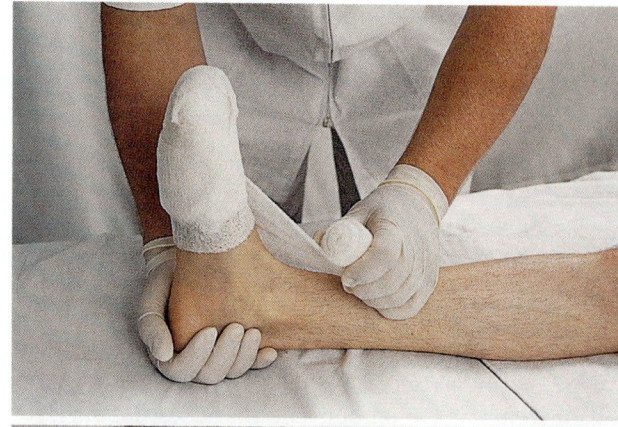

A

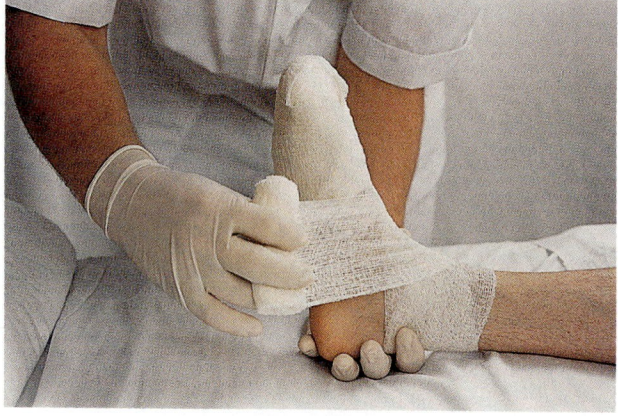

B

Figure 15-2

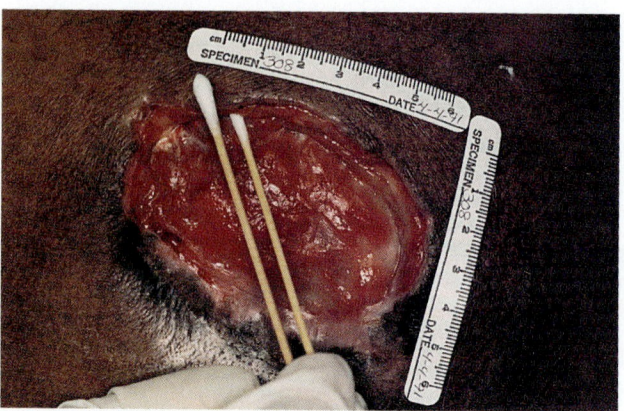

Figure 15-3 Transparent measuring tool.

Sterile dressings

Cleansing solution

Tape, ties, or roller gauze as needed

Waterproof bag

Measuring guide (optional): tape measure or transparent measuring tool (Figure 15-3)

Moisture-proof gown, goggles, and mask (if risk of splashing is present)

Assessment

nurse alert   Review medical orders for type and frequency of dressing changes.

1. Assess size and location of wound to be dressed. **This assists nurse to plan for proper type and amount of supplies needed.**

2. Ask client to rate pain using a scale of 0 to 10. **Client may require pain medication before dressing change to allow drug's peak effect during procedure.**

3. Assess client's knowledge of purpose of dressing change to determine level of support and explanation required.

4. Determine the need for client or family member to participate in dressing wound to prepare client or family member if dressing will be changed at home.

Planning

Expected outcomes focus on preventing infection, promoting healing, pain control, and client and family teaching.

EXPECTED OUTCOMES

1. Client's wound shows evidence of healing by smaller size and less drainage, redness, or swelling.

2. Client reports pain less than 4 (scale of 0 to 10) during and after dressing changes.

3. Client demonstrates correct method of dressing changes.

Implementation

Steps	Rationale

nurse alert If evidence of highly contagious infection is suspected, it may be necessary to place client in a private room (Chapter 3). First postoperative dressings are often changed by the physician. If excessive drainage is noted, the dressing is reinforced (added to) without removing existing dressings (check agency policy). Subsequent changes are done by staff as ordered.

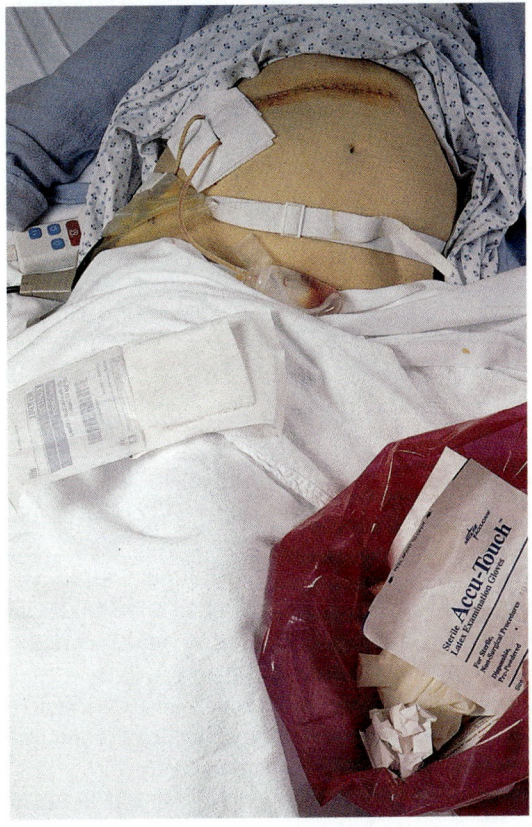

Figure 15-4

1. See Standard Protocol (Chapter 1, p. 5).

2. Expose wound site, preventing unnecessary client exposure. Instruct client not to touch wound or sterile supplies.

3. Place disposable waterproof bag within reach of work area with top folded to make a cuff (Figure 15-4).

4. Remove tape: pull parallel to skin, toward dressing. If over hairy areas, remove in the direction of hair growth.

5. With clean gloves, remove dressings one layer at a time observing appearance and drainage on dressing. Use caution to avoid tension on any drains that are present.

6. Consider client's needs with regard to looking at the wound or drainage.

7. Inspect wound for appearance, size, depth, drainage, integrity (wound edges are together), or granulation tissue.

Provides access to the wound but minimizes unnecessary exposure.

Facilitates safe disposal of soiled dressings.

Reduces stress on suture line or wound edges and reduces irritation and discomfort.

Determine dressings needed for replacement. More or less may be appropriate depending on the degree of saturation. Drains may or may not be sutured in place.

Clients may or may not want to see wound or drainage.

Indicates status of healing.

Steps	Rationale

8. Fold dressings with drainage contained inside and remove gloves inside out. (With small dressings, remove gloves inside out over dressing.) Dispose of gloves and soiled dressings in waterproof bag (Figure 15-5).

Provides containment of soiled dressings and prevents contact of nurse's hands with drainage.

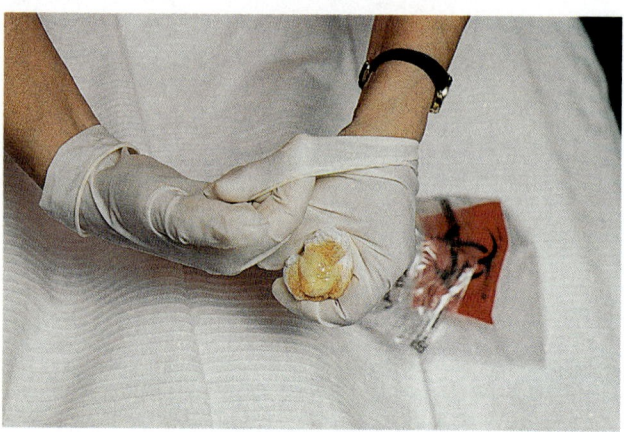

Figure 15-5

9. Create a sterile field with a sterile dressing tray or individually wrapped sterile supplies on overbed table.

Sterile dressings remain sterile while on or within sterile area.

10. Use sterile gloves or no-touch technique with sterile forceps, which maintain sterility of all items in direct contact with the wound (Krasner and Kennedy, 1994).

Sterile gloves may be used for more complex situations with extensive drainage.

11. Cleanse wound using a separate swab for each cleansing stroke and cleaning from least contaminated area to most contaminated (Figure 15-6).

12. Cleanse around drain (if present), using a circular stroke starting near the drain and moving outward (see Skill 20-3).

A 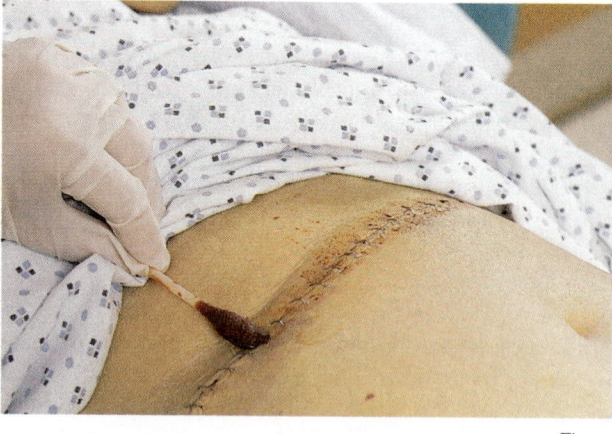 B

Figure 15-6

13. Apply dry sterile dressings to incision or wound site.

Wounds extending around the body or involving a part of the body difficult to reach or wrap may require assistance to cover.

   a. Apply loose woven gauze (fluff gauze sponge or use Kerlix or Supersponge) as contact layer.

Promotes absorption of drainage.

   b. Apply second layer of gauze or thicker absorbent dressing (ABD or Surgi-Pad).

Layering ensures proper coverage and optimal absorption.

Steps	Rationale
14. If worn, remove gloves inside out and dispose of them in a waterproof container.	
15. Secure dressing with tape so that it adheres to 5 to 8 cm (2 to 3 inches) of skin on each side. The ends of tape should be folded under 0.5 to 1 cm on both ends.	Excessive tape irritates skin. Folding under ends of tape facilitates removal with ease and minimal irritation to the skin.
16. See Completion Protocol (Chapter 1, p. 6).	

Evaluation

1. Inspect appearance of wound and compare with previous assessment to identify progress of healing process.
2. Ask client to rate pain using a scale of 0 to 10.
3. Observe client or care giver's ability to perform wound care.

UNEXPECTED OUTCOMES AND RELATED INTERVENTIONS

1. The edges of the wound appear inflamed. Drainage, if visible, is purulent and odorous and has a yellow, green, or brown color, depending on the causative organism.
   a. A contaminated or traumatic wound may show signs of infection early, within 2 to 3 days. A surgical wound infection usually develops on the fourth or fifth day.
   b. Check for evidence of infection: fever, tenderness, and increasing pain at the wound site, and an elevated WBC count.
   c. Wound cultures are usually indicated (see Skill 13.1). Check agency policy.
2. Wound bleeds during removal of dry dressing. This may indicate a slipped surgical suture, a dislodged clot, or erosion of a blood vessel by a drain. Risk of hemorrhage is greatest during the first 24 to 48 hours.
   a. Observe the color and amount of bleeding. Hemorrhage may be serious if the dressing is saturated with bright-red blood (sanguineous). In this case, apply direct pressure immediately and summon help. Continue pressure until bleeding subsides.
   b. Inspect areas where blood may escape along the sides of the dressing and pool beneath client.
   c. Take vital signs for evidence of hypovolemic shock, including decreased blood pressure, increased thready pulse, restlessness, and diaphoresis.

   d. Report findings to the physician. Client may need to return to surgery for hemostasis.
3. Client reports feeling as if something has "given way." There is a sudden increased amount of serosanguineous drainage on the dressing after a sudden strain, such as coughing, vomiting, or sudden movement to sit or stand.
   a. Wound dehiscence (partial or total separation of wound layers) may be associated with obese clients with constant strain on the wound. Cover the wound with a dry dressing, and tape to prevent the incision from further disruption and infection.
   b. If evisceration (total separation of wound layers with protrusion of visceral organs through the wound opening) is apparent, moist sterile dressings must be used to prevent drying of delicate tissues.
   c. Instruct client to lie still until evaluated by physician.
   d. Report to physician immediately. Client will usually require surgical repair.
4. Client is unable to demonstrate application of dressing.
   a. Additional teaching is necessary.
   b. Wounds out of client's reach and vision require family member's assistance.
   c. Personnel resources to assist in wound care include enterostomal therapist, clinical nurse specialist, infection control nurse, and home health nurse.

SAMPLE DOCUMENTATION

1300 Abdominal incision approximately 5 cm long, edges well approximated without inflammation. A 1 cm spot of serous drainage noted at lower end of 4×4. Client denied pain during dressing change.

(See Physical Care/Activity [Wound], Appendix A.)

Skill 15.2 | Changing Moist Dressings
(Wet to Dry or Wet to Damp)

Moist dressings are often used for helping to heal full-thickness wounds that look like craters. Granulation tissue and new capillary networks must form to fill in the defect (Figure 15-7).

Wet-to-dry dressings are used for wounds requiring debridement. The nurse moistens the contact dressing layer that touches the wound surface. The moistened gauze increases the absorptive ability of the dressing to collect exudate and wound debris. This layer dries and adheres to dead cells and debrides the wound when the dressing is removed. An outer absorbent layer is a dry dressing to protect the wound from invasive microorganisms (Johnson, 1992).

Wet-to-damp dressings are appropriate for wounds that are healing with granulation tissue without significant amounts of ischemic or necrotic tissue or large amounts of drainage. Because granulation tissue is fragile and bleeds easily, damp dressings are less likely to result in tissue damage as old dressings are removed. The outermost layer is dry for this type of dressing as well (Krasner, 1991).

The most frequently used solution is normal saline, which is an isotonic solution. Some other solutions may be ordered. Lactated Ringer's solution contains electrolytes that create an environment conducive to tissue growth (Doughty, 1992). Solutions are available in 250 to 1000 cc (ml) containers. At the time the container is opened, the label should be clearly marked with the date and time, and unused portions should be discarded 24 hours after opening. Extended use can harbor growth of microorganisms.

EQUIPMENT
Unsterile and sterile gloves
Sterile dressing set (scissors and forceps)
Sterile drape (optional)
Thin, fine-mesh gauze, dressings, and pads
Sterile normal saline (or prescribed solution)
Protective underpad
Waterproof bag
Moisture-proof gown, goggles, and mask (optional)

Assessment

1. Determine frequency, solution to be used, and location and size of wound to be dressed. **This allows nurse to determine supplies needed. If dressing involves wrapping a foot or leg, assistance may be required.**
2. Review nurses' notes and care plan for a baseline description of wound and drainage characteristics.
3. Assess client's level of comfort, and administer pain medication as needed. **For dressing changes known to be painful, medications may need to be given specifically timed to peak during the procedure.**
4. Assess client's knowledge of purpose of dressing change to determine level of support and explanation required.
5. Assess need for client or family member to participate in dressing wound to prepare client or family member if dressing must be changed at home.
6. Identify clients at risk for delayed wound healing (see Table 15-1).

Planning

Expected outcomes focus on promoting comfort and wound healing.

EXPECTED OUTCOMES
1. Client's wound is free of drainage and is healing, as evident by presence of granulation tissue.
2. Client describes pain less than 4 (scale of 0 to 10) during wet-dry dressing changes.
3. Client (or family) demonstrates wound care procedures to be done at home.

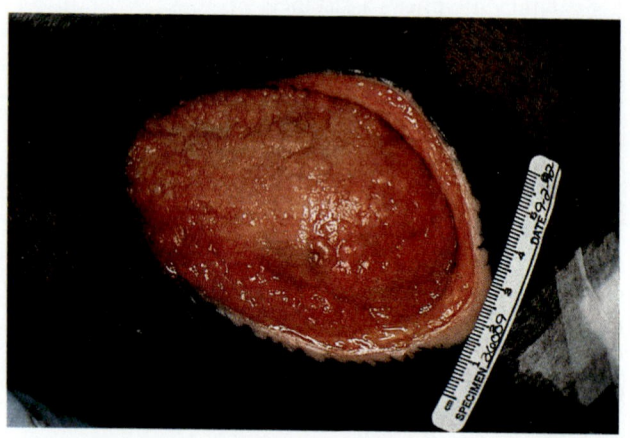

Figure 15-7

Implementation

Steps	Rationale
1. See Standard Protocol (Chapter 1, p. 5).	
2. Make cuff at top of disposable waterproof bag and place within reach of work area.	Cuff prevents contamination of top of outer bag.
3. Place waterproof pad under client where dressing is to be changed to prevent soiling of bed linens.	
4. Untie Montgomery ties (Figure 15-8). If tape is being used, see Skill 15.1, Step 4.	Montgomery ties may be used as indicated to reduce skin irritation from frequent removal of tape.
5. With gloved hand or forceps, lift dressings off, keeping soiled undersurface away from client's sight. If dressing adheres to underlying tissues, gently free dressing and inform client about possible discomfort.	Adherence of dressing should remove drainage and necrotic tissue but not damage new granulation tissue or cause bleeding.
6. Observe character of drainage on dressings, including color, location, and amount. Inspect wound for color, character of drainage, presence and type of sutures, and presence of any drains.	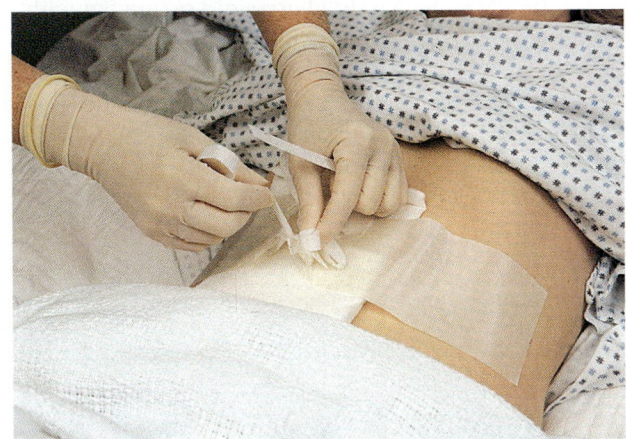
7. Fold dressings with drainage contained inside and remove gloves inside out. (With small dressings, remove gloves inside out over dressing.) Dispose of in prepared waterproof bag.	
	Figure 15-8
8. Prepare sterile dressing supplies by opening packages using sterile technique (see Chapter 14). Arrange for at least one dressing in a plastic container for sterile solution (Figure 15-9), or use a sterile basin. Arrange supplies for convenience.	Moisture is able to saturate paper and increase the risk of contamination with microorganisms from underlying surface.
9. Pour enough prescribed solution over layers of fine-mesh gauze to moisten dressings thoroughly .	
10. Using sterile gloves, cleanse wound with gauze moistened with prescribed solution, moving from least contaminated to most contaminated area.	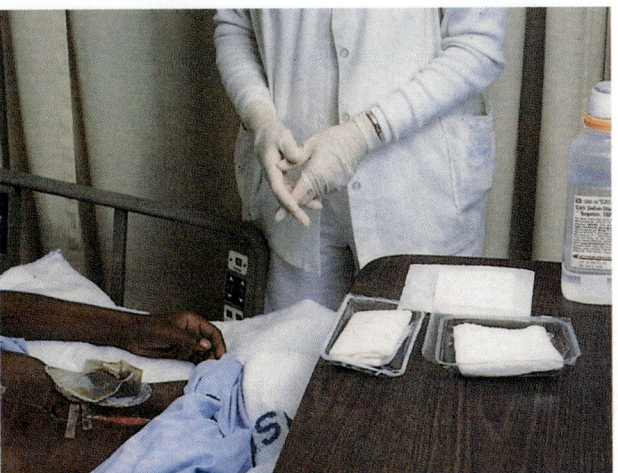
	Figure 15-9

Steps	Rationale
11. Loosely pack moist fine-mesh gauze directly into wound surface so that all surfaces are in contact with wound cavity (Figure 15-10). Moist gauze should not touch intact skin.	Moisture on intact skin may result in maceration and skin breakdown. Some deep wounds may require packing, which involves tucking gauze into the wound cavity.
12. Apply dry sterile gauze lightly over packed wound.	Packing that is too tight creates pressure that decreases circulation and healing. Dry layer pulls moisture from wound.
13. Cover wound with dry ABD pad, Surgi-pad, or gauze. Secure dressings with Montgomery ties.	Dry outer layer prevents entrance of microorganisms.
14. If Montgomery ties are wet or soiled, replace them. a. A protective skin barrier is recommended.	Skin barrier (Stomahesive) protects intact skin from stretch and tension of adhesive tape.
b. Place adhesive so that edges are 5 to 8 cm (2 to 3 inches) apart at the center (Figure 15-11).	
c. Secure dressing by lacing ties across dressing snugly enough to hold dressings secure but without pressure on the skin.	
15. On an extremity, dressing is secured with roller gauze (see Figure 15-1) or Surgiflex elastic net (Figure 15-12).	
16. See Completion Protocol (Chapter 1, p. 6).	

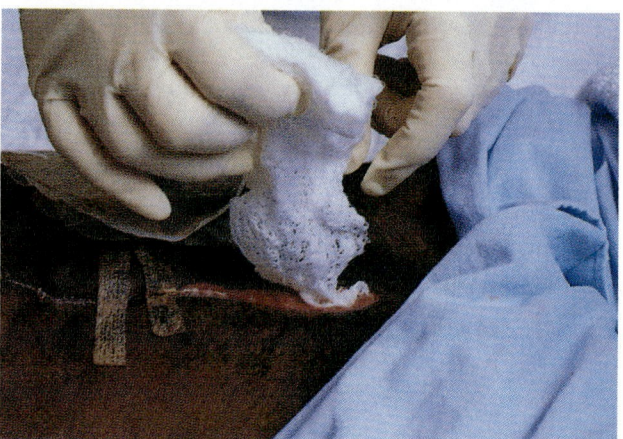

Figure 15-10

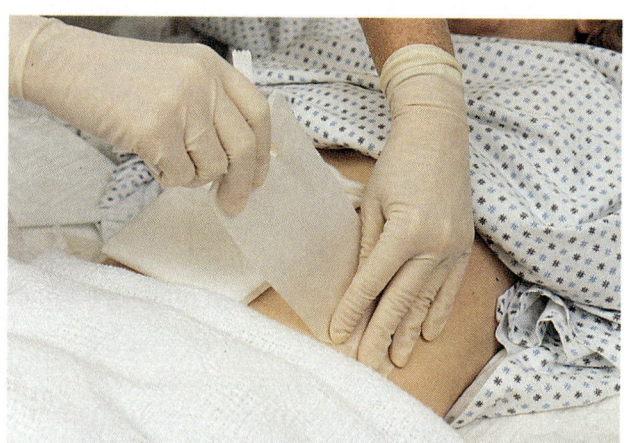

Figure 15-11

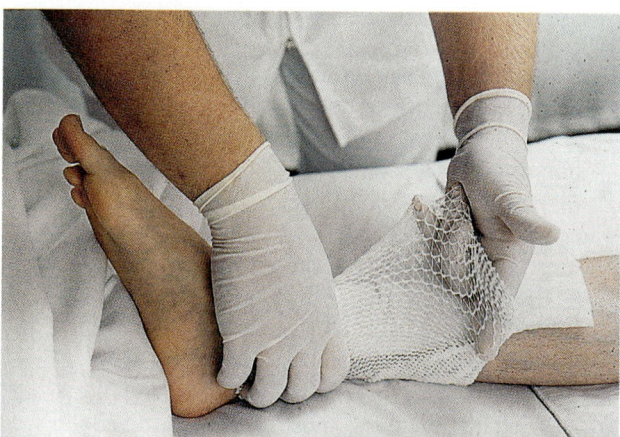

Figure 15-12

Evaluation

1. Inspect the wound for drainage and granulation tissue.
2. Ask client to describe pain (scale of 0 to 10) during wet-dry dressing changes.
3. Observe client demonstrate wound care method in home setting. (Note: In home setting, clean technique may be appropriate.)

UNEXPECTED OUTCOMES AND RELATED INTERVENTIONS

1. Wound eschar toughens.
   a. Report to physician or consult wound care specialist. Eschar may require surgical debridement before resumption of wet-to-dry dressing changes.
   b. Specialists in wound care include enterostomal therapist, clinical nurse specialist, infection control nurse, and home health nurse.
2. Wound drainage increases or becomes purulent, which may indicate infection or dehiscence.
   a. Culture wound (see Skill 13.1).

b. Inspect wound for evidence of inflammation or disruption.
c. Consult physician for appropriate medication if infection is present.
3. Skin around wound margins becomes red and excoriated, which may indicate solution in contact with skin or acidity of wound drainage.
   a. Protect skin from moisture and drainage.
   b. Consult wound care specialist for protective barriers or techniques.

SAMPLE DOCUMENTATION

1000 Wet-to-dry dressing on right ankle changed using normal saline and sterile technique. First layer of gauze had pea-sized spot of light-yellow drainage. Ulceration is 4 cm in diameter, 0.5 cm deep, with pinpoint spots of yellow drainage along the border; erythema noted on surrounding area. Used 1 moist and 1 dry 4×4 gauze and wrapped with Kling gauze. Client denied pain during procedure.

(See Physical Care/Activity [Wound], Appendix A.)

Skill 15.3 | Changing Transparent Dressings

Transparent dressings are thin, self-adhesive elastic films (e.g., Op-site or Tegaderm). This synthetic permeable membrane acts as a temporary second skin, adheres to undamaged skin to contain exudate and minimize wound contamination, and allows the wound surface to "breathe." The nurse is able to assess the wound without removing the film. This dressing conforms well to body contours with less restriction of movement. It promotes a moist environment, which speeds epithelial cell growth, and can be removed without damaging underlying tissues (Krasner, 1992). The film is ideal for small, superficial wounds and as a dressing over an intravenous (IV) catheter site. Transparent dressings may be with or without adhesives and may stay in place up to 7 days, if complete occlusion is maintained.

For best results, these dressings are used on clean, debrided wounds that are not actively bleeding. The film is applied wrinkle free but not stretched over the skin and may be used over another smaller dressing (e.g., Telfa) cut to fit area of wound. Topical medications may be applied over nonadhesive transparent dressings without disturbing the dressing. Nonadhesive transparent dressings will fall off as wound heals. If removal is needed, moisten with normal saline. If approved by physician, the client may shower or bathe with dressing in place.

EQUIPMENT

Clean disposable gloves
Sterile gloves (optional)
Sterile scissors and forceps (optional)
Sterile saline, or other wound cleanser (as ordered)
Transparent dressing (size as needed) and sterile gauze pads (2 × 2)
Waterproof bag for disposal
Moisture-proof gown, goggles, and mask (if risk of splashing is present)

Assessment

Assess location, appearance, and size of wound to be dressed to allow nurse to determine supplies and assistance needed.

Planning

Expected outcomes focus on promoting wound healing.

EXPECTED OUTCOMES

1. Client's wound demonstrates healing, as evidenced by absence of drainage.
2. Skin surrounding the wound remains clean and intact.
3. Client rates pain as less than 4 (scale of 0 to 10).

Implementation

Steps	Rationale
1. See Standard Protocol (Chapter 1, p. 5)	
2. Cuff top of disposable waterproof bag to prevent contamination of outer bag. Place within easy reach of work area.	
3. 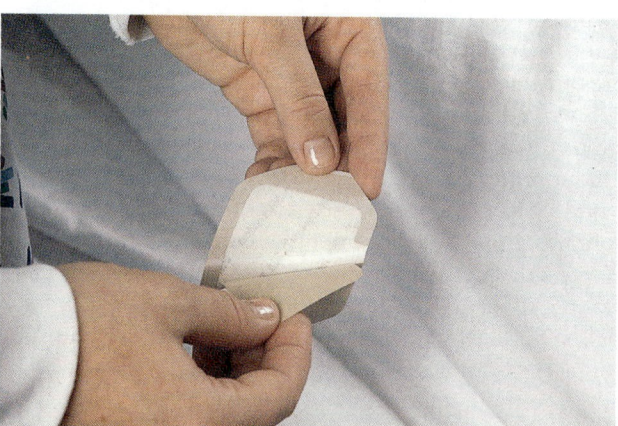 Remove old dressing by pulling back slowly across dressing in direction of hair growth and toward the center.	Reduces excoriation or irritation of skin after dressing removal.
4. Remove disposable gloves by pulling them inside out over soiled dressings and dispose of them in waterproof bag.	
5. Inspect wound for color, odor, and drainage; measure if indicated.	Appearance indicates state of wound healing.
6. Cleanse area gently, swabbing toward area of most exudate, or spray with cleanser (check agency policy and physician preference).	Reduces transmission of organisms from contaminated area to cleaner site.
7. Reapply sterile (or clean) gloves if risk of exposure to body secretions is present.	
8. Dry skin around wound thoroughly with sterile gauze.	Transparent dressing with adhesive backing will not adhere to damp surface. Nonadhesive transparent dressing will cling to moist wound surface.
9. Apply transparent dressing according to manufacturer's directions.	
a. Make sure skin surface is as dry as possible.	Adhesive will not stick to wet skin.
b. Remove paper backing, taking care not to allow adhesive areas to touch each other (Figure 15-13).	Results in wrinkles and may be impossible to use.

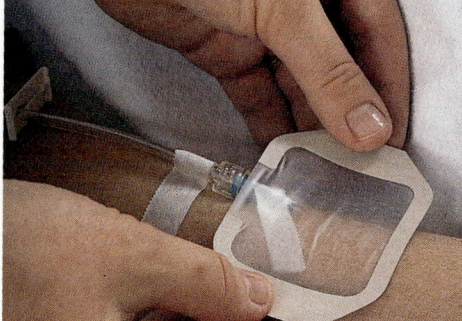

Figure 15-13 **A**, Remove paper backing to expose transparent window. **B**, Remove second side of backing to expose adhesive surface. **C**, Apply over site, and remove edging.

Steps	Rationale

c. Place film smoothly over wound without stretching.

d. Label with date, initials, and time if required by agency policy (Figure 15-14).

10. Remove gloves and discard in waterproof bag.

11. See Completion Protocol (Chapter 1, p. 6).

Wrinkles can provide tunnel for drainage.

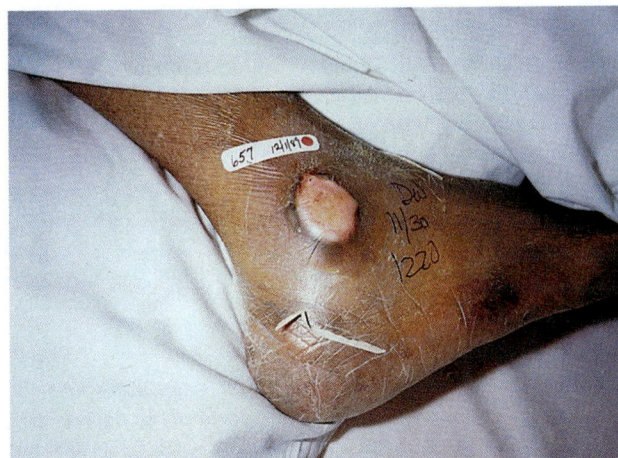

Figure 15-14

Evaluation

1. Inspect condition of wound for drainage and evidence of wound healing.

2. Ask client to rate level of discomfort using a scale of 0 to 10.

UNEXPECTED OUTCOMES AND RELATED INTERVENTIONS

1. Wound becomes infected, as evidenced by fluid accumulation with a white, opaque appearance and erythema of the surrounding tissue.
   a. Remove dressing and obtain a wound culture (see Chapter 13).
   b. Dressing changes may need to be done more frequently.
   c. A different type of dressing may be required.

2. Dressing does not stay in place.
   a. Evaluate size of dressing used for adequate (1 to 1½ inches) margin.
   b. Dry skin more thoroughly before reapplication.

3. Client does not want to see the wound.
   Cover transparent dressing with dry gauze dressing, taking care not to place tape directly on transparent dressing.

4. Wound exudate builds up to cause bulge in dressing.
   a. Change dressing.
   b. Aspirate fluid using small-gauge sterile needle and patch hole with small piece of film.

5. Outer layer of skin tears on removal of dressing.
   a. Adhesive backing may be too strong for the skin of the older adult.
   b. Use nonadhesive-backed transparent dressings.

SAMPLE DOCUMENTATION

1000 Transparent dressing changed. Wound on left thigh is 6×10 cm, with oozing serosanguineous drainage. Area very tender to touch. Client describes pain as 2 (scale 0-10). Refusing medication at this time.

(See Physical Care/Activity [Wound], Appendix A.)

CRITICAL THINKING EXERCISES

1. You are caring for a client who has been taking antibiotics for an infected leg ulcer. It is draining purulent, yellow material. A recent wound culture was negative. Another client has an infected abdominal wound that appears red and swollen. His WBC count is elevated, and he is running a fever. Wound cultures are positive for infective bacteria. Explain how these two individuals can both have infected wounds, although only one has a positive wound culture.

2. Compare and contrast techniques for securing a dressing for the following four clients.
   a. A client with an open wound located on the anterior aspect of the leg
   b. A client with a wound on the palm of the hand
   c. A client with an abdominal wound requiring dressing changes every 2 to 3 hrs
   d. A client with a scalp wound

3. Compare and contrast nursing care measures in response to a client who has experienced a wound dehiscence versus one whose wound has eviscerated. What aspects of care would be similar and different?

4. You are caring for a client with a sacral wound. This is your first observation of the wound, and you note slight redness around the edges; light serous drainage on the old dressing; and depth of 1 cm, size 2 × 3 cm. Discuss how you would determine the status of the wound. Is the wound demonstrating progressive healing?

5. A nurse changes a wet-to-dry dressing on a deep, necrotic foot ulcer. During removal of the packing the client complains of pain. The nurse moistens the packing with normal saline and then finishes removing the packing.
   a. Did the nurse make an appropriate decision? Why or why not?
   b. Under what circumstances would a wet-to-damp dressing be appropriate?

6. Evaluate the following three clients. Each requires a dressing change and currently has a transparent dressing over the wound. Determine how you might need to revise the dressing technique for each client.
   a. A client who does not want to see the wound
   b. An elderly client whose skin tears easily during dressing removal
   c. A client with an infected, draining wound

REFERENCES

Boston L, Rijswijk L: Wound dressings: meeting clinical and biological needs, *Derm Nurs* 3(3):146, 1991.

Doughty DB: Principles of wound healing and wound management. In Bryant R, editor: *Acute and chronic wounds*, St Louis, 1992, Mosby.

Johnson A: A short history of wound dressings, *Ostomy/Wound Manage* 38(2):36, 1992.

Krasner D: Wound care update 91: new packing trends, *Nursing '91* 21(4):50, 1991.

Krasner D: Resolving the dressing dilemma: selecting wound dressings by category, *Plast Surg Nurs* 12(1):22, 1992.

Krasner D, Kennedy KL: Using the no touch technique to change a dressing, *Nursing* 24(9):50, 1994.

ADDITIONAL READINGS

Braden BJ, Bryant R: Innovations to prevent and treat pressure ulcers, *Geriatr Nurs* 11(4):182, 1990.

Cuzzell JZ, Stotts NA: Trial and error yields to knowledge, *Am J Nurs* 90(10):50, 1990.

Faller NA, Lawrence KG: Nursing to promote healing, *Ostomy/Wound Manage* 32:43, 1991.

Hebda PA, Lee CI: Occlusive dressings for surgical and other acute wounds, *Wounds* 4(3):84, 1992.

Motta, GJ: How moisture-retentive dressings promote healing, *Nursing '93* 23(12):26, 1993.

Palamand S, Brenden RA, Reed AM: Intelligent wound dressings and their physical characteristics, *Wounds* 3(4):149, 1991.

Rodeheaver GT: Controversies in topical wound management: wound cleansing and wound disinfection. In Krasner D, editor: *Chronic wound care*, King of Prussia, Pa, 1990, Health Management Publications.

Sussman C: Physical therapy modalities and the wound recovery cycle, *Ostomy/Wound Manage* 28(2):43, 1992.

VanDover D: Topical wound management, *Ostomy/Wound Manage* 32:40, 1991.

Willey T: A decision tree to choose wound dressings, *Am J Nurs* 92(2):43, 1992.

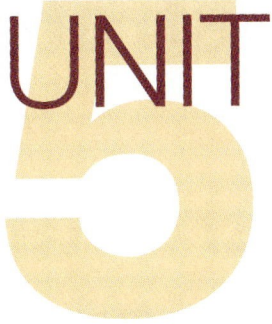

UNIT 5

Administration of Medications

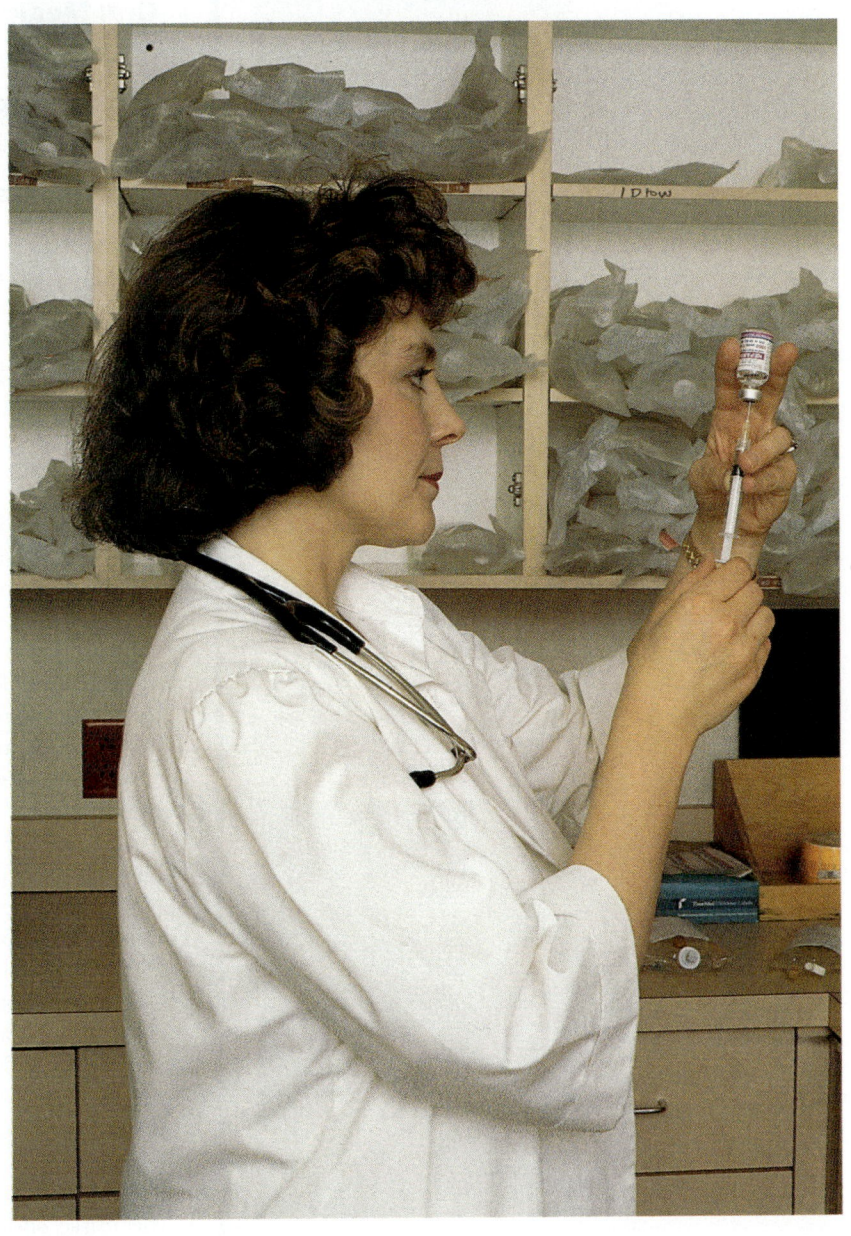

Administration of Non-Parenteral Medications

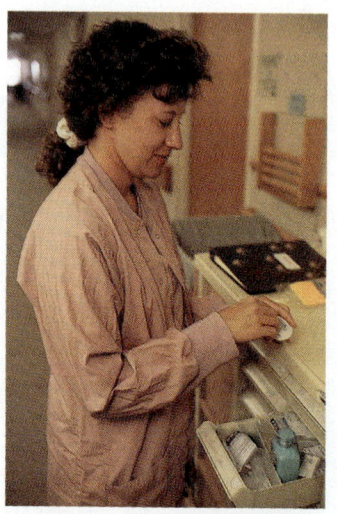

Skill 16.1
Oral Medications

Skill 16.2
Topical Applications

Skill 16.3
Eye/Ear Medications

Skill 16.4
Inhalants

Skill 16.5
Suppositories

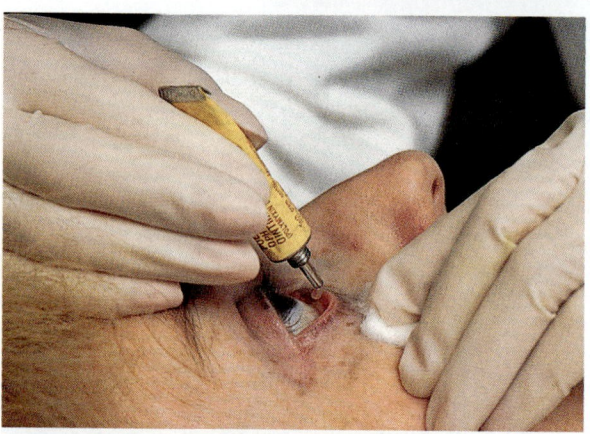

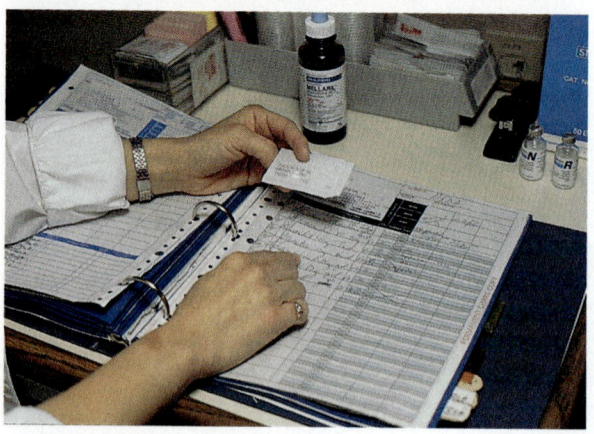

Administration of medications is an interdependent nursing intervention because the nurse shares with the physician and pharmacist the responsibility for ensuring that the right medications are given to the client. Preparing and administering medications require accuracy. The nurse must pay full attention to the procedure. Traditionally, nurses have followed the "five rights" for administration of medications (see box on p. 285).

A physician's order is required for all medications to be administered by the nurse (except in states where Nurse Practice Acts allow advanced practice nurses and nurse practitioners to prescribe in specific situations).

The nurse or a designated unit secretary writes the physician's complete order on the appropriate medication administration record (MAR) (Figure 16-1). The transcribed order includes the client's full name, room, and bed number; date the order is written; drug name and dosage; and time and route of administration. Each time a drug dose is prepared for administration to the client, the nurse refers to the MAR. When transcribing orders, the nurse should be sure names, dosages, and symbols are legible. A registered nurse (RN) is responsible for

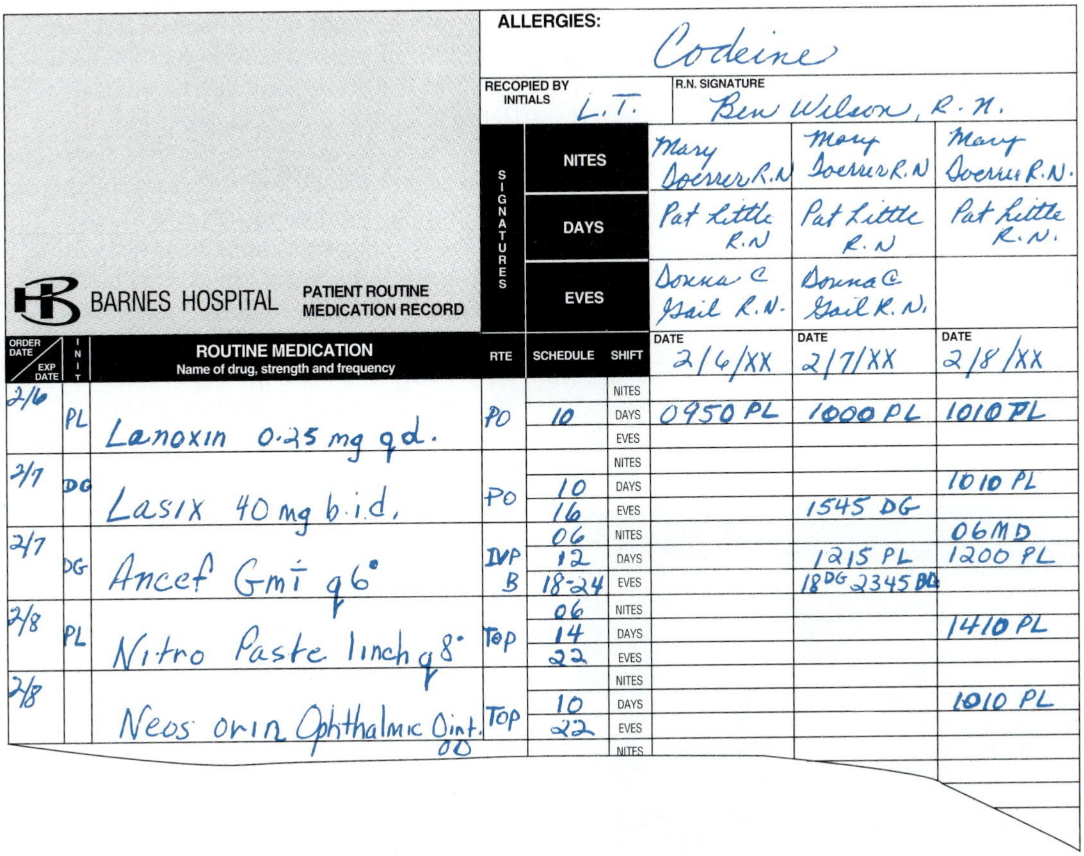

ALLERGIES: *Codeine*			
RECOPIED BY INITIALS *L.T.*	**R.N. SIGNATURE** *Ben Wilson, R.N.*		

S I G N A T U R E S	**NITES**	*Mary Doerrer R.N*	*Mary Doerrer R.N*	*Mary Doerrer R.N.*
	DAYS	*Pat Little R.N*	*Pat Little R.N*	*Pat Little R.N.*
	EVES	*Donna C Gail R.N.*	*Donna C Gail R.N.*	

HB BARNES HOSPITAL PATIENT ROUTINE MEDICATION RECORD

ORDER DATE / EXP DATE	I N I T	ROUTINE MEDICATION Name of drug, strength and frequency	RTE	SCHEDULE	SHIFT	DATE 2/6/XX	DATE 2/7/XX	DATE 2/8/XX
2/6	PL	*Lanoxin 0.25 mg qd.*	PO	10	NITES			
					DAYS	0950 PL	1000 PL	1010 PL
					EVES			
2/7	DG	*Lasix 40 mg b.i.d.*	PO	10 16	NITES			
					DAYS			1010 PL
					EVES		1545 DG	
2/7	DG	*Ancef Gm ī q6°*	IVP B	06 12 18-24	NITES			06 MD
					DAYS		1215 PL	1200 PL
					EVES		18 DG 2345 BD	
2/8	PL	*Nitro Paste 1inch q8°*	Top	06 14 22	NITES			
					DAYS			1410 PL
					EVES			
2/8		*Neos orin Ophthalmic Oint.*	Top	10 22	NITES			1010 PL
						NITES			

Figure 16-1 Medication Administration Record. (Courtesy Barnes Hospital, St. Louis, Mo.)

Five "Rights" for Administration of Medication

- **Right drug**
- **Right dose**
- **Right client**
- **Right route**
- **Right time**

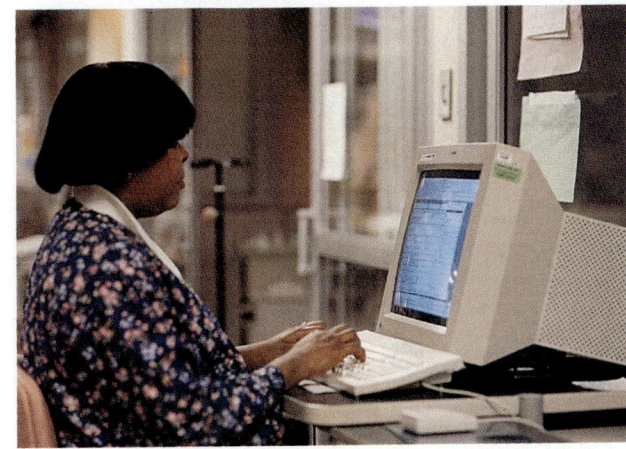

Figure 16-2 Entering medication orders using a computer.

checking and initialing all transcribed orders. Errors in medication administration must be reported to the physician and an incident report filed (see Medication/IV Incident Report, Appendix A).

In some institutions a computer printout lists all currently ordered medications with dosage information. Orders are entered directly into the computer, preventing the need for transcription of orders (Figure 16-2). An RN checks all transcribed orders against the original order for accuracy and thoroughness. If an order seems incorrect or inappropriate, the nurse may consult the physician or pharmacist for clarification. The computer may also be used to record medications given.

CALCULATION OF DOSAGES

The proper administration of medication often depends on the nurse's ability to calculate drug dosages accurately and measure medications correctly. A careless mistake in placing a decimal point or adding a zero to a dosage can lead to a serious or fatal error. With the de-

Approximate Equivalents

$$1 \text{ gr}^* = 60 \text{ mg}$$
$$1 \text{ g} = 1000 \text{ mg}$$
$$1000 \text{ mcg } (\mu g) = 1 \text{ mg}$$
$$1 \text{ kg} = 2.2 \text{ lb}$$
$$1 \text{ mL or ml (1 cc)} = 15\text{-}16 \text{ minims}^*$$
$$5 \text{ mL} = 1 \text{ tsp}\dagger$$
$$3 \text{ tsp} = 1 \text{ tbs}\dagger$$
$$30 \text{ mL} = 1 \text{ oz}\dagger$$
$$1000 \text{ mL} = 1 \text{ L}$$

*Apothecary measure.
†Household measure.

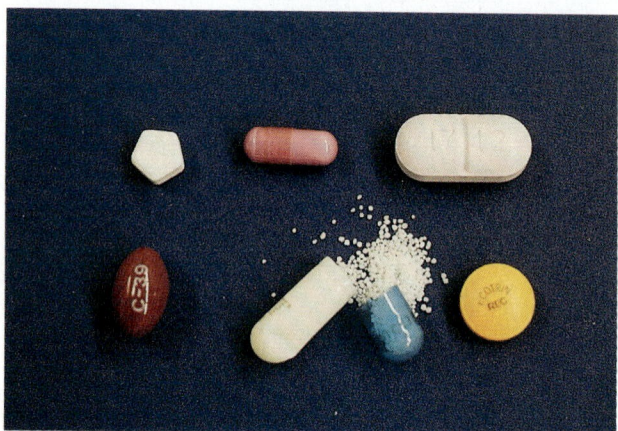

Figure 16-3 Forms of oral medications: *(top row)* unique shape, capsule, scored tablet; *(bottom row)* gelatin-coated liquid, extended-release capsule, enteric-coated tablet.

Dimensional Analysis

Step 1. Identify the starting factor (amount ordered), which is the first item of the equation, and the answer label (tablets, capsules, or ml), which is the last item.

Step 2. Identify appropriate equivalents with a 1:1 ratio (e.g., 1 g = 1000 mg). Set up the equation so that labels can be canceled; e.g., if mg is in the numerator, mg must be in the denominator to cancel.

Step 3. Solve the equation.
  a. Cancel labels first; the answer label should not cancel.
  b. Reduce numbers to lowest terms.
  c. Multiply/divide to solve equation.
  d. Reduce answer to lowest terms, convert to decimal, and round to a measurable quantity.

$$\text{Starting factor} \times \frac{\text{Equivalent}}{\text{Equivalent}} = \text{Answer label}$$

velopment of unit dose, nurses rarely need to convert available units of medication to desired dosages, that is, from metric to apothecary systems (see box below, left).

The metric system is a decimal system organized in units of 10, easily converted by moving the decimal point to the right to multiply and to the left to divide. In the metric system, medications are ordered using grams (g or Gm), milligrams (mg), or micrograms (mcg or μg). The apothecary system is rarely used; apothecary measures include grains (gr), drams, and minims. Household measures, such as teaspoons, may be used for medication administration at home (see box at left) (Gray, 1994).

Medications come in a variety of forms (Figure 16-3). It is important to be able to read labels to determine the name, dose, and expiration date. Tablets are powdered dosage forms compressed into disks of various sizes and colors. They may be enteric coated with materials that do not dissolve until they reach the small intestine. This protects the stomach from irritation, and therefore the tablet should not be crushed. Capsules are powders or liquids encased in a shell that dissolves in the stomach. Many tablets and capsules are marked or coded to aid in product identification. Most oral medications are packaged so that one or two tablets or capsules constitute an average adult dose. When the dose ordered is different from the dose available, calculations are required to confirm the correct amount to give.

Dimensional analysis is becoming a popular method for dosage calculations because it involves simple multiplication and division and does not require algebra. This method involves three steps (see box below, left).

Example 1

Dose ordered: 0.5 g
Tablets available: 0.25 g per tablet

Step 1. The starting factor is 0.5 g.
The answer label is tablets; that is, How many tablets should be given?

Step 2. Formulate the conversion equation:
The equivalent needed is 1 tablet = 0.25 g.

$$0.5 \text{ g} \times \frac{1 \text{ tab}}{0.25 \text{ g}} = \underline{?} \text{ tabs}$$

Cancel labels (g).
NOTE: if properly written, all labels except the answer label will cancel.

Step 3. Solving the equation:
Reduce the numerical values and multiply the numerators and the denominators ($0.5 \div 0.25 = 2$) ($2 \times 1 = 2$).

$$\overset{2}{\cancel{0.5 \text{ g}}} \times \frac{1 \text{ tab}}{\cancel{0.25 \text{ g}}} = 2 \text{ tabs}$$

In some situations, an additional step is needed to convert from one equivalent to another.

Example 2

Dose ordered: 0.5 g
Tablets available: 250 mg per tablet

Step 1. The starting factor is 0.5 g.
The answer label is tablets; that is, How many tablets should be given?

Step 2. Formulate the conversion equation:
The equivalents needed are 1 g = 1000 mg and 1 tab = 250 mg.

$$0.5 \text{ g} \times \frac{1000 \text{ mg}}{1 \text{ g}} \times \frac{1 \text{ tab}}{250 \text{ mg}} = \underline{?} \text{ tabs}$$

Cancel labels (g, mg).

Step 3. Solve the equation:
Reduce the values and multiply the numerators and the denominators (1.0 ÷ 0.5 = 2) (1000 ÷ 250 = 4) (4 ÷ 2 = 2) (2 × 1 = 2).

$$0.5 \text{ g} \times \frac{\overset{4}{\cancel{1000} \text{ mg}}}{\underset{2}{\cancel{1 \text{ g}}}} \times \frac{1 \text{ tab}}{\cancel{250} \text{ mg}} = 2 \text{ tabs}$$

Many medications come in a variety of dosages to facilitate accuracy. The multiple dosages make careful checking of dosages essential. For example, coumadin comes in several dosages (Figure 16-4). Therefore, if a dose of 4.5 mg is ordered, it would require a 2 mg tablet and a 2.5 mg tablet.

Some medications are also available in both tablets or capsules and in liquid form. Liquid forms are appropriate when the client has difficulty swallowing or must be given medications via a nasogastric (NG) tube or gastric (G) tube (see Skill 32.2). Liquid medications include elixirs, suspensions, syrups, and tinctures. Liquids increase the rate of absorption.

Example 3

Dose ordered: Keflex 250 mg PO
Available: 125 mg per 5 ml

Step 1. The starting factor is 250 mg.
The answer label is ml.

Step 2. Formulate the conversion equation:

$$250 \text{ mg} \times \frac{5 \text{ ml}}{125 \text{ mg}} = \underline{\quad} \text{ ml}$$

Cancel labels (mg).

Step 3. Solve the equation:
Reduce and multiply
(250 ÷ 125 = 2) (2 × 5 = 10).

$$\overset{2}{\cancel{250} \text{ mg}} \times \frac{5 \text{ ml}}{\cancel{125} \text{ mg}} = 10 \text{ ml}$$

It is legally advisable only to administer medications personally prepared. Administering a drug prepared by another nurse greatly increases the opportunity for error. The nurse who gives the wrong medication or an incorrect dose is legally responsible for the error. Physicians may order a drug using the trade name, and the pharmacist may dispense it using the generic name. Many drugs have both names on the label. The importance of checking similar names and verifying for the correct drug cannot be overemphasized.

DRUG ACTIONS AND SIDE EFFECTS

Safe and accurate administration of medications requires knowledge of drug actions and side effects in order to exercise good judgment. The nurse must know how to administer medications correctly, evaluate the client's response, and teach the client appropriate information for self-administration. (See standard pharmacology reference books for information about pharmacokinetics, mechanisms of action, effects, tolerance, and interactions.)

Knowledge of the drug action helps to anticipate a drug's effect. This includes onset of drug action, peak (its highest effective concentration), and duration of action (length of time the drug is present in a concentration

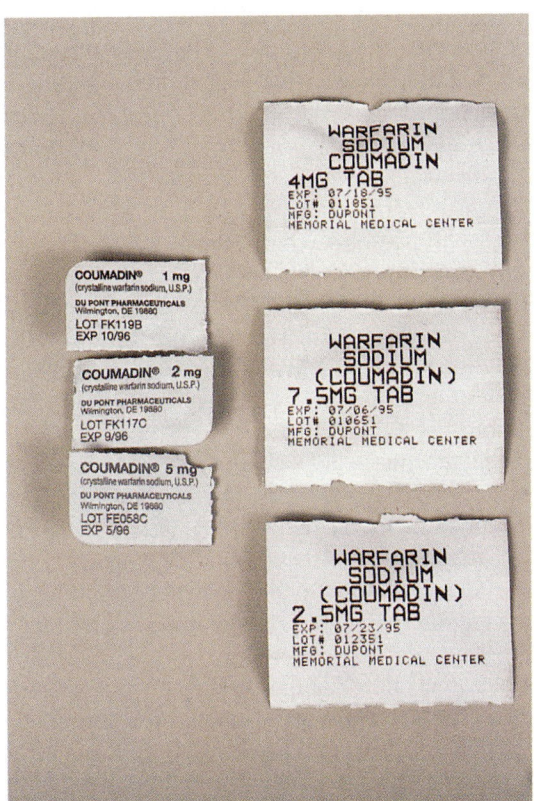

Figure 16-4 Coumadin in 6 strengths.

great enough to produce a response). This information is useful in planning drug administration schedules. Most agencies have standard administration schedules (See Abbreviations and Equivalents, Appendix B) and allow for administration of the drug one-half hour before or after the scheduled time without concern for altering the effectiveness of the medication. Some medications are ordered to be given PRN (as needed) within certain parameters prescribed by the physician.

The therapeutic levels of certain drugs, such as antibiotics, can be monitored by laboratory testing. A blood sample is drawn to identify the peak serum level of a drug, which varies according to the specific drug involved. Blood samples for trough levels, or the lowest serum levels, are usually drawn just before the next scheduled dose of medication. Precise coordination with the laboratory is essential for obtaining meaningful information. These data allow physicians to modify drug dosages.

Desired effects are the expected or therapeutic effects of a drug. Because of a variety of factors, such as age, body weight, metabolism, and hormonal responses to stress, clients may respond differently to the same drugs.

Side effects are unintended and unpleasant drug effects. For example, codeine may result in constipation. Nursing interventions can minimize side effects.

Adverse reactions are potentially harmful or life-threatening effects, such as an allergic response. With repeated administration, clients may develop an allergic response to any drug. Antibiotics cause a high incidence of allergic reactions. Allergic symptoms vary. Common mild allergy symptoms include hives, rashes, and pruritus. Severe or *anaphylactic reactions* are characterized by sudden, severe wheezing and shortness of breath with edema of the pharynx and larynx, which may necessitate emergency resuscitation measures.

An allergic response is always a reason for the client to stop taking the drug and avoid drugs of similar chemical composition (McGovern, 1992). A client with a known history of an allergy to a medication should wear an identification bracelet or medal that identifies specific allergies. This alerts nurses and physicians to allergies if the client is unconscious when receiving medical care. As a precaution, each time the nurse administers medications, allergies should be assessed. It is helpful to determine what type of allergic reaction the client has experienced. Nausea and vomiting usually are not considered an allergic reaction.

Toxic effects, from an accumulation of a drug, may occur in the blood because of impaired metabolism or excretion or after prolonged intake or high doses of medication. Excess amounts of a drug within the body may be life-threatening depending on the drug's action. For example, diazepam (Valium), an antianxiety medication, may cause severe respiratory depression and death at toxic levels.

Table 16-1 Influence of Drug Effects in Older Adults

Drug Effect	Related Interventions
Difficulty swallowing large tablets or capsules; tissue damage related to uncoated medications such as aspirin and potassium chloride	Position client sitting upright. Give full glass of liquid (if unrestricted). Crush tablets and mix with food, or give liquid form if available.
Slowing of drug excretion; overuse and abuse of laxatives by client	Instruct client to increase fluid intake, eat high-fiber foods, and avoid daily use of laxatives.
Longer biotransformation of drugs by the liver with greater risk for drug sensitivity and toxicity	Monitor for signs of liver dysfunction (laboratory tests, jaundice, dark urine). Monitor for contraindications in clients with known liver disease.
Risk of drug accumulation and toxicity related to altered kidney function or renal blood flow	Monitor for renal impairment (decreased urine output) and contraindications/dosage in clients with known renal disease.

Because of changes in the older adult's metabolism and excretion of drugs, the nurse should carefully assess client responses to drug therapy. Consultation with the physician may be appropriate to ensure safe administration (Table 16-1).

CLIENT AND FAMILY TEACHING

The assessment of the client's need for and responses to drug therapy includes a history of drug allergies, medication history (including over-the-counter [OTC] drugs), diet history, client's attitude toward and understanding of drug therapy, and a review of client's current condition.

A well-informed client is more likely to take medications correctly. The nurse can provide information about the purpose of medications, their actions, side effects, dosage schedules, and actions to take in case side or toxic effects develop. Special instructional booklets or leaflets are often available as teaching aids (see box on p. 289).

Clients may alter dosage or the schedule of medications for many reasons. Many clients stop taking medications when symptoms have subsided; regimens involving multiple drugs are confusing; the consequences of not taking medications may be misunderstood; many prescriptions are costly; and some clients fear addiction. A

Basic Guidelines for Drug Safety

1. Keep each drug in its original, labeled container.
2. Labels need to be legible.
3. Discard any outdated medications.
4. Finish a prescribed drug unless otherwise instructed.
5. Do not save a drug for future illnesses.
6. Dispose of drugs by taking them to the pharmacy.
7. Do not place drugs in the trash or within reach of children.
8. Do not give a family member a drug prescribed for another.
9. Refrigerate medications if label indicates this is required.
10. Read labels carefully and follow all instructions.

large percentage of clients who may not comply are older adults, who may have sensory and mobility problems that interfere with the ability to prepare and take medications correctly. Interventions to promote accuracy in self-administration of medication include boxes that have a place for pills for each day of the week and charts to mark off when the medication is taken.

It is important to respect a client's right to refuse a prescribed medication. Often an assessment of the reason for the refusal can result in action that facilitates acceptance of the medication or correction of a potential problem.

The route chosen for administering a drug depends on its properties and desired effect and on the client's physical and mental condition. The nurse is often the best person to judge the route most suitable for a client. Oral administration includes swallowing pills, capsules, or liquids. Sublingual administration involves placing a tablet under the tongue to be dissolved. Buccal administration involves placing the solid medication in the mouth and against the mucous membranes of the cheek until it dissolves. Some drugs are available in a variety of forms, which determine the route of administration. For example, nitroglycerin preparations may be given orally in sustained-release forms, in sublingual tablets, by a transdermal patch, and by injection (Table 16-2).

Nursing Diagnosis

Nursing diagnoses may be identified based on therapeutic effects or side effects of specific prescribed medications.

Ineffective Management of Therapeutic Regimen may be related to a knowledge deficit of the purpose of prescribed medications, the complexity of a drug schedule, or unpleasant side effects. **Health-Seeking Behaviors** is a useful nursing diagnosis when clients have a knowledge deficit and want to learn how to provide self- medication. **Noncompliance** involves a person's informed decision not to adhere to a therapeutic regime of medication administration, which may be related to cultural or spiritual beliefs. Certain medications, such as chemotherapeutic agents, steroids, and anticoagulants, may contribute to **Altered Protection,** in which the client's ability to respond normally to infection or bleeding is decreased. **Sensory/Perceptual Alteration** may be appropriate in relation to eye or ear medications.

Table 16-2 Non-Parenteral Routes of Administration

Route	Advantages/Disadvantages	Comments
Oral (swallowed)	Easy, comfortable, economical; may produce local or systemic effects	Some drugs are destroyed by gastric secretions. Cannot be given if client is NPO, unable to swallow, has gastric suction, or is unconscious or confused and unwilling to cooperate. May irritate lining of gastrointestinal tract, discolor teeth, or have unpleasant taste.
Skin: topical transdermal patches	Provides primarily local effect; painless; limited side effects	Extensive applications may be bulky or cause difficulty in maneuvering. May leave oily or pasty substance on skin; may soil clothing.
Mucous membranes: eyes, ears, nose; vaginal, rectal, buccal, sublingual	Prolonged systemic effects, limited side effects; local application to involved site; readily absorbed, provides rapid relief for respiratory problems	Clients with abrasions may absorb drug too rapidly resulting in excessive systemic effects. Insertion of product may cause embarrassment. Rectal suppositories are contraindicated with rectal surgery or active rectal bleeding.
Inhalation	More invasive, less comfortable; risk of tissue or nerve damage	

Skill 16.1 | Oral Medications

The ability of an oral medication to be absorbed after it is ingested depends largely on its form or preparation. Solutions and suspensions already in a liquid state (Figure 16-5) are absorbed more readily than tablets or capsules. Acidic drugs are absorbed quickly in the stomach. Some drugs are not absorbed until reaching the small intestine. Oral medications are absorbed more easily when administered between meals; when the stomach is filled with food, the contents slow the absorption process. Enteric coatings on some tablets resist dissolution in gastric juices and prevent digestion in the upper gastrointestinal (GI) tract. The coating protects the stomach lining from irritation. Enteric-coated medication should not be crushed or dissolved before administration. When effective absorption in the stomach is required for certain drugs, they should be given at least 1 hour before or 2 hours after meals or antacids.

EQUIPMENT

Medication administration record (MAR) or computer printout
Medication cart (Figure 16-6)
Disposable medication cups
Glass of water, juice, or preferred liquid and drinking straw
Device for crushing or splitting tablets (optional)

Assessment

1. Identify the drug(s) ordered: action, purpose, normal dosage and route, common side effects, time of onset and peak action, and nursing implications. **This allows nurse to anticipate effects of drug and to observe client's response.**
2. Consider the appropriateness of therapy as client's condition changes (e.g., ability to swallow, presence of nausea, vomiting, or diarrhea; reduced peristalsis; gastric suction or feeding tube). **Alterations in GI function alter drug distribution, absorption, and excretion.**
3. Check allergies and replace any missing or faded identification bracelets. **Identification bracelets provide positive client identification.**
4. Assess client's knowledge regarding medications to determine need for drug education and to assist in identifying client's compliance with drug therapy at home.
5. Assess client's preferences for fluids. Maintain fluid restrictions as prescribed. **Fluid intake with medications promotes swallowing and facilitates absorption of medication in the GI tract. Ideally, medications should be taken with 250 ml of fluid.**

Planning

Expected outcomes focus on safe, accurate, and effective drug therapy.

EXPECTED OUTCOMES

1. Client takes medications as prescribed with evidence of improvement in condition (e.g., relief of pain, regular heart rate, stable blood pressure).
2. Client explains purpose of medication and drug dose schedule.

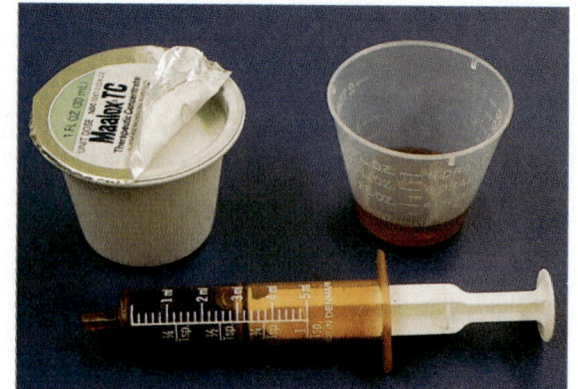

Figure 16-5 **A,** Liquid medication in single-dose package; **B,** liquid measured in medicine cup; **C,** oral liquid medicine in syringe.

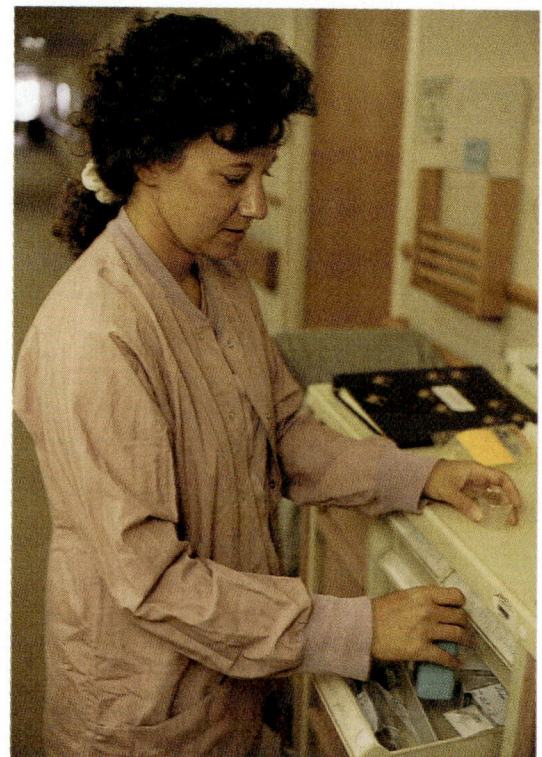

Figure 16-6

Implementation

Steps	Rationale

> **nurse alert** Review five "rights" for administering medications.

1. See Standard Protocol (Chapter 1, p. 5).

Preparing medications

2. Compare medication administration record with scheduled medication list. If discrepancies exist, check against original physician orders.

Physician's order is most reliable source and only legal record of drugs client is to receive. Orders should be checked at least every 24 hours and when client questions a drug order.

3. Unlock medicine drawer or cart (Figure 16-7).

Medications are safeguarded when locked in cabinet or cart.

4. Select correct drug from supply or unit dose drawer and compare label of medication with MAR or computer printout (Figure 16-8).

This comparison of drug name and dose is **the first check for accuracy.**

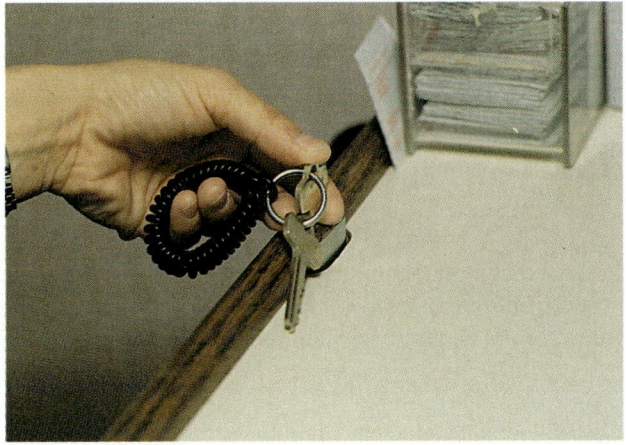

Figure 16-7

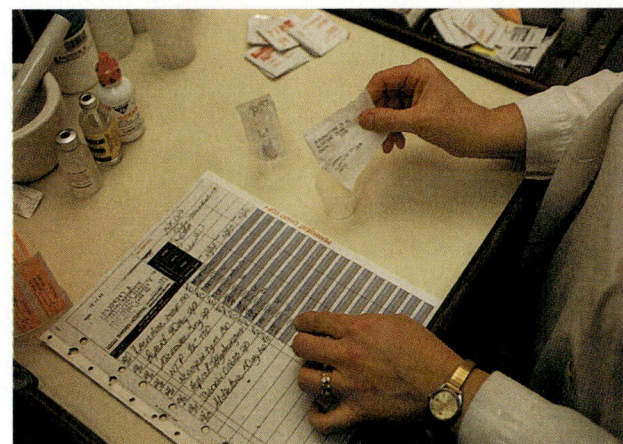

Figure 16-8

5. Check drug dose. If label dose differs from ordered dose, calculate correct amount to give.

Double checking pharmacy calculations reduces risk of error. Some agencies require nurses to check calculations of certain medications with another nurse.

6. To prepare unit dose tablets or capsules, place packaged tablet or capsule directly into medicine cup without removing wrapper. Give medications only from containers with labels that are clearly marked and legible.

Wrapper identifies drug name and dosage, which can facilitate teaching.

7. Check the expiration date of each drug. Return all outdated drugs to pharmacy.

Outdated drugs cannot be safely administered.

8. Place all tablets or capsules requiring preadministration assessments (e.g., pulse rate, blood pressure) in a separate cup.

Serves as a reminder to complete appropriate assessment and facilitates withholding drugs if necessary.

9. Place all other tablets or capsules given to client at same time in one cup.

Steps	Rationale

10. Scored tablets can be broken with gloved hands or cut with a file or cutting device (Figure 16-9). Discard unused portions of divided tablets or capsules.

Prevents accidental mislabeling by placement in the incorrect container.

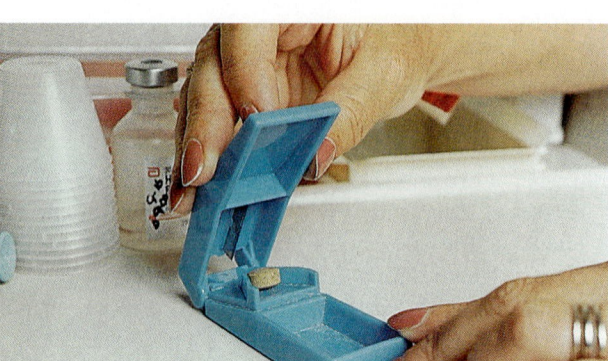

Figure 16-9

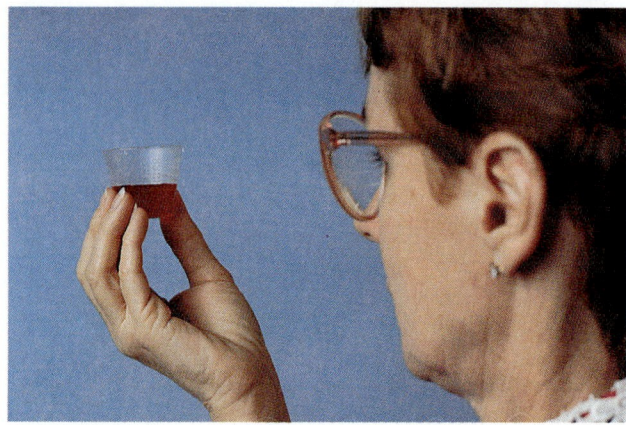

Figure 16-10

11. When preparing liquids, thoroughly mix before administering. Check and discard medications that are cloudy or have changed color.

Liquid medications packaged in single-dose cups need not be poured into medicine cups.

  a. Remove bottle cap from container and place cap upside down.

  b. Hold bottle with label against palm of hand while pouring.

Spilled liquid will not soil or obscure label.

  c. Place medication cup at eye level and fill to desired level (Figure 16-10).

Ensures accurate measurement.

  d. Wipe lip of bottle with paper towel.

Prevents contamination of bottle's contents and prevents bottle cap from sticking.

  e. If giving less than 5 ml of liquids, prepare medication in a sterile syringe without a needle (see Figure 16-5).

Allows more accurate measurement of small amounts.

12. Narcotic preparation. Check narcotic record for previous drug count and compare with supply available. Narcotics may be stored in a computerized locked cart (Figure 16-11).

Controlled substance laws require careful monitoring of dispensed narcotics. In most agencies, co-signature by an RN is required when students administer narcotics.

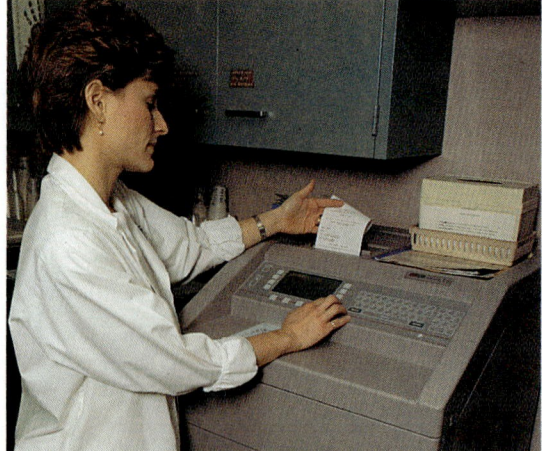

Figure 16-11 Computerized locked cart for narcotics.

Steps	Rationale
13. Compare MAR or computer printout with prepared drug and container, and check expiration date on package.	**Checking label second time reduces error.**
14. Do not leave drugs unattended.	Nurse is responsible for safekeeping of drugs.
Administering medications	
15. Take medications to client at correct time within 30 minutes before or after scheduled time. Stat or single-order medications should be given at time ordered.	Promotes intended therapeutic effect.
16. Identify client.	
a. Compare name on MAR or computer printout with name on client's identification bracelet.	Identification bracelets are made at time of client's admission and are most reliable source of identification.
b. Ask client to state name. (Do not ask, for example, "Are you Mr. Smith?")	Clients easily respond to the incorrect name.
17. Perform necessary preadministration assessment for specific medications (e.g., blood pressure or pulse).	Assessment data determine whether specific medications should be withheld at that time.
18. Discuss the purpose of each medication and its action with client. Allow client to ask any questions about drugs.	Client has right to be informed, and client's understanding of purpose of each medication improves compliance with drug therapy.
19. Assist client to sitting or side-lying position.	Sitting position prevents aspiration during swallowing.
20. Client may want to hold pills or capsule in hand or cup before placing in mouth.	Client can become familiar with medications by seeing each drug. Promotes client's independence.
21. Encourage intake of 250 ml of water or juice.	Choice of fluid promotes client's comfort and can improve fluid intake. Helps client swallow medications and promotes absorption.
22. Administer special forms of medications.	
a. **Sublingual drugs.** Have client place medication under tongue and allow it to dissolve completely. Caution client against swallowing tablet.	Absorbed through blood vessels of undersurface of tongue. If swallowed, drug is destroyed by gastric juices or rapidly detoxified by liver so that therapeutic blood levels are not attained.
b. **Powdered medications.** Mix with liquids at bedside and immediately have client drink.	When prepared in advance, powdered drug forms may thicken, making swallowing difficult.
c. **Lozenges.** Instruct client not to chew or swallow.	These act through slow absorption through oral mucosa, not gastric mucosa.
d. **Effervescent powders and tablets.** Give immediately after dissolving.	Effervescence helps improve unpleasant taste of drug and often has therapeutic value for GI problems.
23. If client is unable to hold medications, place medication cup to the lips and place each tablet or capsule in the mouth, one at a time without rushing.	Promotes swallowing and prevents aspiration.
24. Stay until client has completely swallowed each medication. If concerned about ability or willingness to swallow, ask client to open mouth and inspect for presence of medication.	Nurse assumes responsibility for ensuring that client receives ordered dosage. If left unattended, client may forget to take it, drop it, or intentionally not take dose without nurse's awareness.
25. For certain medications that should not be given on an empty stomach (e.g., aspirin), offer client nonfat snack (e.g., crackers).	Reduces gastric irritation.
26. Replenish stock such as cups and straws, return cart to medicine room, and clean work area.	Well-stocked, clean working space assists other staff in completing duties efficiently.
27. See Chapter 39 for information about discharge teaching.	
28. See Completion Protocol (Chapter 1, p. 6).	

Evaluation

1. Return within appropriate time (60 to 90 minutes) to evaluate client's response to medications, therapeutic benefit, or onset of side effects or allergic reactions.
2. Ask client to discuss drug's purpose and correct regimen.

UNEXPECTED OUTCOMES AND RELATED INTERVENTIONS

1. Client has difficulty swallowing. Most compressed tablets can be crushed and placed in a very small amount of applesauce.
2. Clients with neuromuscular disorders, esophageal strictures, or lesions of the mouth and those who are unresponsive or comatose cannot swallow. (See Skill 32.2.)
3. Tablet or capsule falls to the floor.
   a. Discard it.
   b. Repeat preparation.
   c. Replacement may need to be obtained from pharmacy with unit dose systems.
4. Client exhibits side effects common to medication.
   a. Identify comfort measures that relieve symptoms.
   b. Report severe or intolerable side effects to physician. Dosage or form of medication may be changed.
5. Client experiences allergic response that could be related to medication.
   a. Withhold further doses.
   b. Notify the physician. If symptoms are severe, drugs may be prescribed to counteract adverse effects.
6. Client is unable to explain drug information and is unable or unwilling to remember information about purpose, schedule, or adverse effects.

   a. Identify family member willing to assume responsibility.
   b. Refer to home health agency for follow-up after discharge if needed.
      Examples of learning aids: homemade calendars for each week that contain plastic bags containing medications to take at specific times, egg cartons divided into color-coded sections with medications for day, clock faces for clients who cannot read or see clearly, color coding for drug types (e.g., blue for sedative, red for pain pill).
7. Administration error is made (wrong drug, dose, client, route, or time).
   a. Acknowledge it immediately. Nurses have an ethical and professional responsibility to report the error to the client's physician.
   b. Institute measures to counteract the effects of the error if necessary.
   c. Monitor client for untoward effects according to the drug action and side effects.
   d. Complete medication error form as required by the agency. These reports can assist in preventing additional similar errors. (See Patient/Visitor Incident Report, Appendix A).

SAMPLE DOCUMENTATION

Promptly record actual time each drug was administered on the medication administration record or in the computer. Include initials or signature. (See Medication Administration Record, Appendix A.)

If a drug is withheld, record reason and time the drug normally would have been given in the medication record.

If a narcotic was administered, a record is kept in a separate log (check agency policy).

Skill 16.2 | Topical Applications

Topical administration of medications involves applying drugs locally to skin, mucous membranes, or tissue membranes. This method, as compared with injections, avoids puncturing skin and lessens discomfort, the risk of infection, and tissue injury. The client is unlikely to experience GI disturbances, and the risk of serious side effects is generally low, although serious systemic effects can occur.

Many locally applied drugs such as lotions, patches, pastes, and ointments can create systemic and local effects if absorbed through the skin. Adhesive-backed medicated patches applied to the skin provide sustained, continuous release of medication over several hours or days. Systemic effects from topical agents can occur if the skin is thin, if drug concentration is high, or if contact with the skin is prolonged.

nurse alert To prevent accidental exposure, the nurse must use gloves or applicators. Sterile technique is important if the client has an open wound or impaired skin integrity.

Skin encrustations and dead tissues harbor microorganisms and block contact of medications with the tissues to be treated. Simply applying new medications over previously applied drugs does not offer maximum therapeutic benefit. The skin needs to be cleansed gently and thoroughly with soap and water before applying medications.

EQUIPMENT

Disposable or sterile gloves
Ordered agent (powder, cream, ointment, spray, patch)
Cotton-tipped applicators or tongue blades
Basin of warm water, washcloth, towel, nondrying soap
Sterile dressing, tape
Medication administration record (MAR) or computer
  printout

Assessment

1. Review physician's order for client's name, name of drug, strength, time of administration, and site of application.
2. Review information pertinent to medication: action, purpose, side effects, and nursing implications.
3. Assess condition of client's skin. Note if client has symptoms of skin irritation, for example, pruritus or burning. Cleanse skin if necessary to visualize adequately.
4. Determine whether client has known allergy to topical agent. Ask if client has had reaction to a cream or lotion applied to the skin. **Allergic contact dermatitis is relatively common and can intensify existing dermatologic condition.**

5. Determine amount of topical agent required for application by assessing skin site, reviewing physician's order, and reading application directions carefully (a thin, even layer is usually adequate). **An excessive amount of topical agent can cause chemical irritation of skin, negate drug's effectiveness, or cause adverse systemic effects, for example, decreased white cell counts or decreased immunity.**
6. Determine if client is physically able to apply medication by assessing grasp, hand strength, reach, and coordination. **This is necessary if client is to self-administer drug in the home.**

Planning

Expected outcomes focus on safe, accurate, and effective drug therapy.

EXPECTED OUTCOMES

1. Client applies medications as prescribed with evidence of improvement in condition (e.g., relief of pain, inflammation, and itching).
2. Client self-administers topical medication correctly.
3. Client explains dosage schedule and possible side effects.

Implementation

Steps	Rationale
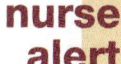 **nurse alert** Review five "rights" for administering medications.	
1. See Standard Protocol (Chapter 1, p. 5).	
2. Topical creams, ointments, and oil-based lotions	
a. In some cases, soaking may be needed using plain warm water and rinsing without soap.	Removes crusting from skin while minimizing inflammation and irritation.
b. Place approximately 1 to 2 teaspoons of medication in palm of gloved hand and soften by rubbing briskly between hands.	Softening of topical agent makes it easier to apply to skin.
c. Once medication is thin and smooth, smear it evenly over skin surface, using long, even strokes that follow direction of hair growth.	Ensures even distribution of medication. Technique prevents irritation of hair follicles.
d. If appropriate, explain to client that skin may feel greasy after application.	Ointments often contain oils.

Steps	Rationale

3. Antianginal (nitroglycerin) ointment

a. Apply desired number of inches of ointment over paper measuring guide (Figure 16-12).
  (1) Antianginal (nitroglycerin) ointments are usually ordered in inches and can be measured on small sheets of paper marked off in 1/2-inch markings.
  (2) Unit dose packages are available. (Warning: one package equals 1 inch; smaller amount should not be measured from this package).

b. Antianginal medication may be applied to the chest area, back, upper arm, or legs. Do not apply on hairy surfaces or over scar tissue. If client complains of headaches, apply ointment farther from head.

c. Apply ointment to skin surface by holding edge or back of the paper wrapper and placing ointment and wrapper directly on the skin (Figure 16-13).

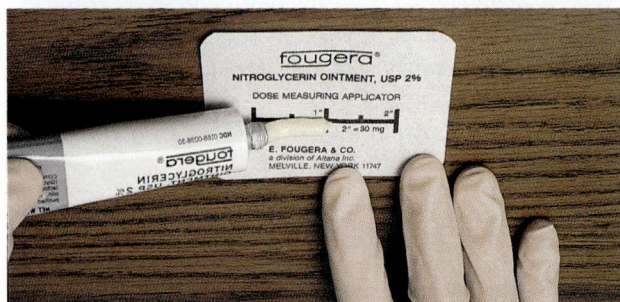

Figure 16-12

Application on hairy surfaces or scar tissue may interfere with absorption. Medication causes vasodilation that may intensify headaches.

Minimizes chance of ointment covering gloves and later touching nurse's hands.

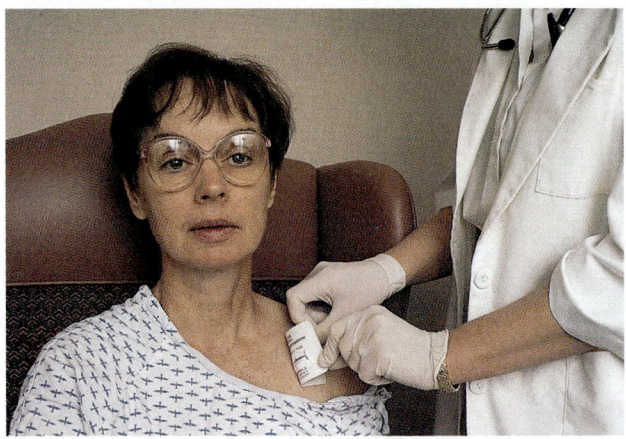

Figure 16-13

d. Do not rub or massage ointment into skin.
e. Date and initial paper and note time.
f. Cover ointment and paper with plastic wrap and tape securely, or follow manufacturer's directions.
g. Remove previous dosage paper.

Massage increases rate of absorption.
Prevents missing doses.
Prevents soiling of clothing.

Prevents overdose that can occur with multiple dosage papers left in place.

4. Transdermal patches (e.g., analgesic, nitroglycerin, nicotine, estrogen) (Figure 16-14).

a. Choose a clean, dry area of the body that is free of hair. Do not attempt to apply the patch on skin that is oily, burned, broken out, cut, or irritated in any way.

b. Carefully remove the patch from its protective covering. Hold the patch by the edge without touching the adhesive edges.

Clients should be cautioned about using alternate forms of medications or drugs when using patches. For example, clients should not smoke while using a nicotine patch. Clients should not apply nitroglycerin ointment in addition to the patch unless specifically ordered to do so by their physician.

Touching only the edges ensures that the patch will adhere and that the medication dosage has not been changed.

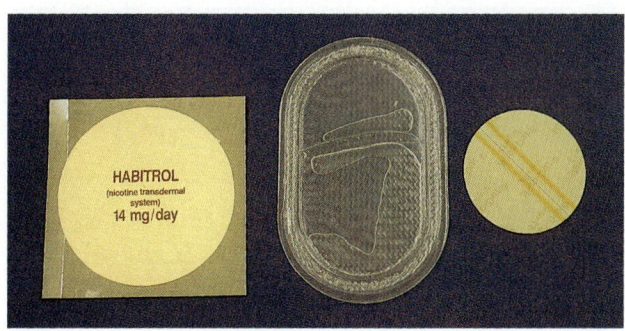

Figure 16-14 A variety of medications are available as skin patches

Steps	Rationale
c. Immediately apply the patch, pressing firmly with the palm of one hand for 10 seconds. Make sure it sticks well, especially around the edges. Date and initial patch and note time.	Visual reminders of dose applications prevent missing doses.
d. Advise clients not to use heating pads anywhere near the site.	Heat increases circulation and the rate of absorption.
e. After appropriate time, remove the patch and fold it so the medicated side is covered and flush down the toilet.	Residual medication can be a hazard to children and pets (Willens, 1994).
f. Avoid previously used sites for at least 1 week.	Minimizes skin irritation.

5. Aerosol spray (e.g., local anesthetic sprays)

a. Shake container vigorously. Mixes contents and propellant to ensure distribution of fine, even spray.	
b. Read container's label for distance recommended to hold spray away from area, usually 15 to 30 cm (6 to 12 inches).	Proper distance ensures fine spray hits skin surface. Holding container too close results in thin, watery distribution.
c. If neck or upper chest is to be sprayed, ask client to turn face away from spray or briefly cover face with towel.	Prevents inhalation of spray.
d. Spray medication evenly over affected site (in some cases, spray is timed for period of seconds).	Entire affected area of skin should be covered with thin spray.

6. Suspension-based lotion

a. Shake container vigorously.	Mixes powder throughout liquid to form well-mixed suspension.
b. Apply small amount of lotion to small gauze dressing or pad, and apply to skin by stroking evenly in direction of hair growth.	Method of application leaves protective film of powder on skin after water base of suspension dries. Technique prevents irritation to hair follicles.
c. Explain to client that area will feel cool and dry.	Water evaporates to leave thin layer of powder.

7. Medicated powder

a. Be sure skin surface is thoroughly dry.	Minimizes caking and crusting of powder.
b. Fully spread apart any skin folds such as between toes or under axilla.	Fully exposes skin surface for application.
c. Dust skin site lightly with dispenser so that area is covered with fine, thin layer of powder.	Thin layer of powder is more absorbent and reduces friction by increasing area of moisture evaporation.
d. Cover skin area with dressing if ordered by physician.	May help prevent agent from being rubbed off skin. Protects clothing from being stained.

Steps	Rationale
e. Instruct client to dispose of applicators, patches, and similar materials into cardboard or plastic disposable containers. f. See Chapter 39 for information about discharge teaching. **8.** See Completion Protocol (Chapter 1, p. 6).	Careful disposal is necessary to ensure the safety of client, others, pets, and children.

Evaluation

1. Inspect condition of skin between applications to determine if skin condition improves.
2. Observe client applying lotion, ointment, or patch.
3. Ask the client or significant other to name the medication and its action, purpose, dosage, schedule, and side effects.

UNEXPECTED OUTCOMES
AND RELATED INTERVENTIONS

1. Skin site may appear inflamed and edematous with blistering and oozing of fluid from lesions, indicating subacute inflammation or eczema that can develop from worsening of skin lesions.

2. Client continues to complain of pruritus and tenderness.
   a. Indicates slow or impaired healing.
   b. Alternate therapies may be needed.
3. Client is unable to explain information about topical application or does not administer as prescribed.
   a. Identify possible reasons for noncompliance.
   b. Explore alternative approaches or options.

SAMPLE DOCUMENTATION

0930 Skin appears dry, red, and flaky on both hands. Client complains of itching. Hydrocortisone cream 1% applied sparingly to affected areas as prescribed.

Skill 16.3 | Eye/Ear Medications

EYE MEDICATIONS

Common eye medications used by clients include OTC preparations such as artificial tears and vasoconstrictors (e.g., Visine, Murine). Many clients receive prescribed ophthalmic drugs for eye conditions, such as glaucoma, and after cataract extraction. Orders may indicate administration to one or both eyes, and abbreviations are often used to indicate the site. The abbreviation for right eye is OD, left eye OS, and both eyes OU.

The eye is extremely sensitive, since the cornea is richly supplied with sensitive nerve fibers that provide a protective mechanism. The conjunctival sac is much less sensitive and thus a more appropriate site for medication instillation. Care must be taken to prevent instilling medication directly onto the sensitive cornea.

Clients receiving topical eye medication should learn correct self-administration of the medication. Clients with glaucoma, for example, usually require lifelong eye drops for control of their disease. At times it may become necessary for family members to learn how to administer eye drops or ointment, particularly immediately after eye surgery, when a client's vision is so impaired that it is difficult to assemble needed supplies and handle applicators correctly.

Eye medications come in a variety of concentrations. Instilling the wrong concentration may cause local irritation to eyes, as well as produce systemic effects. Certain ophthalmic medications (e.g., mydriatics, which dilate the pupil; cycloplegics, which paralyze the ciliary muscles of the eye) temporarily blur a client's vision.

EAR MEDICATIONS

Internal ear structures are very sensitive to temperature extremes, and therefore solutions should be administered at room temperature. Although structures of the outer ear are not sterile, it is wise to use sterile drops and solutions because the eardrum could be ruptured. Introduction of nonsterile solutions into the middle ear can cause serious infection. Forcing solution into the ear or occluding the ear canal with a medicine dropper during administration can cause pressure within the canal and injury to the eardrum.

EQUIPMENT

Medication bottle with sterile eye dropper or ointment tube

Medication administration record or computer printout

Cotton ball or tissue
Warm water and washcloth
Eye patch and tape (optional)
Disposable gloves

Assessment

1. Review physician's medication order, including client's name, drug name, concentration, number of drops (if a liquid), time, and eye/ear.
2. Review information pertinent to medication, including action, purpose, side effects, and nursing implications. **Tell clients receiving mydriatics that vision will be temporarily blurred. Wearing sunglasses reduces photophobia. Clients who receive cycloplegics should temporarily not drive or attempt to perform any activity that requires acute vision.**
3. Assess condition of external eye or ear structures (see Skill 12.4). **This may also be done just before drug instillation to provide a baseline to determine later if local response to medications occurs. This also indicates need to clean area before drug application.**
4. Determine whether client has symptoms of discomfort or hearing or visual impairment. **Occlusion of external ear canal by swelling, drainage, or cerumen can impair hearing acuity and is painful.**
5. Determine whether client has any known allergies to medications.
6. Assess client's level of consciousness and ability to follow directions. **If client becomes restless or combative during procedure, client may require assistance to hold still.**
7. Assess client's knowledge regarding drug therapy and desire to self-administer medication. Assess client's ability to manipulate and hold dropper. **Client's level of understanding may indicate need for health teaching. Motivation influences teaching approach.**

Planning

Expected outcomes focus on relief of symptoms without unpleasant adverse reactions.

EXPECTED OUTCOMES

1. Symptoms (e.g., irritation) are relieved.
2. Client denies unpleasant side effects or adverse reactions.
3. Client describes medication effects and technique of application.
4. Client correctly demonstrates self-instillation of eye drops.

Implementation

Steps	Rationale
nurse alert Review five "rights" for administering medications.	
1. See Standard Protocol (Chapter 1, p. 5).	
2. Compare medication administration record with label of eye/ear medication.	
3. Check client's identification bracelet and ask name.	Ensures correct client receives medication.
4. Explain procedure to client. Clients experienced in self-instillation may be allowed to give drops under nurse's supervision (check agency policy).	Clients often become anxious about medication being instilled into eye because of potential discomfort.
5. Ask client to lie supine or sit back in chair with neck slightly hyperextended.	Position provides easy access to eye/ear for medication instillation. Correct positioning minimizes drainage of eye medication into tear duct.
6. If crusts or drainage is present along eyelid margins or inner canthus, gently wash away from inner to outer canthus. If indicated, soak any crusts that are dried with a damp washcloth for several minutes.	Soaking allows easy removal of crusts. Cleansing from inner to outer canthus avoids introducing microorganisms into lacrimal ducts.
7. Hold cotton ball or clean tissue in nondominant hand on client's cheekbone just below lower eyelid.	Cotton or tissue absorbs medication that escapes eye.

Steps	Rationale

8. With tissue or cotton resting below lower lid, gently press downward with thumb or forefinger against bony orbit, exposing conjunctival sac (Figure 16-15).

Prevents pressure and trauma to eyeball and prevents fingers from touching eye.

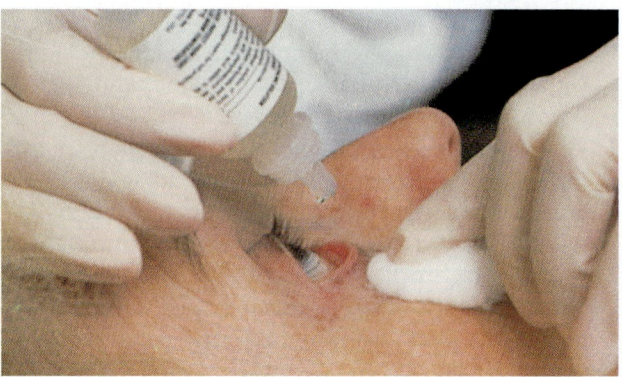

Figure 16-15

9. Ask client to look at ceiling.

Retracts sensitive cornea up and away from conjunctival sac and reduces stimulation of blink reflex.

10. To instill eye drops

a. Rest dominant hand gently on client's forehead, and hold filled medication eyedropper approximately 1 to 2 cm (½ to ¾ inch) above conjunctival sac.

Helps prevent accidental contact of eyedropper with eye, and reduces risk of eye injury and transfer of microorganisms to dropper (ophthalmic medications are sterile).

b. Drop prescribed number of medication drops into conjunctival sac.

Conjunctival sac normally holds 1 or 2 drops. Applying drops to sac provides even distribution of medication across eye.

c. If client blinks or closes eye or if drops land on outer lid margins, repeat procedure.

Therapeutic effect of drug is obtained only when drops enter conjunctival sac.

d. When administering drugs that cause systemic effects, apply gentle pressure to client's nasolacrimal duct with a cotton ball or tissue for 30 to 60 seconds.

Prevents overflow of medication into nasal and pharyngeal passages. Minimizes absorption into systemic circulation.

e. After instilling drops, ask client to close eye gently.

Helps to distribute medication. Squinting or squeezing of eyelids forces medication from conjunctival sac. Avoid pressure directly against client's eyeball.

11. To instill eye ointment

a. Hold ointment applicator above lid margin, and apply thin stream of ointment evenly along inside edge of lower eyelid on conjunctiva from the inner to outer canthus (Figure 16-16).

Distributes medication evenly across eye and lid margin.

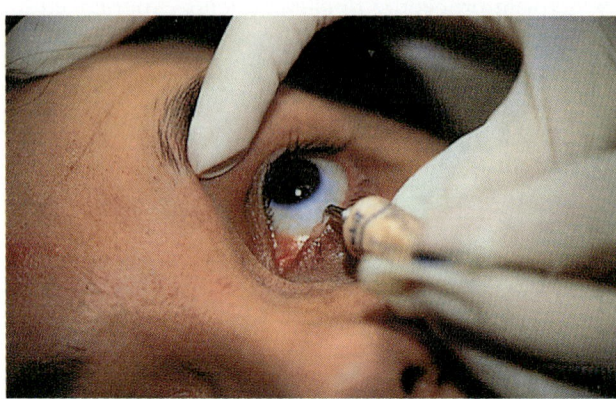

Figure 16-16

Steps	Rationale
b. Ask client to look down.	Reduces blinking reflex during ointment application.
c. Apply thin stream of ointment along upper lid margin on inner conjunctiva.	Distributes medication evenly across eye and lid margin.
d. Have client close eye, and rub lid lightly in circular motion with cotton ball, if rubbing is not contraindicated.	Further distributes medication without traumatizing eye. Avoid pressure directly against client's eyeball.
e. If excess medication is on eyelid, gently wipe it from inner to outer canthus.	Promotes comfort and prevents trauma to eye.
f. If client has eye patch, apply clean one by placing it over affected eye so entire eye is covered. Tape securely without applying pressure to eye.	Clean eye patch reduces chance of infection.

12. To instill ear drops

a. Warm ear drops to body temperature. Hold bottle in hands or place in warm water.	Ear structures are very sensitive to temperature.
b. Position client on side or sitting in a chair, with affected ear facing up.	Position provides easy access to ear for instillation of medication.
c. Straighten ear canal by pulling auricle upward and outward (adult) or down and back (child) (Figure 16-17).	Straightening of ear canal provides direct access to deeper external ear structures.
d. If cerumen or drainage occludes outermost portion of ear canal, wipe out gently with cotton-tipped applicator, taking care not to force wax inward.	Cerumen and drainage harbor microorganisms and can block distribution of medication into canal. Occlusion blocks sound transmission.
e. Instill prescribed drops holding dropper 1 cm (½ inch) above ear canal.	

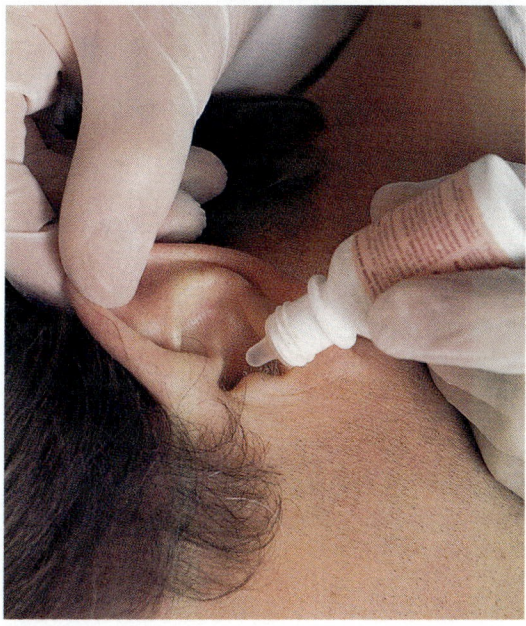

Figure 16-17

f. Ask client to remain in side-lying position 2 to 3 minutes, and apply gentle massage or pressure to tragus of ear with finger.	Allows complete distribution of medication. Pressure and massage move medication inward.
g. If ordered, gently insert a portion of cotton ball into outermost part of canal.	Prevents escape of medication when client sits or stands.
h. Remove cotton after 15 minutes.	Adequate time for drug distribution and absorption.
i. See Chapter 39 for information about discharge teaching.	

13. See Completion Protocol (Chapter 1, p. 6).

Evaluation

1. Observe effects of medication by assessing visual changes and noting any side effects.
2. Note client's response to instillation; ask if any discomfort was felt.
3. Ask client to discuss drug's purpose, action, side effects, and technique of administration.
4. Observe as client demonstrates self-administration of next dose.

UNEXPECTED OUTCOMES AND RELATED INTERVENTIONS

1. Client complains of burning or pain after administration of eye drops.

   Surface of eye should not be touched by eye drops instilled onto cornea or by dropper.
2. Client experiences local side effects, for example, headache, bloodshot eyes, and local eye irritation.

   Drug concentration and client's sensitivity both influence chances of side effects developing.
3. Client experiences systemic effects from eye drops, for example, increased heart rate and blood pressure from epinephrine or decreased heart rate and blood pressure from timolol.

   Systemic absorption through tear duct can cause potentially dangerous effects. Local anesthetics and antibiotics may cause anaphylaxis.
4. Client lacks confidence or ability to instill drops without supervision.
   a. If client is unable to manipulate the dropper or is unable to see, instruct a family member in the technique.
   b. When using OTC eye drops, client should not share with family members to avoid transmission of microorganisms.

SAMPLE DOCUMENTATION

1300 Cyclopentolate ophthalmic 1% solution, 2 drops instilled in each eye. No side effects of tachycardia, drowsiness, or confusion apparent.

Skill 16.4 | Inhalants

Drugs administered with hand-held inhalers are dispersed through aerosol spray, mist, or fine powder to penetrate lung airways. The deeper passages of the respiratory tract provide a large surface area for drug absorption. The alveolar-capillary network absorbs medication rapidly.

Inhaled medications are designed to produce local effects; for example, bronchodilators open narrowed bronchioles, and mucolytic agents liquefy thick mucous secretions. However, since these medications are absorbed rapidly through the pulmonary circulation, most create systemic side effects. For example, isoproterenol (Isuprel) dilates bronchioles and can also cause cardiac dysrhythmias.

Clients who receive drugs by inhalation frequently have chronic respiratory disease, and because clients depend on medications for airway management, they need to know how to administer them safely. It is inappropriate to try to teach a client how to use an inhaler during an episode of shortness of breath, since the client's ability to learn is greatly diminished.

Drugs can be delivered by *metered-dose inhalers* (MDIs), which deliver a measured dose of drug with each push of a canister. Because use of an MDI requires coordination during the breathing cycle, clients may spray only the back of their throats and do not receive a full dose. A device called an *aerochamber* (spacer) fits MDIs and improves a client's ability to deliver a proper dose of medication (Figure 16-18).

EQUIPMENT

Metered-dose inhaler with medication canister
Aerochamber spacer (optional)
Facial tissues (optional)

Assessment

1. Assess client's ability to hold, manipulate, and depress canister and inhaler. **Impairment of grasp or presence of tremors of hands interferes with client's ability to depress canister within inhaler.**

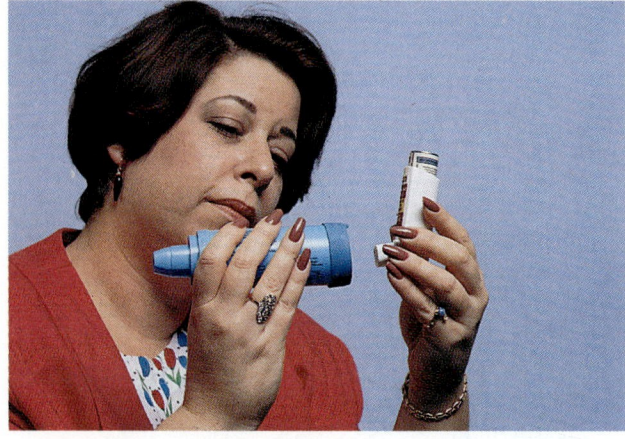

Figure 16-18 Aerochamber for metered-dose inhaler.

2. Assess client's readiness to learn: client asks questions about medication, disease, or complications; requests education in use of inhaler; is mentally alert; participates in own care.
3. Assess client's ability to learn: client should not be fatigued, in pain, or in respiratory distress; assess level of understanding of terms.
4. Assess client's knowledge and understanding of disease and purpose and action of prescribed medications.
5. Identify drug schedule and number of inhalations prescribed for each dose.

Planning

Expected outcomes focus on relief of symptoms and promoting knowledge for self-administration of inhalers.

EXPECTED OUTCOMES

1. Client manipulates mouthpiece, canister, and inhaler correctly and cleans inhaler after use.
2. Client describes proper time during respiratory cycle to inhale spray and number of inhalations for each administration.
3. Client experiences effects of medication within 10 to 15 minutes, which validates proper administration technique.
4. Client lists side effects of medications and criteria for calling health care professional if dyspnea develops.

Implementation

Steps	Rationale
nurse alert Review five "rights" for administering medications.	
1. See Standard Protocol (Chapter 1, p. 5).	
2. Allow client opportunity to manipulate inhaler, canister, and spacer device (aerochamber). Explain and demonstrate how canister fits into inhaler (see Figure 16-18).	Familiarity with equipment enhances learning.
3. Explain what metered dose is, and warn client about overuse of inhaler, including drug side effects.	Client needs to know the dangers of excessive inhalations because of risk of serious side effects. If drug is given in recommended doses, side effects are minimal.
4. Remove mouthpiece cover from inhaler. Shake inhaler well.	Ensures that fine particles are aerosolized.
5. *Without aerochamber (spacer):* Open lips and place inhaler 1 to 2 cm (½ to 1 inch) from mouth with opening toward back of throat. Lips should not touch inhaler (Figure 16-19).	Avoids rapid influx of inhaled medication and subsequent airway irritation.

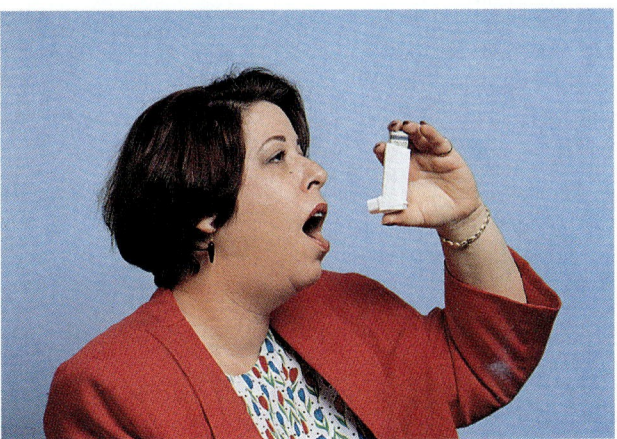

Figure 16-19

Steps	Rationale

6. *With aerochamber (spacer):* Exhale fully, then grasp mouthpiece with teeth and lips while holding inhaler with thumb at the mouthpiece and fingers at the top (Figure 16-20).

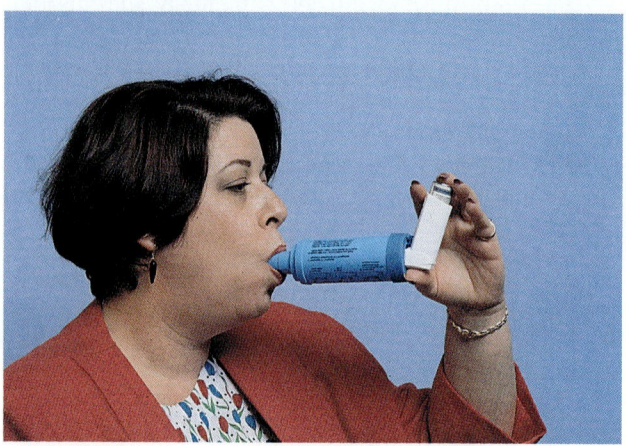

Figure 16-20

7. Press down on inhaler to release medication while inhaling slowly and deeply through mouth.

Medication is distributed to airways during inhalation.

8. Breathe in slowly for 2 to 3 seconds. Hold breath for approximately 10 seconds.

As client inhales, particles of medication are delivered to airway (National Heart, Lung, and Blood Institute, 1991). Holding breath allows tiny drops of aerosol spray to reach deeper branches of airways.

9. Exhale through pursed lips.

Pursed lip breathing keeps small airways open during exhalation.

10. Instruct client to wait 1 minute between puffs. More than one puff is usually prescribed.

First inhalation opens airways and reduces inflammation. Second or third inhalations penetrate deeper airways.

11. If more than one type of inhaled medications are prescribed, wait 5 to 10 minutes between inhalations or as ordered by physician.

Drugs are prescribed at intervals during day to promote bronchodilation and minimize side effects.

12. Explain that client may feel gagging sensation in throat caused by droplets of medication on pharynx or tongue.

Results when inhalant is sprayed and inhaled incorrectly.

13. Instruct client in removing medication canister and cleaning inhaler in warm water.

Accumulation of spray around mouthpiece can interfere with proper distribution during use.

14. Teach client to measure the amount of medication remaining in the canister by immersing it in a large bowl or pan of water (Figure 16-21).

15. See Chapter 39 for implications for discharge teaching.

16. See Completion Protocol (Chapter 1, p. 6).

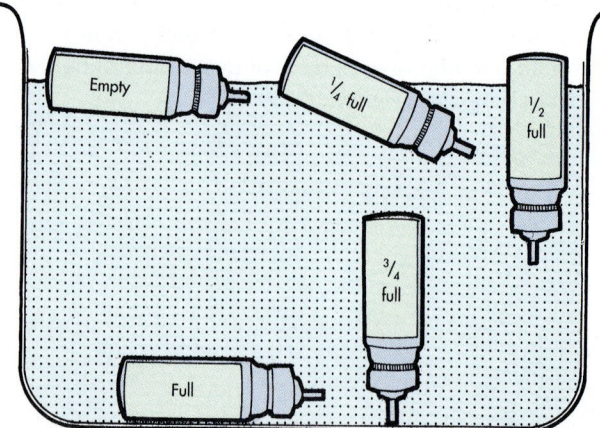

Figure 16-21 A simple method of estimating the amount left in an inhaler canister: a container is filled with water, and the position the canister takes in the water determines the amount remaining.

Evaluation

1. Have client explain and demonstrate steps in use of inhaler.
2. Ask client to explain drug schedule and dose of medication.
3. After medication instillation, assess client's respirations and auscultate lungs.
4. Ask client to list side effects and criteria for calling physician.

UNEXPECTED OUTCOMES AND RELATED INTERVENTIONS

1. Client's breathing pattern is ineffective; respirations are rapid and shallow. Client's need for a bronchodilator more than every 4 hours can signal respiratory problems.
   a. Reassess type of medication or delivery method. Make sure client shakes canister before administration.
   b. Determine fullness of canister, using displacement in water (see Figure 16-21).
   c. Wait adequate time between puffs to allow deeper penetration into the lungs.
   d. Observe if the canister is releasing a spray. If not, the valve may need to be cleaned.

2. Client experiences gags or paroxysms of coughing.
   a. Client may gag or swallow medication if unable to inhale while spray is administered.
   b. Aerosolized particles irritate posterior pharynx.
3. Client is experiencing cardiac dysrhythmias.
   Evidence of side effects from certain medications. Signs and symptoms of overuse of xanthines and sympathomimetic drugs include tachycardia, palpitations, headache, restlessness, and insomnia.
4. Client is unable to depress medication canister because of weakened grasp or presses the canister before or after taking a breath. Both should be done simultaneously for maximum effectiveness.
   a. Client may need practice with assistance for several different steps of procedure before being able to perform each skill independently.
   b. Alternative delivery routes or methods may need to be explored.

SAMPLE DOCUMENTATION

0900 Discussed correct technique for metered-dose inhaler using aerochamber. Client demonstrated correct use and listed the three main side effects of medication without hesitation.

Skill 16.5 | Suppositories (Rectal and Vaginal)

Suppositories come individually packaged in foil wrappers and are usually stored in a refrigerator to prevent melting. *Caution:* Rectal and vaginal suppositories may be stored together in a refrigerator.

After a suppository is inserted into the rectum or vagina, body temperature causes the suppository to melt and be distributed. Clients may prefer self-administering suppositories and are given privacy if capable to self-administer without difficulty.

Drugs administered by rectal suppository exert either a local effect on GI mucosa, such as promoting defecation, or systemic effects, such as relieving nausea or providing analgesia. The rectal route is not as reliable as oral or parenteral routes in terms of drug absorption and distribution. However, the medications are relatively safe, since they rarely cause local irritation or side effects. Rectal medications are contraindicated in clients after rectal surgery or when experiencing active rectal bleeding.

Proper placement is important to promote retention of the medication until it dissolves and is absorbed into the mucosa. Avoid placing a suppository into a mass of fecal material. If necessary, obtain a physician's order to administer a small cleansing enema to evacuate the lower bowel before the suppository is inserted.

EQUIPMENT

Disposable gloves
Suppository insertion
    Suppository (Figure 16-22)
    Lubricant
Vaginal creams or foam instillation (Figure 16-23)
    Vaginal cream or foam in plastic tube or can
    Perineal pad (optional)

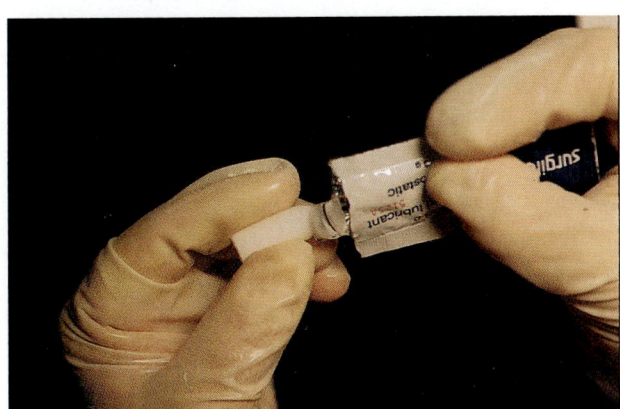

Figure 16-22 Rectal suppository.

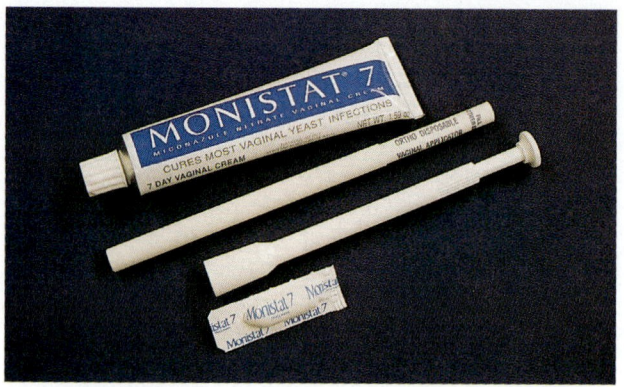

Figure 16-23 Vaginal cream and vaginal suppository with applicator.

Assessment

1. Review physician's order, including client's name, drug name, form (cream or suppository), route, dosage, and time of administration.

2. Review pertinent information related to medication, including action, purpose, side effects, and nursing implications.
3. Inspect condition of external genitalia and vaginal canal or rectum (see Skill 12.8). (May be done just before insertion.)
4. Ask if client is experiencing any symptoms of pruritus, burning, or discomfort.
5. Review client's knowledge of purpose of drug therapy and ability and willingness to self-administer medication.

Planning

Expected outcomes focus on relief of symptoms without unpleasant side effects.

EXPECTED OUTCOMES
1. Client reports relief of symptoms of discomfort.
2. Client has no itching or burning.
3. Client explains purpose of medication, side effects, and steps to use for proper suppository insertion.

Implementation

Steps	Rationale
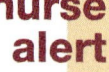 **nurse alert** Review five "rights" for administering medications.	
1. See Standard Protocol (Chapter 1, p. 5).	
2. Vaginal suppository	
a. Assist client to lie in dorsal recumbent position with abdomen and lower extremities covered.	Provides easy access to vaginal canal and allows suppository to dissolve in vagina without leaking out.
b. Be sure vaginal orifice is well illuminated.	Proper insertion requires visualization of external genitalia if not self-administered.
c. Remove suppository from foil wrapper and apply liberal amount of petroleum jelly.	Lubrication reduces friction against mucosal surfaces during insertion.
d. With nondominant gloved hand, gently retract labial folds to expose vaginal orifice.	
e. Insert suppository along posterior wall of vaginal canal entire length of finger (7.5 to 10 cm, or 3 to 4 inches) (Figure 16-24).	Proper placement of suppository ensures equal distribution of medication along walls of vaginal cavity.
f. Wipe away remaining lubricant from around orifice and labia.	
g. Tell client there may be a small amount of discharge that is the color of medication exiting from vaginal canal. Client may wish to use disposable panty liners.	As the medication liquefies at body temperature, it is absorbed; however, small amounts may ooze from the vaginal canal.

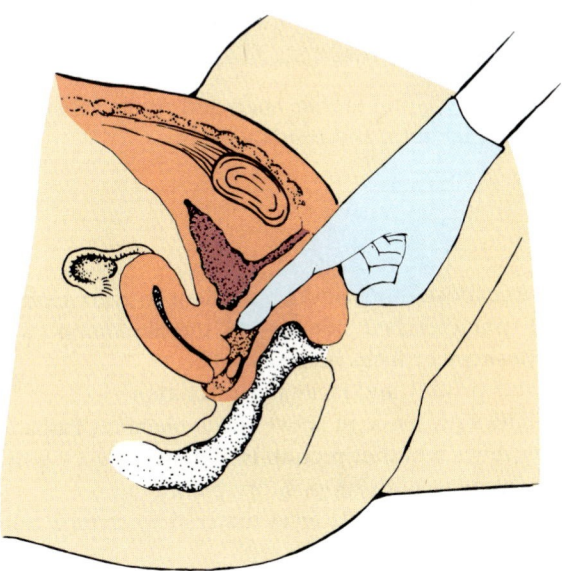

Figure 16-24

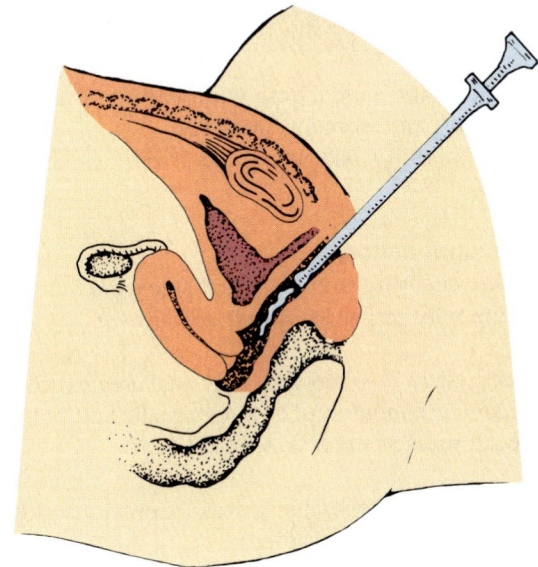

Figure 16-25

Steps	Rationale

3. Cream or foam

a. Fill cream or foam applicator following package directions.

Dose is instilled based on volume in applicator.

b. With nondominant gloved hand, gently retract labial folds to expose vaginal orifice.

c. With dominant gloved hand, insert applicator approximately 5 to 7.5 cm (2 to 3 inches). Push applicator plunger to deposit medication into vagina (Figure 16-25).

d. Withdraw applicator and place on paper towel. Wipe off residual cream from labia or vaginal orifice.

Residual cream on applicator may contain microorganisms.

e. Instruct client who received suppository or cream to remain on her back for at least 10 minutes. Clients may wish to use disposal panty liners.

Medication will be distributed and absorbed evenly throughout vaginal cavity and not be lost through orifice; however, small amounts may ooze from the vaginal canal.

4. Irrigation and douche

a. Place client on bedpan with absorbent pad underneath.

Allows hips to be higher than shoulders and solution will reach posterior fornix of the vagina. Bedpan will collect solution.

b. Be sure fluid is at body temperature, and run fluid through container nozzle.

Body temperature promotes the client's comfort.

c. Gently retract labial folds and direct nozzle toward the sacrum, following the floor of the vagina.

Correct angle allows nozzle access through the cervix into the uterus.

d. Raise the container approximately 30 to 50 cm (12 to 20 inches) above level of vagina. Insert the nozzle 7 to 10 cm (3 to 4 inches). Allow the solution to flow while rotating the nozzle. Administer all the irrigating solution.

Rotating the nozzle allows irrigation of all areas in the vagina.

e. Withdraw the nozzle, and assist the client to a comfortable sitting position.

Remaining solution will drain by gravity.

Steps	Rationale
f. If applicator is used, wash with soap and warm water, rinse, and store for future use.	Vaginal cavity is not sterile. Soap and water assist in removal of bacteria and residual cream.
g. Offer perineal pad when client resumes ambulation.	
5. Rectal suppository	
a. Assist client in assuming a left side-lying Sims' position with upper leg flexed upward.	Position exposes anus and helps client to relax external anal sphincter. Left side lessens the likelihood of the suppository or feces being expelled.
b. Keep client covered with only anal area exposed.	Maintains privacy and facilitates relaxation.
c. Examine condition of anus externally and palpate rectal walls as needed (see Skill 12.8).	Determines presence of active rectal bleeding. Palpation determines whether rectum is filled with feces, which may interfere with suppository placement.
d. Apply clean disposable gloves (if previous gloves were soiled and discarded).	Minimizes contact with fecal material to reduce transmission of infection.
e. Remove suppository from foil wrapper and lubricate rounded end (see Figure 16-22).	Lubrication reduces friction as suppository enters rectal canal.
f. Retract client's buttocks with nondominant hand. Ask client to take slow, deep breaths through mouth and to relax anal sphincter.	Forcing suppository through constricted sphincter causes discomfort.
g. With gloved index finger of dominant hand, insert suppository rounded end first gently through anus, past internal sphincter, and against rectal wall, 10 cm (4 inches) in adults.	
h. Wipe client's anal area and discard gloves by turning them inside out, and dispose of in appropriate receptacle.	Inverting the gloves contains the microorganisms and prevents contamination of other articles.
i. Ask client to remain on side for 5 to 10 minutes or until urge to eliminate is strong.	Prevents expulsion of suppository. Provides sufficient time for the effects of the suppository to reach maximum effectiveness.
j. If suppository contains laxative or fecal softener, place call light within reach so client can obtain assistance to reach bedpan or toilet.	Ability to call for assistance provides client with sense of control over elimination.
k. See Chapter 39 for implications for discharge teaching.	
6. See Completion Protocol (Chapter 1, p. 6).	

Evaluation

1. Ask client about relief of symptoms for which medication was prescribed.
2. Inspect condition of vagina or rectum and external genitalia between applications. Ask about the presence of itching, burning, or discomfort.
3. Ask client to discuss purpose, action, side effects, and method of administration of medication.

UNEXPECTED OUTCOMES AND RELATED INTERVENTIONS

1. Thick, white, patchy, curdlike discharge clings to vaginal walls. Vaginal walls appear bright pink or inflamed, indicating yeast infection.

   a. Female clients often develop vaginal infections requiring topical application of antiinfective agents.
   b. Medications are available in foam, jelly, cream, or suppository form. Medicated irrigations or douches can also be given.
2. Client reports localized pruritus and burning, which usually indicate infection or inflammation.

   Excessive use can lead to irritation of mucous membranes.

SAMPLE DOCUMENTATION

0800 Client complains of constipation. Has not had bowel movement for 3 days. Dulcolax suppository given PR as ordered. Expelled large, hard, dark-brown stool.

States feeling much relieved. Encouraged to drink more fluids, to choose high-fiber foods from menu, and to ambulate as much as possible to prevent further problems.

CRITICAL THINKING EXERCISES

1. While you are preparing medications at the medication cart, a fellow nurse hands you a filled syringe and asks you to give a client pain medication while the nurse cares for another client needing immediate assistance. What should you do, and why?
2. How would you categorize each of the following client reactions?
   a. Sarah complains that she becomes nauseated after taking her oral antibiotic capsules.
   b. Jake has been on a digitalis preparation for 10 days. Today, he states that he is seeing "halos" around lights.
   c. James is being treated for an infection. He has received three doses of oral penicillin. As you enter his room, you note that he is wheezing and having difficulty breathing.
3. Melvin is to receive two enteric-coated aspirin tablets. As you offer the medication to Melvin, he requests that you break the tablets in half so they will be easier to swallow. How should you respond?
4. Mrs. Gomez is to receive 10 mEq of liquid potassium. The bottle is labeled "2 mEq potassium per milliliter." How many cc's of medication should Mrs. Gomez receive?
5. What nursing action(s) are required for each of the following client situations?
   a. Ralph is ordered to receive a ½ inch of nitroglycerin ointment every 12 hours.
   b. While you are administering Chuck's eye medication, he blinks and causes the medication to land on his outer eyelid.
   c. Lola is having difficulty using her inhaler, and you are concerned that she is not receiving the prescribed dose of medication.
6. Mrs. Tubbs is to receive a rectal suppository. What supplies do you need, and how should you position Mrs. Tubbs for this procedure?
7. Melissa has checked to make sure that she has the correct medication, the correct dose, and is administering the dose at the correct time. What else does Melissa need to verify before administering the medication to the client?

REFERENCES

Gray D: *Calculate with confidence,* St Louis, 1994, Mosby.
McGovern K: 10 golden rules for administering drugs safely, *Nursing '92,* March:49-56, 1992.
National Heart, Lung, and Blood Institute: *Guidelines for diagnosis and management of asthma,* National Asthma Education Program, pub no 91-3042, Bethesda, Md, 1991, The Institute.
Willens JS: Giving fentanyl for pain outside the OR, *Am J Nurs,* February:24-28, 1994.

ADDITIONAL READINGS

Clark JB, Queener SF, Karb VB: *Pharmacological basis of nursing practice,* ed 3, St Louis, 1990, Mosby.
Guidry GG et al: Incorrect use of metered dose inhalers by medical personnel, *Chest* 101(1):31, 1992.
Hofford JM: Metered dose inhaler therapy for asthma, bronchitis, and emphysema, *J Fam Pract* 34(4):485, 1992.
Holdcroft C: Efficacy of transdermal nicotine patches for nicotine replacement and smoking cessation, *Nurse Practitioner Am J Primary Health Care* 17(7):46, 1992.
Teplitsky B: Avoiding the hazards of look-alike drug names, *Nursing '92,* January 1992.
Youngkin EQ: Estrogen replacement therapy and the Estraderm transdermal system, *Nurse Practitioner Am J Primary Health Care* 15(5):19, 1990.

chapter 17 | Administration of Injections

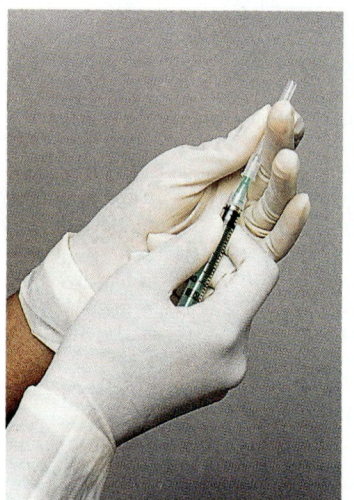

Skill 17.1
Subcutaneous Injections

Skill 17.2
Subcutaneous Heparin

Skill 17.3
Intramuscular Injections

Skill 17.4
Intradermal Injections

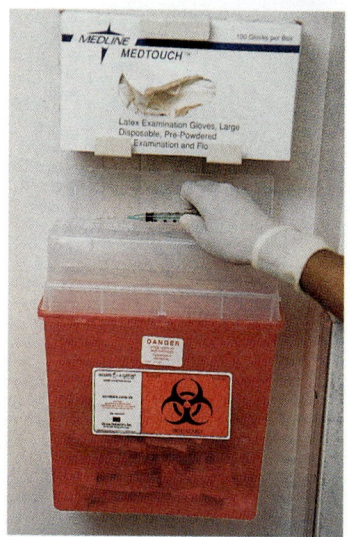

Injections instill medications into body tissues for systemic absorption (see box below). Injected drugs act more quickly than oral medications, and these routes may be used when clients are vomiting, cannot swallow, and/or are restricted from taking oral fluids.

Injections are invasive, and strict aseptic technique is required during preparation and administration to minimize the risk of infection. Injections involve some discomfort. Since risk of tissue or nerve damage exists, site selection is an important nursing concern. The nurse must monitor the client's response closely and be aware of potential side effects or allergic reactions.

SYRINGES

Disposable syringes are packaged separately, with or without a sterile needle. The parts of a syringe are shown in Figure 17-1. Syringes come in various sizes, ranging in capacity from 1 to 50 ml. A 2 to 3 ml syringe is adequate for intramuscular and subcutaneous injections and is marked in tenths (Figure 17-2, *A*). Some syringes have a Luer Lok, which allows the needle to be screwed into

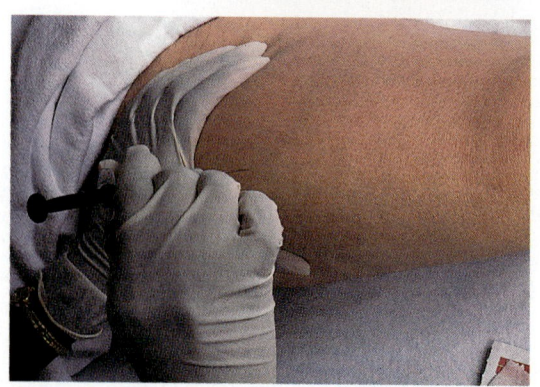

Types of Injections

1. *Subcutaneous* (SQ, SC): injection into tissues just below the dermis of the skin.
2. *Intramuscular* (IM): injection into the body of a muscle.
3. *Intradermal*: injection into the dermis just under the epidermis.

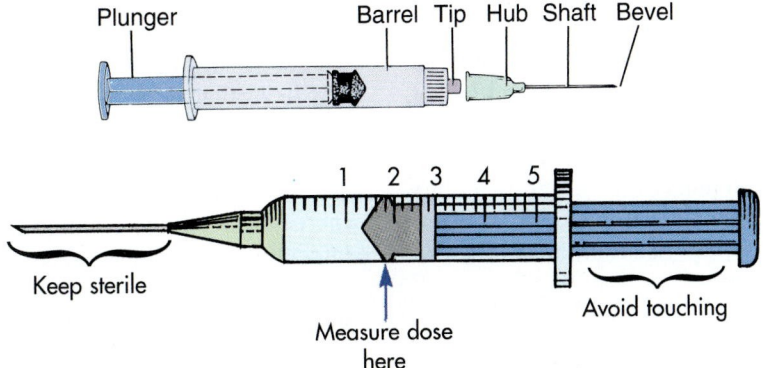

Figure 17-1 Parts of a syringe.

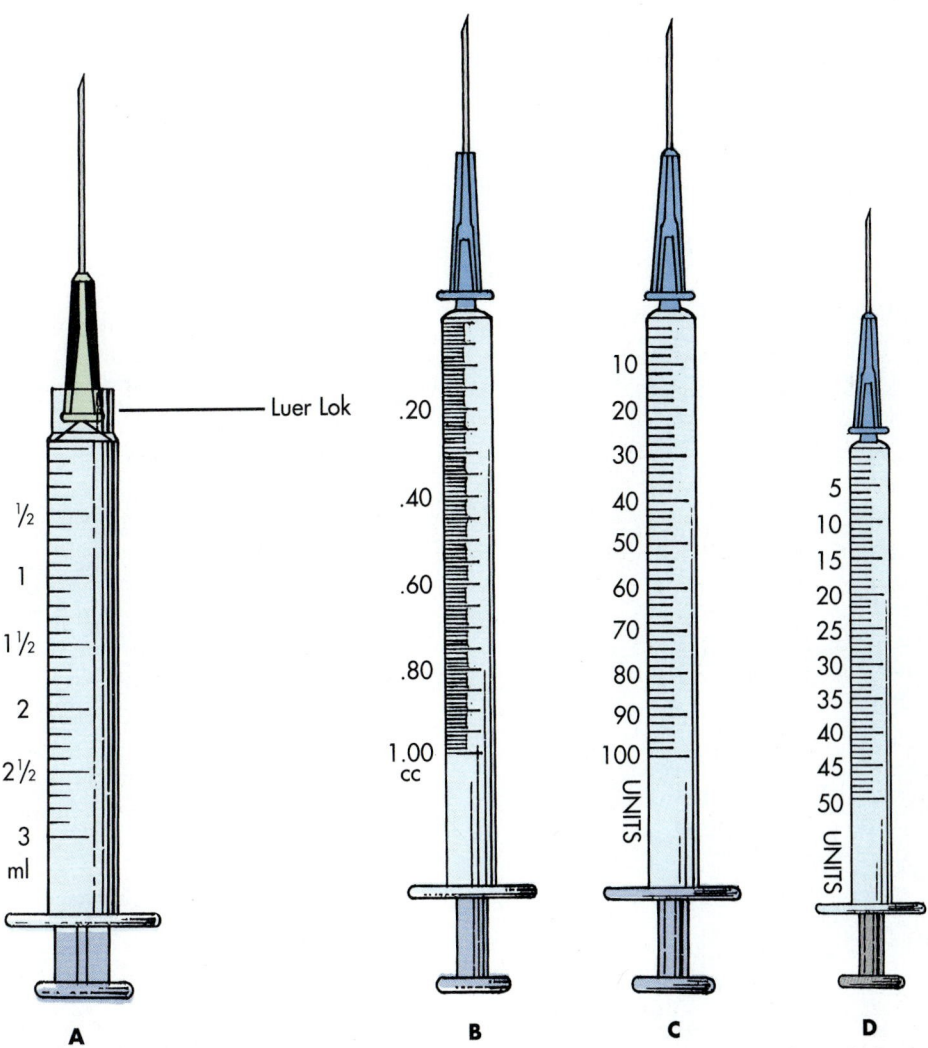

Figure 17-2 Types of syringes. **A,** Syringe with 3 ml capacity is marked in 0.1 (tenths); **B,** tuberculin syringe is marked in 0.01 (hundredths) for doses of less than 1 ml. Insulin syringes marked in units in two sizes: **C,** 100 U; or **D,** 50 U (lo-dose).

place securely. It is unusual to use a syringe larger than 5 ml for injections. Tuberculin (TB) syringes, which are marked in hundredths, are used to measure very small dosages (Figure 17-2, *B*).

Insulin syringes are manufactured to be compatible with insulin, specifically insulin equalling a strength of 100 units per ml. Insulin syringes are marked in units (Figure 17-2, *C* and *D*). Four sizes are available: 100 units (1 ml), 50 units (0.5 ml), 30 units (0.30 ml), and 25 units (0.25 ml). The syringes designed for smaller dosages are easier for diabetic clients with visual problems to read the numbering scales.

NEEDLES

A needle has three parts: the *hub,* which fits onto the tip of the syringe; the *shaft,* which connects to the hub; and the *bevel,* or slanted tip (see Figure 17-1). The nurse may handle the needle hub to ensure a tight fit on the syringe; however, the shaft and bevel must remain sterile.

Needles vary in length from ¼ to 3 inches. Often they are color-coded for ease of selection. Longer needles (1 to 1½ inches) are used for IM injections and shorter needles (⅜ to ⅝ inch) for SQ injections. The nurse may choose the needle length according to the client's size and weight and the type of tissue into which the drug is to be injected. Children and very small, thin adults generally require a shorter needle.

Gauge refers to the diameter of the needle. The smaller the needle gauge number, the larger is the needle diameter (Figure 17-3). For example, a typical 22-gauge 1½-inch needle used for IM injections is larger than a 25-gauge ⅝-inch needle used for SQ injections. The selection of a gauge depends on the viscosity of fluid to be injected.

NEEDLE STICK PREVENTION

Increased concerns about transmission of blood-borne infections from contaminated needle sticks has resulted in special prevention techniques and equipment. Needles are packaged with plastic caps to maintain sterility before the injection. It is recommended that these caps *not* be replaced on the needle after the injection. Special containers for the disposal of "sharps" are readily available on medicine carts and on the walls throughout most agencies. Containers are made so that only one hand needs to be used when disposing of uncapped needles. Keeping the other hand well away from the container prevents accidental injury (Figure 17-4). If it is necessary to delay syringe/needle disposal, as in an emergency, the cap can be replaced using the "scoop" or "one-handed" technique. The cap is placed on a firm surface, and using one hand only, the tip of the needle is placed into it (Figure 17-5).

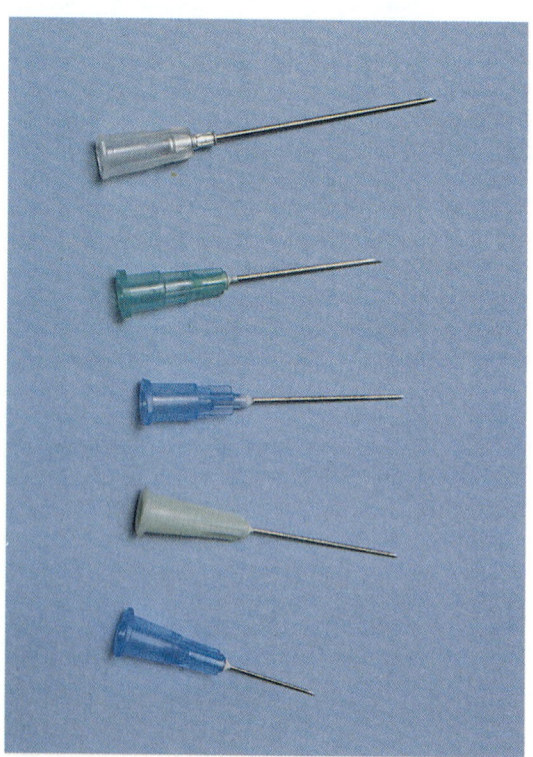

Figure 17-3 Needles *(top to bottom):* 19 gauge, 1½ inch length; 20 gauge, 1 inch length; 21 gauge, 1 inch length; 23 gauge, 1 inch length; and 25 gauge, ⅝ inch length.

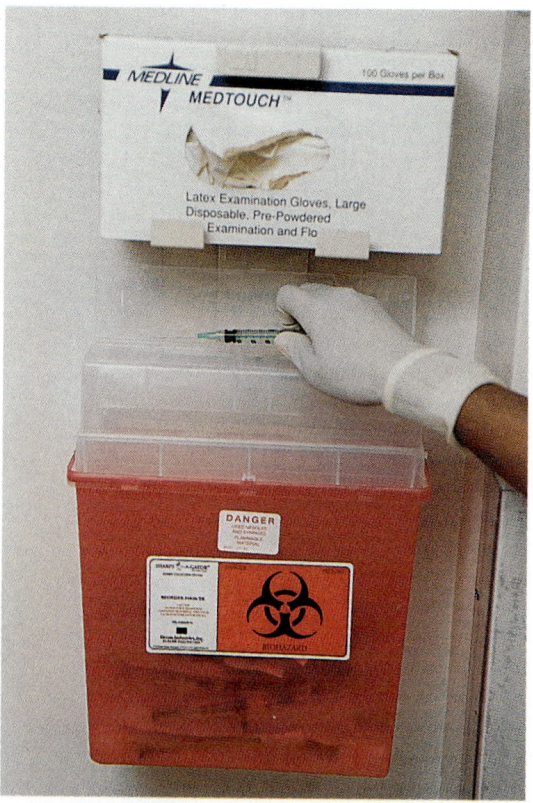

Figure 17-4 Sharps disposal using only one hand.

If a nurse is accidentally stuck with a sterile needle while preparing medication, there is no risk of infection transmission. The contaminated needle must be replaced before proceeding with the injection. If, however, a nurse is injured with a contaminated needle, specific steps must be taken to minimize risk for infection. An incident report is filed, the client is asked to be tested for hepatitis and acquired immunodeficiency syndrome (AIDS), and appropriate follow-up for the nurse is required. (Check agency policy.)

The Centers for Disease Control and Prevention (CDC) and the U.S. Occupational Safety and Health Administration (OSHA) have recommended use of "needleless" devices to reduce the risks to health care workers of needle sticks and sharps injuries (APIC, 1993). Special syringes are designed with a sheath that covers the needle as it is withdrawn from the skin, thus totally eliminating the chance of a needle stick injury (Figure 17-6). The syringe and sheath are disposed of together in a receptacle.

DISPOSABLE INJECTION UNITS

Single-dose, prefilled, disposable syringes are available for some medications. The Tubex and Carpujet injection systems include reusable plastic syringes that hold prefilled, disposable, sterile cartridge-needle units (Figure 17-7). Meperidine (Demerol) and morphine are supplied in sterile cartridges. The nurse slips the cartridge into the syringe, secures it, and expels air from the syringe. With these units the nurse does not have to withdraw medication from a vial and expels excess medication to measure the accurate dose. Most containers have a little more medication than the label indicates; therefore, it is essential to measure the correct volume rather than withdrawing the entire amount in the vial. These syringes also contain some air, which needs to be expelled before giving the injection.

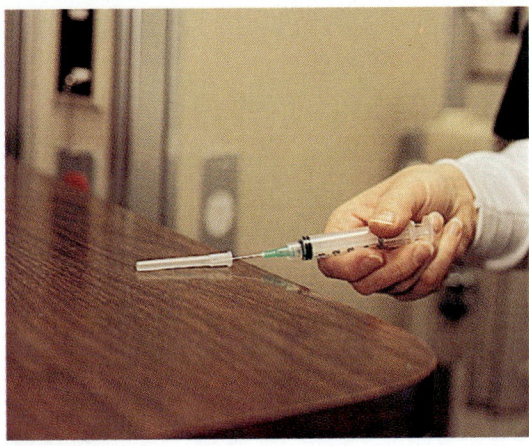

Figure 17-5 The scoop technique to prevent needle stick injuries.

MIXING MEDICATIONS IN SAME SYRINGE

To avoid giving two injections at one time, some medications can be mixed in the same syringe. It is essential that any medications mixed be compatible. Compatibility charts are available in most pharmacology books or the central pharmacy. When mixing medications, observe for changes in the appearance of the solution, which suggests incompatibility. When using multidose vials, it is essential to avoid injecting the vial's contents into medication from another vial or ampule. When mixing medications from a vial and ampule, always prepare the vial first. Then withdraw medication from the ampule.

To mix medications when one of the two is in a prefilled cartridge, draw back on the plunger of the syringe. Remove the needle from the syringe. Fill the syringe with the correct volume of medication from the prefilled cartridge by inserting the cartridge needle into the syringe tip.

PREPARATIONS OF INJECTABLE MEDICATIONS

Ampules contain single doses of injectable medication in a liquid form (Figure 17-8). The fluid enters the syringe

Text continues on p. 318.

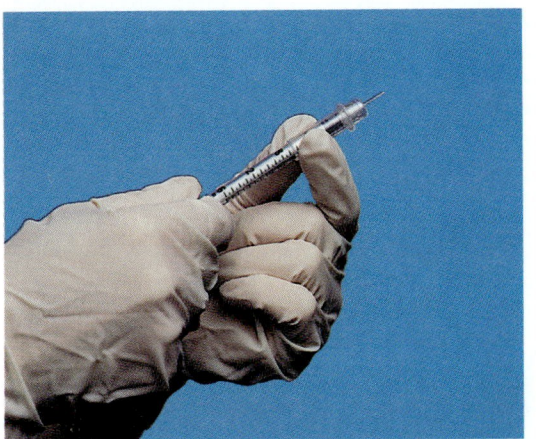

A

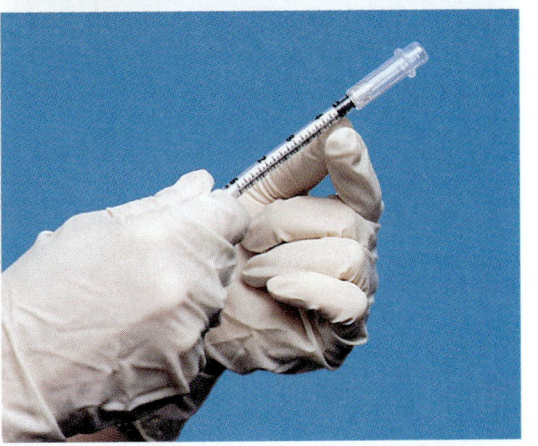

B

Figure 17-6 Needle with plastic guard to prevent needle sticks. **A,** Position of guard before injection. **B,** After injection the guard locks in place, covering the needle.

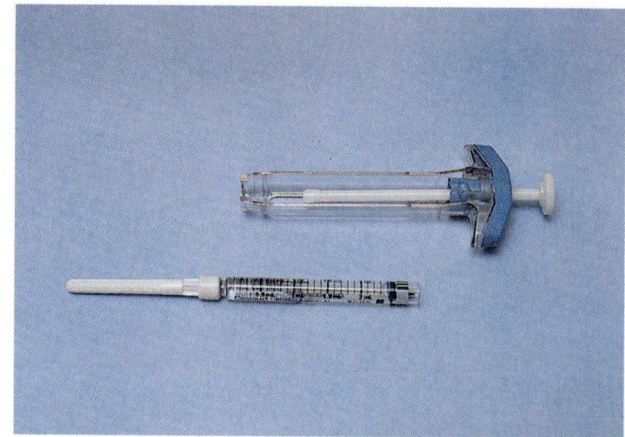
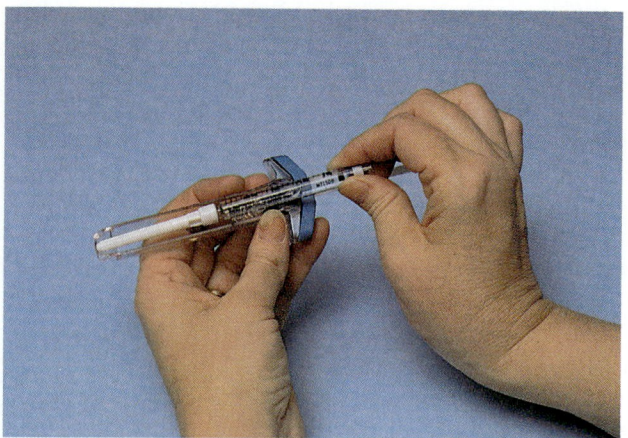
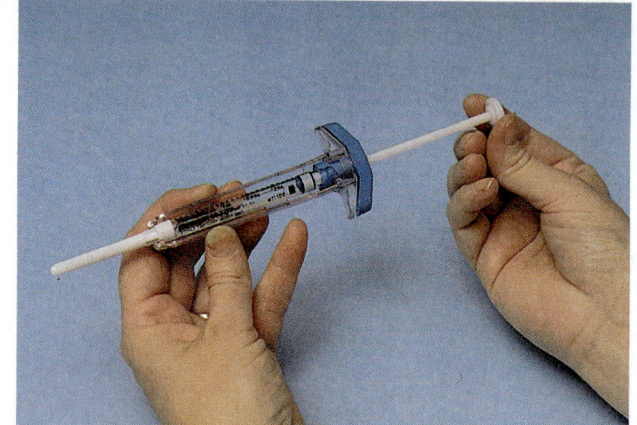

Figure 17-7 **A,** Carpoject syringe and prefilled sterile cartridge with needle. **B,** Assembling the Carpoject. **C,** Cartridge locks at needle end; plunger screws into opposite end.

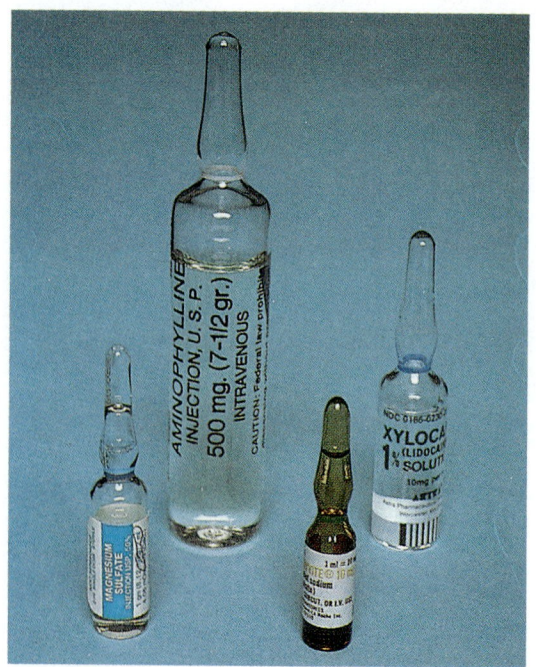

Figure 17-8 Medication in ampules.

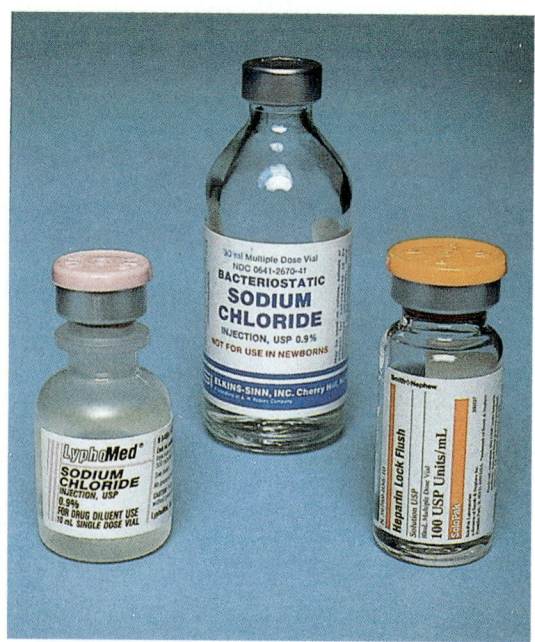

Figure 17-9 Medication in vials. Rubber top must be cleansed with alcohol when vial is reused.

Table 17-1 **Drawing up Medication from an Ampule**

Steps	Rationale
1. Remove fluid from neck of ampule by tapping top of ampule lightly and quickly with finger, quickly moving down in vertical direction or using a swirling motion.	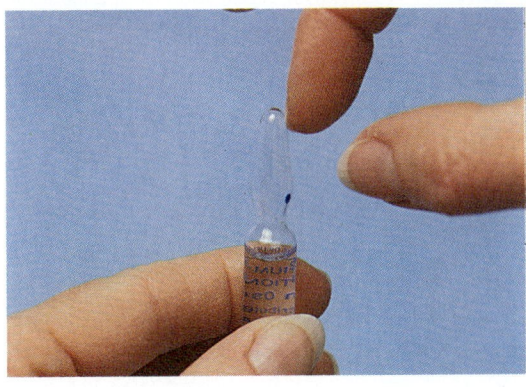
2. Place small gauze pad or unwrapped alcohol swab around neck of ampule.	Protects nurse's fingers from trauma as glass tip is broken off. Avoid wrapping wet alcohol swab around top of ampule, since alcohol may leak into ampule.
3. Break neck of ampule quickly and firmly away from hands. 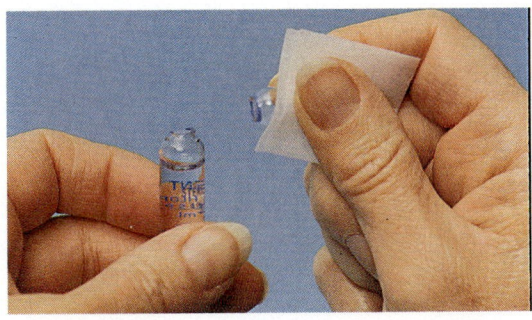	Prevents shattering glass toward or in nurse's fingers or face.
4. Draw up medication. Insert syringe needle into center of ampule opening.	A filter needle may be used for this purpose. If filter needle is not used and it is suspected that glass fragments are in an ampule, discard it and begin again.
5. Aspirate medication from ampule into syringe by gently pulling back on plunger.	Withdrawal of plunger creates negative pressure within syringe barrel, which pulls fluid into syringe.
	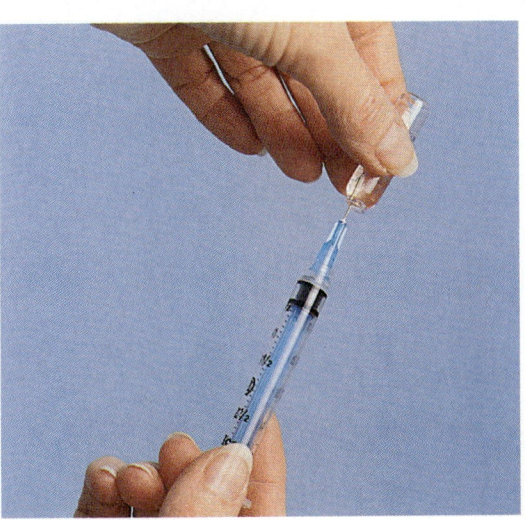

Continued.

6. Alternative for withdrawing medication from an ampule. Keep needle tip below surface of liquid. Tip ampule to bring fluid within reach of needle.

Prevents aspiration of air bubbles.

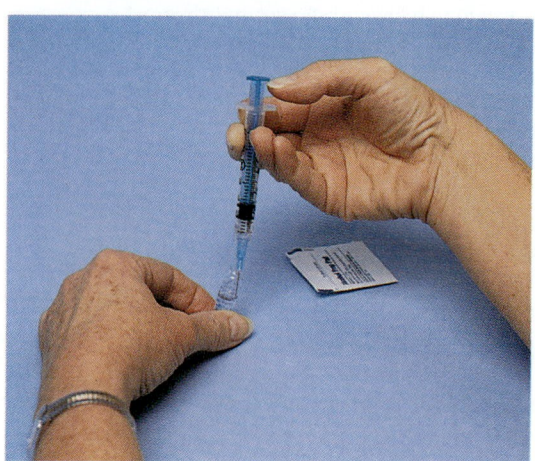

7. If air bubbles are aspirated, remove needle from ampule and hold syringe with needle pointing directly up. Tap side of syringe so that air bubbles rise toward needle. Draw back slightly on plunger, and then push the plunger upward to eject air until 1 drop of fluid is visible on the tip of the needle.

Pulling back on plunger allows fluid within needle to enter barrel so fluid is not expelled. Air at top of barrel and within needle is then expelled.

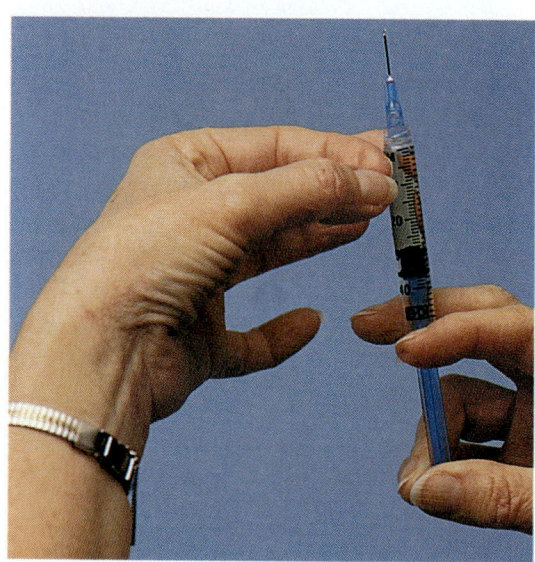

8. If syringe contains excess fluid, hold syringe vertically with needle tip up and slanted slightly toward sink or receptacle, and eject excess fluid into sink. Recheck fluid level in syringe by holding it vertically to measure accurate dose.

Position of needle allows medication to be expelled without it flowing down needle shaft. If necessary, flick sryinge and needle sharply to eliminate fluid from outside of needle.

9. If needle touched rim of ampule, it should be changed. Cover needle with safety cap.

Maintains sterility of needle.

10. Change the needle if irritating medication may be on needle shaft or if needle tip damage or contamination is suspected.

Needle point can be dulled by contact with glass. By changing needle, pain of injection is minimized (Newton, Newton, and Fudin, 1992). New needle also prevents tracking medication through skin and subcutaneous tissues.

11. Dispose of used needles in puncture-proof and leak-proof container.

Table 17-2 **Drawing up Medication from a Vial**

Steps	Rationale
1. Remove cap covering top of unused vial to expose sterile rubber seal, keeping seal sterile. If using a multidose vial that has been used before, firmly wipe off surface of rubber seal with alcohol swab using friction.	Vial comes packaged with cap to maintain sterility of rubber seal. Cap cannot be replaced after removal.
2. Pick up syringe and remove needle cap. Pull back on plunger to draw amount of air into syringe equivalent to volume of medication to be aspirated from vial.	Prevents buildup of negative pressure in vial when aspirating medication.
3. Insert tip of needle through center of rubber seal.	Center of seal is thinner and easier to penetrate.

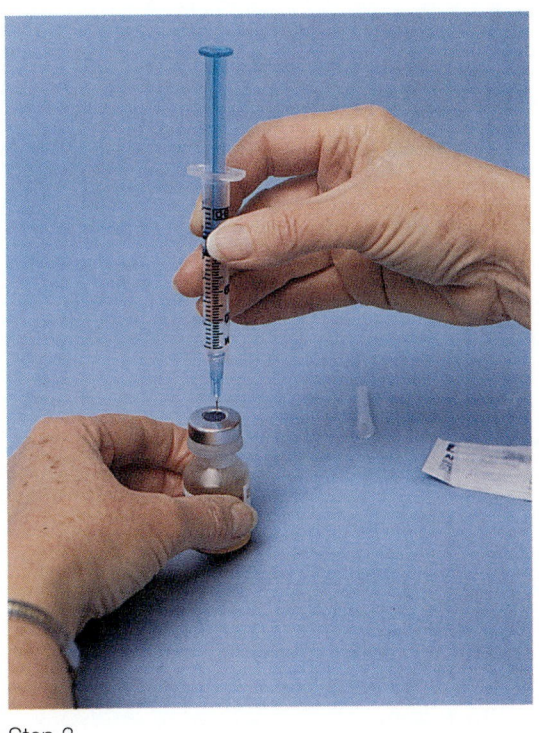

Step 3

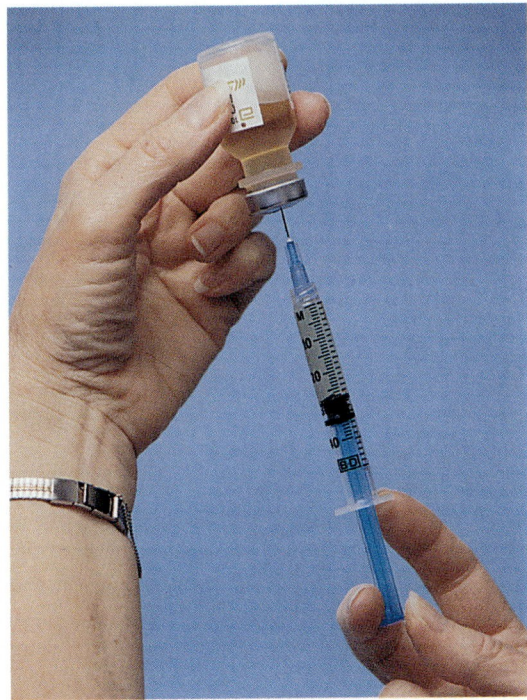

Step 5

Steps	Rationale
4. Inject air into vial, holding on to plunger.	Plunger may be forced backward by air pressure within vial.
5. Invert vial while keeping firm hold on syringe and plunger.	Allows fluid to settle in lower half of container.
6. Keep tip of needle below fluid level.	Prevents aspiration of air.
7. Allow air pressure to fill syringe gradually with medication, or pull back slightly on plunger.	Positive pressure within vial forces fluid into syringe.
8. Tap side of syringe barrel carefully to dislodge any air bubbles, and eject any air remaining at top of syringe into vial.	Accumulation of air displaces medication and may cause dosage errors. Draw up the exact volume of medication.
9. When correct volume is obtained, remove needle from vial by pulling on barrel of syringe.	Pulling plunger rather than barrel causes separation from barrel and loss of medication.
10. Label multidose vial with date, time, and initials.	Check agency policy for expiration regulations.

Table 17-3 **Reconstituting Medications from a Powder**

Steps	Rationale
1. Remove metal cap covering vial containing powdered medication and vial containing diluent.	Cap prevents contamination of rubber seal.
2. Draw up diluent into syringe as before (see Table 17-2, Steps 2 to 9).	Label may specify use of sterile water, normal saline, or special diluent provided with the medication.
3. Insert tip of syringe needle through center of rubber seal of vial of powdered medication. Inject diluent into vial. Remove needle.	Diluent begins to dissolve and reconstitute medication.
4. Withdraw needle and mix medication by gently rolling vial between hands until completely dissolved.	Dry, powdered drugs usually dissolve easily. Shaking vigorously tends to produce bubbles.
5. Once diluent has been added, concentration of medication (mg/ml) determines dose to be given.	

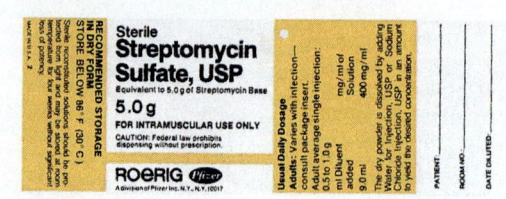

Step 5 Medication label for powdered drug. (From Gray D: *Calculate with confidence*, St. Louis, 1994, Mosby.)

easily with aspiration because no vacuum exists within the ampule.

A vial is a single-dose or multidose container with a rubber seal at the top (Figure 17-9). A cap protects the seal until it is used and cannot be replaced. Vials may contain liquid or dry forms of medications; drugs that are unstable in solution are packaged in dry form. The vial label specifies the liquid to use to dissolve the dry drug and the amount needed to prepare a desired drug concentration. Air must be injected into it to permit easy withdrawal of the solution.

Tables 17-1 through 17-4 describe the steps and rationale for drawing up medications from ampules and vials and reconstituting medication from a powder.

Nursing Diagnosis

Nursing diagnoses may be based on therapeutic effects or side effects of prescribed medications (see Chapter 16, p. 289).

Skill 17.1 | **Subcutaneous Injections (Includes Insulin)**

An SQ injection involves depositing medication into the loose connective tissue underlying the dermis (Figure 17-10). Subcutaneous tissue is not as richly supplied with blood vessels as muscle; thus drugs are absorbed more slowly than those given IM. Drugs given SQ include insulin, heparin, tetanus toxoid, allergy medications, vitamin B$_{12}$, and morphine.

The rate of absorption is affected by anything affecting blood flow to tissues, such as physical exercise or the local application of hot or cold compresses. Conditions such as circulatory shock or occlusive vascular disease impair client's blood flow and may prevent or delay absorption (Newton, Newton, and Fudin, 1992).

Only small doses of medications (0.5 to 1 ml) should be given SQ. The subcutaneous tissue is sensitive to irri-

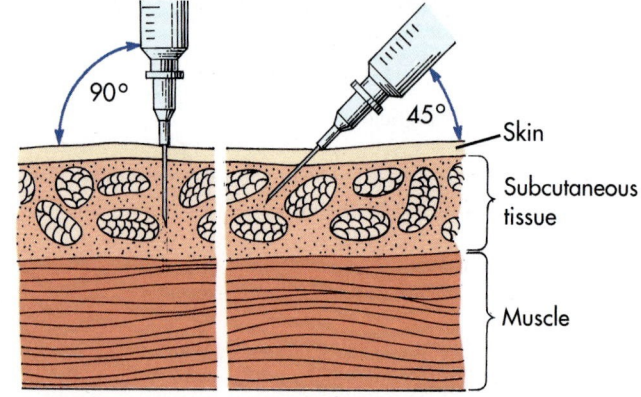

Figure 17-10 Subcutaneous injection. Angle and needle length depend on the thickness of skinfold.

Table 17-4 **Mixing Medications from Vials**

1. Cleanse tops of both vials with alcohol wipe.

2. Take syringe and aspirate volume of air equivalent to first medication's dosage (vial A).

   Air introduced into vial prevents a vacuum when medication is withdrawn.

3. Inject air into vial A, making sure needle does not touch solution. Withdraw needle.

   Prevents cross-contamination.

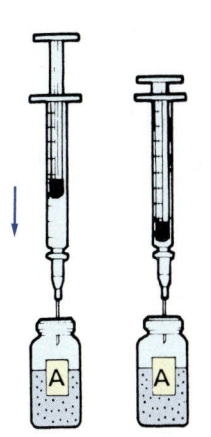

Step 3 Injecting air into vial A.

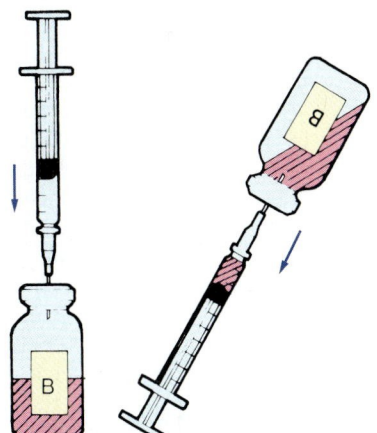

Step 4 Injecting air into vial B and withdrawing dose.

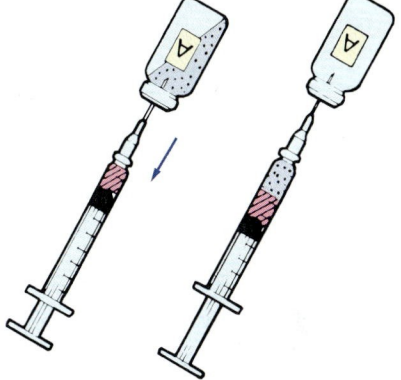

Step 6 Withdrawing medication from vial A; medications are now mixed.

4. Repeat with vial B. Without removing needle from vial B, fill syringe with proper volume of medication from vial.

5. Calculate total volume of medication by adding volume of both prescribed medications.

6. Insert needle of syringe into vial A, being careful not to push plunger and expel medication into vial. Invert vial and carefully withdraw the exact amount of medication required into syringe.

   Exact measurement is essential because medications are now mixed and cannot be readjusted without discarding entire amount and starting again.

---

tating solutions and large volumes of medications. Medications collecting within the tissues can cause sterile abscesses, which appear as hardened, painful lumps.

The sites for SQ injections are shown in Figure 17-11. The best sites include the outer aspect of the upper arms, the abdomen, and the anterior thighs. The upper abdomen is the best injection site for clients with little peripheral subcutaneous tissue. These areas are easily accessible for clients who self-administer medication. Injection sites should be free of infection, skin lesions, scars, bony prominences, and large underlying muscles or nerves.

Body weight influences the depth of the subcutaneous layer and is the criterion for selecting needle length and angle of insertion. Generally, a 25-gauge $\frac{3}{8}$- to $\frac{1}{2}$-inch needle with a medium bevel inserted at a 90-degree angle deposits medication into subcutaneous tissue of a normal-sized client. A $\frac{5}{8}$-inch needle is inserted at a 45-degree angle.

If a client is obese, the skin is pinched, and a longer needle will avoid the fatty tissue at the base of the skinfold. The preferred needle length is one-half the width of the skinfold. A $\frac{7}{8}$-inch needle is the longest needle appropriate for SQ use. In thin clients the shorter needle at a 45-degree angle is appropriate.

SPECIAL CONSIDERATIONS FOR ADMINISTRATION OF INSULIN

Insulin is the hormone used to treat diabetes. Often, clients with diabetes receive a combination of different types of insulin to control their blood sugar levels. Regular, unmodified insulin is a clear solution. The other types

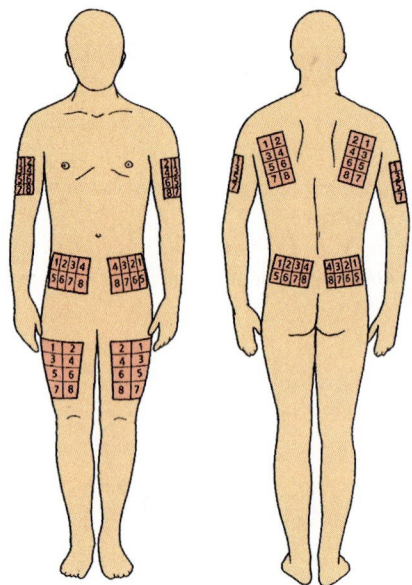

Figure 17-11 Sites recommended for subcutaneous injections.

of insulin are cloudy solutions because of the addition of a protein, which slows absorption. Table 17-5 compares effects of various insulin preparations. General guidelines related to insulin administration are listed in the box at right.

EQUIPMENT

Syringe (1 to 3 ml)
Needle (27 to 25 gauge, 3/8 to 5/8 inch)
Medication
Antiseptic swabs (e.g., alcohol)
For insulin
    Multidose (U-100) vial (Figure 17-12)
    U-100 insulin syringe with needle; 100 units/1 ml, 50
      units/0.5 ml, 30 units/0.30 ml, 25 units/0.25 ml
    Disposable gloves

General Guidelines for Insulin Administration

1. Store insulin in cool, dry place. It does *not* need refrigeration for short-term storage.
2. A variety of insulin preparations are available (Table 17-5). Be certain the correct form is prepared. Clients should consistently use the same form in the hospital as at home.
3. Insulin should be administered as ordered, usually 30 minutes before meals. **Orders may indicate AC breakfast only or AC both breakfast and dinner depending on individual needs.**
4. If client is NPO for diagnostic tests, hold insulin until client can eat. Check with the physician regarding insulin administration before surgery or diagnostic tests.
5. Before administering, review available laboratory results, including serum glucose and blood glucose monitoring (BGM): normal range is 80-120. Abnormal results may indicate need for dosage adjustment. The physician may specify parameters for a sliding scale and when to be called.
6. If a client has received insulin and is unable to eat food, replace it by contacting a dietitian. If oral intake is refused, the physician may order parenteral glucose.
7. When the dose of insulin is being adjusted, watch for signs of hypoglycemia and encourage the client to report symptoms (e.g., weakness, headache, visual disturbances, ataxia).
8. Administer mixed insulin (regular and NPH) within 5 minutes of preparation. Regular insulin binds with NPH, which reduces the action of the regular insulin.
9. When mixing insulin, fill syringe with regular insulin first to prevent transmission of NPH or Lente into the regular insulin (see Table 17-4). Accuracy is essential. Some agencies require that the dose is checked with an RN (see agency policy).
10. Many factors can influence insulin requirements, including dietary intake, level of exercise, stress, and infection.

Table 17-5 Comparison of Insulin Preparations

Action	Preparations	Actions in hours		
		Onset	Peak	Duration
Rapid or short	Regular (Humulin-R, beef, pork)	$^1/_2$-1	2-4	6-8
Intermediate	Humulin-N, NPH	1-2	8-12	24-28
Long	Protamine zinc suspension (PZI)	4-8	14-24	36
	Ultralente			

Modified from Edmunds MW: *Introduction to clinical pharmacology,* St. Louis, 1991, Mosby.

NOTE: Regular insulin can be mixed with any other type of insulin. Lente insulins can be mixed with each other and regular insulin but should not be mixed with any other types of insulin.

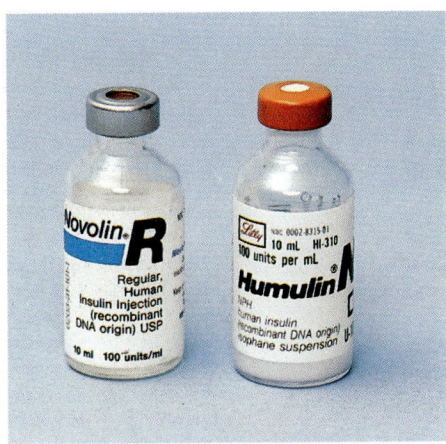

Figure 17-12 Multidose vials of regular (clear) and NPH (cloudy) insulin.

Assessment

1. Review physician's medication order for client's name, drug name, dose, and time and route of administration.
2. Gather information pertinent to drug(s) ordered: action, purpose, time of onset and peak action, normal dosage, common side effects, and nursing implications.
3. Assess for factors that may contraindicate SQ injections, such as circulatory shock or reduced local tissue perfusion.

4. Assess client's medical history, history of allergies, and medication history.
5. Assess client's knowledge regarding medication to be received. **Information may pose implications for client education. Assessment may also reveal drug use problems at home.**
6. Observe client's verbal and nonverbal responses toward injection. Injections can be painful. **Clients may experience considerable anxiety, which can increase pain.**
7. Ask if client prefers to administer own injection if accustomed to doing so. If learning to do own injections, reinforce the learning process (see Chapter 39).

Planning

Expected outcomes focus on safe, effective administration of injection with minimal anxiety and discomfort.

EXPECTED OUTCOMES

1. Client demonstrates improved clinical condition after medication administration.
2. Client denies adverse reactions or side effects by discharge.
3. Client's tissues remain soft and supple at the injection site.

For insulin

4. Client maintains serum glucose levels between 80 and 120.

Implementation

Steps	Rationale
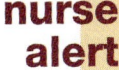 Review five "rights" for administration of medications.	
1. See Standard Protocol (Chapter 1, p. 5).	
2. Before drawing up insulin, gently roll vial in palm of hands. Do not shake.	Resuspends insulin. Exception: do not mix short-acting insulin (ADA, 1995).
3. Prepare medication in syringe.	
4. Select appropriate injection site. Inspect skin's surface over sites for bruises, inflammation, or edema. Palpate site for masses, edema, or tenderness.	
5. Rotate injection site daily. A chart may be kept in nursing Kardex or care plan to keep track of injection sites.	Overuse of a single site can result in tissue damage, which can interfere with drug absorption. Current information suggests that as long as tissues remain healthy, rotating sites may not be as critical (Newton, Newton, and Fudin, 1992).

Steps	Rationale
6. Be sure needle size is correct by grasping skinfold at site with thumb and forefinger. Measure skinfold from top to bottom, and be sure needle is approximately one-half this length.	Ensures that needle will be injected into subcutaneous tissue.
7. Assist client to comfortable position and ask client to relax arm, leg, or abdomen depending on site chosen for injection.	Relaxation of area minimizes discomfort during injection. Promoting client's comfort through positioning and distraction helps reduce anxiety.
8. Talk with client about subject of interest. Keep needle out of line of vision.	Minimizes anxiety.
9. Relocate site using anatomical landmarks (see Figure 17-11).	Correct site avoids injury to underlying nerves, bone, or blood vessels.
10. Cleanse site with an antiseptic swab. Apply swab at center of site and rotate outward in circular direction for about 5 cm (2 inches) (Figure 17-13).	Mechanical action removes microorganisms.
11. Hold swab between fingers of nondominant hand or place near site.	Swab remains readily accessible for when needle is withdrawn.
12. Remove needle cap or sheath from needle by pulling it straight off.	Prevents needle from touching sides of cap and prevents contamination.
13. Hold syringe between thumb and forefinger of dominant hand as if grasping dart (Figure 17-14), or hold syringe across tops of fingertips.	Facilitates quick, smooth injection.

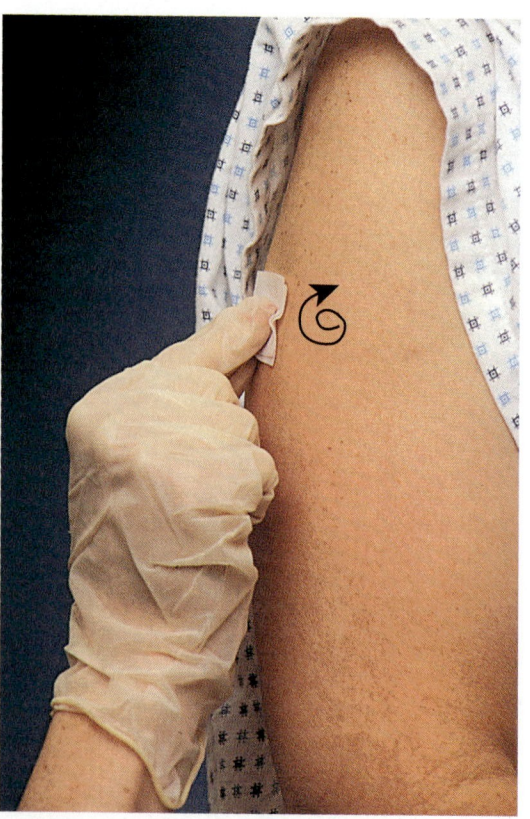

Figure 17-13 Cleansing site with circular motion.

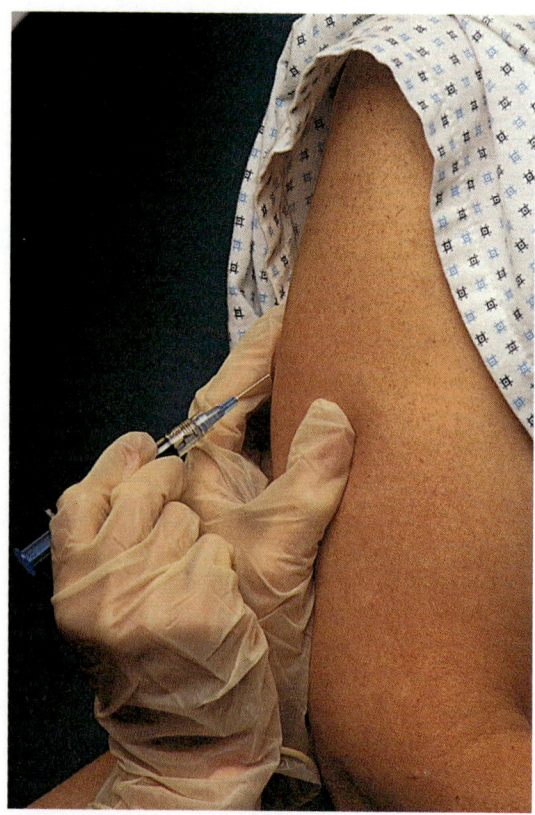

Figure 17-14 Holding syringe as if grasping a dart.

Steps	Rationale

14. *Average-sized client*
    a. Spread skin tightly across injection site. Exception: ADA (1995) recommends clients injecting insulin should lightly grasp fold of skin.
    b. Inject needle quickly and firmly at 90-degree angle.
	Needle penetrates tight skin easier than loose skin.
	
	Quick, firm insertion minimizes discomfort. Ninety-degree angle is easier for clients to learn for self-injection.

15. *Thin client*
    a. Pinch skin at site.
    b. Inject needle quickly and firmly at 45-degree angle.
16. *Obese client*
    a. Pinch skin at site and inject needle below tissue fold.
    b. Angle of insertion may be between 45 and 90 degrees to ensure medication reaches subcutaneous tissue.
        (1) If 5 cm (2 inches) of tissue can be grasped, needle is inserted at a 90-degree angle.
        (2) If 2.5 cm (1 inch) of tissue can be grasped, needle is inserted at a 45-degree angle.
17. After needle enters site, grasp lower end of syringe barrel with nondominant hand. Move dominant hand to end of plunger. Avoid moving syringe (Figure 17-15).
	Pinching and angle ensure that medication reaches subcutaneous tissues rather than muscle.
	
	Obese clients have fatty layer of tissue above subcutaneous layer. Pinching skin elevates subcutaneous tissue.
	
	Movement of syringe may displace needle and cause discomfort.

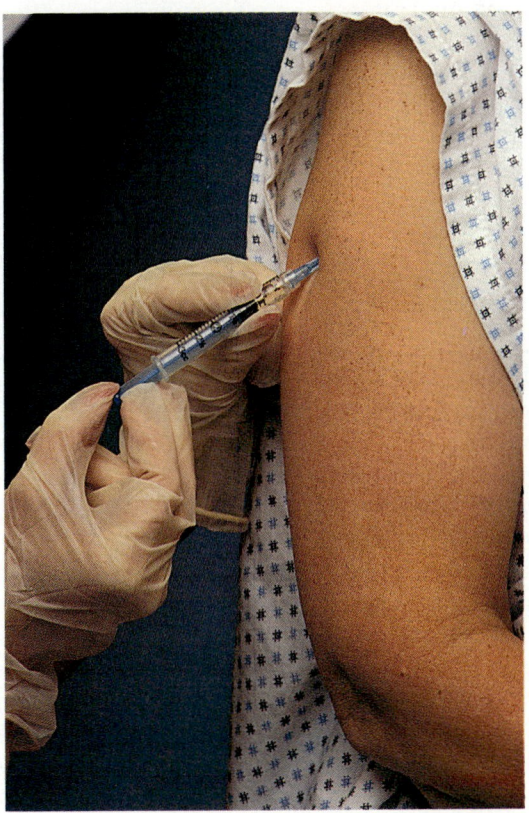

Figure 17-15 Pull back on plunger to aspirate.

Steps	Rationale
18. Unless contraindicated, gently pull back on plunger to aspirate. If blood appears in syringe, withdraw needle, discard medication and syringe properly, and repeat procedure. (ADA [1995] does not recommend clients regularly aspirate.)	Aspiration of blood into syringe indicates IV placement of needle. Aspiration is contraindicated with heparin (see Skill 17.2).
19. If no blood appears, inject medication slowly.	Slow injection reduces pain and trauma.
20. Withdraw needle quickly while placing antiseptic swab gently above or over site.	Supporting tissues around injection site minimizes discomfort during needle withdrawal.
21. Unless contraindicated, massage site lightly.	Stimulates circulation and improves drug distribution and absorption. Massage is contraindicated with insulin.
22. Using one hand, discard uncapped needle and attached syringe in appropriately labeled receptacle.	Prevents injury to client and health care personnel. CDC (1988) warns that capping needles increases risk of needle stick.
23. See Completion Protocol (Chapter 1, p. 6).	

Evaluation

1. Observe client's response to medication 30 minutes after injection to determine effectiveness of drug and undesired side effects.
2. Identify any indications of side effects or adverse reactions.
3. Inspect and palpate injection site for lumps, tenderness, or swelling.

For insulin

4. Monitor blood glucose readings before meals, at bedtime, and when possibility of hypoglycemia is evident.

UNEXPECTED OUTCOMES AND RELATED INTERVENTIONS

1. Client complains of localized pain or continued burning at injection site.
   a. Indicates potential injury to nerve or tissues.
   b. Provide warm or cool compresses for comfort.
2. Client displays signs of urticaria, eczema, pruritus, wheezing, and dyspnea.
   a. Indicates possible allergy.
   b. Report to physician for treatment of symptoms and change medication orders.

SAMPLE DOCUMENTATION

See Medication Administration Record and Diabetic Management Record, Appendix A.

Skill 17.2 | Subcutaneous Heparin

Heparin therapy may be prescribed to provide therapeutic anticoagulation to reduce the risk of thrombus formation in immobilized clients; clients with cardiovascular disease, including after cardiac surgery; and clients with cancer. It is administered SQ, although some clients may receive it IV. Heparin is an anticoagulant that suppresses clot formation; therefore, a major risk of too much medication is bleeding. The site most frequently recommended for heparin injections is the abdomen. Injections should not be given within 2 inches of the umbilicus, which has large umbilical veins that should be avoided. Other sites include the subscapular area and upper ventral or dorsal gluteal areas. Care must be taken not to administer heparin into the muscle, which could result in hematomas, pain, and irritation at the injection site. Muscular areas of the legs and arms, which are more likely to bleed or bruise, should be avoided. Because heparin inactivates prothrombin and prevents formation of thromboplastin, its therapeutic range is measured using a blood test to measure the activated partial thromboplastin time (APTT). The desired therapeutic range is $1\frac{1}{2}$ to $2\frac{1}{2}$ times the normal value. If shorter than 50 seconds, the dose of heparin should be increased; if longer than 100 seconds, the risk of spontaneous bleeding is high (Pagana and Pagana, 1992).

EQUIPMENT

Tuberculin or 1 to 3 ml syringe
2 needles, one of which is $\frac{1}{2}$ to $\frac{5}{8}$ inches, 25 to 26 gauge
Alcohol wipes
Heparin in appropriate concentration
Disposable gloves

Assessment

1. Assess for preexisting conditions that may contraindicate the use of SQ heparin, including kidney disease, liver disease, blood dyscrasias, and chronic ulcerative colitis (McConnell, 1990).
2. Assess APTT levels. If greater than 100 seconds or $2\frac{1}{2}$ times the control, consult with the physician before administering prescribed dose.
3. Inspect possible injection sites for bruising or hardening of tissue. **These sites should be avoided.**

Planning

Expected outcomes focus on preventing clot formation or extension and maintaining tissue integrity.

EXPECTED OUTCOMES

1. Client maintains an APTT at therapeutic levels ($1\frac{1}{2}$ to $2\frac{1}{2}$ times the control value).
2. Client describes symptoms of bleeding to report to the physician.
3. Client lists ways to prevent injuries that could result in bleeding.

Implementation

Steps	Rationale
nurse alert Review five "rights" for administration of medications	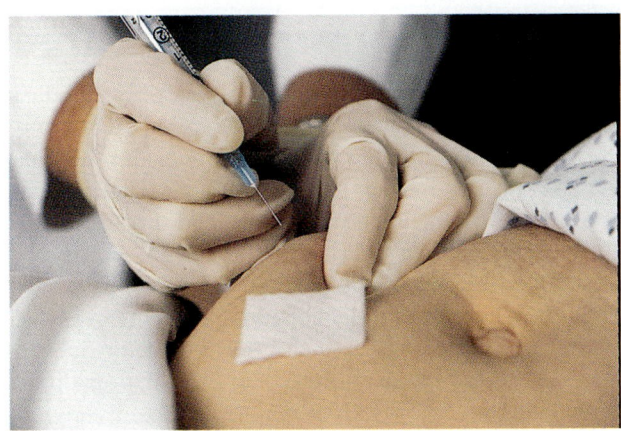 Figure 17-16 Giving SQ heparin in the abdomen.
1. See Standard Protocol (Chapter 1, p. 5).	
2. Draw up heparin in syringe (see Table 17-2).	
3. Change to a new 25- to 26-gauge needle, $\frac{1}{2}$ to $\frac{5}{8}$ inch long.	Reduces the risk of heparin entering tissues during injection.
4. Select appropriate site for administration (see Table 17-5). The lower abdomen between iliac crests and at least 5 cm (2 inches) from umbilicus is preferred. Avoid scarred or bruised tissue.	Avoids areas of muscular activity and decreases risk of capillary bleeding.
5. Cleanse site with an alcohol wipe using circular motion, moving from center outward approximately 5 cm (2 inches). Do not massage. Allow to dry.	Decreases pathogens on the skin and reduces risk of infection.
6. Grasp tissue, creating a tissue roll of $\frac{1}{2}$ inch and insert needle at 90-degree angle (Figure 17-16).	Minimizes tissue injury and hematoma formation.
7. Inject heparin slowly and withdraw needle quickly.	Minimizes discomfort.
8. Apply gentle pressure. Do not massage.	Massage of site increases risk of bruising.
9. Carefully dispose of needle and syringe in a puncture-resistant container.	Minimizes risk of accidental needle stick with contaminated needle.
10. Teach client to use a soft toothbrush and electric razor.	Reduces risk of injury that could cause bleeding.
11. See Completion Protocol (Chapter 1, p. 6).	

Evaluation

1. Monitor APTT for a therapeutic level (1½ to 2 times the control value).
2. Ask client to describe symptoms of bleeding to report to the physician.
3. Ask client to list ways to prevent injuries that could result in bleeding. (Apply to home situation.)

UNEXPECTED OUTCOMES AND RELATED INTERVENTIONS
APTT exceeds 100 seconds.
   a. Hold the dose and notify the physician for dosage adjustment.
   b. Observe for evidence of bleeding (bleeding gums, nosebleed, tarry black stools, hematuria, blood in stools, fall in hematocrit or blood pressure). Notify physician if these occur.
   c. Be prepared to administer protamine sulfate if ordered for the treatment of spontaneous bleeding.

SAMPLE DOCUMENTATION
Document heparin dose, site, and time, using standard medication administration record. (See Medication Administration Record, Appendix A.) In progress notes: 0900 Bruise (4 cm diameter) noted on RLQ, deep purple, soft, and nontender.

Skill 17.3 | # Intramuscular Injections

An injection given by the IM route deposits medication into deep muscle tissue. The vascularity of muscle tissue results in rapid drug absorption, and the muscle has few pain-sensing nerves. A larger volume of drug (up to 4 ml) can be injected because fluid spreads rapidly through the muscle's elastic fibers. The IM site is preferred for irritating drugs or more rapid or stronger effects. In some areas, IM injections are being replaced with the IV route (see Chapter 29). The IV route delivers an exact dose directly into the bloodstream, providing a rapid onset of action within minutes (Newton, Newton, and Fudin, 1992).

IM injections require a longer and larger-gauge needle to penetrate deep muscle tissue. Body weight also influences needle size selection. Generally, for the average adult, a 19- to 23-gauge, 1¼- to 1½-inch needle inserted at a 90-degree angle is appropriate. Older adults, malnourished clients, and children require a smaller needle. Emaciated muscles do not absorb medication well and should be avoided when possible.

Most IM injections involve a volume of 1 to 2 ml; however, a normal well-developed adult client can safely tolerate as much as 5 ml of medication in larger muscles such as the vastus lateralis. Smaller muscles require smaller amounts of medication. Children, older adults, and thin clients should be given no more than 1 ml at a single site (Whaley and Wong, 1995).

SITES FOR INTRAMUSCULAR INJECTIONS
When selecting an IM site, the nurse considers the following. Is the area free of infection or necrosis? Are there local areas of bruising or abrasions? What is the location of underlying bones, nerves, and major blood vessels? What volume of medication is to be given? Each site has certain advantages and disadvantages (see box at right.

Location of an appropriate site for IM injection involves ability to palpate anatomical landmarks accurately and knowledge of underlying nerves and major blood vessels. Presence of excessive fatty tissue may make location of bony structures difficult; with experience, however, accurate site location is achieved. Correct techniques for locating standard IM sites for injection are described in Table 17-6.

Advantages and Disadvantages of Intramuscular Injection Sites

Ventrogluteal. The ventrogluteal muscle is situated deep and away from major nerves and blood vessels and is a safe, relatively painless site for all clients. It is the preferred site for small or debilitated clients.

Vastus lateralis. The vastus lateralis muscle is a desired injection site for adults, children, and infants; however, it has small nerve endings resulting in discomfort after injection. The muscle is thick and well developed in persons by walking.

Dorsogluteal. The dorsogluteal muscle is the traditional site for IM injections; however, it is more dangerous because a risk exists of injuring the underlying sciatic nerve, causing permanent or partial paralysis of the involved leg. There is also risk of piercing major blood vessels. In clients with flabby, sagging tissues the site is difficult to locate. In children the muscle is too small until about 3 years of age.

Deltoid. The deltoid site is easily accessible, and the muscle is relatively small in many adults. The radial and ulnar nerves and brachial artery lie within the upper arm along the humerus. This site should be used only for volumes of 0.1 to 2 ml when other sites are inaccessible because of dressings or casts.

Table 17-6 **Locating Sites for Intramuscular Injections**

Site/steps	Figure

VENTROGLUTEAL SITE

1. Position client on either side with knee bent and upper leg slightly ahead of the bottom leg. Client may also remain supine or may be lying on abdomen. Instruct client to relax muscles to be injected.

2. Palpate the greater trochanter at the head of the femur and the anterior superior iliac spine. To locate the proper site, use the left hand when the client lies on the left side and the right hand when the client lies on the right side.

3. Place the palm of the hand over the greater trochanter and index finger on the anterior superior iliac spine. Point the thumb toward the client's groin and fingers toward the client's head.

4. Spread the middle finger back along the iliac crest toward the buttock as far as possible.

5. The injection site is the center of the triangle formed by your index and middle fingers.

6. Change hands as needed to spread skin taut to give injection. Use dominant hand to give injection.

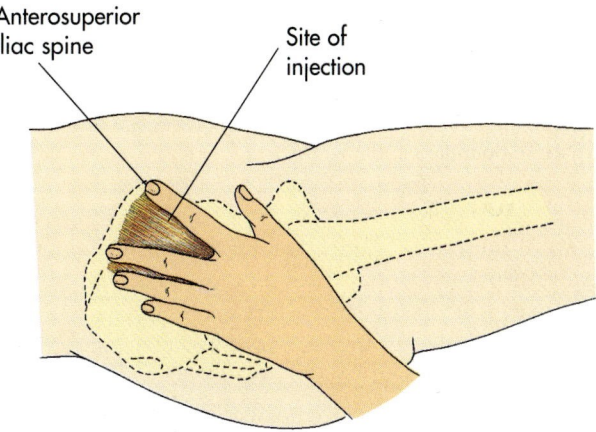

Step 1 Landmarks for ventrogluteal site.

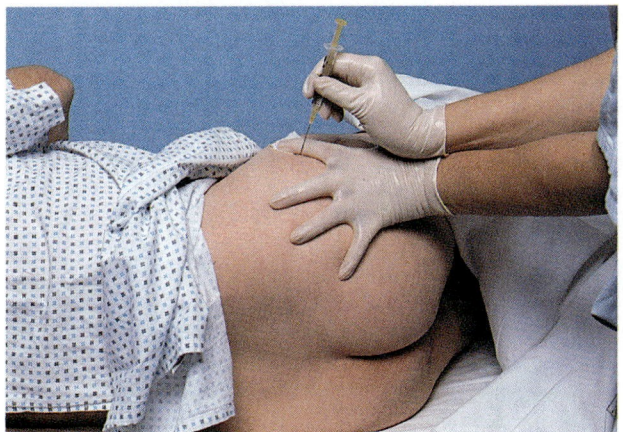

Step 3 Locating IM injection for ventrogluteal site.

VASTUS LATERALIS SITE

1. Client may be lying supine or sitting with site well exposed.

2. Place one hand above the knee and one hand below the greater trochanter of the femur.

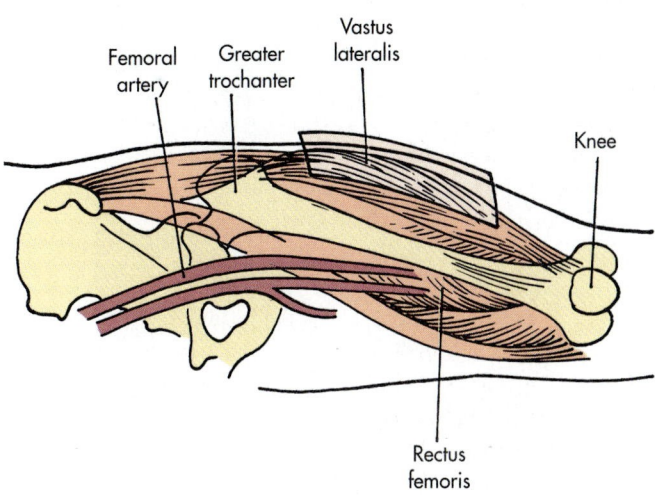

Step 2 Landmarks for vastus lateralis site.

Continued.

Table 17-6 **Locating Sites for Intramuscular Injections—cont'd**

Site/steps	Figure

VASTUS LATERALIS SITE—cont'd

3. Locate the midline of the anterior thigh and the midline of the thigh's lateral (outer) side.

4. The injection site is located within a rectangle formed by these boundaries.

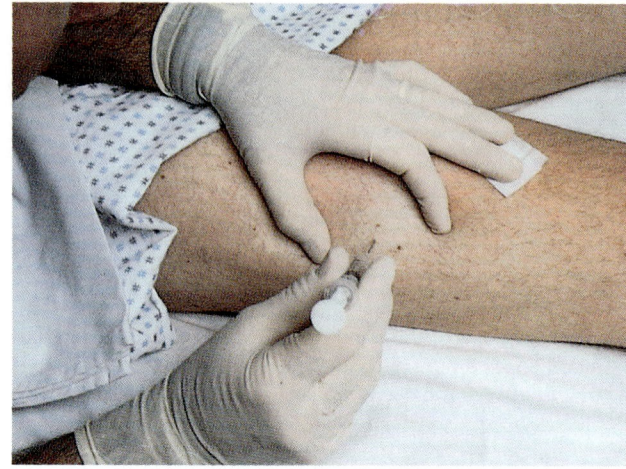

Step 4 Giving IM injection in vastus lateralis site.

DORSOGLUTEAL SITE IN UPPER OUTER QUADRANT OF BUTTOCK

1. Client may lie prone with toes turned medially or in a side-lying position with the upper leg flexed at the hip and knee.

2. Locate the posterosuperior iliac spine and the greater trochanter of the femur, and draw an imaginary line between the two anatomical landmarks.

3. The injection site is above and lateral to the line. The sciatic nerve runs parallel and below the line.

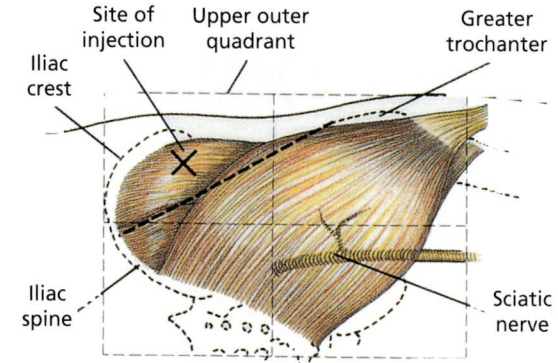

Step 1 Landmarks for dorsogluteal site.

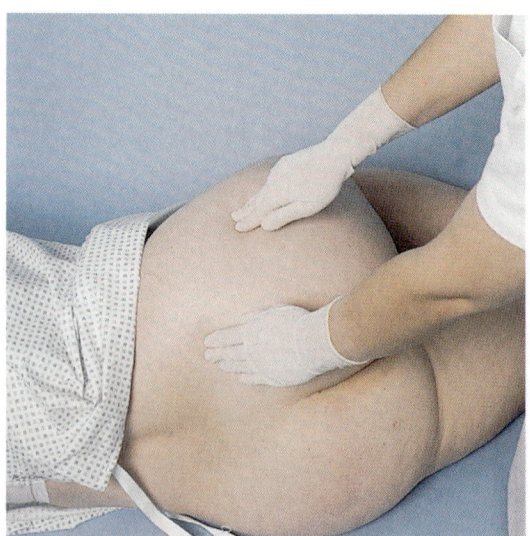

Step 2 Locating right dorsogluteal site (client is on left side).

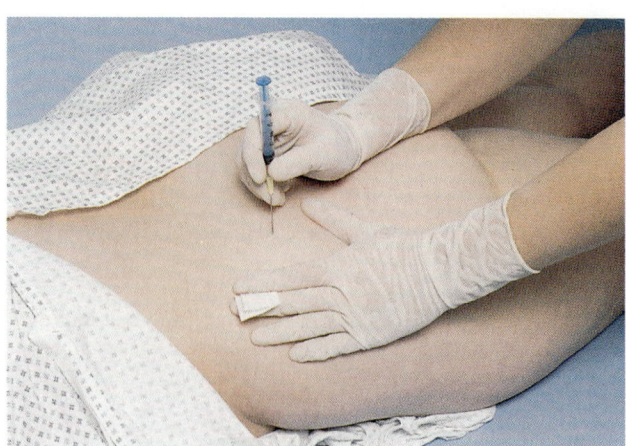

Step 3 Giving IM injection in left dorsogluteal site (client is prone).

Table 17-6 **Locating Sites for Intramuscular Injections—cont'd**

Site/steps	Figure

TO LOCATE DELTOID MUSCLE

1. Client may be sitting or lying down, exposing the upper arm and shoulder. A tight-fitting sleeve should be removed rather than rolled up.

2. Ask client to relax the arm at the side with the elbow flexed.

3. Palpate the lower edge of the acromion process, which forms the base of a triangle.

4. Place four fingers across the deltoid muscle, with the top finger along the acromion process.

5. The injection site is in the center of the triangle, three fingerwidths or 2.5 to 5 cm
(1 to 2 inches) below the acromion process.

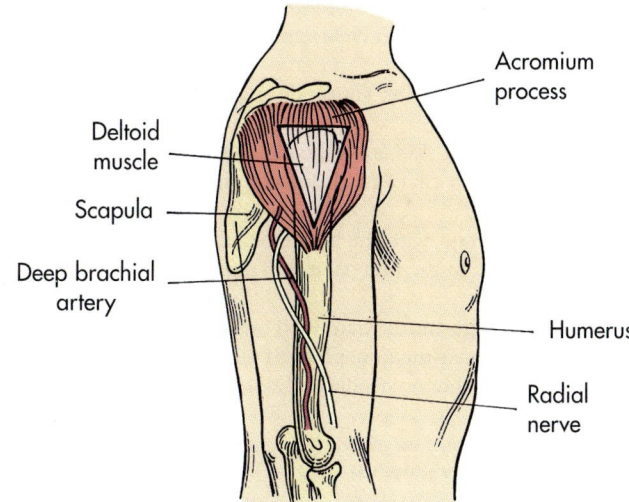

Step 3 Landmarks for deltoid site.

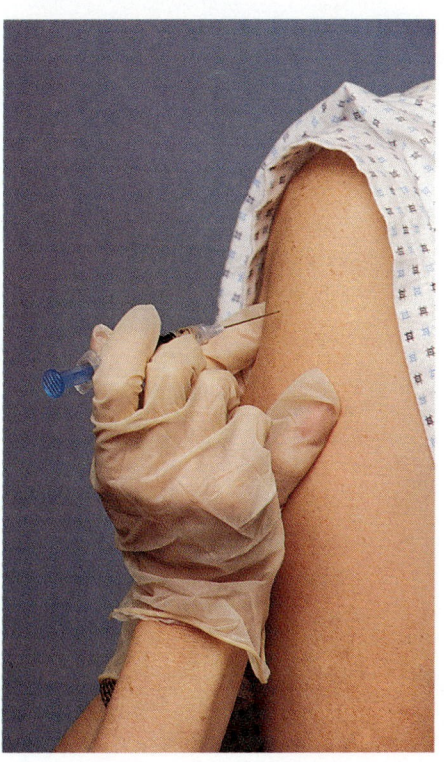

Step 5 Giving IM injection in deltoid site.

The Z-track method of IM injection minimizes tissue irritation by sealing the drug within muscle tissues. It is preferred when irritating preparations, such as iron or Vistaril, are given IM. An IM site in larger, deeper muscles such as the ventrogluteal is selected (Table 17-7).

Using an air lock involves injecting a small volume of air to clear the needle of medication, preventing tracking of the drug through the subcutaneous tissues. This is specifically recommended for iron dextran (Imferon) and DPT vaccine for diphtheria, pertussis (whooping cough), and tetanus toxoid. After preparing the proper dose, 0.2 ml of air is left in the syringe. The needle must be injected so that the air rises to the top. As the injection is completed, air clears the medication from the needle and seals the site (Figure 17-17).

EQUIPMENT

Syringe (1 to 3 ml)
Needle (1 to 1½ inch 22 gauge)
Prescribed medication
Antiseptic (alcohol) swab
Disposable gloves

Table 17-7 **Z-Track Technique**

Steps	Figure

1. Apply a new needle to the syringe after preparing the drug so no solution remains on the outside needle shaft.

2. Draw up 0.2 ml of air to create an air lock.

3. Prepare the site with an antiseptic swab.

4. Pull the overlying skin and subcutaneous tissues approximately 2.5 to 3.5 cm (1 to 1½ inches) laterally to the side.

5. Hold the skin taut with the nondominant hand while placing the needle to the hub deep into muscle.

6. Hold the syringe and aspirate with one hand. If there is no blood return on aspiration, proceed with injection. If blood is aspirated, withdraw needle and start again.

7. Inject the drug and air slowly. The needle remains inserted for 10 seconds to allow the medication to disperse evenly.

8. Release the skin after withdrawing the needle, which leaves a zigzag path that seals the needle track wherever tissue planes slide across each other.

9. Do not massage the injection site. The drug is less likely to escape from the muscle tissue.

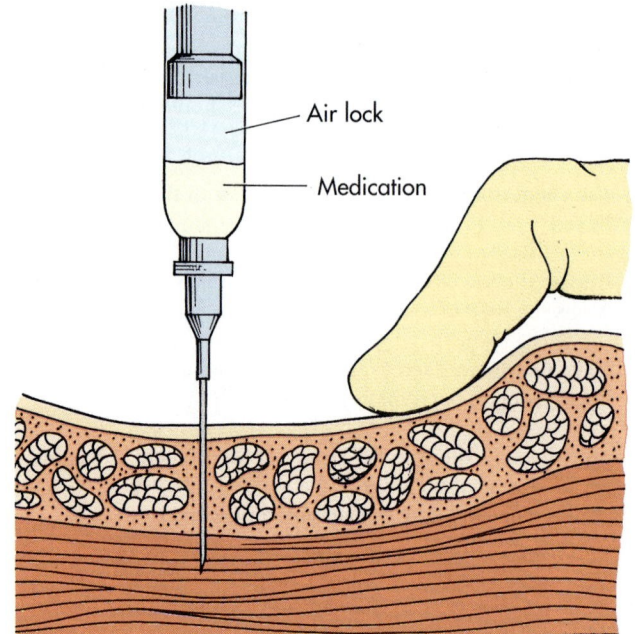

During Injection

Step 2

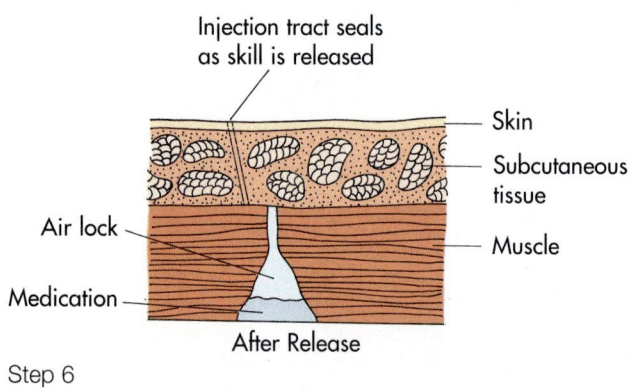

After Release

Step 6

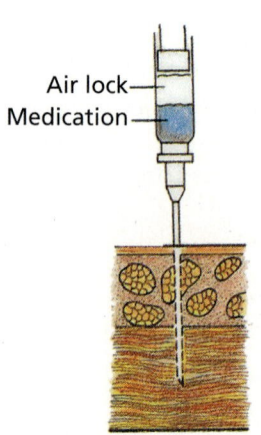 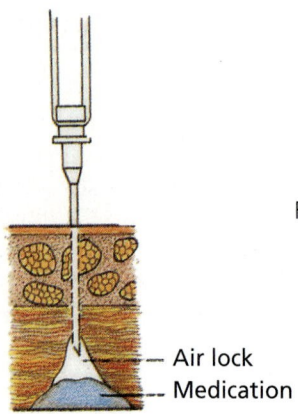

Figure 17-17 Using an air lock.

Assessment

1. Review physician's medication order for client's name, drug name, dose, time, and route of administration.
2. Gather information pertinent to drug(s) ordered: action, purpose, time of onset and peak action, normal dose, common side effects, and nursing implications.
3. Consider factors that may contraindicate IM injection, for example, muscle atrophy, reduced blood flow, or circulatory shock.
4. Assess client's medical history, history of allergies, and medication history.
5. Assess client's knowledge regarding medication and dosage schedule.

6. Observe client's verbal and nonverbal responses toward receiving injection.

Planning

Expected outcomes focus on safe, effective administration of injection with minimal anxiety and discomfort.

EXPECTED OUTCOMES

1. Client demonstrates effects of medication within 30 to 60 minutes.
2. Client has no evidence of adverse effects from medication or injection.

Implementation

Steps	Rationale
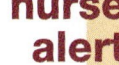 **nurse alert** Review the five "rights" for administration of medications.	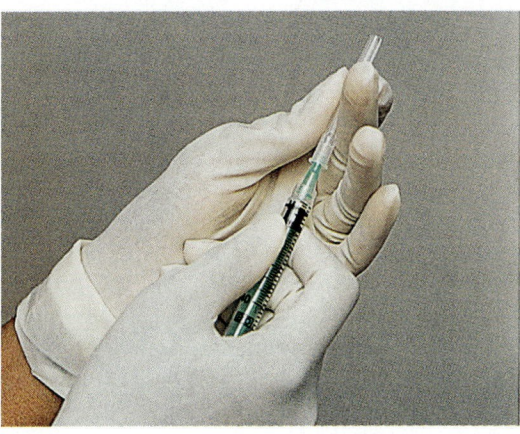
Figure 17-18 Removing protective cap from needle.	
1. See Standard Protocol (Chapter 1, p. 5).	
2. Prepare medication in syringe.	
3. Explain procedure, location of injection site, and how positioning lessens discomfort. Proceed in calm manner.	Allows client to anticipate injection so as to lessen anxiety.
4. Choose appropriate IM injection site by assessing size and integrity of muscle. Palpate for areas of tenderness or hardness. Note presence of bruising or area of infection.	Muscle is soft when relaxed and firm when tense; absence of tenderness or bruising indicates healthy tissue.
5. Assist client to comfortable position, depending on site (see Table 17-6).	Position that reduces strain on muscle minimizes discomfort of injection.
6. Relocate site using anatomical landmarks.	Injection into correct anatomical site prevents injury to nerves, bones, and blood vessels.
7. Cleanse site with an antiseptic swab beginning at the center of the site and moving outward in a circular direction for about 5 cm (2 inches).	Cleansing reduces surface pathogens, reducing risk of infection when skin integrity is broken.
8. Hold swab between fingers of nondominant hand or place near site.	Swab remains readily accessible when needle is withdrawn.
9. Loosen needle cap or sheath carefully with hands braced together to maintain control (Figure 17-18). Remove cap from needle by pulling it straight off.	

Steps	Rationale
10. Hold syringe between thumb and forefinger of dominant hand as if holding a dart, with palm down at 90-degree angle to client's skin.	Needle must be injected at 90-degree angle to enter muscle and so air lock rises to top of medication toward plunger.
11. Position nondominant hand at proper anatomical landmarks and spread skin tightly. If client's muscle mass is small, grasp body of muscle between thumb and fingers.	Taut skin facilitates insertion and reduces discomfort. Ensures that medication reaches muscle mass.
12. After needle enters site, grasp lower end of syringe barrel with nondominant hand and move dominant hand to end of plunger. Slowly pull back on plunger to aspirate. If no blood appears, inject medication slowly. If blood appears in syringe, remove needle and dispose of medication and syringe. Repeat preparation procedure.	Slow injection reduces pain and tissue trauma.

Aspiration of blood into syringe indicates placement of needle in a blood vessel. |
13. Withdraw needle quickly while placing antiseptic swab gently above or over injection.	Support of tissues around injection site minimizes discomfort during needle withdrawal.
14. Massage skin lightly. Place small Band-Aid over puncture site if bleeding is noted.	Massage can stimulate circulation and improve drug distribution.
15. Discard uncapped needle and attached syringe into appropriate receptacle.	Prevents injury to clients and health care personnel. CDC (1988) recommends needles should not be recapped before disposal.
16. See Completion Protocol (Chapter 1, p. 6).	

Evaluation

1. Observe for effects of prescribed IM medication within 30 to 60 minutes.
2. Monitor for adverse effects of medication or IM injection.

UNEXPECTED OUTCOMES AND RELATED INTERVENTIONS

1. Client develops signs and symptoms of allergy or side effects.
   a. Notify physician for treatment of symptoms and to change medication.
   b. Be sure client wears allergy bracelet indicating medications and substances to which client is allergic.
2. Client insists on selecting site using incorrect criteria.
   a. Clients requiring regular injections (e.g., vitamin B_{12}) should learn how to rotate and select sites.
   b. Instruct client and primary care giver how to observe injection sites for complications.

SAMPLE DOCUMENTATION

See Medication Administration Record, Appendix A. Include site used.

Skill 17.4 | Intradermal Injections

Intradermal injections are used for skin testing, such as in tuberculin screening and allergy tests. Because these medications are potent, they are injected into the dermis, where blood supply is reduced and drug absorption occurs slowly. A client may have an anaphylactic reaction if the medication enters the circulation too rapidly. For clients with a history of numerous allergies, the physician may perform skin testing.

Skin testing requires clear identification of injection sites for changes in color and tissue integrity. Intradermal sites should be lightly pigmented, free of lesions, and relatively hairless. The inner forearm and upper back are ideal locations.

A tuberculin or 1 ml syringe with a short (¼- to ½-inch), fine-gauge (26 or 27) needle is used for skin testing. Very small amounts of medication (0.01 to 0.1 ml) are injected intradermally. If a bleb does not appear or if the site bleeds after needle withdrawal, the medication may enter subcutaneous tissues. In this case, skin test results will not be valid.

EQUIPMENT

1 ml tuberculin syringe with 26- or 27-gauge needle
Alcohol swabs
Vial or ampule of skin test solution
Disposable gloves

Assessment

1. Review physician's medication order for client's name, drug name, dose, time, and route of administration.
2. Know information regarding expected reaction when testing skin with specific allergen or medication.
3. Assess client's history of allergies, and know substance to which client is allergic and normal allergic reaction.

4. Check date of expiration for medication vial or ampule.
5. Assess client's knowledge of purpose and reactions of skin testing.

Planning

Expected outcomes focus on safe administration and identification of allergies.

EXPECTED OUTCOMES

1. Client remains free from systemic allergic reaction.
2. Client describes purpose and expected skin reactions.
3. Client observes for skin reaction and notifies health care provider as instructed.

Implementation

Steps	Rationale

nurse alert   Review the five "rights" for administration of medications.

1. See Standard Protocol (Chapter 1, p. 5).	
2. Prepare medication in syringe.	
3. Select appropriate injection site three to four finger-widths below antecubital space and handwidth above wrist. Avoid bruises, areas of inflammation, edema, lesions, or discolorations of forearm.	Injection sites should be free of abnormalities that may interfere with drug absorption. An intradermal site should be clear so results of skin test can be seen and read correctly.
4. Assist client to comfortable position with elbow and forearm extended and supported on flat surface.	Stabilizes injection site for easiest accessibility.
5. Cleanse site with an antiseptic swab beginning at center of the site and rotating outward in a circular direction for about 5 cm (2 inches). Allow to dry.	Mechanical action of swab removes secretions containing microorganisms. Drying prevents antiseptic from affecting test results.
6. Hold swab between fingers of nondominant hand.	Swab remains readily accessible when needle is withdrawn.
7. Remove needle cap or sheath from needle by pulling it straight off.	Preventing needle from touching sides of cap prevents contamination.
8. Hold syringe between thumb and forefinger of dominant hand with bevel of needle pointing up.	Bevel up facilitates correct needle placement.
9. With nondominant hand, stretch skin over site with forefinger or thumb.	Needle pierces tight skin more easily.
10. With needle almost against client's skin, insert it carefully at 5- to 15-degree angle until resistance is felt, and advance needle through epidermis to approximately 3 mm ($\frac{1}{8}$ inch) below skin surface. Needle tip can be seen through skin (Figure 17-19).	

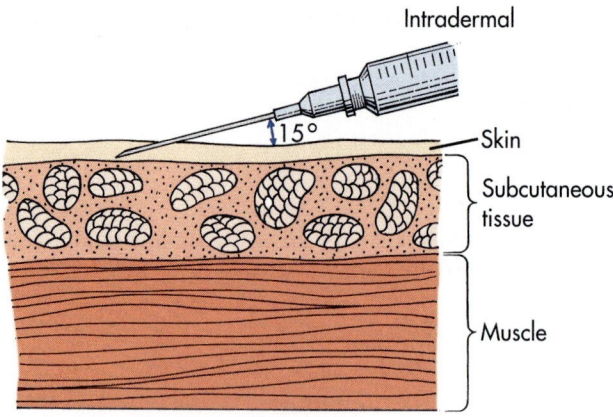

Figure 17-19 Intradermal injection.

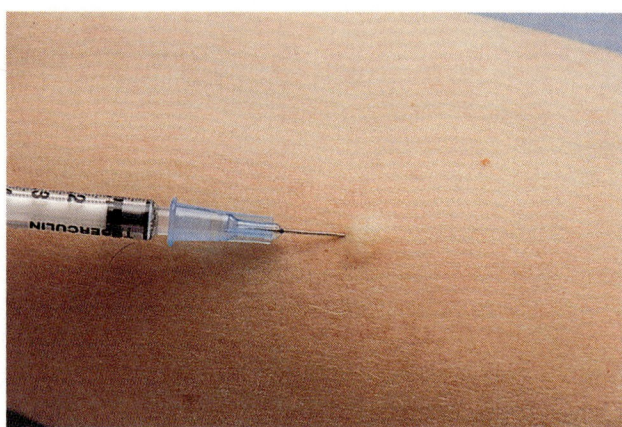

Figure 17-20 Bleb shows correct placement of needle.

Steps	Rationale
11. Inject medication slowly. It is not necessary to aspirate, since dermis is relatively avascular. Normally, resistance is felt. If not, needle is too deep; remove and begin again.	Slow injection minimizes discomfort at site. Dermal layer is tight and does not expand easily when solution is injected.
12. While injecting medication, a light-colored bleb resembling a mosquito bite approximately 6 mm (¼ inch) in diameter forms at site and gradually disappears (Figure 17-20). Minimal bruising may be present.	Medication is in dermis and is eventually absorbed. Bruising is result of minor bleeding from capillaries.
13. Withdraw needle while applying alcohol swab gently over site.	Support of tissue around injection site minimizes discomfort during needle withdrawal.
14. Do not massage site.	Massage may disperse medication into underlying tissue layers and alter test results.
15. Discard uncapped needle and syringe in appropriately labeled receptacle.	Prevents injury to client and health care personnel.
16. Use skin pencil and draw circle around perimeter of injection site. Tell client not to wash off markings around injection site.	Identifies site for testing to be read in 48 to 72 hours.
17. See Completion Protocol (Chapter 1, p. 6).	

Evaluation

1. Observe for any allergic reactions.
2. Have client observe site for raised, reddened, or hard zones that form around test site 48 to 72 hours after injection. This indicates sensitivity to the injected allergen (positive test for tuberculin skin testing).
3. Ask client to describe implications of skin testing and signs of expected skin reaction and hypersensitivity.

UNEXPECTED OUTCOMES
AND RELATED INTERVENTIONS

1. Severe anaphylactic reaction is characterized by dyspnea, wheezing, and circulatory collapse. Onset of al-

lergic reaction may develop within minutes. A negative skin test does not mean client will not react to larger dose.
2. Positive tuberculin reaction is indicated by induration or hardening of skin around 10 mm or more of injection site; read at 48 to 72 hours.
   NOTE: An induration of 5 to 9 mm is doubtful unless known exposure has occurred.
   a. Positive tuberculin test indicates exposure, not active disease.
   b. A person who has contact with an individual with TB and whose initial tuberculin reaction (induration) is more than 5 mm should have a chest x-ray

film and be considered for preventive therapy (American Thoracic Society, 1992).

c. Contacts who initially have negative skin test results should receive a repeat skin test 10 to 12 weeks after the initial test (American Thoracic Society, 1992).

SAMPLE DOCUMENTATION

Record amount, type, and site of testing substance and date and time on medication record. Client should wear allergy identification band listing all substances to which he or she is allergic.

CRITICAL THINKING EXERCISES

1. For the following situations, discuss the type of syringe/needle you would use and where you would administer the injection.
   a. A 26-year-old client requiring a preoperative injection of Demerol 50 mg (1 cc) and Robinul 0.2 mg (1 ml); Ht. 5'2", Wt. 110 lbs.
   b. An 80-year-old client receiving regular insulin 5 units; Ht. 5', Wt. 100 lbs.
   c. A 71-year-old client receiving an iron preparation (2 ml) for anemia; Ht. 5'6", Wt. 180 lbs.
   d. A 45-year-old client requiring an SQ injection of heparin 1000 units (1 ml) for thrombophlebitis; Ht. 5'11", Wt. 170 lbs.
   e. An 18-year-old client receiving skin testing for possible allergies; Ht. 5'4", Wt. 130 lbs.
   f. A 50-year-old client requiring a tetanus toxoid injection (1 ml) after stepping on a nail; Ht. 6'2", Wt. 190 lbs.
2. Discuss how your injection technique would differ for the following clients:
   a. A 51-year-old client, Ht. 5'6", Wt. 64 kg, receiving Demerol 75 mg and Vistaril 25 mg IM for postoperative pain management.
   b. A 72-year-old client, Ht. 5'9", Wt. 91 kg, receiving 35 units of NPH insulin.
   c. A 35-year-old client, Ht. 5'4", Wt. 49 kg, receiving 35 units of NPH insulin.
3. You are preparing to give heparin and insulin SQ to the same client.
   a. Compare and contrast the administration of heparin and insulin via the subcutaneous route, explaining why techniques for these two drugs differ from other types of SQ injections.
   b. What additional data should be gathered before giving either of these injections?
   c. The insulin order is as follows: Regular Humulin insulin 6 units and NPH insulin 22 units SQ at 0730. Describe how you will prepare this insulin order.
   d. If the regular insulin vial were contaminated with NPH insulin, what might the consequence be?
4. What general precautions should you take when administering any type of injection?

REFERENCES

American Diabetes Association: *Position statement: insulin administration, diabetes care,* 18(suppl I):29-32, Jan 1995.
American Thoracic Society: Control of tuberculosis in the United States, *Am Rev Respir Dis* 146(16):1623, 1992.
Association for Practitioners in Infection Control: APIC position paper: prevention of device-mediated blood-borne infections to health care workers, *Am J Infect Control* 21(2):76, 1993.
Centers for Disease Control: Update: universal precautions for prevention of transmission of HIV, hepatitis B virus, and other bloodborne pathogens in health care settings, *MMWR* 37:377, 1988.
Gray D: *Calculate with confidence,* St Louis, 1994, Mosby.
McConnell EA: Administering S.C. heparin, *Nursing '90* 20(12):24, 1990.
Newton M, Newton D, Fudin J: Reviewing the "big three" injection routes, *Nursing '92* 22(2):34-42, 1992.
Pagana KD, Pagana TJ: *Mosby's diagnostic and laboratory test reference tests,* St Louis, 1992, Mosby.
Whaley L, Wong D: *Nursing care of infants and children,* ed 5, St Louis, 1995, Mosby.

ADDITIONAL READINGS

Clark JB, Queener SF, Karl GB: *Pharmacologic basis of nursing practice,* ed 4, St Louis, 1993, Mosby.
Jagger J: Preventing HIV transmission in health care workers with safer needle devices, Sixth International Conference on AIDS, San Francisco, 1990.
Kim MJ et al: *Pocket guide to nursing diagnosis,* ed 4, St Louis, 1991, Mosby.

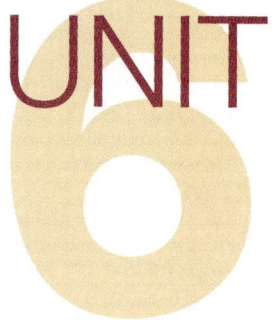

UNIT 6

Perioperative Nursing Care

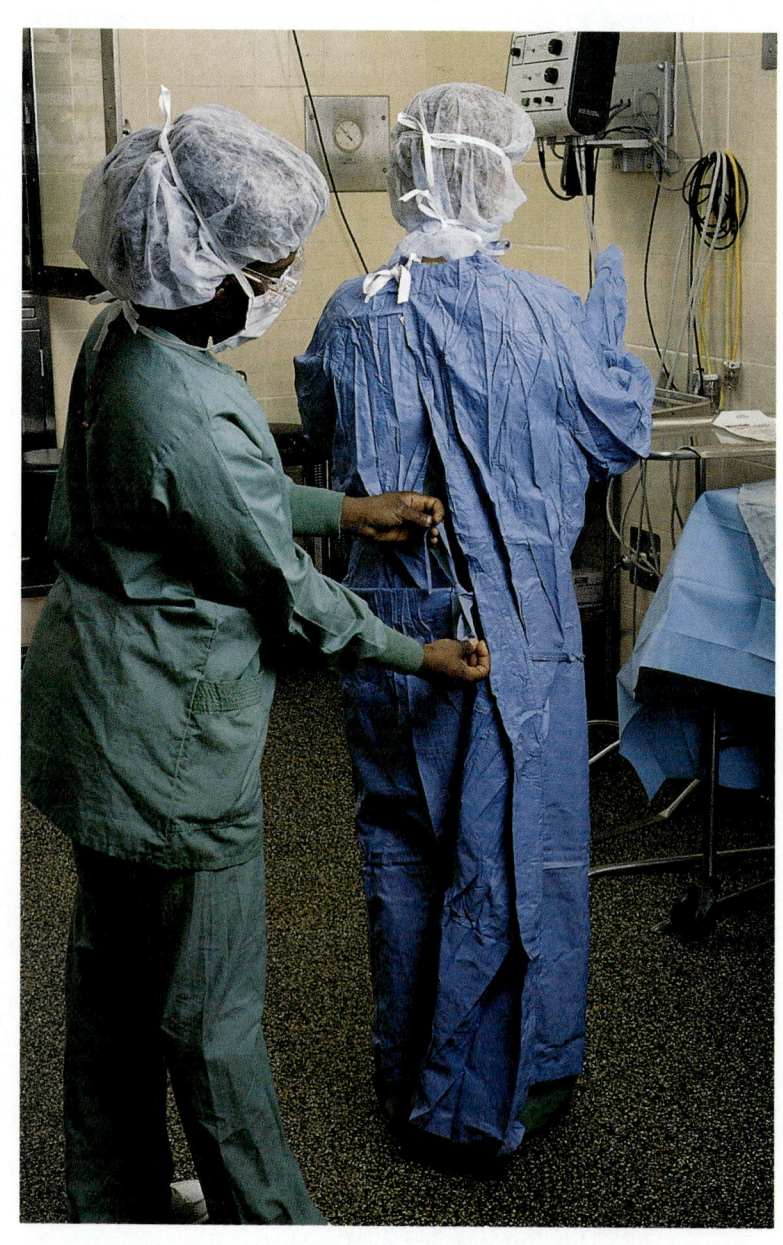

chapter 18

Preparing the Client for Surgery

Skill 18.1
Preoperative Assessment

Skill 18.2
Preoperative Teaching

Skill 18.3
Physical Preparation

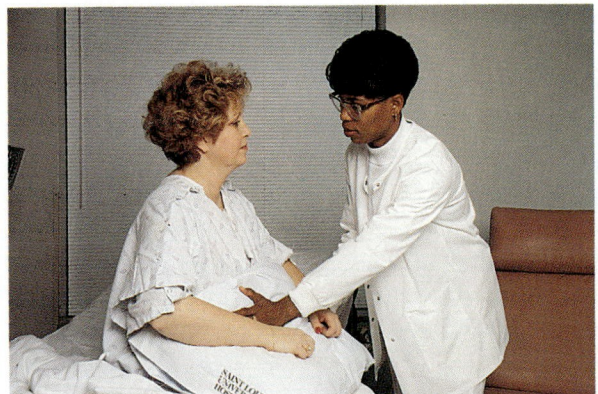

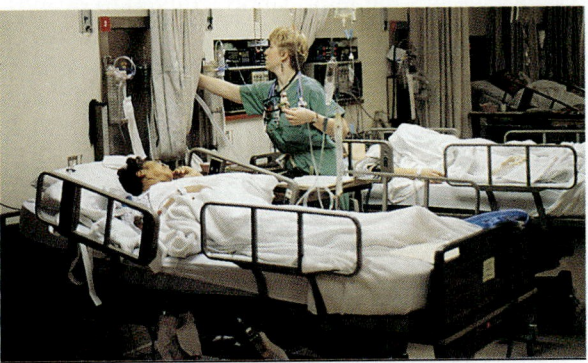

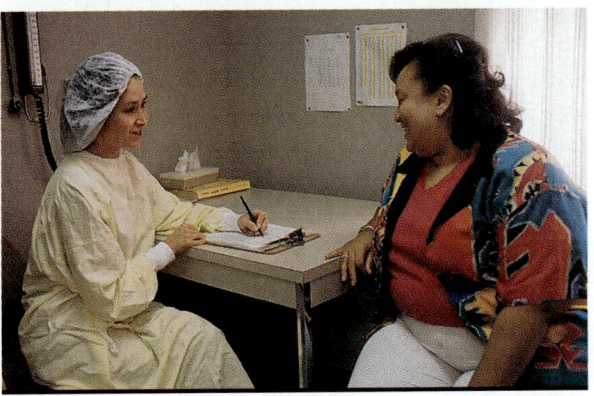

Surgery is a stressful experience, both psychologically and physiologically, for the client. The client has little control over the situation or the outcome. This results in feelings of anxiety, fear, and powerlessness. As with trauma, the surgery itself is a physiological stressor affecting the major body systems. Preoperative care can reduce this stress and place the client in the best condition possible to undergo the surgery. The nurse thoroughly assesses the client's condition, teaches the client and family what to expect, and physically prepares the client for surgery.

For any surgical procedure, it is important for the nurse to complete a thorough preoperative assessment. For clients who have been hospitalized, this may occur the day before surgery. In an outpatient setting, the preoperative assessment may begin several days before surgery and be completed the morning of surgery. Regardless of the setting, the preoperative assessment forms the basis for a plan of care for the client during and after surgery.

Often the client is unsure what to expect and has concerns about the amount of pain or disfigurement involved with surgery. Many clients return home the same day, and the family members may be unsure about their role in the client's recovery. Before the client undergoes surgery, the nurse teaches the client and family what to expect and what they can do to assist in the recovery process.

Physically preparing the client to undergo surgery is an important skill for the nurse. Regardless of the surgery, some safety measures, such as verifying the procedure and consent, are always taken. Other steps, such as urinary catheterization or special laboratory tests, are only completed for specific surgical procedures. This physical preparation minimizes risks of surgery and anesthesia and places the client in the best condition possible for surgery.

Nursing Diagnosis

Nursing diagnoses associated with the surgical experience include **Risk for Infection** related to the surgical wound and **Risk for Injury** related to inadequate identification and communication of risks. The risk for injury is also related to electrical equipment used in the operating room (OR). Psychological factors such as **Knowledge Deficit** and **Anxiety** result when a client is unsure what to expect before, during, and after the surgery. The inability to control the situation often results in **Powerlessness.** During and after surgery with general anesthesia, the client's cough and gag reflexes are suppressed. This results in a risk for **Ineffective Airway Clearance** related to the presence of secretions.

Skill 18.1 | Preoperative Assessment

To identify risks and plan for the client's care during and after surgery, the nurse performs a thorough preoperative assessment of the client's physiological and psychological condition. To provide efficient services, the assessment is frequently begun before the day of surgery and completed 1 to 2 hours before the scheduled time of surgery. This provides time for the nurse to follow up on any unexpected outcomes. Before beginning this assessment, the nurse establishes a trusting relationship with the client. It is not unusual for the client to remember and report facts to the nurse at this time that were not told to the physician earlier. To encourage open communication, the nurse provides privacy and a location free of interruption.

EQUIPMENT
Stethoscope
Blood pressure cuff
Pulse oximeter
Thermometer
Watch/clock
Scale
Preoperative assessment form (Figure 18-1)

Planning

Expected outcomes of the preoperative assessment focus on obtaining accurate information and identifying risk factors related to the intended surgery. Based on this assessment, the nurse establishes a plan of care to limit these risks to the extent possible and properly care for the client during and after surgery.

EXPECTED OUTCOMES
1. Client provides the information required to establish a plan of care.
2. Client assists the nurse in completing the assessment.

Implementation

Steps	Rationale
1. See Standard Protocol (Chapter 1, p. 5).	
2. Obtain a nursing history.	
a. Planned surgery	
b. Condition leading to surgery	
c. Previous hospitalizations	
d. Chronic illnesses	
e. Medication history, including prescription and over-the-counter (OTC)	Client may not report OTC medications unless specifically asked.
f. Previous experience with surgery and anesthesia	
g. Family history of complications from surgery or anesthesia	A family history of reactions to anesthetic agents may indicate a familial condition, malignant hyperthermia, which is life-threatening.
h. Allergies to medications, food, including specific questions about rubber latex	Reactions to latex can be life-threatening, and prevention in sensitized clients requires specific precautions. Many clients do not know that rubber and latex are the same. Using both words will help obtain accurate information (Steelman, 1994).

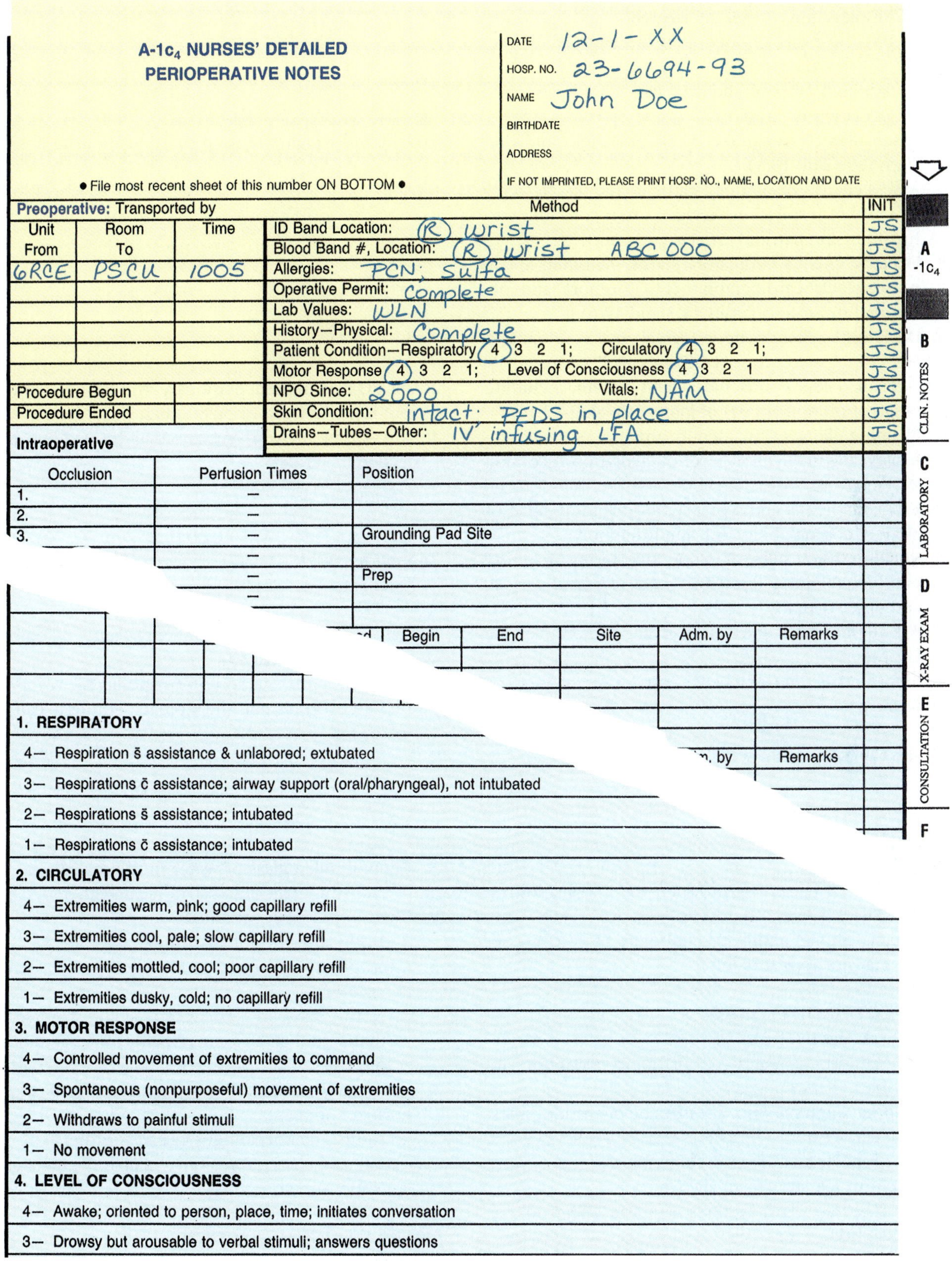

A-1c₄ NURSES' DETAILED PERIOPERATIVE NOTES

DATE _12-1-XX_

HOSP. NO. _23-6694-93_

NAME _John Doe_

BIRTHDATE

ADDRESS

IF NOT IMPRINTED, PLEASE PRINT HOSP. NO., NAME, LOCATION AND DATE

● File most recent sheet of this number ON BOTTOM ●

Preoperative: Transported by			Method	INIT
Unit From	Room To	Time	ID Band Location: (R) wrist	JS
			Blood Band #, Location: (R) wrist ABC 000	JS
6RCE	PSCU	1005	Allergies: PCN; Sulfa	JS
			Operative Permit: Complete	JS
			Lab Values: WLN	JS
			History—Physical: Complete	JS
			Patient Condition—Respiratory ④ 3 2 1; Circulatory ④ 3 2 1;	JS
			Motor Response ④ 3 2 1; Level of Consciousness ④ 3 2 1	JS
Procedure Begun			NPO Since: 2000 Vitals: NAM	JS
Procedure Ended			Skin Condition: intact; PFDS in place	JS
			Drains—Tubes—Other: IV infusing LFA	JS

Intraoperative

Occlusion	Perfusion Times	Position
1.	—	
2.	—	
3.	—	Grounding Pad Site
	—	
	—	Prep

	Begin	End	Site	Adm. by	Remarks

	by	Remarks

1. RESPIRATORY

4— Respiration s̄ assistance & unlabored; extubated

3— Respirations c̄ assistance; airway support (oral/pharyngeal), not intubated

2— Respirations s̄ assistance; intubated

1— Respirations c̄ assistance; intubated

2. CIRCULATORY

4— Extremities warm, pink; good capillary refill

3— Extremities cool, pale; slow capillary refill

2— Extremities mottled, cool; poor capillary refill

1— Extremities dusky, cold; no capillary refill

3. MOTOR RESPONSE

4— Controlled movement of extremities to command

3— Spontaneous (nonpurposeful) movement of extremities

2— Withdraws to painful stimuli

1— No movement

4. LEVEL OF CONSCIOUSNESS

4— Awake; oriented to person, place, time; initiates conversation

3— Drowsy but arousable to verbal stimuli; answers questions

A
-1c₄

B

CLIN. NOTES

C

LABORATORY

D

X-RAY EXAM

E

CONSULTATION

F

Figure 18-1 (Courtesy University of Iowa Hospitals and Clinics.)

Steps	Rationale
i. Physical and mental impairment j. Prostheses (e.g., dentures, hearing aid, pacemaker, artificial eye) k. Smoking, alcohol, and drug use l. Occupation	
3. Assess client's weight (see Skill 7.3), height, and vital signs (see Skill 10.1).	Height and weight are used to calculate drug dosages.
4. Assess client's respiratory status, including character and rate of respirations, oxygen saturation, ability to breathe lying flat, and chest x-ray report.	
5. Evaluate client's circulatory status, including apical pulse, electrocardiographic (ECG) report, and peripheral pulses (see Skills 11.3 and 12.6).	
6. Determine client's neurological status, including level of consciousness (LOC) (see Skill 12.9).	
7. Evaluate client's musculoskeletal system, including range of motion (ROM) of joints (see Skill 12.10).	If the ROM is limited, extra care will be needed to prevent injury related to positioning in surgery.
8. Examine client's skin; identify any breaks in skin integrity and determine level of hydration (see Skill 23.1).	If skin is thin, broken, or bruised, extra padding will be needed in surgery.
9. Evaluate client's emotional status, including level of anxiety, coping ability, and family support.	
10. Review the results of laboratory tests, including complete blood count (CBC), electrolytes, urinalysis, and other diagnostic tests.	Laboratory work provides an assessment of major body systems.
11. Ask client if he or she has an advanced directive (see Chapter 38).	Advanced directives protect client's rights by communicating client's desires.
12. Identify the time of client's last intake of food or drink.	With client under general anesthesia, the esophageal sphincter relaxes and the stomach contents can be aspirated.
13. See Completion Protocol (Chapter 1, p. 6).	

Evaluation

1. Determine if client has provided the information requested.
2. Evaluate client's ability to cooperate (e.g., eye contact, answers appropriately).

UNEXPECTED OUTCOMES AND RELATED INTERVENTIONS

1. Client reports having a cold or upper respiratory infection.
   Notify surgeon and anesthesiologist/nurse anesthetist.
2. Client reports an allergy to rubber latex.
   a. Remove all latex from client's room.
   b. Post a latex precautions sign on the door or stretcher.
   c. Notify surgeon, anesthesiologist/nurse anesthetist, and OR nurse (Steelman, 1994).

3. Client drank a glass of water in the morning.
   Notify anesthesiologist/nurse anesthetist.
4. Client reports recent chest pain.
   Notify anesthesiologist/nurse anesthetist.
5. Appropriate laboratory tests were not ordered or completed.
   Notify surgeon and anesthesiologist/nurse anesthetist, and make arrangements for tests to be completed.
6. Chest x-ray report, ECG, or laboratory tests show abnormal findings.
   Notify anesthesiologist/nurse anesthetist.
7. Client has a blister/abrasion/boil near the incision site.
   Notify surgeon.

SAMPLE DOCUMENTATION

Routine documentation involves completion of the preoperative portion of the nurses' detailed perioperative notes (see Figure 18-1).

Skill 18.2 | **Preoperative Teaching**

Preoperative client teaching involves assisting a client to understand and mentally prepare for the surgical experience (Iowa Intervention Project, 1992). Clients and their families are often very anxious about impending surgery. This anxiety increases heart rate and blood pressure during surgery, which can lead to bleeding and complications. Postoperatively, this high anxiety can lead to negative psychological and physiological outcomes. Preoperative information about the sensations that will be experienced has been shown to decrease the distress associated with surgery (Horsley and Pelz, 1981). Therefore, by teaching the client preoperatively, the nurse can make a significant contribution to the success of surgery and the client's postoperative recovery.

EQUIPMENT
Stretcher or bed
Pillow
Incentive spirometer
Preoperative education flow sheet (Figure 18-2)

Assessment

1. Determine client's previous experiences with surgery and anesthesia. **This information indicates the amount of information that the client and family need as well as any aspects of the surgical experience that may be especially stressful for the client.**
2. Determine client and family's understanding of surgery. **This information determines if correction of misunderstanding is necessary.**
3. Identify the client's cognitive level, language, and culture. **These factors may alter the client's ability to understand the meaning of surgery.**

4. Assess client's anxiety related to surgery. **This information directs the nurse to provide additional emotional support and indicates the client's readiness to learn (Rakel, 1992).**

Planning

Based on the preoperative assessment, the nurse plans preoperative teaching. A private area free of distractions is needed. The best learning method for the client should be selected. In many settings, a videotape and written materials are available to assist the nurse. Whenever possible, the family should be present. Later, they serve as coaches and assist the client in performing exercises. Expected outcomes of preoperative teaching focus on reducing the anxiety level of the client and family and demonstrations of their understanding of key information and specific skills necessary to prevent complications.

EXPECTED OUTCOMES
1. Client demonstrates eye contact and asks and answers questions appropriately.
2. Client correctly performs breathing exercises and leg exercises.
3. Family identifies the location of the waiting room.
4. Family verbalizes the ability to care for client at home.
5. Family provides emotional support for client preoperatively.
6. Client and family have appropriate coping skills.

Implementation

Steps	Rationale
1. See Standard Protocol (Chapter 1, p. 5).	
2. Inform client and family of date, time, location of surgery, and where to wait.	Accurate information helps reduce the stress associated with surgery.
3. Inform client and family about the anticipated length of time of surgery.	
4. Answer questions client and family ask.	
5. Describe preoperative routines (e.g., intravenous [IV] therapy, urinary catheterization, enema, hair removal, laboratory tests, transport to OR).	
6. Describe preoperative medications.	

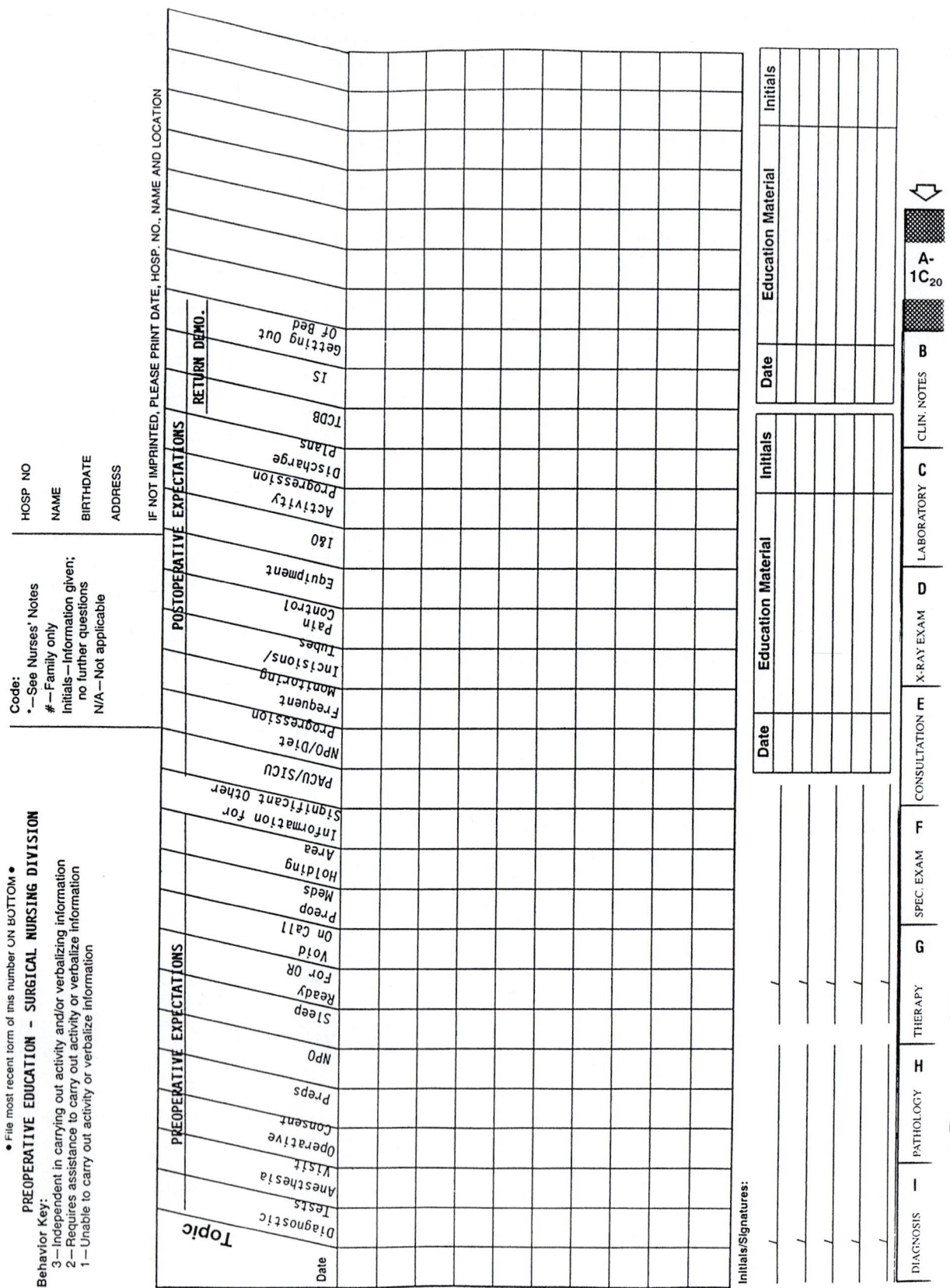

Figure 18-2 *TCDB* = turn, cough, and deep breathe; *IS* = incentive spirometry. (Courtesy University of Iowa Hospitals and Clinics.)

Steps	Rationale

7. Review which routine medications are to be discontinued before surgery.

Some medications are discontinued before surgery. For example, anticoagulants may increase bleeding and are usually discontinued before surgery. Insulin dosages are usually adjusted because of the reduced intake of food preoperatively.

8. Describe intraoperative sensations (e.g., blood pressure cuff tightening, ECG leads, cool room, beep of monitor).

Describing what sensations client will experience has been shown to reduce distress associated with the experience (Horsley and Pelz, 1981).

9. Describe pain control methods. Many clients have a patient-controlled anesthesia (PCA) pump (see Chapter 21).

Clients are fearful of postoperative pain. Explaining pain management techniques will reduce this fear.

10. Describe what client will experience postoperatively (e.g., frequent vital signs, turning, catheters, drains, tubes).

11. Instruct client in splinting. Hold pillow to abdomen for support while sitting up or coughing (Figure 18-3).

12. **Instruct client on turning and sitting up.**
    a. Flex knees.
    b. Splint incision with left arm and pillow (Figure 18-4).
    c. Push on the mattress with right arm and swing feet over the edge of the bed.

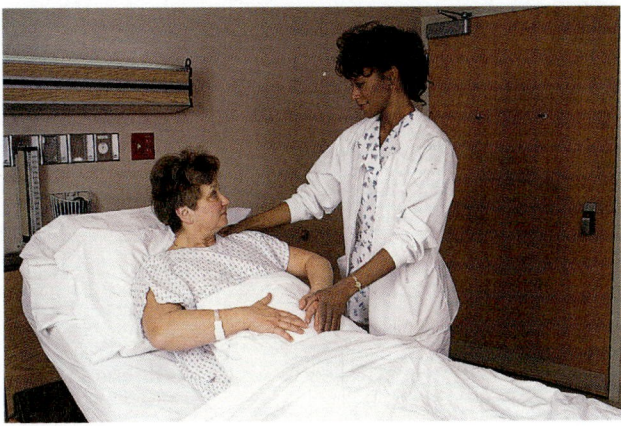

Figure 18-3

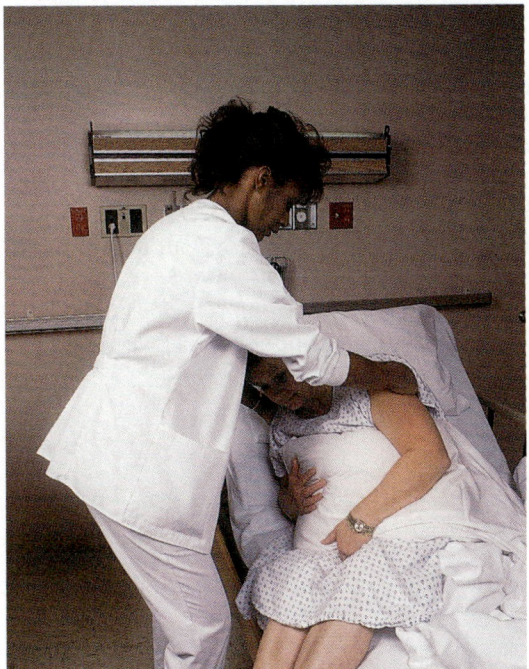

Figure 18-4

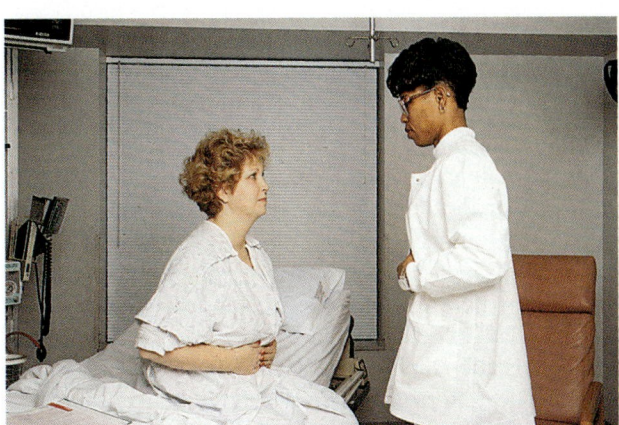

Figure 18-5

Steps	Rationale
13. Instruct client in deep breathing and coughing (Figure 18-5). a. Assist client to sitting position. b. Instruct client to place palms of hands over the lower border of the rib cage with third fingers touching. c. Have client take slow, deep breaths and feel fingers separate. d. Have client hold the breath for 3 seconds and exhale through the mouth as if blowing out a candle. e. Instruct client to cough forcefully. f. Have the client practice several times. g. Instruct client to perform turn, cough, and deep breathing every 2 hours.	Client may be unable or reluctant to deep breathe because of weakness or pain, resulting in secretions remaining in the base of the lungs. This collection of secretions increases the risk of pulmonary complications such as pneumonia.
14. Instruct client in use of an incentive spirometer (Figure 18-6). a. Position in semi-Fowler's position. b. Instruct client to exhale completely, then place mouthpiece so that lips completely cover it and inhale slowly, maintaining constant flow through unit. c. After maximum inspiration, client should hold breath for 2 to 3 seconds, then exhale slowly.	Encourages deep breathing and loosens secretions in lung bases. Promotes optimum lung expansion. Promotes complete inflation of lungs and minimizes atelectasis. 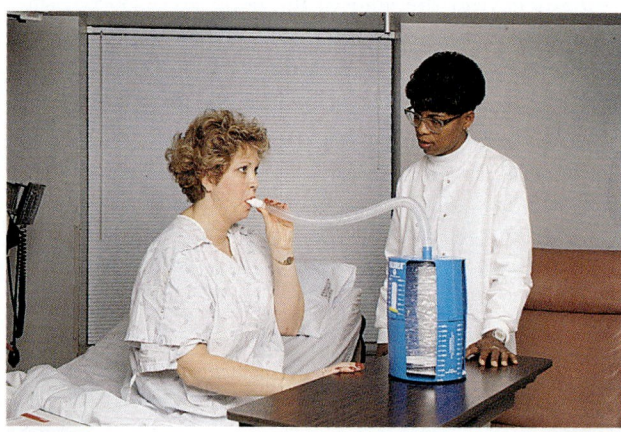 Figure 18-6
d. Instruct client to breathe normally for a short period, then repeat process.	Prevents hyperventilation and fatigue.
15. Instruct client on three leg exercises. a. Rotate each ankle in a complete circle. b. Instruct client to draw imaginary circles with the big toe five times. c. Alternate dorsiflexion and plantar flexion while instructing client to feel calf muscles tighten and relax. Repeat five times (Figure 18-7). d. Instruct client to alternate flexing and extending knees. Repeat five times (Figure 18-8). e. Instruct client to alternate straight leg raises. Repeat five times.	Leg exercises encourage circulation in the lower extremities and reduce the risk of circulatory complications such as an embolism.

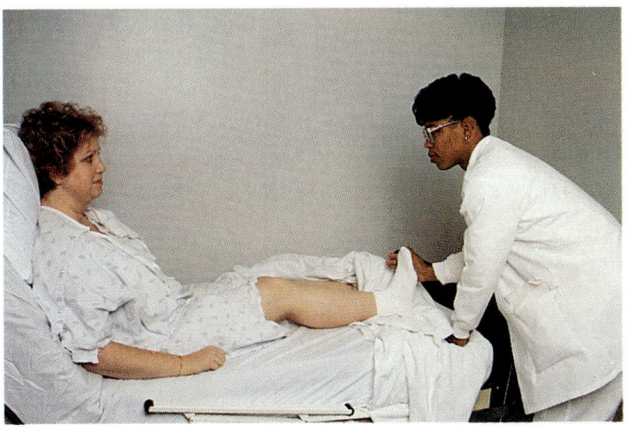

Figure 18-7

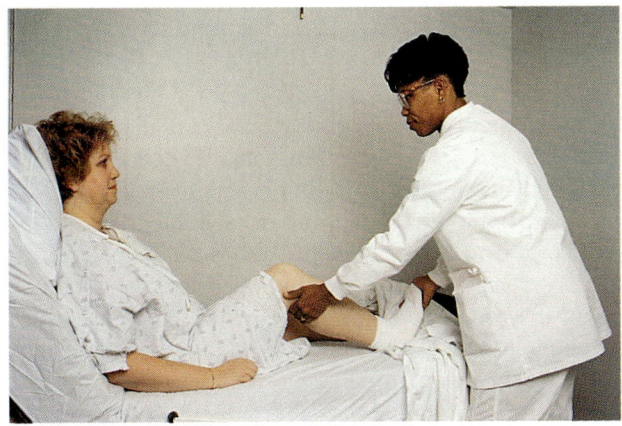

Figure 18-8

Steps	Rationale

   f. Instruct client to perform these three leg exercises every 2 hours while awake.

16. Verify that client's expectations of surgery are realistic. Correct expectations as needed.

17. Reinforce therapeutic coping strategies. If ineffective, encourage alternatives.

18. See Completion Protocol (Chapter 1, p. 6).

Evaluation

1. Ask client to repeat key information.
2. Ask client to demonstrate splinting, deep breathing, and leg exercises.
3. Ask family to identify location of the waiting room.
4. Ask family if they are able to care for client at home after discharge.
5. Observe the level of emotional support family provides client.
6. Observe client and family coping strategies.

UNEXPECTED OUTCOMES AND RELATED INTERVENTIONS

1. Client identifies an incorrect date, time, or location of surgery.

    Provide the correct information verbally and in writing for client and family.

2. Client questions the importance of not drinking the morning of surgery.

    Explain that under anesthesia, the fluid can come up from the stomach and go into the lung.

3. Client is withdrawn.

   a. Explain that it is normal to feel anxious about surgery.

   b. Ask how client feels about the surgery.

4. Client incorrectly performs breathing exercises.

   a. Explain the correct breathing technique.

   b. Explain the importance of postoperative breathing.

   c. Instruct client to repeat the demonstration.

5. Family verbalizes anxiety about care for client at home.

   a. Explain that these feelings are normal.

   b. Provide written instructions.

   c. Provide a telephone number for contact if there are further questions.

6. Family indicates that they are unable to care for client at home.

    Contact physician and discuss the alternative of a home health care referral.

SAMPLE DOCUMENTATION

Routine documentation involves completion of preoperative education flow sheet (Figure 18-2).

Skill 18.3 | # Physical Preparation

Physical preparation of the client for surgery involves providing care immediately before surgery and verification of required procedures/tests and documentation in the client's record (Iowa Intervention Project, 1992). This preparation minimizes the risks of infection and injury related to surgery. Specific steps are taken to prepare every client, which depend on the type of surgery being performed and the risks involved. For example, antiembolism stockings may be used for adult clients undergoing surgery that will last several hours and require a long period of immobilization afterward. The bowel may need to be prepped or an enema given for abdominal surgery on or near the intestine. It is important to check the physician's orders to determine what steps are needed for the surgical client. Regardless of the type of surgery, the goal of physical preparation is to place the client in the best condition possible to minimize the risks of the surgery that is planned.

EQUIPMENT

Hospital gown
IV bag, tubing, catheter, tourniquet, alcohol swab, and tape
Antiembolism stockings
Sequential compression device
Clippers, gloves, disposable towel
Antimicrobial soap, sponge, water, gloves, and towels
Preoperative checklist (Figure 18-9).

Assessment

The preoperative assessment forms the basis for physical preparation of the client for surgery (see Skill 18.1).

Planning

Based on the preoperative assessment and the preparations ordered by the physician, the nurse determines the timing of the physical preparation of the client. The nurse provides a private area with access to a restroom.

EXPECTED OUTCOMES

1. Client cooperates during preparatory measures (e.g., IV starting, laboratory tests).
2. Client undergoes measures to reduce the risk of infection (e.g., preoperative antibiotics, skin preparation).

Implementation

Steps	Rationale
1. See Standard Protocol (Chapter 1, p. 5).	
2. Assist client to put on hospital gown and remove personal items.	
3. Instruct client to remove makeup, nail polish, hairpins, and jewelry.	During and after surgery, the skin is assessed to determine tissue perfusion. (In some settings, clients are allowed to have a ring taped and to remove polish from only one nail.)
4. Ensure that money and valuables have been locked up or given to a family member.	
5. Verify that client's identification and blood band are correct and legible.	In outpatient settings, these bands are applied at this time.
6. Ensure that client has had nothing to eat or drink during the last 8 hours.	Under general anesthesia, the sphincters in the stomach relax, and contents can reflux into the esophagus and into the trachea. (Some settings now use a shorter time frame.)
7. Verify that client has taken medications as instructed.	
8. Ensure that a medical history and physical examination results are in client's record.	
9. Verify that surgical consent is complete (Figure 18-10).	
10. Ensure that necessary laboratory work, ECG, and chest x-ray studies have been completed.	

A-1c PREOPERATIVE/PREPROCEDURAL CHECKLIST

● File with other A-1c's of same date. ●

PROCEDURE: _____

DATE OF PROCEDURE: _____

1. Place initials in appropriate box: YES, NO, N/A (not applicable, or was not ordered). Each item must have an entry.
2. Explain any "No." This can be done in the space after the item or in the "Comments" section. Use back of form, if needed.
3. To give more information on any item, use the space after the item. If more space needed, use the "Comments" section or back of form.

DATE

HOSP. NO.

NAME

BIRTHDATE

ADDRESS

IF NOT IMPRINTED, PLEASE PRINT DATE, HOSP. NO., NAME AND LOCATION

YES	NO	N/A	
			Special Information (e.g., blind, O$_2$, combative)
			Preoperative orders written.
			(If "NO", Dr. _____ notified at _____ date/time.)
			Consent complete and in medical record.
			Allergies (or NKA) labelled on cover of medical record.
			Specify Allergies:
			Isolation label on cover of medical record. Specify type:
			Ordered lab results in medical record.
			Urinalysis results in medical record.
			Chest x-ray completed. (Report in medical record: Yes _____ No _____)
			EKG in medical record.
			Type and cross/screen (circle) done. Date drawn:
			History and physical in medical record.
			Forms complete and in medical record:
			1. Nursing documentation with assessment, VS, and wt./ht.
			2. IV Solution Administration Cardex.
			3. Medication Administration Cardex.
			Addressograph plate on cover of medical record. All volumes to procedure, if required.
COMMENTS:			
			Blood band on patient and legible. Specify location _____ and blood band # _____
			Identification band on patient and legible. Specify location:
			Bathed and in proper attire.
			Nail polish, makeup, and hairpins removed.
			Jewelry removed. Specify item(s) removed and disposition:
			Prosthesis removed: hearing aid, dentures, eye glasses, contact lenses (circle).
			Other: Disposition:
			Anti-embolism stockings on.
			Sequential compression device sleeves on and controller to OR.
			NPO since:
			Teaching completed and documented.
			Preps/tests completed as ordered. Specify:
			Voided/catheterized (circle). Time:
			Medication(s) given.
			Medication(s)/article(s) sent with patient. Specify:
COMMENTS:			

Date	Initials	Signature and Title of Individuals Filling Out Form
Date	Initials	Signature of RN Sending Patient to Procedure

41006/4-93/H7528

THE UNIVERSITY OF IOWA HOSPITALS AND CLINICS

Figure 18-9 (Courtesy University of Iowa Hospitals and Clinics.)

G-2d₂ CONSENT FOR OPERATION OR PROCEDURE

(See reverse for Monitored Telephone Call)

DATE

HOSP. NO.

NAME

BIRTHDATE

ADDRESS

● File most recent sheet ON BOTTOM ●

IF NOT IMPRINTED, PLEASE PRINT DATE, HOSP. NO., NAME AND LOCATION

1. I hereby authorize Doctors _____ , and such other associates
(Attending and Resident Physician[s]/Dentist[s])
as may be selected by the attending doctor to perform upon _____
(Myself or Name of Patient)
the following operation/procedure: _____
(Technical name, followed by description in lay language)

_____

_____

_____

_____

_____

2. In the event developments indicate that further operations/procedures may be necessary, I authorize the physicians to use their own judgment and do whatever they deem advisable during the operation/procedure for the patient's best interests, except the following: _____

_____
(List any exclusions. If none, write "none.")

_____

3. I consent to the administration of such anesthetics as may be considered necessary or advisable by the anesthetist, with the exception of: _____

_____
(List any exclusions. If none, write "none.")

4. The nature of my condition, the nature and purpose of the operation/procedure, possible alternative methods of treatment, the risks involved, and the possible consequences and complications have been explained to me by Doctor _____ . My questions concerning the operation/procedure and its possible outcome have been answered to my satisfaction.

5. I am aware that the practice of dentistry, medicine, and surgery is not an exact science and acknowledge that no guarantees have been made to me by anyone concerning the results of the operation/procedure.

6. Any tissues surgically removed may be disposed by the Hospital in accordance with accustomed practice, including use in research studies, except as follows: _____

_____
(If none, write "none.")

Signature: _____
(Patient or person authorized to consent for patient)

I declare that I have personally explained to _____ the nature of the patient's
(Patient or Representative)
condition, the procedures to be undertaken, the risks involved, and the alternatives, as set forth in 1 and 4 above,

on_____at_____a.m. _____
(Date)   (Time) p.m.
(Signature of Physician/Dentist)

—Continued On Reverse—

29365/7-84/H1575   **THE UNIVERSITY OF IOWA HOSPITALS AND CLINICS**

Figure 18-10 (Courtesy University of Iowa Hospitals and Clinics.)

Steps	Rationale

11. Check that blood transfusions are available as needed.
12. Ask client if he or she has an advanced directive. If so, place it in client's record.
13. Assess and record client's heart rate, blood pressure, respiratory rate, oxygen saturation, and temperature.
14. Administer enemas if ordered (see Skill 8.4).

    Enemas are used when surgery is near the lower intestine.

15. Instruct client to void.
16. Start an IV line; refer to unit standards or physician's orders (see Skill 29.1).
17. Administer preoperative medications as ordered (see Chapters 17 and 29).

    To be most effective, preoperative antibiotics should be administered within 2 hours preoperatively (Classen et al., 1992).

18. **Apply antiembolism stockings.**

    Antiembolism stockings promote circulation during periods of immobilization, reducing the risk of an embolism (Coleridge-Smith, 1991).

    a. Measure client while standing, from gluteal fold to the floor, circumference of largest part of the calf.
    b. With the client lying down, invert the stocking and slip it over the foot (Figure 18-11, *A* to *C*).
    c. With the foot raised, ease the stocking snugly over the leg (Figure 18-11, *D*).

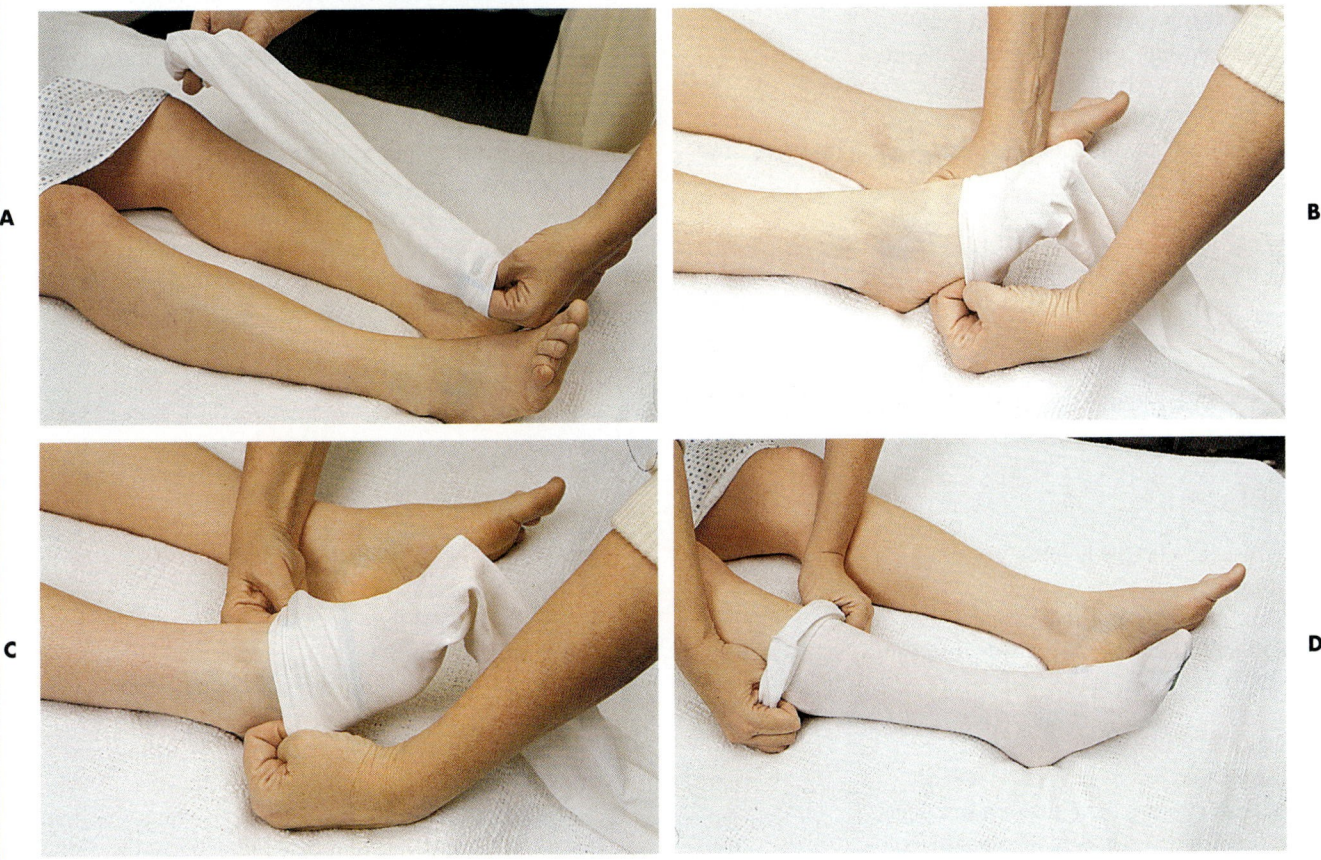

Figure 18-11

Steps	Rationale

19. Apply sequential compression stockings if ordered.

 a. Measure around the largest part of the thigh.
 b. Wrap stockings around the leg, starting at the ankle, with the opening over the patella (Figure 18-12).
 c. Attach the stockings to the insufflator, and verify that the intermittent pressure is between 35 to 45 mm Hg.

Sequential compression stockings promote circulation by sequentially compressing the legs from the ankle upward (Scurr, Coleridge-Smith, and Hasty, 1987).

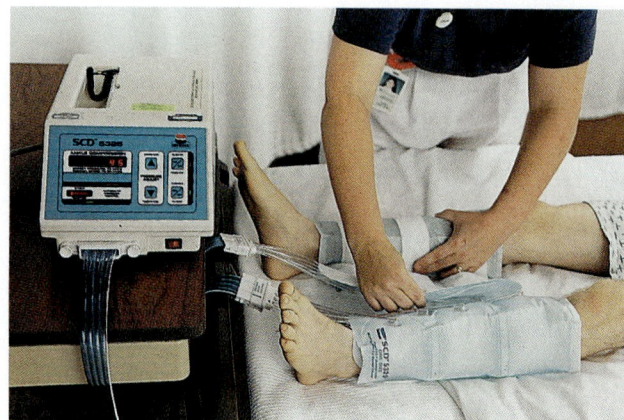

Figure 18-12

20. Clip hair at incision site.
 a. Inspect the general condition of the skin.
 b. Explain the purpose of hair removal to client.
 c. Apply towels along skin edges.
 d. Clip hair with an electric clippers.
 e. Remove hair with disposable towels.
21. Insert a urinary catheter if ordered.
22. Remove contact lenses, eyeglasses, hairpieces, and dentures.

23. Place a cap on client's head.

24. Assist client onto stretcher for transport to OR.
25. See Completion Protocol (Chapter 1, p. 6).

If abrasions or signs of skin infection are present, the risk of surgical wound infection increases. If hair removal is necessary, clipping the morning of surgery has been associated with the lowest infection rates. Shaving increases the risk of infection (Jepsen and Bruttomesso, 1993).

See Skill 34-1.

Eyeglasses and hearing aids are needed for communication and decrease feelings of powerlessness. They should be left in place as long as possible before surgery. In some settings, the dentures are left in place.

The cap contains and protects the hair during surgery. Plastic or reflective caps reduce heat loss during surgery.

Some ambulatory surgery clients walk to OR.

Evaluation

1. Observe client's level of cooperation during preparation.
2. Ask client to assist with measures to reduce the risk of infection (preoperative antibiotics, skin preparation).

UNEXPECTED OUTCOMES AND RELATED INTERVENTIONS

1. Client reports having eaten breakfast.
    Notify surgeon and anesthesiologist/nurse anesthetist.

2. Client refuses to go to surgery until contacting a family member.
    a. Notify surgeon.
    b. Assist client to contact family member.
3. Consent is incomplete.
    Notify surgeon and anesthesiologist/nurse anesthetist.
4. Client did not follow instructions regarding medications.
    Notify surgeon.
5. Client has a reaction to a preoperative medication.
    a. Discontinue the medication.

b. Treat the reaction as per policy in the setting.

c. Notify surgeon.

6. Client is scheduled to be discharged postoperatively and does not have an accompanying adult.

a. Notify surgeon and anesthesiologist/nurse anesthetist.

b. Assist client in contacting someone to provide care at home.

SAMPLE DOCUMENTATION

Preoperative physical preparation is frequently documented in a form called a preoperative checklist (see Figure 18-9).

CRITICAL THINKING EXERCISES

1. Deronda is scheduled for abdominal surgery in the morning. After you teach Deronda about incentive spirometry, she states that she does not have a cold and doesn't understand why this is necessary.

a. How should you respond to Deronda's comment?

b. Following your explanation, Deronda appears anxious and asks if you think she is going to have problems after surgery. Again, how would you respond to Deronda?

2. Evaluate each of the following situations. For each, decide if further action is required on the part of the nurse. If so, what action is required?

a. While you are preparing to give Mr. Brooks his preoperative medication, he states that he wishes he could have two aspirin tablets for his arthritis pain. Upon further questioning, you learn that he takes 6 to 8 aspirin tablets daily for chronic arthritis pain.

b. While reviewing Sondra's chart before her surgery, you note that her last documented complete blood count was 4 days ago, even though a CBC was ordered for this morning.

c. Mrs. White states that the evening nurse told her she would be left in the recovery room after her surgery until she was fully awake.

d. You have just completed Margarita's preoperative teaching, including abdominal splinting, deep breathing, and leg exercises.

e. Mr. Blackfoot has just been given his preoperative medication, which included a narcotic analgesic. His call light is within reach and his wife is at his bedside.

3. The nurse is preparing Mr. Perez for surgery. She performed a brief physical assessment; asked about Mr. Perez's allergies and medication history; obtained his current height and weight and vital signs; made certain the operative permit was accurate and signed; and had Mr. Perez remove all clothing and put on a hospital gown, remove his dentures, and empty his bladder. The nurse also explained to the family where they could wait while Mr. Perez was in surgery and recovery. Evaluate the nurse's preparation of Mr. Perez. Have any important aspects of Mr. Perez's preoperative care been missed? If so, what?

REFERENCES

Classen DC et al: The timing of prophylactic administration of antibiotics and the risk of surgical wound infection, *N Engl J Med* 326(5):281, 1992.

Coleridge-Smith PH: Deep vein thrombosis: effect of graduated compression stockings on distention of the deep veins of the calf, *Br J Surg* 78:724, 1991.

Horsley JA, Pelz DC: *Structured preoperative teaching,* New York, 1981, Grune & Stratton.

Iowa Intervention Project: *Nursing interventions classification,* St Louis, 1992, Mosby.

Jepsen OB, Bruttomesso KA: The effectiveness of preoperative skin preparations: an integrated review of the literature, *AORN J* 58(3):477, 1993.

Rakel B: Interventions related to patient teaching. In GM Bulechek, McCloskey JC, editors: Symposium on nursing interventions, *Nurs Clin North Am* 27(2):397, 1992.

Scurr JH, Coleridge-Smith PD, Hasty JH: Regimen for improved effectiveness of intermittent pneumatic compression in deep vein thrombosis prophylaxis, *Surgery* 102(5):816, 1987.

Steelman V: *Latex sensitivity,* videotape AV 9311-01, Covington, Ga, 1994, Bard.

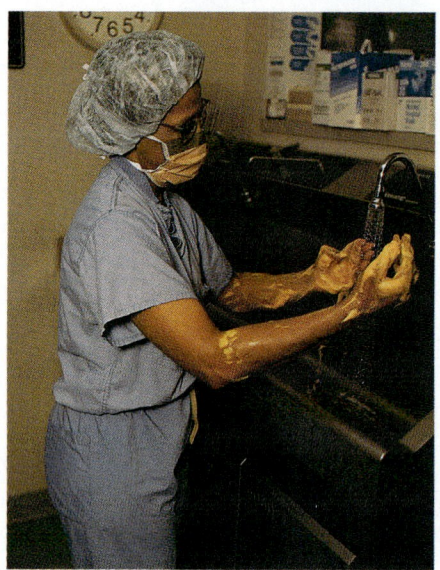

chapter 19

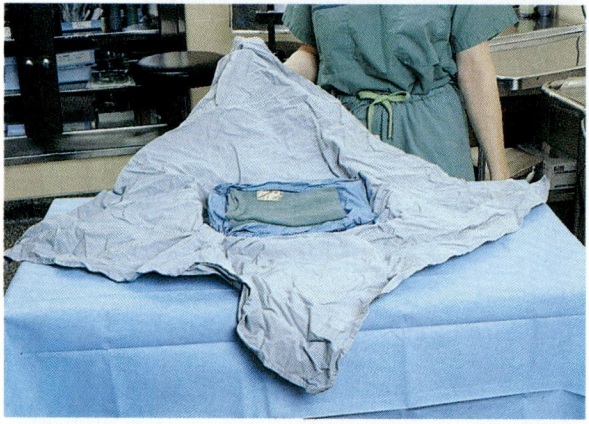

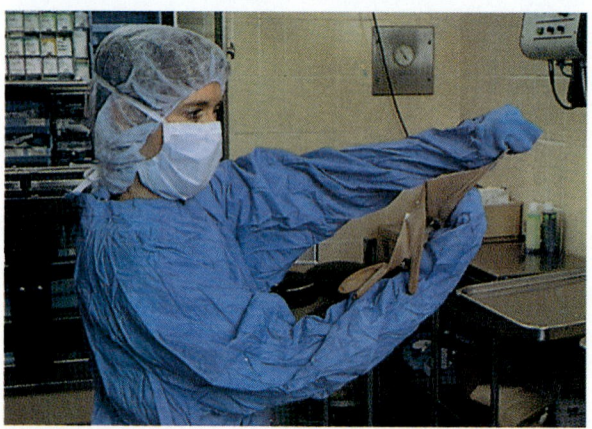

Intraoperative Techniques

Skill 19.1
Surgical Hand Scrub

Skill 19.2
Applying Gown and Gloving

The intraoperative phase starts when the client enters the operating room (OR) suite and ends with admission to the postanesthesia care unit or recovery area. During this intraoperative phase, the perioperative nurse applies the nursing process to coordinate each client's care, keeping in mind safety, comfort, and support.

Members of the surgical team include the surgeon and assistant(s), certified registered nurse anesthetist (CRNA) and/or physician anesthesiologist, circulating nurse, and scrub nurse or surgical technologist. A few examples of more specialized team members include a cardiopulmonary perfusionist, blood (cell) saver technologist, or orthopedic technician.

The perioperative nurse assumes one of two roles in the OR. The *circulating nurse* is always a registered nurse (RN) and is considered to be the charge nurse in the room (AORN, 1994c). The circulator assists the scrubbed personnel by linking the team to the unsterile environment and assumes responsibility and accountability for the delivery of safe, quality client care (see box on p. 353).

The *scrub nurse,* who may be an RN, LPN, or surgical technologist, passes instruments and supplies to the surgeons and assistants and maintains the sterile field (see box on p. 353). Both the circulating and the scrub nurses monitor for and enforce strict adherence to the principles of aseptic technique (see Chapter 14), ensuring optimum client protection against contamination of microorganisms during the surgical procedure.

It is essential that perioperative nurses fully understand and follow the principles of aseptic technique and are willing to develop a sterile conscience. A sterile conscience requires knowledge of the principles of aseptic technique, self-discipline, good communication skills to identify, address, and correct any breaks in sterile technique, and the maturity to overcome personal preferences (Perry and Potter, 1994).

Role of the Circulating Nurse

- Organizes and prepares operating room before start of case; checks to see equipment works properly.
- Gathers supplies for case and opens sterile supplies for scrub nurse.
- Counts sponges, "sharps," and instruments with scrub nurse before incision is made.
- Sends for client at appropriate time.
- Conducts preoperative client assessment, including:
    Explains role and identifies client.
    Reviews medical record and verifies procedure and consents.
    Confirms client's allergies, NPO status, laboratory values, electrocardiogram (ECG), and x-ray studies.
- Safely transfers client to operating table, and positions client according to surgeon's preference and procedure type.
- Applies conductive pad to client if electrocautery used; may prep client's skin; may apply ECG electrodes for local case.
- Explains briefly what he or she and the scrub nurse are doing.
- Assists surgical team by tying gowns and arranging tables.
- Assists anesthesiologist during induction and extubation.
- Continuously monitors procedure for any breaks in aseptic technique or to anticipate needs of the team; opens additional sterile supplies for scrub nurse.
- Handles surgical specimens per institutional policy.
- Documents on perioperative nurses' notes.
- Performs sponge, sharp, and instrument counts with scrub nurse at beginning of wound closure.

Role of the Scrub Nurse

- Assists circulating nurse in preparing OR.
- Performs surgical hand scrub and wears sterile gown and gloves.
- Sets up sterile field with procedure-appropriate supplies and instruments, verifying all are in working order.
- Performs sponge, "sharp," and instrument counts with circulating nurse before incision.
- Gowns and gloves surgeons and assistants as they enter the OR.
- Assists surgeons with sterile draping of client.
- Keeps sterile field orderly and monitors progress or procedure and any breaks in aseptic technique.
- Passes instruments and supplies to surgeons and assistants.
- Handles surgical specimens per institutional policy.
- Constantly monitors location of all sponges and sharps in the field and performs closing sponge, sharp, and instrument counts with circulating nurse.

If any question exists about sterility, the item must be considered to be unsterile. A sterile gown that touches the floor while being put on is discarded and exchanged for a new one; the surgeon who touches an unsterile area with a gloved hand changes the affected glove; the scrub nurse who accidentally touches the faucet with one hand while rinsing rescrubs. These are all examples of following one's sterile conscience and being committed to safe, quality client care.

Although not directly related to aseptic technique, most clients who undergo surgery are unfamiliar with the OR environment and what to expect. The perioperative nurse must assess and document the client's emotional status and understanding of the surgical procedure to be performed. The client's need for more support and information may be defined in most instances by a request for more information but may appear as an inappropriate or exaggerated behavior such as hostility, apathy, or denial.

Nursing Diagnosis

Risk for Infection is the most appropriate nursing diagnosis for clients undergoing invasive procedures. When the surgical procedure involves an incision or entrance into a sterile body cavity, such as the bladder, prevention of infection is a major nursing responsibility. Even when aseptic technique is followed, some clients will have a greater-than-average risk for infection (see Chapters 15 and 20).

Anxiety related to a knowledge deficit regarding OR procedures is another major focus for the perioperative nurse. Nurses need to provide support and information as they prepare clients for surgery.

Skill 19.1 Surgical Hand Scrub

The surgical hand scrub is an essential skill to achieving surgical asepsis. Although the skin cannot be sterilized, the number of microorganisms can be greatly reduced by chemical, physical, and mechanical means. The surgical hand scrub (AORN, 1994b):

- Removes debris and transient microorganisms from the nails, hands, and forearms
- Reduces the resident microbial count to a minimum
- Inhibits rapid/rebound growth of microorganisms

Antimicrobials such as Betadine, Hibiclens, and Septisol improve removal of bacteria from hands and arms (Perry and Potter, 1994).

Surgical attire (scrubs) should be worn in the OR to reduce the chance for contamination from personnel to clients, and vice versa. Fingernails should be short, clean, and free of polish and/or artificial nails, which can harbor bacteria and fungi (AORN, 1994b). All rings, watches, and bracelets are removed before the surgical scrub.

The AORN recommends a 5- to 10-minute hand scrub with an approved antimicrobial agent for all surgical procedures. The institution should standardize the surgical hand scrub procedure for all staff using either the anatomical timed scrub or the counted stroke method (AORN, 1994b) (see agency policy). Some procedures require a vigorous hand wash but not necessarily a surgical scrub. Some examples of clean procedures are laryngoscopy, esophagoscopy, and proctoscopy.

EQUIPMENT

Deep sink with foot or knee controls for dispensing water and soap
Antimicrobial agent (approved by institution)
Surgical scrub brush with plastic nail file
Paper mask and cap or hood
Sterile towel
Proper scrub attire
Protective eye wear

Assessment

1. Determine type and length of time for hand wash or scrub (check agency policy).
2. Remove bracelets, rings, and watches.
3. Inspect fingernails, which must be short and free of polish and/or artificial nails or tips.
4. Inspect skin and cuticles of hands and arms for abrasions, cuts, or open lesions.

Planning

Expected outcomes should focus on prevention of infection resulting from breaks in aseptic technique.

EXPECTED OUTCOME

Client does not develop signs of surgical wound infection.

Implementation

Steps	Rationale
1. Put on surgical shoe covers, cap or hood, face mask, and protective eye wear.	
2. Turn water on using knee control and adjust to comfortable temperature.	
3. Wet hands and arms, keeping arms flexed with hands pointed upward, allowing the water to flow off at the elbows.	
4. Rinse hands and arms, keeping arms flexed with hands pointed upward, allowing the water to flow off at the elbows.	Water runs from fingertips to elbows by gravity, thus keeping the hands the cleanest part of the upper extremity.
5. Clean under nails of both hands with file under running water, then discard file (Figure 19-1).	Removes dirt and organic materials that harbor a large number of microorganisms.
6. Wet brush and apply antimicrobial agent. Scrub the nails of one hand with 15 strokes (Figure 19-2). Scrub the palm, each side of thumb and fingers, and the posterior side of the hand with 10 strokes each (Figure 19-3). The arm is mentally divided into thirds, and each third is scrubbed 10 times (Perry and Potter, 1994). Some agencies may scrub by time rather than 10 strokes.	
7. Discard brush; flex arms and rinse from fingertips to elbows in one continuous motion, allowing water to run off at elbow (Figure 19-4).	
8. Turn off water with foot or knee control and back into room with hands elevated in front and away from body.	

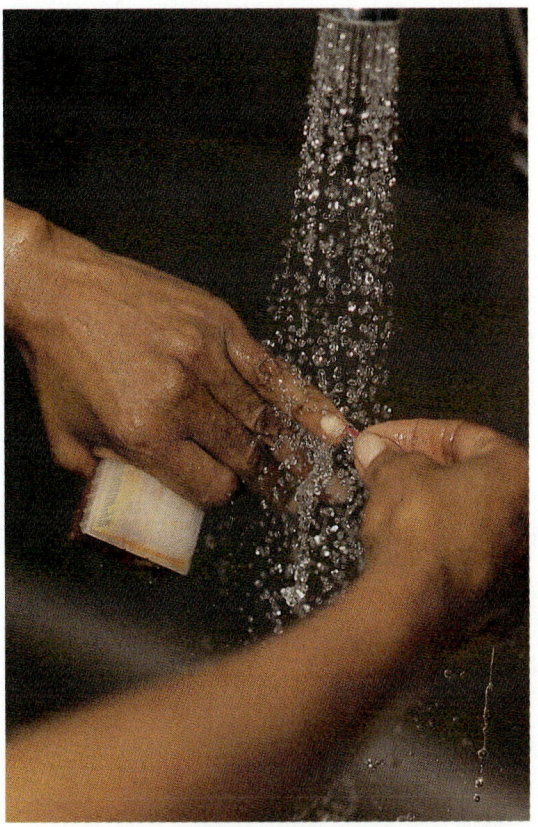

Figure 19-1

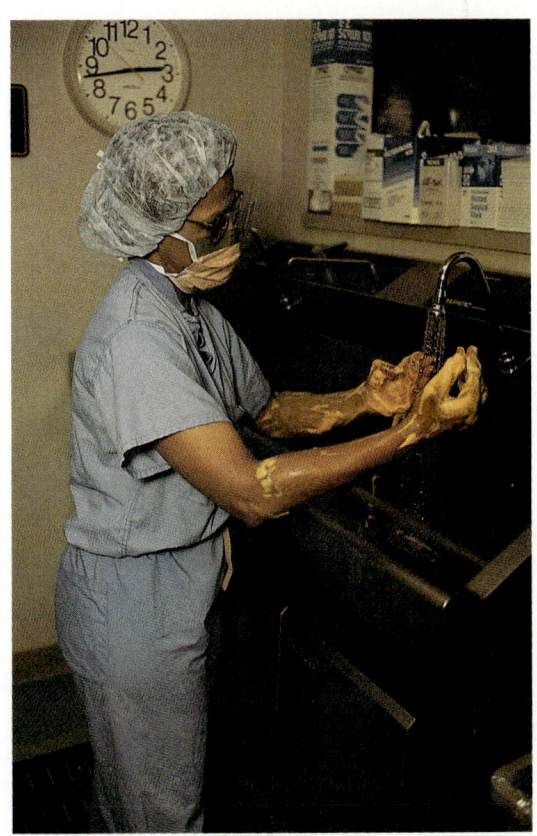

Figure 19-2

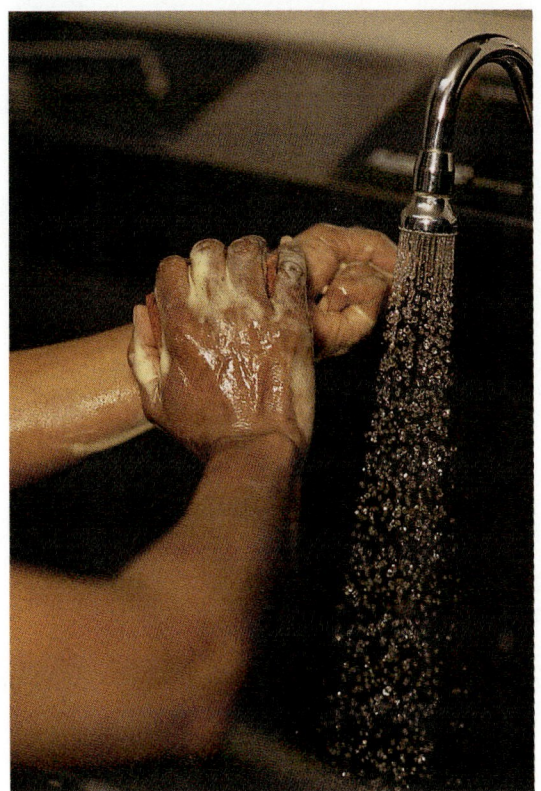

Figure 19-3

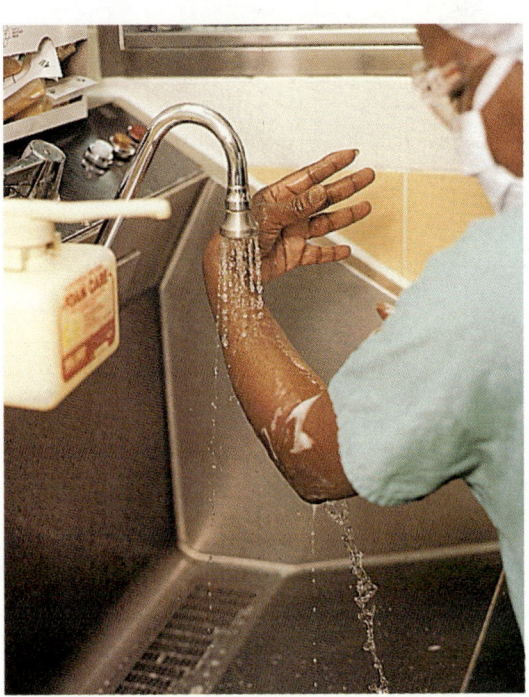

Figure 19-4

Steps	Rationale
9. Go to sterile setup and grasp sterile towel, taking care not to drip water on the sterile field (Figure 19-5). Using a sterile towel, dry one hand thoroughly, moving from fingers to elbow in a rotating motion (Figure 19-6).	Dry from cleanest (hands) to least clean (elbows).
10. Transfer sterile towel to opposite end (Figure 19-7), and repeat Step 9 for other hand.	Avoids transfer of microorganisms from elbow to opposite hand.
11. Drop towel into linen hamper or into circulating nurse's hands.	

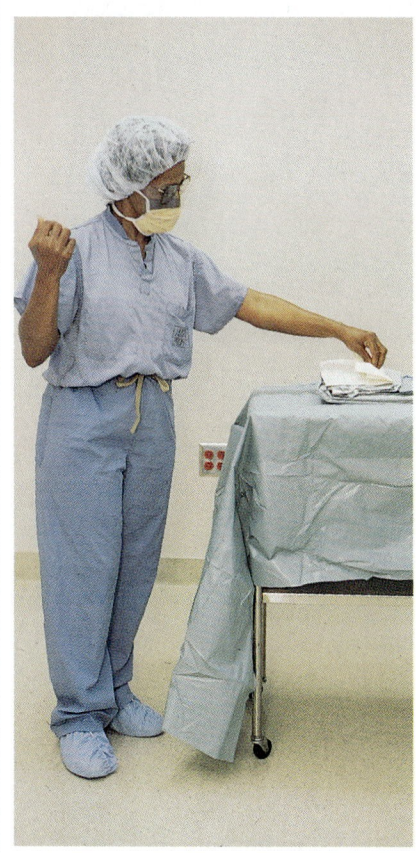

Figure 19-5

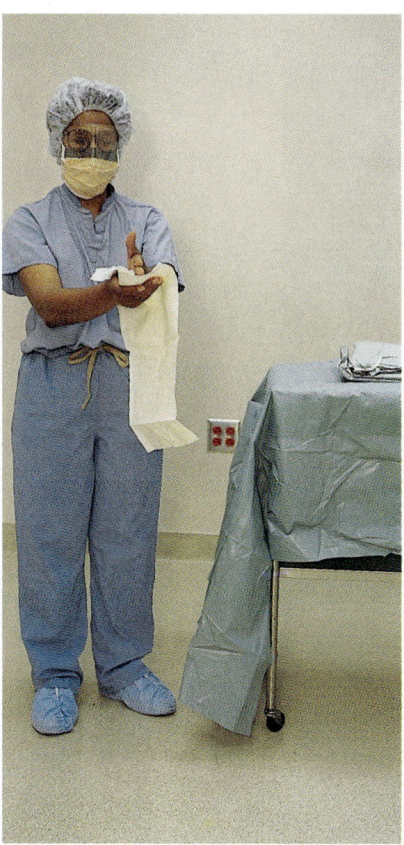

Figure 19-6

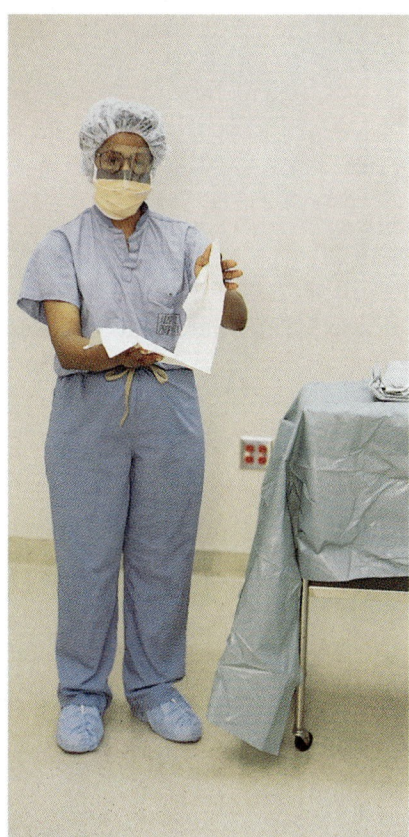

Figure 19-7

Evaluation

Monitor postoperative client for signs of surgical wound infection, including redness, tenderness, and purulent drainage.

UNEXPECTED OUTCOME AND RELATED INTERVENTIONS

Client develops postoperative surgical wound infection. Interventions should be individualized to client situation (e.g., wound care, antibiotic therapy).

Skill 19.2 | Applying Sterile Gown and Closed Gloving

Immediately following a surgical scrub, a sterile gown should be applied, followed by application of sterile gloves. All members of the surgical team that will work around the sterile field must prepare in this manner before entering the sterile field. Once applied, the surgical gown is considered sterile in front from chest to waist or table level. The sleeves are considered sterile from 5 cm (2 inches) above the elbow to fingertips. The back of the gown is no longer considered sterile.

Surgical gowns should cover all garments worn underneath. All sterile gowns and drapes made of materials that are free of tears, punctures, strain, and abrasion, provide an effective barrier against microorganisms passing between unsterile and sterile areas (AORN, 1994a).

Nursing personnel should use the closed-glove method when initially entering the sterile field. If a glove becomes contaminated during the surgery, the circulating nurse, wearing protective unsterile gloves, grasps the outside of the glove and pulls off the glove inside out, leaving the stockinette cuff in place. Another sterile team member can assist in regloving, or the open-glove method can be used. If both the scrub nurse's gloves become contaminated, it is recommended to regown and reglove using the closed-glove method.

EQUIPMENT

Package of proper-sized sterile gloves
Sterile pack containing sterile gown
Clean, flat, dry surface (table or Mayo stand) on which to open gown and gloves
Surgical cap, mask, eyewear, and footwear
Protective eye wear

Assessment

1. Select proper size and type of sterile gloves. Proper fit ensures care of handling supplies.
2. Select proper size and type of sterile surgical gown.

Planning

Expected outcome focuses on prevention of infection resulting from breaks in aseptic technique.

EXPECTED OUTCOME

Client does not develop signs of surgical wound infection.

Implementation

Steps	Rationale
1. Perform surgical hand scrub (see Skill 19.1). Nurse will have protective garments applied.	
2. Have circulating nurse open sterile gown and glove package on a clean, dry, flat surface (Figure 19-8; see Skill 14.2).	
3. Enter operating suite after surgical scrub (see Skill 19.1), keeping elbows bent and hands above waist. Pick up gown (folded inside out) from sterile package, grasping the inside surface of gown at the collar.	Prevents hands from touching contaminated object.
4. Lift folded gown directly upward and away from the table.	
5. Locate neckband and with both hands; grasp the inside front of gown just below neckline.	Clean hands may touch inside of gown without contaminating outer surface.
6. Allow gown to open, keeping at arm's length away from body with the inside of gown toward body (Figure 19-9). Do not touch outside of gown or allow it to touch the floor.	Outside of gown remains sterile.
7. Slip both arms into armholes simultaneously (do not allow hands to move through cuff opening), keeping hands at shoulder level.	
8. Have circulating nurse pull on gown by reaching inside arm seams. Gown is pulled on, leaving sleeves covering hands.	

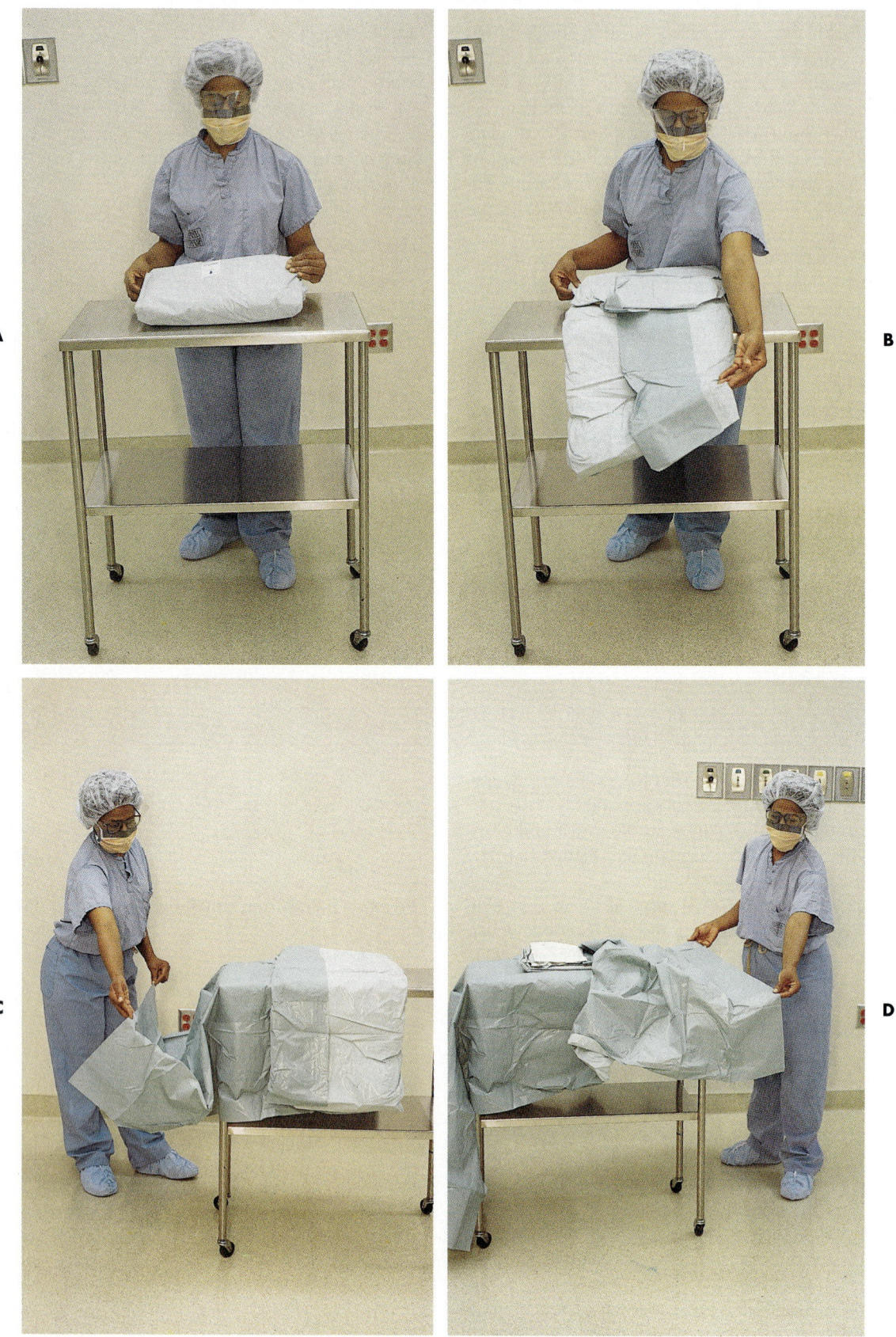

Figure 19-8

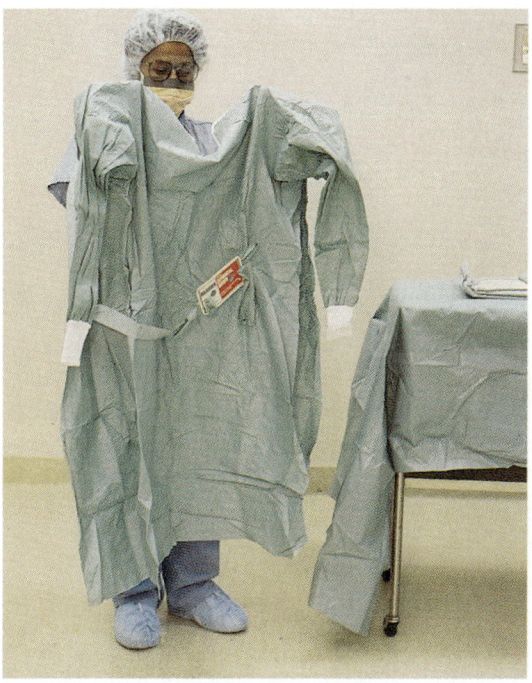

Figure 19-9

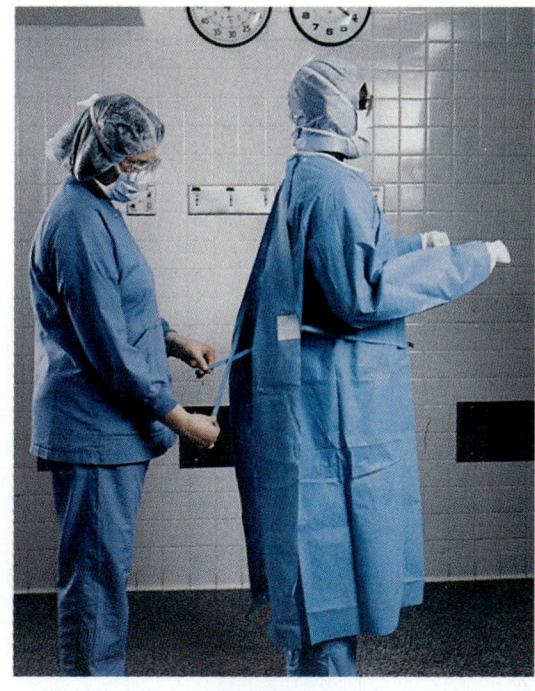

Figure 19-10

Steps	Rationale
9. Have circulating nurse tie gown at neck and waist (Figure 19-10). If wrap around gown, sterile flap is not touched until sterile gloves have been applied.	
10. Apply gloves using the closed-glove method.	
a. With hands covered by gown cuffs and sleeves, open inner sterile glove package (Figure 19-11,*A*).	Hands remain clean, and sterile gown cuff will touch sterile glove surface.
b. Grasp folded cuff of glove for dominant hand with the nondominant hand.	Sterile gown touches sterile glove.
c. Extend dominant forearm forward with palm up, and place palm of glove against palm of dominant hand. Gloved fingers point toward elbow.	Open end of glove is positioned for application over cuff-covered hand.
d. Grasp cuff edges with thumb and forefingers of dominant hand. Grasp back of glove cuff with nondominant hand, and turn cuff over dominant hand (Figure 19-11, *B*). Extend fingers into glove and pull glove over cuff.	
e. Glove nondominant hand in same manner with gloved, dominant hand (Figure 19-11, *C* and *D*). Keep hand inside sleeve. Be sure fingers are fully extended into both gloves.	
11. For wraparound gown:	
a. Grasp sterile waist tie with gloved hands and untie.	Front of gown is sterile.
b. Pass tie to another sterile team member, who stands still, or wrap tie in sterile towel and pass to circulating nurse. Keep gown tie in left hand (Figure 19-12).	

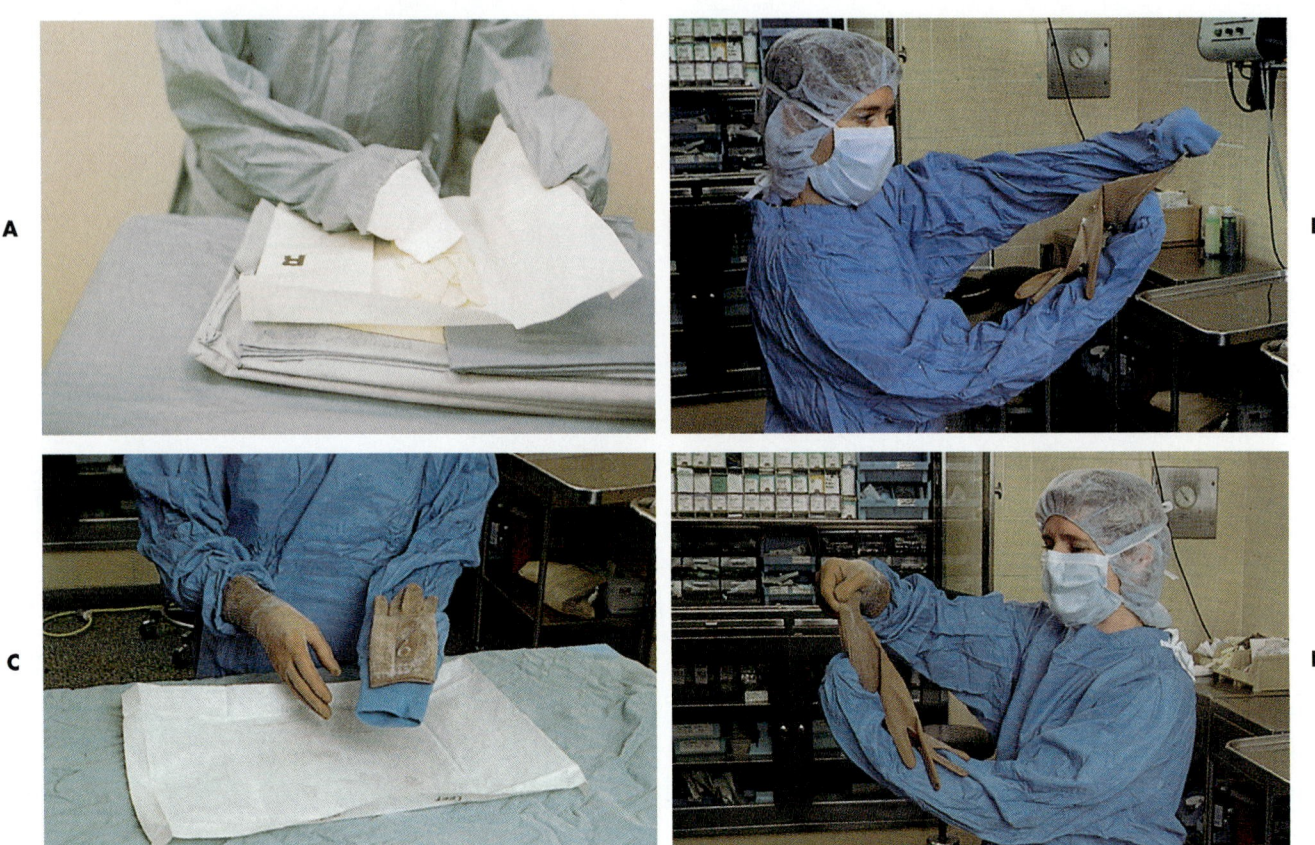

Figure 19-11

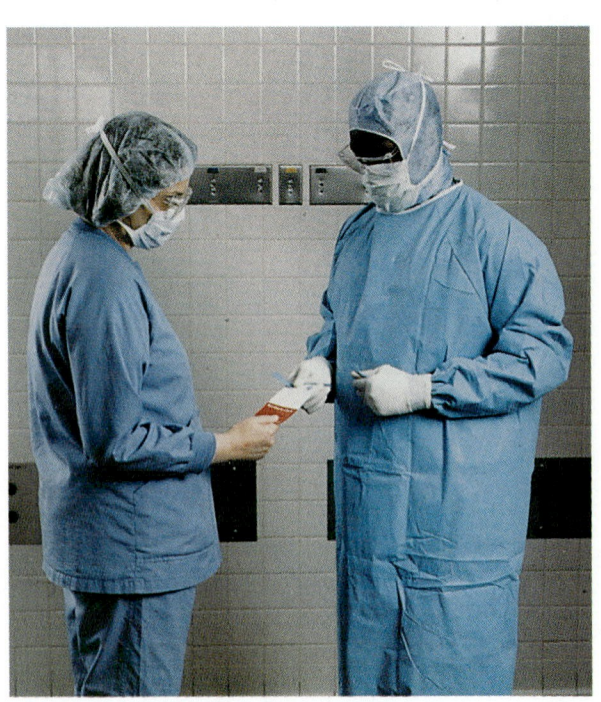

Figure 19-12

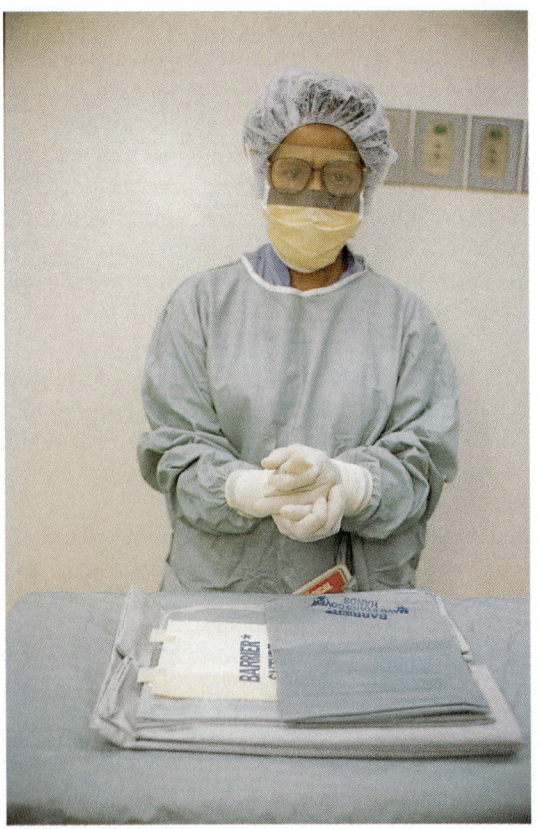

Figure 19-13

Steps	Rationale

c. Allowing margin of safety, turn to the left one-half turn, covering back with extended gown flap. Retrieve tie only from team member, and secure both ties in place.

12. Stand so as to maintain sterility (Figure 19-13).

Evaluation

Monitor postoperative client for signs of surgical wound infection; inspect wound and palpate for tenderness.

UNEXPECTED OUTCOME AND RELATED INTERVENTIONS

Client develops postoperative surgical wound infection. Interventions should be individualized to client situation (e.g., wound care, antibiotic therapy).

SAMPLE DOCUMENTATION

1000 48 hr postop; surgical wound incision clean, dry, and well approximated without redness, tenderness, edema, or drainage. Client remains afebrile; complains of only slight discomfort around suture line.

CRITICAL THINKING EXERCISES

1. The circulating nurse and scrub nurse function differently in the operating room; however, they share an important responsibility. What is that responsibility, and why is it important?

2. You are teaching a nursing student how to perform a surgical hand scrub. As you finish scrubbing and start rinsing your hands, the student asks why you are holding your hands in an upward position, since water is running down to your elbows. How would you answer the student's question?

3. Lucia is the scrub nurse. Upon requesting another package of sterile sutures from the circulating nurse, Lucia notes that the package touches an unsterile part of her table when it is delivered to her. She leaves the package unopened and requests another package of sutures from the circulating nurse.

   a. What does Lucia's action represent?
   b. What consequence could have occurred if Lucia had not acted as she did?

4. You are the circulating nurse for Mr. Armeed's surgery. As the OR technician pulls on his sterile gloves, he comments that they feel tight. Is any intervention appropriate on your behalf? Why or why not?

5. Label each of the following functions according to the roles of the circulating and scrub nurses.
   C - Role of circulating nurse
   S - Role of scrub nurse
   B - Role of both the circulating and scrub nurse

   a. Performs sponge and instrument counts before surgeon makes incision.
   b. Checks to verify that all surgical instruments are properly working.
   c. Opens sterile packages during the surgery.
   d. Assists client with transfer to the operating room table.
   e. Handles surgical specimens according to agency policy.
   f. Sets up sterile field.
   g. Continually monitors for breaks in sterile technique.

REFERENCES

Association of Operating Room Nurses: Recommended practices for protective barrier materials for surgical gowns and drapes. In *AORN standards and recommended practices for perioperative nursing,* Denver, 1994a, AORN.

Association of Operating Room Nurses: Recommended practices for surgical hand scrubs. In *AORN standards and recommended practices for perioperative nursing,* Denver, 1994b, AORN.

Association of Operating Room Nurses: Statement on mandate for the registered nurse as circulator in the operating room. In *AORN standards and recommended practices for perioperative nursing,* Denver, 1994c, AORN.

Perry A, Potter P: *Clinical nursing skills and techniques,* ed 3, St Louis, 1994, Mosby.

ADDITIONAL READINGS

Atkinson L: *Berry and Kohn's operating room technique,* ed 7, St Louis, 1994, Mosby.

Meeker M, Rothrock J: *Alexander's care of the patient in surgery,* ed 10, St Louis, 1995, Mosby.

Caring for the Postoperative Client

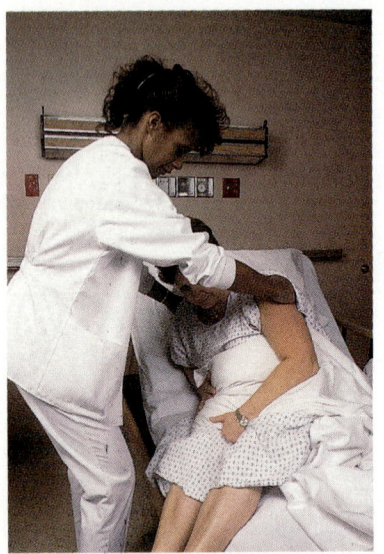

Skill 20.1
Providing Postanesthesia Care

Skill 20.2
Providing Comfort Measures

Skill 20.3
Providing Wound Care

Skill 20.4
Monitoring and Measuring Drainage

Skill 20.5
Removing Staples and Sutures

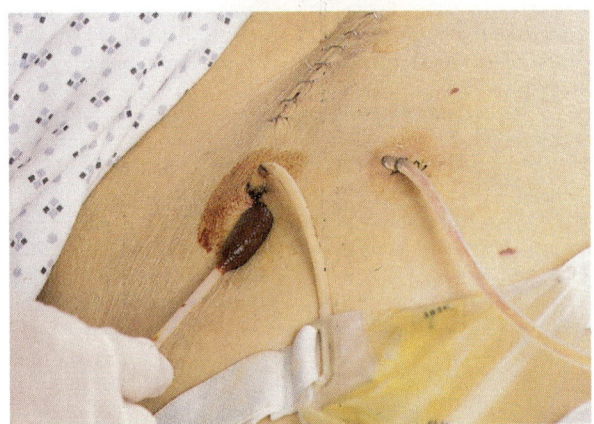

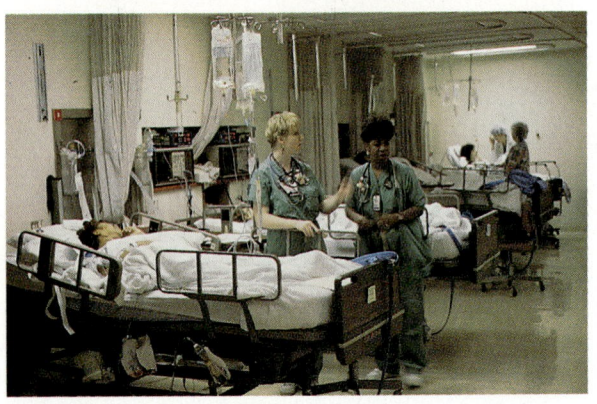

The care of postoperative clients may be divided into two phases, the immediate postanesthesia recovery and the convalescent phase. Phase I extends from the time the client leaves the operating room (OR) to the time of transfer from the postanesthesia room (PAR) to the nursing division. This phase requires 2 or more hours. Phase II, the convalescent phase, involves several days or weeks for the initial healing process. The client with a chronic medical condition, such as chronic respiratory disease or diabetes, may require even longer.

Cost-containment measures and reimbursement policies have dramatically changed routines for surgical procedures. Many surgical procedures that once required an overnight hospital admission are not reimbursed by insurance for inpatient services. Newer equipment, such as laser and laparoscopy, are less invasive and also decrease the need for inpatient admission. Many clients are admitted the morning of surgery rather than receiving inpatient preparation for surgery (Kratz, 1993). The current trend involves more ambulatory outpatient surgery and shorter hospitalizations to achieve cost containment. In addition, clients often recover better at home.

Postanesthesia care units (PACUs), in many respects, are critical care units that require professional nurses with specific education and experience to recognize and help manage anesthesia-related and surgery-related complications (ASPAN Standards, 1992).

The client is accompanied to the PACU by a member of the anesthesia care team, who provides a verbal report, including postoperative status (e.g., vital signs, oxygen saturation, allergies, hearing aids); length of anesthesia and technique (general, regional, or local); anesthesia, muscle relaxant, narcotic, and reversal agents used; vital signs; intravenous (IV) fluids or blood products used in surgery; presence of drains; estimated blood loss and replacement; and complications that occurred during surgery (ASPAN Standards, 1992).

Preoperative orders typically are canceled by surgery, in which case postoperative orders may include a statement to "Continue all preoperative orders." Postoperative orders usually specify frequency of vital signs and special assessments, types of IV fluids and infusion rate, postoperative medications, fluids or foods allowed by mouth, level of activity or type of positioning, intake and output, laboratory tests or x-ray studies to be done, and special interventions such as dressing changes, an immobilizing device, or an incentive spirometer.

The immediate postoperative recovery phase requires frequent assessments for potentially life-threatening complications resulting from anesthesia or surgery. It is important to emphasize the ABCs: *A* is for airway, *B* is for breathing, and *C* is for circulation (Table 20-1). All postoperative clients have a tendency to be hypoxic and should be supplemented with oxygen (Lubarsky and Gallager, 1990).

Size, location, and depth of wound influence type and

Table 20-1 **Complications of Anesthesia**

Condition	Interventions
AIRWAY	
Mechanical obstruction: decreased level of consciousness and muscle relaxants resulting in flaccid muscles and tongue blocking airway	Hyperextend neck; pull mandible forward; use nasal or oral airway; encourage deep breathing.
Retained thick secretions: irritation from anesthesia; anticholinergic medications: history of smoking	Suction; encourage coughing.
Laryngospasm: stridor from excessive secretions or airway irritation	Provide positive-pressure ventilation with oxygen, small dose of muscle relaxant, and intubation.
Laryngeal edema: allergic reaction, irritation from endotracheal tube, fluid overload	Administer oxygen, antihistamines, steroids, sedatives, and intubation.
Bronchospasm: preexisting asthma, anesthetic irritation (expiratory wheeze)	Administer bronchodilators as ordered.
Aspiration: vomiting from hypotension, accumulated gastric secretions and delayed gastric emptying, pain, fear, position changes	Position on side; suction airway; administer antiemetic as ordered.
BREATHING: HYPOVENTILATION/HYPOXEMIA	
Central nervous system depression: anesthesia, analgesics, muscle relaxants (respiratory rate shallow)	Encourage to cough and deep breathe; use mechanical ventilator; administer narcotic antagonist, muscle relaxant reversal agent; reposition; give analgesic; loosen cast or dressings; provide nasogastric intubation.
Mechanical restriction: obesity, tight cast or dressings, abdominal distention, pain	
CIRCULATION	
Hypovolemia: blood loss, dehydration	Elevate legs; give oxygen, IV fluids, or blood replacement; administer vasopressors; monitor intake and output, stimulation, hemoglobin and hematocrit
Hypotension: Anesthesia/drug effects, spinal anesthesia may cause vasodilation; narcotics	
Cardiac failure: preexisting cardiac disease; circulatory overload; excessive/too-rapid fluid replacement	Provide digitalization, diuretics; monitor electrocardiogram (ECG).
Cardiac arrhythmias: hypoxemia; myocardial infarct; hypokalemia, hypothermia; imbalance of potassium, calcium, magnesium	Provide IV fluid replacement; monitor ECG, urine output; identify and treat cause.
Hypertension: pain, distended bladder, preexisting hypertension, vasopressor drugs	Compare to preoperative baseline; identify and cause.
Compartment syndrome: pressure from edema causing enough compression to obstruct arterial and venous circulation resulting in ischemia, permanent numbness, loss of function; forearm and lower leg most common sites	Elevate extremity, apply ice, remove or loosen bandage or cast to relieve compression; if left untreated, amputation may be required.

Table 20-2 Expected Drainage from Tubes and Catheters

Substance	Amount	Characteristics
Urine	>60 ml/hour 500-700ml/24 hours for 1 to 2 days postoperatively 1500-2500 ml/24 hours thereafter	Clear yellow; after urinary tract surgery, bright-red tinged Gynecological surgery may involve instillation of a dark-blue dye into bladder to detect leakage; urine appears dark blue, changing to green 6-8 hours postoperatively as it is eliminated.
Nasogastric tube or gastrostomy	Up to 1500 ml	Gastric contents yellow-green, watery, with mucus; bloody after gastric surgery
Wound drainage, Hemovac, Jackson-Pratt drain, chest tube drainage	Variable with procedure	Bloody
T tube	500 ml	Bright yellow to dark green: bile

Modified from Lewis SM, Collier IC: *Medical-surgical nursing: assessment and management of clinical problems,* ed 3, St Louis, 1992, Mosby.

amount of drainage. It is important to know what type of drainage is expected (Table 20-2). Nurses can estimate drainage by counting the number of saturated gauze sponges. Hemorrhage is loss of large amounts of blood either externally or internally in a short time and will result in shock if uncontrolled. Arterial bleeding is bright red and gushes forth in waves related to heart rhythm; or if a vessel is very deep, flow will be steady. Venous bleeding is dark red and flows smoothly. Capillary bleeding is oozing of dark-red blood; self-sealing controls this bleeding. Some bloody drainage is expected through chest tubes. Bloody drainage exceeding 100 to 200 ml per hour must be reported.

Many physicians prefer reinforcement with additional dressings only, since changing dressings immediately postoperatively can disrupt wound edges and aggravate drainage. Some surgical wounds have gauze dressings or are covered with a clear, transparent dressing. Some are left open to air (OTA).

Nursing Diagnosis

High-risk nursing diagnoses are appropriate relating to the prevention of complications of surgery and anesthesia. Some incisional pain is expected and can increase the risk for postoperative complications. Risk for **Ineffective Airway Clearance** related to incisional pain and increased secretions secondary to general anesthesia and history of smoking could be appropriate. This directs interventions of pain control and removal of secretions from the airway. Risk for or actual **Altered Breathing Pattern** related to sedation secondary to general anesthesia could be appropriate for clients who need stimulation to promote respiratory effort and tend to hypoventilate. **Risk for Aspiration** related to depressed cough/gag reflex secondary to anesthesia focuses interventions on prevention of airway obstruction. **Impaired Physical Mobility** related to incisional pain is useful when the focus of increasing mobility is facilitated by adequate pain control. Risk for **Decreased Cardiac Output** may be used to identify the risk for hemorrhage caused by slipping of suture, inadequate clotting, or excessive blood or fluid loss for any reason. **Fluid Volume Deficit** is also related to excessive loss of fluid and blood from wound drainage or from inadequate fluid replacement. Risk for **Altered Tissue Perfusion** related to venous stasis or vessel trauma may be indicated after surgery of the legs, abdomen, pelvis, and major blood vessels. This is also appropriate when blood coagulation studies indicate increased coagulation and when clients are immobilized, have chronic hypoxia, or use oral contraceptives containing estrogen.

Risk for Infection related to surgical incision (specify location) is appropriate when the client has lowered resistance to infection for any reason. Conditions such as obesity, advanced age, impaired circulation, diabetes, immunosuppression, radiation, smoking, poor cellular nutrition, very deep wounds, or wounds healing by secondary intention result in increased risk of infection. **Risk for Altered Health Maintenance** related to inadequate knowledge of postoperative self-care may be appropriate for clients who have not had surgery previously or who require an extended convalescence because of the nature of the surgery. Teaching needs should be considered for all postoperative clients. **Risk for Injury** related to altered (visual, auditory, kinesthetic, or tactile) perception may be appropriate when surgery or anesthesia alters a client's ability to receive and interpret information.

| Skill 20.1 | **Providing Immediate Postoperative Care in Postanesthesia Care Unit** |

The first phase of postoperative care takes place during the immediate recovery period, which extends from the time the client leaves the OR to the time the client has stabilized in the recovery room (RR) or Postanesthesia Care Unit (PACU) and has been transferred to the nursing division.

The first 1 to 2 hours are the most critical for assessing aftereffects of anesthesia, including airway clearance, cardiovascular complications, temperature control, and neurological function. The client's condition can change rapidly, and assessments must be timely, knowledgeable, and accurate. Quick judgment regarding the most appropriate interventions is essential. The client is usually considered ready for discharge to the general unit when specific standardized criteria are met. REACT is one of several scoring systems for assessment. It uses parameters of *r*espiration, *e*nergy, *a*lertness, *c*irculation, and *t*emperature (Table 20-3). A score of 10 indicates a fully recovered client.

Recovery from ambulatory surgery requires the same assessments; however, the depth of general anesthesia may be less because the surgery is less involved and of shorter duration. Some clients have only IV sedation, for which less monitoring is usually required. As soon as the client is stable and alert, instructions for home care are given to the client and care giver. Demonstrations and written instructions are provided. Encourage the client

not to drive and to postpone making important decisions for 24 hours. Adequate support for home care must be established.

EQUIPMENT

Stethoscope, sphygmomanometer, pulse oximeter, cardiac monitor, thermometer
Oxygen equipment such as mask, oxygen regulator and tubing, and positive-pressure delivery system
Suction equipment
Dressing supplies
Warmed blanket or active rewarming device
Emergency equipment
Emergency medications

Assessment

1. Review client's condition during operative procedure, including range of vital signs, blood volume or fluid loss, fluid replacement, type of anesthesia, type of airway and size, and extent of surgical wound. **This determines client's general status and allows nurse to anticipate need for special equipment, nursing care, and activities in PACU.**

2. On client's arrival in PACU, obtain report from circulating nurse and anesthesiologist or nurse anesthetist that provides review of client's physiological status

Table 20-3 **Postanesthesia Recovery Scoring System (REACT)**

Category	Criterion	Score*
Respiration	Requires ventilator	0
	Artificial airway; spontaneous respirations	1
	Spontaneous respirations; rate <10 without support	2
Energy	Does not move legs, even with stimulation	0
	Moves legs, cannot keep head up	1
	Moves legs, can keep head up	2
Alertness	Awakens when vigorously stimulated	0
	Awakens when gently stimulated	1
	Usually awake, dozes occasionally	2
Circulation	Systolic blood pressure (BP) <80, pulse weak	0
	Systolic BP between 80 and preoperative level, pulse strong	1
	Systolic BP at or above preoperative resting level, pulse strong	2
Axillary temperature	<35° C (95° F)	0
	35° C (95° F) to 35.5° C (95° F to 96° F)	1
	>35.5° C (96° F)	2

*Scoring: fully recovered, 10; some residual effects of anesthesia, 9; continuous close monitoring required, 8 or less.

and baseline data to determine any change in condition.

3. Consider the effects of the client's type of surgery and anesthesia and restrictions to movement. **This information influences type of assessments nurse initiates, type of complications to observe for, and specific nursing interventions.**

Planning

Expected outcomes focus on early detection of complications from surgery or anesthesia and adequate pain control by the time of transfer (usually 1 to 2 hours).

EXPECTED OUTCOMES

1. Client's airway remains clear, and respirations are deep, regular, and within normal limits by the time of transfer.
2. Client's blood pressure, pulse, and temperature remain within previous baseline or normal expected range by the time of transfer.
3. Dressings are clean, dry, and intact by discharge from recovery.
4. Intake and output are within expected parameters by discharge from recovery.
5. Client reports relief of discomfort after analgesia or other pain relief measures by the time of transfer from the immediate recovery area (usually 1 to 2 hours).
6. Client's postoperative assessments are within expected normal postoperative parameters.

Implementation

Steps	Rationale
1. See Standard Protocol (Chapter 1, p. 5).	
2. As client enters RR or PACU on stretcher, immediately attach oxygen tubing to regulator and check IV flow rates. Connect any drainage tubes to intermittent suction.	Inhaled oxygen promotes tissue oxygenation during recovery from anesthesia. IV fluids maintain circulatory volume and provide route for emergency drugs. Drainage tubes must remain patent to prevent pressure within wound cavity.
3. Compare vital signs with client's preoperative baseline. Continue assessing vital signs at least every 5 to 15 minutes until stable.	Vital signs can reveal respiratory depression, cardiac irregularity, hypotension, or hypothermia.
4. Maintain airway after general anesthesia.	
a. If client is supine, elevate head of bed slightly, support neck extension, and turn head to side unless contraindicated. Initially, client may need to be reminded to breathe (Figure 20-1).	Opens airway while client has decreased level of consciousness (LOC).
b. Suction artificial airway and oral cavity if secretions accumulate (see Skill 30.3). Assist client to spit out oral airway (Figure 20-2) as gag reflex returns.	Indicates client can clear airway independently.
5. Call client by name in normal tone of voice. If there is no response, attempt to arouse client by touching or gently moving a body part. Explain that surgery is over and you are in the RR.	Determines client's LOC and ability to follow commands. Assists client to be oriented to place.
6. Encourage client to cough and deep breathe every 15 minutes (see Skill 18.2).	Promotes lung expansion, elimination of inhalation anesthetic, and expectoration of mucous secretions.
7. Inspect color of nail beds and skin. Palpate for skin temperature.	Indicators of peripheral tissue perfusion.
8. Assess closely for potential cardiovascular complications of anesthesia (see Table 20-1).	

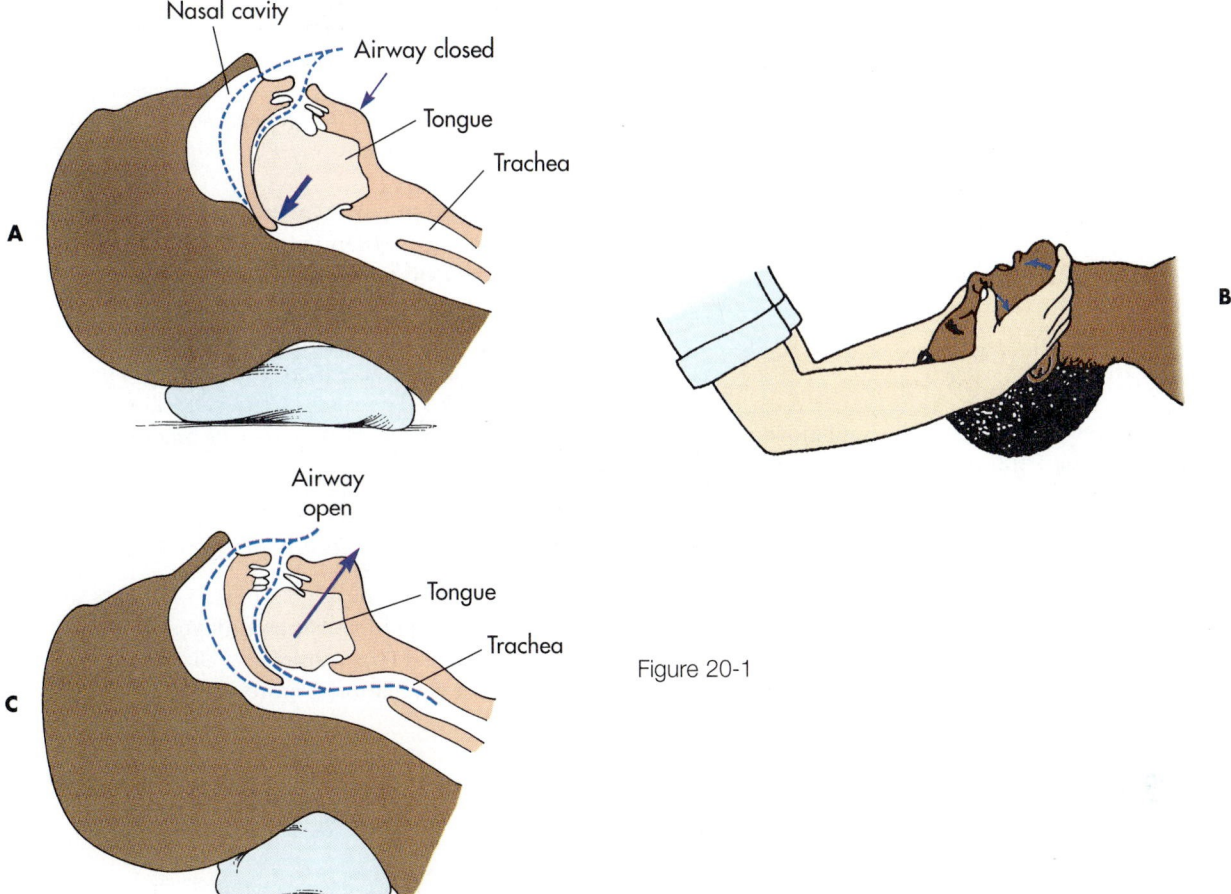

Figure 20-1

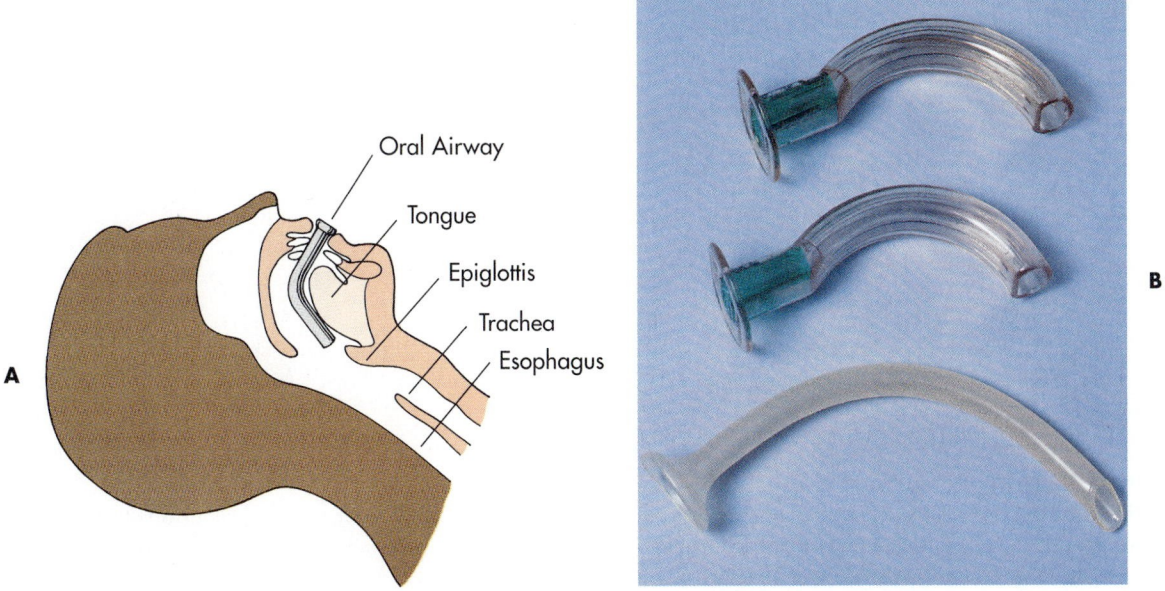

Figure 20-2 **A**, Oral airway in place. **B**, Oral airways *(top* and *middle); nasal airway (bottom).*

Steps	Rationale
9. Provide care after spinal anesthesia. a. Monitor for hypotension, bradycardia, and nausea and vomiting.	Blockade of sympathetic nervous system may result in vasodilation of major vessels and systemic hypotension.
b. Maintain adequate IV infusion.	Maintains blood pressure by increasing fluid volume and fills temporarily expended vascular space.
c. Keep client flat and maintain position.	Minimizes risk of post–spinal anesthesia headache from leakage of spinal fluid at injection site, with increased pressures induced by elevation of upper body. (Incidence of headache is less with use of smaller-gauge spinal needles [Lewis and Collier, 1992].)
d. Clients are observed in PACU until movement has been regained. Inform client that loss of extremity sensation and that movement is temporary and usually requires several hours to be restored to normal.	Clients often fear permanent loss of function.
e. Assess level of sensation and mobility in lower extremities. Following IV sedation, drowsiness will be apparent.	Spinal block should be set within 20 minutes of onset. However, if level of anesthesia moves above sixth thoracic vertebra (T6), respiratory distress may require mechanical ventilation (Figure 20-3).

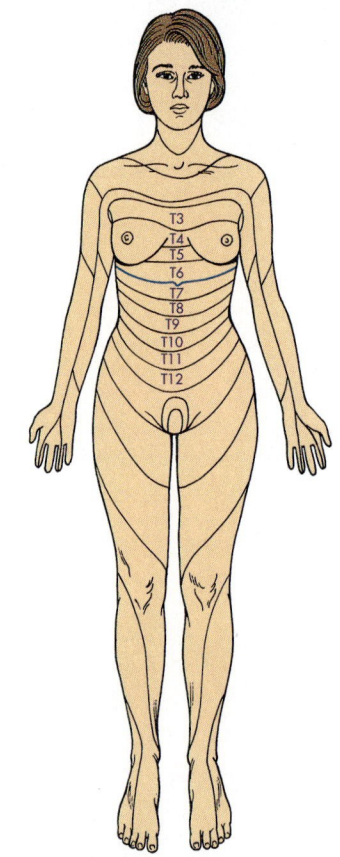

Figure 20-3

Steps	Rationale
10. Monitor drainage. a. Observe dressing and drains for any evidence of bright-red blood. Also, look underneath client for any pooling of bloody drainage.	Hemorrhage from a surgical wound is most likely within first few hours, indicating inadequate hemostasis during surgery. As a dressing becomes saturated, blood may ooze down client's side and collect under client.

Steps	Rationale
b. Inform physician of unexpected bloody drainage, and reinforce dressing as indicated. Monitor for decreased blood pressure and increased pulse.	Dressing maintains hemostasis and absorbs drainage. First dressing changes usually occur 24 hours postoperatively and are done by the surgeon unless otherwise ordered.
c. Inspect condition and contents of any drainage tubes and collecting devices. Note character and volume of drainage (see Skill 20.4).	Determines drainage tube patency and extent of wound drainage.
d. Observe amount, color, and appearance of urine from indwelling Foley catheter (if present).	Urine output of less than 30 ml/hr may indicate decreased renal perfusion or altered renal function (see Table 20-2).
e. If nasogastric (NG) tube is present, assess drainage. If not draining, check placement (see Skill 31.1) and irrigate if necessary with normal saline (see Skill 32.2).	Maintains patency of tube to ensure gastric decompression. Expected drainage may be dark or pale, yellow, green, and 100 to 200 ml/hr. Bloody drainage may be expected after some surgeries.
f. Monitor IV fluid rates. Observe IV site for signs of infiltration.	Provides adequate hydration and circulatory function.
11. Promote comfort.	
a. Provide mouth care by placing moistened washcloth to lips, swabbing oral mucosa with dampened swab, or apply petrolatum to lips.	Mouth may be dry from nothing-by-mouth (NPO) status and preoperative anticholinergics such as atropine.
b. Provide a warm blanket or active rewarming therapy to promote warmth and minimize shivering.	General anesthesia impairs thermoregulation, the OR environment is cold, and exposure of the body cavity may result in internal heat loss. Shivering can increase oxygen consumption and predispose client to arrhythmias and hypertension (Einhorn and Chant, 1994).
12. Assess pain as client awakens, including quality, severity, and location. Do not assume postoperative pain is incisional pain.	Pain may not be directly related to the surgical procedure, for example, chest pain (myocardial infarction/pulmonary emboli) or muscle pain (trauma from positioning). Referred pain (in shoulder) often occurs after a laparoscopy.
13. Provide pain medication as ordered and when vital signs have stabilized (see Chapter 21).	Clients in pain often have increased blood pressure and occasionally decreased blood pressure. Pain medication can influence anesthesia effects.
14. Explain client's condition to the client, and inform of plans for transfer to nursing division or discharge to home.	
15. When stabilized, contact anesthesiologist to approve transfer to clinical unit or release to home (see Table 20-3).	A physician is responsible for authorizing transfer or discharge.
16. Before discharge to home from the ambulatory surgery unit (ASU), provide verbal and written instructions (Figure 20-4).	Clients and home care providers must be aware of potential complications and follow-up care.
a. Do not drive for 24 hours.	
b. Avoid important legal decisions for 24 hours.	
c. Care for surgical site.	
d. Restrict activities.	
e. Control pain.	
f. Plan for follow-up visit.	
17. See Completion Protocol (Chapter 1, p. 6).	

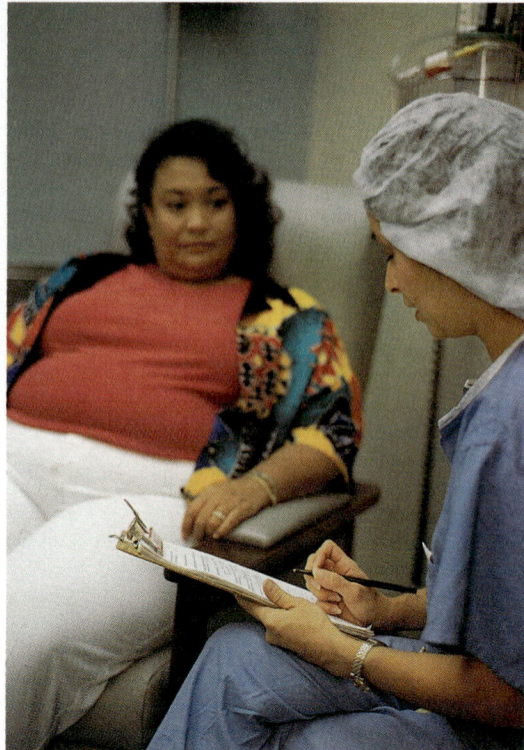

Figure 20-4

Evaluation

1. Observe respirations: rate, depth and rhythm. Auscultate breath sounds.
2. Compare all blood pressure, pulse, and temperature readings with client's baseline and expected normal values.
3. Inspect dressings for drainage.
4. Measure intake and output. Urine output is at least 30 to 50 ml/hr.
5. Ask client to rate pain on scale of 0 to 10, and determine location and characteristics.
6. Conduct physical assessments according to client's unique type of surgery for example:
   a. Craniotomy—neurological assessment (see Skill 12.9)
   b. Neck surgery—airway status (see Skill 12.5)
   c. Vascular surgery—circulation and bleeding (see Skill 12.6)
   d. Orthopedic surgery—immobility or positioning (see Chapters 26 and 27).

UNEXPECTED OUTCOMES AND RELATED INTERVENTIONS

These include alterations from effects of anesthesia or surgical complications.

1. Client exhibits respiratory depression (pulse oximetry less than 92, respiratory rate less than 10 and/or shallow).

   a. Administer oxygen.
   b. Encourage deep breathing every 5 to 15 minutes.
   c. Position to promote chest expansion (on side or semi-Fowler's).
   d. Administer prescribed medications (epinephrine, muscle relaxant, or narcotic reversal agent).
2. Client exhibits respiratory obstruction (abnormal lung sounds, snoring, stridor or crowing sounds, wheezing).
   a. Reposition to open airway.
   b. Administer oxygen.
   c. Encourage to cough and deep breathe.
   d. Suction if needed (see Skill 30.3).
   e. Notify anesthesiologist if unresponsive to interventions; may need to be reintubated if severe.
3. Client exhibits signs of hypovolemia related to internal or incisional hemorrhage.
   a. Client's legs should be elevated enough to maintain a downward slope toward the trunk of the body. The head should not be lowered past flat position, which would increase respiratory effort and potentially decrease cerebral perfusion.
   b. Administer oxygen.
   c. Increase rate of IV fluid or administer blood products.
   d. Monitor blood pressure and pulse every 5 to 15 minutes.

   e. Apply pressure dressings as follows.
      (1) *Abdominal dressing.* Cover bleeding area with several thicknesses of gauze compresses, and place tape 7 to 10 cm (3 to 4 inches) beyond width of dressing with firm even pressure on both sides close to bleeding source. Maintain pressure as entire dressing is taped to maximize pressure at the source of bleeding.
      (2) *Dressing on extremity.* Apply roller gauze, pressing gauze compress over bleeding site. Tape must *not* be continued around entire extremity. Assess frequently to ensure blood flow to distal tissues, and identify compartment syndrome resulting from edema that creates sufficient pressure to cause ischemia (see Unexpected Outcome 4).
      (3) *Dressing in neck region.* Assess every 5 to 15 minutes for evidence of airway obstruction.
   f. Client should remain NPO, since it may be necessary to return to surgery for control of bleeding.
   g. Report to physician present status of client's bleeding control, time bleeding was discovered, estimated blood loss, nursing interventions (including effectiveness of applied pressure bandage), apical and distal pulses, blood pressure, LOC, and signs of restlessness.

4. Client complains of severe incisional pain (see Chapter 21).
   a. The earliest symptom of compartment syndrome is pain unrelieved by analgesics. Other symptoms include numbness, tingling, pallor, coolness, and absent peripheral pulses. The physician should be notified, the extremity elevated to improve venous return, and ice applied to minimize edema (Lewis and Collier, 1992).
   b. Nurse should administer analgesics before the pain is severe. It is not necessary to wait for client to request pain medication.
   c. Pain can sometimes lower blood pressure; thus analgesia may restore vital signs to normal. Monitor vital signs carefully.
   d. For clients with patient-controlled analgesia (PCA), be sure client is using device correctly.
5. Client has hypothermia (temperature less than 34.5° C [94° F]) resulting from effects of anesthesia or loss of body heat from surgical exposure. Shivering can increase oxygen consumption and predispose client to arrhythmias and hypertension.
   a. Use warm blankets or active rewarming device.
   b. Monitor temperature every 30 to 60 minutes.

> **nurse alert** In an emergency situation, document interventions and evaluation as reported to physician, including maintenance of airway and bleeding control, distal pulses, vital signs, IV line, LOC, oxygenation or hypoxia, and anxiety level.

SAMPLE DOCUMENTATION

1300 Abdominal dressing saturated with bright-red blood and pad under client saturated, 12×20 cm area. Dressing reinforced with pressure dressing. BP 110/60, pulse 98, respirations 22. Client alert. Oxygen administered at 3 L/nasal cannula, IV infusing with lactated Ringer's at 150 ml/hour. Dr J. notified. Client is NPO. Warm blanket applied.

Skill 20.2	**Providing Comfort Measures During Phase II (Convalescent Phase)**

Phase II of postoperative recovery is the convalescent period. This period extends from the time the client is discharged from the RR or PACU to the time the client is discharged from the hospital. Clients who have outpatient surgery undergo convalescence at home. Nursing care needs to be individualized depending on the type of surgery, preexisting medical conditions, the risk or development of complications, and the rate of recovery. Teaching promotes the client's independence, educates the client about any limitations, and provides resources needed for the client to achieve an optimal state of wellness.

EQUIPMENT
Postoperative bed (recliner in ASU)
Stethoscope, sphygmomanometer, thermometer
IV fluid poles
Emesis basin
Washcloth and towel
Waterproof pads
Equipment for oral hygiene
Pillows
Facial tissue
Oxygen equipment
Suction equipment (to suction airway)
Dressing supplies
Intermittent suction (to connect to NG or wound drainage tubes)
Orthopedic appliances (if needed)

Assessment

1. Obtain phone report from nurse in PACU. A preliminary report allows nurse to prepare hospital room with necessary supplies and equipment for client's special needs.
2. On arrival, assist with transfer and complete initial assessment. Review chart to identify type of surgery, preoperative medical risks, and baseline vital signs. **Data provide baseline to detect any change in client's condition.**
3. Review surgeon's postoperative orders.

Planning

Expected outcomes focus on prevention of complications, maintenance of pain control adequate for recovery activities, and teaching to promote optimal wellness.

EXPECTED OUTCOMES

1. Client's breath sounds remain clear by discharge.
2. Client's vital signs remain within normal limits compared with preoperative baseline.
3. Client describes pain as less than 3 (scale 1 to 10) while engaged in moderate activity by discharge.
4. Fluid balance is evident by intake and output records.
5. Normal bowel sounds present after bowel surgery or general anesthesia within 48 to 72 hours postoperatively.
6. Incisional wound edges are well approximated; no drainage is noted.
7. Client (or care giver) describes plans for coping with stress of surgery (altered function or body image).
8. Client (or care giver) describes evidence of complications that should be reported to physician by discharge.
9. Client (or care giver) describes or demonstrates incision care and activity restriction and plans follow-up visit.

Implementation

Steps	Rationale
1. See Standard Protocol (Chapter 1, p. 5).	
Initial postoperative care	
2. Prepare bed in high position (level with the stretcher), with sheet folded to side with room for a stretcher to be easily placed beside bed (Figure 20-5) (see Skill 6.1).	Arrangement of equipment ensures smooth transfer process.
3. Assist transport staff to move client from stretcher to bed (see Skill 5.5).	
4. Attach any existing oxygen tubing, position IV fluids, check IV flow rate, and check drainage tubes (Foley catheter or wound drainage).	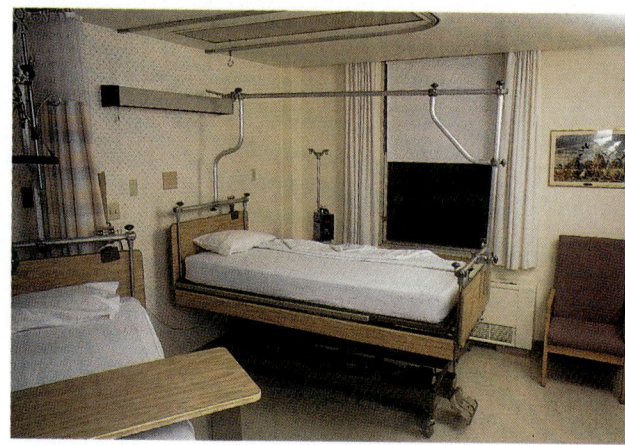 Figure 20-5
5. Take vital signs and compare findings with vital signs in recovery area as well as client's baseline values. Continue monitoring as ordered.	During transfer, client's status may change. Movement of client and pain level can influence stability of vital signs.
6. Maintain airway. If client remains sleepy or lethargic, keep head extended and support in side-lying position (see Skill 5.1). 	Minimizes chances of aspiration and obstruction of airway with tongue.
7. Encourage coughing and deep breathing (see Skill 18.2).	Anesthesia, medications, and intubation irritate airways, resulting in secretions and atelectasis (Figure 20-6).
8. If NG tube is present, check placement (see Skill 31.1) and connect to proper drainage device. Connect all drainage tubes to appropriate suction device as indicated, and secure to prevent tension.	Transfer and movement may dislodge tube, which would interfere with drainage.
9. Assess client's surgical dressing for appearance and presence and character of drainage. Unless contraindicated by physician, outline drainage along the	Hemorrhage is most likely to occur on the day of surgery. Dressing should be clean, dry, and intact.

Steps	Rationale

edges with a pen and reassess in 1 hour for increase. If no dressing present, inspect condition of wound (see Skill 20.3).

10. Assess client for bladder distention. If Foley catheter is present, check placement and be sure it is draining freely and properly secured. Client may have continuous bladder irrigations or suprapubic catheter for urinary drainage (see Chapter 34).

11. Measure all sources of fluid intake and output (including estimated blood loss during surgery).

Altered fluid and electrolyte balance is a potential complication of major surgery (see Chapter 36).

12. Describe the purpose of equipment and frequent observations to client and significant others.

Unfamiliar sights (equipment, client's appearance) can be anxiety provoking.

13. Position client for comfort, maintaining correct body alignment. Avoid tension on surgical wound site.

Reduces stress on suture line. Helps client relax and promotes comfort.

14. Place call light within reach and raise side rail. Instruct client to call for assistance to get out of bed.

Promotes client's safety as effects of anesthesia continue to diminish.

15. Assess the need for pain medication based on client's level of discomfort and last time analgesic was given. PCA may be used for pain control (see Skill 21.3).

Client should be medicated freely every 3 to 4 hours during the first 24 to 48 hours. Adequate pain control is needed to permit client to participate with breathing exercises, coughing, and ambulation.

Continued postoperative care

16. Assess vital signs every 4 hours or as ordered.

Temperature above 38° C (100.4° F) in the first 48 hours may indicate atelectasis, the normal inflammatory response, or dehydration. Elevation above 37.7° C on the third day or after may indicate wound infection, pneumonia, or phlebitis (Lewis and Collier, 1992). Altered blood pressure and/or pulse may indicate cardiovascular complications (see Table 20-1).

17. Provide oral care every 2 hours as needed (see Skill 6.3). If permitted, offer ice chips.

Medication given preoperatively, such as atropine (anticholinergic), makes mouth dry. Oral care and ice chips promote comfort.

18. Encourage to turn, cough, and deep breathe every 2 hours.

Benefits clients with history of smoking, pneumonia, with chronic obstructive pulmonary disease (COPD), or confined to bed rest.

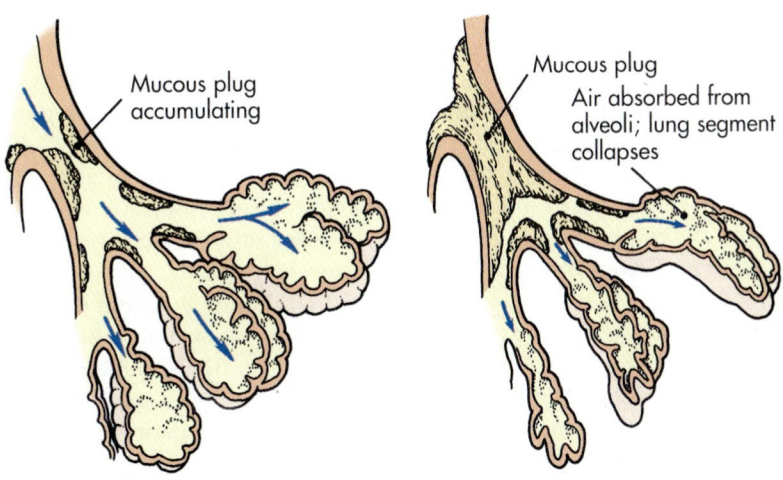

Mucous plug accumulating

Mucous plug
Air absorbed from alveoli; lung segment collapses

Figure 20-6 (Modified from Lewis SM, Collier IC: *Medical-surgical nursing: assessment and management of clinical problems,* ed 3, St. Louis, 1992, Mosby.)

Steps	Rationale

19. Encourage use of incentive spirometer as ordered (see Skill 18.1).

20. If no urinary drainage system is present, explain that voiding within 8 hours postoperatively is expected. Male clients may void successfully if allowed to stand.

After spinal or epidural anesthesia, risk for urinary retention is increased. Many clients are unable to feel the urge to void. If client is unable to void and bladder is distended, catheterization may be required.

21. Promote ambulation and activity as ordered. Assess vital signs before and after activity to assess tolerance. Clients often are encouraged to be up in a chair the evening of surgery or the following morning and progress to walking in room or hallway.

Ambulation is the most significant nursing intervention to prevent postoperative complications. Mobility promotes circulation, lung expansion, and peristalsis. Sudden position changes can cause postural hypotension.

22. Progress from clear liquids to regular diet progressively as tolerated if nausea and vomiting do not occur.

Nausea and vomiting are associated with anesthesia and surgery. IV fluids are usually discontinued when oral intake is tolerated. Some clients must be NPO for several days until bowel sounds are heard.

23. If possible, include client and family in decision making and answer questions as they arise.

Promotes client's sense of control and independence and improves self-esteem.

24. Provide opportunity for clients who must adjust to a change in body appearance or function to verbalize feelings.

Radical surgery (mastectomy, colostomy), amputation, or inoperable cancer may result in anxiety and depression. The grief response to loss of a body organ (e.g., the uterus) is common and should be expected.

25. Discuss plans for discharge with client and care givers, including wound care, medications, activity restrictions, and complications that warrant notifying the physician. Clarify follow-up appointments and encourage quick access to emergency telephone numbers.

26. See Completion Protocol (Chapter 1, p. 6).

Evaluation

1. Auscultate breath sounds.
2. Obtain vital signs.
3. Ask client to describe pain (scale 1 to 10) after moderate activity.
4. Evaluate intake and output records.
5. Auscultate bowel sounds.
6. Inspect incision (wound edges well approximated, no drainage is noted).
7. Ask client to describe ability to cope with stress of surgery (altered function or body image).
8. Ask client (or care giver) to indicate complications that should be reported to the physician by discharge.
9. Have client (or care giver) describe incision care, activity restrictions, and plans for follow-up visit.

UNEXPECTED OUTCOMES AND RELATED INTERVENTIONS

1. Bowel sounds are absent or decreased. Client experiences nausea and vomiting. Client is unable to pass flatus, and abdomen is hard and distended.
   Paralytic ileus is a common complication after bowel surgery. Intestinal motility may return slowly.
   a. Report to physician.
   b. Placement of an NG tube may be required (see Chapter 31).
2. Client has fluid volume excess or deficit and risk for electrolyte imbalance.
   a. Report to physician.
   b. See Chapter 36.

SAMPLE DOCUMENTATION

Third postoperative day after abdominal surgery:

1800 Client vomited 300 ml dark-green mucus ×2 since 1600. Abdomen firm and distended. No bowel sounds heard. Not passing flatus. Rates pain at 7 (scale 1-10). Demerol 50 mg given IM. Instructed not to eat or drink anything.

1910 Vomited 200 ml dark-green material and c/o being "very nauseated." Abdominal pain now rated at 6 (scale 1-10). Dr. K notified. NG tube inserted and connected to low intermittent suction as ordered with return of 400 ml dark-green material within 15 minutes. Phenergan 5 mg given IM for nausea.

1950 Resting comfortably. Denies nausea. Pain now rated at 4 (scale 0 to 10).

Skill 20.3 | Providing Surgical Wound Care

Proper wound care is necessary to promote healing after a surgical incision. Risk of local or systemic infection, impaired circulation, and breakdown of tissue is directly influenced by the ability of the dermal layer to heal. Factors that influence wound healing include age, nutrition, circulation, chronic illness, and drug therapy (see box below).

The stages of healing and interventions related to dressings are described in Chapter 15. Types of healing include healing by primary intention and healing by secondary intention. Healing by *primary intention* is expected when the edges of a clean surgical incision remain close together, tissue loss is minimal or absent, and the client is not at risk for developing an infection. The skin cells quickly regenerate, capillary walls stretch across under the suture line to form a smooth surface as they join, and inflammation is absent or minimized. A healing ridge can be palpated beneath the incision, extending about 1 cm on each side between day 5 and day 9 after surgery. If no ridge is apparent, the risk of dehiscence (separation) is increased by the eighth postoperative day (Bryant, 1992).

Healing by *secondary intention* often accompanies traumatic open wounds with tissue loss, jagged edges, and granulation tissue gradually filling in the area of the scar. This process is typical of severe laceration or massive surgical intervention with skin loss. The risk of infection is directly related to the length of time it takes for the body surface to be covered with an intact skin covering.

When drainage is expected within the wound, a Penrose drain (Figure 20-7) may be used to help prevent complications. This type of drain is a soft tube that may be "advanced" or pulled out in stages as the wound heals from the inside out. A safety pin is inserted through this drain, not the skin, to prevent the tubing from moving into the wound. Nursing interventions protect skin surfaces in direct contact with the drainage, especially if it is irritating to the skin. Other types of drains are described in Skill 20-4.

Meticulous handwashing and infection control procedures relating to wound care limit the risk of nosocomial infection. Antiseptic swabs are used to clean, beginning at the cleanest area to avoid transmitting microorganisms from one area to another. The presence of wound exudate is an expected stage of epithelial cell growth. After the third postoperative day, increasing inflammation and a temperature above 38° C (100.4° F) with or without apparent drainage indicate possible wound infection. Wound infection, particularly from aerobic organisms, is often accompanied by a fever that spikes in the afternoon or evening and returns to near-normal levels in the morning.

Intermittent high fever accompanied by shaking chills and diaphoresis suggests septicemia, a systemic infection with microorganisms in the bloodstream. The source of microorganisms may be the wound site, a urinary infection, phlebitis, or peritonitis (Table 20-4). Wound culture reveals the type of organisms causing infection. Sensitivity reports indicate which antibiotics will be effective for the specific microorganism present.

EQUIPMENT
Clean gloves
Sterile gloves
Waterproof underpad, if needed
Dressing supplies (unless incision is OTA)

Factors that Influence Healing of an Incision

1. With increasing age, blood vessels become less elastic, collagen tissue is less pliable, and scar tissue is tighter.
2. Inadequate nutrition, including proteins, carbohydrates, lipids, vitamins, and minerals, delays tissue repair and increases risk for infection. Nutrition requirements can double in presence of infection.
3. Obese client has greater risk for wound infection and dehiscence or evisceration. Fatty tissue has less vascularization, which decreases transport of nutrients and cellular elements required for healing.
4. Tissue repair is negatively influenced by a hematocrit value below 33% and a hemoglobin value below 10 g/dl. Oxygen delivery is decreased with both. Oxygen release to tissues is reduced in smokers.
5. Diabetes alters tissue perfusion and interferes with release of oxygen to tissues. Uncontrolled hypoglycemia interferes with phagocytosis of the leukocytes.
6. Radiation therapy results in vascular scarring and fibrosis within 4 to 6 weeks and influences tissue healing. Chemotherapy depresses bone marrow function and resistance to infection.
7. Long-term steroid therapy may reduce inflammatory response and interfere with wound healing.

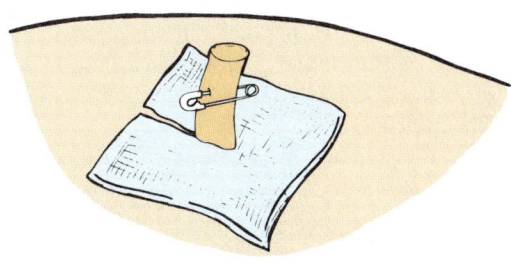

Figure 20-7 Penrose drain with drain dressing

Disposable waterproof bag
Gown, if risk of spray
Goggles, if risk of spray

Assessment

1. Identify the wound's location, its size (measure depth, length, width), type of incision, presence of drains, and type of dressing.
2. Review documentation related to healing of the incision, including approximation of wound edges and drainage from wound (amount, color), to provide basis for comparison. **Amount decreases as healing takes place; serous drainage is clear; presence of small amounts is normal; bright-red drainage indicates fresh bleeding; purulent drainage is thick and yellow, pale green, or white.**
3. Review culture reports to identify presence of pathogenic organisms (Table 20-4).
4. Assess client's comfort level and identify symptoms of anxiety. Administer prescribed analgesic 30 to 45 minutes before changing dressing if appropriate. **Discomfort may be related directly to wound or indirectly to muscle tension and immobility. Anxiety may result from outcome of surgery, awaiting pathology reports, anticipation of pain, or other factors.**
5. Identify client's history of allergies. **Known allergies suggest application of a sample of prescribed antiseptic as skin test and avoidance of certain types of tape.**

Planning

Expected outcomes focus on prevention and early detection of infection.

Implementation

Table 20-4 **Some Common Pathogenic Organisms that Cause Wound Infections**

Microorganism	Possible Sources/Comments
GRAM POSITIVE	
Staphylococcus aureus	Skin infections, pneumonia, urinary tract infections. Methicillin resistant *S. aureus* (MRSA) is a common nosocomial infection resistant to many antibiotics and very difficult to treat.
Streptococcus faecalis	Genitourinary infection, common infection in surgical wounds.
GRAM NEGATIVE	
Pseudomonas aeruginosa	Urinary tract infection
Klebsiella/Enterobacter	Peritonitis
Proteus species	
Escherichia coli	

Modified from Lewis SM, Collier IC: *Medical-surgical nursing: assessment and management of critical problems*, St Louis, 1992, Mosby.

EXPECTED OUTCOMES

1. Client's incision shows wound edges well approximated and absence of drainage.
2. Wound drain, if present, is patent and intact. Skin around drain is free of irritation.
3. Client verbalizes pain at less than 4 (scale 0 to 10).

Steps	Rationale
1. See Standard Protocol (Chapter 1, p. 5).	
2. Form cuff on waterproof bag and place it near bed.	
3. Remove dressing, pulling tape toward suture line.	Prevents tension on suture line.
4. Inspect dressing for drainage. A small amount of serous drainage is normal. Enclose small, soiled dressings within gloves before discarding in waterproof bag. Otherwise, discard directly into appropriate receptacle.	
5. Inspect incision for inflammation and healing and describe appearance to client. In some cases, client may want to see incision. Provide a mirror if necessary.	Inflammation is evidenced by pink area and slight swelling, which confirms increased circulation to enhance healing. Incision edges should be well approximated and may be stapled or closed with visible or subcutaneous sutures.

Steps	Rationale

6. Open sterile supplies for dressing and antiseptic swabs using aseptic technique. Position for easy access without reaching over the sterile field.

7. Put on sterile gloves.

8. Cleanse the suture line from top to bottom. Discard the antiseptic swab (Figure 20-8).

Avoids introducing microorganisms from surrounding skin into the incision.

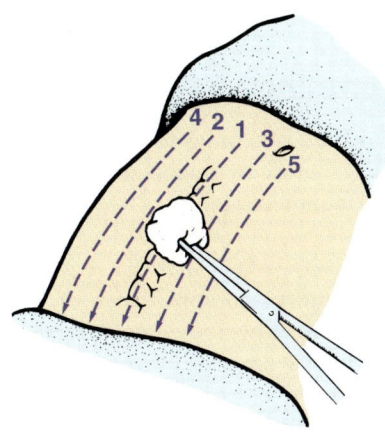

Figure 20-8

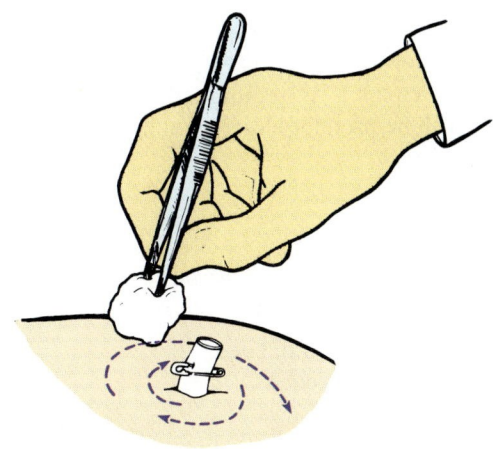

Figure 20-9

9. Then cleanse the skin along each side of the incision using a single, sterile antiseptic swab for each stroke.

10. To cleanse a drain site, use a circular stroke starting with the area immediately next to the drain and moving out from the drain (Figure 20-9).

11. Apply dry, sterile dressing and secure with tape with ends folded under 0.5 cm (¼ inch).

Facilitates removal of tape with minimal trauma to skin.

12. See Completion Protocol (Chapter 1, p. 6).

Evaluation

1. Inspect dressing at the beginning of each shift and periodically as necessary.
2. If drain is present, inspect skin integrity. Drainage may be irritating to skin.
3. Ask client to describe pain (scale of 0 to 10) and indicate quality, location, and factors that intensify or relieve it.

UNEXPECTED OUTCOMES AND RELATED INTERVENTIONS

Client develops increased tenderness and pain at wound site

   a. Monitor for temperature above 37.7° C (100° F) and increased white blood cell count.

   b. Observe for purulent drainage; a culture and sensitivity assists in identifying infectious microorganisms and appropriate antibiotic therapy (see Skill 13.1).

   c. Institute interventions to increase resistance to infection and promote healing.

SAMPLE DOCUMENTATION

0930 Abdominal dressing changed. Two 4 × 4 saturated with serosanguineous drainage at site of Penrose drain. Area of ABD 3 cm diameter also noted. Sutures intact. Three 4 × 4 and ABD applied and secured with nylon tape. Client describes pain as 3 (scale 0 to 10) and denies need for analgesic. Resting comfortably on right side.

Skill 20.4 Monitoring and Measuring Drainage Devices

When drainage may interfere with healing, a drain may be inserted directly through the suture line into the wound or through a small stab wound near the suture line into the wound. Two common types of drainage devices are portable, self-contained suction units that connect to drainage tubes within the wound and provide constant low-pressure suction to remove and collect drainage without wall suction. When the container is one-half to two-thirds full, it should be emptied and reset to apply suction. A Jackson-Pratt drain (Figure 20-10) is used when small amounts (100 to 200 ml) of drainage are anticipated. A Hemovac drainage system (Figure 20-11) can be used for larger amounts (up to 500 ml) of drainage.

EQUIPMENT

Measuring container (size varies)
Alcohol sponge
Gauze sponges
Sterile specimen container, if needed
Sterile dressings, if drain needed
Gloves

Assessment

1. Identify presence of closed wound drain or type of drainage system when client returns from surgery. **System may include one straight tube or a Y-tube arrangement with two tube insertion sites and one drainage container.**
2. Inspect for tube patency by observing drainage movement through tubing in direction of the reservoir, and look for intact connection sites.

Planning

Expected outcomes focus on promoting wound healing and comfort by maintaining adequate suction and preventing infection.

EXPECTED OUTCOMES

1. Quantity and appearance of wound drainage remain within expected guidelines based on type of surgery.
2. Client's drainage device is properly located and intact.
3. Client denies discomfort from presence of drainage device.

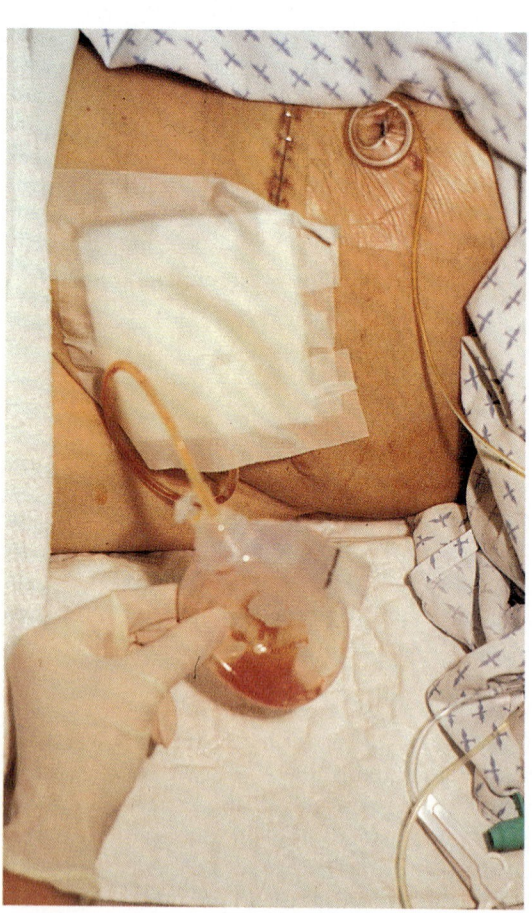

Figure 20-10

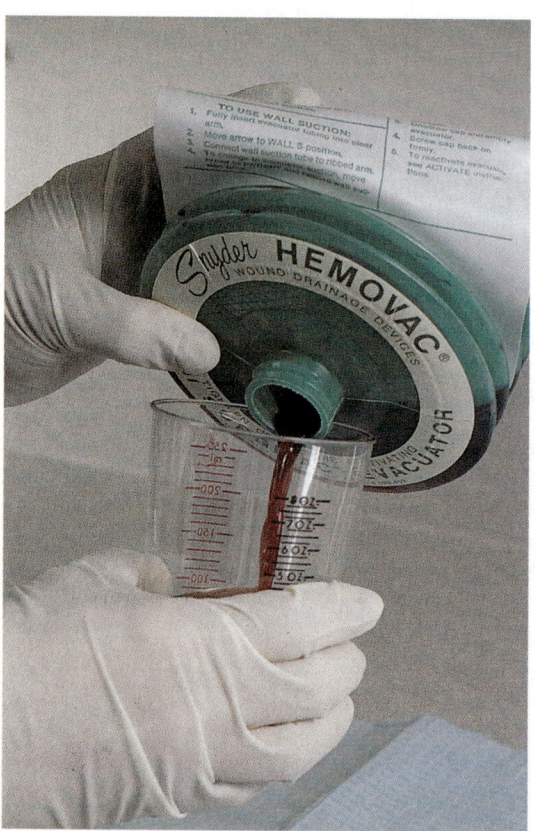

Figure 20-11

Implementation

Steps	Rationale

 nurse alert To prevent cross-infections, Centers for Disease Control and Prevention (CDC, 1985) recommendations include maintaining individualized equipment for drainage collection.

1. See Standard Protocol (Chapter 1, p. 5).

2. Empty Hemovac, VacuDrain, or Constavac.
 a. Open plug on port for emptying drainage reservoir, and slowly squeeze two flat surfaces together, tilting container in that direction.
 b. Drain contents into sterile measuring container (see Figure 20-11).
 c. Place container on a flat surface and press downward until bottom and top are in contact (Figure 20-12).

Vacuum is broken and reservoir pulls air in until chamber is fully expanded.

Prevents splashing of contaminated drainage.

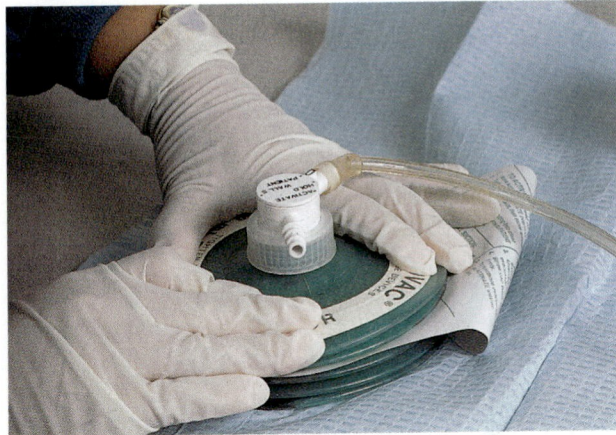
Figure 20-12

 d. Hold surfaces together with one hand, cleanse opening and plug with other hand, and immediately replace plug.
 e. Check for patency of drainage tubing and absence of tension on tubing.

Compression of surface of Hemovac creates vacuum.

Facilitates wound drainage and prevents pressure and trauma to tissues.

3. Empty Hemovac with wall suction.
 a. Attach Hemovac to wall suction. Connect graduated adaptor to emptying port and then to wall suction tubing.
 b. Set suction level as prescribed or on *low* if physician does not specify suction level.
 c. Attach tubing with graduated connector to open port and secure with tape.

Steps	Rationale

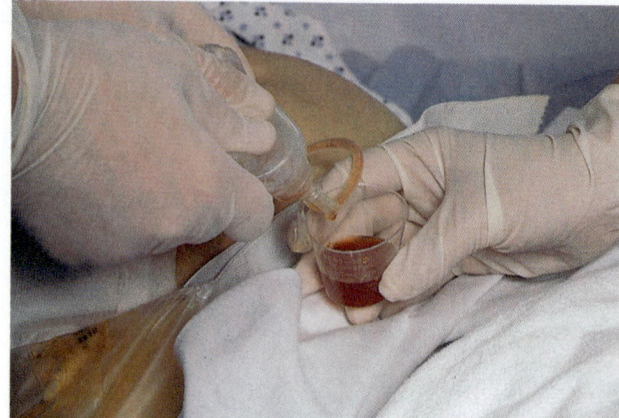

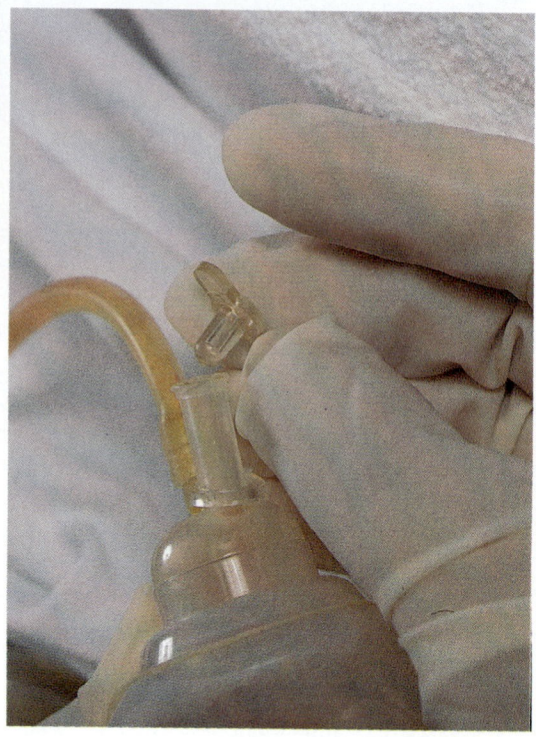

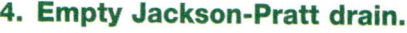
Figure 20-13

4. Empty Jackson-Pratt drain.

a. Open port on the end of bulb-shaped reservoir.

b. Hold bulb over drainage container to empty drainage (Figure 20-13). Compress bulb to reestablish vacuum (see Figure 20-10, p. 378).

c. Cleanse ends of emptying port with alcohol sponge. Replace cap immediately.

d. Note characteristics of drainage; measure volume and discard by flushing down the commode.

e. Proceed with inspection of skin and dressing change using drain sponges. Place the bulk of the dressings below the drain, depending on client's usual position.

Drainage may be irritating to skin and may cause skin breakdown. Application of protective barrier may be indicated.

f. Instruct client about anticipated postoperative drainage, expected progress of wound healing and drainage volume, and estimated date of removal of drain as volume diminishes.

Unexplained bloody drainage is worrisome to any client. Knowing what to expect reduces anxiety.

g. Instruct client to keep drain lower than waist level when ambulating, sitting, and lying down.

Facilitates drainage.

h. Instruct client not to pull or tug on tubing; secure drain below incision to dressing with tape and safety pin.

5. Remove drains (Penrose, Jackson-Pratt, Hemovac).

a. Remove dressings, discard in receptacle, and clean the area around the drain (see Skill 15.1).

b. If removing a Jackson-Pratt or Hemovac drain, release the suction on the drainage device by opening the drainage port.

Continued suction increases the tension required for drain removal and the risk of tissue damage and bleeding.

c. Inform client that there will be a pulling sensation as the drain is removed.

Gains cooperation and alleviates anxiety.

d. Place a disposable drape adjacent to the area to receive the drain after removal.

Allows immediate enclosure of drain and prevents spread of microorganisms.

e. Clip and remove the suture if present (see Skill 20.5). Remove clean gloves and put on sterile gloves.

Steps	Rationale

f. Grasp the drain with sterile forceps or sterile gloved fingers and gently remove the drain. Inform client that momentary increased tension is felt just before completion of the removal.

Jackson-Pratt drains have a wide flat area (Figure 20-14) that must be pulled through the stab wound with more force.

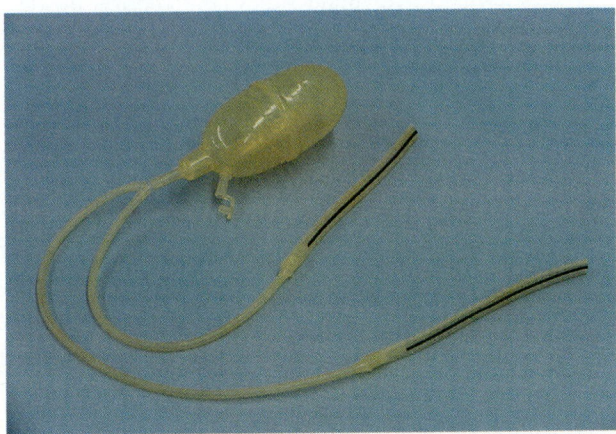

Figure 20-14

g. Immediately cover the stab wound with a 4×4 dressing.

Some drainage may continue for a few hours.

h. Instruct client to notify you if dressing becomes saturated with drainage.

Dressing may need to be changed.

6. See Completion Protocol (Chapter 1, p. 6).

Evaluation

1. Routinely empty container every 8 hours and sooner if half to two-thirds full. Compare amount and characteristics of drainage with what is expected to determine patency of tubing and functioning of drainage evacuator.
2. Inspect wound for drainage around the tubing, which may indicate obstruction of drainage system.
3. Ask client to describe level of comfort in relation to drainage tubing.

UNEXPECTED OUTCOMES AND RELATED INTERVENTIONS

1. Drainage is not accumulating in drainage system.
   a. Position tubing to enhance gravity flow and eliminate kinks or pressure on tubing.
   b. Gently "milk" tubing to release any clots that may have blocked tubing.
2. Drainage containers should expand slowly. If rapid expansion occurs:
   a. Check all connections for leakage.
   b. Tape or otherwise eliminate leaks in system.
3. Excessive amount of bright bloody drainage accumulates over a short time (e.g., 4 hours). Drainage that is bright red in large amounts may indicate hemorrhage.
   a. Drainage container is routinely emptied every 8 hours and more frequently if container is more than half full.
   b. Drainage is usually greatest during the first postoperative day and gradually decreases each shift. After 2 to 3 days, when it is minimal, whole system can be removed.
   c. Drainage appears very red at first and later changes to lighter color.
   d. Report excessive bright-red drainage to the surgeon.
   e. Keep client NPO, since it may be necessary to return to surgery for suturing of a bleeding vessel.
4. Wound infection develops as evidenced by unexpected purulence or foul odor.
   a. Initiate collection of diagnostic specimen for culture and sensitivity.
   b. Assess for additional indications of infection, including fever, elevated white blood count, redness, swelling, and increasing pain.
   c. Report findings to physician.
5. Pain can result from manipulation of drainage device or accumulation of drainage within the wound. After a time, infection accompanied by inflammation and edema may increase pain.
   a. Secure tubing to minimize irritation from moving or pulling at the insertion site.
   b. Report unrelieved increasing pain to the physician.

SAMPLE DOCUMENTATION

Emptying drain and dressing change:

1300 Dark-red drainage (700 ml) emptied from Hemovac and dressing changed around insertion site. Site is pink. Quarter-sized spot of serosanguineous drainage noted. Drain is securely sutured with one stitch. 4×4 drain dressings applied over drain site. Client reports no discomfort with dressing change.

Amount of drainage is usually documented on the intake and output sheet as well (see Intake and Output Summary, p. 109).

Drain removal:

1020 Hemovac drain and 1 suture removed as ordered. Site pink (1 cm around perimeter), covered with 4×4. Client reports no discomfort. No drainage apparent on dressing.

Skill 20.5 Removing Staples and Sutures (Including Applying SteriStrips)

Sutures are threads used for closure of a surgical wound both within tissue layers in deep wounds and for the skin layer. The client's history of wound healing, site of wound, tissues involved, and the purpose of the sutures determine the closure material selected. Deep sutures may be a material that is absorbed or an inert wire that remains indefinitely. Sutures are available in silk, steel, cotton, linen, wire, nylon, and Dacron. Skin sutures that are removed may be interrupted or continuous. *Interrupted* sutures are separate stitches, each with its own knot (Figure 20-15, *A*). A *continuous* suture is one long "thread" that spirals along the entire suture line at evenly spaced intervals. The surface appearance is very similar to a line of interrupted sutures, except that each section crossing the incision line does not have knot (Figure 20-15, *B*). Another type of continuous stitch is *blanket* continuous suture. This spirals along the incision with each turn pulled over to one side. The suture is looped around the thread of the previous stitch before making the next turn in spiral (Figure 20-15, *C*).

When appearance and minimal scarring are important, very fine Dacron or subcutaneous sutures beneath the skin are used. An obese client with abdominal surgery may have retention (wire) sutures covered with rubber tubing to provide greater strength (Figure 20-15, *D*). Wire sutures are usually removed by the physician.

Staples are made of stainless steel wire, are quick to use, and provide ample strength. They are popular for skin closure of abdominal incisions and orthopedic surgery when appearance of the incision is not critical (Figure 20-16). The time of removal is based on the stage of incisional healing and extent of surgery. Sutures and staples are generally removed within 7 to 10 days after surgery if healing is adequate. Retention sutures are left in place longer (14 days or more). Leaving sutures in too long makes removal more difficult and increases the risk of infection. The physician determines the time for removal of sutures or staples.

Routinely, every other suture or staple is removed first, with the rest removed if the incision remains securely closed. If any sign of suture line separation is evident during the removal process, the remaining sutures are left in place and a description is documented and reported to the physician. In some cases, these sutures are left to be removed several days to a week later.

EQUIPMENT

Disposable waterproof bag
Sterile suture removal set (forceps and scissors) or sterile staple remover
Sterile applicators or antiseptic swabs
Steristrips (optional)
Clean gloves
Sterile gloves (optional)

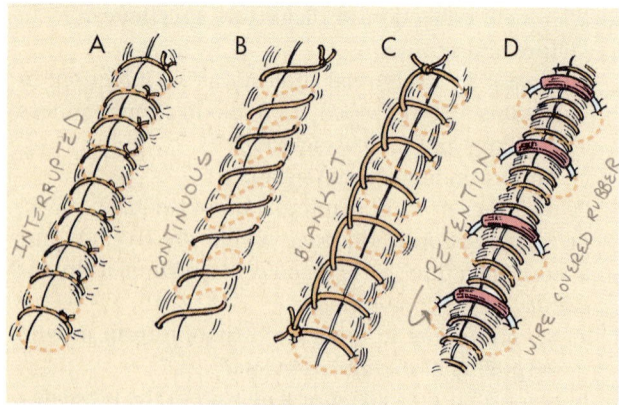

Figure 20-15

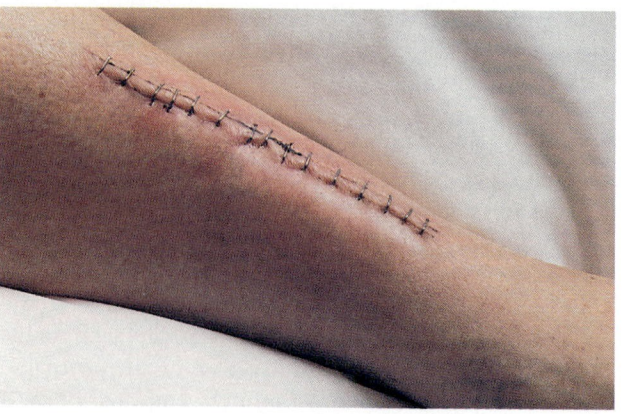

Figure 20-16

Assessment

1. Review physician's orders for specific directions related to suture or staple removal, including which sutures are to be removed.
2. Check for allergies to antiseptic solutions or tape.
3. Consider conditions that may interfere with healing, including advanced age, cardiovascular disease, diabetes, immunosuppression, radiation, obesity, smoking, poor cellular nutrition, very deep wounds, and infection.

Planning

Expected outcomes focus on maintaining skin integrity, preventing infection, and promoting comfort.

EXPECTED OUTCOMES

1. Client's incision is intact with edges well approximated after suture/staple removal.
2. Client describes pain as less than 2 (scale 0 to 10) during suture removal.
3. Client demonstrates ability to perform self-care related to promoting wound healing by discharge.

Implementation

Steps	Rationale
1. See Standard Protocol (Chapter 1, p. 5).	
2. Prepare sterile field with suture or staple removal instruments, sterile antiseptic swabs, and Steristrips.	
3. Remove dressing, and discard dressing enclosed in clean gloves. If dressing is too large, dispose of in proper receptacle. Remove gloves and dispose in same receptacle.	Enclosing soiled dressings within gloves prevents transmission of microorganisms.
4. Inspect wound for approximation of wound edges and absence of drainage and inflammation (redness, warmth, swelling).	Presence of these findings may indicate need for delay of suture/staple removal.
5. Apply sterile gloves if required.	Use of sterile instruments can provide adequate protection from infection when incision is healing well. If drainage is anticipated, such as with drain removal, sterile gloves are advisable.
6. Cleanse sutures or staples and healed incision with antiseptic swabs.	Softens dry crusting and facilitates gentle removal.
7. Remove staples.	
a. Place lower tips of staple remover under first staple (Figure 20-17, *A*).	
b. Squeeze handles together all the way (without lifting).	Releases the ends of staple from the skin with minimal suture line pressure and pain.
c. When both ends of staple are visible, gently lift it away from skin surface. If necessary, alter the angle and remove one end at a time (Figure 20-17, *B*).	

A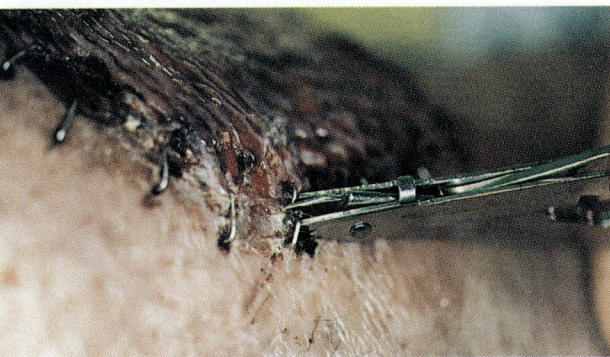
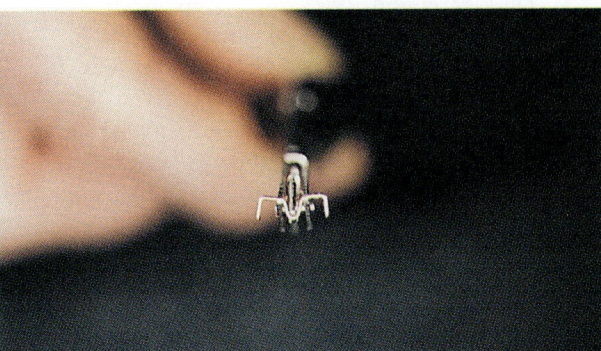 B

Figure 20-17

Steps	Rationale

d. Release handles of staple remover over container.

e. Repeat steps for every other staple.

f. Assess for healing ridge and secure approximation of incision edges before remaining staples are removed.

Allows staple to drop into container.

Minimizes risk of separation of wound edges.

If edges separate, staple removal should be discontinued.

8. Remove interrupted sutures.

a. Hold scissors in dominant hand and forceps (clamp) in nondominant hand. Note position of indented tip of scissors (Figure 20-18).

b. Grasp knot of suture with forceps and gently pull while slipping tip of scissors under suture near skin (Figure 20-18, *A*).

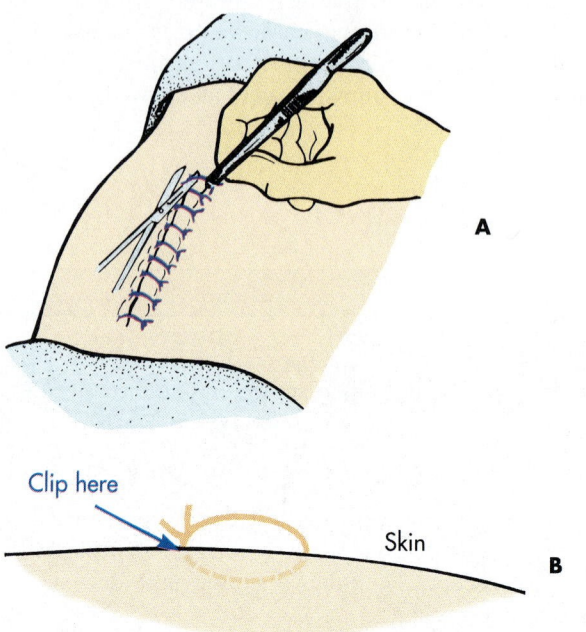

Figure 20-18

c. Snip suture as close to skin as possible and pull the suture through from the other side (Figure 20-18, *B*).

d. Gently remove suture and place it on sterile gauze.

e. Repeat steps until every other suture has been removed.

f. Assess for healing ridge and secure approximation of incision edges before remaining sutures are removed.

Portion of the suture on the skin's surface harbors microorganisms and debris, which could lead to infection if pulled through the underlying tissue.

If edges separate, suture removal should be discontinued.

9. Remove continuous sutures (see Figure 20-15, *B*, p. 382).

a. Snip suture close to skin surface at end distal to knot.

b. Snip second "suture" on same side.

c. Grasp knot and gently pull with continuous smooth action, removing suture from beneath the skin. Place suture on gauze.

d. Grasp and lift next suture, and snip with tip of scissors close to skin.

e. Grasp suture and gently remove loop of suture.

f. Repeat these steps until the end knot is reached. Cut the last one and remove it by grasping and pulling the knot.

Avoids tension to suture line.

Steps	Rationale

10. Remove blanket continuous suture (see Figure 20-15, *C*, p. 382).
  a. Cut the suture opposite the looped blanket edge.
  b. Remove each "suture" by grasping at the looped end.

11. Apply SteriStrips.
  a. Gently cleanse suture line with antiseptic swab.
  b. Using a strong light, carefully inspect incision to be sure all sutures are removed.
  c. When skin is dry, cut Steristrips to allow strips to extend 4 to 5 cm (1½ to 2 inches) on each side of the incision (Figure 20-19).
  d. Apply light dressing if drainage is apparent or if clothing may rub and irritate the suture line, or the incision may be left open to air (OTA).
  e. Inform client to take showers rather than soak in bathtub according to physician's preference.

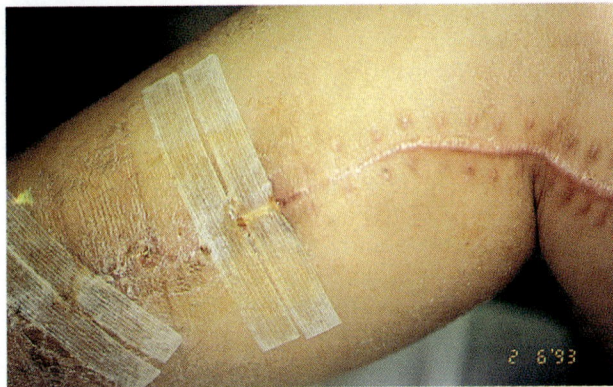

Figure 20-19

Steristrips are not removed and are allowed to fall off gradually.

12. Review local and systemic indications of infection. Instruct client to notify physician if these occur after discharge.

13. Inform client to minimize abdominal strain during defecation, and show how to support the incision with pillow or bath blanket.

Minimizes tension on sutures and discomfort.

14. Encourage good nutrition (protein, vitamins).

Enhances healing process.

15. Encourage ambulation.

Promotes circulation and healing.

16. Follow physician's instructions for limiting activity.

Heavy lifting, driving, and stair climbing may need to be avoided for a time.

17. Provide written instructions as well as verbal instructions, allowing opportunity to answer questions as they arise.

18. See Completion Protocol (Chapter 1, p. 6).

Evaluation

1. Inspect incision for approximation of wound edges.
2. Ask client to rate pain using a scale of 0 to 10.
3. Ask client to explain self-care guidelines before discharge.

UNEXPECTED OUTCOMES AND RELATED INTERVENTIONS

Predisposition to delayed wound healing includes diabetes, immunosuppression, radiation, wound stress, inadequate cellular nutrition and tissue oxygenation, obesity, smoking, depth of wound, and length of surgical procedure.

1. Client exhibits wound dehiscence (separation of wound or incision edges).
  a. Client reports feeling something "gave way."
  b. Increased serosanguineous drainage is noted.
2. Evisceration is seen, involving protrusion of visceral organs through wound opening. This is a serious emergency because blood supply to tissues may be compromised when organs protrude.
  a. Organs must be kept moist by applying sterile towels that have been saturated in warm sterile saline.
  b. Notify surgeon so that surgical intervention can be arranged.

SAMPLE DOCUMENTATION

1030 Wound edges well approximated. Healing ridge palpated. Sutures removed from abdominal incision, and Steristrips applied and left OTA. No redness, swelling, or drainage. Client instructed to shower, avoid tension on incision, and avoid heavy lifting.

CRITICAL THINKING EXERCISES

1. Carla is a 44-year-old client entering the recovery room after a surgical procedure for which she received a spinal anesthetic. How will your immediate postoperative care differ for Carla compared to a client receiving a general anesthetic?

2. Identify specific assessment areas unique to the following postoperative clients.
   a. A 56-year-old client who had a craniotomy for a brain tumor.
   b. A 72-year-old client who had a radical neck dissection for cancer.
   c. A 65-year-old client who had a femoral-popliteal bypass of the left leg.
   d. A 20-year-old client who had an open-reduction, internal fixation of the right femur.

3. Mr. Carlson is a 58-year-old male brought to the postanesthesia care unit after knee surgery.
   a. Mr. Carlson is returned to your surgical unit. The recovery room nurse gives the following report: "BP 148/76, P 88, R 12; Received two units of whole blood in surgery; Alert and oriented; Has received Demerol 100 mg total for pain; IV Ringer's Lactate infusing at 125 cc/hr in right forearm; Dressing intact with a 2 × 2 cm spot of bright red drainage; Hemovac in place." What additional information should you obtain from the recovery room nurse?
   b. You perform the following initial nursing care measures: "BP 150/78, P 90, R 12, T 98° F. O_2 at 3L/nasal cannula, IV infusing at 125 cc/hr, IV site patent, Hemovac emptied of 40 cc bright red drainage, outlined drainage on knee dressing (2 × 2 area), explained equipment and nursing care measures to family." Before leaving the room, you reevaluate. Determine if any essential nursing care measures have been omitted.
   c. Six hours after Mr. Carlson returns to his room, you measure 150 cc of bright red drainage from the Hemovac and note that drainage on the dressing has increased in size. Mr. Carlson is complaining of severe incisional pain unrelieved by the morphine he has been receiving. What additional assessment data should you obtain before calling the physician?
   d. While waiting for the physician to return your call, what should you be doing for the client?
   e. Mr. Carlson is returned to surgery to repair a bleeder. Five days later, you note that there is no drainage in the Hemovac. What should you do?

4. Connie is a 48-year-old female recovering from an abdominal hysterectomy.
   a. Connie refuses to ambulate. How would you handle the situation?
   b. On the third postoperative day, Connie calls you into her room complaining of more pain than usual in her abdominal incision. She states, "It sure seems more tender than it did before." What nursing action would you take at this time?

5. Which clients are at increased risk for diminished wound healing and/or wound infection?
   a. An 80-year-old diabetic client with an abdominal incision
   b. A 45-year-old client after open reduction of an arm fracture
   c. A 50-year-old client after removal of a lung (received radiation therapy 4 weeks earlier)
   d. A 30-year-old client after abdominal surgery (history of long-term steroid therapy)
   e. A 44-year-old female after removal of the thyroid gland (Ht. 5'6", Wt. 130 lbs)
   f. A 27-year-old male after an emergency appendectomy
   g. A 17-year-old client with a large leg wound caused by a car accident (hemoglobin 8 g/dl, hematocrit 29%)
   h. A 12-year-old child requiring sutures for a large jagged wound on the chin

REFERENCES

American Society of Post Anesthesia Nurses: *Standards of post anesthesia nursing practice,* Richmond, 1992, ASPAN.

Bryant R: *Acute and chronic wounds: nursing management,* St Louis, 1992, Mosby.

Centers for Disease Control: *Guidelines for prevention of surgical wound infections,* Atlanta, 1985, Hospital Infection Control Programs, US Department of Health and Human Services.

Einhorn GW, Chant P: Practical points: postanesthesia care unit dilemmas: prompt assessment and treatment, *J Post Anesth Nurs* 9(1):28, 1994.

Kratz A: Preoperative education: preparing patients for a positive experience, *J Post Anesth Nurs* 8(4):270, 1993.

Lewis SM, Collier IC: *Medical-surgical nursing: assessment and management of clinical problems,* ed 3, St Louis, 1992, Mosby.

Lubarsky DA, Gallager CJ: *Board stiff,* Boston, 1990, Butterworth.

ADDITIONAL READINGS

Association of Operating Room Nurses: *Standards and recommended practices for perioperative nursing,* Denver, 1990, The Association.

Doughty DB: Principles of wound healing and wound management. In Ruth Bryant, editor: *Acute and chronic wounds,* St Louis, 1992, Mosby.

Holtzclaw BJ: Temperature problems in the postoperative period, *Crit Care Nurs Clin North Am* 2:589, 1990.

Huddleston VB: Pulmonary problems, *Crit Care Nurs Clin North Am* 2:527, 1990.

Joint Commission on Accreditation for Health Care Organizations: *Accreditation manual for hospitals,* Chicago, 1993, The Commission.

Kim MJ, McFarland GK, McLane AM: *Pocket guide to nursing diagnoses,* ed 5, St Louis, 1993, Mosby.

Lepczyk M, Raleigh EH, Rowley C: Timing of preoperative patient teaching, *J Adv Nurs* 15:300, 1990.

McConnell EA: Assessing abdominal pain in the postoperative patient, *Nursing '90* 20:86, 1990.

Meeker MH, Rothrock JC: *Alexander's care of the patient in surgery,* ed 10, St Louis, 1995, Mosby.

Neelon VJ: Postoperative confusion, *Crit Care Nurs Clin North Am* 2:579, 1990.

Phipps WJ, Long BC, Weeds NF, Cassmeyer VL: *Medical-surgical nursing: concepts and clinical practice,* ed 4, St Louis, 1991, Mosby.

Rodeheaver GT: Controversies in topical wound management: wound cleansing and wound disinfection. In Krasner D, editor: *Chronic wound care,* King of Prussia, Pa, 1990, Health Management Publications.

Sussman C: Physical therapy modalities and the wound recovery cycle, *Ostomy/Wound Manage* 28(2):43, 1992.

VanDover D: Topical wound management, *Ostomy/Wound Manage* 32:40, 1991.

chapter
21

Pain Management

Skill 21.1
Nonpharmacological Pain Management

Skill 21.2
Pharmacological Pain Management

Skill 21.3
Patient-Controlled Analgesia (PCA)

Skill 21.4
Epidural Analgesia

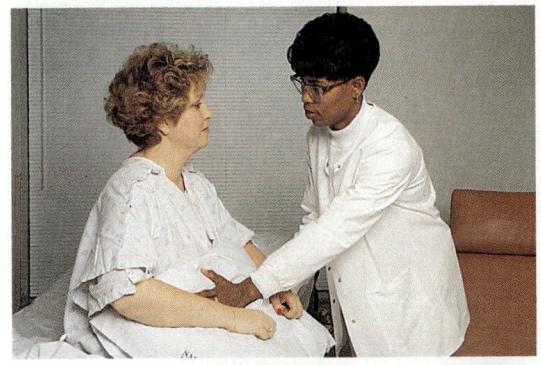

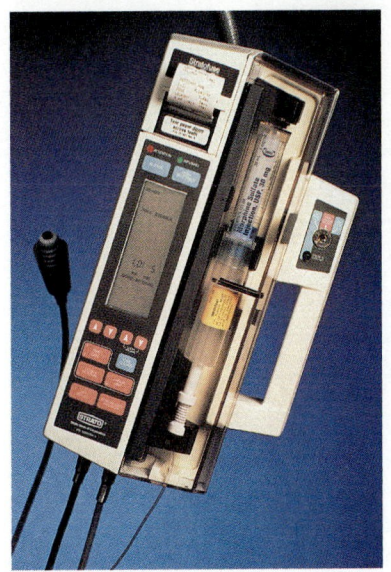

Pain can be described as an unpleasant sensory, perceptual and emotional experience resulting from tissue damage. It may be caused by disease, trauma, surgery, or certain therapeutic procedures (Lewis and Collier, 1992). It is influenced by the individual's psychosocial, economic, and cultural experiences and varies in ways that often make it difficult for others to comprehend (McFarland and McFarlane, 1993).

Pain is classified as either acute or chronic. These classifications are differentiated according to onset, duration, and cause. *Acute pain* usually has a sudden onset and is limited in duration to less than 6 months. Acute pain is usually obvious, confined to a distinct area, decreases over time, and eventually is completely relieved (Lewis and Collier, 1992). *Chronic pain* is a continuous or regularly recurring pain that extends for more than 6 months. It is less easily differentiated, and defining characteristics are less obvious. Suffering tends to increase over time, and complete relief is unlikely (McFarland and McFarlane, 1993). Chronic pain may serve as a constant reminder of a threat to function and possibly to life itself. Clients may become anxious, frustrated, and depressed, and life may begin to revolve around the pain affecting every aspect of the person's life (Lewis and Collier, 1992).

Managing a client's discomfort can be a challenging and rewarding experience when the nurse is skilled and knowledgeable about a variety of management options. Since freedom from pain is not always a realistic option, the goal of pain management may need to be pain control rather than pain relief. In 1992 the Agency for Health Care Policy and Research (AHCPR) issued a guideline for effective pain management for clients with acute pain after surgery, medical procedures, or trauma (AHCPR, 1992). This guideline is designed to help care givers, clients, and their families to understand the assessment and treatment of acute pain in both adults and children and has four major goals:

1. Reduction of incidence and severity of client's postoperative or posttraumatic pain
2. Education of clients about the need to communicate unrelieved pain so that they can receive prompt evaluation and effective treatment
3. Enhancement of client comfort and satisfaction
4. Decrease in postoperative complications to achieve shorter stays after surgical procedures

The flow chart (Figure 21-1) offers a guide for decision making about acute pain management. It must be emphasized that pain is a unique experience for each client, and multiple strategies may be needed for successful management. No single therapy can provide relief for all clients all the time. The AHCPR guidelines advocate a range and combination of approaches to pain management, including nonpharmacologic (Table 21-1) and pharmacologic interventions (Table 21-2).

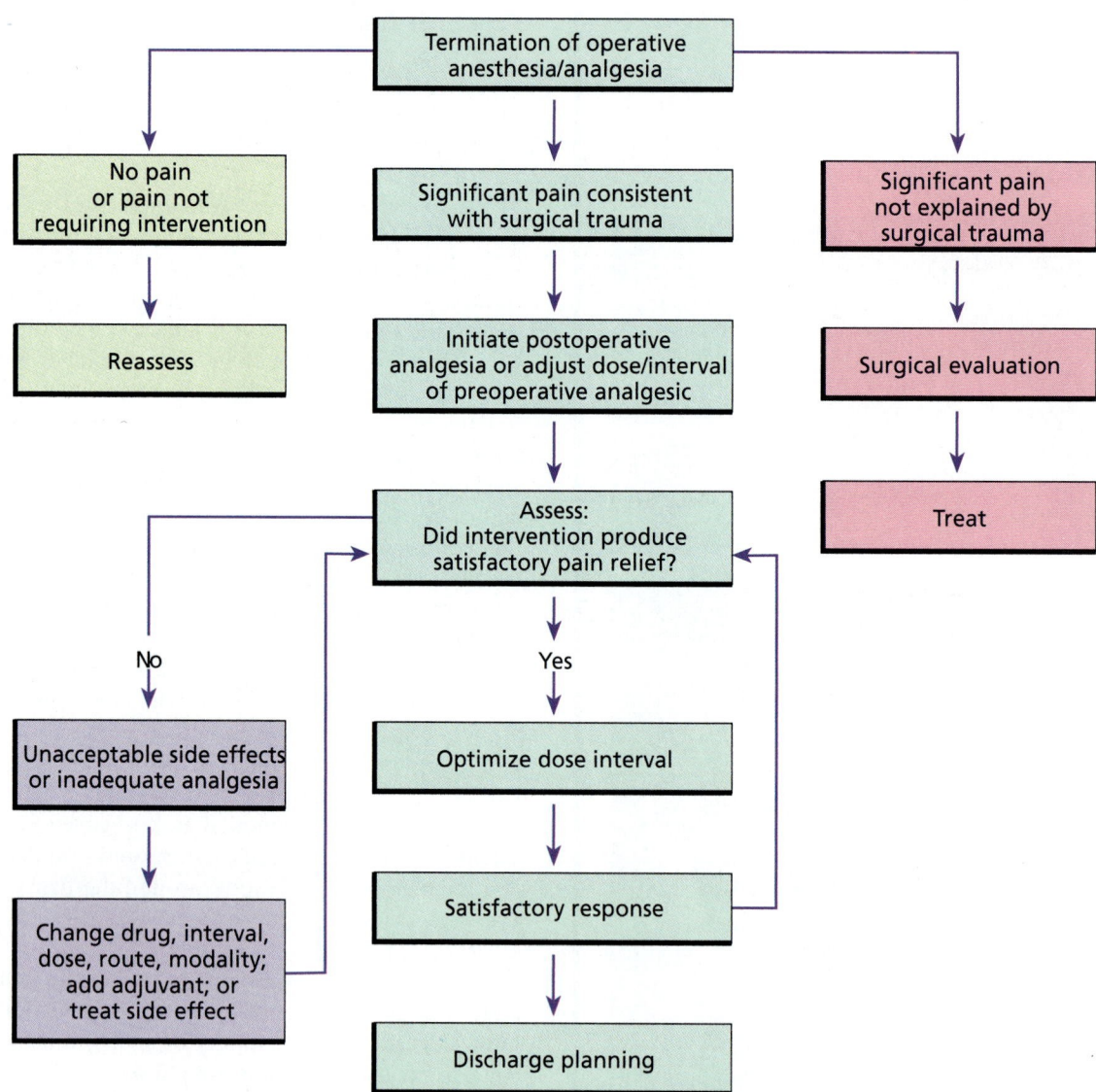

Figure 21-1 Pain treatment flow chart: postoperative phase. (From Acute pain management guideline panel. Acute pain management: Operative or medical procedures and trauma, *Clinical practice guideline,* AHCPR Pub No 92-0032, Rockville, Md, AHCPR, Public Health Service, USDHHS, Feb. 1992.)

Table 21-1 **Nonpharmacological Interventions for Pain**

Interventions	Comments
Progressive muscle relaxation	Reduces mild to moderate pain. Use as an adjunct to analgesics for clients interested in relaxation. Requires 3-5 minutes of staff time for instruction.
Music	Simple relaxation. Best taught preoperatively. Both client preferred and "easy listening" music effective for mild to moderate pain.
Biofeedback	Effective in reducing mild to moderate pain and operative site muscle tension. Requires skilled personnel and special equipment.
Imagery	Effective for reduction of mild to moderate pain. Requires skilled personnel.
Education	Effective for reduction of all types of pain. Should include sensory and procedural information and instruction aimed at reducing activity-related pain. Requires 5-15 minutes of staff time.
Massage	Effective for reduction of mild to moderate discomfort. May be firm, gentle, or light stroking of the body part involved or the opposite extremity. Requires 3-10 minutes of staff time.
Cold or heat applications	Selection of heat vs. cold varies with the situation. Moist heat relieves stiffness of arthritis, and cold applications reduce acute pain associated with inflammation associated with arthritis (Ceccio, 1990).
Transcutaneous electrical nerve stimulation (TENS)	Effective in reducing mild to moderate pain by stimulating the skin with mild electrical current. Electrodes are placed over or near the site of pain. Requires special equipment (Figure 21-2).

Nursing Diagnosis

Impaired Physical Mobility related to pain applies to clients who have limited independent physical movement resulting from painful conditions. Other nursing diagnoses may include **Anxiety, Ineffective (Individual) Coping,** or **Powerlessness** when pain compromises a client's emotional resources. **Pain** and **Chronic Pain** are nursing diagnoses in which the focus of care is on pain control rather than the client's response to pain.

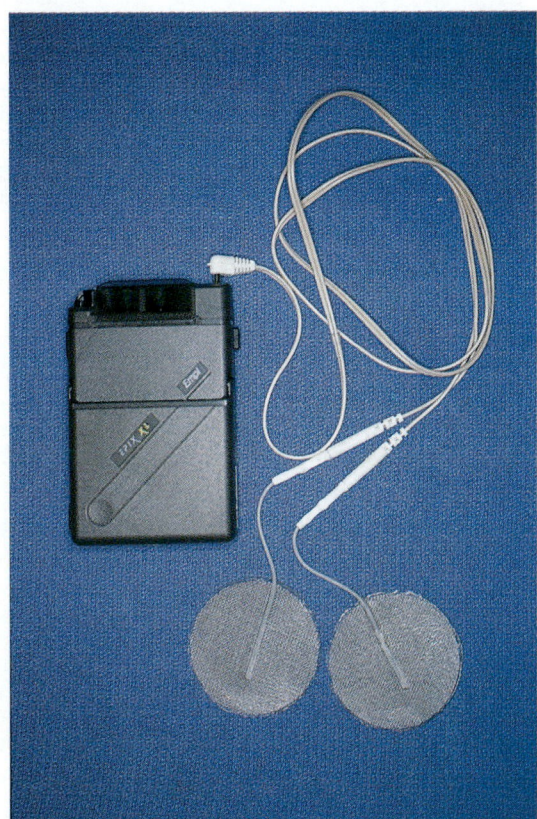

Figure 21-2 Transcutaneous electrical nerve stimulation (TENS) unit.

Table 21-2 **Pharmacological Interventions**

Pharmacological agents	Route	Comments
Nonsteroidal antiinflammatory drugs (NSAIDs)	Oral	Effective for mild to moderate pain. Begin preoperatively. May mask fever.
	Parenteral	Effective for moderate to severe pain.
Narcotics	Oral	As effective as parenteral in appropriate doses. Route of choice as soon as oral medication is tolerated.
	Transdermal patch	Noninvasive and relatively stable plasma drug level.
	Intramuscular	Has been the standard parenteral route, but injections are painful and absorption unreliable. Avoid this route when possible.
	Intravenous	Parenteral route of choice after major surgery. Suitable for titrated bolus or continuous administration, including PCA.
	Patient-controlled analgesia (PCA)	Intravenous or subcutaneous routes recommended. Good steady level of analgesia. Requires special infusion pumps and staff education.
	Epidural	When suitable, provides good analgesia. Risk of respiratory depression. Requires careful monitoring.

Modified from Pharmacologic interventions. In Acute Pain Management Guideline Panel: *Acute pain management in infants, children and adolescents: operative or medical procedures and trauma,* Clinical practice guideline, AHCPR pub no 92-0032, Rockville, Md, 1992, Public Health Service, US Department of Health and Human Services, AHCPR.

Skill 21.1 | Nonpharmacological Pain Management

Controlling pain and promoting comfort are two of the most important aspects of nursing practice. All clients experience some form of physical or emotional discomfort or pain, and attention to providing comfort needs to be considered in every client interaction. When possible, the nurse should design interventions to achieve satisfactory pain relief using nonpharmacologic pain relief measures.

Assessment

1. Identify factors that cause discomfort/pain. Alterations in comfort may be acute (postoperative, associated with labor of childbirth, traumatic wounds, burns) or chronic (associated with cancer, migraine headaches, low back pain).
2. Assess factors that influence tolerance of discomfort/pain. **Fatigue, loneliness, anxiety, and fear are examples of influences that significantly reduce client's ability to cope with pain.**
3. Assess client's perception of the discomfort/pain.
   a. *Onset:* sudden or gradual
   b. *Precipitating factors:* position, movement, inability to move, edema, constricting dressings, tubes or drains, invasive procedures, or distended bladder
   c. *Quality:* ask, "What is your discomfort like?" If client is unable to describe it, suggest examples such as sharp, dull, burning, nagging, stabbing, aching, throbbing, or crushing. Assessment is more

accurate if clients describe the sensation with their own words.
   d. *Region:* localized, radiating, or generalized. Have client point to area of body affected.
   e. *Severity:* rate on a scale as established by agency policy (0 to 10 where 0 = no pain and 10 = worst pain)
   f. *Duration:* constant or intermittent

Table 21-3 **Physiological and Psychological Responses to Acute and Chronic Pain**

Mild to Moderate Acute Pain	Severe Acute Pain	Chronic Pain
Tachycardia	Decreased heart rate	Fatigue
Tachypnea	Rapid/irregular rate	Insomnia
Increased blood pressure	Respirations	Anorexia
Diaphoresis	Decreased blood pressure	Weight loss
Increased serum glucose	Weakness	Depression
Dilated pupils	Nausea/vomiting	Anger
Pallor	Muscle tension	Hopelessness
	Stoicism	Despair
	Powerlessness	Fear
		Anxiety
		Isolation

Table 21-4 **Behavioral Indicators of Pain**

Motor	Affective
Facial Expression	Moaning
Posture	Crying
Gait	Withdrawal
Decreased activity level	Irritability
Guarding	Restlessness
Muscle tension	

Modified from Lewis SM, Collier IC: *Medical-surgical nursing: assessment and management of clinical problems,* ed 3, St Louis, 1992, Mosby.

4. Assess physiological and psychological responses to acute or chronic pain (Table 21-3). **Signs of sympathetic nervous system stimulation (fight or flight) are often, but not always, present. Persons with chronic pain are less likely to show overt physical responses because of physiological adaptation, and psychological distress is often evident.**

5. Assess behavioral responses to pain (Table 21-4). **Nonverbal behavior may be useful in describing pain experienced by clients.**

6. Assess environment for factors that may aggravate the client's perception or tolerance of pain. Environmental factors that may intensify discomfort include noise, bright light, interrupted sleep patterns, or lack of privacy.

7. Assess affected body part by inspection, palpation, auscultation, or percussion as indicated. **Further assessment may suggest the nature of the pain and appropriate interventions.**

8. Determine what relieves the discomfort or what the client believes will help. Consider physician's orders regarding activity, oral intake, and prescribed medication.

Planning

Adequate management may be pain reduction rather than elimination. What is tolerable varies from client to client.

EXPECTED OUTCOMES

1. Client rates pain less than 4 (scale 0 to 10).
2. Client identifies factors that increase pain.
3. Client asks for repositioning at least three times.
4. Client ambulates three times a day with pain level rated as less than 4 (scale 0 to 10) by second postop day.

Implementation

Steps	Rationale
1. See Standard Protocol (Chapter 1, p. 5).	
2. Remove or reduce painful stimuli.	
a. Reposition using pillows as needed for support and prevent pressure areas.	Repositioning reduces stimulation of pain and pressure receptors.
b. Reapply dressings if wet or constricting (see Skill 15.2).	Clean, dry dressings minimize irritation to surrounding tissues and improve circulation.
c. Reapply or adjust equipment as needed: blood pressure (BP) cuff, intravenous (IV) armboard, Ace bandages, tubes, or drains.	
3. Reduce or eliminate factors that increase the pain experience.	Fear or anxiety may cause muscle tension and vasoconstriction, which intensify the pain experience.
a. Relate acceptance and acknowledge the reality of the pain experience.	
b. Explain the cause of pain (if known), providing accurate information.	
4. Assist client to splint painful area using firm pressure over a bath blanket or pillow during coughing, deep breathing, and turning (see Skill 18.2).	Splinting reduces pain by minimizing muscle movement.
5. Massage painful area gently or firmly.	Cutaneous stimulation alters conscious awareness of pain.

nurse alert Do not massage in the presence of abnormal reactive hyperemia. Massage may cause tissue damage (see Chapter 23).

Steps	Rationale
6. Encourage relaxation using imagery, progressive relaxation, or deep rhythmical breathing (see Chapter 9).	
7. Direct client's attention to something else that increases pain tolerance. Possible distractions include: a. Singing or music b. Praying c. Describing pictures d. Discussing pleasant memories 8. See Completion Protocol (Chapter 1, p. 6).	The reticular activating system (RAS) in the brain, which is essential for concentration, inhibits painful stimuli if a person receives sufficient or excessive sensory input. With meaningful sensory input a person can ignore the pain. Pleasurable stimuli also increase endorphins, which relieve pain.

Evaluation

1. Ask client to rate pain using a scale of 0 to 10. Assess location and characteristics of pain.
2. Ask client what intensifies or alleviates pain.
3. Observe client's position, mobility, relaxation, and ability to rest and sleep.
4. Ask client to rate pain using a scale of 0 to 10 before and after ambulation.

UNEXPECTED OUTCOME AND RELATED INTERVENTIONS

Client continues to display nonverbal behaviors reflecting pain.

Discomfort that is unrelieved or is worse may indicate need for additional diagnostic, medical, or surgical intervention.

SAMPLE DOCUMENTATION

0700 Client continues to describe pain in left foot at 6 (scale 0 to 10). Repositioned with foot elevated and gentle massage of ankle and knee for 5 minutes. Body more relaxed, and client expressed relief with pain now at 3 (scale 0 to 10). Refused pain medication at this time.

Skill 21.2 | Pharmacological Pain Management

Analgesics are the most common method of pain relief. There are, however, misconceptions about the dangers and effects of analgesics. Concerns about addiction and misinformation about client behaviors in relation to pain have resulted in inadequate management of pain until recently.

Nonnarcotic analgesics and nonsteroidal antiinflammatory drugs (NSAIDs) provide relief for mild to moderate pain, such as associated with arthritis, minor surgery and dental procedures, and low back problems. These act primarily on peripheral receptors to diminish transmission of pain stimuli. Most inhibit the synthesis of prostaglandins at the site of injury.

Narcotic analgesics are used for severe pain, such as malignant pain, and are given orally or by injection acting on higher centers of the brain and modifying perception of and reaction to pain. Opiates may cause respiratory depression and result in side effects such as nausea, vomiting, constipation, and drowsiness.

Sedatives, antianxiety agents, and muscle relaxants are adjuncts often prescribed to minimize responses to pain and other signs and symptoms associated with pain such as depression and nausea. These drugs can cause drowsiness and impaired coordination, judgment, and mental alertness.

EQUIPMENT

Prescribed medication
Necessary administration device (see Chapter 17)
Narcotic control sheet (for controlled substances only)

Assessment

1. Perform complete assessment as for Skill 21.1.
2. Determine time of administration of previously administered medications, including dose, length of time, and degree of relief experienced.
3. Determine if client has allergies to medications.
4. Determine analgesics prescribed, route, and frequency. Nonnarcotics can be alternated with narcotics. Injectable medications act within 1 hour; oral medications may require up to 2 hours to take effect.

Planning

Expected outcomes focus on return to optimal functioning with minimal side effects.

EXPECTED OUTCOMES
1. Client rates pain less than 4 (scale 0 to 10).
2. Client identifies factors that increase pain.
3. Client asks for repositioning at least three times.
4. Client ambulates three times a day with pain level rated as less than 4 (scale 0 to 10).

Implementation

Steps	Rationale
1. See Standard Protocol (Chapter 1, p. 5).	
2. Administer analgesics:	
a. As soon as pain occurs	
b. Before it increases in severity	
c. Before pain-producing procedures or activities	
3. Include nonpharmacologic pain control measures in addition to analgesics (see Skill 21.1).	Increases effectiveness of pain control.
4. Identify expected time for peak effects and usual duration of action of analgesics.	Effects vary depending on the type of medication used.
5. Coordinate nursing care measures to maximize effectiveness (i.e., encourage to turn, cough, and deep breathe while medication effects are best).	
6. See Completion Protocol (Chapter 1, p. 6).	

Evaluation

1. Ask client to rate pain using a scale of 0 to 10. Assess location and characteristics of pain.
2. Ask client what intensifies or alleviates pain.
3. Observe client's position, mobility, relaxation, and ability to rest and sleep.
4. Ask client to rate pain using a scale of 0 to 10 before and after ambulation.

**UNEXPECTED OUTCOME
AND RELATED INTERVENTIONS**
See Skill 21.1

SAMPLE DOCUMENTATION
0800 Client complains of severe aching pain in lower back, 9 on scale of 0 to 10. Unable to obtain relief in any position, lying, sitting or standing. Morphine 10 mg given IM. Positioned on side with legs supported and back in alignment.
0845 Is relaxed now and drowsy. Pain now described as 6 (scale 0 to 10). Encouraged to rest.

Skill 21.3 | Patient-Controlled Analgesia (PCA)

PCA is based on the theory that clients are the best judges of their pain; it allows them to take active roles in controlling that pain (Kresl, 1988). PCA allows clients to self-administer small, frequent doses of IV narcotics such as morphine as they feel the need.

The equipment used includes a portable infusion pump with a timing device that can be set to limit the amount and frequency of medication. Most are battery operated, have locking doors to prevent tampering, and have digital readouts that describe functions and store information about the amount of medication actually used.

PCA enables a client to self-administer prescribed doses of analgesic intermittently on demand or through the continuous infusion feature. Both features may be used simultaneously to control severe pain. Clients must be able to understand the use of the PCA equipment and be physically able to locate and press the button to deliver the dose. Instructions are best given when the client is not experiencing intense pain or sedated from anesthesia. If surgery is the reason for PCA analgesia, teaching should be done preoperatively. The client should be aware that the analgesia may not eliminate all discomfort but will allow reasonable comfort to allow rest and movement with minimal pain.

Not all clients are suitable candidates for PCA. Older adults and debilitated and cognitively impaired clients should be carefully assessed before initiating therapy. In addition, PCA is not appropriate for clients with a history of narcotic addiction or abuse, neurological disease, hypovolemia, or impaired renal or pulmonary function (Kresl, 1988). Several models of PCA devices are available; therefore the nurse must read the manufacturer's guide to obtain specific guidelines.

EQUIPMENT

PCA system and tubing (Figure 21-3)
Prescribed medication in a 30 ml vial (e.g., morphine, 1 mg/ml) (Preparations vary with pump design.)
Tape

Assessment

1. Check physician's orders for prescribed medication, dosage, and lockout settings. Verify that client is not allergic to prescribed medication.
2. Verify patency of the IV site and compatibility with the solution currently infusing. Other medication and blood transfusions are not compatible. If necessary, start another IV infusion.
3. Determine client's physical ability to manipulate PCA device and cognitive ability to understand directions.

Planning

Planning focuses on proper use of PCA device and adequate pain control without oversedation.

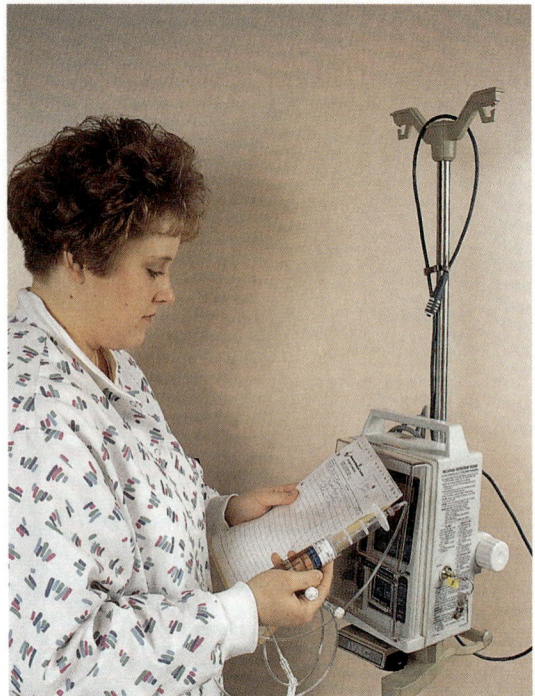

Figure 21-3

EXPECTED OUTCOMES

1. Client demonstrates how to operate PCA device correctly.
2. Client describes pain control level as less than 4 (scale 0 to 10).
3. Client remains cooperative and responsive to verbal instructions.
4. Client maintains respirations of greater than 12 per minute.

Implementation

Steps	Rationale
1. See Standard Protocol (Chapter 1, p. 5).	
2. Teach the client before the therapy is initiated, including:	Ensures client understands how to manipulate device and implications of therapy.
a. The advantages of self-initiated control of medication delivery.	
b. How to initiate a dose of medication using the control button.	
c. That the lockout feature prevents risk of overdose.	
d. Possible side effects, based on the medication prescribed.	
e. To notify the nurse if relief is not being obtained, severity or location of pain changes, alarms sound, or questions arise.	

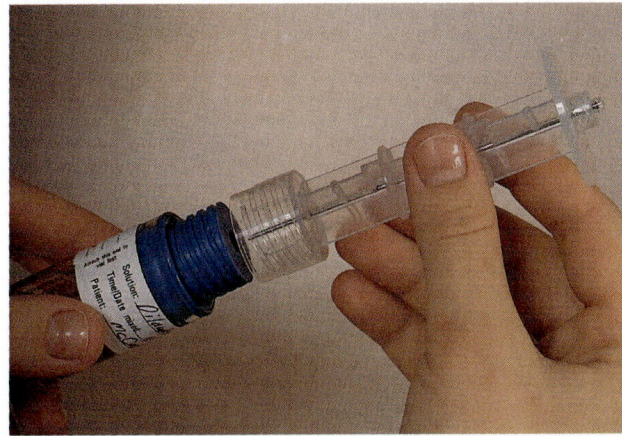

Figure 21-4

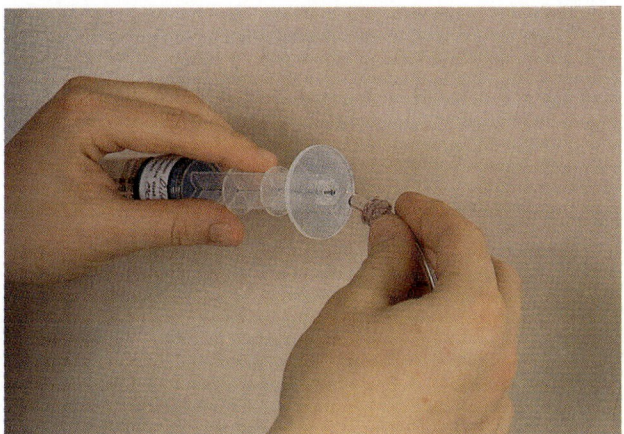

Figure 21-5

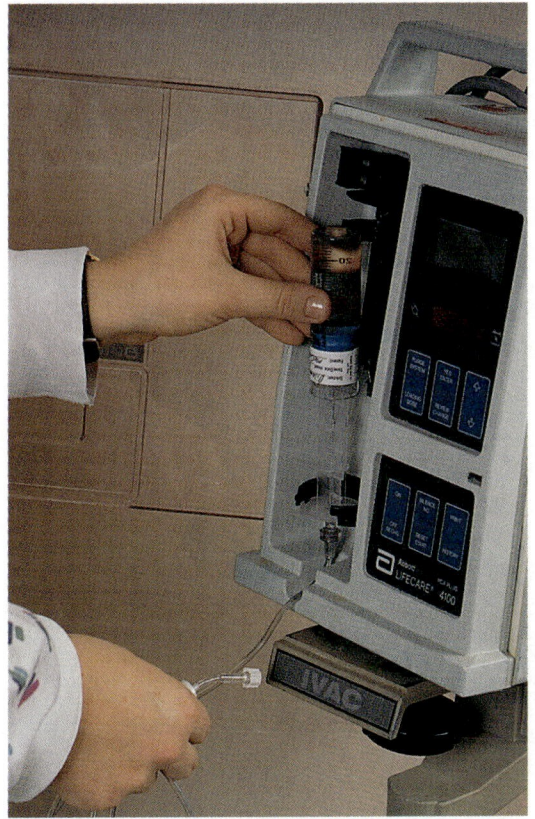

Figure 21-6

Steps	Rationale

3. Prime the unit.
   a. Remove protective caps from prefilled vial and connect to plunger (Figure 21-4). Eject air from the vial.
   b. Attach PCA tubing to the vial (Figure 21-5).
   c. Flush the tubing as far as the Y branch and clamp the tubing.
4. Insert the vial into the drive mechanism of the pump (Figure 21-6).
   a. Insert key and open door.
   b. Pinch the spring-loaded lever, and clamp vial securely in place until it clicks. Close door.
5. Transport equipment to client's room and plug into electrical outlet.

   Battery backup is intended for transport only.

6. Verify client identity by checking identification band and asking client to state name.

   Following the five "rights" is essential for client safety.

Steps	Rationale

7. Attach assembly to client's IV tubing.
   a. If client has maintenance fluids running, clamp off fluids and disconnect from connecting tubing, being sure to maintain sterility.
   b. Remove protective cap from Y site on PCA tubing and attach maintenance fluids.
   c. Prime tubing.
   d. Insert PCA tubing directly into hub of intracath or connecting tubing.
   e. Open slide clamps on both PCA tubing and tubing for IV maintenance fluids.
   f. Secure with tape.
   g. Remove gloves and wash hands.
   h. Place control device within easy reach of client.
8. Reinforce previous teaching of proper use of PCA pump. Assist client to self-administer initial dose by pressing button (Figure 21-7).
9. Encourage client to self-administer medication without delay whenever discomfort is felt.
10. Instruct family to support and assist client, but not to administer medication independently while client is sleeping.
11. See Completion Protocol (Chapter 1, p. 6).

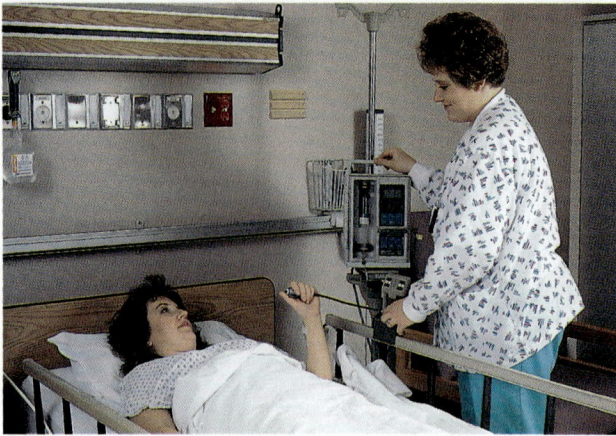

Figure 21-7

VOLUME DELIVERED will display as each dose is delivered. LOCKOUT INTERVAL will display until allotted time has passed. Repeating instructions reinforces learning.

Effectiveness and appropriate dosage are able to be determined only with participation of client. Oversedation can occur.

Evaluation

1. Observe client manipulate control button.
2. Ask client to describe pain control level using a scale of 0 to 10. Compare to the number representing this individual client's satisfactory comfort level.
3. Observe client's ability to cooperate and respond to verbal instructions.
4. Evaluate client's respiratory rate regularly.

nurse alert   If pump is discontinued before syringe is completely empty, waste must be witnessed by another RN, noting date, time, amount wasted, and reason. Federal regulations specify guidelines for recording use and waste of controlled substances in the Controlled Substances Act.

UNEXPECTED OUTCOMES AND RELATED INTERVENTIONS

1. Client does not achieve adequate comfort level.
   a. Physician may need to adjust the dosage parameters.
   b. Use other pain-relieving interventions (e.g., positioning, relaxation, distraction).

2. The venipuncture site shows evidence of infiltration or inflammation.
   Restart a new IV site.
3. Client is too sedated and unable to participate in recovery activities (turning, coughing, deep breathing, ambulation). Adverse reactions to medication occur, including hypotension, dizziness, nausea, vomiting, constipation, or shallow respirations at a rate less than 12 per minute.
   a. Determine how frequently the pump has been used and total dose administered.
   b. Dosage parameters may need to be adjusted by the physician.
4. Client is unable to manipulate device to maintain pain control.
   a. Repositioning of the PCA button may help.
   b. Alternative form of analgesia may be required.

SAMPLE DOCUMENTATION

Record drug, dose, time started, and lockout time. Many institutions have a separate flow sheet for PCA documentation (Figure 21-8).
1500 Client reports abdominal pain at level of 5. Sleeping at intervals. IV infusing in left forearm, no signs of infiltration. Morphine 8 mg infused in last 4 hours.

MEMORIAL MEDICAL CENTER
Springfield, Illinois
PATIENT CONTROLLED ANALGESIA (PCA)
FLOW SHEET

Drug Used: [X] Morphine 1mg/ml-30ml [ ] Morphine 5mg/ml-30ml [ ] Other ___ mg/ml-30ml

Instructions: - Record one syringe only per flow sheet. Syringes must be changed q 48-72 h, tubing q 72 h.
- Chart all appropriate information q 4 h.

Date	10-15-XX	10/15	10/15	10/15
Time		1300	1700	2100
Mode: P=PCA / C=Continuous / P+C=PCA+Cont.		PCA+C	PCA+C	PCA+C
PCA Dose (mg)		2 mg	2 mg	2 mg
Lockout Interval (min)		15	15	15
Continuous Dose (mg/hr)		2 mg	2 mg	2 mg
4 hr. Limit		8 mg	8 mg	8 mg
Loading Dose (mg)		4 mg		
TOTAL DELIVERED		4 mg	8 mg	6 mg
Tubing Change				
Sedation Level		2	3	2
Analgesic Level		3	2	2
RN Initial		RM	RM	RM
RN Signature		R. Martinez, RN		

Sedation Level
1=wide awake 4=mostly sleeping
2=drowsy 5=awaken only when aroused
3=dozing intermittently

Analgesic Level
1=asleep 4=pain
2=comfortable 5=bad pain
3=mild discomfort 6=very bad pain

Record of waste & Spoilage

Date	Quantity	Describe in Detail	Signature #1	Signature #2

Return carbon copy to pharmacy

16756
Order #7408

Figure 21-8 (Courtesy Memorial Medical Center, Springfield, Ill.)

Skill 21.4 | Epidural Analgesia

The administration of narcotics into the epidural space has become an increasingly popular technique for managing acute postoperative pain. Epidural narcotic infusions may also be used to control chronic pain, especially for clients with cancer. An epidural narcotic infusion reduces the total amount of narcotic required to control pain while producing fewer side effects.

The epidural space is located between the vertebral column and the dura mater, the outermost protective layer of the spinal cord. When a narcotic is injected into the epidural space, it diffuses slowly into the cerebrospinal fluid (CSF) of the subarachnoid space, where it binds to opiate receptors located on the dorsal horn of the spinal cord. The binding of the narcotic on the dorsal horn results in a block of pain impulse transmission to the cerebral cortex.

The anesthesiologist or nurse anesthetist places a catheter into the epidural space, usually in the lower lumbar region, to administer analgesics. Usually, opiates such as morphine sulfate or fentanyl citrate (Sublimaze) are used. When the epidural catheter is intended for short-term use, it does not need to be sutured in place and exits from the insertion site on the back (Figure 21-9). A catheter utilized for long-term use, however, is tunneled under the subcutaneous tissue and exits on the side of the body or the abdomen (Figure 21-10). Tunneling reduces the risk of infection and dislodging of the catheter. In both cases the catheter is secured with a sterile occlusive dressing (Figure 21-11).

Although the use of epidural narcotics for control of pain has many advantages for the client, it also requires astute nursing observation and care. The epidural catheter poses a threat to client safety because of its anatomical location, its potential for migration through the dura, and its proximity to spinal nerves and vessels. In many hospitals, anesthesiologists and nurse anesthetists are the only health care professionals who may initiate an epidural narcotic infusion or administer a bolus. Some hospitals have nurses who have successfully completed a certification program that enables them to initiate the epidural narcotic infusion or administer a bolus once the catheter has been placed (review agency policy).

EQUIPMENT
Gloves
Bolus medication:
    10 to 12 ml syringe
    Filter needle
    20-gauge 1-inch needle
    Povidone-iodine swabs
    Prediluted preservative-free narcotic as prescribed by physician

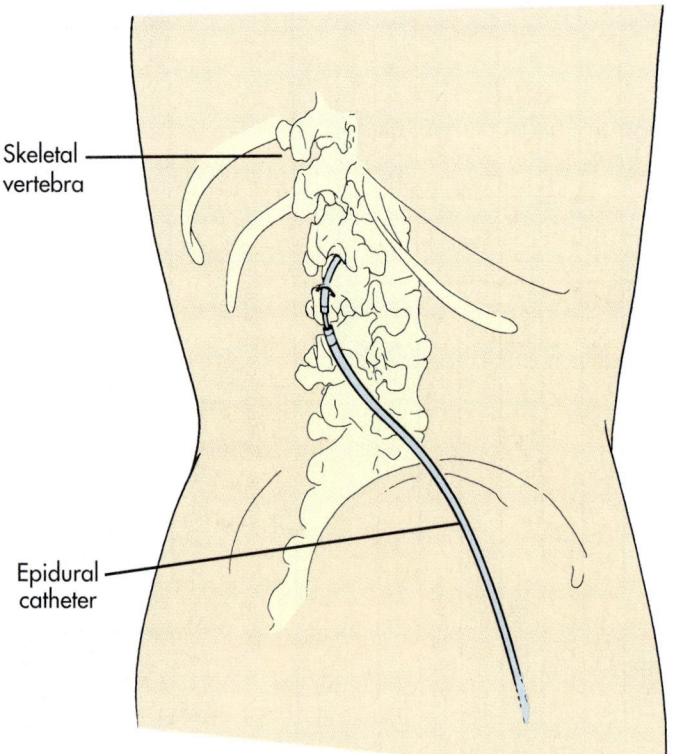
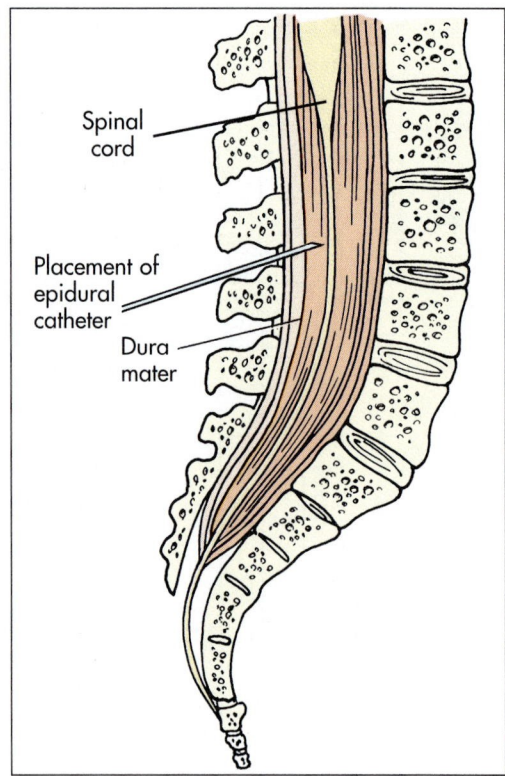

Skeletal vertebra

Epidural catheter

Spinal cord

Placement of epidural catheter

Dura mater

Figure 21-9 Epidural catheter.

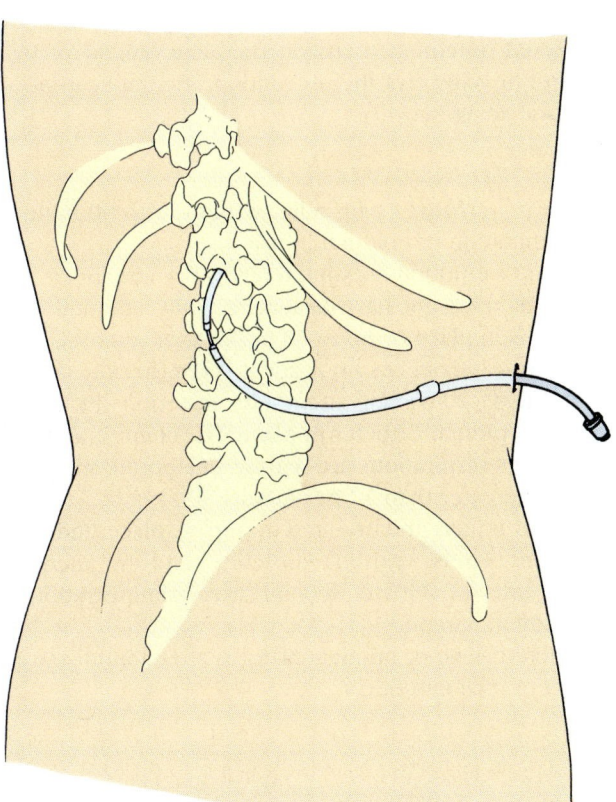

Figure 21-10 Tunneled epidural catheter.

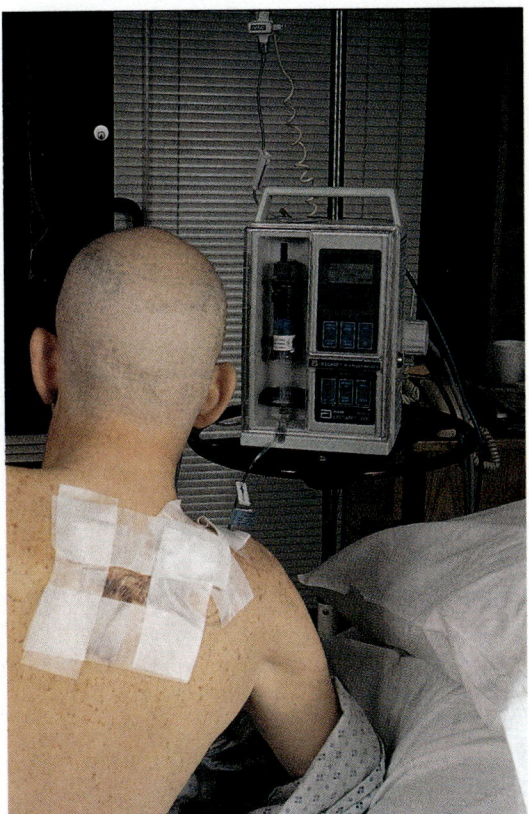

Figure 21-11 Epidural catheter taped in place.

Label (for injection port)
Continuous infusion:
    Prediluted preservative-free narcotic as prescribed by physician and prepared for use in IV infusion pump (usually prepared by pharmacy)
    Infusion pump
    Infusion pump–compatible IV tubing *without* Y ports
    Tape
    Label (for tubing)

Assessment

1. Assess client's comfort level (see Skill 21.1). Certain conditions make epidural analgesia the method of choice for clients experiencing pain: postoperative states, trauma, and advanced cancer.
2. Assess client's nonverbal response. Signs of sympathetic nervous stimulation are often, but not universally, seen in clients experiencing acute pain of mild to moderate intensity or superficial pain (Donovan, 1990; McCaffery and Ferrell, 1992). **Clients with chronic pain often do not show overt signs and symptoms of acute pain.**
3. Assess characteristics and intensity of pain (see Skill 21-1, Assessment) to allow client to describe pain. Pain is primarily a subjective experience. **Objective indicators are not as reliable as client's expression of pain (McCaffery, 1992).**

4. Assess sedation level of client, including level of consciousness (LOC), to establish a baseline before first dose. **The first sign of altered respiratory function from opioid use is most often a change in LOC (Wild and Coyne, 1992).**
5. Check rate, depth, and pattern of respirations to establish a baseline. **Slow, shallow, and irregular respirations are signs of respiratory depression, which may occur as late as 24 hours after epidural injection (Wild and Coyne, 1992).**
6. Check blood pressure to establish a baseline. Small drop in blood pressure may be seen in the first hour after epidural injection. **Hypotension after opioid use usually results, however, from a decreased circulating catecholamine level that was elevated in response to pain (Wild and Coyne, 1992).**
7. Assess mobility and motor/sensory function (see Chapter 12) before assisting client into or out of bed. Check for motor weakness and numbness and tingling of lower extremities (paresthesias) to prevent injury from falling that may occur from weakness, sedation, or postural hypotension. **In addition, rapid onset of motor weakness is indication that epidural catheter may have migrated across dura into subarachnoid space (Wild and Coyne, 1992); if catheter puts pressure on spinal nerves, paresthesias can result (Chalupka and Gillon-Allard, 1989).**

8. Check to see if epidural catheter is secured to client's skin. **Prevents dislodging or migration of catheter.**

9. Assess epidural catheter insertion site for redness, warmth, tenderness, swelling, and drainage. **Local inflammation and a superficial skin infection at the insertion site are the most common infections resulting from epidural catheters (Wild and Coyne, 1992). Purulent drainage is a sign of infection. Clear drainage may indicate puncture of the dura, causing narcotic to be delivered into subarachnoid space or causing CSF leak. Bloody drainage may indicate catheter entered a blood vessel.**

10. If continuous infusion, check infusion pump for proper calibration and operation to ensure client will obtain prescribed analgesic dose.

11. If continuous infusion, check patency of IV tubing. **IV tubing must be patent for medication to reach epidural space.**

12. Check client's history of drug allergies to avoid placing client at risk for allergic reaction.

Planning

Expected outcomes focus on the achievement of pain control or relief and the prevention of complications of epidural analgesia.

EXPECTED OUTCOMES

1. Client verbalizes pain relief within 30 to 60 minutes of initiation of epidural infusion.
2. Client's epidural dressing remains dry and intact.
3. Client does not have headache while epidural catheter is in place or up to 72 hours after removal.
4. Client experiences no redness, warmth, exudate, tenderness, or swelling at catheter insertion site during time epidural catheter in place. The client is afebrile.
5. Client's respirations are regular, unlabored, and equal to or greater than 12 per minute.
6. Client is alert and oriented to person, place, and time.
7. Client voids without difficulty and in adequate amounts of 250 to 500 ml after administration of epidural narcotic.
8. Client has no or minimal pruritus after administration of epidural narcotic.

Implementation

Steps	Rationale
1. See Standard Protocol (Chapter 1, p. 5).	
2. Administer bolus injection.	
a. Attach "epidural line" label close to injection cap on epidural catheter.	Labeling helps to ensure narcotic analgesic is administered into correct line and into epidural space.
b. Using a large syringe, draw up prediluted preservative-free narcotic solution through a filter needle.	A large volume of fluid permits narcotic to contact the optimal number of receptors (Wild and Coyne, 1992). Preservative may be toxic to neural tissue and could result in nerve damage (Williams, Beaulauier, and Seal, 1990). Filter needle removes any microscopic glass particles.
c. Change from filter needle to regular 20-gauge needle.	Changing to regular needle is necessary to allow medication to be injected.
d. Clean injection cap with povidone-iodine. (Do *not* use alcohol.)	Cleaning agent prevents introduction of microorganisms during needle insertion. Alcohol causes pain and is toxic to neural tissue.
e. Dry the injection cap with sterile 2×2 gauze.	
f. Insert needle into injection cap. Aspirate.	Aspiration of clear fluid of less than 1 ml is indicative of epidural catheter placement. More than 1 ml of clear fluid or bloody return means catheter may be in subarachnoid space or in a vessel (Williams, Beaulauier, and Seal, 1990).
g. If less than 1 ml clear fluid returns, inject drug slowly (see Chapter 29). (Do not inject if more than 1 ml or a bloody return. Notify anesthesiologist/nurse anesthetist.)	Slow injection helps prevent client discomfort by lowering the pressure exerted by fluid as it exits the catheter (Wild and Coyne, 1992).

Steps	Rationale

h. Remove needle from injection cap.

i. Dispose of uncapped needle and syringe in "sharps" container.

Prevents accidental needle sticks.

3. Administer continuous infusion.

a. Attach "epidural line" label to IV tubing connected to epidural catheter. Use tubing without Y ports.

b. Attach container of diluted preservative-free narcotic to infusion pump tubing and prime.

Tubing should be filled with solution and free of air bubbles to avoid air embolus.

c. Attach proximal end of tubing to pump and distal end to epidural catheter. Tape all connections. Start infusion. (See Chapter 29 for use of infusion pump.)

Infusion pump propels fluid through tubing. Taping maintains a secure, closed system to help prevent infection.

d. Check infusion pump for proper calibration and operation.

Maintains patency and ensures client is receiving proper dose and pain relief.

4. See Completion Protocol (Chapter 1, p. 6).

Evaluation

1. Ask client if pain is relieved.
2. Inspect epidural dressing for dryness and intactness.
3. Ask client if headache is present. Note nonverbal expression.
4. Assess catheter insertion site for redness, warmth, exudate, tenderness, or swelling.
5. Assess rate, depth, and pattern of respirations. (When infusion started or if a bolus is given, check respiratory rate, depth, and pattern every 15 minutes for 2 hours, then every 30 minutes for 2 hours, then every 1 hour for 1 hour, then every 2 hours.)
6. Assess LOC and orientation.
7. Assess client's voiding pattern and amount. If voiding in amounts less than 150 ml and is experiencing frequency, palpate for bladder distention.
8. Ask client if pruritus is present.

UNEXPECTED OUTCOMES AND RELATED INTERVENTIONS

1. Client's respirations decrease to 6 per minute and are shallow. Client is not easily aroused with verbal stimulation.
   a. Follow institution's policy, which may include:
      (1) Administer naloxone (Narcan), 0.4 mg IV.
      (2) Stop epidural infusion.
      (3) Notify anesthesiologist/nurse anesthetist.
      (4) Assess respiratory rate, rhythm, and depth every 15 minutes for 2 hours, every 30 minutes for 2 hours, every hour for 1 hour, then every 2 hours.
   b. Do not give other narcotics or central nervous system depressants except as prescribed by the anesthesiologist/nurse anesthetist responsible for epidural analgesia.

2. Client states pain is not controlled.
   a. Check infusion pump for malfunction if receiving a continuous infusion.
   b. Check tubing for kinks.
   c. Teach client other pain management strategies that may supplement or enhance pharmacologic intervention (e.g., imagery, distraction, relaxation).
   d. Explain that pain relief begins within 30 to 60 minutes after epidural injection and may last between 6 and 24 hours.
3. Client experiences redness, warmth, tenderness, swelling, or exudate at catheter insertion site. Client is febrile.
   Notify anesthesiologist/nurse anesthetist.
4. Client complains of headache. Clear drainage is present on epidural dressing or more than 1 ml can be aspirated from catheter.
   a. Stop infusion or bolus injection.
   b. Notify anesthesiologist/nurse anesthetist.

SAMPLE DOCUMENTATION

Many agencies have an epidural analgesic flow sheet (Figure 21-12).

0800 2000 μg fentanyl in 500 ml 0.9 normal saline infusing at 15 ml per hour into epidural catheter via infusion pump. Respiratory rate 10 with moderate depth and regular pattern. States abdominal surgical pain relieved.

1000 Respiratory rate 6 with shallow depth and periods of apnea. Arouses with verbal stimulation. Epidural infusion stopped. Narcan 0.2 mg IV push given. Anesthesiologist notified.

1005 Respiratory rate 8, shallow depth, and regular pattern. Alert.

1020 Respiratory rate 12, moderate depth, regular pattern. Rates abdominal surgical pain a 4 on a 0 to 10 scale.

MEMORIAL MEDICAL CENTER
Springfield, Illinois

EPIDURAL ANALGESIA FLOW SHEET

Analgesic Drug Used:

✓ Duramorph (_____mcg/ml)
✓ Fentanyl (_10_ mcg/ml)
_____ Hydromorphone (_____mcg/ml)
_____ Sufentanil (_____ mcg/ml)

Device In Use:

_____ Abbott PCA (mcg units)
_____ Bard PCA (ml units)

Date	5/3	5/3													
Time	09	13													
Mode: B = Bolus / P = PCA / C = Continuous / P+C = PCA + Continuous	P+C	P+C													
Manual Bolus by MD (Drug/Dose)	3mcg	—													
Volume in Bag	100	60													
Volume Infused	—	40													
Concentration	0.0	0.0	0.0	0.0	0.0	0.0	0.0	0.0	0.0	0.0	0.0	0.0	0.0	0.0	0.0
PCA Dose (ml)	1.0	1.0													
Delay (min)	20	20													
Basal Rate	10	10													
One Hour Limit	13	13													
Sedation Level	2	3													
Analgesic Level	7	3													
Complications	—	—													
Initials	JD	JD													
RN Signature	J Davenport, RN														

Sedation Level
1=wide awake   4=mostly sleeping
2=drowsy   5=awakens only when aroused
3=dozing intermittently

Analgesic Level
1 2 3 4 5 6 7 8 9 10
no   worst
pain   pain
                          imaginable

Complications
1=nausea   5=headache
2=vomiting   6=respiratory depression
3=pruritis   7=ileus
4=unable to void

Record of Waste & Spoilage				
Date	Quantity	Describe in Detail	Signature #1	Signature #2

White copy to chart   Yellow copy to Pharmacy   Pink copy to Anesthesia Pain Service   Page 1 of 1

Figure 21-12 (Courtesy Memorial Medical Center, Springfield, Ill.)

CRITICAL THINKING EXERCISES

1. Determine whether the following situations represent acute or chronic pain. Identify the criteria by which you make your decision. If there are insufficient data to determine the classification, determine what additional information would be necessary.
   a. A 50-year-old female with c/o intermittent low back pain of 10 months' duration
   b. A 44-year-old client with abdominal pain of 1 week's duration that abates after meals c/o sweating and palpitations during the painful episodes
   c. A child c/o a toothache since breakfast 4 hours ago; his pulse is fast
   d. A 34-year-old c/o intermittent headaches, insomnia, and depression
   e. A 63-year-old with c/o pain in her legs unrelieved by aspirin
   f. A 17-year-old male with persistent knee pain after a football injury 8 months ago
2. Pam is a 55-year-old client who has just returned from the postanesthesia care unit after a left modified radical mastectomy. The surgeon has prescribed a PCA pump, and Pam can receive Morphine 10 mg every 10 minutes up to a maximum of 160 mg/4 hrs.
   a. After connecting Pam to the PCA pump you assess her to determine teaching requirements regarding the PCA system. What factors will determine the extent of teaching needed?
   b. Pam turns on the call light and tells you she is not getting pain relief. Even after pushing the button for Morphine, she still has pain rated as 8 on a scale of 0 to 10. What steps will you take to improve pain control?
   c. Two hours later you note that Pam's respirations have decreased from 16 to 8/minute. She is drowsy but responds to verbal stimulus. What will you do with this information, if anything? Explain your action or nonaction.
3. After having an orthopedic surgical procedure, Mr. Nelson is complaining of severe leg pain rated as 7 on a scale of 0 to 10. He can have Demerol 75 mg IM q 3-4 hrs. You realize that Mr. Nelson has not had his morning bath, his dressing needs changing, and the surgeon has ordered ambulation tid beginning this morning. Outline your plan of care.
4. Assuming that all of the following clients require pain management, determine those who would be candidates for a PCA device.
   a. A 91-year-old client who is alert and oriented
   b. A 45-year-old client with known history of morphine addiction
   c. A 70-year-old client with severe rheumatoid arthritis and Parkinson's disease
   d. A 50-year-old client who is hypoventilating secondary to a head injury
   e. A 78-year-old client after a colon resection; oriented in all three spheres
   f. A 35-year-old client on renal dialysis due to kidney failure
5. You are caring for a 55-year-old male who had abdominal surgery 3 days ago. He is complaining of pain rated as a 4 on a scale of 0 to 10. How will you decide if pharmacological pain management is appropriate for this client?

REFERENCES

Agency for Health Care Policy and Research: Acute Pain Management Guideline Panel: *acute pain management in infants, children and adolescents: operative or medical procedures and trauma,* Clinical practice guideline, AHCPR pub no 92-0032, Rockville, Md, 1992, Public Health Service, US Department of Health and Human Services, AHCPR.

Ceccio CM: Heat vs cold as treatment for arthritic pain, *RN* 53:83, 1990.

Chalupka S, Gillon-Allard B: Home care: when your patient has an epidural catheter, *RN* 52(12):70, 1989.

Donovan MI: Acute pain relief, *Nursing Clin North Am* 25(4):851, 1990.

Kresl JS: Patient controlled analgesia: a new system for pain management, *AORN J* 48(3), 1988.

Lewis SM, Collier IC: *Medical-surgical nursing: assessment and management of clinical problems,* ed 3, St Louis, 1992, Mosby.

McCaffery M: RN's assessment is critical in pain control, *Am Nurse* 42(2):4, 12, 1992.

McCaffery M, Ferrell BR: How vital are vital signs, *Nursing '92* 22(1):42, 1992.

McFarland GK, McFarlane EA: *Nursing diagnosis and intervention,* ed 2, St Louis, 1993, Mosby.

Wild L, Coyne C: The basics and beyond: epidural analgesia, *Am J Nurs* 92(4):26, 1992.

Williams AR, Beaulauier KE, Seal DL: Chronic cancer pain management with the Du Pen epidural catheter, *Cancer Nurs* 13(3):176, 1990.

ADDITIONAL READINGS

Brockopp DY et al: Postoperative pain: getting a grip on the facts, *Nursing* 24(6): 49, 1994.

Cohen MR: Preventing errors associated with P.C.A. pumps, *Nursing* 23(4):17, 1993.

Lyons MJ, Stuart T: An epidural narcotics program for general care units, *Nurs Manage* 22(8):33, 1991.

McCready M, MacDavitt K, O'Sullivan KK: Children and pain, easing the hurt: *Orthop Nurs* 10(6): 33, 1991.

McShane F: Epidural narcotics: mechanism of action and nursing implications, *J Post Anesth Nurs* 7(2):155, 1992.

Perry AG, Potter PA: *Clinical nursing skills and techniques,* ed 3, St Louis, 1994, Mosby.

Slack J, Faut-Callahan M: Pain management, *Nursing Clin North Am* 26(2):463, 1991.

Tucker SM: *Patient care standards: nursing process, diagnosis, outcome,* ed 5, St Louis, 1991, Mosby.

Watt-Watson JH, Donovan MI: *Pain management: nursing perspective,* St Louis, 1992, Mosby.

Woodin LM: Cutting postop pain, *RN* 56(8):26, 1993.

Therapeutic Use of Heat and Cold

Skill 22.1
Moist Heat

Skill 22.2
Dry Heat

Skill 22.3
Cold Compresses and Ice Bags

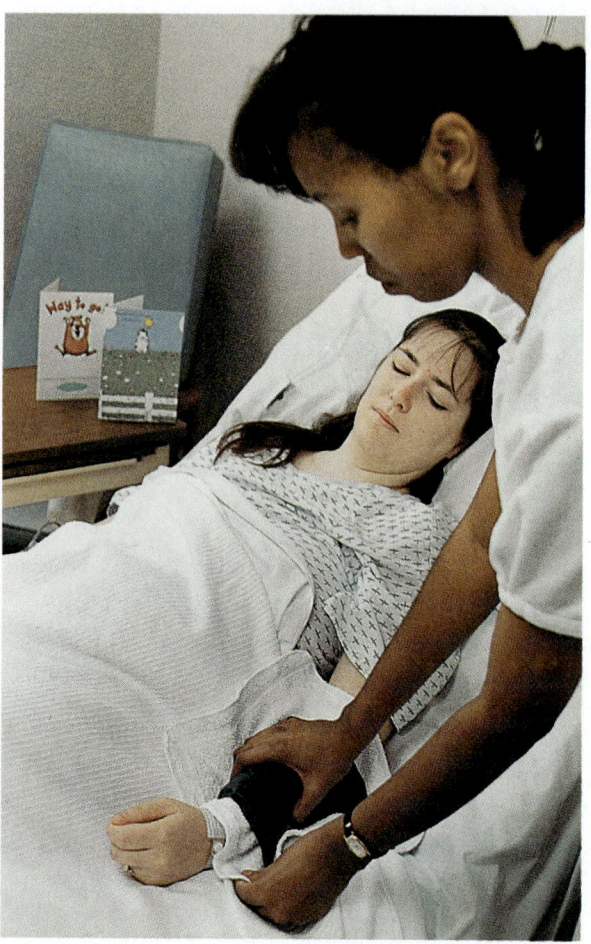

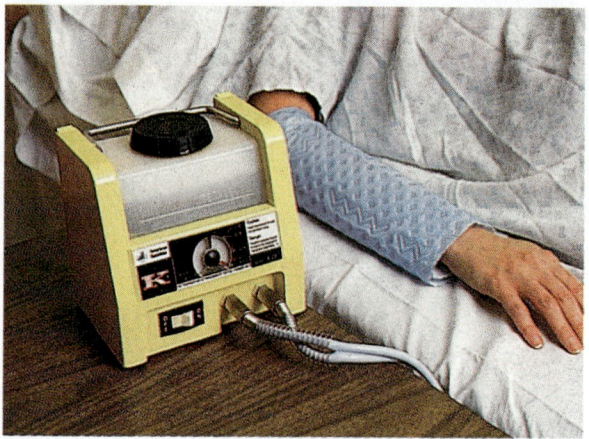

There are both benefits and risks to the therapeutic use of heat and cold. The local benefits of hot treatments are the healing, decreased pain, and increased mobility when venous congestion in tissue is prevented. Local heat improves circulation and prevents congestion through increased delivery of nutrients and removal of wastes when vasodilation occurs. Local cold therapy reduces bleeding and inflammation by means of vasoconstriction (Table 22-1).

The risks involved in hot and cold therapies are burns, dehydration, chilling, and ischemia. The central reason for these risks follows: moist hot and cold treatments penetrate deeply into tissue layers and change body temperature rapidly. Dry treatments penetrate superficially but retain their temperature longer. Systemically, heat treatments cause loss of body heat through vasodilation, whereas cold applications result in the conservation of body heat through vasoconstriction and piloerection.

In addition, risks of injury from hot and cold treatments are great because sensory receptors adapt, preventing awareness of the temperature change before tissue damage occurs. Certain clients are at greater risk for such injury: clients who are very young or elderly, clients with any actual risk for skin impairment, and clients with a localized inflammation in the area of intended treatment. It is important to verify safe temperatures (Table 22-2).

Table 22-1 **Therapeutic Effects of Heat and Cold Applications**

Therapy		Physiological response	Therapeutic benefit	Examples of conditions treated
Heat		Vasodilation	Improves blood flow to injured body part, promotes delivery of nutrients and removal of wastes, lessens venous congestion in injured tissues.	Inflamed or edematous body part; new surgical wound; infected wound; arthritis, degenerative joint disease; localized joint pain, muscle strains; low back pain, menstrual cramping; hemorrhoidal, perianal, and vaginal inflammation; local abscesses
		Reduced blood viscosity	Improves delivery of leukocytes and antibiotics to wound site.	
		Reduced muscle tension	Promotes muscle relaxation and reduces pain from spasm or stiffness.	
		Increased tissue metabolism	Increases blood flow; provides local warmth.	
		Increased capillary permeability	Promotes movement of waste products and nutrients.	
Cold		Vasoconstriction	Reduces blood flow to injured body part, prevents edema formation, reduces inflammation.	Immediately after direct trauma such as sprains, strains, fractures, muscle spasms, after superficial laceration or puncture wound; after minor burn; when malignancy is suspected in area of injury or pain; after injections; for arthritis, joint trauma
		Local anesthesia	Reduces localized pain.	
		Reduced cell metabolism	Reduces oxygen needs of tissues.	
		Increased blood viscosity	Promotes blood coagulation at injury site.	
		Decreased muscle tension	Relieves pain.	

Nursing Diagnosis

Reasons for implementing hot and cold therapies may include **Pain** or **Impaired Tissue Integrity** related to an inflammatory process. When using these treatments, there is a **Risk for Injury** or a **Risk for Impaired Tissue Integrity**. Each of these risks may be related to **Altered Peripheral Tissue Perfusion** or **Tactile Sensory/Perceptual Alterations**. The nurse will want to teach about hot and cold treatments if the client has a **Knowledge Deficit** about these therapies, especially if the treatments are to be used at home.

Table 22-2 **Temperature Ranges for Hot and Cold Applications**

Temperature	Centigrade range	Fahrenheit range
Very hot	41° to 46° C	105° to 115° F
Hot	37° to 41° C	98° to 105° F
Warm	34° to 37° C	93° to 98° F
Tepid	26° to 34° C	80° to 93° F
Cool	18° to 26° C	65° to 80° F
Cold	10° to 18° C	50° to 65° F

Skill 22.1 | Moist Heat

Moist heat therapy is implemented by immersing a body part in a warmed solution. Whirlpool (Figure 22-1), soaks, and sitz baths are such treatments. Also, moist heat is delivered by placing a clean or sterile gauze or towel in a warmed solution and then applying it to the skin or open wound. Such a treatment is called a compress. These compresses are clean when the skin is intact. If skin is broken, sterile supplies and technique must be used. Commercially packaged, sterile, premoistened compresses are available. They are heated with a special infrared lamp. An aquathermia pad can be placed over a compress as a controlled means to maintain heat during an application.

Care must be taken to protect the skin from maceration and burns. Also, maintaining the temperature of the treatment is important, as is protecting the client from chilling (McConnell, 1993).

EQUIPMENT

All moist heat
    Bath blanket
    Warmed prescribed solution
    Dry bath towel
Clean compress
    Clean gauze dressings or towel
    Clean basin
    Waterproof pad
    Ties, tape, or pin
    Aquathermia (optional) (see Figure 22-3)
Sterile compress
    Sterile gauze dressings
    Sterile basin
    Waterproof pad

    Sterile towel or pad
    Clean gloves
    Hazardous waste bag
    Sterile cotton-tipped swabs
Soak or sitz bath
    Basin (clean or sterile)
    Sitz bath (water temperature: 37° to 41°C or 98° to 105°F)
    Bath thermometer
    Hazardous waste bag

Assessment

Inspect the client's skin and/or wound area to be treated. Note intactness, color, temperature, and sensitivity to touch. Observe or palpate for visible or underlying inflammation, including redness, edema, drainage, and amount of pain on a scale of 0 to 10. **This information provides a baseline to assess benefits or adverse effects both during and after the treatment.**

Planning

Expected outcomes focus on decreasing pain and other signs of inflammation, preventing burns and promoting healing.

EXPECTED OUTCOMES

1. Client reports decreased levels of pain 30 minutes after the treatment.
2. Client's wound remains stable or is improved.
3. Client's skin is intact 30 minutes after the treatment.

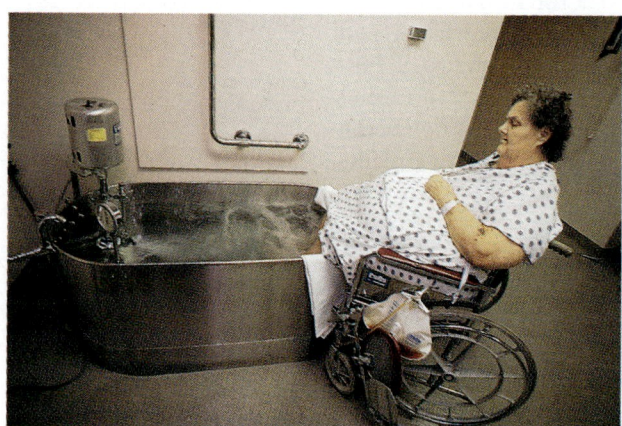

Figure 22-1 Whirlpool moist heat therapy.

Implementation

Steps	Rationale
1. See Standard Protocol (Chapter 1, p. 5).	
2. Provide warmth using bedclothes or bath blanket.	Prevents chilling by preventing heat loss.
3. Apply clean compress or soak to intact skin.	
a. Place waterproof pad under treatment area.	
b. Pour solution into clean basin.	
c. Test solution temperature using sensitive part of hand or wrist.	Prevents burns by ensuring proper temperature.
d. Place gauze or towel into solution, wring out excess solution, and apply lightly to skin. Alternately, assist client to position body part into solution.	
e. Apply compress to intact or open skin. Every 5 minutes, change compress or maintain temperature with aquathermia.	
4. Apply sterile compress to open area using preheated, premoistened sterile compress heater.	

nurse alert   Use gloves when treatment involves nonintact skin or potential exposure to blood or body fluids.

Steps	Rationale
a. Place up to 10 packages of sterile compresses into container (follow manufacturer's directions).	
b. Put cover on, turn on, and wait until red light is on.	Signifies compress is at proper temperature.
c. Remove bottom compress and take to bedside.	
d. Remove dressings and dispose of them and gloves.	
e. Put on sterile gloves. Place sterile compress lightly over area.	
f. Cover sterile towel, pad, or bath towel with aquathermia (optional).	Steps 10 through 14 maintain constant temperature of treatment (McConnell, 1991).
5. Provide sitz bath to intact skin.	Sitz bath may be disposable type or special device with circulating water and temperature controls (Figure 22-2).
a. Set sitz bath under toilet seat, hang bag on intravenous (IV) pole nearby, and connect tubing into sitz bath.	
b. Test clean solution temperature using bath thermometer.	
c. Pour solution into sitz bath bag.	
d. Fill sitz bath one-third full with solution from bag.	
e. Assist client to sit in solution.	
6. Provide sitz bath to open skin.	
a. Set sitz bath under toilet seat, hang bag on IV pole nearby, and connect tubing into sitz bath.	

Steps	Rationale

b. Test sterile solution temperature by pouring small amount over back of hand.

c. Pour solution into sitz bath bag.

d. Fill sitz bath one-third full of solution from the bag.

e. Remove dressing and dispose of it and gloves properly.

f. Assist client to sit in solution.

g. Every 5 minutes, stand client, pat skin dry, run heated solution into sitz bath, check temperature, and assist client to sit in solution.

7. Cover compress or basin or wrap cover around client on sitz bath. Cover and technique to handle it should be clean or sterile as appropriate.

nurse alert   Aquathermia temperature should not exceed 105° F. Do not use pins with aquathermia.

8. Tape or tie in place.

9. **Apply soak to intact or open skin.**

a. Every 10 minutes, empty solution and replace with new.

b. Reimmerse area being treated.

10. Every 5 to 10 minutes, assess client for tolerance of treatment.

11. Remove treatment after 20 minutes or no more than 30 minutes.

12. See Completion Protocol (Chapter 1, p. 6).

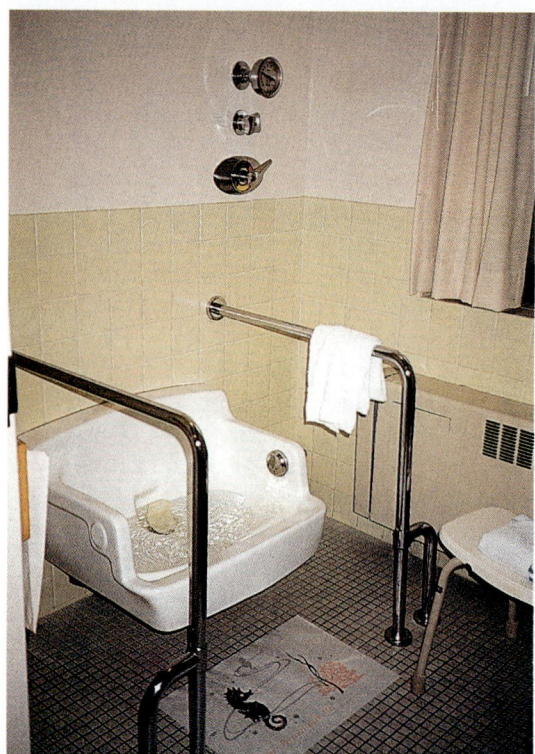

Figure 22-2

Evaluation

1. Ask client to report pain level 30 minutes after the treatment. Assess pain using a 0 to 10 scale.

2. Observe wound and/or skin, after multiple applications, for changes in redness, edema, size of impairment, and drainage.

3. Inspect client's skin after 30 minutes for intactness, redness, and blisters.

UNEXPECTED OUTCOMES AND NURSING INTERVENTIONS

1. Client reports increased pain level.

a. Ensure the proper temperature of solution.

b. Assess skin for impairment and report to physician.

2. Client's wound or skin impairment, after multiple applications, has increased redness, edema, size, and/or amount of drainage.

a. Report to physician.

b. In collaboration with other health team members, evaluate effectiveness of concurrent therapies and consider alternative treatments.

3. Client develops red, broken, and/or blistered skin.

a. Discontinue treatments and report to physician.

b. Reduce the temperature of treatments for clients more susceptible to temperature changes.

SAMPLE DOCUMENTATION

1000 Warm clean compress to left thigh for complaint of pain. Client states 7 on scale of 0 to 10. Skin intact, pink, no blisters. States feels touch of hand.

1030 Discontinued warm compress to left thigh. States pain 1 on scale of 0 to 10.

Skill 22.2 | **Dry Heat**

Dry heat can be applied directly to the skin with an aquathermia pad or a heating pad (Figure 22-3). It is important to protect the client from burns, skin dryness, and loss of body fluids through diaphoresis.

EQUIPMENT
Aquathermia pad
   Set to 43°-46° C (110°-115° F)
Heating pad
   Set to low or medium
Bath towel
Ties or tape

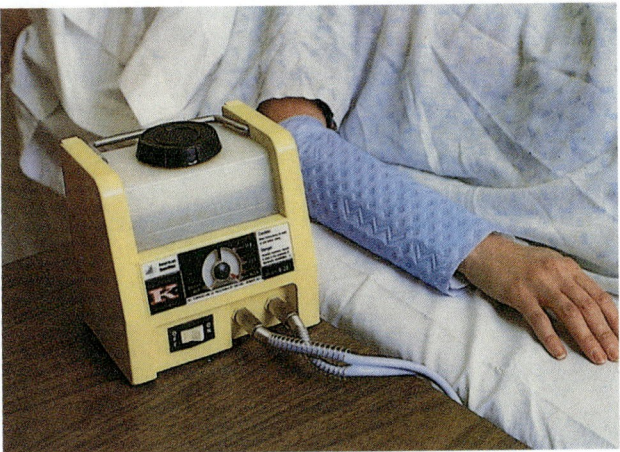

Figure 22-3

nurse alert Avoid using high setting on heating pad. Avoid placing heat source under any body part. Aquathermia pad should be placed on a table. Avoid using pins with heating pads or aquathermia. Avoid using heat treatments on clients who have elevated temperatures.

Assessment

1. Ask client to report level of pain on a scale of 0 to 10.
2. Assess range of motion (ROM) of client's body part.
3. Assess client's skin for intactness, color, temperature, sensitivity to touch, dryness, and any signs of underlying inflammation, including edema or redness.
4. Assess client's skin for blisters and excessive dryness.

Planning

Expected outcomes focus on comfort, improved mobility, and preventing burns.

EXPECTED OUTCOMES

1. Client reports decreased pain 30 minutes after the treatment.
2. Client is able to increase ROM of the body part 30 minutes after the treatment.
3. Client's skin remains intact.
4. Client's tissues are less red and edematous after treatments.

Implementation

Steps	Rationale
1. See Standard Protocol (Chapter 1, p. 5).	
2. Turn pad or aquathermia on.	
3. Apply aquathermia and cover area to be treated with bath towel.	Prevents burns by providing insulation between skin and pad.
4. Apply heating pad. If uncovered, cover with pillowcase.	
5. Place pad over area to be treated.	
6. Secure with ties or tape.	
7. Assess client's skin every 5 minutes for response to treatment.	
8. Remove treatment after 15 to 20 minutes.	
9. See Completion Protocol (Chapter 1, p. 6).	

Evaluation

1. Ask client to report pain level on a scale of 0 to 10. Ask again in 30 minutes.
2. Observe client's ROM to body part treated.
3. Inspect client's skin for intactness, any increased redness or temperature, blisters, dryness, and decreased sensitivity to touch, immediately and 30 minutes after the treatment.
4. After several treatments, observe client's tissues for redness and edema.

UNEXPECTED OUTCOMES AND RELATED INTERVENTIONS

1. Client reports increased pain and decreased ability to move the body part treated.
   a. Remove the treatment and examine client for burns and increased inflammation. Report to physician.
   b. Reduce temperatures for susceptible client.
   c. Check for proper function of equipment.

2. Client's skin is broken, red, dry, blistered, and insensitive to touch.
   a. Remove the treatment. Notify physician.
   b. In collaboration with other health team members, consider treatment for the problem.
3. Client's tissues become more red and edematous.
   a. Remove the treatment. Report to physician.
   b. In collaboration with other health team members, evaluate current therapies and consider new ones.

SAMPLE DOCUMENTATION

1000 Aquathermia at 110° F to right forearm IV infiltration site for complaint of pain level 5 on a scale of 0 to 10, edema 6.5 cm diameter. Area sensitive to touch, no redness noted.

1020 Aquathermia removed. Edema area 6.5 cm right forearm, slightly reddened, sensitive to touch.

1030 States pain level right forearm 2 on a scale of 0 to 10. Area of edema 4.5 cm diameter, sensitive to touch, no redness, blisters, broken areas.

Skill 22.3 | Cold Compresses and Ice Bags

Cold treatments are most therapeutic immediately after injury to tissues. For instance, a bruise can be arrested and the edema and pain of a sprain prevented most effectively if a cold treatment is applied right away.

Cold treatments can be delivered by means of a compress or an ice bag or pack. Most often, compresses are gauze pieces or towels soaked in cooled or iced solutions and placed on a body part. These compresses are usually clean. However, if the area to be treated has broken skin, sterile technique and supplies must be used. Ice bags and packs are a means of cooling tissues without moistening the skin. They are available in many shapes and sizes to mold to different parts of the body. Disposable bags and packs are available.

Care must be taken to prevent maceration and ischemia of the skin and tissues. Clients can become chilled during these treatments.

EQUIPMENT

Ice bag or pack
  Ice bag or pack
  Towel or pillowcase
  Cloth ties or tape
  Clean gloves if blood or body fluids are present
  Water and ice if needed
  Waterproof pad
Cold compress
  Gauze or towel
  Clean basin
  Prescribed solution at 15° C or 59° F

  Clean gloves if blood or body fluids are present
Bath towel or absorbent pad
Bath thermometer

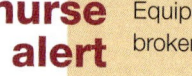 **nurse alert** Equipment must be sterile if skin is broken.

Assessment

1. Assess client's level of pain on a scale of 0 to 10.
2. Inspect the wound for bleeding and edema.
3. Inspect the surrounding tissues for color, temperature, intactness, and sensitivity to touch. Maintain the injured part in a state of immobilization and good alignment.

Planning

Expected outcomes center on decreased pain and bleeding while preventing tissue maceration and ischemia.

EXPECTED OUTCOMES

1. Client reports a decreased level of pain.
2. Client's wound has a minimal level of bleeding and edema after 30 minutes.
3. Client's surrounding tissues are slightly pale and cool.
4. Client's surrounding tissues remain intact.

Implementation

Steps	Rationale

1. See Standard Protocol (Chapter 1, p. 5)

2. Apply cold compress (Figure 22-4).
   a. Remove compress from freezer 5 to 10 minutes before use.

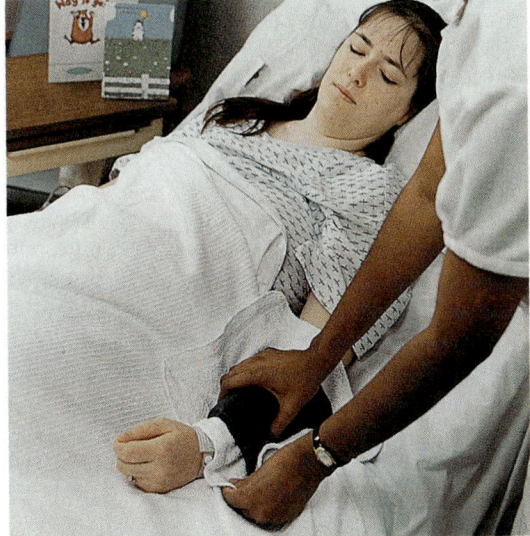

Figure 22-4

   b. Wrap in soft material (pillowcase or washcloth).
   c. Place compress on area to be treated.
   d. Cover with towel or absorbent pad.

Prevents ischemia by ensuring proper temperature.

3. Apply ice bag or pack.
   a. Fill bag with water, then empty.
   b. Fill bag two-thirds full with ice or pack.
   c. Express air from bag.
   d. Secure closure.
   e. Wipe bag dry.
   f. Cover bag with towel or pillowcase.
   g. Apply bag snugly over area.
4. Secure with ties or tape as needed.
5. Lift compress or bag to inspect condition of skin every 5 minutes.
6. Check condition of ice and refill bag or pack as needed. Can be done when checking condition of skin every 5 minutes.
7. Remove treatment after 20 to 30 minutes.

8. Apply electrically controlled cooling device.
   a. Wrap cool water flow pad around body part (Figure 22-5).
   b. Make sure all connections are intact and temperature is set. (See agency policy or physician's order.)
   c. Instruct client to call if unable to tolerate cold sensation.
9. See Completion Protocol (Chapter 1, p. 6).

Prevents maceration by testing for leaks

Prevents maceration and ischemia by keeping moisture and cold off skin.

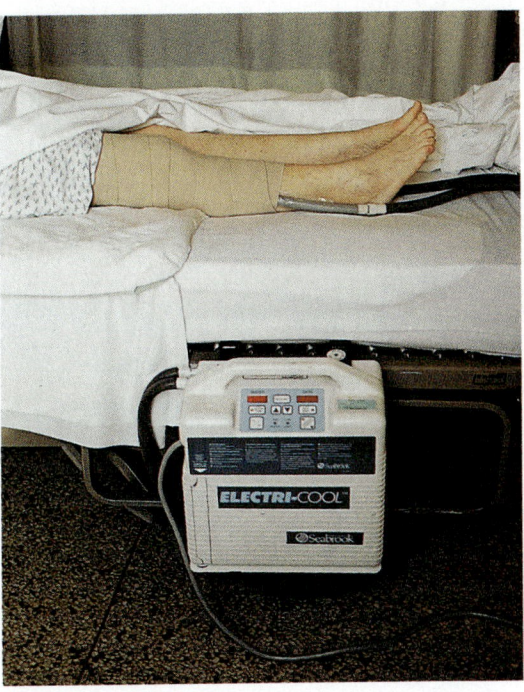

Figure 22-5

Evaluation

1. Ask client to report pain level on a scale of 0 to 10.
2. Inspect wound for bleeding and edema immediately. Inspect again after 30 minutes.
3. Palpate surrounding tissues for excessive pallor, coldness, breaks or maceration, and sensitivity to touch immediately. Reevaluate in 30 minutes.

UNEXPECTED OUTCOMES AND NURSING INTERVENTIONS

1. Client reports increased pain, and there is increased bleeding and edema immediately or after 30 minutes.
   a. Remove treatment. Apply pressure for bleeding.
   b. Report to physician.
2. Immediately after treatment or 30 minutes later, the surrounding tissues are paler (even blue), colder, with skin breaks and decreased sensitivity to touch.
   a. Discontinue treatment.
   b. Report to physician if symptoms persist for 30 minutes.

SAMPLE DOCUMENTATION

0900 Ice bag to right ankle measuring 27 cm at level of medial and lateral malleolus. States pain 3 on a scale of 0 to 10, redness extending 1 cm around site, no bleeding noted. Surrounding tissues pink, warm, intact. States feels touch of hand.

0930 Ice bag removed from right ankle. Surrounding tissues pale, cool. States feels touch of hand.

1000 Right ankle measuring 26 cm at level of medial and lateral malleolus. No bleeding, redness noted. Surrounding tissues pink, warm, intact. States feels touch of hand.

CRITICAL THINKING EXERCISES

1. As the nurse caring for the following clients, how would you respond in each case?
   a. Jorge is being treated with warm, moist compresses for a back injury that resulted in a muscle strain. After the placement of the compress on Jorge's back he flinches and complains that the compress is stinging.
   b. Ellen has a deep vein thrombosis in her left lower leg, to which an aquathermia pad has been applied. When repositioning the pad you note that she has turned up the temperature to 108° F and has pinned the pad in place to prevent it from slipping off her leg.
   c. Mrs. Chinn is ordered to have sitz baths four times each day following rectal surgery.
2. Should heat or cold treatment be used for each of the following clients?
   a. Maria just sprained her ankle when she got out of her car.
   b. Harry's IV site is pale and cold from an infiltrated IV.
   c. Ruby's joints are painful from rheumatoid arthritis.
   d. Lucinda's injection site is swollen and red.
   e. Mr. Lau is suffering from low back pain.
3. Tia is being treated with ice compresses to her leg until her fracture can be surgically repaired.
   a. What is the rationale for this treatment?
   b. For what reasons would you remove the ice compresses, other than for assessment purposes?
   c. What precautions should you take to prevent Tia from developing a cold burn?

REFERENCES

McConnell EA: Using an aquathermia pad safely, *Nursing '91* 21(12):72, 1991.

McConnell EA: Giving your patient a sitz bath, *Nursing '93* 23(12), 1993.

ADDITIONAL READINGS

Bayles FH: Heat and cold injury guide, *Health You* 7(1):34, 1991.

McConnell EA: Clinical do's and don't's: how to apply an ice bag, ice collar, or ice glove, *Nursing '92* 22(7):18, 1992.

Nanneman D: Thermal modalities: heat and cold. A review of physiologic effects with clinical applications, *Am Assoc Occupat Health Nurs* 39(2):70, 1991.

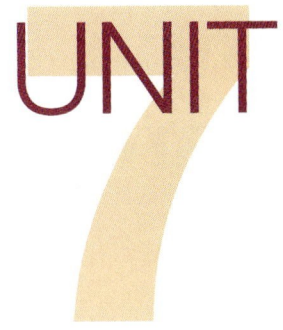

UNIT 7

Managing Immobilized Clients

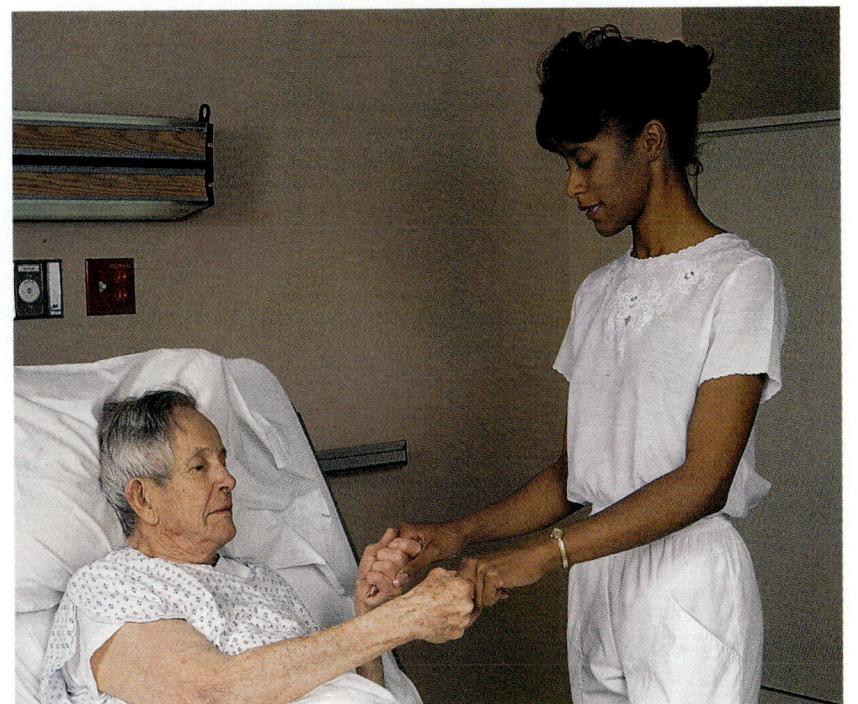

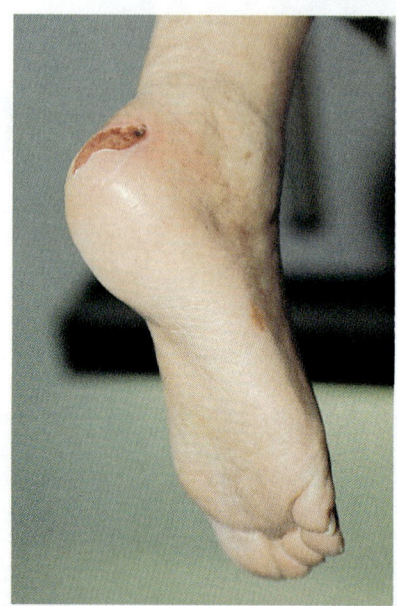

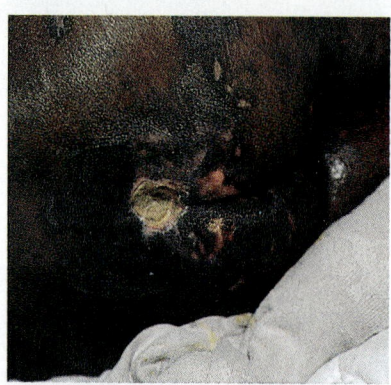

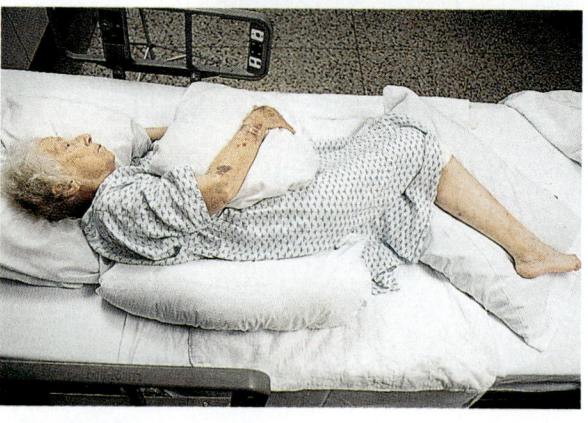

chapter 23

Pressure Ulcer Care

Skill 23.1
Risk Assessment and Prevention Strategies

Skill 23.2
Cleaning and Topical Applications

Pressure ulcers are defined as "localized areas of tissue necrosis that develop when soft tissue is compressed between a bony prominence and an external surface for a prolonged period of time" (National Pressure Ulcer Advisory Panel [NPUAP], 1989). Formerly called decubitus ulcers (from the Latin meaning "to lay down"), it is now known that these ulcers develop when clients are in positions other than bed rest. Pressure ulcers can occur when clients are in the sitting position. Pressure points over bony prominences where pressure ulcers develop in sitting and lying positions are shown in Figures 23-1 and 23-2. Some of the most common sites are the sacrum, heels, elbow, lateral malleoli, greater trochanters, and ischial tuberosities (Meehan, 1994). Three elements are the cornerstone of pressure ulcer development (1) intensity of pressure (Landis, 1930; capillary closing pressure 32), (2) duration of pressure (Koziak, 1959; sustained pressure), and (3) tissue tolerance (Husain, 1953; Trumble, 1930). Many risk factors such as friction, shear, poor nutrition, altered sensory perception, incontinence, and moisture have been proposed (Bergstrom, Demuth, and Braden, 1987). Using the web of causation, Oot-Giromini (1993) recently proposed a new conceptual framework to view pressure ulcers. This model (Figure 23-3) involves the concept of synergism where the whole is greater than the sum of its parts. This model also considers personal wellness (e.g., activities of daily living, medical diagnosis, coping abilities, attitudes, desire to participate in health regimens) and socioeconomic variables (e.g., living conditions, income, support systems, ability to purchase needed supplies, knowledge of care givers, availability and affordability of help outside the home, rural or urban setting, personal value systems). The complex interrelationship among the multiple factors rather than the individual factors is emphasized.

Pressure ulcers are an important health concern.

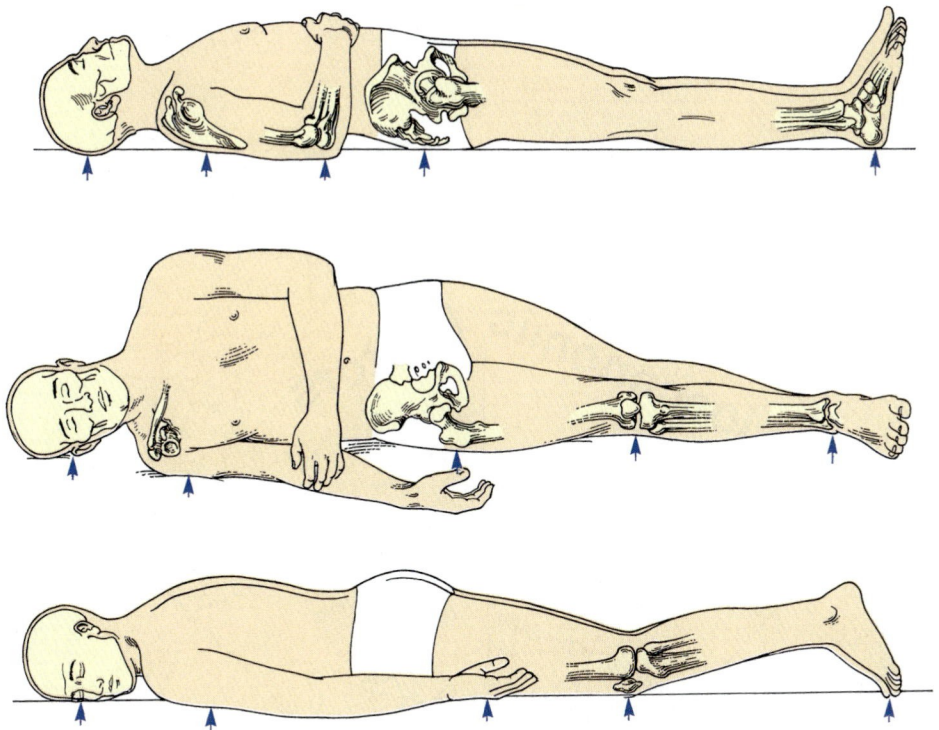

Figure 23-1 Pressure points in lying positions.

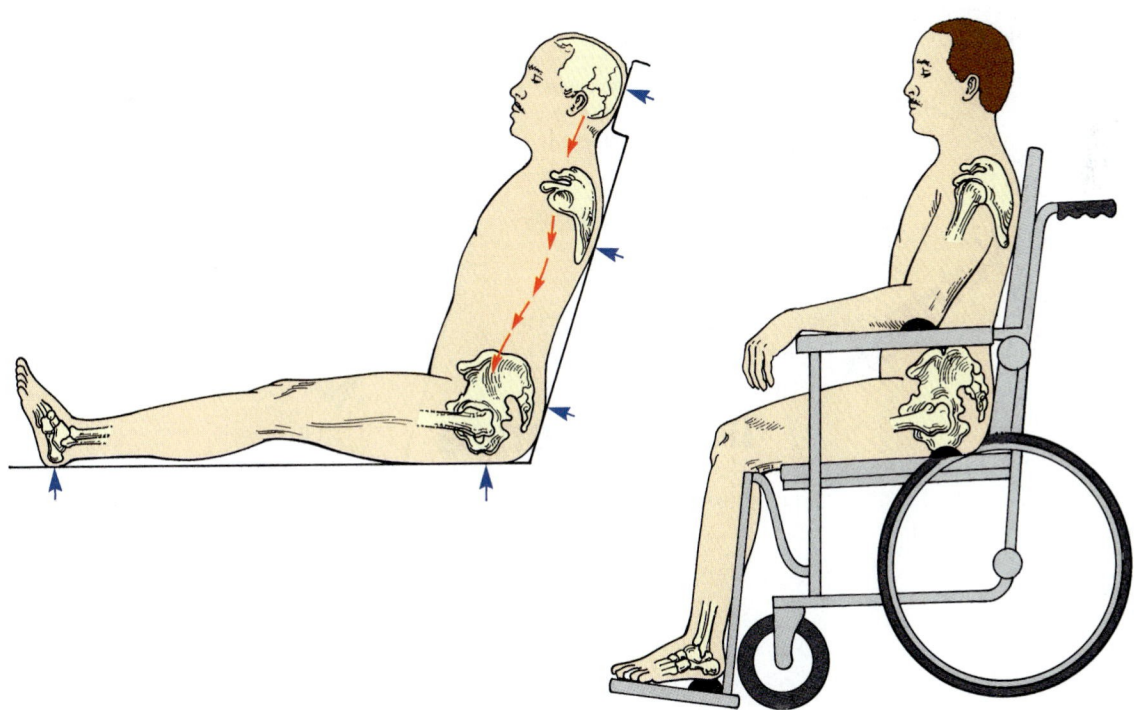

Figure 23-2 Pressure points in sitting positions.

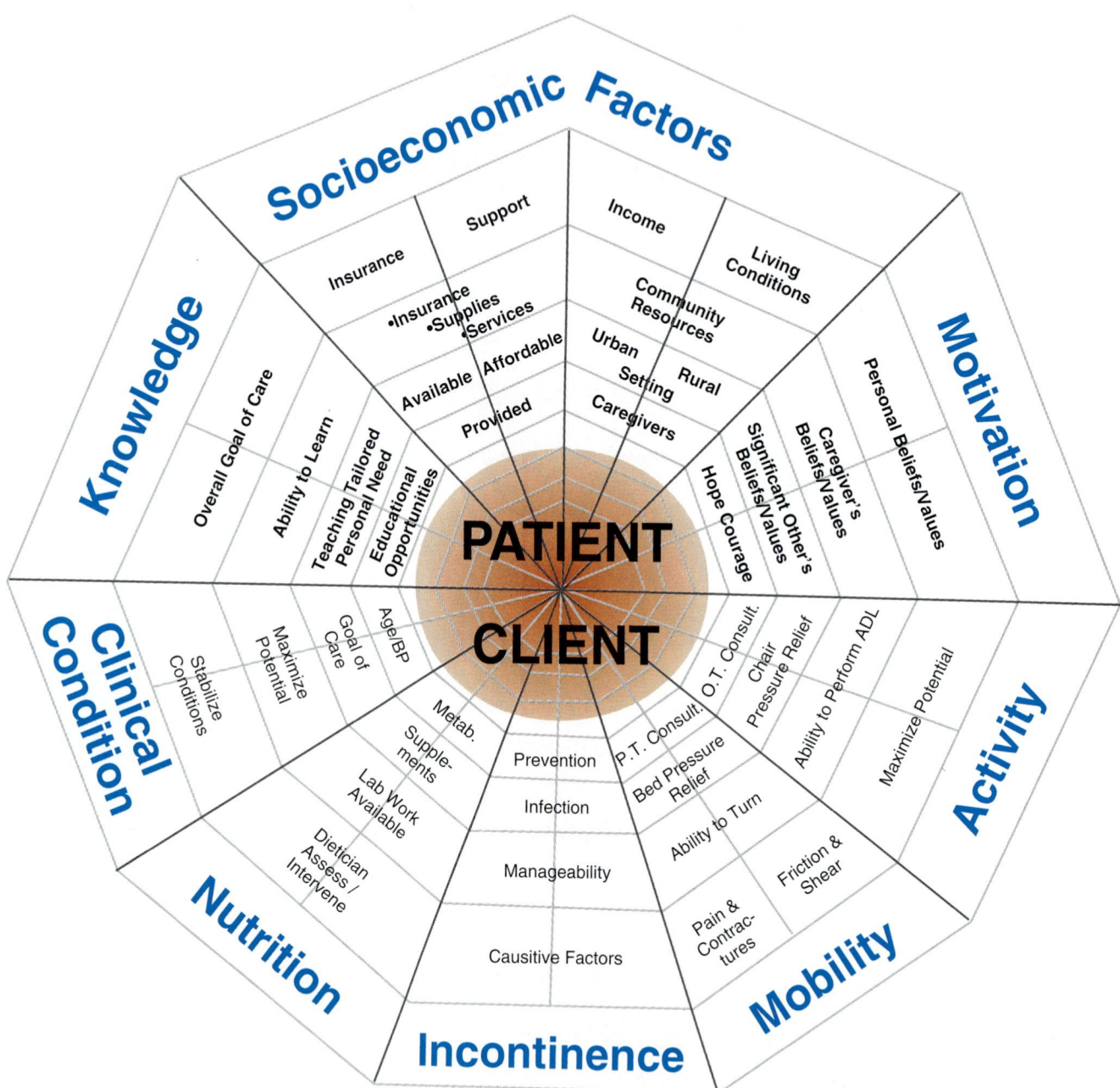

Figure 23-3 Web of causation for pressure ulcers. (©1992 Barbara Oot-Giromini. Reprinted with permission.)

Prevalence rates vary among various client settings, hospital care, and long-term care and have been reported between 3% and 23% (Allman, 1989; Langemo et al., 1989; Leshem and Skelskey, 1994; McKnight's Survey, 1992; Meehan 1994). Prevalence rate in the home care setting is reported at 19% (Hanson et al., 1993). Research has shown that treatment costs for pressure ulcers is 2.5 times greater than prevention costs (Oot-Giromini et al., 1989). Every effort must be made to identify clients at risk for pressure ulcers and prevent their occurrence.

Nursing Diagnosis

Nursing diagnoses that are associated with prevention of pressure ulcers include **Risk for Impaired Skin Integrity,** such as clients on prolonged bed rest. **Impaired Skin Integrity** related to physical immobilization and/or altered circulation is appropriate for clients who have skin breakdown. Related nursing diagnoses using the web of causation model might include **Impaired Physical Mobility** associated with pain; decreased strength and endurance; prolonged bed rest or external devices such as casts, splints, braces, or tubing; **Incontinence; Altered Nutrition: Less than Body Requirements; Altered Peripheral Tissue Perfusion; Altered Body Temperature;** and **Hyperthermia.**

Skill 23.1 | Risk Assessment and Prevention Strategies

Pressure ulcer risk assessment should be done systematically (Agency for Health Care Policy and Research [AHCPR], 1992; NPUAP, 1990). An assessment tool that is validated for a specific type of client population is recommended. There are several published pressure ulcer risk assessment tools, including the Norton scale, Gosnell scale, and Braden scale (Tables 23-1 to 23-3, pp. 420 to 424). Each tool identifies risk factors (five to eight items) that are ranked with a number. The client's risk assessment score is obtained by adding the individual number given for each risk factor. Interpretation of the meaning of the numerical score differs with each scale. A low score on the Braden or Norton scales indicates a client at high risk for skin breakdown. A high numerical score on the Gosnell scale indicates high risk for skin breakdown. Therefore, it is important to always identify which risk assessment scale is being used when reporting a risk assessment score. Once a client is identified to be at risk for developing pressure ulcers, prevention strategies proposed by AHCPR (1992) and summarized by NPUAP (1992) in pressure points should be implemented (see box on pp. 424 to 425). Further information about these two Panels can be obtained by contacting them (see box on p. 425).

EQUIPMENT
Risk assessment tool
Client's documentation record
AHCPR booklet: *Preventing Pressure Ulcers: A Patient's Guide*

Assessment

1. Select which pressure ulcer risk assessment tool will be used in your client setting (see Tables 23-1 to 23-3). **A validated risk assessment tool is recommended by AHCPR and NPUAP.**

2. Identify client's risk for pressure ulcer formation by assessing the factors for each client according to the selected tool. This information will yield a risk assessment score. Compare the obtained score for client with the established scores that indicate high risk for skin breakdown with the selected risk assessment tool. **"To prevent pressure ulcers, individuals at risk must be identified so that risk factors can be reduced through intervention"** (AHCPR, 1992a).

3. Assess condition of client's skin, especially over areas at high risk for breakdown such as bony prominences. Indicators other than color, such as temperature, "orange peel" pore appearance, firmness or tightness, and hardness, may be helpful in early assessment of clients with dark skin (Graves, 1990; Maklebust and Sieggreen, 1991). **"Skin inspection is fundamental to any plan for preventing pressure ulcers"** (AHCPR, 1992a).

4. Assess client's and support person's understanding of risks for pressure ulcers and knowledge of skin care. **"Patient and family are integral to prevention and management of pressure ulcers"** (AHCPR, 1992a).

Planning

Expected outcomes focus on identifying clients at risk for skin breakdown and beginning nursing actions to prevent skin breakdown.

EXPECTED OUTCOMES
1. Client's skin remains intact.
2. Client cooperates with mobility/range of motion activities.
3. Client achieves adequate nutritional status.
4. Client and/or support person can state strategies to prevent skin breakdown.

Implementation

Steps	Rationale

1. See Standard Protocol (Chapter 1, p. 5).
2. Inspect once a day.

"Skin inspection provides the information essential for designing interventions to reduce risk and for evaluating the outcomes of those interventions" (AHCPR, 1992).

3. Cleanse skin with warm water and a mild cleansing agent.

Hot water and soap can dry and irritate the skin.

4. Apply moisturizers after bathing and do not massage reddened bony prominences (AHCPR, 1992; Olson, 1989.

Prevents drying of skin. Massage may lead to tissue trauma.

5. Maintain adequate humidity in environment.

Environmental factors, such as low humidity (less than 40%), can dry the skin.

6. Manage incontinence (see Skill 8.2).

Skin exposed to moisture from incontinence is more susceptible to injury (Table 23-4, p. 426, lists interventions designed to reduce the risk of pressure ulcer development resulting from tube-feeding–related diarrhea).

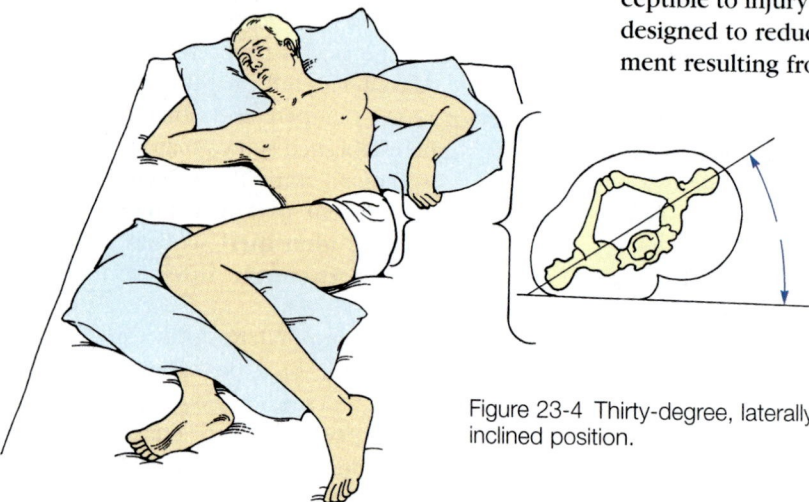

Figure 23-4 Thirty-degree, laterally inclined position.

7. Turn and reposition: (AHCPR, 1992).
   a. Perform full position changes every 2 hours.

Prolonged, unrelieved pressure on an area can lead to skin breakdown (Knox et al., 1994).

   b. Use 30-degree lateral position (Figure 23-4) rather than side-lying position directly on the trochanter.

Higher pressures when positioned directly on the trochanters can lead to their breakdown.

   c. Perform small shift of body weight changes every 15 minutes.

Relief of pressure is needed at shorter intervals to prevent tissue breakdown, especially for clients in the sitting position.

   d. When needed, use pillow bridging (Figure 23-5).

Use of pillows will prevent direct contact between bony prominences.

8. Keep head of bed at less than 30 degrees, except as required for care (e.g., feeding).

Limiting the amount of time that the head of the bed is elevated will reduce tissue injury from shearing forces.

9. Use protective devices and support surfaces (see Chapter 24).

Pressure-reducing devices can decrease the incidence and severity of pressure ulcers. (Flemister, 1991; Johnson et al., 1991; Lazzara and Buschmann, 1991).

10. Encourage range of motion and ambulation (see Chapters 25 and 28).

Improving mobility and activity levels can reduce risk of pressure ulcers.

11. Evaluate client's nutritional status (see Chapter 7) (Kaminski et al., 1989). Nutritional assessment of clients with a pressure ulcer includes review of

"Assessment of nutritional intake and nutritional support is suggested to maintain skin integrity and prevent pressure ulcers" (AHCPR, 1992a, p. 21). Malnutrition is

| Steps | Rationale |

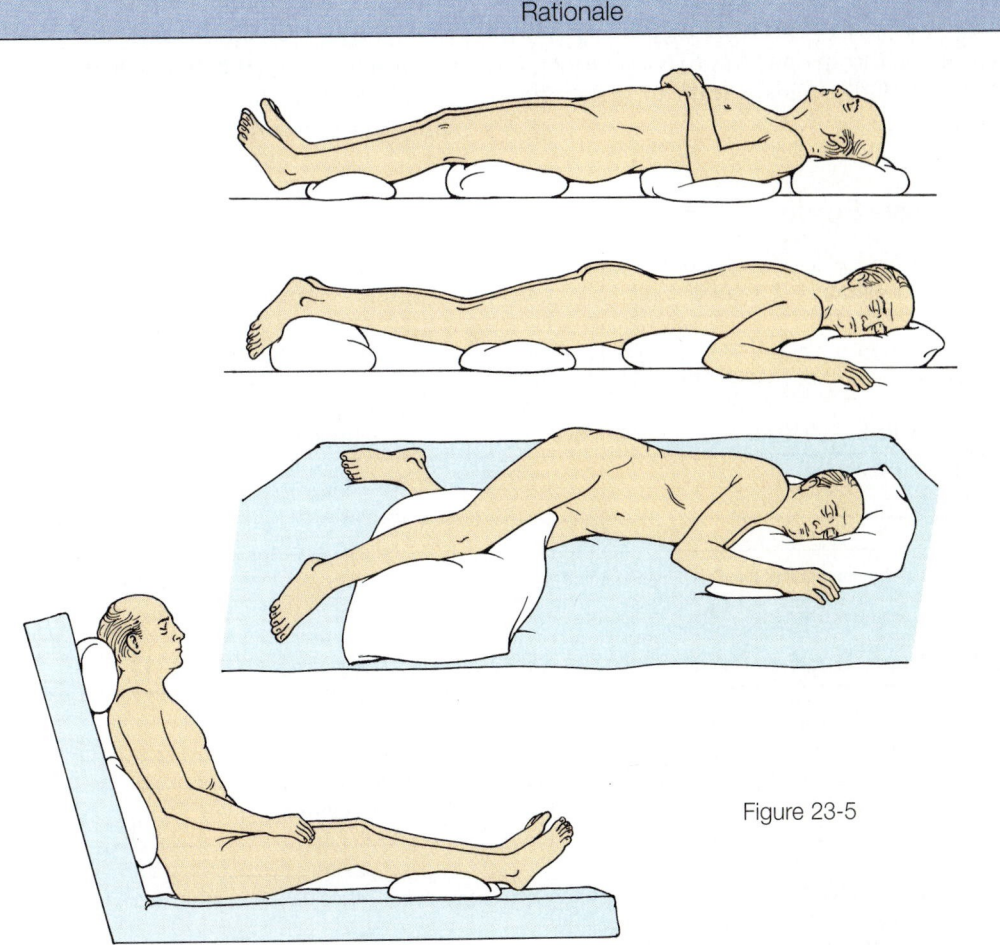

Figure 23-5

weight pattern and serum albumin and total lymphocyte laboratory values. Clinically significant malnutrition is present if serum albumin is less than 3.5 mg/dl, total lymphocyte count less than 1800 mm³, or weight loss greater than 15%. This should be done at least every 3 months. Also observe the mouth and skin for signs of vitamin or mineral deficiencies (see box on p. 426).

12. Provide patient and support person education about pressure ulcer risk and prevention (Maklebust and Magnan, 1992). Use of the AHCPR booklet *Preventing Pressure Ulcers: A Patient's Guide* (AHCPR, 1992b) can be a helpful teaching tool (Ayello, 1993) (Table 23-5, p. 427).

13. See Completion Protocol (Chapter 1, p. 6).

a risk factor for formation of pressure ulcers. Stage of pressure ulcer correlates with serum albumin levels (Bergstrom et al., 1994).

"Effective pressure ulcer prevention depends on the coordinated efforts of health care professionals in hospital settings and continued implementation of preventive interventions by family and the patient in the home" (AHCPR, 1992b).

Evaluation

1. Inspect skin over pressure areas for signs of skin breakdown.
2. Monitor client's level of mobility.
3. Monitor client's nutritional status.
4. Ask client or significant other to state prevention strategies.

UNEXPECTED OUTCOME AND RELATED INTERVENTIONS

Client's risk of skin breakdown increases.

Consider increasing the frequency of turning schedules. Reevaluate currently used pressure-relieving products for additional changes needed because of client's increasing risk of skin breakdown. Consider a consultation with a specialist in the care of pressure ulcers, such as a certified enterostomal therapy nurse (CETN). Consider a meeting with the multidisciplinary team to revise the client plan of care.

SAMPLE DOCUMENTATION

1500 Norton risk assessment scale done on admission. Client score = 12, therefore client is at high risk for skin breakdown. Client inspection reveals intact skin. Pressure ulcer prevention points protocol implemented.

Table 23-1 **Norton Scale**

Name	Date	Physical condition		Mental condition		Activity		Mobility		Incontinent		Total score
		Good	4	Alert	4	Ambulant	4	Full	4	Not	4	
		Fair	3	Apathetic	3	Walk/help	3	Slightly limited	3	Occasional	3	
		Poor	2	Confused	2	Chairbound	2	Very limited	2	Usually/urine	2	
		Very Bad	1	Stupor	1	Bed	1	Immobile	1	Doubly	1	

Modified from Centre for policy on ageing, London, England. Used with permission.

Table 23-2 **Gosnell Scale: Pressure Sore Risk Assessment (Part 1)**

I.D. _____

Age _____ Sex _____

Height _____ Weight _____

Date of Admission _____

Date of Discharge _____

Medical Diagnosis:

  Primary _____

  Secondary _____

Nursing Diagnosis:

_____

Instructions: Complete all categories within 24 hours of admission and every other day thereafter. Refer to the accompanying guidelines for specific rating details.

DATE	Mental status*	Continence*	Mobility*	Activity*	Nutrition*	Total score
	1. Alert 2. Apathetic 3. Confused 4. Stuporous 5. Unconscious	1. Fully Controlled 2. Usually Controlled 3. Minimally Controlled 4. Absence of Control	1. Full 2. Slightly Limited 3. Very Limited 4. Immobile	1. Ambulatory 2. Walks with Assistance 3. Chairfast 4. Bedfast	1. Good 2. Fair 3. Poor	

PRESSURE SORE RISK ASSESSMENT MEDICATION PROFILE

Medication	Dosage	†Frequency	Route	Date Begun	Date Discon.

*See Part 3, p. 422, for guidelines for rating.

†If PRN, record pattern past 48 hours.

Table 23-2 **Gosnell Scale: Pressure Sore Risk Assessment—cont'd (Part 2)**

	Vital Signs				Diet	24-Hour Fluid Balance		Color 1. Pallor 2. Mottled 3. Pink 4. Ashen 5. Ruddy 6. Cyanotic 7. Jaundice 8. Other	General skin appearance			Interventions		
									Moisture 1. Dry 2. Damp 3. Oily 4. Other	Temperature 1. Cold 2. Cool 3. Warm 4. Hot	Texture 1. Smooth 2. Rough 3. Thin/Transp 4. Scaly 5. Crusty 6. Other			
Date	T	P	R	BP	Diet	Intake	Output					No	Yes	Describe

Vital signs: The temperature, pulse, respiration, and blood pressure to be taken and recorded at the time of every assessment rating.

Skin appearance: A description of observed skin characteristics: color, moisture, temperature, and texture.

Diet: Record the specific diet order.

24-hour fluid balance: The amount of fluid intake and output during the previous 24-hour period should be recorded.

Interventions: List all devices, measures, and/or nursing care activity being used for the purpose of pressure sore prevention.

Medications: List name, dosage, frequency, and route for all prescribed medications. If a PRN order, list the pattern for the period since last assessment.

Comments: Use this space to add explanation or further detail regarding any of the previously recorded data, patient condition, etc.

   or

   Describe anything that you believe to be of importance but not accounted for previously.

NOTE: For any item marked "other," please describe.

If any signs of pressure, etc., on bony prominences or other body parts are observed, please describe in detail the location, color, temperature, moisture, texture, and size and any other pertinent items.

Continued.

Used with permission of Davina Gosnell, RN, PhD.

Table 23-2 Gosnell Scale: Pressure Sore Risk Assessment—cont'd (Part 3)

GUIDELINES FOR NUMERICAL RATING OF THE DEFINED CATEGORIES

Rating	1	2	3	4	5
MENTAL STATUS An assessment of one's level of response to the environment.	**ALERT** Oriented to time, place, and person. Responsive to all stimuli and understands explanations.	**APATHETIC** Lethargic, forgetful, drowsy, passive, and dull. Sluggish, depressed. Able to obey simple commands. Possibly disoriented to time.	**CONFUSED** Partial and/or intermittent disorientation to TPP. Purposeless response to stimuli. Restless, aggressive, irritable, anxious, and may require tranquilizers or sedatives.	**STUPOROUS** Total disorientation. Does not respond to name, simple commands, or verbal stimuli.	**UNCONSCIOUS** Nonresponsive to painful stimuli.
CONTINENCE The amount of bodily control of urination and defecation.	**FULLY CONTROLLED** Total control of urine and feces.	**USUALLY CONTROLLED** Incontinent of urine and/or of feces not more often than once every 48 hours or has Foley catheter and is incontinent of feces.	**MINIMALLY CONTROLLED** Incontinent of urine or feces at least once every 24 hours.	**ABSENCE OF CONTROL** Consistently incontinent of both urine and feces.	
MOBILITY The amount and control of movement of one's body.	**FULL** Able to control and move all extremities at will. May require the use of a device but turns, lifts, pulls, balances, and attains sitting position at will.	**SLIGHTLY LIMITED** Able to control and move all extremities but a degree of limitation is present. Requires assistance of another person to turn, pull, balance, and/or attain a sitting position at will but self-initiates movement or requests for help to move.	**VERY LIMITED** Can assist another person, who must initiate movement via turning, lifting, pulling, balancing and/or attaining a sitting position (contractures, paralysis may be present).	**IMMOBILE** Does not assist self in any way to change position. Is unable to change position without assistance. Is completely dependent on others for movement.	
ACTIVITY The ability of an individual to ambulate.	**AMBULATORY** Is able to walk unassisted. Rises from bed unassisted. With the use of a device such as cane or walker is able to ambulate without the assistance of another person.	**WALKS WITH HELP** Able to ambulate with assistance of another person, braces, or crutches. May have limitation of stairs.	**CHAIRFAST** Ambulates only to a chair, requires assistance to do so or is confined to a wheelchair.	**BEDFAST** Is confined to bed during entire 24 hours of the day.	
NUTRITION The process of food intake.	Eats some food from each basic food category every day and the majority of each meal served or is on tube feeding.	Occasionally refuses a meal or frequently leaves at least half of a meal.	Seldom eats a complete meal and only a few bites of food at a meal.		

Table 23-3 **Braden Scale For Predicting Pressure Sore Risk**

Patient's Name ———————————— Evaluator's Name ———————————— Date of Assessment

SENSORY PERCEPTION Ability to respond meaningfully to pressure-related discomfort	1. Completely Limited Unresponsive (does not moan, flinch, or grasp) to painful stimuli due to diminished level of consciousness or sedation. OR Limited ability to feel pain over most of body surface.	2. Very Limited Responds only to painful stimuli. Cannot communicate discomfort except by moaning or restlessness. OR Has a sensory impairment which limits the ability to feel pain or discomfort over 1/2 of body.	3. Slightly Limited Responds to verbal commands, but cannot always communicate discomfort or need to be turned. OR Has some sensory impairment that limits ability to feel pain or discomfort in 1 or 2 extremities.	4. No Impairment Responds to verbal commands. Has no sensory deficit that would limit ability to feel or voice pain or discomfort.	
MOISTURE Degree to which skin is exposed to moisture	1. Constantly Moist Skin is kept moist almost constantly by perspiration, urine, etc. Dampness is detected every time patient is moved or turned.	2. Very Moist Skin is often, but not always, moist. Linen must be changed at least once a shift.	3. Occasionally Moist Skin is occasionally moist, requiring an extra linen change approximately once a day.	4. Rarely Moist Skin is usually dry, linen only requires changing at routine intervals.	
ACTIVITY Degree of physical activity	1. Bedfast Confined to bed.	2. Chairfast Ability to walk severely limited or nonexistent. Cannot bear own weight and/or must be assisted into chair or wheelchair.	3. Walks Occasionally Walks occasionally during day, but for very short distances, with or without assistance. Spends majority of each shift in bed or chair.	4. Walks Frequently Walks outside the room at least twice a day and inside room at least once every 2 hours during waking hours.	
MOBILITY Ability to change and control body position	1. Completely Immobile Does not make even slight changes in body or extremity position without assistance.	2. Very Limited Makes occasional slight changes in body or extremity position but unable to make frequent or significant changes independently.	3. Slightly Limited Makes frequent though slight changes in body or extremity position independently.	4. No Limitations Makes major and frequent changes in position without assistance.	

Continued.

Table 23-3 **Braden Scale For Predicting Pressure Sore Risk—cont'd**

Patient's Name _____ Evaluator's Name _____ Date of Assessment [ ]

NUTRITION *Usual* food intake pattern	1. Very Poor Never eats a complete meal. Rarely eats more than 1/3 of any food offered. Eats 2 servings or less of protein (meat or dairy products) per day. Takes fluids poorly. Does not take a liquid dietary supplement. OR Is NPO and/or maintained on clear liquids or IVs for more than 5 days.	2. Probably Inadequate Rarely eats a complete meal and generally eats only about 1/2 of any food offered. Protein intake includes only 3 servings of meat or dairy products per day. Occasionally will take a dietary supplement. OR Receives less than optimum amount of liquid diet or tube feeding.	3. Adequate Eats over half of most meals. Eats a total of 4 servings of protein (meat, dairy products) each day. Occasionally will refuse a meal, but will usually take a supplement if offered. OR Is on a tube feeding or TPN regimen that probably meets most of nutritional needs.	4. Excellent Eats most of every meal. Never refuses a meal. Usually eats a total of 4 or more servings of meat and dairy products. Occasionally eats between meals. Does not require supplementation.
FRICTION AND SHEAR	1. Problem Requires moderate to maximum assistance in moving. Complete lifting without sliding against sheets is impossible. Frequently slides down in bed or chair, requiring frequent repositioning with maximum assistance. Spasticity, contractures, or agitation leads to almost constant friction.	2. Potential Problem Moves feebly or requires minimum assistance. During a move skin probably slides to some extent against sheets, chair, restraints, or other devices. Maintains relatively good position in chair or bed most of the time but occasionally slides down.	3. No Apparent Problem Moves in bed and in chair independently and has sufficient muscle strength to lift up completely during move. Maintains good position in bed or chair at all times.	

©1988 Barbara Braden and Nancy Bergstrom. Used with permission.   Total Score [ ]

Pressure Ulcer Prevention Points

I. Risk assessment
1. Consider all bed-bound or chair-bound persons, or those whose ability to reposition is impaired, to be at risk for pressure ulcers.
2. Select and use a method of risk assessment, such as the Norton Scale or the Braden Scale, that ensures systematic evaluation of individual risk factors.
3. Assess all at-risk patients at the time of admission to health care facilities and at regular intervals thereafter.
4. Identify all individual risk factors (decreased mental status, moisture, incontinence, nutritional deficits) to

direct specific preventive treatments. Modify care according to the individual factors.

II. Skin care and early treatment
1. Inspect the skin at least daily, and document assessment results.
2. Individualize bathing frequency. Use a mild cleansing agent. Avoid hot water and excessive friction.
3. Assess and treat incontinence. When incontinence cannot be controlled, cleanse skin at time of soiling, use a topical moisture barrier, and select underpads or briefs that are absorbent and provide a quick drying surface to the skin.

National Pressure Ulcer Advisory Panel (NPUAP), 1989.

Pressure Ulcer Prevention Points—cont'd

4. Use moisturizers for dry skin. Minimize environmental factors leading to dry skin such as low humidity and cold air.
5. Avoid massage over bony prominences.
6. Use proper positioning, transferring, and turning techniques to minimize skin injury caused by friction and shear forces.
7. Use dry lubricants (cornstarch) or protective coverings to reduce friction injury.
8. Identify and correct factors compromising protein/calorie intake, and consider nutritional supplementation/support for nutritionally compromised persons.
9. Institute a rehabilitation program to maintain or improve mobility/activity status.
10. Monitor and document interventions and outcomes.

III. Mechanical loading and support surfaces
1. Reposition bed-bound persons at least every 2 hours, chair-bound persons every hour.
2. Use a written repositioning schedule.
3. Place at-risk persons on a pressure-reducing mattress/chair cushion. Do not use donut-type devices.
4. Consider postural alignment, distribution of weight, balance and stability, and pressure relief when positioning persons in chairs or wheelchairs.
5. Teach chair-bound persons, who are able, to shift weight every 15 minutes.
6. Use lifting device (e.g., trapeze or bed linen) to move rather than drag persons during transfer and position changes.

7. Use pillows or foam wedges to keep bony prominences such as knees and ankles from direct contact with each other.
8. Use devices that totally relieve pressure on the heels (e.g., place pillows under the calf to raise the heels off the bed).
9. Avoid positioning directly on the trochanter when using the side-lying position (use the 30-degree lateral inclined position).
10. Elevate the head of the bed as little (maximum 30-degree angle) and for as short a time as possible.

IV. Education
1. Implement educational programs for the prevention of pressure ulcers that are structured, organized, comprehensive, and directed at all levels of health care providers, patients, family, and care givers.
2. Include information on:
   a. Etiology of and risk factors for pressure ulcers
   b. Risk assessment tools and their application
   c. Skin assessment
   d. Selection/use of support surfaces
   e. Development/implementation of individualized programs of skin care
   f. Demonstration of positioning to decrease risk of tissue breakdown
   g. Accurate documentation of pertinent data
3. Include built-in mechanisms to evaluate program effectiveness in preventing pressure ulcers.

Pressure Ulcer Resources

Agency for Health Care Policy and Research (AHCPR)
Publications Clearinghouse
PO Box 8547
Silver Springs, MD 20907
1 800 358 9295

"The Agency for Health Care Policy and Research (AHCPR) was established in December 1989 under Public law 101-238 (Omnibus Budget Reconciliation Act of 1989) to enhance the quality, appropriateness, and effectiveness of health care services and access to these services. AHCPR carries out its mission by conducting and supporting general health services research, including medical effectiveness research, facilitating development of clinical practice guidelines, and disseminating research findings and guidelines to health care providers, policy makers, and the public.

"The legislation also established within AHCPR the Office of the Forum of Quality and Effectiveness in Health Care (the Forum). The Forum has primary responsibility for facilitating the development, periodic review, and updating of clinical practice guidelines. The guidelines will assist practitioners in the prevention, diagnosis, treatment, and management of clinical conditions."

Copies of the clinical guidelines and patient guides are available free of charge from them.

National Pressure Ulcer Advisory Panel (NPUAP)
SUNY at Buffalo
Beck Hall
3435 Main Street
Buffalo, NY 14214
716 881 3558

"The National Pressure Ulcer Advisory Panel (NPUAP) is an independent, not-for-profit organization that provides multi-disciplinary leadership for improved outcomes in pressure ulcer prevention and management through education, legislation and research. Formed in 1987, the NPUAP is comprised of fifteen leading authorities on pressure ulcer prevention and management."

Copies of Pressure Ulcer Prevention points printed on a buff card suitable for posting on a nursing unit are available free of charge from them.

Table 23-4 **Measures to Reduce Risk of Pressure Ulcers: Practical Management of Loose Bowel Movements Related to Tube Feeding***

Possible cause(s)	Treatment
Antibiotic use	Lactobacilli per feeding tube (2 packets tid $\times$ 3 doses)
Lactose intolerance	Use lactose-free liquid diet
Choleretic diarrhea	Questran, 1 g q6–8h and/or
	Titralac tabs, 2 q6–8h
Mild enterotoxigenic pathogens	Pepto-Bismol, 30 ml q6–8h
Severe enterotoxigenic pathogens with WBCs in stool-on Gram stain	Selected antibiotic per stool culture and sensitivity testing
Insufficient fiber	Fiber supplement, 3 g q6–8h
Idiopathic	Lomotil, Imodium, paregoric (Warning: This may cause reactive constipation.)

From Bergstrom N et al: *Treatment of pressure ulcers,* AHCPR pub no 95-0652, Rockville, Md, 1994, DHHS, PHS, AHCPR.
*Any or all treatments may be indicated. tid, Three times daily; q, every; h, hours; WBCs, white blood cells.

Sample Nutritional Assessment Guide for Patients With Pressure Ulcers

Patient Name: _____ Date: _____ Time: _____

To be filled out for all patients at risk on initial evaluation and every 12 weeks thereafter, as indicated. Trends will document the efficacy of nutritional support therapy.

PROTEIN COMPARTMENTS
Somatic:
Current weight (kg) _____
Previous weight (kg) _____ (_____ date)
Percent change in weight _____

Height (cm) _____
Height/weight _____
Current body mass index (BMI) _____ [wt/(ht)^2]
Previous BMI _____ (_____ date)
Percent change in BMI _____
Visceral:
Serum albumin _____
 (normal $\geq$ 3.5 mg/dl)
Total lymphocyte count (TLC) _____ (optional)
 (white blood cell count $\times$ percent lymphocytes/100)

 Guide to TLC:
 • Immune competence $\geq$1800 mm^3
 • Immunity partly impaired <1800 but $\geq$ 900 mm^3
 • Anergy $\leq$900 mm3

STATE OF HYDRATION
24-hour intake _____ ml   24-hour output _____ ml
NOTE: Thirst, tongue dryness in non-mouth-breathers and tenting of cervical skin may indicate dehydration. Jugular vein distention may indicate overhydration.

ESTIMATED NUTRITIONAL REQUIREMENT
Estimated nonprotein   Estimated
 calories (NPC) _____/kg   protein _____(g/kg)
         Actual
Actual NPC _____/kg   protein _____(g/kg)

RECOMMENDATIONS/PLAN
1.
2.
3.
4.

From Bergstrom N et al: *Treatment of pressure ulcers,* AHCPR pub no 95-0652, Rockville, Md, 1994, DHHS, PHS, AHCPR.

Table 23-5 **Care of Pressure Ulcers by Risk Factors**

Risk factor	Preventive actions
Bed or chair confinement	Inspect skin at least once a day.
	Bathe when needed for comfort or cleanliness
	Prevent dry skin.
	For client in bed:
	Change position at least every 2 hours.
	Use a special mattress that contains foam, air, gel, or water.
	Raise the head of bed as little and for as short a time as possible.
	For client in a chair:
	Change position every hour.
	Use foam, gel, or air cushion to relieve pressure.
	Reduce friction by:
	Lifting rather than dragging when repositioning.
	Using cornstarch on skin.
	Avoid use of donut-shaped cushions.
	Participate in a rehabilitation program.
Inability to move	Clients confined to chairs should be repositioned every hour if unable to do so themselves.
	For client in a chair who is able to shift his or her own weight, change position at least every 15 minutes.
	Use pillows or wedges to keep knees or ankles from touching each other.
	When in bed, place pillow under legs from midcalf to ankle to keep heels off the bed.
Loss of bowel or bladder control	Clean skin as soon as soiled.
	Assess and treat urine leaks.
	If moisture cannot be controlled:
	Use absorbent pads and/or briefs with a quick-drying surface.
	Protect skin with a cream or ointment.
Poor nutrition	Eat a balanced diet.
	If a normal diet is not possible, talk to health care provider about nutritional supplements.
Lowered mental awareness	Choose preventive actions that apply to client with lowered mental awareness. For example, if the client is confined to chair, refer to the specific preventive actions outlined in first risk factor.

Modified from Agency for Health Care Policy and Research (AHCPR): *Preventing pressure ulcers: a patient's guide,* pub no 92-0048, Rockville, Md, 1992b, US Department of Health and Human Services, Public Health Sevice.

Skill 23.2	**Cleaning and Topical Applications for Pressure Ulcers**

Treatment of clients with pressure ulcers requires a holistic approach that uses the expertise of several multidisciplinary health care professionals. Besides the nurse, this can include the physician, physical therapist, occupational therapist, nutritionist, and pharmacist (Rodeheaver et al., 1994). Aspects of pressure ulcer treatment include the local care of the wound, which is described in this skill, and supportive measures such as adequate nutrients and relief of pressure (see Skill 23.1).

A thorough description of the pressure ulcer (Table 23-6) provides the basis for the decision-making tree (Figure 23-6) for the treatment plan (Maklebust and Sieggreen, 1991). Principles of local wound care include debridement, cleansing, and dressing application. Removal of necrotic tissue is necessary to rid the ulcer of a source of infection, enable visualization of the wound bed to stage the ulcer accurately, and to provide a clean base necessary for healing (Rodeheaver et al., 1994). Methods

Table 23-6 **Staging of Pressure Ulcers**

Definition

Stage I

Nonblanchable erythema of intact skin; the heralding lesion of skin ulceration. Individuals with darker skin, discoloration of the skin, warmth, edema, induration, or hardness may also be indicators (Bergstrom et al., 1994).

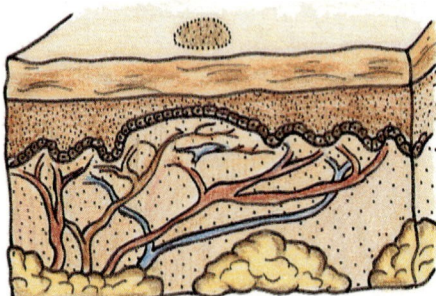 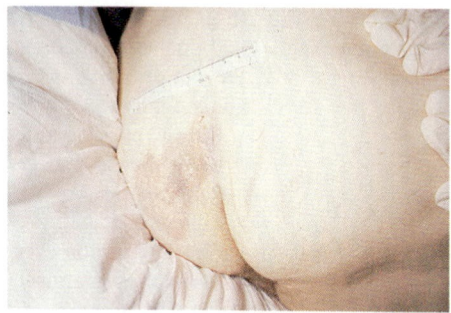

Stage II

Partial-thickness skin loss involving epidermis and/or dermis. The ulcer is superficial and presents clinically as an abrasion, blister, or shallow crater.

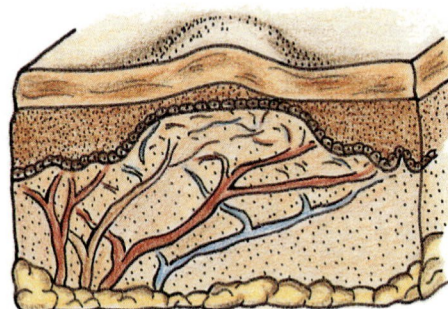 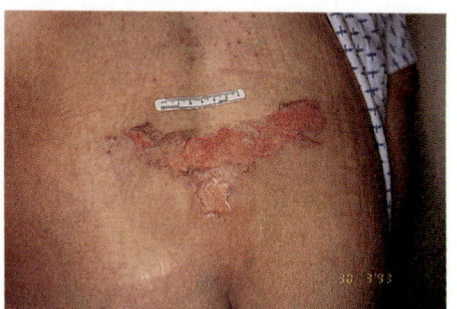

Stage III

Full-thickness skin loss involving damage or necrosis of subcutaneous tissue that may extend down to, but not through, underlying fascia. The ulcer presents clinically as a deep crater with or without undermining of adjacent tissue.

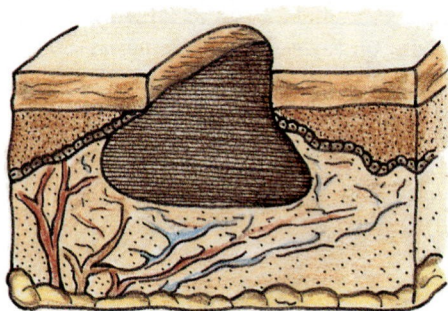 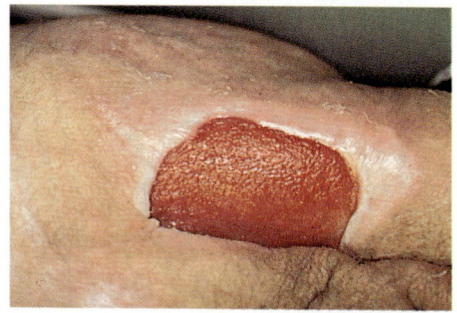

Stage IV

Full-thickness skin loss with extensive destruction, tissue necrosis, or damage to muscle, bone, or supporting structures, for example, tendon or joint capsule. (NOTE: Undermining and sinus tracts may also be associated with stage IV pressure ulcers.)

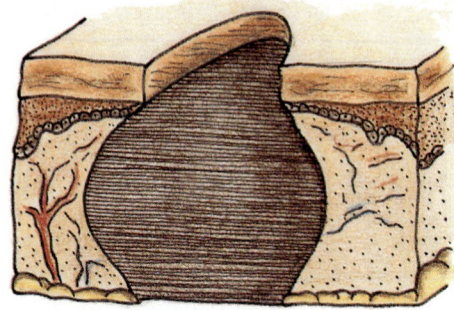 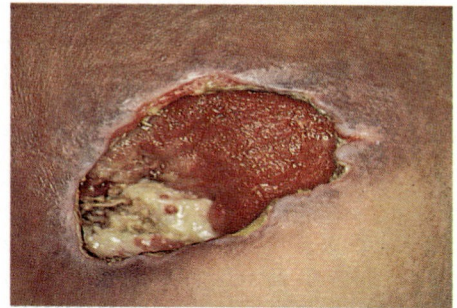

Staging definitions recognize these assessment limitations:

1. Identification of stage I pressure ulcers may be difficult in patients with darkly pigmented skin.
2. When eschar is present, accurate staging of the pressure ulcer is not possible until the eschar has sloughed or the wound has been debrided.

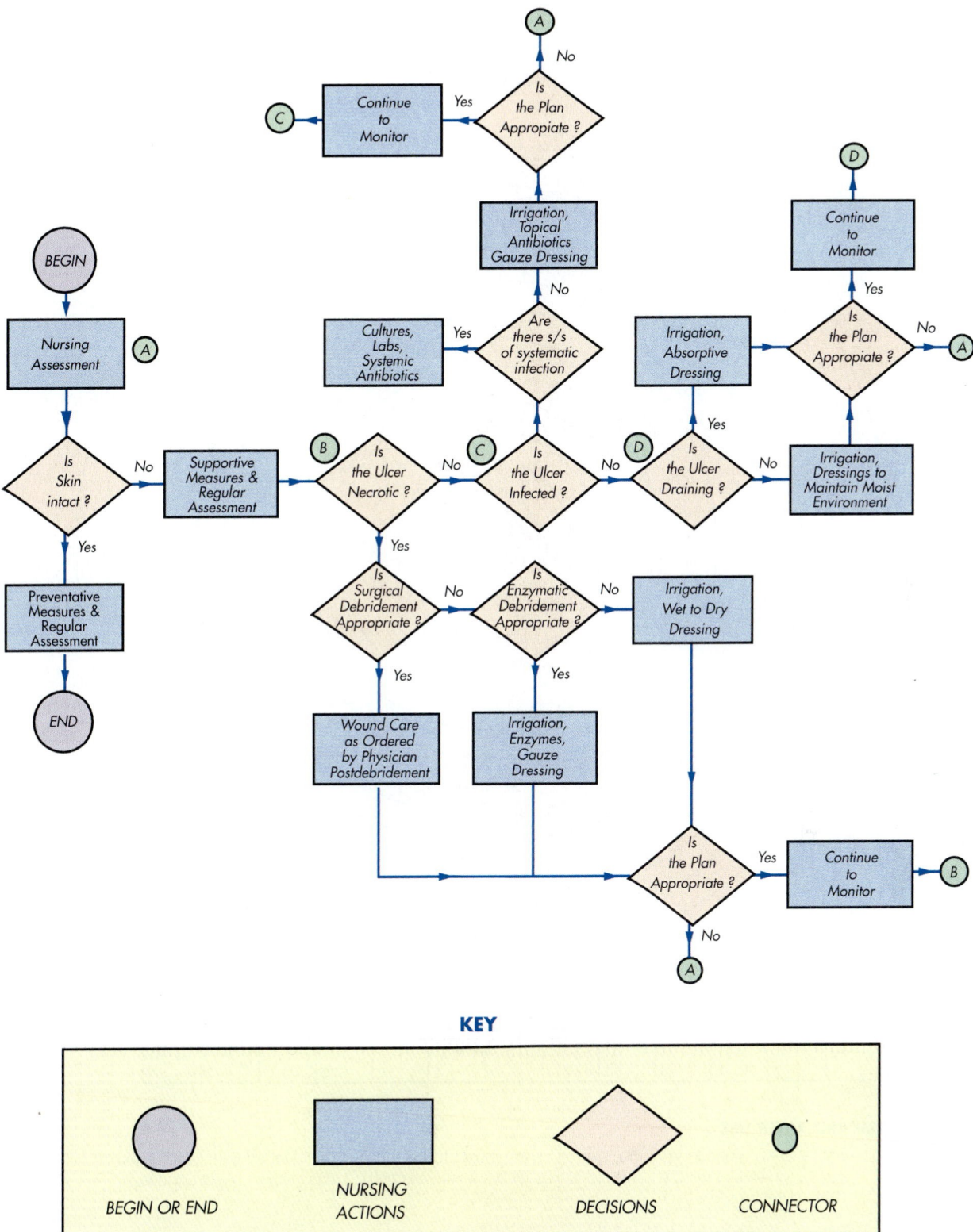

KEY

BEGIN OR END   NURSING ACTIONS   DECISIONS   CONNECTOR

Figure 23-6 Pressure ulcers: a decision tree for local wound care. (Modified from Maklebust J and Sieggreen M: *Pressure ulcers: guidelines for prevention and nursing management*, West Dundee, Ill, 1991, SN Publications.)

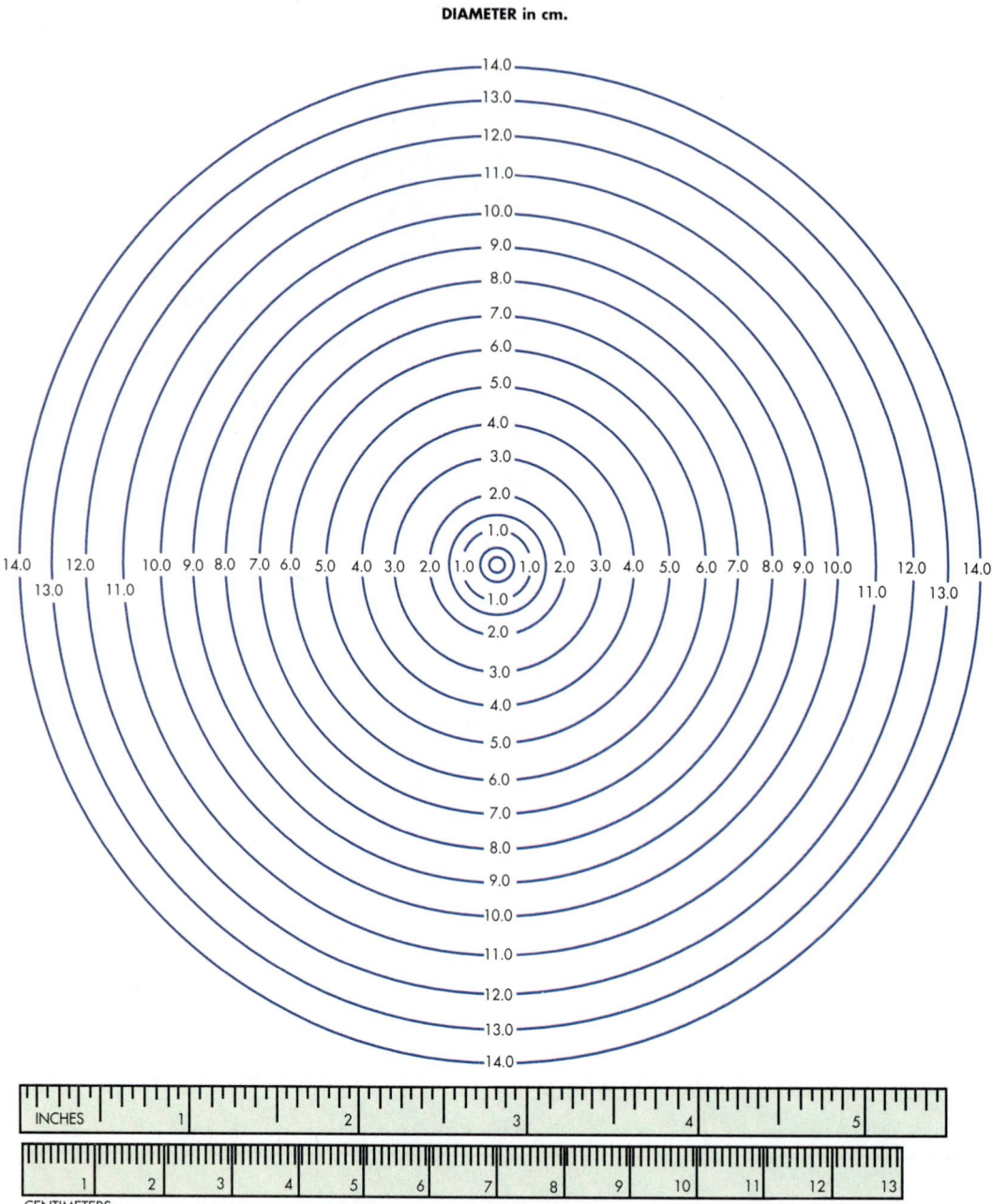

DISCARD AFTER USE

Figure 23-7 Measuring guide. Center over wound to be measured. (Modified from Maklebust J and Sieggreen M: *Pressure ulcers: guidelines for prevention and nursing management,* West Dundee, Ill, 1991, SN Publications.)

of debridement include mechanical, autolytic, chemical/enzymatic, and surgical. Pressure ulcers should be cleansed with solutions such as normal saline or commercial wound cleansers that will not damage fibroblasts and healing tissue. To avoid tissue trauma, care must be taken not to use pressure forces above 15 psi in cleaning or irrigating the pressure ulcer. The choice of dressing depends on the characteristics of the ulcer identified during the pressure ulcer assessment and the goal of the treatment plan. It will change as the ulcer heals. For example, for a necrotic wound, a membrane dressing may be used initially to debride the wound by autolysis. Afterward, pressure ulcers staged III or IV that had large amounts of exudate would require a dressing with absorptive ability. *Clean* dressings, rather than sterile dressings, can be used to treat pressure ulcers (Bergstrom et al., 1994).

All pressure ulcers are colonized; therefore, swab cultures should not be used to diagnose wound infection. Quantitative bacterial cultures of the wound fluid or of the soft tissue is recommended by AHCPR (1994) (Bergstrom et al., 1994).

The new AHCPR pressure ulcer treatment guidelines (1994) recommend that *clean* gloves be used when doing pressure ulcer care. "One set of gloves can be used on the same patient with multiple pressure ulcers. When treating multiple ulcers on the same patient attend to the most contaminated ulcer last (e.g., in the perianal region). Remove gloves and wash hands between patients" (Bergstrom et al., 1994).

Besides local wound treatment, other methods such as electromagnetic energy have been used to foster ulcer healing (Itoh et al., 1991). Education (Maklebust and Magnan, 1992) and understanding of the client and experience of the support person are helpful (Baharestani, 1994). The AHCPR treatment guidelines released in December 1994 are an additional resource for clinicians to use for client care management (Bergstrom et al., 1994).

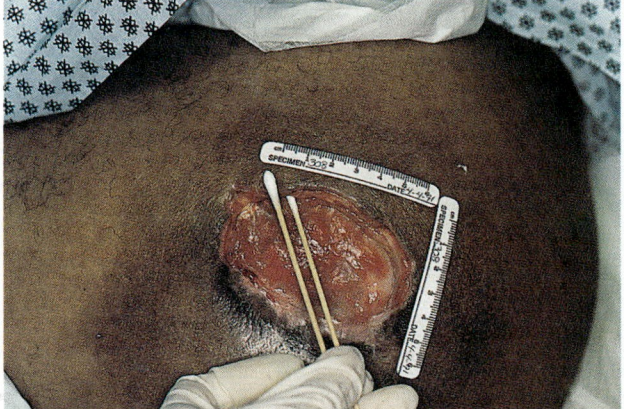

Figure 23-8 Measuring depth of pressure ulcer.

EQUIPMENT

Disposable gloves (clean)
Plastic bag for dressing disposal
Tracing film, wound measuring device (Figures 23-7 and 23-8), cotton tip applicators
Topical agent as ordered
Cleansing agent/solution
Wash basin, washcloths, towels
Dressing
Skin protectant
Tape, if needed
Irrigating syringe and needle if needed
Documentation record
AHCPR *Consumer Guide: Pressure Sore Treatment*

Table 23-7 **Oral and Cutaneous Signs of Vitamin or Mineral Deficiencies***

Clinical signs (by site)	Deficiency(ies)
ORAL CAVITY	
Cheilosis and angular stomatitis	Vitamin B_2
Glossitis (i.e., pink or magenta discoloration with loss of villi)	Multiple B vitamins
EYES	
Scleral changes	Vitamin A
Bitot's spots	Vitamin A
FACE	
Seborrhea-like dryness and redness of nasolabial fold and eyebrows	Zinc
UPPER EXTREMITIES	
Purplish blotches on lightly traumatized areas (from capillary fragility and subepithelial hemorrhages)	Vitamin C
Extreme transparency of skin of hands ("cellophane skin")	Vitamin C
ABDOMEN/BUTTOCKS	
Waxy, perifollicular hyperkeratosis	Vitamin A
LOWER EXTREMITIES	
Superficial flaking of epidermis, large flakes of dandruff	Essential fatty acids
Cracks in skin between islands of hyperkeratosis:	
Pigmented	Nicotinamide (niacinamide)
Nonpigmented	Vitamin A

From Bergstrom N et al: *Treatment of pressure ulcers,* AHCPR pub no 95-0652, Rockville, Md, 1994, DHHS, PHS, AHCPR.
*These manifestations may be seen in disease processes other than vitamin deficiencies. If the cause is in fact a deficiency, clinical improvement should be evident 4 weeks after supplementation is begun.

PRESSURE SORE STATUS TOOL   NAME_____

Complete the rating sheet to assess pressure sore status. Evaluate each item by picking the response that best describes the wound and entering the score in the item score column for the appropriate date.

Location: Anatomic site. Circle, identify right (**R**) or left (**L**) and use "**X**" to mark site on body diagrams:

_____ Sacrum & coccyx	_____ Lateral ankle	
_____ Trochanter	_____ Medial ankle	
_____ Ischial tuberosity	_____ Heel Other Site _____	

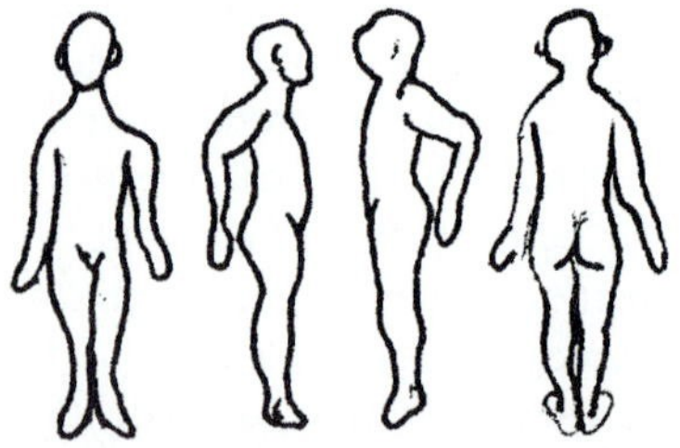

Shape: Overall wound pattern; assess by observing perimeter and depth.
Circle and <u>date</u> appropriate description:

_____ Irregular	_____ Linear or elongated
_____ Round/oval	_____ Bowl/boat
_____ Square/rectangle	_____ Butterfly Other Shape _____

Item	Assessment	Date	Date	Date
		Score	**Score**	**Score**
1. Size	1 = Length x width < 4 sq cm 2 = Length x width 4 -16 sq cm 3 = Length x width 16.1 - 36 sq cm 4 = Length x width 36.1 - 80 sq cm 5 = Length x width > 80 sq cm			
2. Depth	1 = Non-blanchable erythema on intact skin 2 = Partial thickness skin loss involving epidermis &/or dermis 3 = Full thickness skin loss involving damage or necrosis of subcutaneous tissue; may extend down to but not through underlying fascia; &/or mixed partial & full thickness &/or tissue layers obscured by granulation tissue 4 = Obscured by necrosis 5 = Full thickness skin loss with extensive destruction, tissue necrosis or damage to muscle, bone or supporting structures			
3. Edges	1 = Indistinct, diffuse, none clearly visible 2 = Distinct, outline clearly visible, attached, even with wound base 3 = Well-defined, not attached to wound base 4 = Well-defined, not attached to base, rolled under, thickened 5 = Well-defined, fibrotic, scarred or hyperkeratotic			
4. Under-mining	1 = Undermining < 2 cm in any area 2 = Undermining 2-4 cm involving < 50% wound margins 3 = Undermining 2-4 cm involving > 50% wound margins 4 = Undermining > 4 cm in any area 5 = Tunneling &/or sinus tract formation			
5. Necrotic Tissue Type	1 = None visible 2 = White/grey non-viable tissue &/or non-adherent yellow slough 3 = Loosely adherent yellow slough 4 = Adherent, soft, black eschar 5 = Firmly adherent, hard, black eschar			
6. Necrotic Tissue Amount	1 = None visible 2 = < 25% of wound bed covered 3 = 25% to 50% of wound covered 4 = > 50% and < 75% of wound covered 5 = 75% to 100% of wound covered			

c 1990 Barbara Bates-Jensen

Figure 23-9 Bates-Jensen Pressure Sore Assessment Tool. (Courtesy Barbara Bates-Jensen.)

Item	Assessment	Date	Date	Date
		Score	Score	Score
7. Exudate Type	1 = None or bloody 2 = Serosanguineous: thin, watery, pale red/pink 3 = Serous: thin, watery, clear 4 = Purulent: thin or thick, opaque, tan/yellow 5 = Foul purulent: thick, opaque, yellow/green with odor			
8. Exudate Amount	1 = None 2 = Scant 3 = Small 4 = Moderate 5 = Large			
9. Skin color Surrounding Wound	1 = Pink or normal for ethnic group 2 = Bright red &/or blanches to touch 3 = White or grey pallor or hypopigmented 4 = Dark red or purple &/or non-blanchable 5 = Black or hyperpigmented			
10. Peripheral Tissue Edema	1 = Minimal swelling around wound 2 = Non-pitting edema extends < 4 cm around wound 3 = Non-pitting edema extends $\geq$ 4 cm around wound 4 = Pitting edema extends < 4 cm around wound 5 = Crepitus &/or pitting edema extends $\geq$ 4 cm			
11. Peripheral Tissue Induration	1 = Minimal firmness around wound 2 = Induration < 2 cm around wound 3 = Induration 2-4 cm extending < 50% around wound 4 = Induration 2-4 cm extending $\geq$ 50% around wound 5 = Induration > 4 cm in any area			
12. Granulation Tissue	1 = Skin intact or partial thickness wound 2 = Bright, beefy red; 75% to 100% of wound filled &/or tissue overgrowth 3 = Bright, beefy red; < 75% & > 25% of wound filled 4 = Pink, &/or dull, dusky red &/or fills $\leq$ 25% of wound 5 = No granulation tissue present			
13. Epithelializtion	1 = 100% wound covered, surface intact 2 = 75% to <100% wound covered &/or epithelial tissue extends >0.5cm into wound bed 3 = 50% to <75% wound covered &/or epithelial tissue extends to <0.5cm into wound bed 4 = 25% to < 50% wound covered 5 = < 25% wound covered			
TOTAL SCORE				
SIGNATURE				

PRESSURE SORE STATUS CONTINUUM

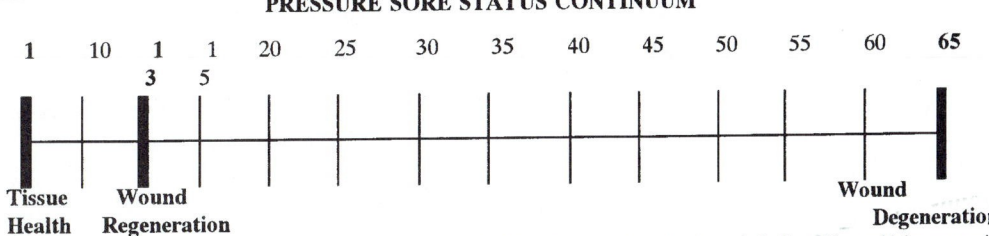

Plot the total score on the Pressure Sore Status Continuum by putting an "X" on the line and the date beneath the line. Plot multiple scores with their dates to see-at-a-glance regeneration or degeneration of the wound.   *Continued.*

c 1990 Barbara Bates-Jensen

Figure 23-9, cont'd.

PRESSURE SORE STATUS TOOL

Instructions for use

<u>General Guidelines:</u>

Fill out the attached rating sheet to assess a pressure sore's status after reading the definitions and methods of assessement described below. Evaluate once a week and whenever a change occurs in the wound. Rate according to each item by picking the response that best describes the wound and entering that score in the item score column for the appropriate date. When you have rated the pressure sore on all items, determine the total score by adding together the 13-item scores. The HIGHER the total score, the more severe the pressure sore status. Plot total score on the Pressure Sore Status Continuum to determine progress.

<u>Specific Instructions:</u>

1.   **Size:** Use ruler to measure the longest and widest aspect of the wound surface in centimeters; multiply length x width.

2.   **Depth:** Pick the depth, thickness, most appropriate to the wound using these additional descriptions:

    1 =   tissues damaged but no break in skin surface.
    2 =   superficial, abrasion, blister or shallow crater. Even with, &/or elevated above skin surface (e.g., hyperplasia).
    3 =   deep crater with or without undermining of adjacent tissue.
    4 =   visualization of tissue layers not possible due to necrosis.
    5 =   supporting structures include tendon, joint capsule.

3.   **Edges:** Use this guide:

Indistinct, diffuse	=	unable to clearly distinguish wound outline.
Attached	=	even or flush with wound base, <u>no</u> sides or walls present; flat.
Not attached	=	sides or walls <u>are</u> present; floor or base of wound is deeper than edge.
Rolled under, thickened	=	soft to firm and flexible to touch.
Hyperkeratosis	=	callous-like tissue formation around wound & at edges.
Fibrotic, scarred	=	hard, rigid to touch.

4.   **Undermining:** Assess by inserting a cotton tipped applicator under the wound edge; advance it as far as it will go without using undue force; raise the tip of the applicator so it may be seen or felt on the surface of the skin; mark the surface with a pen; measure the distance from the mark on the skin to the edge of the wound. Continue process around the wound. Then use a transparent metric measuring guide with concentric circles divided into 4 (25%) pie-shaped quadrants to help determine percent of wound involved.

5.   **Necrotic Tissue Type:** Pick the type of necrotic tissue that is <u>predominant</u> in the wound according to color, consistency and adherence using this guide:

White/gray non-viable tissue	=	may appear prior to wound opening; skin surface is white or gray.
Non-adherent, yellow slough	=	thin, mucinous substance; scattered throughout wound bed; easily separated from wound tissue.
Loosely adherent, yellow slough	=	thick, stringy, clumps of debris; attached to wound tissue.
Adherent, soft, black eschar	=	soggy tissue; strongly attached to tissue in center or base of wound.
Firmly adherent, hard/black eschar	=	firm, crusty tissue; strongly attached to wound base <u>and</u> edges (like a hard scab).

c 1990 Barbara Bates-Jensen

Figure 23-9, cont'd.

6.   **Necrotic Tissue Amount**: Use a transparent metric measuring guide with concentric circles divided into 4 (25%) pie-shaped quadrants to help determine percent of wound involved.

7.   **Exudate Type**: Some dressings interact with wound drainage to produce a gel or trap liquid. Before assessing exudate type, gently cleanse wound with normal saline or water. Pick the exudate type that is <u>predominant</u> in the wound according to color and consistency, using this guide:

Bloody	=	thin, bright red
Serosanguineous	=	thin, watery pale red to pink
Serous	=	thin, watery, clear
Purulent	=	thin or thick, opaque tan to yellow
Foul purulent	=	thick, opaque yellow to green with offensive odor

8.   **Exudate Amount**: Use a transparent metric measuring guide with concentric circles divided into 4 (25%) pie-shaped quadrants to determine percent of dressing involved with exudate. Use this guide:

None	=	wound tissues dry.
Scant	=	wound tissues moist; no measurable exudate.
Small	=	wound tissues wet; moisture evenly distributed in wound; drainage involves $\leq$ 25% dressing.
Moderate	=	wound tissues saturated; drainage may or may not be evenly distributed in wound; drainage involves > 25% to $\leq$ 75% dressing.
Large	=	wound tissues bathed in fluid; drainage freely expressed; may or may not be evenly distributed in wound; drainage involves > 75% of dressing.

9.   **Skin Color Surrounding Wound**: Assess tissues within 4cm of wound edge. Dark-skinned persons show the colors "bright red" and "dark red" as a deepening of normal ethnic skin color or a purple hue. As healing occurs in dark-skinned persons, the new skin is pink and may never darken.

10.   **Peripheral Tissue Edema**: Assess tissues within 4cm of wound edge. Non-pitting edema appears as skin that is shiny and taut. Identify pitting edema by firmly pressing a finger down into the tissues and waiting for 5 seconds, on release of pressure, tissues fail to resume previous position and an indentation appears. Crepitus is accumulation of air or gas in tissues. Use a transparent metric measuring guide to determine how far edema extends beyond wound.

11.   **Peripheral Tissue Induration**: Assess tissues within 4cm of wound edge. Induration is abnormal firmness of tissues with margins. Assess by gently pinching the tissues. Induration results in an inability to pinch the tissues. Use a transparent metric measuring guide with concentric circles divided into 4 (25%) pie-shaped quadrants to determine percent of wound and area involved.

12.   **Granulation Tissue**: Granulation tissue is the growth of small blood vessels and connective tissue to fill in full thickness wounds. Tissue is healthy when bright, beefy red, shiny and granular with a velvety appearance. Poor vascular supply appears as pale pink or blanched to dull, dusky red color.

13.   **Epithelialization**: Epithelialization is the process of epidermal resurfacing and appears as pink or red skin. In partial thickness wounds it can occur throughout the wound bed as well as from the wound edges. In full thickness wounds it occurs from the edges only. Use a transparent metric measuring guide with concentric circles divided into 4 (25%) pie-shaped quadrants to help determine percent of wound involved and to measure the distance the epithelial tissue extends into the wound.

Figure 23-9, cont'd.

Assessment

1. Assess client's level of comfort and need for pain management. **Client pain interferes with assessment process.**
2. Assess condition of client's skin, especially over areas at high risk for breakdown, such as bony prominences. **Bony prominences are the most common sites for pressure ulcer development.**

3. Assess each of the client's pressure ulcers. Consider using either the Bates-Jensen Pressure Sore Assessment Tool (Bates-Jensen, 1990) (Figure 23-9, pp. 432 to 435) or Ayello (1992) Assessment Mnemonic (see the box on p. 437). **A complete description of the pressure ulcer is necessary to determine appropriate treatment plan. Pressure ulcers should be reassessed weekly (Bergstrom et al., 1994).**

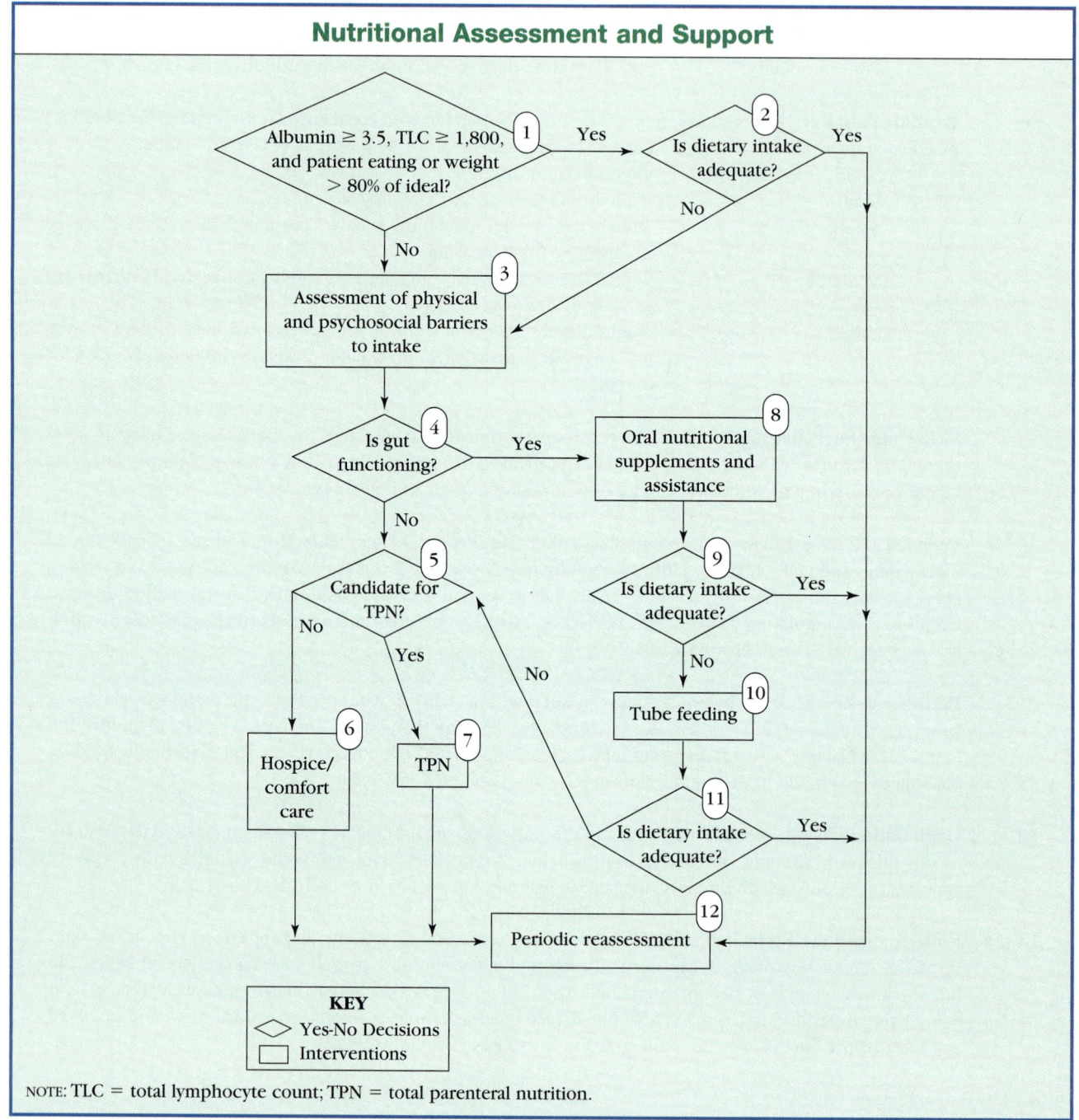

Figure 23-10 (From Bergstrom N et al: *Treatment of pressure ulcers,* AHCPR pub no 95-0652, Rockville, Md, 1994, DHHS, PHS, AHCPR.)

4. Assess client's nutritional status at least every 3 months. Clinically significant malnutrition is present if weight loss is greater than 15%, serum albumin less than 3.5 mg/dl, or total lymphocyte count less than 1800 mm^3 (Bergstrom et al., 1994). Also observe the mouth and skin for signs of vitamin or mineral deficiencies) (Table 23-7; Figure 23-10). **Malnutrition is a risk factor for pressure ulcers. Low serum albumin levels have been correlated with pressure ulcer stages (Maklebust, 1994) (Figure 23-10).**

5. Assess client's and support person's understanding of pressure ulcers treatment(s). **Client and support person need to participate in the plan of care.**

Planning

Expected outcomes focus on healing of the ulcer and nursing actions to prevent further skin breakdown.

EXPECTED OUTCOMES

1. Client's pressure ulcer heals.
2. Client/support person demonstrates knowledge of treatment plan and prevention.

Ayello's Assessment Mnemonic

A natomical location, age	**A** Chronic wounds heal slower.
S ize, shape, stage	**S** Staging of the wound will help in selecting the appropriate healing treatments and dressing. Measuring guides can assist in determining the length and width of the ulcer. A sterile cotton-tipped application can be used to measure the depth of the ulcer.
S inus tract	**S** Gently use a sterile cotton-tipped applicator tip to locate any sinus tracts.
E xudate	**E** Wound drainage must be contained to protect the surrounding skin.
S epsis	**S** Systemic infections must be treated. Routine swab culturing of pressure ulcers for local infection is not recommended (Maklebust, 1994).
S urrounding skin	**S** Protect the surrounding skin from breakdown from moisture.
M argins, maceration	**M** Identity condition of wound margins and if they are contracting. Evaluate for maceration; if present, institute measures to protect skin.
E rythremia, epithelization, eschar	**E** Evaluate for wound healing, as evidenced by these changes in the ulcer. Erythremia in client's with dark skin tone is best assessed with good lighting. Skin may have a purplish hue (Graves, 1990).
N ecrotic, nose, neovascularization	**N** Necrotic tissue must be removed to stage and heal the ulcer.
T issue bed, tenderness to touch, tension, temperature, treatments	**T** Identify tissue bed and prior ulcer treatment and medicate for pain (Bergstrom et al., 1994).

Courtesy Elizabeth Ayello.

Implementation

Steps	Rationale
1. See Standard Protocol (Chapter 1, p. 5). 	
2. Consider selecting pressure ulcer management based on identified stage and other factors. Principles of local wound care: a. Debride wound. b. Clean wound. c. Dress wound. d. Relieve pressure.	The use of a decision tree may be useful in determining pressure ulcer care (see Figure 23-6).
3. Remove any necrotic tissue in the pressure ulcer (see physician's orders).	Necrotic tissue provides a source for infection; a clean wound base free of devitalized tissue is necessary for healing.
4. Wound healing and treatment protocols The débridement method that is most appropriate and consistent with overall client goals should be selected.	
a. Mechanical: wet to dry dressings	Removes eschar by the mechanical force of pulling out the tissue from the wound bed. As a nonselective method of debridement, it can injure healthy tissue.
b. Autolytic: membrane dressings	A readily available selective method of debridement that is effective for small wounds. Increased bacterial growth can occur beneath the dressing. Use is contraindicated in infected pressure ulcers.
c. Chemical/enzymatic: (1) Santyl (collagenase) (2) Travase (sutilains) (3) Panafil (papain) (4) Granulex (trypsin, balam Peru, and castor oil) (5) Elase (fibrinolysin and desoxyribonuclease)	Easily applied and cost-effective selective method of debridement. Crosshatching of the pressure ulcer with use of these products is recommended. It is important to know the specific application, technique, effects, and storage of each of these products because they differ from each other.
d. Surgical debridement	A rapid selective method of removing necrotic tissue. It is expensive and includes risks associated with anesthesia.
5. Cleaning the pressure ulcer Use an appropriate cleansing solution such as normal saline or commercially available wound cleansers (Wright and Orr, 1993).	Avoid using solutions that harm new granulation tissue and kill fibroblasts and therefore interfere with wound healing (Table 23-8) (Bergstrom et al., 1994).

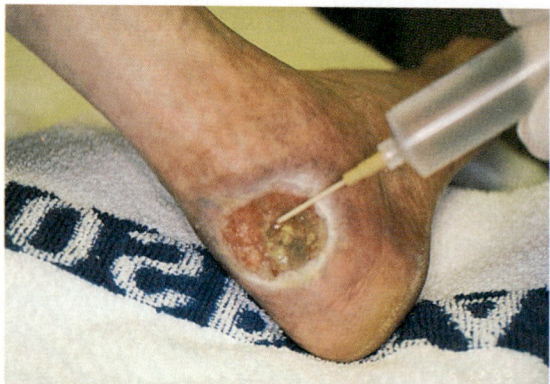

Figure 23-11 Wound irrigation.

Steps	Rationale
6. Ulcers that are irrigated should be done with equipment that has a pressure of 4 to 15 psi. An example is a 35 ml syringe and 19-gauge needle (Figure 23-11).	High-pressure systems above 15 psi should not be used because they can cause trauma to the tissue (Bergstrom et al., 1994).
7. Appropriate dressing Select appropriate dressing (see boxes on pp. 440 to 442) (see Chapter 15) based on the pressure ulcer assessment. Some of these dressings are transparent films and membranes, hydrocolloids, absorption, foam, hydrogels, gauze, and alginates.	Dressings should keep the ulcer bed moist and the skin around the ulcer dry. Different dressings are needed to achieve the various goals of pressure ulcer management. Monitor dressings applied near the anus to make sure they are intact. Loosely fill the wound cavity with dressing to eliminate dead space. Do not overpack the wound (Bergstrom et al., 1994).
8. Provide patient and support person education about pressure ulcer risk and prevention. Use AHCPR *Preventing Pressure Ulcers: A Patient's Guide* or AHCPR *Consumer Guide: Pressure Sore Treatment* (Ayello, 1993).	Client and family need to know correct prevention and treatment information and care techniques.
9. Implement nursing interventions to minimize pressure ulcers.	Treating pressure ulcers goes beyond just the local wound care. It also requires a multidisciplinary approach that uses the resources of many health care professionals (Bergstrom et al., 1994).
10. See Completion Protocol (Chapter 1, p. 6).	

Table 23-8 **Common Antiseptic Solutions**

Solutions	Actions	Considerations
Acetic acid	Effective against *Pseudomonas aeruginosa* Effective against gram positive and gram negative microorganisms	Toxic to fibroblasts in standard dilutions Color of wound exudate is changed; therefore can give false assurance that infection has been eliminated
Sodium hypochlorite solutions Dakin's solution Chloramine-T (Chlorazene)	Effective against *Staphylococcus, Streptoccus* Dissolves necrotic tissue Controls odors	Toxic to fibroblasts in normal dilutions Can cause bleach irritations to surrounding skin Surrounding skin must be protected to minimize chance of skin breakdown
Hydrogen peroxide	Little bactericidal action in wounds Provides nonselective mechanical cleansing Provides some nonselective debridement by effervescent action	Toxic to fibroblasts can cause ulceration of newly formed tissue Don't use to pack sinus tracts; air embolisms have been reported Don't use for forceful irrigation; subcutaneous emphysema has been reported
Povidone-iodine preparations	Broad-spectrum effectiveness when used on intact skin	Toxic to fibroblasts in normal dilutions Not always effective in infected wounds Questionable value in treating chronic wounds Iodine toxicity such as thyrotoxicosis has been reported when used in large wounds for a long period of time

Modified from Bryant RA: *Acute and chronic wounds,* St. Louis, 1992, Mosby.

Transparent Adhesive Dressings: Critical Clinical Features

- Support autolytic debridement of wounds with dry eschar
- Help prevent infection because of hydrophobic outer surface. Studies have shown that bacteria do not penetrate the membrane; however, bacteria may migrate into the wound from the surrounding skin.
- Maintain moist wound surface
- Provide some degree of insulation because of the fluid layer retained next to the wound surface
- Provide a nonadherent surface against wound bed and so do not traumatize the wound with removal; adhesives may damage fragile intact skin surrounding wound with removal

INDICATIONS FOR USE
- Partial-thickness wounds
- Dry necrotic wounds requiring débridement

CONTRAINDICATIONS TO USE
- Exudative wounds
- Wounds with sinus tracts (unless used with packing)
- Friable skin surrounding the lesion

GUIDELINES FOR USE
- Must have border of intact dry skin; shaving and defatting of skin improves seal
- Frequency of change based on exudate accumulation or loss of secure seal

From Bryant RA: *Acute and chronic wounds,* St Louis, 1992, Mosby,

Hydrocolloid Wafer Dressing: Critical Clinical Features

- Support autolytic débridement, especially for wounds with slough or a combination of necrosis and exudate
- Prevent secondary infection; reduce infection rates compared with conventional dressings
- Provide limited to moderate absorption, depending on thickness and formula of specific dressing
- Maintain moist wound surface
- Provide insulation of wound
- Do not adhere to wound bed and so protect from traumatic removal; may traumatize fragile surrounding skin and so must be carefully removed

INDICATIONS FOR USE
- Partial-thickness wounds (stage II)
- Shallow full-thickness wounds (stage III); considered the dressing of choice for venous ulcers, in conjunction with compression
- Granulating stage IV ulcers with minimal-moderate exudate

CONTRAINDICATIONS TO USE
- Heavily exudative wounds
- Wounds with undermining or sinus tracts, unless used with some type of packing
- Infected wound
- Fragile surrounding skin

GUIDELINES FOR USE
- Edges need to be secured with tape
- Frequency of change based on amount of exudate: typical frequency every 3 to 5 days. Dressing should be changed for wrinkling, or if edges loosen or dressing leaks.
- Yellowish odorous exudate is normal when dressing is removed.

From Bryant RA: *Acute and chronic wounds,* St Louis, 1992, Mosby.

Nonadhesive Semipermeable Polyurethane Foam Dressings: Critical Clinical Features

- Support autolytic débridement in exudative wounds but not in dry wounds
- Provide minimal to moderate absorption of wound exudate
- Maintain moist wound surface
- Insulate wound surface
- Nonadherent surface provides atraumatic removal

INDICATIONS FOR USE

- Full-thickness wounds with moderate amounts of exudate (stage III or granulating stage IV). For wounds with depth or dead space, use with packing.
- As secondary dressing to provide additional absorption and some protection against contaminants, because of repellent surface

CONTRAINDICATIONS TO USE

- Partial-thickness wounds with no exudate
- Full-thickness wounds with dry eschar
- Wounds with sinus tracts, unless used with packing

GUIDELINES FOR USE

- May need to protect intact skin around wound from maceration with skin sealant, for example.
- Must secure wafer with elastic bandage, wrap bandage, or tape. More difficult to use in sacral area.
- Dressing change frequency depends on exudate; typical frequency is every 2 to 5 days.

From Bryant RA: *Acute and chronic wounds,* St Louis, 1992, Mosby.

Absorption Dressings: Critical Clinical Features

- Support autolytic débridement as long as moist wound surface is maintained
- Absorb large volumes of exudate, up to 20 times weight of each dressing
- Eliminate dead space
- Maintain moist wound surface when used correctly

INDICATIONS FOR USE

- Wounds with moderate to large amounts of exudate (stages III and IV)
- Wounds with sinus tracts. NOTE: Narrow sinus tracts are probably best managed with ribbon gauze packing.
- Wounds with a combination of necrosis and exudate

CONTRAINDICATIONS TO USE

- Wounds with minimal exudate. NOTE: Absorption dressings that are placed in the wound in a *moist* state may be used for wounds with minimal exudate that require packing.
- Wounds covered with dry eschar; these wounds must be débrided before a filler dressing can be used.
- Partial-thickness wounds (stage II)

GUIDELINES FOR USE

- *Copolymer starch dressings* are applied to the wound in moist form, and so they may be used for wounds with minimal exudate as well as for wounds with large amounts of exudate. They are usually changed daily; the wound is flushed and then lightly packed with the dressing.
- *Dextranomer bead dressings* are applied to the wound in dry or paste form, and so they are appropriate only for exudative wounds. The frequency of dressing change depends on amount of exudate but is usually once or twice a day. Tight packing of the wound is contraindicated because dressings are designed to swell with exudate.
- *Calcium alginate dressings* are applied to the wound in dry form, and so they are appropriate only for exudative wounds; if used for less exudative wounds, they should be moistened with saline. These dressings are available in standard-size dressings as well as ribbons for packing sinus tracts. They are effective for shallow exudative wounds as well as for deep wounds.
- All dressings require a *cover dressing.* The cover dressing provides protection from environmental contaminants and some degree of insulation; it should be selected based on wound location and amount of protection needed. For example, a gauze cover dressing may be sufficient for a trochanteric ulcer, whereas a sacral ulcer in an incontinent client may require a waterproof secondary dressing such as transparent adhesive dressings or semipermeable polyurethane foam dressings with waterproof tape.

From Bryant RA: *Acute and chronic wounds,* St Louis, 1992, Mosby.

Gel Dressings: Critical Clinical Features

- Support autolytic débridement because of moisturizing effects
- Granulate form can be used to fill dead space
- Provide limited absorption of exudate
- Maintain moist wound surface
- Nonadherent surface provides atraumatic removal

INDICATIONS FOR USE
- Partial-thickness wounds, best managed with sheet form
- Full-thickness wounds, usually best managed with granulate form
- Can be used to support autolytic débridement

CONTRAINDICATIONS TO USE
- No contraindications; must match appropriate form of gel dressing to wound

GUIDELINES FOR USE
- *Granulate form* is used to lightly pack full-thickness wound. Provides minimal to moderate absorption; frequency of dressing change depends on the amount of exudate. Usual frequency is once or twice a day.
- *Sheet form* is most appropriate for partial-thickness wounds. Sheet gels made primarily of water can macerate the surrounding skin, and so they should be cut to fit the lesion. Frequency of dressing change is usually every other day, depending on the volume of exudate. Sheet gels made primarily of water must be monitored carefully and changed frequently enough to prevent dehydration of the dressing. When these dressings are used to support autolytic débridement of eschar, more frequent dressing changes are usually required.
- Cover dressings are selected based on the amount of protection needed.

From Bryant RA: *Acute and chronic wounds,* St Louis, 1992, Mosby.

Synthetic Barrier Dressing: Critical Clinical Features

- Provides for absorption of exudate
- Maintains moist wound surface
- Provides some degree of insulation
- Provides for atraumatic removal

INDICATIONS FOR USE
- Partial-thickness wounds, with tape or secondary dressing for security
- Full-thickness wounds with exudate

CONTRAINDICATIONS TO USE
- Wounds with dry eschar
- Wounds with sinus tracts

GUIDELINES FOR USE
- Secondary dressing is changed as needed, depending on the volume of exudate.
- Synthetic barrier dressing is changed once or twice a week.

From Bryant RA: *Acute and chronic wounds,* St Louis, 1992, Mosby.

Gauze Dressings: Critical Clinical Features

- Support autolytic débridement if applied moist and kept moist
- Provide absorption of exudate
- Can be used as filler dressing to pack sinus tracts
- Must be used with appropriate solutions or gels to maintain moist wound surface

INDICATIONS FOR USE
- Exudative wounds
- Wounds with dead space or sinus tracts
- Wounds with combination of exudate and necrotic tissue

CONTRAINDICATIONS TO USE
- Partial-thickness wounds, unless used with topical agent that maintains moist wound surface
- Dry wounds covered with necrotic tissue, unless used with debriding agents or solutions

GUIDELINES FOR USE
- Mesh gauze should be used against the wound surface, as opposed to cotton-filled sponges. Fine mesh is recommended as opposed to coarse mesh because fine mesh is less likely to damage the wound with removal.
- Wounds should be packed lightly; tight packing compromises blood flow, may be painful, and delays wound closure.
- Narrow sinus tracts are best managed with narrow ribbon gauze.
- Moisturizing agents must be added to the gauze to prevent trauma and promote healing; the one exception is hypertonic saline gauze, which is intended for heavily exudative wounds and is placed into the wound dry.
- Topical agents used with gauze should be selected based on assessment of wound status; for example, noncytotoxic agents should be used for clean proliferating wounds.
- Frequency of dressing change depends on the amount of exudate.
- Moist gauze is placed *into* the wound but kept off the surrounding skin to prevent maceration.

From Bryant RA: *Acute and chronic wounds,* St Louis, 1992, Mosby.

Evaluation

1. Reevaluate the pressure ulcer for evidence of healing.
2. Evaluate client's and support person's knowledge of treatment of pressure ulcers and risk prevention for further ulcers.

UNEXPECTED OUTCOMES AND RELATED INTERVENTIONS

Client's pressure ulcer does not heal.
  a. Reassess the pressure ulcer.
  b. Consider implementing a change in the local wound care products being used. For example, would a different category of dressing be more effective?
  c. Evaluate if measures to reduce pressure need to be increased. Consider client's nutritional status and if additional nutritional measures are needed.
  d. Consider a consultation with a specialist in pressure ulcer care, such as a CETN.
  e. Consider having a meeting with the multidisciplinary team to discuss and review client's plan of care.

SAMPLE DOCUMENTATION

2300 Sacral stage III pressure ulcer is 2 by 3 cm irregular shape. Pale pink subcutaneous tissue visible, no drainage present. Wound edges are rolled, surrounding skin is intact. Wound cleansed with normal saline and hydrocolloid dressing applied. Client and family have read AHCPR booklets, *Preventing Pressure Ulcers: A Patient's Guide* and *Pressure Sore Treatment* and are practicing positioning techniques.

CRITICAL THINKING EXERCISES

1. What important factors place each of the following clients at increased risk for the development of pressure ulcers?
  a. Mary is an 89-year-old client who is being treated for weight loss, fatigue, and dehydration.
  b. Ralph is a 78-year-old client transferred to the hospital from a geriatric center. He is incontinent of urine and stool. He is disoriented and is in restraints to prevent falling out of bed.
  c. Joe, a 59-year-old diabetic client, is on complete bed rest following a blood clot in his lower leg.
2. Provide at least three interventions to decrease the risk of pressure ulcer development that would apply to all three of the above clients.
3. You are caring for an elderly male client who is on continuous tube feedings. While assessing his chart, you note the following data:

Gosnell Scale: Pressure Sore Risk Assessment

Mental status	3
Continence	4
Mobility	3
Activity	3
Nutrition	1

  a. What conclusions can be drawn from this data?
  b. What aspects of this client's status, if any, decrease his risk for pressure ulcer development?
4. When assessing Martha, an elderly client with a pressure ulcer on her coccyx, you note that there is a transparent dressing over the ulcer. On further inspection you determine that the ulcer crater is filled with serous fluid. How should you respond, and why?

REFERENCES

Agency for Health Care Policy and Research (AHCPR): *Pressure ulcers in adults: prediction and prevention,* pub nos 92-0047 and 92-0050, Rockville, Md, 1992a, US Department of Health and Human Services, Public Health Service.

Agency for Health Care Policy and Research (AHCPR): *Preventing pressure ulcers: a patient's guide,* pub no 92-0048, Rockville, Md, 1992b, US Department of Health and Human Services, Public Health Service.

Allman RM: Epidemiology of pressure sores in different populations, *Decubitus* 2(20):30, 1989.

Ayello EA: Teaching the assessment of patients with pressure ulcers, *Decubitus* 5(4):53, 1992.

Ayello EA: A critique of the AHCPR's "Preventing pressure ulcers: a patient's guide" as a written instructional tool, *Decubitus* 6(3):44, 1993.

Baharestani MM: The lived experience of wives caring for their frail, home bound, elderly husbands with pressure ulcers, *Adv Wound Care* 7(3):40, 1994.

Bates-Jensen B: New pressure ulcer status tool, *Decubitus* 3(3):14, 1990.

Bergstrom N, Demuth PJ, Braden B: A clinical trial of the Braden scale for predicting pressure sore risk, *Nurs Clin North Am* 22(2):417, 1987.

Bergstrom N et al: *Treatment of pressure ulcers,* AHCPR pub no 95-0652, Rockville, Md, 1994, US Department of Health and Human Services, Public Health Service, Agency for Health Care Policy and Research.

Bryant RA: *Acute and chronic wounds,* St Louis, 1992, Mosby.

Flemister BG: A pilot study of interface pressure with heel protectors used for pressure reduction, *J ET Nurs* 18:158, 1991.

Graves DJ: Stage I in ebony complexion, *Decubitus* 3(4):4, 1990 (letter).

Hanson D et al: The prevalence and incidence of pressure ulcers in home care: are patients at risk? *J Home Health Care* 5(3):25, 1993.

Husain T: An experimental study of some pressure effects on tissues, with reference to the bedsore problem, *J Pathol Bacteriol* 66:347, 1953.

Itoh M et al: Accelerated wound healing of pressure ulcers by pulsed high peak power electromagnetic energy (Diapulse), *Decubitus* 4(1):24, 1991.

Johnson G, Daily C, Franciscus V: A clinical study of hospital replacement mattresses, *J ET Nurs* 18:153, 1991.

Kaminski MV, Pinchocofsky-Devin G, Williams SD: Nutritional management of decubitus ulcers in the elderly, *Decubitus* 2(4):20, 1989.

Knox DM, Anderson TM, Anderson PS: Effects of different turn intervals on skin of healthy older adults, *Adv Wound Care* 7(1):48, 1994.

Koziak M: Etiology and pathology of ischemic ulcers, *Arch Phys Med Rehabil* 40:62, 1959.

Landis EM: Micro-injection studies of capillary blood pressure in human skin, *Heart* 15:209, 1930.

Langemo DK et al: Incidences of pressure sores in acute care, rehabilitation, extended care, home health and hospice in one locale, *Decubitus* 2(2):42, 1989.

Lazzara DJ, Buschmann MT: Prevention of pressure ulcers in elderly nursing home residents: are special support surfaces the answer? *Decubitus* 4(4):42, 1991.

Leshem OA, Skelskey C: Pressure ulcers: quality management, prevalence, and severity in a long-term care setting, *Adv Wound Care* 7(2):50, 1994.

Maklebust J: Highlights: AHCPR guideline for pressure ulcer treatment, *Clinical Symposium on Pressure Ulcer Wound Management,* Nashville, Tenn, October 1994.

Maklebust J, Magnan MA: Approaches to patient and family education for pressure ulcer management, *Decubitus* 5(4):18, 1992.

Maklebust J, Sieggreen M: Pressure ulcers: guidelines for prevention and nursing management, West Dundee, Ill, 1991, S-N Publications.

Meehan M: National Pressure Ulcer Prevalence Survey, *Adv Wound Care* 7(3):27, 1994.

McKnight's Survey: Data watch: pressure sores, *McKnight's Long Term Care News* 26, 1992.

National Pressure Ulcer Advisory Panel: Pressure ulcer prevalence, cost and risk assessment: consensus development conference statement, *Decubitus* 2(2):24, 1989.

Olson B: Effects of massage for prevention of pressure ulcers, *Decubitus* 2(4):32, 1989.

Oot-Giromini BA: Pressure ulcer prevalence, incidence and associated risk factors in the community, *Decubitus* 6(5):24, 1993.

Oot-Giromini BA et al: Pressure ulcer prevention versus treatment: comparative product cost study, *Decubitus* 2(3):52, 1989.

Panel for Urinary Incontinence Guideline: *Urinary incontinence in adults,* AHCPR pub no 920038, Rockville, Md, 1992, Agency for Health Care Policy and Research, Public Health Service, US Department of Health and Human Services.

Rodeheaver G et al: Wound healing and wound management: focus on debridement, *Adv Wound Care* 7(1):22, 1994.

Trumble HC: The skin tolerance for pressure and pressure sores, *Med J Aust* 2:724, 1930.

Wright RW, Orr R: Fibroblast cytotocity and blood cell integrity following exposure to dermal wound cleaners, *Ostomy/Wound Manage* 39(7):33, 1993.

Young L: Pressure ulcer prevalence and associated patient characteristics in one long-term care facility, *Decubitus* 2(2):52, 1989.

ADDITIONAL READINGS

Hess CT: *Nurse's clinical guide: wound care,* Springhouse, Pa, 1995, Springhouse.

International Association for Enterostomal Therapy: *Standards for pressure ulcer care,* Irvine, Calif, 1987, The Association.

Krasner D, editor: *Chronic wound care: a clinical source book for health care professionals,* King of Prussia, Pa, 1990, Health Management.

Shea JD: Pressure sores: classification and management, *Clin Orthop* 112:89, 1975.

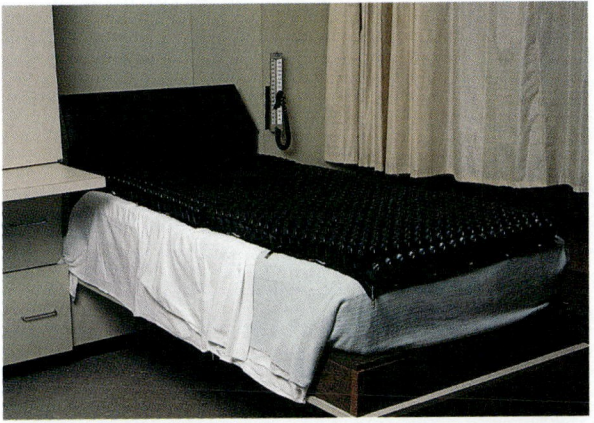

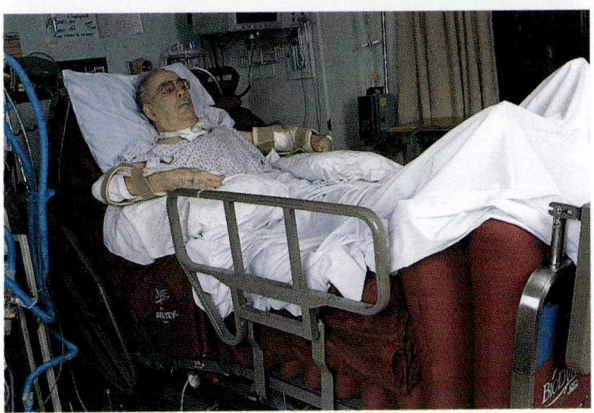

chapter 24

Special Mattresses and Beds

Nurses have at their disposal a variety of special mattresses and beds to use as adjuncts to their care. These support surfaces have differing purposes, including pressure reduction, pressure relief, rotation, and support of the morbidly obese client. These support surfaces are used in acute, rehabilitative, long-term, and home care settings.

Pressure reduction or relief is a common nursing concern in the immobile or bedridden client. According to Bryant (1992), 12 to 32 mm Hg is considered the normal pressure exerted on the capillaries. High capillary pressures (greater than 32 or even lower in the compromised client) lead to cellular ischemia and tissue damage. In a normal healthy adult, high capillary pressures stimulate a shifting of body weight to relieve pressure on the affected tissue. Repositioning distributes pressure among tissues, avoiding tissue compression and subsequent ischemia. When immobility prevents these natural shifts in weight, the client's tissue becomes compressed between his or her skeletal structure and the bed. This compression decreases circulating blood supply, leading to tissue anoxia and damage.

For clients with restricted mobility, those with chronic diseases, and elderly clients, pressure management is a significant nursing concern because these clients lack the ability to reposition themselves. Special support mattresses and beds are frequently used to reduce or relieve pressure on tissues. Support surfaces designed for uses other than pressure management include the Rotokinetic bed and the bariatric bed. The Rotokinetic bed (see Figure 24-5, p. 452) provides skeletal alignment with constant side-to-side 60- to 90-degree rotation. This rotating motion provides some pressure relief while stimulating body systems. The bariatric bed, also called an obesity bed, is wider and sturdier than standard hospital beds. It is useful in the care of the morbidly obese patient because it accommodates weights of 700 pounds.

Nursing Diagnosis

Multiple conditions (e.g., cerebrovascular accident [CVA], head injury, multiple sclerosis, chronic illness) may limit mobility and necessitate the use of specialty beds. When a client has limited physical movement, as in **Impaired Physical Mobility,** pressure reduction/relief or rotational beds may lessen the effects of immobility. Clients with actual or high risk for **Impaired Skin Integrity** may benefit from the use of pressure reduction/relief surfaces to counteract the combined effects of immobility and pressure. In situations where skin breakdown has occurred, **Risk for Infection** must be considered since the skin serves as the body's first line of defense against bacterial invasion.

Psychological factors such as **Anxiety** and **Fear** may surface, especially with the use of kinetic beds. In particular, the constant turning and rigid structure of the Rotokinetic bed may contribute to sympathetic stimulation, restlessness, increased tension, and apprehension. A sense of **Hopelessness** (passivity, lack of involvement) may be experienced if clients interpret the use of the specialty bed as a "worsening" in their condition.

Skill 24.1   Using a Support Surface Mattress

Support surfaces are widely used to reduce pressure on tissues underlying bony prominences. They may be used as a replacement mattress, actually replacing the standard hospital mattress, or as an overlay that rests on top of the hospital mattress.

Foam and air are the two prevalent types of support surfaces. A foam mattress overlay (Figure 24-1), commonly called an egg crate because of its appearance, is designed with foam peaks. The egg crate is used for client comfort, since it has minimal pressure reduction capabilities.

Foam replacement mattresses are denser, thicker, and more resilient to weight and actually decrease pressure to a much greater degree than the foam overlay.

These replacement mattresses have built-in foam, gel, or fluid sections that can be customized to a specific client's need.

The air mattress overlay rests over the mattress. It may be inflated once by the use of a blower, or it may use a pressure cycling device to inflate and deflate intermittently the air pressure among various segments of the mattress (Figure 24-2). Another available option is an air mattress that replaces the conventional mattress. These mattresses may also be fully integrated into the bed (see Skill 24.2).

Use of support surfaces simply aids in pressure reduction. Clients still must be repositioned regularly to avoid complications of immobility such as pulmonary congestion and contractures.

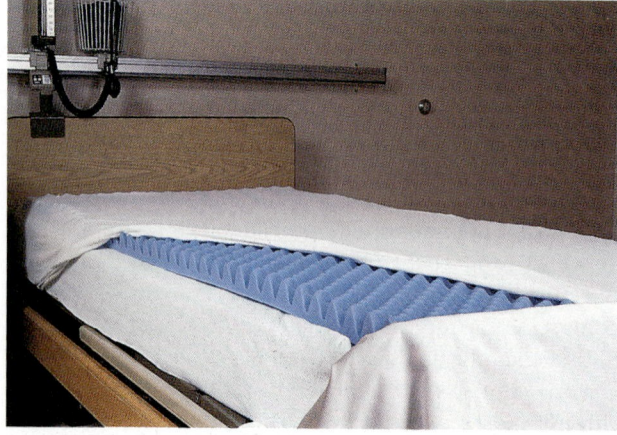

Figure 24-1 "Egg-crate" foam overlay is primarily for comfort.

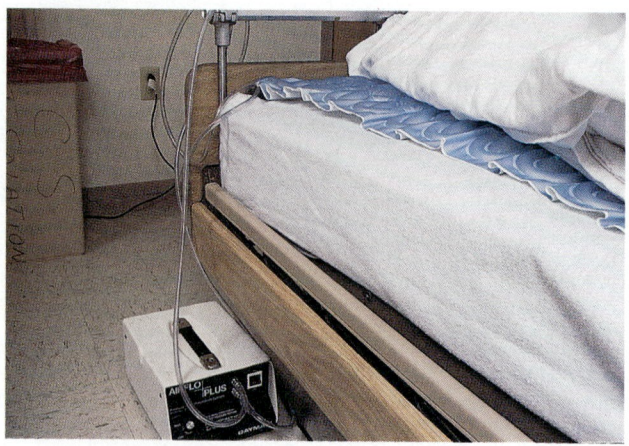

Figure 24-2

EQUIPMENT

Mattress support surface of choice:
Foam or air overlay
Foam or air mattress
Sheets

Assessment

1. Determine client's risk for pressure ulcer formation. Immobile clients are particularly vulnerable.
2. Carefully inspect the skin for erythema, induration, and blistering, especially over bony prominences. **These data provide a baseline to determine changes in client's skin.**
3. Assess client's level of comfort and presence of pain.

Implementation

4. Assess client's understanding of purposes of support surfaces.

Planning

Expected outcomes focus on maintenance of skin integrity and client comfort.

EXPECTED OUTCOMES

1. Client's skin remains intact without evidence of abnormal reactive hyperemia or mottling.
2. Existing pressure ulcers show evidence of healing by formation of granulation tissue.
3. Client rates comfort as a 4 (scale of 0 to 10).

Steps	Rationale
1. See Standard Protocol (Chapter 1, p. 5).	
2. Apply support surface to bed (bed may be occupied or unoccupied).	
a. Foam mattress replacement Remove the mattress and replace with foam mattress. Remove cushions as needed in areas of high risk for breakdown (e.g., heels). Apply sheet. Avoid wrinkles.	Pressure reduction surface reduces pressure in direct contact with the skin.
b. Foam mattress overlay (see Figure 24-1) Apply directly over hospital mattress. Leave thin protective covering in place. Apply sheet. Avoid wrinkles.	Foam egg crate surface is primarily for comfort. It minimally reduces pressure in direct contact with the skin.
c. Air mattress replacement Remove standard hospital mattress and replace with air mattress. Use blower to inflate to the appropriate pressure. Apply sheet. Avoid wrinkles. Limit the use of incontinent pads.	Air pressures may vary among manufacturers. Air pressure is necessary to distribute client's weight. Often a company representative will assist with this process to ensure appropriate use of the device.
nurse alert Avoid use of sharp objects near mattress.	Air loss secondary to tears and multiple layers decreases the effectiveness of the mattress.
d. Air mattress overlay (see Figure 24-2) Apply deflated overlay over hospital mattress. Use supplied flaps or clips to secure mattress. Use blower or continuous inflation device to inflate mattress to the desired pressure. Apply sheet. Avoid wrinkles. Check cycling on continuous cycling unit. Avoid use of sharp objects near mattress.	Intermittent cycling inflates portions of the mattress at a time that alternates pressure against the skin.
3. Position client over support surface as frequently as condition warrants to minimize pressure. Perform range of motion (ROM) exercises every shift.	Supportive surfaces only minimize pressure. Repositioning is needed to relieve pressure (see Skill 5.1) and to facilitate removal of secretions from the airways (see Skill 18.3, Step 13). ROM exercises are needed to prevent contractures (see Skill 25.1).
4. See Completion Protocol (Chapter 1, p. 6).	

Evaluation

1. Inspect condition of skin every 8 hours to determine changes in skin and effectiveness of support mattress.
2. Inspect client's pressure ulcers for evidence of granulation tissue.
3. Ask client to rate comfort on a 0 to 10 scale.

UNEXPECTED OUTCOMES AND RELATED INTERVENTIONS

1. Client develops localized areas of abnormal reactive hyperemia for longer that 30 minutes, mottling, swelling, and tenderness with evidence of breakdown. Existing pressure ulcers fail to heal or increase in size.
   a. Revise turning schedule for more frequent position changes.
   b. Avoid prolonged exposure on any one side.
   c. Keep skin clean and dry. Keep linens free of wrinkles.

   d. Notify physician. Advancement of existing pressure ulcers may be related to infection, nutritional deficiencies, or an exacerbation of other systemic factors.
   e. Evaluate need for alternative therapy (see Skill 23.2).
2. Client expresses or demonstrates discomfort.
   a. Evaluate air level of surface.
   b. Evaluate need for alternative surface.
   c. Reposition client more frequently.
   d. Unless contraindicated, provide back massage. Do not massage reddened areas, since this may contribute to skin breakdown.
3. Support surface develops a leak.
   Take corrective action in accordance with institutional policies.

SAMPLE DOCUMENTATION

1000 Foam pressure reduction overlay applied to bed. Client's skin dry and intact without erythema.

Skill 24.2 | Using an Air Suspension Bed

Air suspension beds are useful in promoting skin integrity in the immobile or bedridden client. These beds reduce the effects of shear, friction, maceration, and pressure. Air-filled cushions support and redistribute weight. Each cushion may be inflated to varying degrees of firmness to give adequate support yet minimize pressure on the bony prominences (Lovell and Anderson, 1990). A controlled amount of air is continually lost through the surface of the bed cushions. This air loss has a drying effect on the skin, which decreases the effects of maceration without dehydrating the client. Special high-air-loss cushions may also be used to draw moisture from a certain area.

As with conventional hospital beds, air suspension beds adjust to a variety of positions. In addition, these

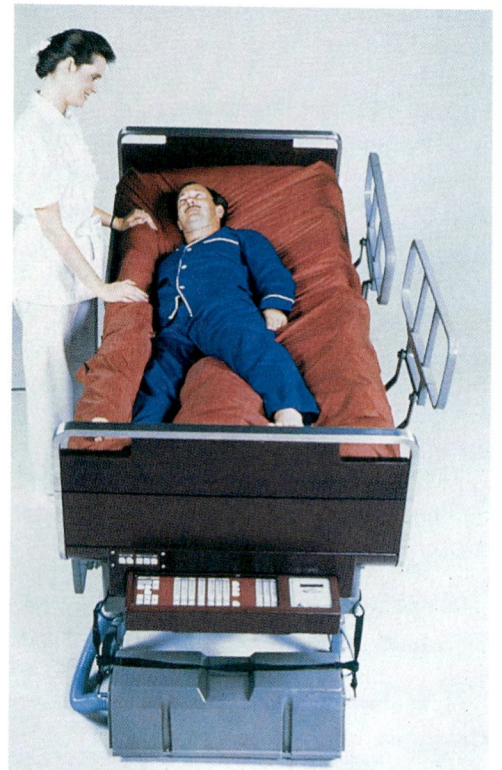

Figure 24-4 Air suspension bed. (Courtesy Kinetic Concepts, Inc. [KCI], San Antonio, Tex.)

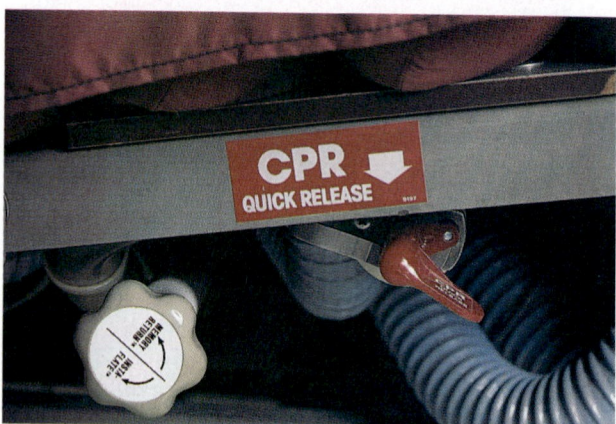

Figure 24-3

beds have cardiopulmonary resuscitation (CPR) switches (Figure 24-3), which permits immediate deflation to provide a hard surface for chest compressions. Scales may be built into the bed for ease in weighing. A battery system is necessary to maintain inflation during interruptions of power or during transport. Some air suspension beds provide gentle movement (approximately 30 degrees), which is believed to facilitate capillary circulation.

EQUIPMENT
Air suspension bed (Figure 24-4)
Gortex sheet (supplied by distributor)
Disposable bed pads, if indicated

Assessment

1. Determine client's risk for pressure ulcer formation. **Immobile clients are particularly vulnerable.**

2. Carefully inspect the skin for erythema, especially over bony prominences. **These data provide a baseline to detect changes in client's skin.**
3. Assess client's level of comfort and presence of pain.
4. Assess client's understanding of the air suspension bed.

Planning

Expected outcomes focus on the maintenance of skin integrity and comfort for the patient.

EXPECTED OUTCOMES
1. Client's skin remains intact without evidence of abnormal reactive hyperemia or mottling.
2. Existing pressure ulcers show evidence of healing by formation of granulation tissue.
3. Client rates comfort as a 4 (scale of 0 to 10).
4. Client remains alert and oriented.

Implementation

Steps	Rationale
1. See Standard Protocol (Chapter 1, p. 5).	
2. Transfer client onto air suspension bed using appropriate transfer techniques.	Appropriate transfer techniques reduce the risk of injury.
3. Turn bed on by depressing switch.	
4. Position client and perform ROM exercises routinely.	The bed minimizes pressure on skin. Frequent turning and exercising are needed to prevent joint deformity and skin breakdown.
5. Activate maximum inflation switch for turning, positioning bedpan, or other procedures. Release maximum inflation when procedure concluded.	Maximum inflation hardens the bed, thus eliminating pressure relief. Firm surface necessary for turning and other procedures.
nurse alert Activate CPR switch to quickly deflate the bed in an emergency (see Figure 24-3).	CPR switch deflates the bed within seconds to allow a firm surface for chest compressions.
6. See Completion Protocol (Chapter 1, p. 6).	

Evaluation

1. Inspect condition of skin every 8 hours to determine changes in skin and effectiveness of air suspension mattress.
2. Inspect client's pressure ulcers for evidence of granulation tissue.

3. Ask client to rate comfort on a 0 to 10 scale.
4. Observe client's level of consciousness and orientation.

UNEXPECTED OUTCOMES AND RELATED INTERVENTIONS

1. Client develops areas of breakdown, or existing areas of breakdown worsen.
   a. Evaluate and revise turning schedule as needed.
   b. Avoid prolonged exposure on any one side.
   c. Keep skin clean and dry and linens wrinkle free.
   d. Notify physician. Advancement of existing pressure ulcer may be related to tissue necrosis, infection, nutritional deficiencies, or exacerbation of other systemic factors. Surgical débridement may be required.
   e. Evaluate need for alternative therapy.
2. Client experiences restlessness or nausea or becomes disoriented because of constant flotation.
   a. Reposition patient for comfort.
   b. Notify physician. Symptomatic treatment may be required while adjusting to the bed.
   c. If unable to adjust to flotation, evaluate the need for alternative support mattress.
3. Bed malfunctions.
   Follow institutional policies to obtain replacement. Client may need to be transferred to hospital bed in the interim.

SAMPLE DOCUMENTATION

1000 Client transferred onto air suspension bed without injury. Skin warm, dry and intact without erythema or breakdown. Denies dizziness. Rates comfort as an 8 on a scale of 0 to 10.

Skill 24.3 | Using an Air Fluidized Bed

Air fluidized beds provide pressure relief, eliminate shear and friction, and decrease moisture (Bryant, 1992). These beds consist of a high, rigid, boxlike bed frame through which warm air currents continuously circulate silicone beads. The bed takes on fluid properties, making a very soft, conforming surface for the client to "float" on. The client's torso and pelvic regions are engulfed by the bed's surface as the body floats on the fluidized bed. Although the floating sensation is awkward for many clients, fluidization keeps capillary closing pressures well below the normal 32 mm Hg.

The beads absorb moisture from the sheet, keeping the client dry (Lovell and Anderson, 1990). For this reason, the nurse must continually assess the client's fluid and electrolyte status. Air fluidized beds, as with air suspension beds, are equipped with an emergency switch to be used to harden the bed. Conventional fluidized beds do not allow for head-of-bed position changes. Foam wedges are used to elevate the head of the bed. The weight of the bed structure makes transport extremely difficult.

A physician's order is required for third-party payment.

EQUIPMENT

Air fluidized bed
Foam positioning wedges
Filter sheet (supplied by the distributor)

Assessment

1. Determine client's risk for pressure ulcer formation. Immobilized clients are particularly vulnerable.
2. Carefully inspect the skin for evidence of pressure and impending breakdown. **These data provide a baseline to determine changes in client's skin.**
3. Review client's serum electrolytes.
4. Assess client's and family member's understanding of the purposes of and response to the air fluidized bed.

Planning

Expected outcomes focus on maintenance of skin integrity and adequate electrolyte balance and the client's comfort.

EXPECTED OUTCOMES

1. Client's skin remains intact without evidence of abnormal reactive hyperemia or mottling.
2. Client maintains adequate hydration, good skin turgor, moist mucous membranes. Temperature and serum electrolytes are within normal limits.
3. Client demonstrates a decrease in tension, apprehension, and restlessness in response to flotation.

Implementation

Steps	Rationale

nurse alert Review manufacturer's instructions. (Company representative may be in attendance.) Premedicate client 30 minutes before transfer if needed. Obtain additional personnel as needed.

Ensures proper and safe use of bed.

Promotes comfort during transfer for those clients in moderate to severe pain.

Aids in ensuring client's safety. Company representatives ensure proper functioning of bed.

1. See Standard Protocol (Chapter 1, p. 5).
2. Transfer client onto air fluidized bed using appropriate transfer techniques (see Chapter 5). A slide or lift may be used.

A slide or lift is needed to maneuver client over the rigid sides of the bed.

3. Depress *on* switch to begin fluidization; regulate temperature.

Fluidization relieves pressure on the skin.

4. Position client and perform ROM exercises routinely. Foam wedges are needed to place client in a Fowler's position.

Positioning and ROM exercises are necessary to prevent pulmonary complications and contractures.

5. Use fluidization switch to harden bed for turning, positioning bedpans, and other procedures. Remember to reactivate fluidization after procedure.

When fluidization is stopped, the bed becomes firm, allowing for ease in positioning. Reactivation of fluidization is necessary to minimize pressure.

nurse alert Activate CPR switch when resuscitation is necessary.

Allows for hard surface to perform manual chest compressions.

6. See Completion Protocol (Chapter 1, p. 6).

Evaluation

1. Inspect condition of skin every 8 hours to determine changes in skin and effectiveness of air fluidized therapy.
2. Observe moisture of client's skin and mucous membranes and skin turgor.
3. Monitor client's temperature and laboratory serum electrolytes.
4. Assess client's emotional response to flotation.

UNEXPECTED OUTCOMES AND RELATED INTERVENTIONS

1. Client develops areas of breakdown, or existing areas of breakdown worsen.
   a. Evaluate and revise turning schedule as needed.
   b. Keep skin clean and dry.
   c. Reevaluate the client's risk factors affecting wound healing.
   d. Notify physician. Advancement of existing pressure ulcer may be related to tissue necrosis, infection, nutritional deficiencies, or other systemic factors.

2. Client experiences agitation or restlessness related to flotation.
   a. Reposition for comfort.
   b. Provide reassurance and emotional support. Encourage client to verbalize concerns.
   c. Notify physician. Symptomatic treatment may be necessary while adjusting to constant flotation.
   d. If unable to adjust to flotation, evaluate the need for alternative measures.
3. Client's skin and mucous membranes are dehydrated and serum electrolytes are abnormal related to the temperature and evaporative effects of the bed.
   a. Evaluate nutritional and fluid status, including intake and output.
   b. Increase fluid intake unless contraindicated.
   c. Collaborate with physician for other treatment modalities.
4. The filter sheet tears, expelling small sandlike particles in the air.
   a. Cover the puncture site to prevent particles from getting on client and wounds.

b. Promptly follow the institution's policy to obtain a replacement. Client may need to be transferred to another bed while corrective measures are taking place.

SAMPLE DOCUMENTATION
1000 Client transferred onto air fluidized bed without injury. Skin warm, dry, and intact. A 3 cm reddened area noted on right scapula. Rates comfort as a 9 on a scale of 0 to 10.

Skill 24.4 | Using a Rotokinetic Bed

The Rotokinetic bed is used to maintain skeletal alignment while providing movement. It is used in the care of spinal cord–injured and multitrauma clients. The support structure of the bed outlines the body parts and maintains proper alignment when secured properly. The bed rotates from side to side at a 60- to 90-degree angle every 7 minutes. Turning angles may be adjusted to meet the client's needs. Constant rotation prevents pressure ulcer development and stimulates body systems. It is recommended that the bed stay in the rotation mode for at least 20 hours a day. There is an emergency gatch that can quickly interrupt rotation when needed.

The constant motion may lead to sensory distress for the client. This may be associated with the constant kinetic stimulation, the limited visual field, and inner ear disequilibrium. The nurse must be mindful of these complications and provide necessary emotional support.

A physician's order is required for third-party payment.

EQUIPMENT
Rotokinetic bed with support packs, bolsters, and safety straps (Figure 24-5)
Top sheet
Pillowcases for bolsters

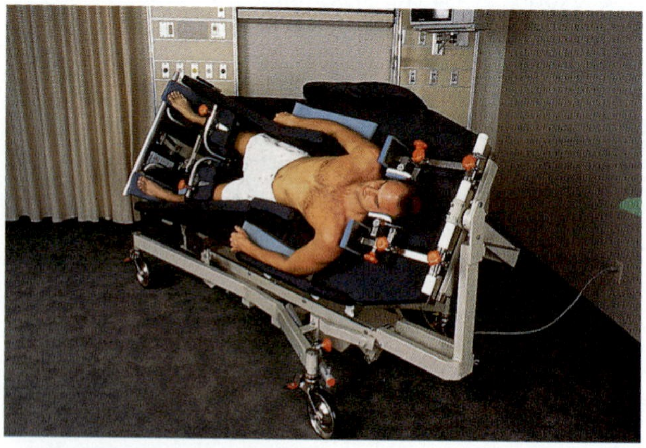

Figure 24-5 Rotokinetic bed. (Courtesy Kinetic Concepts, Inc. [KCI], San Antonio, Tex.)

Assessment

1. Determine clients who require complete immobilization and continuous skeletal alignment.
2. Carefully inspect the skin for evidence of pressure.
3. Assess the client's level of consciousness, orientation, and anxiety.
4. Assess client's breath sounds, blood pressure, height, and weight.
5. Assess the client's and family member's understanding of and response to the rotokinetic bed.

Planning

Expected outcomes are concerned with maintaining skin integrity and proper body alignment, promoting client comfort, decreasing client's anxiety, preventing pulmonary congestion, and maintaining skin integrity.

EXPECTED OUTCOMES
1. Client's skin remains intact without evidence of abnormal reactive hyperemia or mottling.
2. Existing pressure ulcers show evidence of healing by formation of granulation tissue.
3. Client's musculoskeletal system is properly aligned and free of contractures.
4. Client rates comfort as greater than 4 (scale of 0 to 10).
5. Client's breath sounds improve from baseline assessment or remain clear to auscultation.
6. Client remains alert, oriented, and cooperative.
7. Client denies nausea or dizziness.
8. Client's blood pressure remains consistent with baseline vital signs.

Implementation

Steps	Rationale

nurse alert Review manufacturer's instructions. (Company representatives may be in attendance.) Premedicate client 30 minutes before transfer if needed. Obtain additional personnel as needed.

Promotes safe use of the bed.

Promotes comfort during transfer.
Ensures client safety. Company representative to ensure proper functioning of the bed.

1. See Standard Protocol (Chapter 1, p. 5).
2. Place Rotokinetic bed in horizontal position and remove all bolsters, straps, and supports. Close posterior hatches.
3. Unplug electrical cord. Lock gatch.
4. Maintaining proper alignment, transfer client to Rotokinetic bed.
5. Secure thoracic panels, bolsters, head and knee packs, and safety straps.
6. Cover client with top sheet.
7. Plug bed in.
8. Have company representative set rotational angle as ordered by the physician. May gradually increase rotation.

9. Set full rotation as soon as client is able to tolerate it.
10. To stop bed, permit bed to rotate to desired position, and push knob in. To stop quickly, release gatch and manually maneuver bed to desired position. Push knob in.
11. See Completion Protocol (Chapter 1, p. 6).

Prevents accidental rotation during transfer.
Reduces risk of further tissue injury during transfer.

Maintains proper alignment and prevents sliding during rotation.

Rotational angle is determined by the physician based on the client's overall condition and tolerance to constant motion. Gradually increasing rotation may prevent nausea and dizziness.
Provides optimal benefit of bed.
Manual rotation may cause nausea or dizziness if done too rapidly. Bed should be stopped for no longer than 30 minutes at a time.

Evaluation

1. Inspect condition of skin (sacrum, elbows, heels, occiput, axillae, and ears) and musculoskeletal alignment every 4 hours to determine changes in skin and effectiveness of rotokinetic therapy.
2. Inspect client's pressure ulcers for evidence of granulation tissue.
3. Observe alignment and range of motion of all joints.
4. Ask client to rate comfort on a 0 to 10 scale.
5. Auscultate lung sounds every shift and compare with baseline.
6. Determine client's level of orientation once per shift while on the bed.
7. Frequently ask whether client is experiencing nausea or dizziness.
8. Monitor blood pressure for orthostatic hypotension.

UNEXPECTED OUTCOMES AND RELATED INTERVENTIONS

1. Client develops areas of breakdown, or existing areas of breakdown worsen.

   a. Evaluate rotation schedule because bed should stay in rotation for 20 hours a day to prevent breakdown.
   b. Keep skin clean and dry. Change linen on bolsters as needed.
2. Client experiences orthostatic hypotension.
   a. If severe drop in blood pressure, stop rotation. Notify physician. Monitor vital signs every 5 minutes.
   b. For less severe blood pressure changes, decrease the rotational angle. Gradually increase the rotational angle as client adjusts to rotation.
3. Client becomes disoriented, confused, or uncooperative related to sensory/perceptual distortion.
   a. Reorient client to person, place, and time.
   b. Provide audio simulation via radio or tape recorder.
   c. Provide TV secured to bed frame.
   d. Hang mirror on ceiling so that client may view surroundings.

e. Notify physician. Symptomatic treatment for motion sickness may be helpful.

4. Client develops crackles in lung fields.
   a. Have client cough and deep breathe every 2 hours.
   b. Notify physician. Incentive spirometry or other treatment measures may be warranted.

5. Bed malfunctions or fails to rotate.
   a. Ensure safety of client.
   b. Follow institutional policies to correct situation. Client may need to be transferred to conventional hospital bed in the interim.

SAMPLE DOCUMENTATION

1000 Transferred to Rotokinetic bed. Alignment maintained during transport. Bolsters, thoracic panels, head pack, and safety straps securely positioned. Initial rotation begun at 30 degrees. Client tolerating rotation without nausea, dizziness, or blood pressure changes.

Skill 24.5 | Using a Bariatric Bed

The bariatric bed is used in the care of the morbidly obese client. These beds are sturdier and wider than conventional beds yet can be maneuvered through standard doorways. These beds are capable of supporting weights of up to 700 pounds, contain an adjustable head of bed, and contain in-bed scales. Bariatric beds provide a safer environment for the patient and reduce risk of injury to the staff while positioning the obese client.

A disadvantage of this bed is the lack of pressure reduction in the mattress. This is especially a concern for the obese client who is at risk for skin impairment related to physical immobility. For this reason, pressure relief surfaces such as foam or air overlays are usually used with these beds.

A physician's order is required for third-party payment.

EQUIPMENT
Bariatric bed
Pressure relief overlay
Sheets
Overhead frame (optional)

Assessment

1. Determine client's need for bed based on height and weight. **Morbidly obese clients who have the potential for independent positioning with assistance of a stable surface will benefit from the use of a bariatric bed.**
2. Assess condition of skin. Note condition of skin between skinfolds. Note potential pressure sites.

Planning

Expected outcomes are concerned with safety, maximum independence, and maintaining skin integrity.

EXPECTED OUTCOMES
1. Client achieves as much independent positioning as possible.
2. Client remains free of injury.
3. Client's skin remains intact without abnormal reactive hyperemia.

Implementation

Steps	Rationale
nurse alert Review manufacturer's instructions. Obtain additional personnel as needed for transfer.	Promotes safe and correct use of bed. Ensures safety of client and staff during transfer.
1. See Standard Protocol (Chapter 1, p. 5).	
2. Transfer client to bed using appropriate transfer techniques.	Proper transfer techniques reduce the risk of injury.
3. Position client. Place hand controls and trapeze bar within reach.	Encourages maximum independence and mobility.
4. See Completion Protocol (Chapter 1, p. 6).	

Evaluation

1. Observe client's ability to manipulate the bed and change positions independently.
2. Assess client's risk for injury and comfort level.
3. Inspect client's skin every 8 hours for evidence of breakdown.

EXPECTED OUTCOMES AND RELATED INTERVENTIONS

1. Client is unable to operate bed independently.
   a. Assist client as needed.
   b. Consult physician regarding physical therapy or occupational therapy evaluation to increase mobility or to provide facilitative devices.
2. Client develops areas of skin breakdown, or existing areas worsen.
   a. Reevaluate need for support surface in use.
   b. Evaluate turning schedule. May need to change or shift position more frequently than every 2 hours.

SAMPLE DOCUMENTATION

1000 Transferred to bariatric bed without injury. Client demonstrated use of hand controls and trapeze bar. Skin without erythema or evidence of breakdown.

CRITICAL THINKING EXERCISES

1. What aspects of client care remain the same regardless of the type of support-surface mattress applied to the bed?
2. Charles is a 72-year-old bedridden client on an air suspension bed. He has a pressure ulcer on his coccyx.
   a. Are there any bed adjustments you should make to place Charles on the bedpan?
   b. The existing pressure ulcers are not healing. Identify how you would revise nursing care.
3. Aside from skin inspection, what additional assessment information should you gather when caring for a client placed on an air fluidized bed?
4. Identify safety precautions for transferring a client to any type of support bed.
5. During transfer of a client to a Rotokinetic bed, the nurse obtains the client's blood pressure, asks questions about nausea, and determines the client's level of orientation. Discuss the reason for this assessment.
6. Mr. Wills is a 55-year-old client hospitalized for abdominal surgery. He is 70 inches tall and weighs 410 lbs. He is unable to turn himself after surgery. He is placed on a Bariatric bed. Under what circumstances would use of the Bariatric bed not be advised?

REFERENCES

Bryant RA: *Acute and chronic wounds: nursing management,* St Louis, 1992, Mosby.
Lovell HN, Anderson C: Put your patient on the right bed, *RN* 53(5):66, 1990.

ADDITIONAL READINGS

Ceccio CM: Understanding therapeutic beds, *Orthop Nurs* (9)3:57, 1990.
Krasner D: *Chronic wound care: a clinical source book for health care professionals,* King of Prussia, Pa, 1990, Health Management.
Frantz R, Xakellis G, Arteaga M: The effects of prolonged pressure on skin blood flow in elderly patients at risk for pressure ulcers, *Decubitus* 6(6):16, 1993.
Maklebust J, Sieggreen M: *Pressure ulcers: guidelines for prevention and nursing management,* West Dundee, Ill, 1991, S-N Publications.
Thomason S, Hawley G, Wurzel J: Speciality support surfaces: a cost containment perspective, *Decubitus* 6(6):32, 1993.

chapter 25

Promoting Range of Motion

Skill 25.1
Range of Motion Exercises

Skill 25.2
Continuous Passive Motion Machine

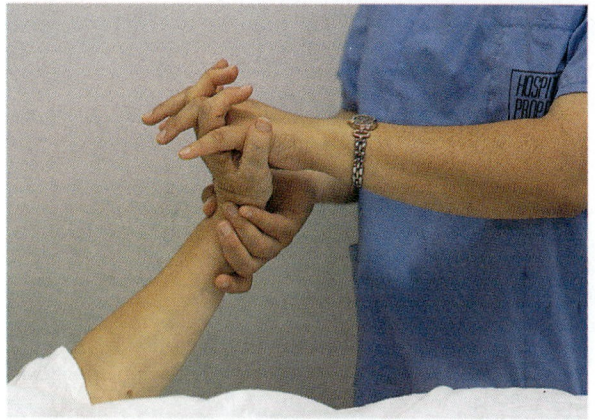

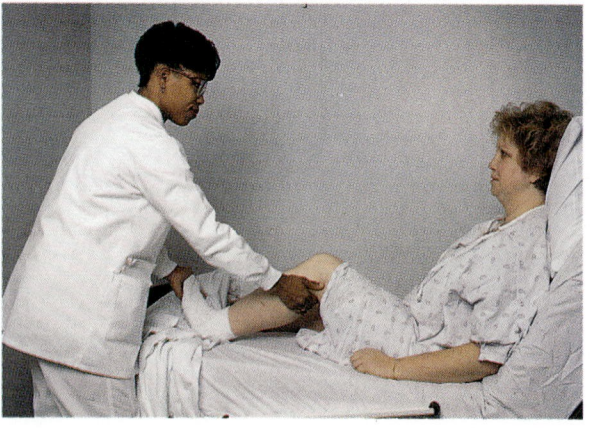

The range of motion of a joint is the maximum movement that is possible for that joint. Each person's range is determined by genetic inheritance, developmental patterns, the presence or absence of disease, and the person's normal amount of physical activity.

Range of motion (ROM) exercises have a number of purposes: (1) to restore, maintain, or increase the tone and strength of the muscles; (2) to maintain or increase the flexibility of the joints; (3) to maintain or promote the growth of bones through application of physical stressors; and (4) to improve the functioning of other body systems, such as the cardiovascular and gastrointestinal systems.

Being hospitalized is a disruption in a person's mobility and may lead to an altered health status. Each system may then be at risk for impairment. Examples of medical conditions that can alter mobility are musculoskeletal conditions such as fractured extremities or muscle sprains, neurological conditions such as spinal cord trauma, degenerative neurological conditions such as myasthenia gravis, and head injuries. Some clients may not actually be immobilized by an injury or musculoskeletal problem but are prescribed bed rest or restricted ambulation for therapeutic conditions or infectious problems (Perry and Potter, 1994).

Regardless of whether the causes of immobility are permanent or temporary, the immobilized client must receive some type of exercise to prevent excessive muscle atrophy and joint contracture. The total amount of activity required to prevent physical disuse syndrome is only about 2 hours for every 24-hour period, and this activity must be scheduled throughout the day to prevent the client from remaining inactive for long periods (Perry and Potter, 1994).

Nurses need to assess clients for individual mobility levels. If the client is mobile and can move about freely, the client can independently perform activities of daily living (ADLs) and ROM exercises. If the client is partially immobile or unable to move about freely (paraplegic, quadriplegic), the nurse or a mechanical device is needed to assist the client with ROM exercises.

Nurses are responsible for assessing the need for and implementing interventions to prevent complications associated with immobility. Frequent interventions used to prevent complications include coughing and deep-breathing exercises, frequent repositioning and turning to prevent problems with skin integrity, upper and lower extremity exercises to prevent contracture of the muscles, adequate hydration, and well-balanced meals to maintain muscle strength and endurance. It is important to initiate ROM exercises early. The client will profit by actively participating in the level of care, which decreases length of stay and the risk for further impairment in body functions (Beare and Myers, 1994).

Nursing Diagnosis

Risk for Impaired Physical Mobility is appropriate when the inability to move independently could result in the development of contractures or decreased strength and endurance. **Altered Health Maintenance** may be related to lack of knowledge or difficulty following through with prescribed ROM exercises.

Skill 25.1 | Range of Motion Exercises

Range of motion exercises may be active, passive, or active assisted. They are *active* if the client is able to perform the exercise independently and *passive* if the exercises are performed for the client by someone else. *Active-assisted* exercises are done by a client with only some assistance by the nurse. A client who is weak or partially paralyzed may be able to move a limb partially through ROM. In this case the nurse can help the client perform active-assisted ROM exercises by helping the client finish the full ROM. Another form of active-assisted exercise is when a client uses the strong arm to exercise the weaker or paralyzed arm (Perry and Potter, 1994). The nurse should always encourage the client to be as independent as possible. Active ROM exercises should be encouraged and supervised every day by the nurse. Active ROM exercises can be incorporated into the client's ADLs (Table 25-1).

Passive ROM exercises should be performed by the nurse only if the client is unable to perform the activity (e.g., exercising the lower extremities in a paraplegic client). Passive ROM exercises help maintain joint function but do not exert enough muscle tension to maintain muscle tone (Perry and Potter, 1994).

Passive ROM can also be performed mechanically by a continuous passive motion (CPM) machine. Many orthopedic surgeons routinely order a knee CPM machine postoperatively for a total knee arthroplasty (replacement). ROM machines are also used for continuous passive motion specifically to the hip, ankle, shoulder, wrist, and fingers. These types of CPM machines are used less frequently and are not discussed in this book. CPM machines must be applied correctly to the client to obtain correct flexion and extension. The knee CPM machine is discussed in full detail in Skill 25.2.

EQUIPMENT
No mechanical or physical equipment is needed.

Assessment

1. Review client's chart for physician orders, medical diagnosis, past medical history, and client's progress. **The nurse must know client's history and physician's specific order to determine appropriate ROM exercises.**
2. Assess client's readiness to learn. Explain all rationale for the ROM exercises and what specific exercises will be performed. **This allows client time to express questions and concerns before the implementation begins.**
3. Assess client's level of comfort (scale 0 to 10) before exercising. **This information determines if client will be able to perform the ROM exercises without further discomfort or if an analgesic will be required before the exercises are performed.**
4. Assess for activity/mobility. **This information determines whether specific ROM activities can be performed without added risk to client's existing health status.**

Planning

Expected outcomes focus on client's physical and emotional ability to perform exercises.

Table 25-1 Incorporating Active ROM Exercises into Activities of Daily Living

Joint exercised	Activity of daily living	Movement
Neck	Nodding head yes	Flexion
	Shaking head no	Rotation
	Moving right ear to right shoulder	Lateral flexion
	Moving left ear to left shoulder	Lateral flexion
Shoulder	Reaching to turn on overhead light	Extension
	Reaching to bedside stand for book	Extension
	Scratching back	Hyperextension
	Rotating shoulders toward chest	Abduction
	Rotating shoulders toward back	Adduction
Elbow	Eating, bathing, shaving, grooming	Flexion, extension
Wrist	Eating, bathing, shaving, grooming	Flexion, extension, hyperextension, abduction, adduction
Fingers and thumb	All activities requiring fine motor coordination (e.g., writing, eating, hobbies)	Flexion, extension, abduction, adduction, opposition
Hip	Walking	Flexion, extension, hyperextension
	Moving to side-lying position (knee flexed)	Flexion, extension, abduction
	Moving from side-lying position (knee extended)	Extension, adduction
	Rolling feet inward	Internal rotation
	Rolling feet outward	External rotation
Knee	Walking	Flexion, extension
	Moving to and from a side-lying position	Flexion, extension
Ankle	Walking	Dorsiflexion, plantar flexion
	Moving toe toward head of bed	Dorsiflexion
	Moving toe toward foot of bed	Plantar flexion
Toes	Walking	Extension, hyperextension
	Wiggling toes	Abduction, adduction

EXPECTED OUTCOMES

1. Client experiences less pain (on a scale of 0 to 10) after taking pain medication.
2. Client verbalizes how to incorporate ROM exercises into ADLs.
3. Client assists with or performs ROM exercises independently and correctly two times daily by time of expected discharge. The client lists all incorrect activities performed at the time of the exercises.
4. Client verbalizes to significant other how to perform active-assisted ROM exercises.
5. Significant other correctly performs passive ROM on client by discharge.

Implementation

Steps	Rationale

1. See Standard Protocol (Chapter 1, p. 5).

2. 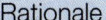 Wear gloves (only if there is wound drainage or skin lesions).

3. Assist the client to a comfortable position, preferably sitting or lying down.

4. When performing active-assisted or passive ROM exercises, support joint by holding distal and proximal areas adjacent to joint (Figure 25-1), by cradling distal portion of extremity (Figure 25-2), or by using cupped hand to support joint (Figure 25-3).

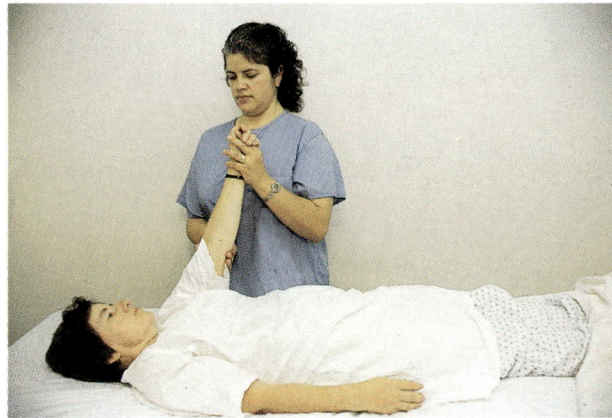

Figure 25-1

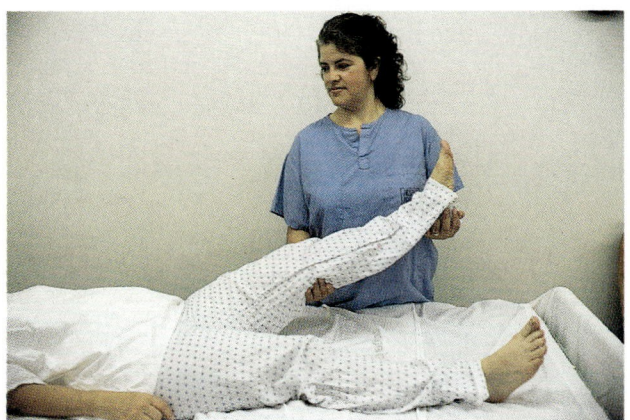

Figure 25-2

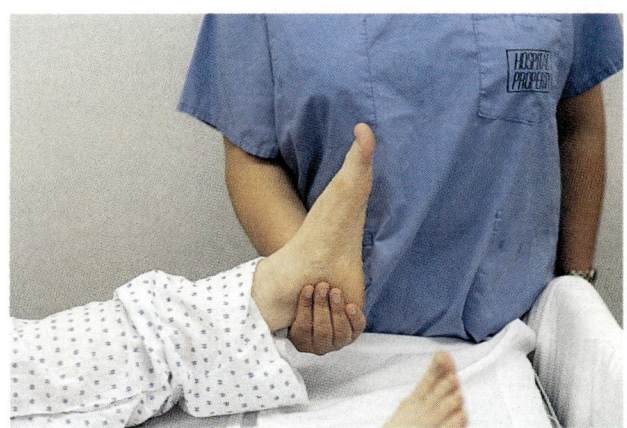

Figure 25-3

5. Begin following exercises in sequence outlined. Each movement should be repeated five times during exercise period.

It is easiest to perform exercises in head-to-toe format.

nurse alert Discontinue exercise if client complains of discomfort or if there is resistance or muscle spasm. Ranges are measured in degrees (e.g., ROM: 45°).

a. **Neck**
   (1) *Flexion:* Bring chin to rest on chest (ROM: 45°) (Figure 25-4).

Adequate ROM in all directions permits satisfactory visual fields and increased level of independence. If flexion contracture of neck occurs, client's neck is permanently flexed with chin toward or actually touching chest. Ultimately, client's total body alignment is altered, visual field is changed, and overall level of independent functioning is decreased.

Steps	Rationale

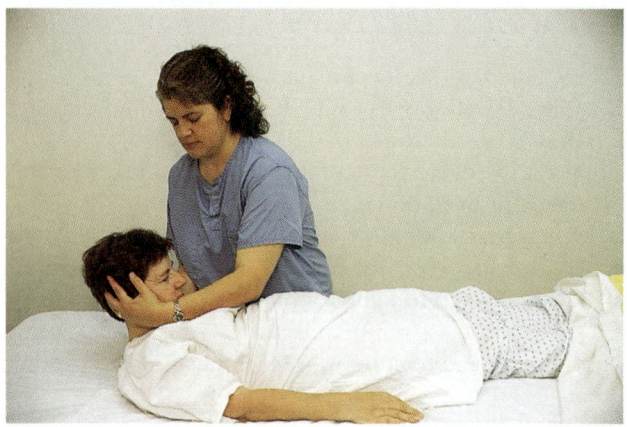

Figure 25-4

(2) *Extension:* Return head to erect position (ROM: 45°).

(3) *Hyperextension:* Bend head as far back as possible (ROM: 10°) (Figure 25-5).

(4) *Lateral flexion:* Tilt head as far as possible toward each shoulder (ROM: 40° to 45°) (Figure 25-6, *A*).

(5) *Rotation:* Rotate head in circular motion (ROM: 360°) (best done in sitting position) (Figure 25-6, *B*).

(6) Turn head side to side (Figure 25-6, *C*).

b. **Shoulder**

(1) *Flexion:* Raise arm from side position forward to above head (ROM: 180°) (Figure 25-7, *A*).

(2) *Extension:* Return arm to position at side of body (ROM: 180°).

(3) *Hyperextension:* Move arm behind body, keeping elbow straight (ROM: 45° to 60°) (Figure 25-7, *B*).

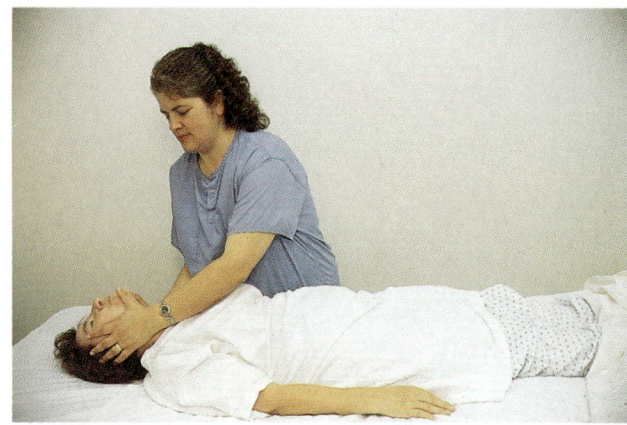

Figure 25-5

Exercising shoulder actively increases power of deltoid muscle and facilitates use of crutches or a walker.

A frozen shoulder makes it impossible to reach overhead and makes dressing difficult.

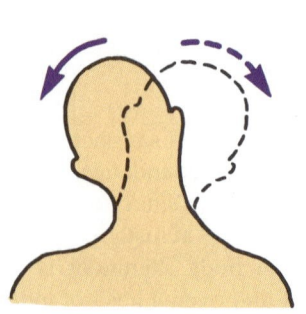

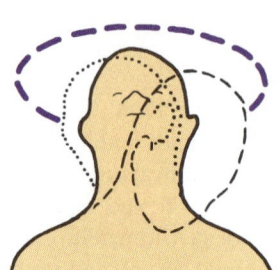

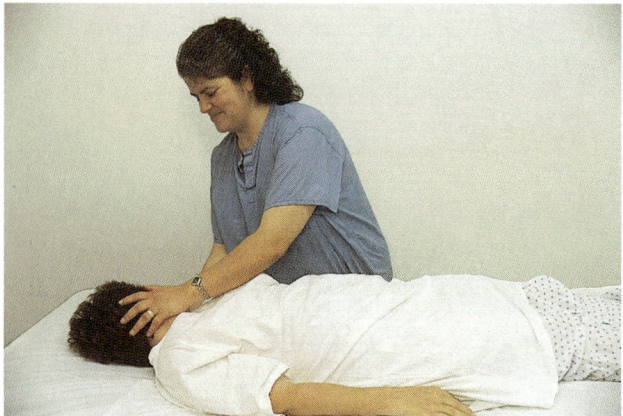

A   B   Figure 25-6   C

Steps	Rationale

(4) *Abduction:* Raise arm to side to position above head with palm away from head (ROM: 180°) (Figure 25-8, *A*).

(5) *Adduction:* Lower arm sideways and across body as far as possible (ROM: 320°) (Figure 25-8, *B*).

(6) *External rotation:* With elbow flexed, move arm until thumb is upward and lateral to head (ROM: 90°) (Figure 25-9, *A*).

(7) *Internal rotation:* With elbow flexed, rotate shoulder by moving arm until thumb is turned inward and toward back (ROM: 90°) (Figure 25-9, *B*).

(8) *Circumduction:* Move arm in full circle. Circumduction is a combination of all movements of ball-and-socket joint (ROM: 360°) (Figure 25-10).

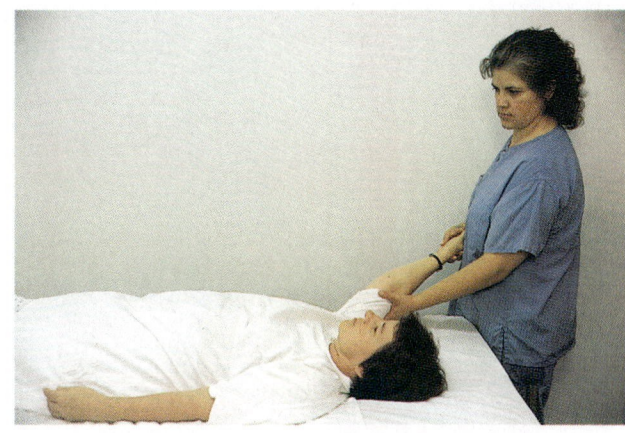

A

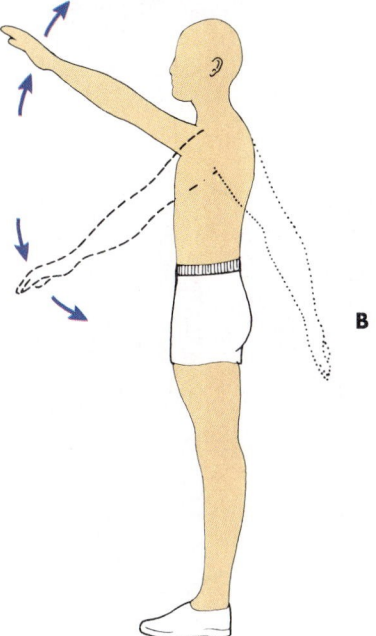

B

Figure 25-7

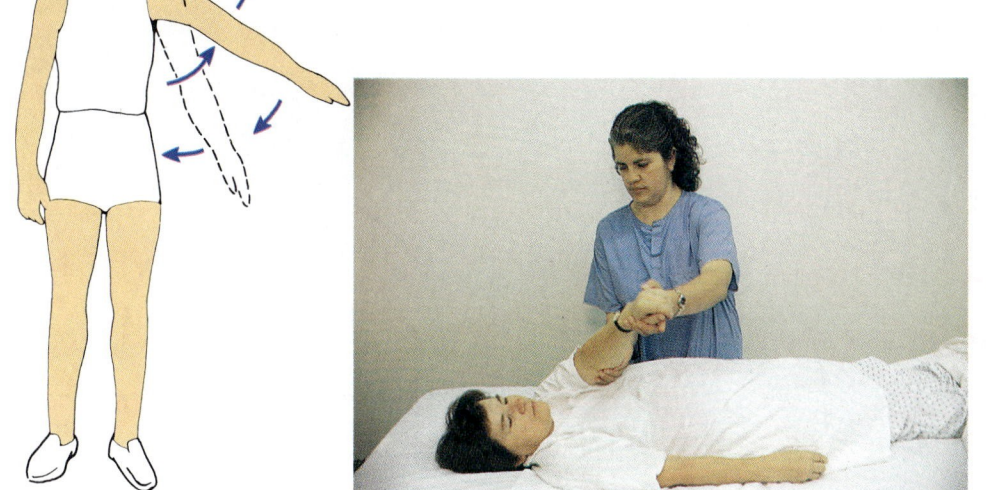

Figure 25-8

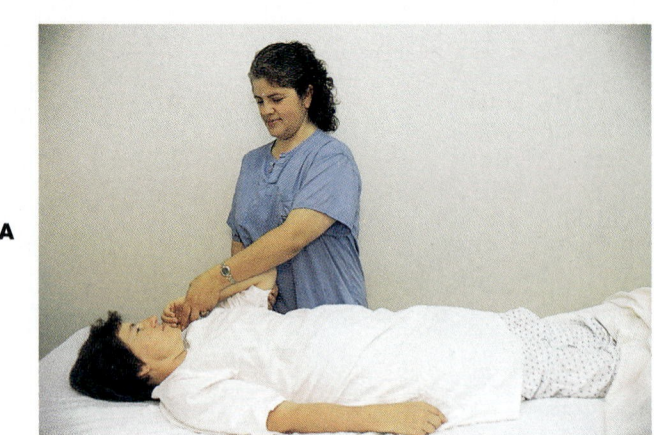
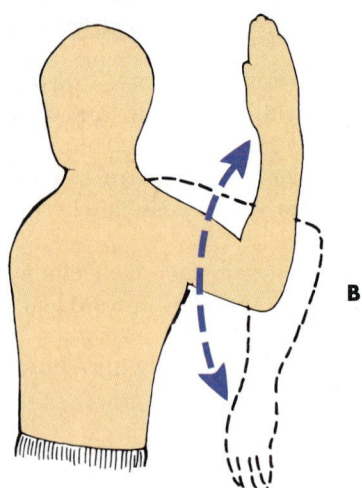

Figure 25-9

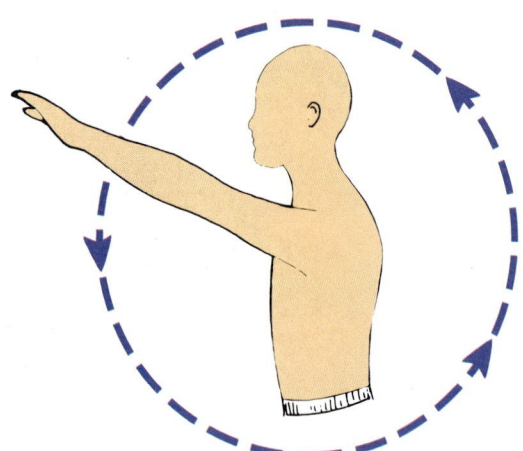

Figure 25-10

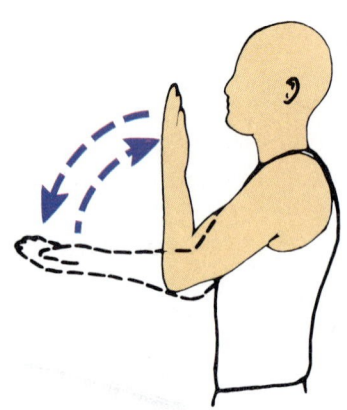

Figure 25-11

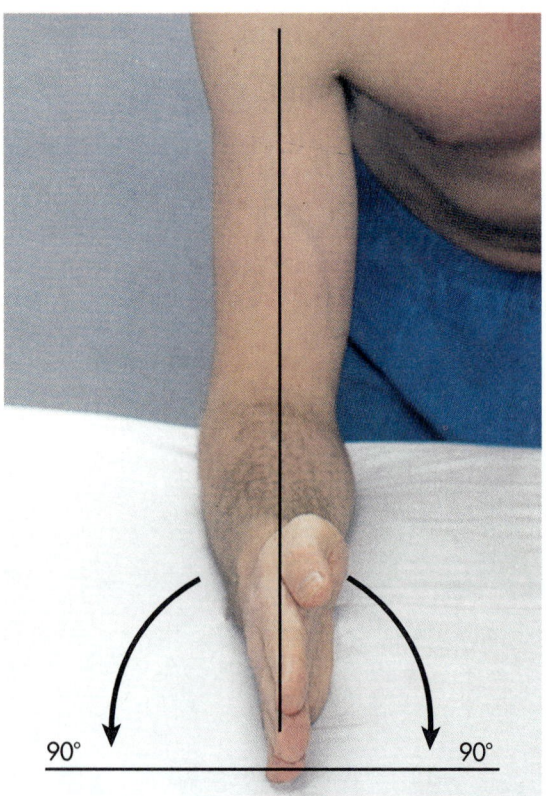

Supination   Pronation

Figure 25-12 (From Mourad LA: *Orthopedic disorders*, Mosby's Clinical Nursing Series, St. Louis, 1991, Mosby.)

Steps	Rationale

c. **Elbow**
  (1) *Flexion:* Bend elbow so that lower arm moves toward its shoulder joint and hand is level with shoulder (ROM: 150°) (Figure 25-11).
  (2) *Extension:* Straighten elbow by lowering hand (ROM: 150°) (Figure 25-11).
  (3) *Hyperextension:* Bend lower arm back as far as possible (ROM: 10° to 20°).

Elbow fixed in full extension or full flexion is very disabling and limits client's independence.

d. **Forearm**
  (1) *Supination:* Turn lower arm and hand so that palm is up (ROM: 70° to 90°) (Figure 25-12).
  (2) *Pronation:* Turn lower arm so that palm is down (ROM: 70° to 90°) (Figure 25-12).

Forearm rotates from supination to pronation.

e. **Wrist**
  (1) *Flexion:* Move palm toward inner aspect of forearm (ROM: 80° to 90°) (Figure 25-13, *A*).

If wrist becomes fixed in even slightly flexed position, client's grasp is weakened. Wrist strength is necessary to be able to use crutches.

  (2) *Extension:* Move palm so fingers, hands, and forearm are in the same plane (ROM: 80° to 90°).
  (3) *Hyperextension:* Bring dorsal surface of hand back as far as possible (ROM: 80° to 90°) (Figure 25-13, *B*).
  (4) *Abduction (radial flexion):* Bend wrist medially toward thumb (ROM: up to 30°) (Figure 25-14, *A*).
  (5) *Adduction (ulnar flexion):* Bend wrist laterally toward fifth finger (ROM: 30° to 50°) (Figure 25-14, *B*).

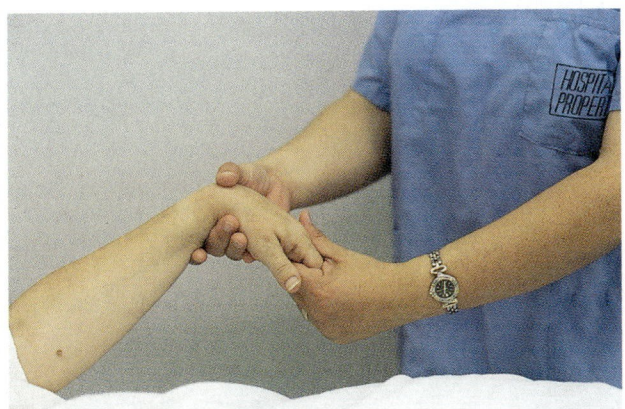

A

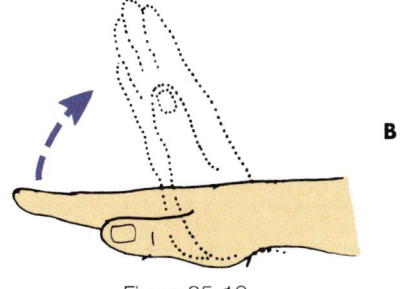

B

Figure 25-13

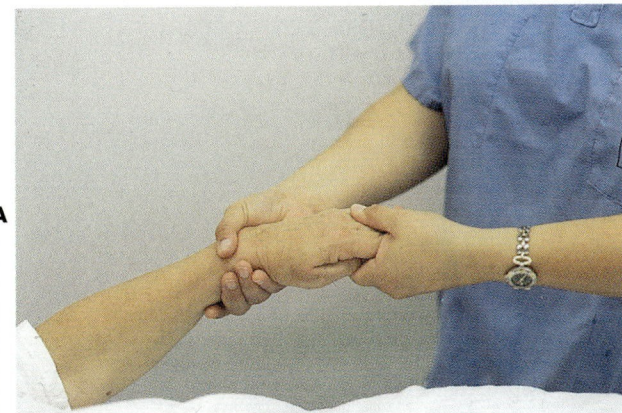

A

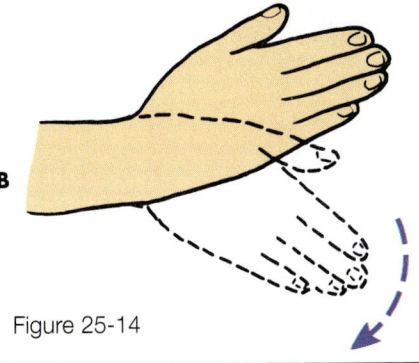

B

Figure 25-14

Steps	Rationale

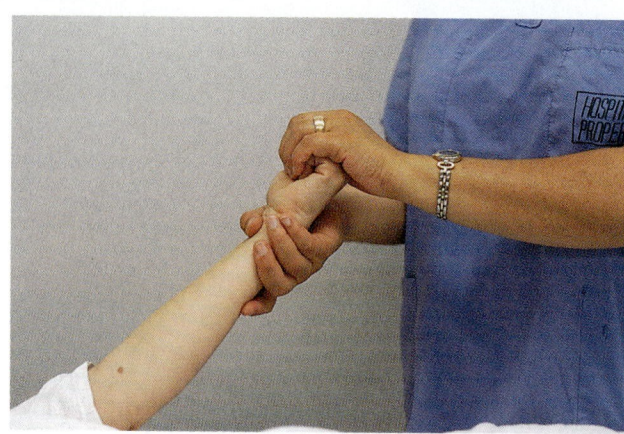

Figure 25-15

f. **Fingers**
   (1) *Flexion:* Make fist (ROM: 90°) (Figure 25-15).

   (2) *Extension:* Straighten fingers (ROM: 90°).

   (3) *Hyperextension:* Bend fingers back as far as possible (ROM: 30° to 60°) (Figure 25-16).
   (4) *Abduction:* Spread fingers apart (ROM: 30°) (Figure 25-17).
   (5) *Adduction:* Bring fingers together (ROM: 30°) (Figure 25-17).

Flexibility of fingers and thumb is necessary to grasp items (e.g., holding onto a crutch or using feeding utensils).

If not stretched into extension, natural tendency is for flexion. (In between ROM sessions, client with cerebrovascular accident (CVA) may need a firm device placed in hand to prevent full flexion.)

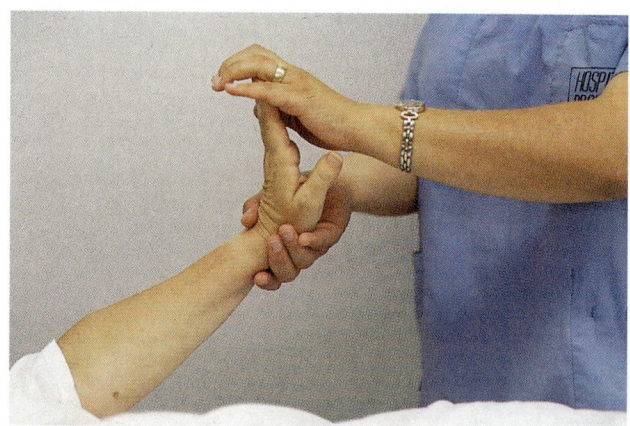

Figure 25-16

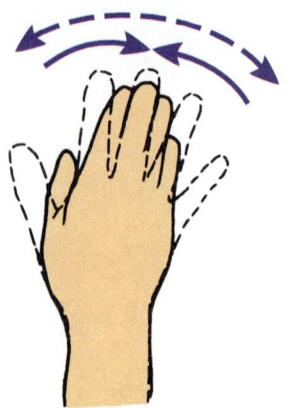

Figure 25-17

Steps	Rationale

g. **Thumb**

(1) *Flexion:* Move thumb across palmar surface of hand (ROM: 90°) (Figure 25-18, *A*).

(2) *Extension:* Move thumb straight away from hand (ROM: 90°).

(3) *Abduction:* Extend thumb laterally (usually done when placing fingers in abduction and adduction) (ROM: 30°).

(4) *Adduction:* Move thumb back toward hand (ROM: 30°).

(5) *Opposition:* Touch thumb to each finger of same hand (Figure 25-18, *B*).

Flexibility of thumb maintains coordination for fine motor activities.

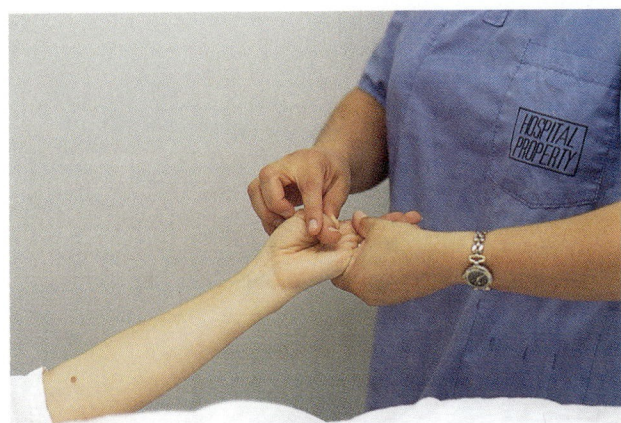
A

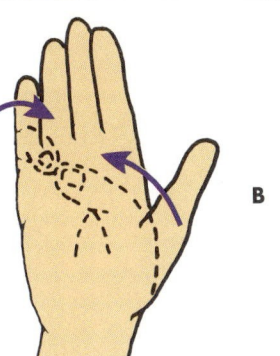
B

Figure 25-18

h. **Hip**

(1) *Flexion:* Move leg forward and up (ROM: 90° to 120°) (Figure 25-19).

(2) *Extension:* Move leg back beside other leg (ROM: 90° to 120°).

(3) *Hyperextension:* Move leg behind body (best done standing or lying on abdomen) (ROM: 30° to 50°) (Figure 25-20).

(4) *Abduction:* Move leg laterally away from body (ROM: 30° to 50°) (Figure 25-21).

(5) *Adduction:* Move leg back toward medial position and beyond if possible (ROM: 30° to 50°) (Figure 25-21).

(6) *Internal rotation:* Turn foot and leg toward other leg (ROM: 90°) (Figure 25-22).

(7) *External rotation:* Turn foot and leg away from other leg (ROM: 90°).

(8) *Circumduction:* Move leg in circle (ROM: 360°) (Figure 25-23).

Adequate ROM in lower extremities (i.e., hip, knee, ankle, foot) allows client to walk with stable gait.

Contracture of hip can cause unsteady gait or difficulty ambulating.

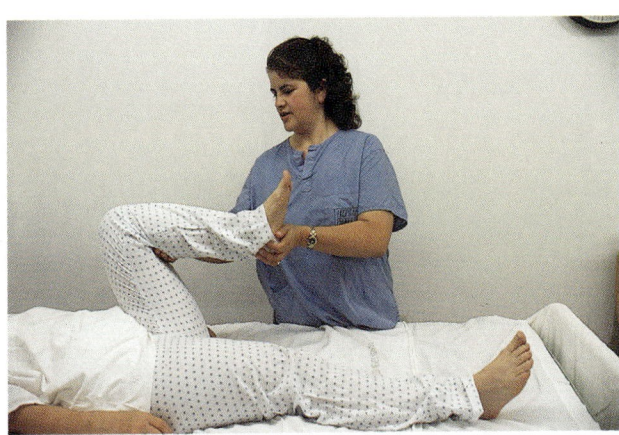
Figure 25-19

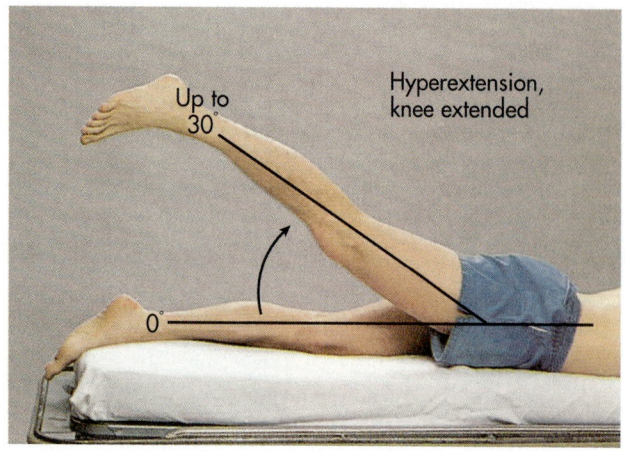

Figure 25-20 (From Mourad LA: *Orthopedic disorders,* Mosby's Clinical Nursing Series, St. Louis, 1991, Mosby.)

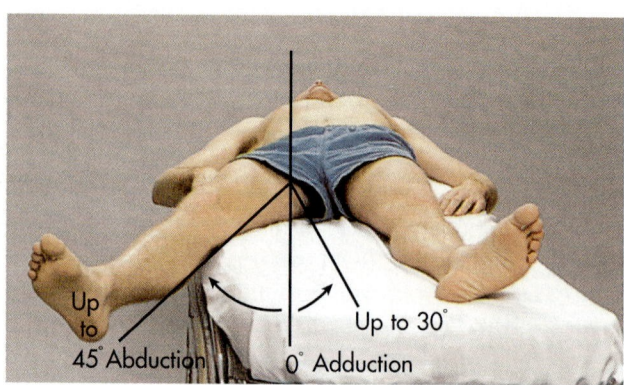

Figure 25-21 (From Mourad LA: *Orthopedic disorders,* Mosby's Clinical Nursing Series, St. Louis, 1991, Mosby.)

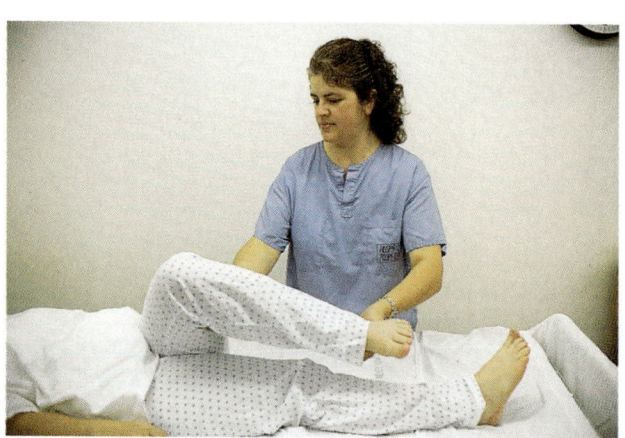

Figure 25-22

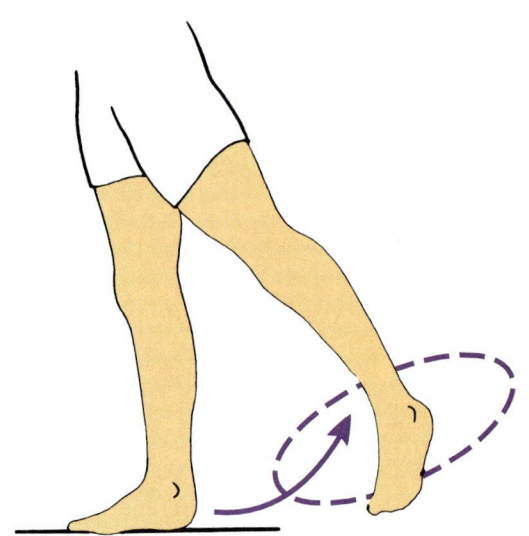

Figure 25-23

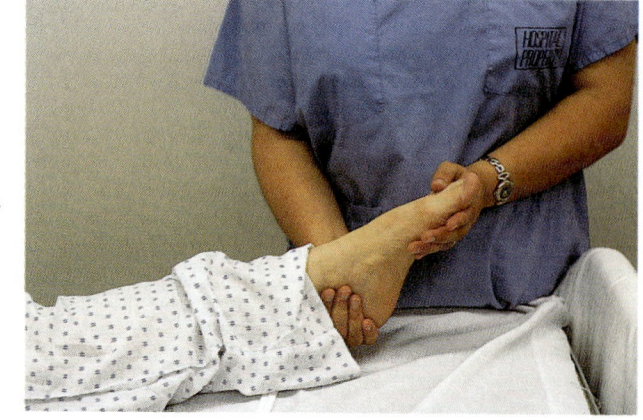

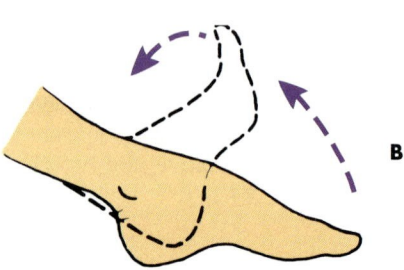

Figure 25-24

Steps	Rationale

  i. **Knee**
  (1) *Flexion:* Bring heel toward back of thigh (done with hip flexion) (ROM: 120° to 130°).
  (2) *Extension:* Return leg to straight position on bed (ROM: 120° to 130°).

Stiff knee can result in severe disability, degree of which depends on position in which knee is stiffened. If knee is fixed in full extension, client must sit with leg thrust straight out in front. If knee is fixed in any flexed position, client limps when walking or may be unable to "touch down" with foot.

  j. **Ankle**
  (1) *Plantar flexion:* Move foot so toes are pointed downward (ROM: 45° to 50°) (Figure 25-24, *A*).
  (2) *Dorsal flexion:* Move foot so toes are pointed upward (ROM: 20° to 30°) (Figure 25-24, *B*).

Deformity of ankle can impair client's ability to walk.

  k. **Foot**
  (1) *Inversion:* Turn sole of foot medially (ROM: 10° or less) (Figure 25-25).
  (2) *Eversion:* Turn sole of foot laterally (ROM: 10° or less) (Figure 25-25).
  (3) *Flexion:* Curl toes downward (ROM: 30° to 60°).
  (4) *Extension:* Straighten toes (ROM: 30° to 60°).
  (5) *Abduction:* Spread toes apart (ROM: 15° or less).
  (6) *Adduction:* Bring toes together (ROM: 15° or less).

Adequate ROM of foot permits steady gait and stable base of support.
Adequate ROM in lower extremities allows client to walk.

6. See Completion Protocol (Chapter 1, p. 6).

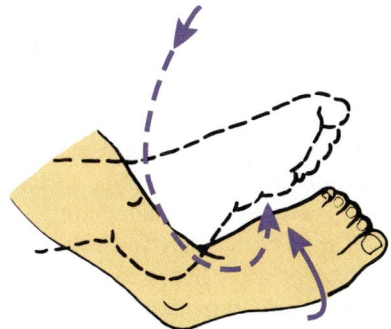

Figure 25-25

Evaluation

1. Ask client to rate any discomfort on a scale from 0 to 10.
2. Ask client to demonstrate active ROM exercises during selected ADLs.
3. Observe client perform ROM activities.
4. Observe client perform active-assisted ROM exercises.
5. Observe significant other perform passive ROM exercises on client.

UNEXPECTED OUTCOMES AND RELATED INTERVENTIONS

1. Client experiences discomfort with ROM exercises.
   a. Reposition client to a comfortable position.
   b. Premedicate client 30 minutes before ROM exercises begin, if necessary.
2. Client cannot perform ROM exercises correctly.
   a. Assess if joint is capable of ROM (presence of prior injury or contracture).
   b. Demonstrate specific exercises to client thoroughly.
   c. Provide illustrations to client regarding specific ROM exercises.
3. Client is extremely anxious regarding exercises to be performed.
   a. Provide further emotional support to client.
   b. Teach use of progressive relaxation.
   c. Review problem-solving process.

SAMPLE DOCUMENTATION

0900 Client able to correctly perform hip flexion >90 degrees 5 times without sign of fatigue.

1300 Client incorrectly performed hip flexion exercises. Client reinstructed on correct technique; was able to correctly perform hip flexion exercises >90 degrees 5 times without signs of fatigue. Client verbalized understanding of the correct and incorrect way to perform the specific ROM exercises.

Skill 25.2 Continuous Passive Motion (CPM) Machine (for Patient with Total Knee Replacement)

The CPM machines are designed to exercise many different joints, including the hip, ankle, shoulder, wrist, and fingers. These specific machines are used less frequently in the hospital and more often in outpatient physical therapy or home health settings and therefore are not discussed in this chapter. The most common CPM used in the hospital setting is the knee CPM. The knee CPM is discussed here in detail.

The purpose of the CPM machine is to mobilize the knee joint early enough and thoroughly enough to prevent contracture, muscle atrophy, venous stasis, and thromboembolism. Passive movement of the joint can replace more strenuous exercises during the first few postoperative days. Properly used, the CPM can decrease complications and shorten a client's hospital stay (Maier, 1986).

The electronically controlled CPM machine flexes and extends the knee to a desired degree and at a set speed as ordered by the physician. There are many different brands and models. They differ slightly, but each includes a full-length leg cradle hinged at the knee and ankle, a foot support, a motor controller, an electric plug, and an on/off switch. The foot support and the cradle frame adjust to fit the length of the client's thigh and calf. The frame is metal or plastic. Sheepskin or liners are available from most manufacturers. Velcro straps attached to the liner loosely strap the leg to the cradle. When the device is turned on, the frame slides slowly back and forth, gently moving the joint through preset ROM (Birdsall, 1986).

Continuous passive motion (CPM) may be initiated on the day of surgery or on the first postoperative day, according to individual surgeon's preference. If initiated on the day of surgery, heavier wound drainage should be expected (Johnson, 1993).

Before the CPM can be adjusted, it is applied to the client's affected lower extremity. This process will take two hospital personnel because the CPM is heavy and weighs approximately 20 to 25 pounds. Using two hospital personnel will (1) prevent damage to the client's knee and (2) prevent unnecessary strain on the staff's backs.

EQUIPMENT
CPM machine and sheepskin that is applied to the CPM (Figure 25-26).

Assessment

1. Check the machine for electrical safety.
2. Assess the setup of the machine before placing on bed: check the stability of the frame, the flexion/extension controls, speed controls, and the on/off switch. **This ensures that all pieces of the equipment are operational and will prevent damage to the client's knee.**
3. Assess the client for comfort before and during use. **This determines if the client will be able to tolerate the CPM at the ordered flexion and extension.**
4. Assess the client's ability and willingness to learn about the CPM machine.

Planning

Expected outcomes focus on activity tolerance, physical mobility, and skin integrity.

Expected Outcomes

1. Client increases length of time in CPM machine by 2 hours every day with no evidence of increased heart rate or increased blood pressure.
2. Client increases flexion 10 degrees daily, starting at 0 degrees extension and 40 degrees flexion. (By discharge, the client should have increased flexion to almost 90 degrees.)
3. Client maintains intact skin throughout use of CPM.

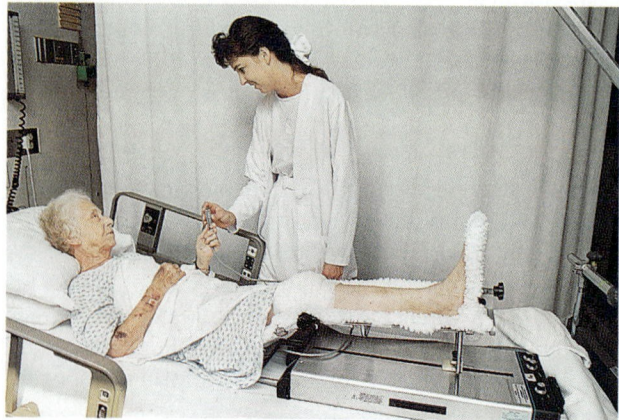

Figure 25-26

Implementation

Steps	Rationale

1. See Standard Protocol (Chapter 1, p. 5).
2. 🖐 Wear gloves (if wound drainage is present).

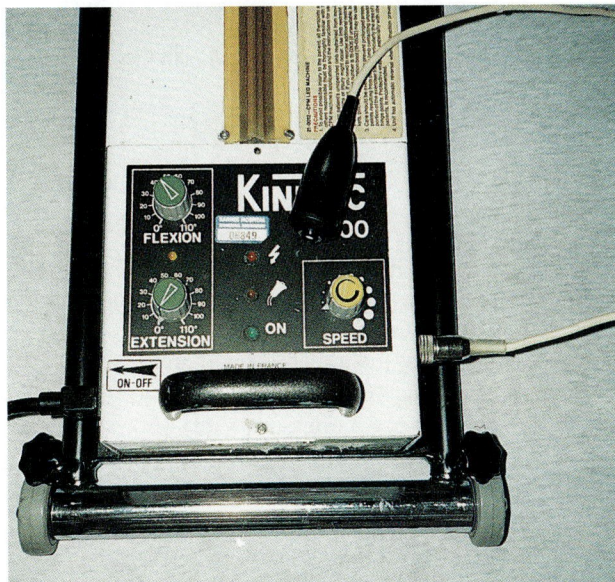

Figure 25-27

3. Test all CPM controls to make sure they are functional (Figure 25-27).

Testing equipment first saves time for nurse and client. A malfunctioning machine can cause damage to client's knee and may increase client's pain.

4. Stop the machine in full extension.

This position allows correct fit of client's leg.

5. Place client's leg in the machine, being sure to support above, below, and at knee.

Two nurses perform this step to prevent damage or injury to client or nurse.

6. Fit CPM machine to client by lengthening and shortening appropriate section of the CPM frame.

Ensures a proper fit.

7. Align client's knee joint (bend of the knee) with the machine knee hinge, then position the client's knee 2 cm below knee joint line of the CPM.

This is extremely important because if the client's new knee is not properly aligned, the knee may be damaged.

8. Center client's leg in the machine to avoid pressure on the knee joint.
   Adjust the foot support to approximately 20 degrees of dorsiflexion to prevent footdrop.

Footdrop is an abnormal condition caused by damage of the peroneal nerve and can cause abnormal gait.

9. When client's leg is in correct position, secure the Velcro straps across lower extremity (thigh) and top of foot (Figure 25-28).

Correct placement of the thigh and foot strap prevents friction and skin breakdown.

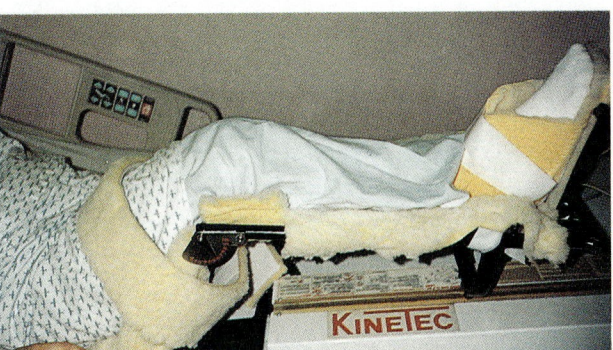

Figure 25-28

Steps	Rationale
10. Start CPM machine. Watch at least two full cycles of 40 degrees flexion and 0 degrees extension.	Ensures that CPM machine is fully operational at the pre-set flexion and extension modes.
11. Make sure client is comfortable. Provide client with the on/off switch. Instruct to use only if CPM seems to be malfunctioning.	Allows client to stop the machine if the degree of flexion/extension or speed changes, creating intolerable discomfort.
12. See Completion Protocol (Chapter 1, p. 6).	

Evaluation

1. Ask client to keep a log of when the CPM machine is in use, with times and dates.
2. Observe client at the initial onset of an increase in the flexion of the machine.
3. Observe skin every 2 hours for signs of breakdown.

UNEXPECTED OUTCOMES AND RELATED INTERVENTIONS

NOTE: Because of new insurance guidelines regarding length of stay in the hospital, most clients are discharged in a relatively short period of time. If the client needs additional physical therapy to maintain function of the new knee replacement and to increase flexion, client may be placed in a temporary rehabilitation facility or be sent home with a CPM machine.

1. Client cannot increase flexion by 10 degrees daily.
   a. Increase activities throughout the day to improve muscle strength (e.g., ambulation, physical therapy exercises).
   b. Give "time out" periods throughout the day to rest the leg.
2. Client experiences increased pain when in CPM machine.
   a. Provide analgesic as prescribed.
   b. Release leg out of CPM until pain subsides.
3. Client develops reddened areas on heel from foot support.
   a. Readjust foot in CPM machine every 2 hours.
   b. Pad the foot support more.
   c. Loosen straps and check skin every 2 hours.

SAMPLE DOCUMENTATION

1000 Functional CPM applied to client's left leg. Client able to tolerate 0 degrees extension and 40 degrees flexion at slow speed. Prescribed analgesic offered to client and given 2 TC#3 tablets. Areas of skin assessed for breakdown. Skin dry and intact.

1200 Client tolerating CPM well at 0-40 degrees. Stated the TC#3 tablets took care of his pain in the left knee. Skin assessed for breakdown, top of left foot slightly red under CPM foot strap. Foot repositioned in CPM and strap readjusted to a secure but loose position. Reassessment will be done in 1 hour.

CRITICAL THINKING EXERCISES

1. Critique the following situation. Is the ROM procedure appropriate for this situation? Mr. Johnson is a 68-year-old who had a recent stroke. His wife is performing full range of motion to the left side, which is weak. Mr. Johnson has full ROM on the right side.
2. Mr. Marshall is a 65-year-old client hospitalized for pneumonia. He has a history of arthritis. During morning care, Mr. Marshall completes the following activities. Determine what aspects of range of motion have been completed during these activities.
   a. Walking to the vanity
   b. Brushing teeth
   c. Gargling
   d. Washing face, neck, arms, torso
   e. Washing perineal area and thighs
   f. Standing and putting on new pajamas
   g. Combing hair
3. Differentiate between active, passive, and active-assisted range of motion in the following situations.
   a. The nurse observes a client going through hip range of motion.
   b. A paraplegic client performs range of motion to his lower extremities.
   c. The nurse performs range of motion on a comatose client.
   d. A client with a total knee replacement is receiving range of motion via a machine.
   e. The physical therapist assists the client in performing full range of motion to a partially paralyzed extremity.
4. You are caring for a client who has had a total knee replacement. The surgeon has prescribed a CPM machine for continuous range of motion. Identify two essential procedural steps that prevent damage or injury to the client during application of the device.

REFERENCES

Beare P, Myers J: *Principles and practice of adult health nursing,* ed 2, St Louis, 1994, Mosby.

Birdsall C: How do you use the continuous passive motion device? *Am J Nurs* 86(6):657, 1986.

Johnson RL: Total shoulder arthroplasty, *Orthop Nurs* 12(1):14, 1993.

Maier P: Take the work out of range of motion exercises, *RN* 49(9), 1986.

Mourad L: *Orthopedic disorders,* St Louis, 1991, Mosby.

Perry A, Potter P: *Clinical nursing skills and techniques,* ed 3, St Louis, 1994, Mosby.

ADDITIONAL READINGS

Diehm S: CPM devices . . . continuous passive motion, *J Burn Care Rehabil* 9(5):498, 1988.

Dugan MC: PROM: where a little movement means a lot, *Nurs Manage* 23(5):92, 1992.

Garrett B, Lavender D: Continuous passive motion CQI project, *Nurs Admin Q* 17(4):41, 1993.

Glick OJ: Intervention related to activity and movement, *Nurs Clin North Am* 27(2):541, 1992.

Oagley C: Basic ROM exercises for forearm and wrist, *Patient Care* 26(4):104, 1992.

Rush K, Ouellet L: Mobility: a concept analysis, *J Adv Nurs* 18(3):486, 1993.

Smith J: Applying the continuous passive motion device, *Orthop Nurs* 9(3):54, 1990.

Strang EL, Johns JL: Nursing care of the patient treated with continuous passive motion following total knee arthroplasty, *Orthop Nurs* 3(6):27, 1984.

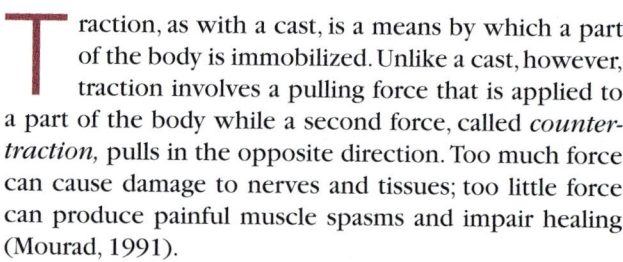

chapter 26

Traction

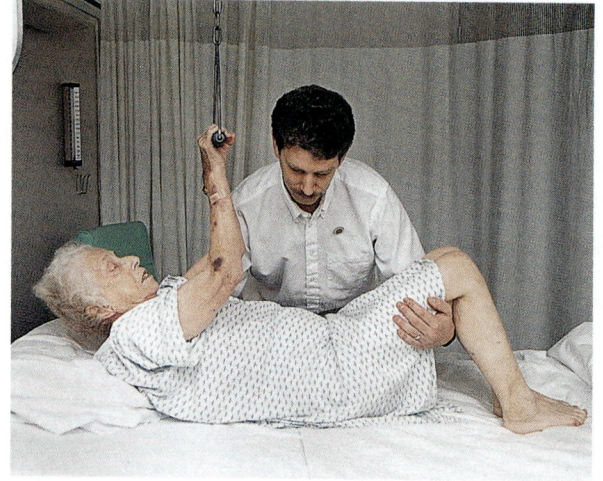

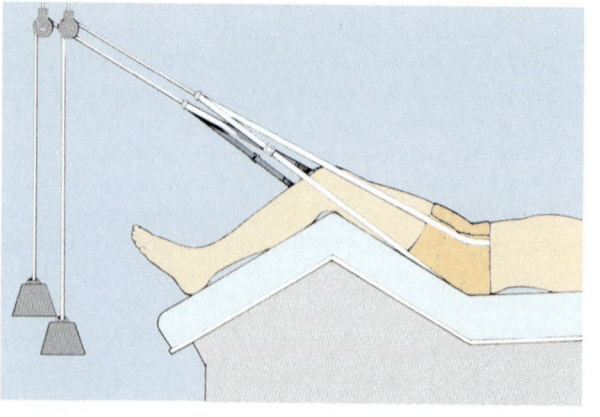

Traction, as with a cast, is a means by which a part of the body is immobilized. Unlike a cast, however, traction involves a pulling force that is applied to a part of the body while a second force, called *countertraction,* pulls in the opposite direction. Too much force can cause damage to nerves and tissues; too little force can produce painful muscle spasms and impair healing (Mourad, 1991).

The pulling force of traction is provided through a system of pulleys, ropes, and weights attached to the client; the countertraction is often achieved by elevating the foot or head of the bed and therefore is supplied by the client's body. In *balanced* traction, the amount of force in the traction is equal to the amount of force in the countertraction. A *suspension* is a mechanism that suspends a body part by using traction equipment, but it does not involve a pulling force. However, traction may be added to a suspension. In *straight* or *running* traction, the traction force pulls against the long axis of the body, and the countertraction is supplied by the client's body. In a *suspension* or *balanced* traction, the affected part is supported by a sling, hammock, or the body and partly by a system of weights attached to an overhead frame with pulleys and ropes (Mourad, 1991).

Traction is prescribed for one or more of the following general uses: (1) correction of deformities, (2) gradual correction or improvement of a joint contracture, (3) treatment of a dislocation, (4) reduction of a fracture, (5) treatment of disease processes of the musculoskeletal system, (6) preoperative and postoperative positioning and alignment, and (7) general immobilization of specific areas of the body (Hilt and Cogburn, 1980). The two general types of traction are skin traction and skeletal traction.

The particular type of traction applied to the client is determined by the physician with regard to (1) the client's injury or condition, (2) the traction's purpose, (3) the client's age, (4) the client's weight, (5) the condition of the skin tissues to be placed in traction, and (6) the length of time the client will need to be kept in traction (Thompson et al., 1993).

The client must be prepared both physically and emotionally for the traction. The need for a specific traction is determined by the client's history, the physical examination, and x-ray results. The skin surfaces involved in the specific traction are examined carefully for open areas, bruises, rashes, and scars. The injury or deformity is assessed, and a complete neurovascular assessment is done. The chest, abdomen, and head are examined appropriately if one of these areas is to be placed in traction.

The physician discusses the benefits and risks of the proposed traction with the client and significant others for informed consent and to relieve anxiety or concerns. A sedative may be administered if ordered. The traction may be applied in the client's room, in the surgical suite, or in the recovery room, depending on the type of traction and the client's condition. Skin traction (also referred to as Buck's traction when placed on the lower part of the leg) may be applied by the physician, nurse, or other orthopedic technician. If applied by the nurse or technician, the traction is to be checked by the physician as soon as possible for the client's safety and to determine the accuracy of the traction setup and direction of pull. The physician orders the amount of weight applied, whether the traction can be intermittent (only for skin traction) or whether the traction can be off at night (orders may be "in 2 hours, out 2 hours at night"), and other special considerations that are to be followed while the client is in the specific traction (Mourad, 1991).

Clients in traction often must stay in bed for weeks or even months. Nursing care involves supporting activities of daily living (ADLs), maintenance of the traction, and prevention of problems related to immobility such as pressure sores. Although there are many types of traction for different parts of the body, five general principles usually apply for all types of traction: (1) maintain the established line of pull, (2) prevent friction, (3) maintain countertraction, (4) maintain continuous traction unless ordered otherwise, and (5) maintain correct body alignment (Beare and Myers, 1994).

Older adults are particularly prone to the development of broken skin integrity when they are bedridden and not repositioned frequently. This tendency results from a decreased amount of subcutaneous fat and skin that is less elastic, thinner, drier, and more fragile than that of a younger adult.

Nursing Diagnosis

Nursing diagnoses for clients in traction focus on comfort and prevention of complications. **Anxiety** related to pain and/or immobility is appropriate when the traction results in muscle spasms or if immobilization creates nervous tension. **Risk for Impaired Skin Integrity** and **Risk for Impaired Gas Exchange** are appropriate if traction is maintained continuously for weeks. All nursing diagnoses related to immobility also need to be considered.

Skill 26.1 | Maintaining Skin Traction

Skin traction (Figure 26-1) is the application of a light pulling force directly to the skin and soft tissue that indirectly pulls on the skeletal system. The amount of force that can be exerted is limited by the tolerance of the skin; the weight is usually 5 pounds. Skin traction may be continuous (following fracture of an extremity or hip to provide traction and relieve muscle spasm) or intermittent (for back discomfort such as to relieve sciatic pain). Skin traction is used for shorter periods than skeletal traction and is a potential source of skin irritation and pressure problems. The more weight applied to the traction, the greater is the chance of skin breakdown. It may be contraindicated for clients with skin problems such as ulcers, dermatitis, burns, or abrasions. Elderly clients and those with diabetes or poor circulation are at increased risk (Burrell, 1992).

The most common type of adult skin traction is Buck's traction. Other common types of skin traction that can be used, but are not discussed here, include: Alvik traction, Hamilton-Russell traction, Bryant's traction, and Cortels traction. The purpose of skin traction is to relieve muscle spasms, restrict movement, and provide proper alignment in cervical disk diseases, pelvic fractures, and spinal deformities (Swager, 1993). Skin traction can also be used for the preoperative immobilization of a fractured hip, as is the case with Buck's traction (Osborne and DiGiacomo, 1987).

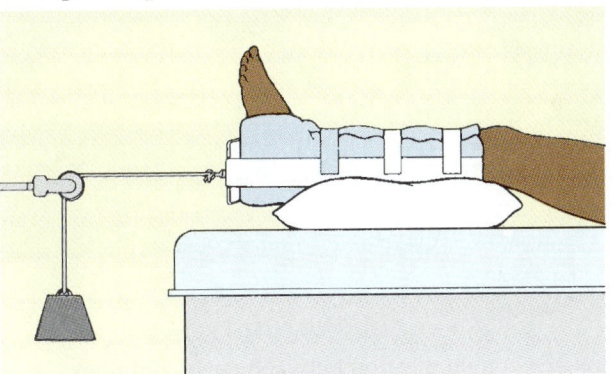

Figure 26-1

EQUIPMENT

Overhead frame
Traction bar
Cross clamp and pulley
Rope
Buck's traction boot
5-pound weight

Assessment

1. Assess client's position in bed. Client should be supine, perpendicular to the ends of the bed, with the affected limb in proper body alignment. **This ensures proper application of the skin traction.**
2. Assess client's need for analgesics before procedure begins. **This decreases client's discomfort while applying skin traction.**
3. Assess traction setup: (weights hanging freely, ordered amount of weight applied, ropes moving freely through pulleys, all knots tight in ropes and away from pulleys). **This ensures accurate function of traction.**

4. Assess affected limb for skin breakdown and pressure sores before applying skin traction.
5. Assess neurovascular status of extremity distal to the traction, including skin color and temperature, capillary refill, sensation, presence of pulses, and client's ability to move digits. **This provides necessary baseline information and detects neurovascular complications.**
6. Assess client's ability and willingness to cooperate.

Planning

Expected outcomes focus on client's mobility, comfort level, breathing, skin integrity, and nutrition.

EXPECTED OUTCOMES

1. Client moves all extremities independently by date of discharge.
2. Client verbalizes a sense of comfort after repositioning and administration of analgesics.
3. Skin under traction boot remains clear of pressure and breakdown.

Implementation

Steps	Rationale
1. See Standard Protocol (Chapter 1, p. 5).	
2. Position client so that affected leg is halfway between edge of the bed and middle of the bed.	Ensures proper alignment of Buck's traction.
3. Raise height of the bed to provide proper body mechanics for nurse.	Prevents injury to nurse's lower back.
4. Explain procedure to client.	Alleviates anxiety.
5. Apply foam boot to client's affected leg.	
6. Apply cross clamp and pulley to overhead frame (Figure 26-2).	
7. Apply rope to boot and through pulley.	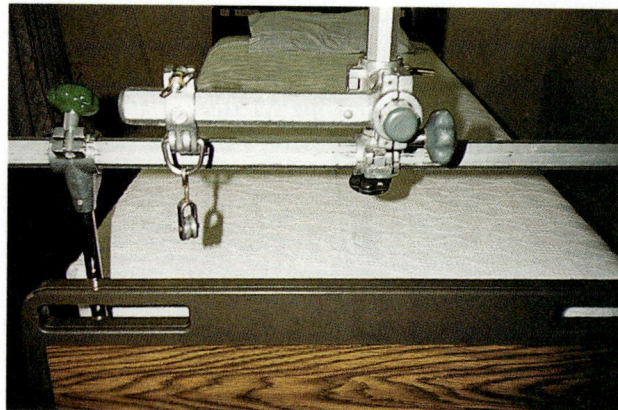 Figure 26-2
8. Tie rope to weight and hang weight gradually and gently at end of the bed.	
9. Ask client if position is comfortable.	Ensures communication between client and nurse.
10. See Completion Protocol (Chapter 1, p. 6).	

Evaluation

1. Observe client's use of trapeze and overhead frame with unaffected limbs to reposition self correctly.
2. Ask client to rate discomfort on a scale of 0 to 10.
3. Inspect skin tissues for signs of pressure, color changes, edema, or tenderness.

UNEXPECTED OUTCOMES AND RELATED INTERVENTIONS

1. Client complains of increased pain after Buck's traction is applied.
   a. Take the traction off (if allowed by physician), reposition client, and then reapply the traction.
   b. Administer analgesics as prescribed.
2. Client has reddened areas on leg under Buck's traction boot.
   a. Take foam boot off for 1 hour to relieve pressure if ordered by physician.
   b. Foam boot should always be applied securely (nurse should be able to insert one finger between client's skin and Buck's traction boot). Recheck correct tightness frequently.
   c. Increase skin checks to every hour.
   d. Apply protective barrier agent (e.g., Aloe Vista) to affected limb for protection against breakdown.

SAMPLE DOCUMENTATION

0900 Buck's traction applied to client's left leg by RN and then rechecked by physician. Client tolerated application of Buck's traction and stated no pain medication needed.

1100 Client assessed for comfort. States he is "hurting a lot." Medicated with 5 mg morphine sulfate IM. Buck's boot taken off. Skin assessed and no breakdown evident. Buck's reapplied. Client repositioned. No skin breakdown noted to heels, coccyx, or back.

1200 Client reassessed for comfort. Verbalized that pain medication helped and that pain is almost gone. Client resting comfortably at present.

Skill 26.2 | Skeletal Traction Assessment and Care

Skeletal traction (Figure 26-3) is the application of a force directly to bone that provides a strong, steady, continuous pull. The use of such devices as pins, wires, or tongs inserted into bone enables direct longitudinal pull. Skeletal traction is always applied by the physician under sterile technique. A local anesthetic is given to the client before pin insertion to provide comfort. A Steinmann pin and Kirschner wire (Figure 26-4) are used for pin insertion for balanced-suspension skeletal traction. The traction force itself is applied to a traction bow that is attached to the wire or pin. The attachments can withstand the stress of up to 40 pounds of weight for extended periods (6 to 8 weeks) (Burrell, 1992). Uses of skeletal traction include fractures of the femur below the trochanter, fractures of the cervical spine, and some fractures of the bones of the arm or ankle. The purpose is to immobilize bones for longer periods to allow healing.

External fixation is a frequently used form of skeletal traction involving one of a variety of frames of apparatuses to hold pins drilled into or through bones (Figure 26-5). External fixation frames have been used for skull and facial fractures, ribs, all bones of the upper and lower extremities, and pelvic bones. Frames may fit on one side of a bone or bones or may be attached to pins on either side of an injured limb (Perry and Potter, 1994). Usually a client is discharged with an external fixator and must be taught specific guidelines for care of the device at home (e.g., pin care, assessment of pin sites, assessment of apparatus for displacement).

EQUIPMENT

Skeletal traction
   Sterile gloves
   Sterile Kirschner wire tray
   Local anesthetic (1% to 2% lidocaine)
   Drill
   Skin preparation solution (Betadine scrub)
   Ropes
   Pulleys
   Weights
   Weight holders
   Felt
   Antiseptic ointment
Pin care supplies
   Sterile applicators
   Sterile normal saline
   Hydrogen peroxide (in 1:1 mixture with normal saline)
   Sterile container
   Disposable gloves

Assessment

1. Observe client's nonverbal behavior and response to traction, and answer questions. **This alleviates anxiety toward pending application of skeletal traction.**
2. Assess client for level of pain. **Use as baseline for future comparisons.**

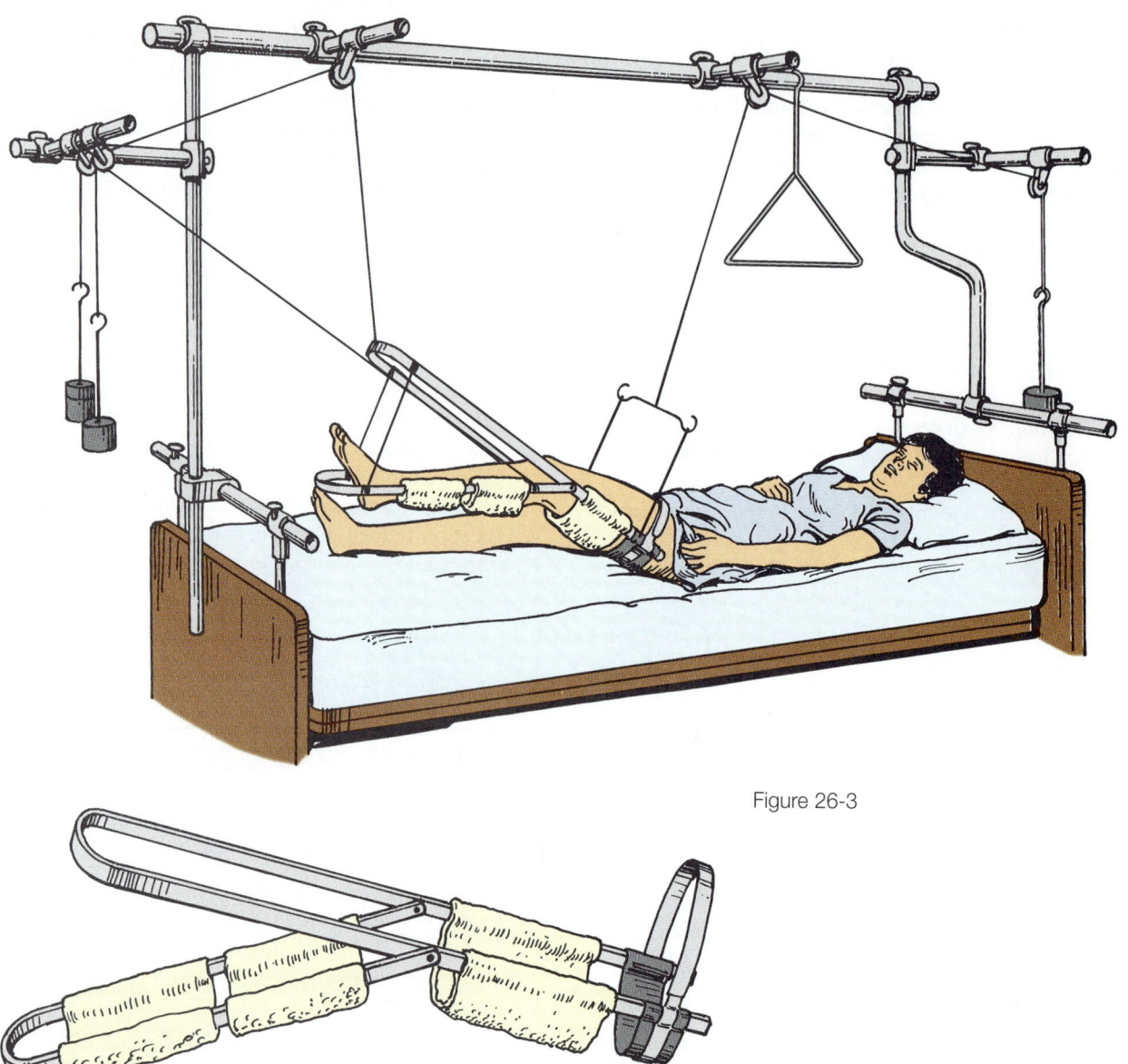

Figure 26-3

3. Assess neurovascular status of extremity distal to the traction, including skin color and temperature, capillary refill, sensation, presence of pulse, and ability to move digits. **This provides necessary baseline information and detects neurovascular complications.**
4. Assess equipment. **Making sure all pieces of equipment are operational promotes client's safety.**
5. Assess client's mobility. **This determines client's ability to participate in repositioning and ADLs.**
6. Assess pin sites for redness, edema, discharge, or odor. **This determines presence of infection.**

Planning

Expected outcomes focus on client's anxiety level, self-care abilities, comfort and mobility level, and infection risks.

Expected Outcomes

1. Client repositions self with assistance.
2. Client retains strength and endurance in unaffected extremities.
3. Skin around pin sites shows no evidence of redness, swelling, or drainage.
4. Client experiences a decrease in the amount of discomfort.
5. Client performs ADLs independently to all unaffected areas.

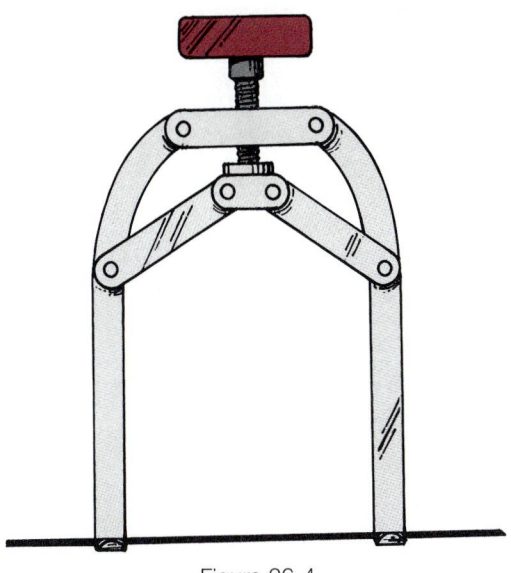

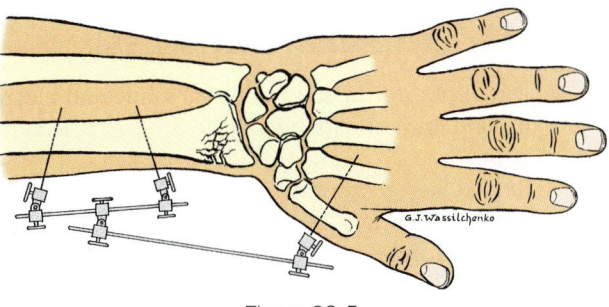

Figure 26-5

Figure 26-4

Implementation

Steps	Rationale
1. See Standard Protocol (Chapter 1, p. 5).	
2. Administer sedative as ordered.	
3. Position client in bed as requested by physician. Client will often be supine with head slightly elevated.	Ensures proper alignment of traction.
4. Explain procedure to client, emphasizing importance of maintaining counterbalance and position.	Decreases anxiety.
5. Provide for privacy.	Decreases embarrassment.
6. Obtain all equipment necessary and assist physician in applying the skeletal traction (if done at the bedside).	Assisting physician decreases the time needed to apply skeletal traction. Nurse is present at bedside to provide comfort and reassure client.
7. Assess client's reaction to skeletal traction, including anxiety and pain, before physician leaves.	Assures client that physician is available to make adjustments if increased pain is occurring. Gives client opportunity to ask questions to physician.

nurse alert Weights on skeletal traction are **NOT** to be removed without a physician's order.

8. Provide pin care.	
a. Prepare 1:1 mixture of normal saline/hydrogen peroxide in sterile container.	Aseptic technique reduces infection transmission.
b. Dip sterile applicator into saline/hydrogen peroxide mixture. Place applicator next to pin site, and clean around pin and outward away from pin site. Throw away applicator. (Repeat twice, using a new, sterile applicator each time.)	Removes crust from pin site. Crust can obstruct drainage and lead to bacterial buildup (Jones-Walton, 1991).
c. Perform Step b on other pin site.	Cleaning pin site completely on one side of leg and then the other side prevents cross-contamination.

Steps	Rationale
d. Dip applicator in sterile normal saline and clean around pin site to remove hydrogen peroxide residue. e. Repeat Step d on other pin site. 9. Change linen. a. When changing linen, change from top to bottom. Remove soiled linen, starting at the top, and at the same time, replace clean linen. b. When ready to slide linen under client, instruct client to use hands on trapeze to lift upper body off the bed and to use unaffected leg to lift lower part of body off the bed. 10. Every 4 to 8 hours, check the four "P's" of traction maintenance. a. Pounds—Is the correct weight in place? b. Pull—Is the direction of pull aligned with the long axis of bone? c. Pulleys—Is the rope riding over the pulley and gliding smoothly? d. Pressure—Is every clamp and connection tight? 11. See Completion Protocol (Chapter 1, p. 6).	Removing hydrogen peroxide prevents skin irritation. This procedure requires two personnel—one on each side of the bed. Two personnel have more control over keeping linen straight, and procedure is done more quickly. Lifting body off of bed provides an area of clearance while linen is being changed.

Evaluation

1. Observe client reposition self in bed using overhead frame and trapeze bar.
2. Observe client using trapeze, upper extremities, and the unaffected lower extremity for active range of motion and to maintain proper body alignment.
3. Observe pin sites every shift.
4. Evaluate the amount of pain on a scale of 0 to 10.
5. Observe client participating in ADLs.

UNEXPECTED OUTCOMES AND RELATED INTERVENTIONS

1. Client has increased pain in affected leg.
   a. Ask physician to assess skeletal traction for correct placement.
   b. Obtain order for stronger analgesic.
   c. Reposition client for comfort as much as possible, maintaining proper alignment of traction.
2. Client develops infection at pin site.
   a. Alert physician.
   b. Administer any prescribed antibiotics.
   c. Continue pin site care every shift.
3. Client experiences withdrawn behavior because of extensive length of stay at hospital.
   a. Allow client to verbalize feelings concerning traction.
   b. Provide emotional support through social services and pastoral care.
   c. Allow client time to vent frustrations.
   d. Allow client time to ask questions freely.
   e. Reevaluate pain management. (Withdrawn behavior follows unrelieved pain.)

SAMPLE DOCUMENTATION

1000 Balanced-suspension skeletal traction applied to left leg by Dr. Brown, assisted by S. Jones RN, 26 lb of weights hanging freely at end of bed. Client was premedicated with Demerol 75 mg and Vistaril 25 mg IM as ordered and tolerated the application of the balanced-suspension skeletal traction with minimal discomfort. Pin sites cleaned using aseptic technique with $\frac{1}{2}$ hydrogen peroxide and $\frac{1}{2}$ normal saline mixture. Pin sites without redness, edema, or bleeding. Dorsalis pedal pulse present. Brisk capillary refill in all toes. Positive sensation and movement of left foot. At end of procedures, client is lying quietly with respirations even and unlabored and denies pain.

CRITICAL THINKING EXERCISES

1. You are preparing to apply skin traction to a 46-year-old female with back pain. You observe the client lying on her right side with her legs flexed.
   a. What adjustments should you make in the client's position before traction application?
   b. What additional assessments should you conduct before applying the skin traction?
   c. After you apply the skin traction, the client begins to complain of increased back pain. What should you do?
2. You are caring for Mr. Conley, a 42-year-old male admitted with a traumatic fracture of the femur. He is in balance-suspension skeletal traction. As you enter the room, you notice that the weights are touching the floor, the HOB is elevated to 30°, and the leg is externally rotated. Is there anything wrong with this situation?
3. You are teaching pin care to a client's wife. Critique her procedure.
   a. Uses 1:1 mixture of normal saline/hydrogen peroxide.
   b. Dips sterile applicator into solution and cleans around pin, moving outward.
   c. Dips applicator into solution and cleans other pin site.
   d. Obtains new applicator and repeats steps b and c.
   e. Removes hydrogen peroxide from each pin site using applicator dipped in normal saline.
4. In caring for the client with balanced-suspension skeletal traction, how would changing bed linens differ from changing the linen for a client in skin traction?

REFERENCES

Beare P, Myers J: *Principles and practice of adult health nursing,* ed 2, St Louis, 1994, Mosby.

Burrell L: *Adult nursing in hospital and community settings,* East Norwalk, Conn, 1992, Appleton & Lange.

Hilt N, Cogburn S: *Manual of orthopedics,* St Louis, 1980, Mosby.

Jones-Walton P: Clinical standards in skeletal traction pin site care, *Orthop Nurs* 10(2):12, 1991.

Mourad L: *Orthopedic disorders,* St Louis, 1991, Mosby.

Osborne J, DiGiacomo I: Traction: a review with diagnosis and interventions, *Orthop Nurs* 6(4):13, 1987.

Perry A, Potter P: *Clinical nursing skills and techniques,* ed 3, St Louis, 1994, Mosby.

Swager J: Musculoskeletal care. In Buxbaum B, Mauro E, Norris C, editors: *Illustrated manual of nursing practice,* ed 2, Springhouse, Pa, 1993, Springhouse.

Thompson J et al: *Mosby's manual of clinical nursing,* ed 3, St Louis, 1993, Mosby.

ADDITIONAL READINGS

Barratt JB, Bryant BH: Fractures: types, treatment, perioperative implications, *AORN J* 52(4):755, 1990.

Jones IH: Making sense of—traction, *Nurs Times* 86(23):39, 1990.

Jones-Walton P: Effects of pin care in adults with extremity fracture treated with skeletal traction and external fixation, *Orthop Nurs* 7(4):29, 1988.

Morris L et al: Special care for skeletal traction, *RN* 51(2):24, 1988.

Nichol D: Preventing infection—patients with skeletal pins, *Nurs Times* 99(13):78, 1993.

Nussman D, Pools R: Rescue and recovery in traumatic hip dislocation, *Am J Nurs* 91(11): 34, 1991.

Smith A, Young-Johnson J: *Nurse's guide to clinical procedures,* Philadelphia, 1990, Lippincott.

Strength D: Musculoskeletal system. In Hogstel Mo: *Clinical manual of gerontological nursing,* St Louis, 1992, Mosby.

Styrcule L: Traction—basics. Part 1, *Orthop Nurs* 13(2):71, 1994.

Styrcule L: Traction—basics. Part IV, *Orthop Nurs* 13(5):59, 1994.

chapter 27

Cast Care

Skill 27.1
Cast Application

Skill 27.2
Cast Removal

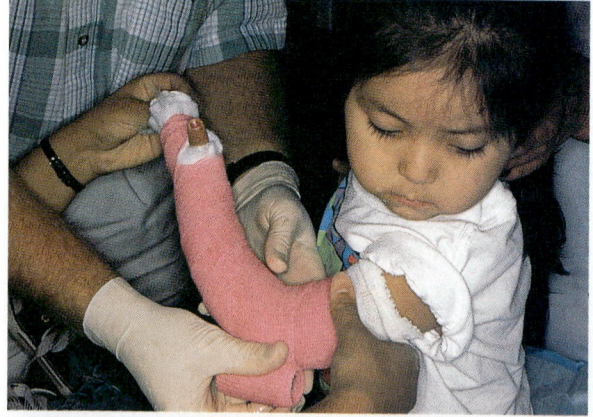

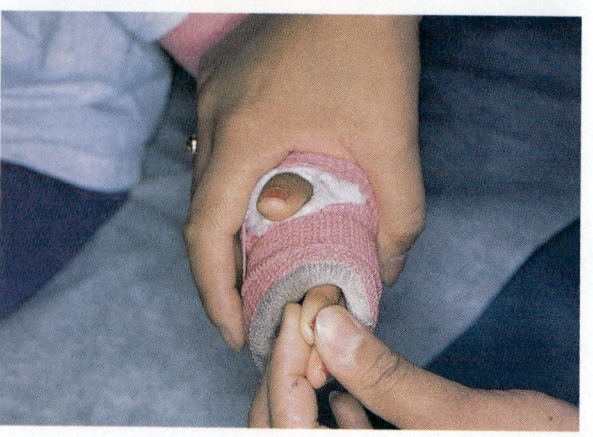

A cast is an immobilization device applied externally to hold injured or deformed musculoskeletal tissues in proper position to promote healing. A cast prevents movement of injured tissues. Therefore, correct application of the cast, with tissue structures in optimal position for healing, is imperative. Casts are used in many different ways (Figure 27-1). The use and application materials required depends on the anatomical area involved.

One of two types of cast materials, plaster of Paris or synthetic, may be used. The type of cast material selected depends on physician preference, number of cast changes anticipated, and type of musculoskeletal injury. Plaster of Paris is composed of open-weave cotton covered with calcium sulfate crystals. This material molds easily during application and requires 48 hours to dry before weight bearing or external pressure can be applied. During the period of drying, the cast must be well supported on firm surfaces to avoid indentations. Lifting the cast is accomplished by supporting the joints above and below the casted area. This prevents injury to underlying soft tissues. This material is supplied in open-weave cotton rolls of varying widths. This type of cast is heavier when compared with the synthetic cast. Synthetic casting materials are composed of polyester and cotton covered with a polyurethane resin that is activated by water. This cast sets very quickly, in approximately 15 minutes, and can withstand pressure or weight bearing in 30 minutes (Table 27-1). Material for this cast is also supplied in rolls of varying widths. Different colors of this casting material are also available, ranging from fluorescent pink to navy blue. Colors are often more appealing to children and aid in maintaining the appearance of the cast (Figure 27-2).

When caring for clients with casts, it is important to understand the techniques for cast removal. This procedure consists of removing the cast and padding, followed by skin care to the affected area. The cast is removed by use of a mechanical device such as a cast saw (Figures 27-3 and 27-4). The saw is noisy, but the procedure is painless because the saw will not cut the skin. It is nec-

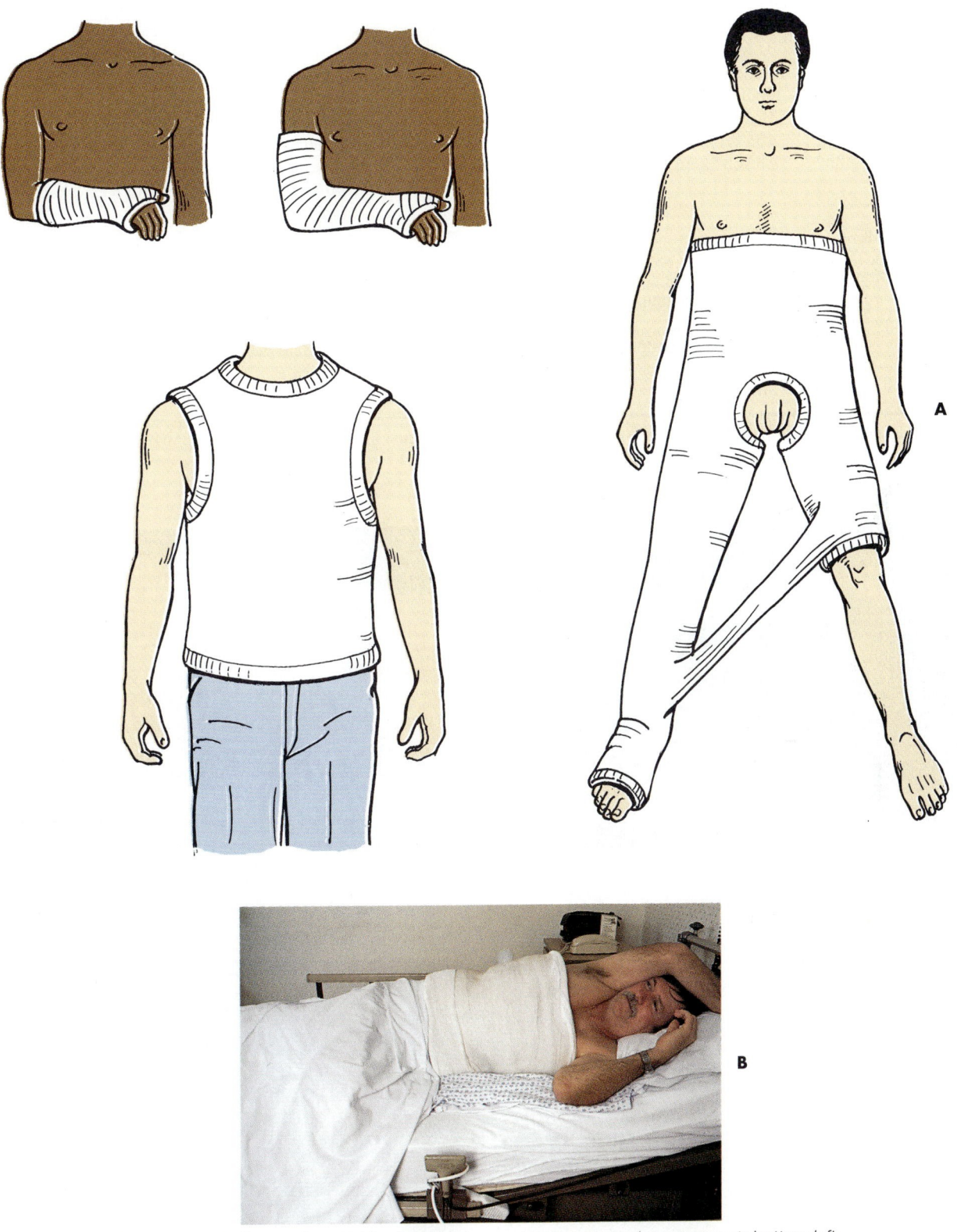

Figure 27-1 **A,** Types of casts. *Top left,* short arm cast; *top center,* long arm cast; *bottom left,* plaster body jacket cast; *far right,* one and one-half hip spica cast. **B,** Client in body cast.

Table 27-1 **Comparison of Casting Materials**

	Plaster of Paris	Synthetic
Indications	Unstable fractures, edema, frequent cast changes	Stable fractures, long-term cast
Drying time	At least 24 hours	7-15 minutes; can be weight bearing in 30 minutes
Drying method	Air dry	Air dry
Radiolucent	Minimal	Yes
Weight of cast	Heavy	Lightweight
Durability	Can crumble and flake	Very durable
Bathing/immersibility	Must be kept from moisture	Can be immersed, as in swimming and bathing; *must be thoroughly dried after exposure to water*
Choice of colors	No	Yes
Surface area	Smooth	Rough
Allergic reactions	Possible	Possible
Molding	Greater moldability	Limited moldability
Special equipment	None	May need special cast saw for cast removal
Padding	Natural fiber padding and stockinette	Synthetic nonabsorbent lining
Cost	Inexpensive (usually requires more rolls)	Expensive
Strength	Strong	Stronger than plaster of Paris

Modified from Slye D, Theis L: *An introduction to orthopaedic nursing: an orientation module,* Pitman, New Jersey, 1991, Anthony J Jannetti.

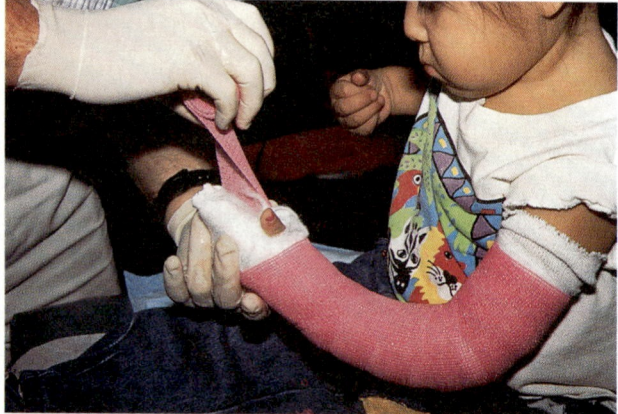

Figure 27-2

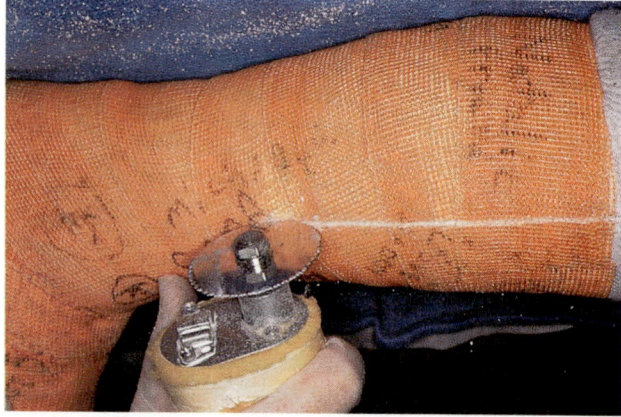

Figure 27-3

essary, however, to prepare the client adequately for cast removal. A small child or confused adult may require gentle restraint during removal to avoid any injury.

Nursing Diagnosis

Nursing diagnoses associated with cast application include **Bathing/Hygiene Self-Care Deficit, Dressing/Grooming Self-Care Deficit,** and **Toileting Self-Care Deficit,** in which clients with a cast applied to an extremity or body portion (body spica cast) experience difficulty in performing activities of daily living (ADLs). These clients are also at a high risk for **Impaired Skin Integrity** relating to the skin condition before, during, and after cast application. Rash, irritation, pruritus, and

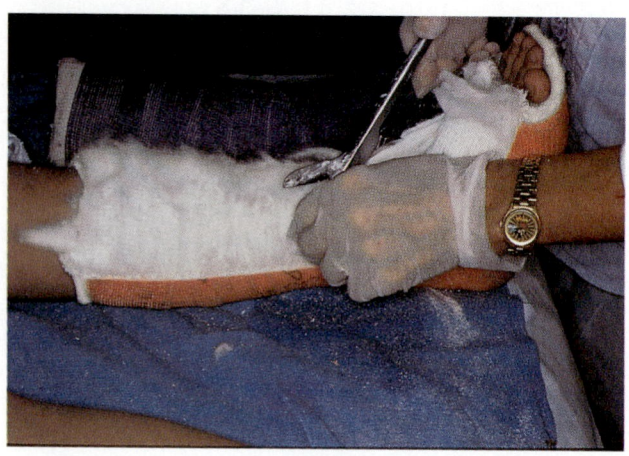

Figure 27-4

skin breakdown may occur. Because of the rigidity of the cast and the inflammatory process that accompanies injury, **Risk for Peripheral Neurovascular Dysfunction** should be considered.

When a client is at home with a cast, **Impaired Home Maintenance Management** is a possibility, depending on the client's degree of independence, self-care, and assistance required. **Knowledge Deficit** regarding cast care is important in these clients, especially regarding contact with water, restrictions in activity, and positioning. **Pain** may be a significant concern in fractures and musculoskeletal injuries. Finally, if the cast is on a lower extremity or torso, **Risk for Injury** or **Impaired**

Physical Immobility may be appropriate as a result of gait disturbances or the client's need for ambulatory assistive devices.

Nursing diagnoses associated with cast removal include **Anxiety,** in which clients are concerned about how the procedure is performed, and **Impaired Skin Integrity** resulting from pressure points within the cast, previous skin conditions before the casting, or presence of surgical incisions under the cast. **Knowledge Deficit** regarding cast removal should also be considered. This is especially true for the small child and the confused client.

Skill 27.1 | Cast Application, Assessment, and Care

This skill includes assessment parameters before, during, and after cast application, including peripheral neurovascular status. Assisting with the application of the cast is also discussed. It is important to follow guidelines for care after application in respect to pressure and weight bearing.

EQUIPMENT (MAY BE ON CAST CART) (FIGURE 27-5)

Plaster cast
Plaster rolls: sizes 2, 3, 4, or 6 inch
Padding material (felt, sheet wadding, Webril, stockinette, or other material)
Gloves, apron, or protective cover
Plastic-lined bucket or basin
Water warmed at time of application
Cart, chair, or fracture table scissors
Paper or plastic sheets
Synthetic cast
Synthetic rolls: 2, 3, or 4 inch
Pail with water to dampen rolls

Padding materials (sheet wadding, stockinette, Webril)
Gloves, apron, or protective cover
Elastic bandages or cast cutter (to trim edges of cast, if needed)

Assessment

1. Assess client's health status, focusing on factors that may affect wound healing, such as diabetes, poor nutritional status, or steroid medication use. **Healing of the injured tissues may be slower in these clients, or additional nutritional supplements may be required.**
2. Assess client's ability to cooperate and level of understanding concerning the casting procedure (see box on p. 484).
3. Assess condition of the skin that will be under the cast. Specifically, note any areas of skin breakdown, rashes present, or incisional wound.
4. Assess neurovascular status of the area to be casted. Specifically, note presence or absence of motor and sensory function, skin color, temperature, and capillary refill. Compare to opposite or surrounding tissues. **Changes in neurovascular status may occur after casting, possibly further compromising already injured tissues. It is important to note the baseline neurovascular status so that these changes, if they occur, can be readily assessed.**
5. Assess client's pain status using a scale of 0 to 10.
6. Determine the extent to which client will be able to use the casted body part.

Planning

Expected outcomes focus on skin integrity, comfort, self-care, mobility, prevention of neurovascular complications, and maintenance of cast integrity.

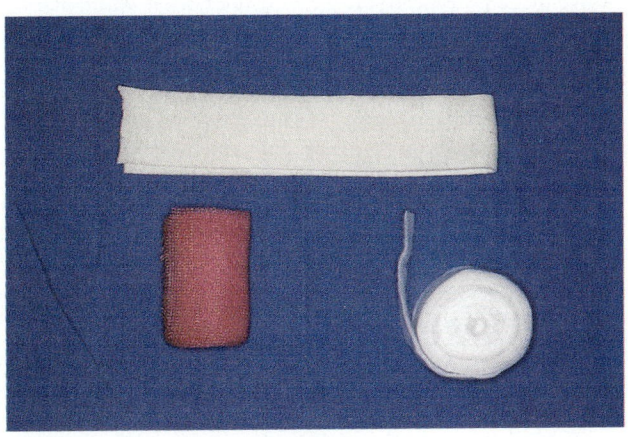

Figure 27-5

Casts

So now you or a member of your family is wearing a cast. The cast is only one of several devices used to promote the healing of broken bones. Doctors also use traction and pins, or a combination of these three, to help heal broken bones. The cast has the advantage of being less expensive, requiring little care on your part, and allowing you to move around. The cast also encloses and immobilizes the broken bone and injured soft tissues to prevent movement that could cause further injury and to keep the bone in place for proper healing.

Your cast may be made of plaster or of a synthetic material such as fiberglass. Although the plaster cast is heavy, the doctor can mold a plaster cast more easily for a close fit over severe injuries. The synthetic cast is lightweight and easier to move around, making it good for elderly clients. Your cast has a name. If it covers your forearm or lower leg, it is a **short arm** or **short leg** cast. A **long leg** cast covers the whole leg, and a **hanging** cast covers the whole arm and forearm. The **body** cast encircles the chest and abdomen, whereas the **Minerva** cast covers the chest, neck, and head with openings for the ears, face, and arms. The cast that covers the hips and one or both legs is the **hip spica** or **spica** cast.

THINGS TO WATCH FOR

Your cast will be warm at first because of the setting process. However, warm areas on the cast later on may indicate infection, and you should notify your doctor at once.

You should watch for increased pain or soreness under the cast, particularly around bony prominences such as the wrist or ankle, that is not relieved by repositioning the body. Check the skin color and temperature periodically. When the tip of a finger or the big toe that protrudes from the cast is squeezed until it is white, the pink color should return within 2 to 4 seconds. If skin color does not return within 4 to 6 seconds or if the skin is red, blue, white, or discolored, notify your doctor. If fingers or toes are cool, cover them. If they do not warm up in 20 minutes, call your doctor. Call your doctor immediately if any of these other symptoms occur:

- An increase in swelling
- A tingling or burning sensation
- An inability to move muscles around the cast
- A foul odor around the edges of the cast
- Any drainage, which may show through the cast
- Any cracks or breaks in the cast

Modified from Mourad L: *Orthopedic disorders,* St Louis, 1991, Mosby.

Home Cast Care

THE FIRST 24 HOURS

Your cast needs at least 24 hours to dry if it is plaster. Avoid handling it as much as possible. When you do have to move the cast, such as when you change your body position, use only the palms of your hands and support the cast under your joints. You want to avoid putting indentations in the cast that will put pressure on the skin inside. You may use a fan placed 18 to 24 inches from the cast to aid its drying in the first 24 hours. You should be sure to expose the whole cast for drying, and do not cover it with linen for the first 24 hours.

Keep the cast and extremity above the level of the heart for at least 48 hours by propping your cast up on firm pillows. Put ice directly over the fractured area for 24 hours, but be sure to enclose the ice in a plastic bag to keep the cast dry. Move the parts of your body above and below the cast regularly to aid circulation and relieve stiffness. Massaging the joints and extremities around the cast will also improve circulation.

HOW TO CARE FOR YOUR CAST

If you have a plaster cast, do not get the cast wet because it will lose its strength. To keep the cast clean and dry, you should cover it with plastic when bathing, using the toilet (if it is a spica cast), or going out in rain or snow. You may use a

damp cloth and scouring powder to clean soiled spots on the cast. Be sure to brush away plaster crumbs or other objects from the edges of the cast, but do not remove any padding.

If you have a synthetic cast and you do not have any wounds under the cast, your doctor may allow you to bathe and swim with it. You should use only a small amount of mild soap around your cast and should rinse under your cast thoroughly. If you swim in a pool or a lake, be sure to rinse both the inside and outside of the cast to flush out any dirt and chemicals. Dry your cast and stockinette thoroughly each time they get wet to avoid excess moisture on your skin. Use a towel to blot moisture off the cast, then dry it with a hair dryer set on low. When your cast does not feel cold and damp, it is dry.

Skin care is very important during the time a cast is worn. Do not insert objects under the cast, because you could scrape the skin or add pressure and cause an infection or sore under the cast. You should use powders and lotions only outside the cast so that the skin stays clean and soft. Powder inside a cast can cake and cause sore areas.

Do not walk on a leg cast for the first 48 hours. If you are allowed to walk on it, be sure to walk on the walking heel. If your arm is in a cast, be sure to use your sling for support and comfort.

Modified from Mourad L: *Orthopedic disorders,* St Louis, 1991, Mosby.

EXPECTED OUTCOMES

1. Client's exposed skin distal to cast is warm, pink, with capillary refill less than 3 seconds.
2. Integrity of the cast is maintained until removal.
3. Client has edema of 1 plus or less and demonstrates less than 25% decrease in active range of motion (ROM) of affected extremity after cast application.
4. Client verbalizes satisfactory pain control after anal-gesic administration 20 to 30 minutes before the procedure.
5. Client requires minimal assistance with ADLs when an extremity is casted.
6. Client verbalizes correct activities related to cast care.
7. Client demonstrates proper cast care (see box on p. 484).

Implementation

Steps	Rationale
1. See Standard Protocol (Chapter 1, p. 5).	
2. Position client and injured extremity as desired, depending on type of cast to be used and area to be casted.	The parts to be casted must be supported and in optimal alignment.
3. Prepare skin that will be enclosed in the cast. Change any dressing (if present), and cleanse the skin with mild soap and water.	Assists in maintaining skin integrity.
4. Assist with application of padding material. Avoid wrinkles or uneven thicknesses.	Decreases complications to the skin and prevents pressure points under the cast.
5. Hold body part or parts to be casted *or* assist with preparation of casting materials.	Support of body part may require application of slight manual traction.
a. Plaster cast: Mark the end of the roll by folding one corner of the material under itself. Hold plaster roll under water in a plastic-lined bucket or basin until bubbles stop, then squeeze slightly and hand roll to person applying the cast.	Once dampened, the end of the casting tape may be difficult to find. Dampened plaster rolls are unrolled and molded to fit the extremity or body part to be casted.
b. Synthetic cast: Submerge cast roll in lukewarm water for 10 to 15 seconds. Squeeze to remove excess water.	Submersion in water initiates the chemical reaction, which will eventually result in hardening of the cast.
6. Continue to hold the body parts as necessary or to supply additional rolls of casting tape as needed.	Thickness of the plaster determines strength of the cast.
7. Provide walking heel, brace, bar, or other material to stabilize the cast as requested by the physician.	After cast has dried, ambulation may be permitted with partial weight bearing on the affected extremity. This is facilitated by the use of a walking heel or sole. Bars or wooden posts may be used to stabilize a spica cast. Braces are often incorporated into a cast to assist in joint motion and mobility.
8. Assist with "finishing" the cast by folding the edge of the stockinette down over the cast to provide a smooth edge. A dampened plaster roll is unrolled over the stockinette to hold it in place.	Smooth edges decrease the chance for irritation to the skin or tissue injury.
9. Using scissors, trim the cast around fingers, toes, or the thumb as necessary.	The cast should not restrict joint movement or constrict circulation.
10. After casting, the casted tissues are elevated on cloth-covered pillows or placed in a sling. Avoid complete encasing of the cast.	Pillows or other soft areas prevent indentation or other undesirable hardening of the cast. Covering of the cast delays drying.

Steps	Rationale

nurse alert Client with wet large-limb or wet spica cast requires three people to assist in turning and transfer. Proper assistance prevents undue pressure on cast and prevents client injury.

11. Assist client with transfer to stretcher or wheelchair for return to unit, or prepare for discharge.	Additional personnel may be required to transfer client safely, especially with client in a spica or other large body cast. Pillows, restraints, and side rails may also be needed to maintain principles of safe client transport.
12. Clean used equipment and return to usual storage area.	Expedites use of equipment for the next client and maintains principles of infection control.
13. Explain to client the need to keep cast exposed until drying is complete and the use of elevation or ice.	Casts must dry from the inside out for thorough drying. Elevation and application of ice assist in decreasing edema formation.
14. Have client turn every 2 to 3 hours when a body jacket or a hip spica cast is applied.	Avoids indentation and prevents continuous pressure to one area.
15. See Completion Protocol (Chapter 1, p. 6).	

Evaluation

1. Inspect exposed skin and assess capillary refill by pressing on toe or finger if the cast is on an extremity (Figure 27-6).
2. Inspect condition of the cast. Palpate the temperature of tissues around the casted area for warmth.
3. Observe for edema of tissues distal to the cast for signs of vascular compromise (whitish or bluish coloration).
4. Observe client for signs of pain or anxiety (hyperventilation, tachycardia, blood pressure increases).
5. Observe client performing ADLs and ROM.
6. Ask client to describe cast care.
7. Observe client perform cast care.

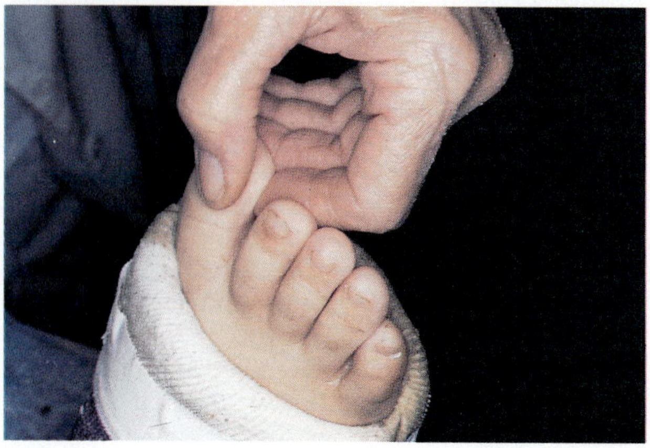

Figure 27-6

UNEXPECTED OUTCOMES AND RELATED INTERVENTIONS

1. Client experiences impaired physical mobility related to the cast.
   a. Assist client with ROM exercises every 3 to 4 hours.
   b. Teach isometric exercises.
2. Client complains of pain after application of the cast.
   a. Assess description, amount, type, and severity.
   b. Reposition casted extremity or client. Adjust elevation of pillows as necessary.
   c. Apply ice bags as needed.
   d. Administer analgesics as ordered to maintain client's comfort level.
   e. Perform neurovascular checks.
   f. Assess tightness of the cast by checking with fingers around the edges and checking with client.
3. Client develops compartmental syndrome, a condition in which increased pressure within a limited space compromises the circulation and function of tissues within that space (Masten and Krugmire, 1978).
   a. Assess for severe pain (usually more severe than explained by injury).
   b. Assess change in neurovascular status, such as numbness, tingling, or decreased movement in distal skin and tissues.
   c. Assess for pulse in area distal to casted extremity (pulselessness develops late in the syndrome).
4. Client is unable to describe cast care.
   a. Reinforce the rationale for correct skin care measures with the cast.
   b. Reinstruct client concerning cast care.

SAMPLE DOCUMENTATION

0900 Left long arm synthetic cast applied and left arm placed in shoulder sling by Dr. Miller. Capillary refill of left index finger is 2 seconds. Client able to move all fingers of left hand, fingers warm to touch, nail beds pink, no swelling noted. No complaints of pain or discomfort at this time.

0930 Left long arm cast intact and sling readjusted. Capillary refill of left index finger unchanged. Client moves all fingers of left hand, fingers warm to touch, denies any numbness or tingling present. No edema noted. Denies any pain or discomfort.

Skill 27.2 | Cast Removal

This skill includes gathering the equipment necessary for cast removal, adequate client preparation, and providing skin care to the casted area after cast removal. After cast removal, the client may experience tenderness, soreness, or muscle weakness. Gait imbalance may be present because of the loss of the cast's weight.

EQUIPMENT

Cast saw (Figure 27-7)
Plastic sheets or paper
Cold water enzyme wash
Skin lotion
Basin, water, washcloth, towels
Scissors

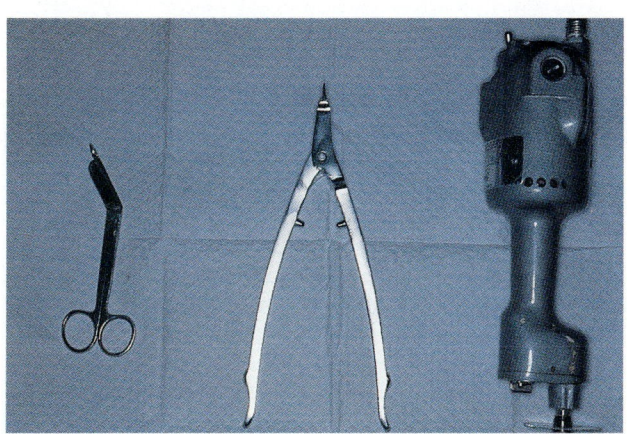

Figure 27-7

Assessment

1. Assess client's understanding and ability to cooperate with cast removal. **Cast removal may require a cast saw. Client needs to understand that the saw is noisy but does not cut skin.**
2. Assess client's readiness for cast removal (physician's orders, x-ray results, physical findings).
3. Ask if client feels itching or irritation under the cast. **Skin breakdown may be present.**

Planning

Expected outcomes focus on skin integrity of the underlying skin and client understanding of the cast removal procedure.

EXPECTED OUTCOMES

1. Client is able to verbalize the sensations and procedural steps involved in cast removal.
2. Client is able to describe and demonstrate levels of activity and weight-bearing limitations.
3. There is no underlying tissue damage after cast removal.
4. Client can describe skin care measures and perform ADLs as appropriate.

Implementation

Steps	Rationale
nurse alert Proper positioning techniques prevent accidental injury to the skin during cast removal.	
1. See Standard Protocol (Chapter 1, p. 5).	

Steps	Rationale
2. Describe the physical sensations to expect during cast removal (vibration of cast saw and generation of heat).	Knowledge of the procedure decreases level of anxiety.
3. Describe the expected appearance of the extremity.	Skin under cast becomes scaly, and dead cells that normally slough off accumulate.
4. Explain the loud noise of the cast saw.	
5. Assist with positioning of client.	Prevents injury.
6. Stay with client, and explain progress of procedure as cast is removed.	
7. Inspect tissues underlying the cast after removal.	
8. If skin is intact, apply cold water enzyme wash (if available) to skin and leave on for 15 to 20 minutes. Mild soap and water may also be used. Do not scrub the skin.	Enzyme washes assist in dissolving dead cells and fatty deposits.
9. Gently wash off enzyme wash. Immerse tissues in basin or tub, if possible, to assist in dead cell removal.	
10. *Pat* extremity dry and apply thin coat of skin lotion.	Rubbing may further traumatize the tissues.
11. Explain and write out skin care procedures after cast removal to client (see box below).	Provides ongoing home care instruction for client and family.
12. Obtain physician's order to perform active and passive ROM, and clarify level of activity allowed.	After immobilization, the involved joints and muscles will be weak and ROM may be limited. Activity must be resumed slowly.

Skin Care After Cast Removal

Instructions on skin care and strategies to relieve the pain, edema, and muscle weakness should be given in writing prior to discharge.

INSTRUCTIONS RELATED TO SKIN CARE
- Wash the areas with full-strength cold water wash solution with enzymes such as Woolite or Delicare. Apply the solution liberally and leave in place for at least 20 minutes. The enzymes in the solution loosen dead cells and help emulsify fatty or crusty lesions but cause no skin irritation.
- After 20 minutes, immerse the area in warm water and gently wash away all the debris. Caution client not to rub or scrub the skin areas but to gently rinse off the areas with a soft cloth.
- Rinse with clear warm water and **pat** dry.
- Apply a moisturizing skin lotion, gently massaging it in to help maintain the integrity of the cells.
- Instruct client to repeat the above steps in 24 hours, after which the area should need no special care.

INSTRUCTIONS FOR RELIEVING EDEMA
- Apply ice bags if the edema is marked.
- Wrap (or have the edematous tissues wrapped) from distal to proximal areas with elastic bandages.
- Elevate the affected tissues for the next 24 hours.

INSTRUCTIONS FOR TENDERNESS, SORENESS, OR PAIN
- Take prescribed nonnarcotic analgesic every 3 to 4 hours to build a therapeutic blood level, and continue the medication for 24 to 48 hours.
- Immerse the part or entire body in warm water and gently exercise muscles under water.
- Begin to reuse affected tissues and muscles slowly to avoid frank pain. Explain that usually it takes twice as long to regain full function because the part was in the cast. Thus, it would take 8 weeks to regain full function of a part that was in a cast for 4 weeks.
- Perform prescribed muscle exercises with 5 to 10 repetitions every 4 hours to aid in regaining muscle strength. If muscle soreness persists, continue intake of prescribed nonnarcotic analgesic and preexercise soaking in warm water. Soreness should lessen as the muscle regains strength.

From Mourad L: *Orthopedic disorders,* St Louis, 1991, Mosby.

Steps	Rationale
13. Assist in transfer of client for return to unit or discharge.	
14. Clean all equipment. Dispose of cast and materials according to universal precautions.	Prevents spread of infection.
15. See Completion Protocol (Chapter 1, p. 6).	

Evaluation

1. Ask client to describe cast removal procedure.
2. Ask client to explain and demonstrate activity level and ROM exercises prescribed.
3. Inspect underlying skin for pressure areas, erythema (redness), or other signs of irritation or trauma.
4. Observe client perform skin care.

UNEXPECTED OUTCOMES AND RELATED INTERVENTIONS

1. Client becomes very tense and is unable to cooperate during the cast removal.
   a. Offer reassurance and support.
   b. Reexplain the cast removal procedure and expected sensations during removal.
2. Client experiences edema, pain, and difficulty moving affected tissues after removal of cast.
   a. Assess neurovascular status of involved tissues.
   b. Assess the type, length, site, amount, and severity of the pain, including onset.
   c. Assess ability to perform active and passive ROM.
   d. Contact physician with findings.
3. Client has scratch on underlying skin.
   a. Inspect skin edges and severity of scratch.
   b. Cleanse area and apply water-soluble lotion or ointment as ordered.
4. Client is unable to explain self-care measures or skin care.
   a. Reassure client as necessary.
   b. Reinstruct client in self-care after cast removal.
   c. Instruct client in skin care measures, including gentle cleansing of the casted area (avoid scrubbing) and patting the area dry (avoid rubbing). Apply a water-soluble lotion or ointment to any scratches as ordered.

SAMPLE DOCUMENTATION

1000 Left long arm cast removed without difficulty. Skin dry, intact. Left arm soaking in basin of enzyme wash, rinsed.
1030 Skin on left arm remains dry, lotion applied.

CRITICAL THINKING EXERCISES

1. Casts are made of plaster or synthetic materials.
   a. What advantages do synthetic casts have over plaster casts?
   b. Given the advantages of synthetic casts, for what reasons might a plaster cast be more appropriate?
2. Robert has just had a full-length leg cast applied. When assessing him an hour later you note that his toes on the casted limb are pale and cold. His toes on the noncasted limb are warm and pink.
   a. What might this finding represent, and how should you respond?
   b. You have taught Robert how to care for his plaster cast at home. What statement by Robert would indicate that he needs more teaching?
      (1) "I should not use sharp objects to scratch beneath my cast."
      (2) "If I develop consistent pain beneath the cast I should report it to my doctor."
      (3) "I can shower with my cast as long as I use a hair dryer afterward to dry it out."
      (4) "I can use a damp cloth and scouring powder to clean soiled spots off my cast if it gets dirty."
3. You are preparing the equipment to remove Sarah's arm cast. When you remove the cast saw from the drawer, Sarah becomes apprehensive and asks if there is another way to remove the cast than with a saw.
   a. What is the best explanation you can provide Sarah about removal of her cast with a cast saw?
   b. After removing the cast you note that Sarah's skin is dry and flaking. What should Sarah be taught about her skin?
   c. Sarah wants to know if she will be able to use her arm the same as she did before she fractured it. How should you answer Sarah?

REFERENCES

Matsen FA, Krugmire RB: Compartmental syndromes, *Surg Gynecol Obstet* 147:943, 1978.
Mourad L: *Orthopedic disorders,* St Louis, 1991, Mosby.
Slye D, Theis L: *An introduction to orthopaedic nursing: an orientation module,* Pitman, New Jersey, 1991, Anthony J Jannetti.

ADDITIONAL READINGS

Lewis CB, Knortz KA: *Orthopedic assessment and treatment of the geriatric patient,* St Louis, 1993, Mosby.
Proehl JA: Compartment syndrome, *J Emerg Nurs* 14:284, 1988.
Wise LB: A comparison of orthopedic casts: breaking the mold, *MCN Am J Matern Child Nurs* 11(3):174, 1986.

chapter 28

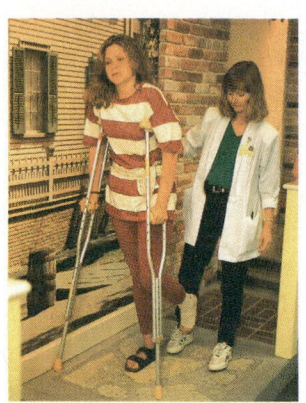
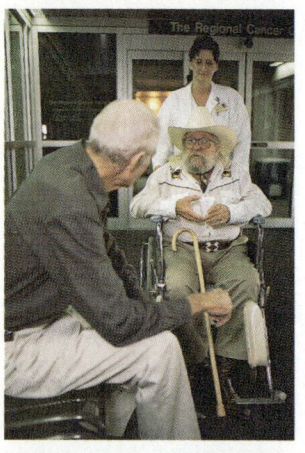
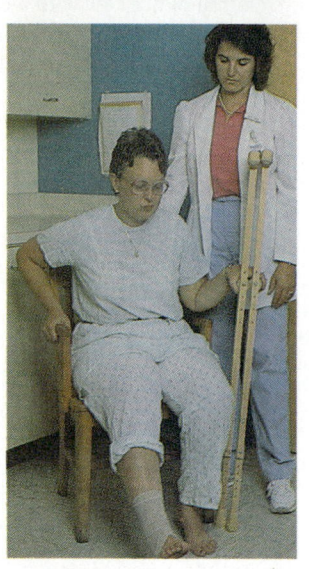

Assistive Devices for Ambulation

Skill 28.1
Teaching Use of Cane, Crutches, and Walker

Several ambulation aids are available to assist the client with mobility and to maintain stability, either with or without weight bearing on an injured lower extremity. The most common of these aids are canes, crutches, and walkers.

An assistive device may be ordered to increase stability, to support a weak extremity, or to reduce the load on weight-bearing structures such as hips, knees, or ankles. These devices range from standard canes, which provide minimal support, to crutches and walkers, which can be used by clients who are unable to bear complete weight on their lower extremities. Selection of the appropriate device depends on the client's age, diagnosis, muscular coordination, and ease of maneuverability. Use of assistive devices may be temporary, such as during recuperation from a fractured extremity or orthopedic surgery, or permanent, as with a client with paralysis or permanent weakness of the lower extremities (Perry and Potter, 1994).

Canes are lightweight, easily movable devices that reach about waist high and are made of wood or metal. Canes help maintain balance by widening the base of support. They are indicated to assist clients with hemiparesis or minor knee or hip injuries or to ease strain on weight-bearing joints. Canes are not recommended for clients with bilateral leg weakness; crutches or walkers are more appropriate. Three types of canes are typically used. The *standard* cane (Figure 28-1, *A*) provides the least support and is used by clients requiring only slight assistance to walk. It has a half-circle handle, which allows it to be hooked over chairs. The *T-handle* cane (Figure 28-1, *B*) has a straight shaft and a bent, shaped handle with grips, which makes it easier to hold. It provides greater stability than the standard cane and is especially useful for clients with hand weakness. The *quad* cane (four legs) (Figure 28-2) or tripod (pyramid cane) provides a wide base of support. This type of cane is useful

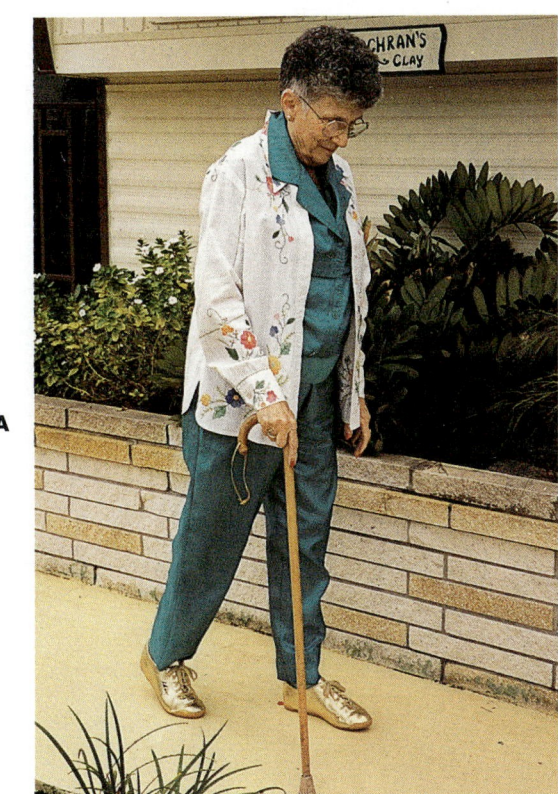
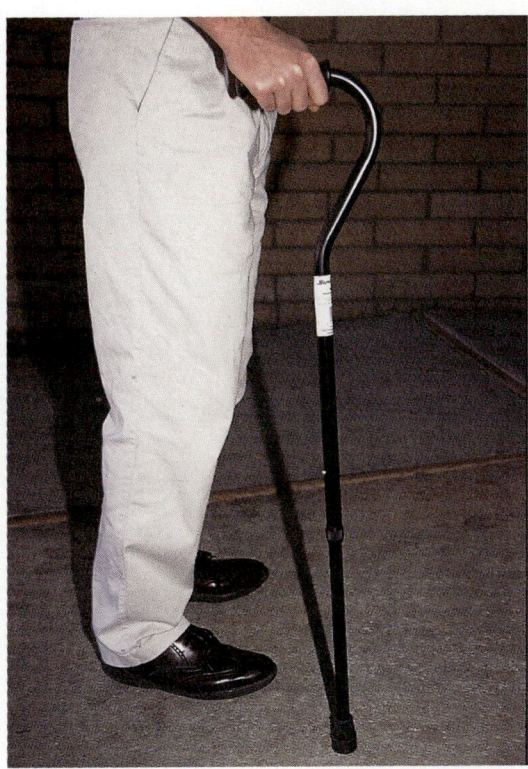

Figure 28-1 **A,** Standard cane. **B,** T-handle cane.

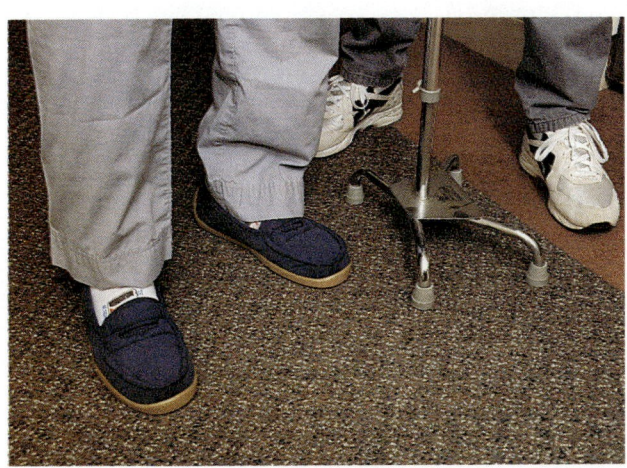

Figure 28-2 Quad cane (four legs).

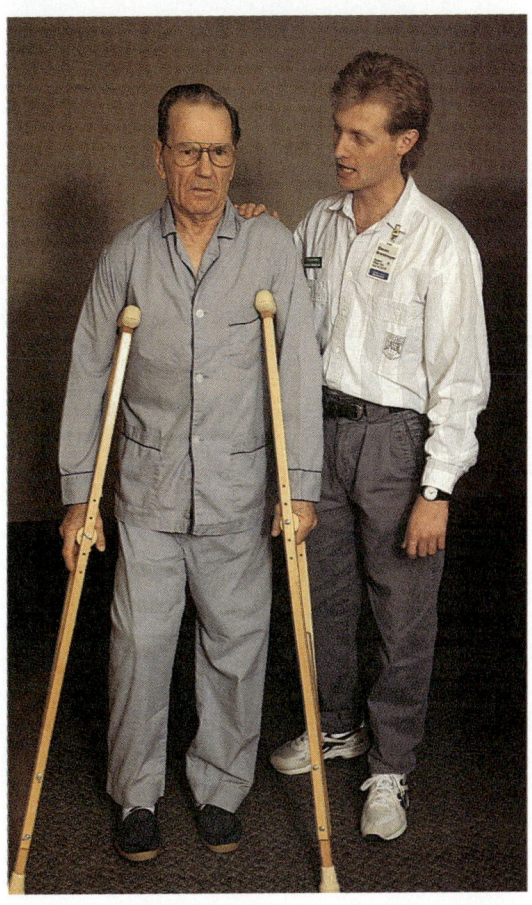

Figure 28-3 Axilary crutches.

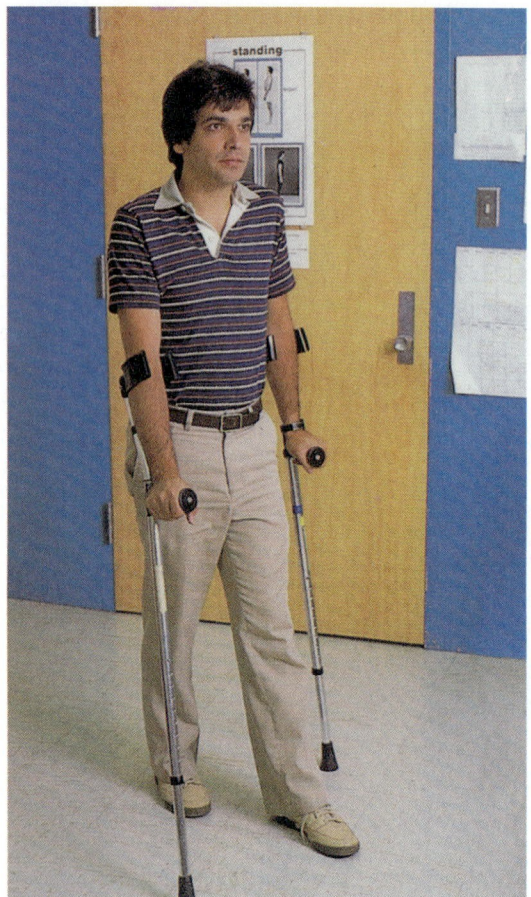

Figure 28-4 Lofstrand crutches.

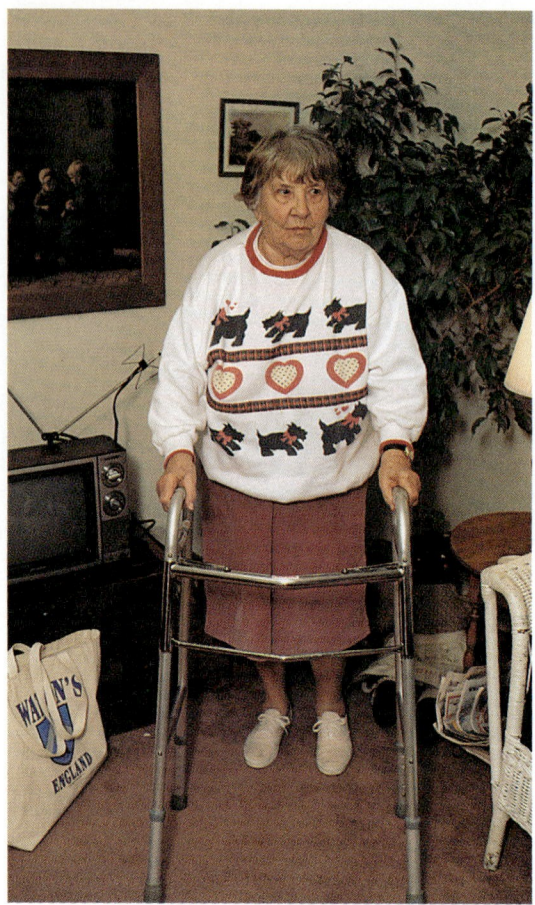

Figure 28-5 Standard walker.

for clients with unilateral or partial paralysis. It also has the advantage in that it stands alone, freeing the arms to help the client rise from a chair (Joyce and Kirby, 1991). Metallic canes are heavier than their wooden counterparts and are frequently adjustable, which is not possible with wooden canes.

A **crutch** is a wooden or metal staff that reaches from the ground almost to the axilla. Crutches are used to support weight from one or both legs. They are used by clients who must transfer more weight to their arms than is possible with canes. There are three types of crutches: the axillary, the Lofstrand or Canadian, and the platform crutch. The *axillary* crutch is frequently used by clients of all ages on a short-term basis (Figure 28-3). The *Lofstrand* crutch has a handgrip and a metal band that fits around the client's forearm. Both the metal band and the handgrip are adjusted to fit the client's height (Figure 28-4). This type of crutch is useful for clients with a permanent disability, such as paraplegic clients. The metal arm band stabilizes and assists in guiding the crutch. The metal arm band offers one other advantage. First, the encircling arm band allows clients to use their hands for other activities, such as opening doors, without dropping the crutches. Second, the anterior opening of the band

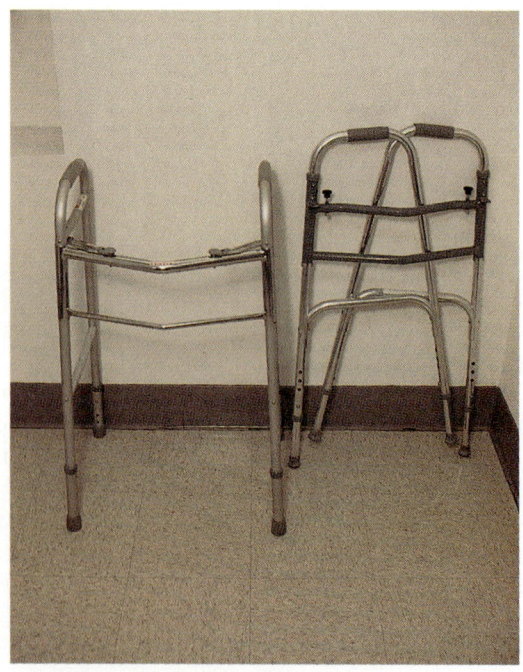

Figure 28-6 Walker can be folded for easier transport and storage.

allows clients to free themselves of the crutches if a fall occurs. The *Canadian* crutch is similar to the Lofstrand, but it has an additional cuff for the upper arm to give added support. The *platform* crutch is used by clients who are unable to bear weight on their wrists. It has a horizontal trough on which the clients can rest their forearms and wrists and a vertical handle for the clients to grip (Joyce and Kirby, 1991).

A **walker** is an extremely light, movable device, about waist high, consisting of a metal frame with handgrips, four widely placed sturdy legs, and one open side. Because it has a wide base of support, the walker provides great stability and security. A walker can be used by a client who is weak or who has balance problems (Figure 28-5). Besides the standard walker, other models are available, for example, a foldable version that is easier to transport and store (Figure 28-6), one with a fold-down seat, and one with wheels on the front legs. Walkers with wheels are useful for clients who have difficulty lifting the walker as they walk because of limited balance or endurance. The disadvantage, however, is that the walker can roll forward when weight is applied (Joyce and Kirby, 1991).

Nursing Diagnosis

Nursing diagnoses associated with teaching the use of assistive devices include **Health-Seeking Behaviors** or **Knowledge Deficit** related to a client's unfamiliarity with use of the assistive device. **Risk for Injury** related to unsteady gait while using an assistive device suggests additional assistance and practice are needed. **Impaired Physical Mobility** related to limited range of motion (ROM) or decreased muscle strength, control, or coordination may be appropriate after traumatic injury or surgery. **Activity Intolerance** related to weakness and fatigue from prolonged bed rest is appropriate when activity alters vital signs (pulse, respirations, blood pressure).

| Skill 28.1 | Teaching Use of Cane, Crutches, and Walker |

Assistive devices (canes, crutches, walkers) are usually recommended for clients who cannot bear full weight on one or more joints of the lower extremities. Other indications for their use are instability, poor balance, or pain in weight bearing. Nurses are expected to supervise clients to use their assistive devices correctly (Phipps et al., 1995).

When partial or touch-down weight bearing is permitted, ambulation is similar to that for non–weight bearing, but either limb can be advanced initially. Partial weight bearing more closely approximates normal walking; joints and muscles are used as for walking normally except that less weight is placed on the affected limb. Muscle-strengthening exercises such as knee-and-foot flexion and walking in parallel bars help the client increase strength and confidence before using an assistive device.

Rubber tips on the ends prevent slipping when using any of the aids. Teaching to lift rather than slide the device lessens the possibility of catching the tips, which could cause the user to lose balance, trip, or fall. Personnel should attend to clients when using an assistive device until they are assured that the client's understanding and strength are sufficient for safe solo ambulation. Observing unaccompanied clients on their walks may reveal a need for attendance and/or additional or continued reminding about the amount of weight permitted or the distance covered. One of the pleasures of being a member of the health profession is assisting clients in regaining mobility with an assistive device after trauma to a foot, leg, knee, or hip, then "graduating" to unassisted walking and moving when possible (Mourad and Droste, 1993).

CANES

Canes primarily increase the person's security and balance by increasing the base of support. Canes also absorb or take the body weight when necessary for mobility during partial weight-bearing periods. Instruction for use of cane-assisted ambulation is required to assess the client's balance, strength, and confidence (Mourad and Droste, 1993). When canes are unilaterally used, they are most often used opposite the weak or injured side and are advanced forward with the injured or affected limb.

CRUTCHES

Persons using one or two crutches as aids for ambulation are seen every day. The user's proficiency varies with age, condition, degree or extent of injury, musculoskeletal functions, and so on. Use of crutches may be a temporary aid for persons with sprains, in a cast, or following surgical treatments; or crutches may be routinely and continuously used for those with congenital or acquired musculoskeletal anomalies, neuromuscular weakness, or paralysis; or they may be used after amputations.

Placing the crutches in an easily accessible location is the first requirement when used to rise to a standing position. Accessible sites are on the back or side of the chair or upright against a near cabinet or wall. The handrests of the crutches may be used for bracing while rising if the chair is solid and heavy enough to preclude tipping, and if only one arm is to be used with the crutches for bracing while rising. If the chair is lightweight, both armrests should be used for even bracing while rising, then the crutches are placed for ambulating. When sitting down or rising, the client should be instructed to use either both armrests or one armrest and both crutches together as one rest to maintain balance. Balance can be lost or chairs can be tipped from uneven or one-sided pressure.

Crutch walking can successfully increase a client's mobility. It is important to take precautions to be certain that the condition of the client, crutches, and environment provides assurances for safety, skill, and comfort (Mourad and Droste, 1993).

WALKER

Constructed of aluminum or metallic alloys, walkers are lightweight aids strong enough to withstand prolonged use. Heights are adjustable for individual needs. The use of a walker facilitates partial or full weight bearing. Before using a walker, the client should understand the specific amount of weight bearing permitted or non–weight bearing to be maintained and how to use and care for the walker. Demonstrating the technique to be used for a particular client is beneficial, because techniques vary for non–weight bearing on one extremity vs. partial weight bearing. For both walking activities, the assistant supports the client to prevent loss of balance, tipping, or uneven balance on the walker. The affected limbs should be referred to as "left or right" or "strong or weak," not as "good or bad," because those words are physiologically distressing to many persons (Mourad and Droste, 1993).

EQUIPMENT

Cane
Axillary crutches
Safety belt (gait belt) (Figure 28-7)
Walker

Assessment

1. Review client's chart, including medical history, previous activity level, and current activity order. **This reveals client's current and previous health status.**
2. Assess client's physical readiness: vital signs and orientation to time, place, and person. **Baseline vital signs offer a means of comparison after exercise. Level of orientation may reveal risk for fall.**
3. Assess ROM and muscle strength or the presence of foot deformities. **This determines if client is able to ambulate safely.**
4. Assess client for any visual, perceptual, or sensory deficits. **This determines if client can use assistive device safely.**

5. Assess environment for potential threats to client safety (e.g., bed brake on, bed in low position, objects not in pathway). Make sure floor is dry and area is well lighted.
6. Assess client for discomfort. **This determines if client needs prescribed analgesic before exercise.**
7. Assess client's understanding of technique of ambulation to be used. **This allows client to verbalize concerns.**
8. Determine optimal time for ambulation.

Planning

Expected outcomes focus on improving mobility, minimizing activity intolerance, preventing risk for injury, minimizing fatigue, and improving client's knowledge.

EXPECTED OUTCOMES

1. Client demonstrates correct use of assistive device.
2. Client ambulates without episode of injury.
3. Client rates pain/discomfort as 4 or less on a scale of 0 to 10 during ambulation.
4. Client performs activities without excessive changes in vital signs.
5. Client independently performs all hygiene, eating, and toileting activities using assistive device safely.

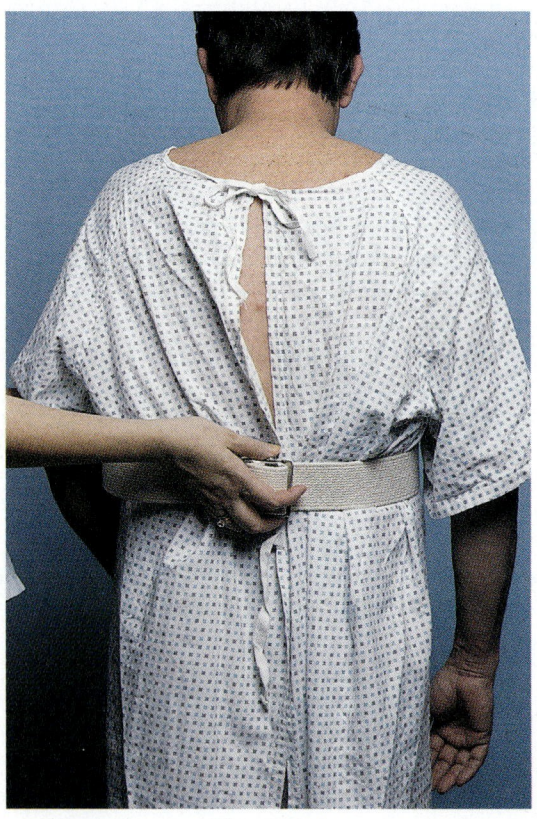

Figure 28-7

Implementation

Steps	Rationale
1. See Standard Protocol (Chapter 1, p. 5).	
2. Prepare client for procedure.	
a. Explain reasons for exercise and demonstrate specific gait technique to client or care giver.	Teaching and demonstration enhance learning, reduce anxiety, and encourage cooperation.
b. Decide with client how far to ambulate.	Determines mutual goal.
c. Schedule ambulation around client's other activities.	Avoids client fatigue.
d. Place bed in low position.	Reduces risk of injury.
e. Slowly assist client from a lying to a sitting or standing position. Assist client to stand stationary until balance is maintained. Check blood pressure as appropriate.	Prevents orthostatic hypotension.
3. Make sure that the assistive device is the appropriate height.	Wrong height causes client to expend more energy, experience greater discomfort, and feel unable to achieve adequate weight transmission through the arms (Hale et al., 1990).
4. Make sure assistive device has rubber tips.	Rubber tips increase surface tension and reduce the risk of the assistive device slipping.

> **nurse alert**   Make sure that surface client will walk on is clean, dry, and well lighted. Remove objects that might obstruct the pathway.

Steps	Rationale
5. Apply safety belt if unsure of client's stability. Safety belt encircles client's waist and has space for nurse to hold while client walks. Assist client to standing position and observe balance. If client appears weak or unsteady, return client to bed. Grasp safety belt in middle of client's back (see Figure 28-7) or place hands at client's waist if safety belt is not available.	Providing constant contact by nurse reduces risk of fall or injury.
6. Cane	
a. Client should hold cane on uninvolved side 4 to 6 inches (10 to 15 cm) to side of foot. Cane should extend from greater trochanter to floor. Allow approximately 15 to 30 degrees elbow flexion (Figure 28-8).	Offers most support when on stronger side of body. Cane and weaker leg work together with each step. If cane is too short, client will have difficulty supporting weight and be bent over and uncomfortable. As weight is taken on by hands and affected leg is lifted off floor, complete extension of elbow is necessary.
b. Assist client in ambulating with cane. (Same steps are taught whether standard or quad canes are used.)	
c. Begin by placing cane on the side opposite the involved leg (Figure 28-9).	Provides added support for the weak or impaired side.
d. Place cane forward 6 to 10 inches (15 to 25 cm), keeping body weight on both legs.	Distributes body weight equally.
e. Move involved leg forward, even with the cane (Figure 28-10).	
f. Advance uninvolved leg past cane (Figure 28-11).	Aligns client's center of gravity. Returns client body weight to equal distribution.
g. Move involved leg forward, even with uninvolved leg.	
h. Repeat these steps.	

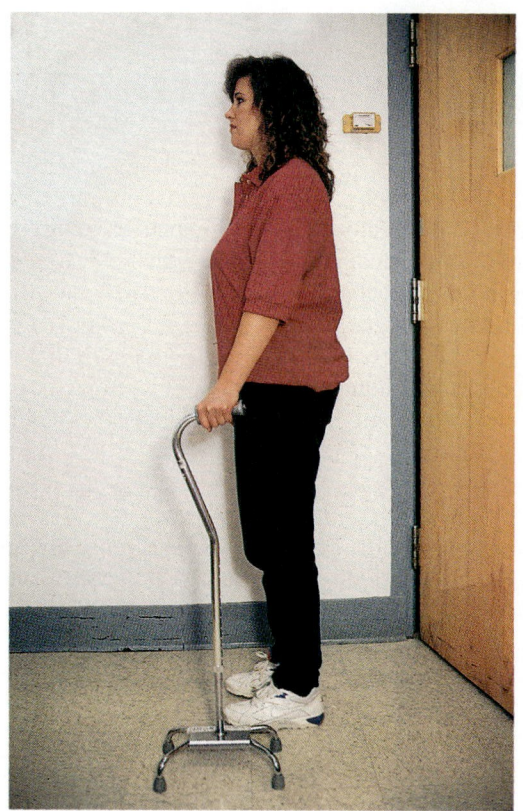

Figure 28-8

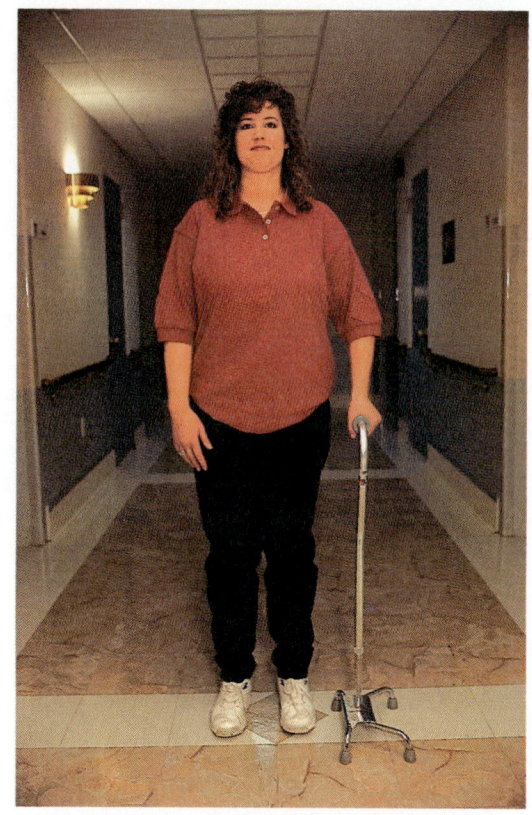

Figure 28-9

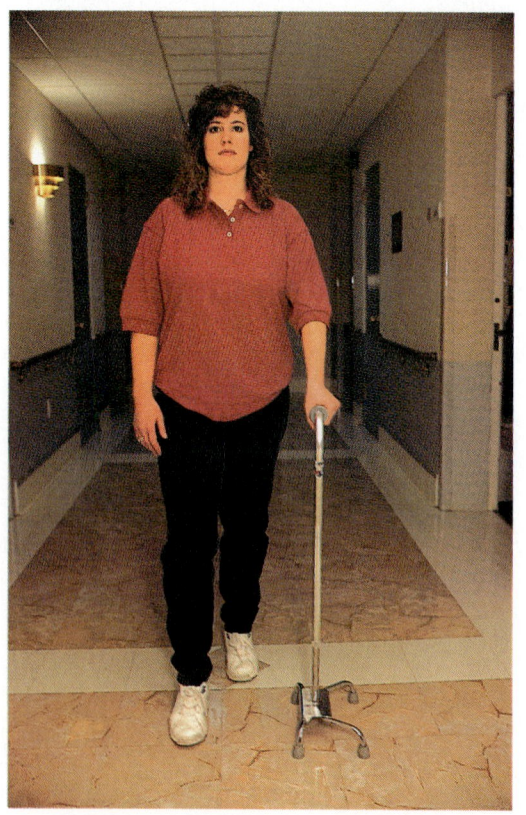

Figure 28-10

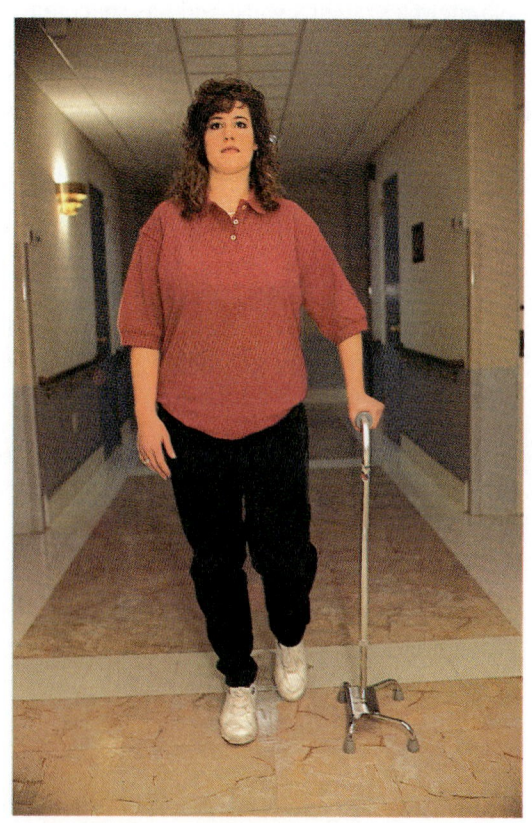

Figure 28-11

Steps	Rationale

7. Crutches

a. Crutch measurement includes three areas: client's height, distance between crutch pad and axilla, and angle of elbow flexion. Measurements may be taken with client standing or lying down.

    (1) *Standing.* Position crutches with crutch tips at point 4 to 6 inches (10 to 15 cm) to side and 4 to 6 inches in front of client's feet. Position crutch pads 1 ½ to 2 inches (4 to 5 cm) below axilla. Two or three fingers should fit between top of crutch and axilla (Figure 28-12). Instruct client to report any tingling or numbness in upper torso. This may mean crutches are being used incorrectly or that they are wrong size.

    (2) *Supine.* Crutch pad should be 3 to 4 finger widths under axilla, with crutch tips positioned 6 inches (15 cm) lateral to client's heel (Figure 28-13).

Measurement promotes optimal support and stability. Radial nerves that pass under axilla are superficial. If crutch is too long, it can cause pressure on axilla. Injury to nerve causes paralysis of elbow and wrist extensors, commonly called crutch palsy. If crutch is too long, shoulders are forced upward and client cannot push body off the ground. If ambulation device is too short, client will be bent over and uncomfortable.

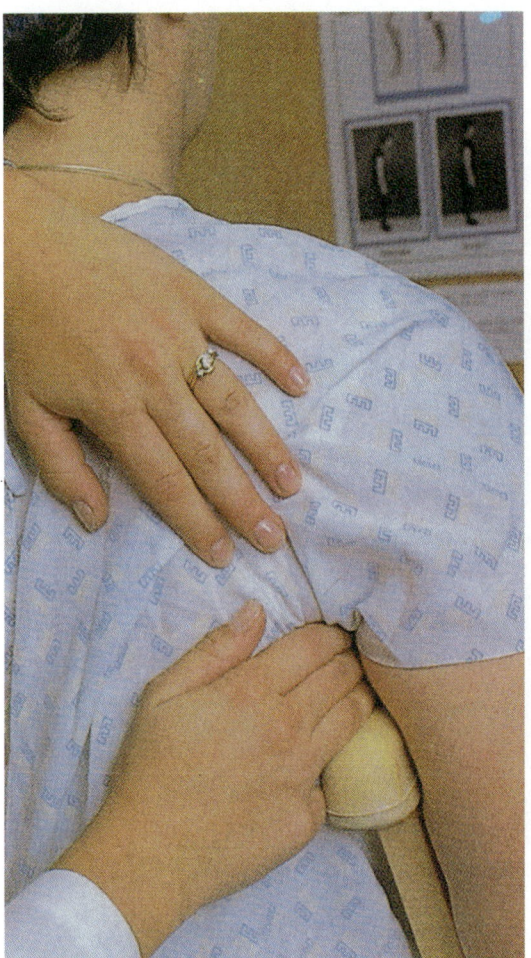

Figure 28-12

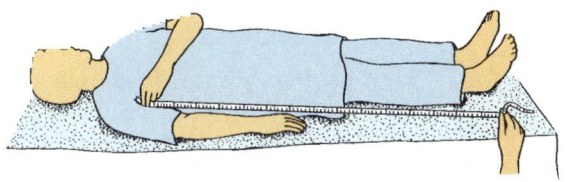

Figure 28-13

Steps	Rationale

(3) Elbow flexion is verified with goniometer (Figure 28-14). Handgrip should be adjusted so that client's elbow is flexed 15 to 30 degrees.

Low handgrips cause radial nerve damage. High handgrips cause client's elbow to be sharply flexed, and strength and stability of arms are decreased.

b. To use crutches, client supports self with hands and arms. Therefore, strength in arm and shoulder muscles, ability to balance body in upright position, and stamina are necessary. Type of gait client uses in crutch walking depends on amount of weight client is able to support with one or both legs.

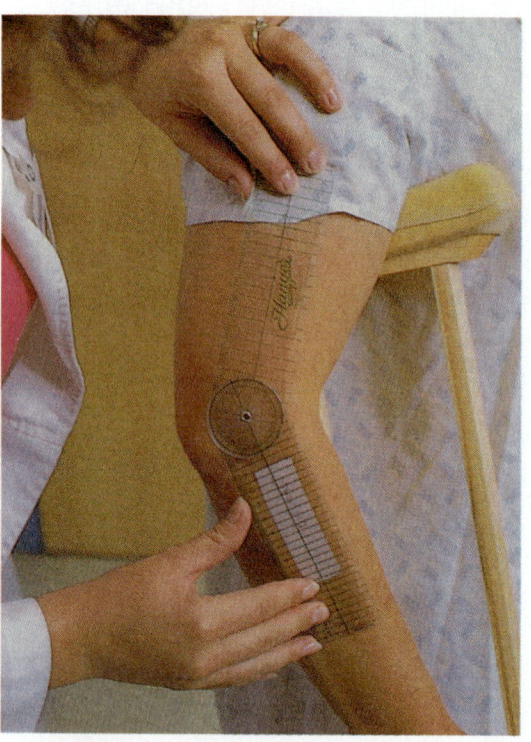

Figure 28-14

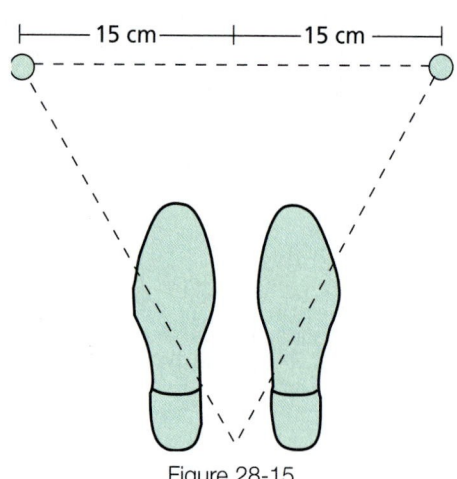

Figure 28-15

Choose appropriate crutch gait.

(1) *Four-point gait*

(a) Begin in tripod position (Figure 28-15). Crutches are placed 6 inches (15 cm) in front and 6 inches to side of each foot. Posture should be erect head and neck, straight vertebrae, and extended hips and knees.

Most stable of crutch gaits because it provides at least three points of support at all times. Requires weight bearing on both legs. Often used when client has paralysis, as in spastic children with cerebral palsy (Whaley and Wong, 1995). May also be used for arthritic clients. Improves client's balance by providing wider base of support.

Steps	Rationale

(b) Move right crutch forward 4 to 6 inches (10 to 15 cm) (Figure 28-16, *A*).

(c) Move left foot forward to level of left crutch (Figure 28-16, *B*).

(d) Move left crutch forward 4 to 6 inches (Figure 28-16, *C*).

(e) Move right foot forward to level of right crutch (Figure 28-16, *D*).

(f) Repeat sequence.

Crutch and foot position are similar to arm and foot position during normal walking.

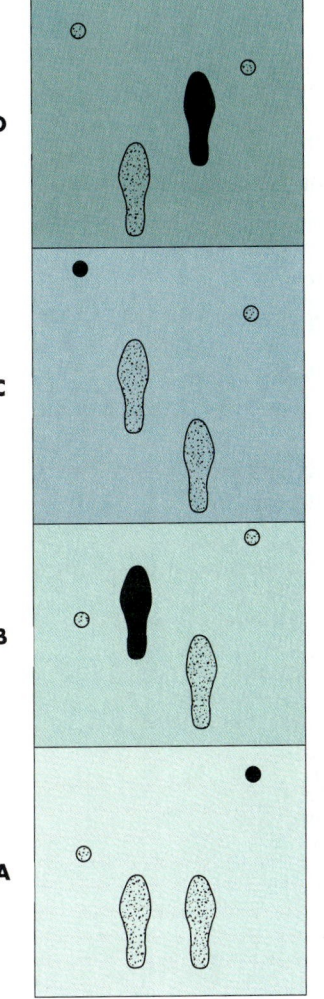

Figure 28-16   Figure 28-17

(2) *Three-point gait*

    (a) Begin in tripod position.

    (b) Advance both crutches and affected leg (Figure 28-17).

    (c) Move stronger leg forward.

    (d) Repeat sequence.

(3) *Two-point gait*

    (a) Begin in tripod position.

Requires client to bear all weight on one foot. Weight is borne on uninvolved leg, then on both crutches. Affected leg does not touch ground during early phase of three-point gait. May be useful for client with broken leg or sprained ankle.

Improves client's balance by providing wide base of support.

Requires at least partial weight bearing on each foot. Is faster than the four-point gait. Requires more balance because only two points support body at one time.

Improves client's balance by providing wider base of support.

Steps	Rationale
(b) Move left crutch and right foot forward (Figure 28-18).	Crutch movements are similar to arm movement during normal walking.
(c) Move right crutch and left foot forward.	
(d) Repeat sequence.	
(4) *Swing-to gait*	Frequently used by clients whose lower extremities are paralyzed or who wear weight-supporting braces on their legs.
	This is the easier of the two swinging gaits. It requires the ability to bear body weight partially on both legs.
(a) Move both crutches forward.	
(b) Lift and swing legs to crutches, letting crutches support body weight.	
(c) Repeat two previous steps.	
(5) *Swing-through gait*	Requires that client have the ability to sustain partial weight bearing on both feet.
(a) Move both crutches forward.	Increases client's base of support so that when the body swings forward, client is moving the center of gravity toward the additional support provided by crutches.
(b) Lift and swing legs through and beyond crutches.	
(6) *Climbing stairs with crutches*	
(a) Begin in tripod position.	Improves client's balance by providing wider base of support.
(b) Client transfers body weight to crutches (Figure 28-19).	Prepares client to transfer weight to unaffected leg when ascending first stair.

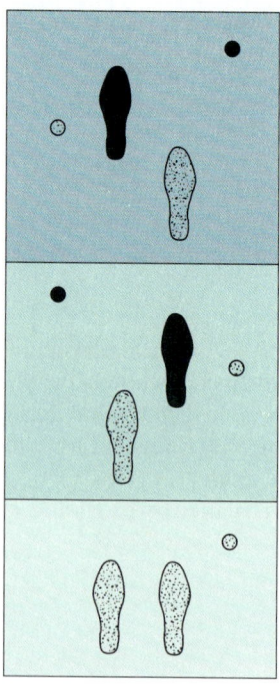

Figure 28-18

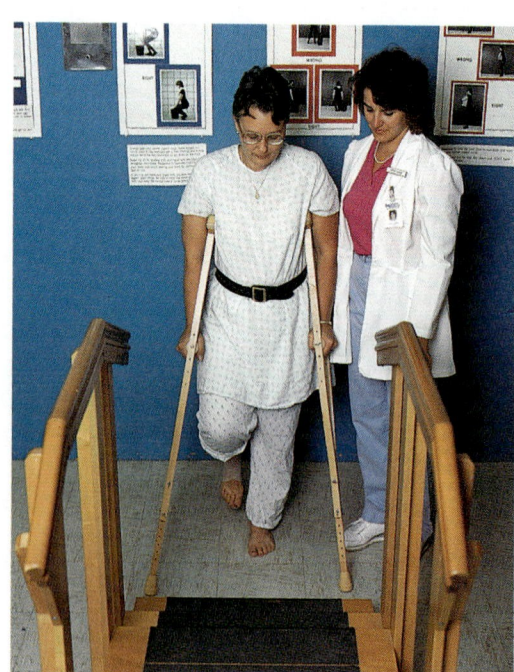

Figure 28-19

Steps	Rationale

(c) Client advances unaffected leg to stair (Figure 28-20).

Crutch adds support to affected leg. Client then shifts weight from crutches to unaffected leg.

(d) Both crutches are aligned with unaffected leg on stairs (Figure 28-21).

Maintains balance and provides wide base of support.

(e) Repeat sequence until client reaches top of stairs.

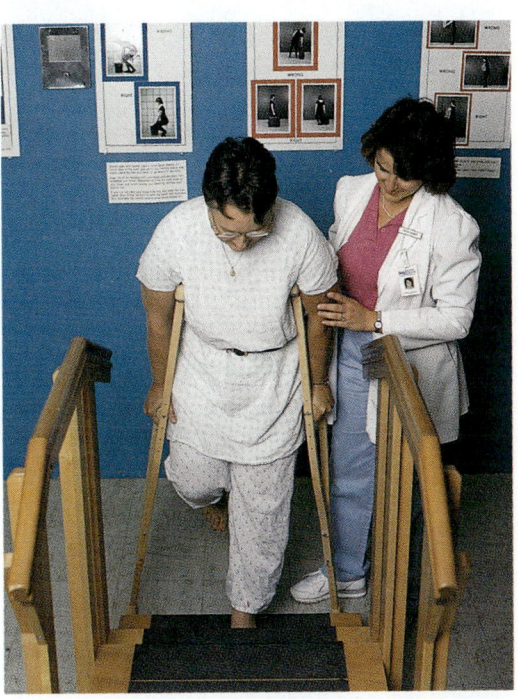

Figure 28-20

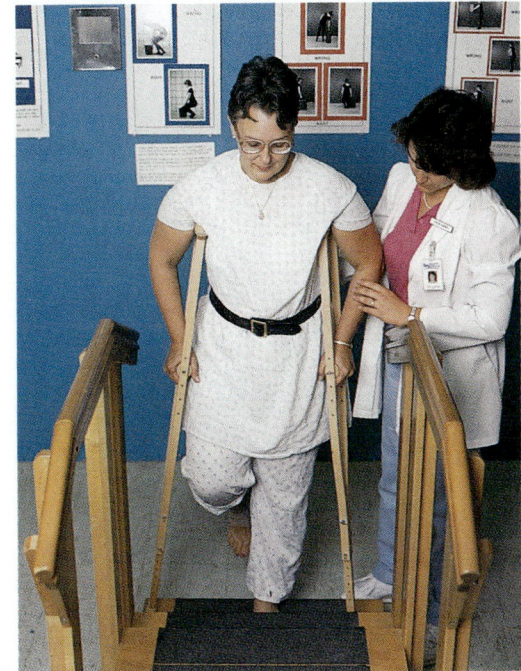

Figure 28-21

(7) *Descending stairs with crutches*

   (a) Begin in tripod position.

Improves client's balance by providing wider base of support.

   (b) Client transfers body weight to unaffected leg (Figure 28-22).

Prepares client to release support of body weight maintained by crutches.

   (c) Move crutches to stair below, and instruct client to begin to transfer body weight to crutches (Figure 28-23) and move affected leg forward.

Maintains client's balance and base of support.

   (d) Client moves unaffected leg to stair below and aligns with crutches (Figure 28-24).

Maintains balance and provides base of support.

   (e) Repeat sequence until client reaches bottom step.

c. Teach client to sit in a chair.

   (1) Transfer both crutches to the same hand and transfer weight to crutches and unaffected leg.

   (2) Grasp arm of chair with free hand and lower into chair (Figure 28-25).

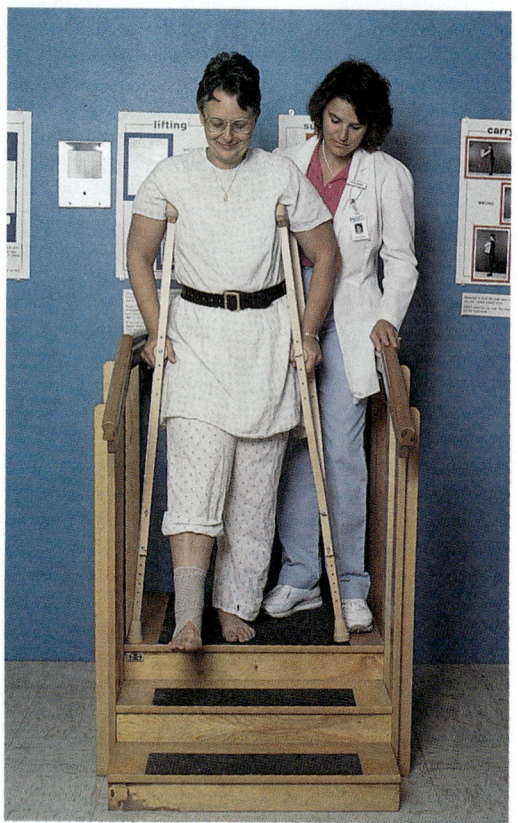

Figure 28-22

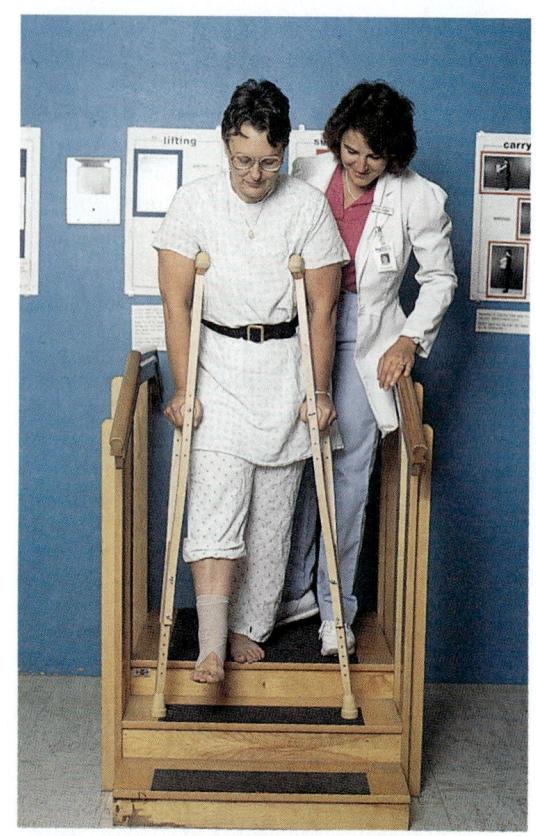

Figure 28-23

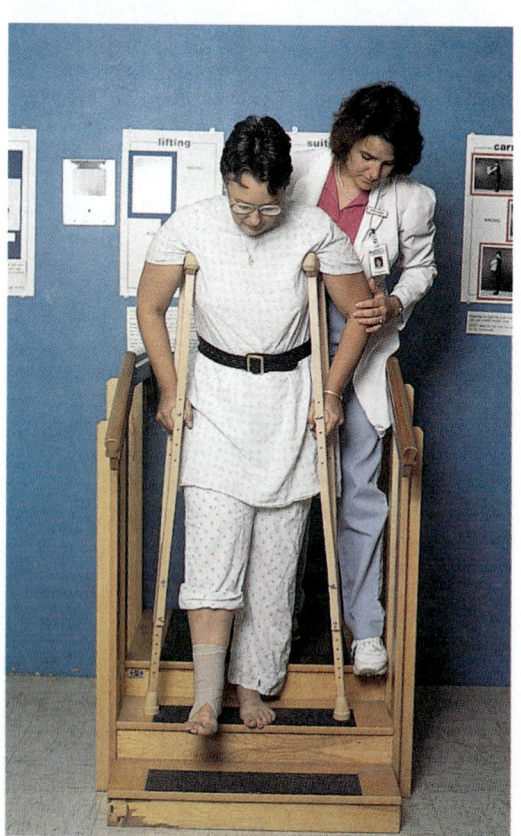

Figure 28-24

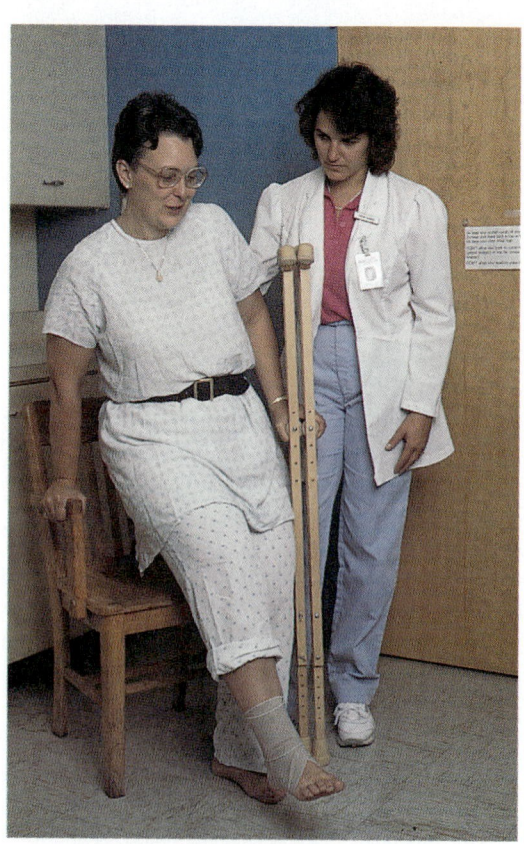

Figure 28-25

Steps	Rationale

8. Walker

a. Upper bar of walker should be slightly below client's waist. Elbows should be flexed at approximately 15 to 30 degrees when standing with walker, with hands on handgrips.

b. Assist client in ambulating.

Walkers do need to be picked up and moved forward. Client must have sufficient strength to be able to move walker. A four-wheeled walker, which does not have to be picked up, is not as stable and may cause injury. Client balances self before attempting to walk.

(1) Have client stand in center of walker and grasp handgrips on upper bars.

(2) Lift walker, moving it 6 to 8 inches (15 to 20 cm) forward, making sure all four feet of walker stay on the floor. Take a step forward with either foot. Then follow through with the other foot (Figures 28-26 and 28-27). If there is unilateral weakness after walker is advanced, instruct client to step forward with the weaker leg, support self with the arms, and follow through with the uninvolved leg. If client is unable to bear full weight on the weaker leg after advancing walker, have client swing the stronger leg through while supporting weight on hands.

Provides broad base of support between walker and client. Client then moves center of gravity toward the walker. Keeping all four feet of the walker on the floor is necessary to prevent tipping of the walker.

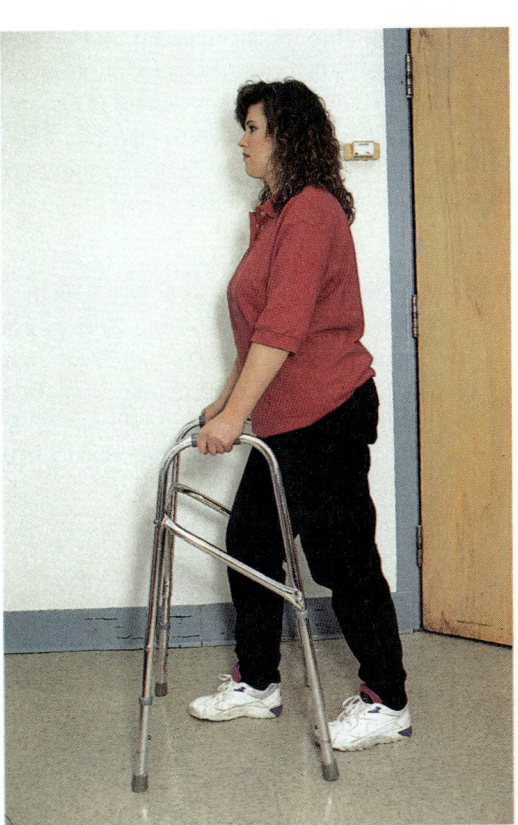

Figure 28-26

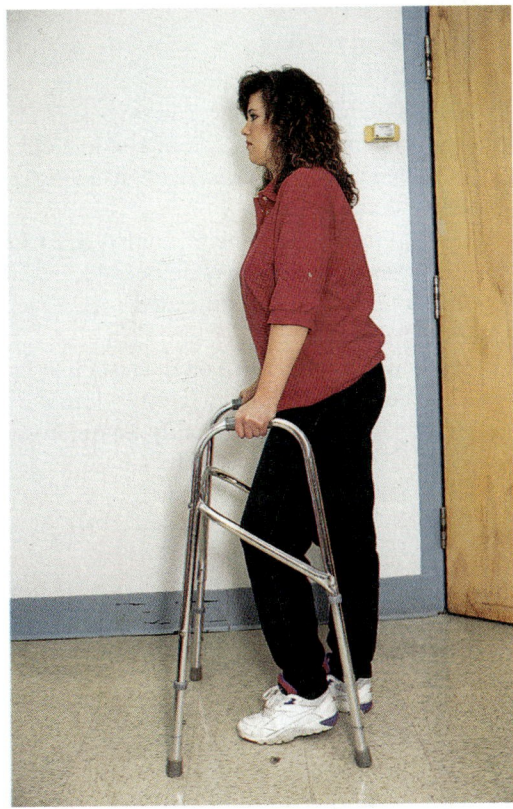

Figure 28-27

Steps	Rationale
9. Have client take a few steps with the assistive device being used. If client is hemiplegic (one-sided paralysis) or has hemiparesis (one-sided weakness), stand next to client's unaffected side. Then support client by placing arm closest to client on safety belt or around client's waist and other arm around inferior aspect of client's upper arm.	Providing constant contact by nurse reduces the risk of fall or injury.
10. Take a few steps forward with client. Then assess for strength and balance.	Ensures client has satisfactory strength and balance to continue.
11. If client becomes weak or dizzy, return to bed or chair, whichever is closer.	Allows client to rest.
12. See Completion Protocol (Chapter 1, p. 6).	

Evaluation

1. Observe client using assistive device.
2. Inspect hands and axillae for injury caused by using assistive device.
3. Ask client to rate level of discomfort after ambulating.
4. Monitor client for increased heart rate, blood pressure, respirations, or shortness of breath during and after ambulation.
5. Ask client/family about the ease with which hygiene, eating, and toileting activities are performed using assistive device.

UNEXPECTED OUTCOMES AND RELATED INTERVENTIONS

1. Client is unable to ambulate correctly.
   a. Reassess client for correct fit of assistive device.
   b. Have added assistance nearby to ensure safety.
   c. Reassess comfort level.
   d. Reassess muscle strength in uninvolved extremities. Alternative device may be needed.
2. Client became dizzy and lightheaded.
   a. Call for assistance.
   b. Have client sit or lie down on nearest chair or bed.
   c. Assess client's vital signs.
   d. Allow client to rest thoroughly before resuming activity.
   e. Ask if client is ready to continue.

SAMPLE DOCUMENTATION

Cane

0900 Client able to ambulate 20 feet correctly using quad cane and standby assist of one. Client requested pain pills. Rates pain in right knee at 6 (scale 0 to 10). Client returned to bed. Side rails up × 4.

0910 Prescribed analgesic given. Resting quietly in bed.

Crutches

0900 Client able to ambulate 40 feet correctly using axillary crutches and standby assist of one. Gait slow and steady. Client then able to ambulate up and down stairs correctly using axillary crutches, standby assistance of two needed to steady gait. Client voiced no complaints of pain. Returned to bed. Side rails up × 4. Client instructed not to get out of bed without assistance of hospital personnel. Client voiced understanding.

Walker

0900 Client able to ambulate 20 feet correctly using walker. Became dizzy and lightheaded. Client assisted to chair with assistance of two personnel. Vital signs: BP 126/70, P 78, R 18. Client rested 5 minutes and then continued ambulating back to bed. Side rails up × 4. Vital signs: BP 124/80, P 72, R 16. Client denies dizziness or discomfort.

CRITICAL THINKING EXERCISES

1. How might teaching the use of crutches vary for an older adult client?

2. Mrs. Gilbert has a sprained left ankle and is learning to use a cane. During ambulation, you observe her bent over with her right elbow fully extended when her left leg is lifted from the floor. What conclusions can you make based on these observations? Are any adjustments required?

3. Marshall is a 60-year-old male with a fractured left femur. The physician has prescribed non–weight-bearing crutch walking. Marshall has a history of an inner ear condition, which causes occasional dizziness. Discuss which type of crutch gait would be most appropriate, and explain the rationale for your selection.

4. You are assisting a client with walker ambulation. You are approximately 50 feet from the nurse's station and the client's room. Suddenly the client complains of lightheadedness.
   a. What would you do first?
   b. Once safety is assured, what additional data should you collect, and why?

REFERENCES

Hale J, Clark A, Harrison R: Guidelines for prescription walking frames, *Physiotherapy* 76(2):118, 1990.

Joyce B, Kirby L: Canes, crutches, and walkers, *Am Fam Physician* 443(2):535, 1991.

Mourad L, Droste M: *The nursing process in care of adults with orthopedic conditions,* ed 3, Albany, N.Y. 1993, Delmar.

Perry A, Potter P: *Clinical nursing skills and techniques,* ed 3, St Louis, 1994, Mosby.

Phipps W, et al: *Medical-surgical nursing: concepts and clinical practice,* ed 5, St. Louis, 1995, Mosby.

Whaley L, Wong D: *Nursing care of infants and children,* ed 4, St Louis, 1995, Mosby.

ADDITIONAL READINGS

Angelucci D, Todaro A, Reno A: When our patients get up is our decision, *RN* 54 (3):19, 1991.

Beare P, Myers J: *Principles and practice of adult health nursing,* St Louis, 1994, Mosby.

Clarkson H, Bhambhani Y: Complications from using axillary crutches, *Can J Rehabil* 3(4):233, 1990.

Corwin D, Miller C: Get your patient off on the right foot, *RN* 53(11):44, 1990.

Deathe A: Canes, crutches, walkers, and wheelchairs: a review of metabolic energy expenditure, *Can J Rehabil* 5(4):217, 1992.

Hall J, Clarke E: An evaluation of crutches, *Physiotherapy* 77(3):156, 1991.

Lane P, LeBlanc R: Crutch walking, *Orthop Nurs* 9(5):31, 1990.

LeBlanc M, Carlson L, Nausenberg T: A quantitative comparison of four experimental axillary crutches, *J Prosthet Orthot* 5(1):40, 1993.

Simpson C, Pirrie L: Walking aids: a survey of suitability and supply, *Physiotherapy* 77(3):231, 1991.

Weaver C: Terminology: assisted gaits, *Clin Manage* 12(1):32, 1992.

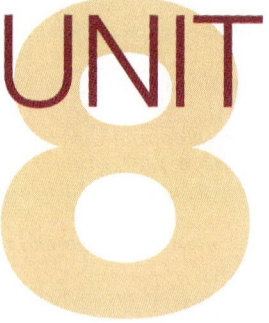

UNIT 8

Managing Complex Nursing Interventions

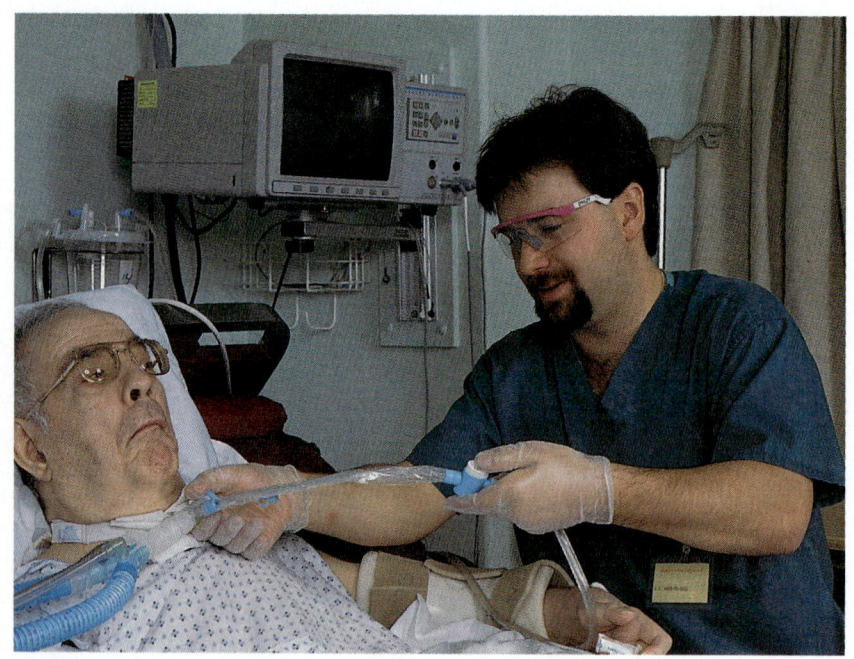

chapter
29

Intravenous Therapy

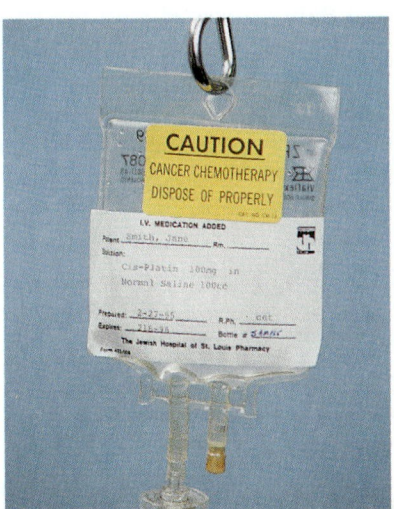

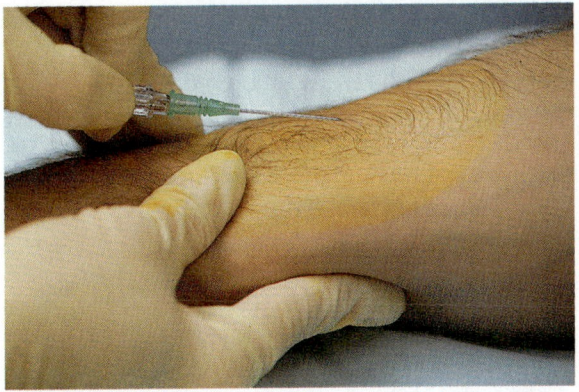

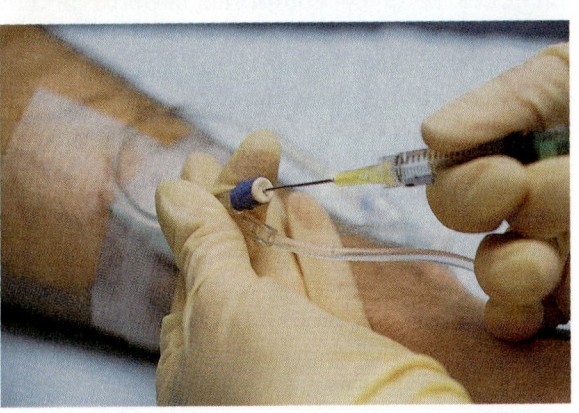

Delivery of infusion therapy is an essential element in the treatment of clients and requires a nurse's professional accountability as well as skill. The nurse applies the nursing process when assessing and choosing the most appropriate vascular access site and device, preparing the client, using proper insertion technique, and closely monitoring the infusion until the completion of therapy. Because of the extensive use of intravenous (IV) therapy, the professional nurse plays a primary role in safely and efficiently delivering IV medications and fluids as well as protecting the client from the potential complications associated with IV therapy.

Nurses should follow institutional policy and procedure when managing IV therapy. Individual practitioners should know the various Nurse Practice Act regulations in their state regarding care and insertion of IV devices for short-duration and long-duration therapy. These may vary from state to state.

National standards guide nursing practice in safeguarding the client, the nurse, and the institution. The Intravenous Nurses Society (INS) Standards of Practice outlines nurses' scope of responsibility in the practice and education in the specialty area of IV therapy. INS stan-

507

dards and standards set forth by the Oncology Nursing Society (ONS) and the American Society for Parenteral and Enteral Nursing (ASPEN) have been developed to ensure quality client care in this high-technology arena (LaRocca and Otto, 1994).

A nurse must be highly skilled with IV therapy. An IV device is invasive, increasing the risk of infection. Pain is associated with any IV insertion. A client's previous experience with IV therapy also affects how the nurse approaches care. The nurse's skill and expertise directly influence the client's response to the initiation of therapy.

Assessment of a client who requires IV therapy should be comprehensive. The nurse considers anatomy and physiology, fluid and electrolyte balance, chemistry, pathophysiology, and the client's response to illness. Assessment also extends to the observation of the client's venous anatomy of the upper extremities, assessment of mobility or immobility, and previous attempts or experiences of IV therapy. The goal of all IV therapy is to restore, prevent, or correct fluid and electrolyte imbalance without complications associated with the delivery of IV medications or fluids.

Nursing Diagnosis

Nursing diagnoses for clients receiving IV therapy may include **Risk for Infection** related to an invasive procedure. The client with an IV line is also at risk for **Impaired Skin Integrity.** For the client receiving IV therapy for correction of fluid and electrolyte imbalance or with potential or existing alterations in regulatory mechanisms of hydration, actual or potential **Fluid Volume Excess** or actual or potential **Fluid Volume Deficit** may be appropriate.

Psychological factors such as **Fear** related to the client's previous experience with IV therapy or perceived **Pain** associated with the actual procedure may result in apprehension or fright. Tension and **Anxiety** may cause sympathetic stimulation, resulting in venous constriction, making venipuncture more difficult and painful. Fear of venipuncture may result in the autonomic nervous system response of vasovagal reaction, resulting in syncope, bradycardia, and peripheral vascular collapse.

| Skill 29.1 | # Basic IV Insertion Techniques (Intermittent and Continuous Infusion) |

To maintain fluid and electrolyte balance, isotonic, hypotonic, or hypertonic fluids can be delivered through a variety of IV methods using continuous or bolus infusion. IV therapy also provides access to the venous system to deliver various medications in emergent and nonemergent situations and to infuse blood or blood products. Reliable access for IV administration is one of the most essential features of current medical care (Maki, 1991).

Successful delivery of peripheral IV therapy depends on client preparation, vein selection, selection of an appropriate catheter, and skilled catheter insertion. Numerous vascular access devices are available for use (Table 29-1). Since potential for exposure to blood-borne pathogens is high during insertion and care of IV devices, adherence to asepsis and universal precautions is required (see Chapters 3 and 14).

EQUIPMENT (Figure 29-1)
Tourniquets
Disposable gloves
Prepping agent(s) (70% alcohol, povidone-iodine, tincture of iodine)
IV fluids (if applicable)
Tubing (if applicable)
Heparin stopper or PRN adapter (intermittent infusion)
3 ml syringe

Flush solution (e.g., sterile normal saline [NS] or heparin)
Transparent membrane dressing
Sterile 2 × 2 pad with Betadine ointment
IV pole
Appropriate IV catheter (gauge appropriate to type of solution infused) (Table 29-1)

Assessment

1. Assess client's previous or perceived experience with IV therapy and arm placement preference. **This determines level of emotional support and instruction necessary.**

2. Determine if client is to undergo any planned surgeries. **This allows nurse to place an adequate-size catheter (i.e., 18 or 16 gauge for surgery) and avoids placement in an area that will interfere with medical procedures.**

3. Assess client's activities of daily living (ADLs). **This ensures placement will not impair therapy or interfere with mobility and improves client's comfort and tolerance of IV therapy.**

4. Assess the type and duration of IV therapy as ordered by the physician. **This assists in selection of an appropriate access device and early placement of**

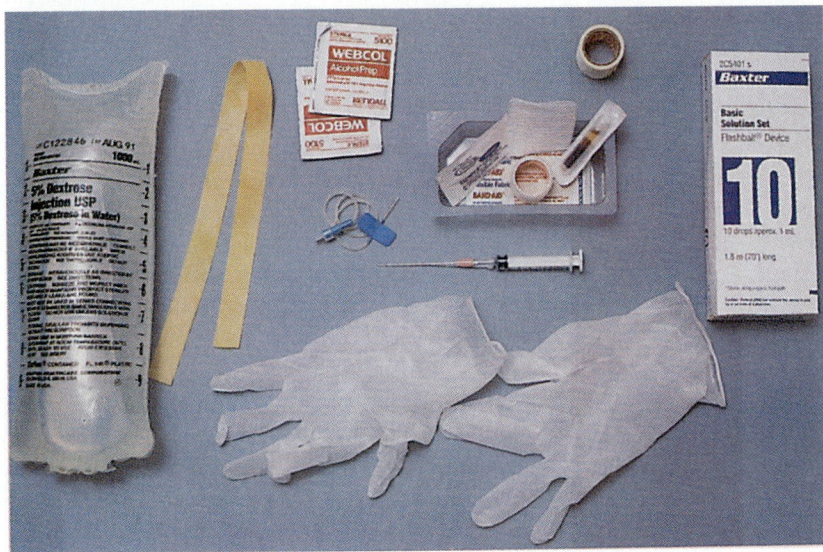

Figure 29-1 Equipment for starting IV therapy.

Table 29-1 **IV Access Device Options**

Type	Use
Winged infusion butterfly catheter	One-time infusion, IV push administration

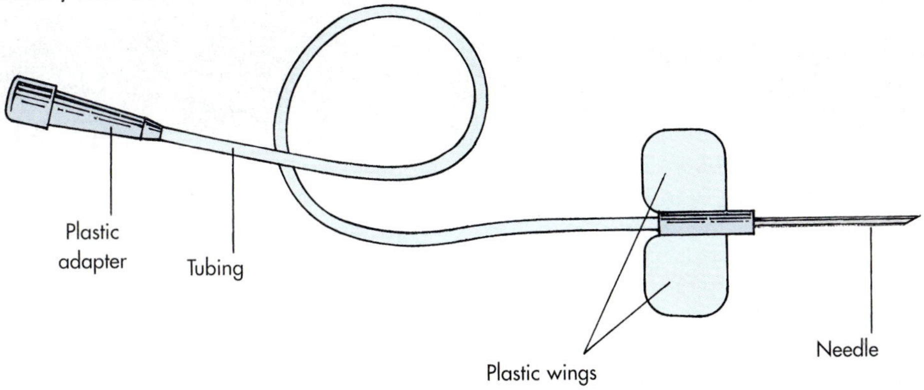

Plastic adapter Tubing Plastic wings Needle

Short, over-the-needle catheter (ONC) (less than 3 inches [7.5 cm])	Continuous infusion, intermittent infusion, short–term duration (less than 1 week)

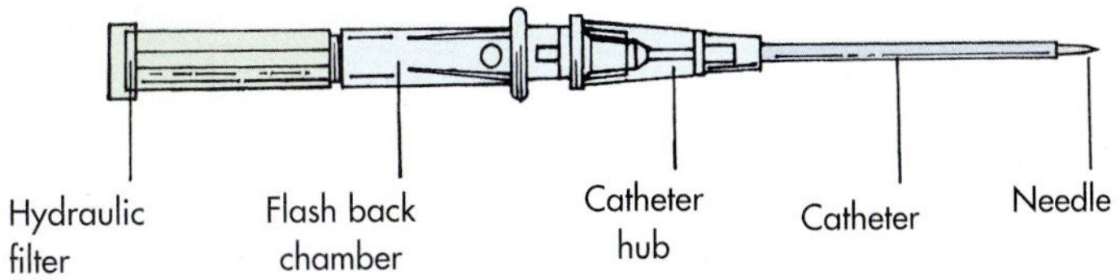

Hydraulic filter Flash back chamber Catheter hub Catheter Needle

Peripheral midline 6-inch (15 cm) catheter	Nonhyperosmolar therapy lasting 1 to 6 weeks

Catheter adapter Sleeve Needle hub Flow control plug end style Catheter Collar Needle

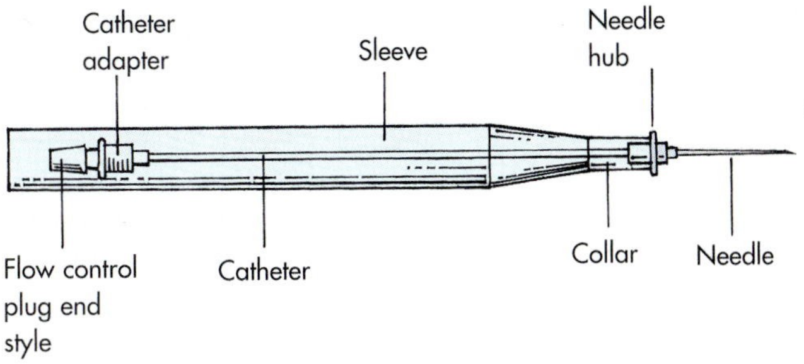

Peripherally inserted central venous catheter, tunneled or implanted access device	Hyperosmolar therapy lasting 1 to 6 weeks or longer

longer-term infusion devices and minimizes multiple venipunctures.

5. Assess laboratory data and client's history of allergies. **This may reveal information that affects insertion of devices, such as fluid volume deficit or allergy to iodine or adhesive.**

Planning

Expected outcomes focus on minimal complications from IV therapy, minimal discomfort to the client, restoration of normal fluid and electrolyte balance, and client's ability to verbalize complications that require immediate nursing intervention.

EXPECTED OUTCOMES

1. Client achieves a normal level of fluid volume as evidenced by body weight within client's range, client's hemodynamic status is normal, and client's electrolyte level stays within a normal range.
2. Client is free of complications from IV therapy as evidenced by positive blood return from the IV device and the absence of pain, swelling, or redness during and after the infusion.
3. Client verbalizes comfort and minimal restrictions to ADLs during IV therapy.
4. Client identifies one symptom of infiltration (e.g., swelling), phlebitis (e.g., tenderness), and IV occlusion (e.g., stoppage of flow).
5. Client has appropriate serum level of titrated drug.

Implementation

Steps	Rationale
1. See Standard Protocol (Chapter 1, p. 5).	
2. Assist client in techniques to minimize anxiety: visual imagery, deep breathing, and not looking at the site. Explain steps of procedure.	Assists in minimizing apprehension, sympathetic nervous system stimulation, and possible vasovagal reaction to venipuncture.
3. Prepare equipment and prime tubing, maintaining sterility of closed system (see Skill 29.2).	
4. Apply tourniquet 4 to 6 inches (10 to 15 cm) above the proposed insertion site (Figure 29-2).	Tourniquet should be tight enough to impede venous return but *not* occlude arterial flow.

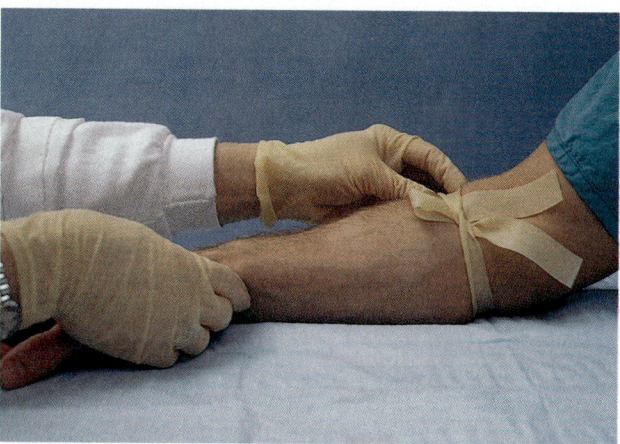

Figure 29-2 Tourniquet application.

Steps	Rationale
5. Select the vein.	
a. Use the most distal site in the nondominant arm, if possible (Figure 29-3).	Venipuncture should be performed distal to proximal, which increases the availability of other sites for future IV therapy.
b. Avoid areas that are painful to palpation.	
c. Select a vein large enough for catheter placement.	Prevents interruption of venous flow while allowing adequate blood flow around the catheter.

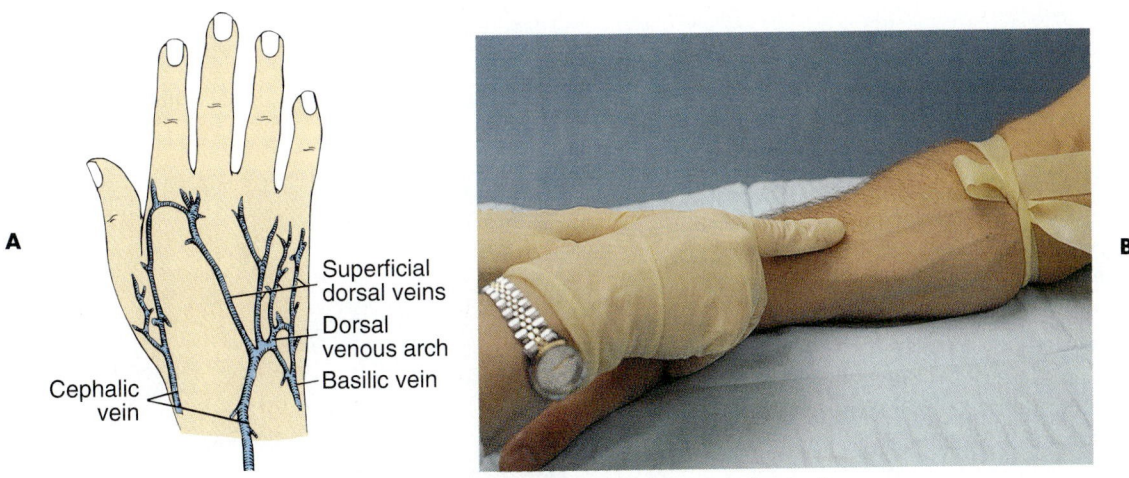

Figure 29-3 **A,** Veins in hand. **B,** Actual distended veins in arm.

Steps	Rationale
d. Choose a site that will not interfere with client's ADLs or planned procedures.	
e. Palpate the vein, feeling for resiliency, softness, fullness, and a "spongy" feeling.	Vein is accessed easily with less chance of infiltration.
f. Avoid sites distal to previous venipuncture site, sclerosed or hardened cordlike veins, infiltrated site or phlebitic vessels, or bruised areas.	Such sites cause infiltration of newly placed IV line.
g. Avoid fragile dorsal veins in older adult and vessels of surgically compromised arm (mastectomy or fistula).	
6. Release tourniquet temporarily and carefully. Clip arm hair with scissors. Avoid shaving the area.	Hair impedes venipuncture or adherence of the dressing. Shaving can cause microabrasions and predispose client to infection.
7. Reapply tourniquet. Ask client to clench and open fist several times. If veins do not enlarge from engorgement:	
a. Lower arm in dependent position.	Causes veins to fill more quickly.
b. Apply warm packs to arm for 10 to 20 minutes.	Heat causes vasodilation.
c. Rub or stroke client's arm or hand toward the tourniquet.	Promotes venous filling.
d. *Option:* Apply a blood pressure cuff instead of tourniquet, and inflate to level just below client's diastolic pressure (e.g., if client's diastolic is 80, inflate to 70). Maintain inflation at that pressure until the completion of venipuncture. (Observe circulation to arm carefully.)	Distends veins.

nurse alert In clients with sclerosed vessels or veins that are prominent without a tourniquet (e.g., older adult client with congestive heart failure [CHF]), application of a tourniquet may increase venous pressure and distention and make venipuncture more difficult.

Steps	Rationale

8. Cleanse the insertion site using a circular motion, moving from the insertion site outward in concentric circles. Use 70% alcohol, povidone-iodine, or tincture of iodine and allow to dry (Figure 29-4). Reprep the skin if touched after preparation.

Drying prevents chemical reactions between agents.

9. Stabilize the vein by pulling the skin taut opposite the direction of the venipuncture.
10. Tell client that he or she will feel a sharp, quick stick. Puncture the skin and vein using a direct or indirect approach, holding the catheter at a 20- to 30-degree angle (Figure 29-5).

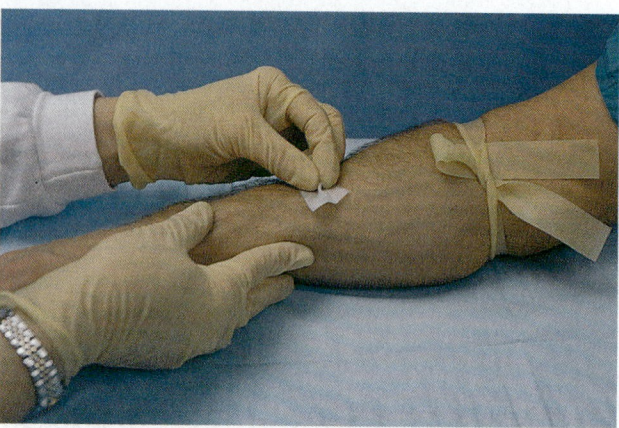

Figure 29-4 Cleanse insertion site with antiseptic prep.

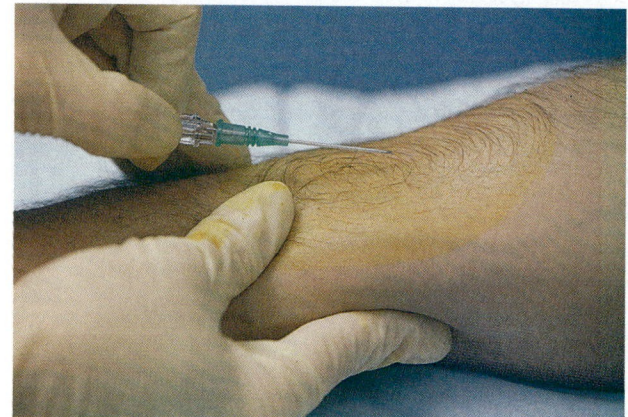

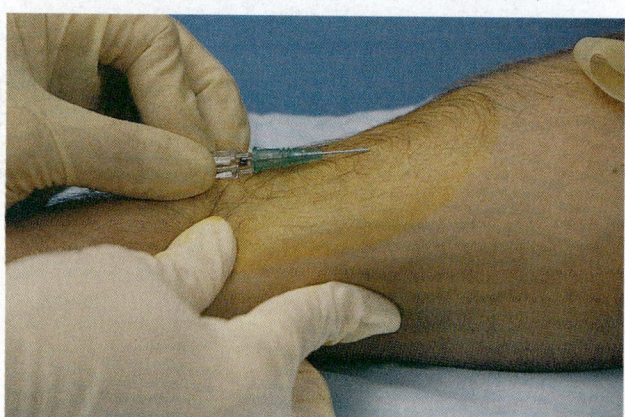

Figure 29-5 **A,** Puncture skin with catheter at 20- to 30-degree angle. **B,** Enter vein with bevel pointing up.

11. Observe for a "flashback" of blood in the catheter's stylet, lower the catheter until almost flush with the skin, and slowly advance another ⅛ to ¼ inch.

Allows for full penetration of the vein wall, placement of the catheter in the vein's inner lumen, and easy advancement of the catheter off the stylet.

12. Release the tourniquet (or blood pressure cuff).

Restores venous return.

13. Push the catheter off the stylet using a one-handed or two-handed technique (Figure 29-6).
14. After catheter is fully advanced, apply pressure with index finger of nondominant hand 1¼ inches (3 cm) above the insertion site and remove the stylet.

Obstructs venous flow, minimizing blood loss, and reduces exposure when removing the stylet.

15. Connect IV tubing (Figure 29-7) primed with fluid or attach injection cap, maintaining sterile technique.

16. **Intermittent infusion**
Hold the cannula firmly with nondominant hand. Insert prefilled syringe containing flush solution into injection cap. Flush injection cap slowly with flush solution. Withdraw the syringe while still flushing.

"Positive-pressure flushing" allows fluid to displace the removed needle, creates positive pressure in the catheter, and prevents reflux of blood during flushing. Stabilizing the cannula prevents accidental withdrawal or dislodgement.

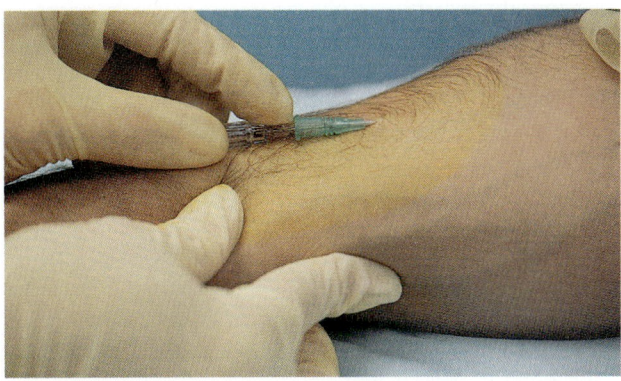

Figure 29-6 Push catheter off stylet using one-handed technique.

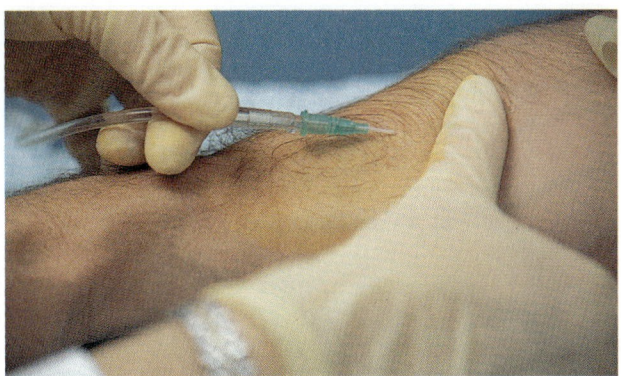

Figure 29-7 Connect IV tubing.

Steps	Rationale

17. **Continuous infusion**

Begin the infusion by opening the slide clamp or adjusting the roller clamp of the IV tubing.

Initiates flow of fluid through IV catheter, preventing clotting.

18. Tape the IV catheter (Figure 29-8). Place narrow piece ($\frac{1}{2}$ inch) of tape under hub of catheter with adhesive side up and cross tape over hub.

Place tape only on the catheter, *never* over the insertion site. Secure the site to allow easy visual inspection and early recognition of infiltration and phlebitis. Avoid applying tape around the extremity.

Securing the catheter and tubing prevents movement and tension on the device, reducing mechanical irritation and possible phlebitis or infection.

Taping around extremity could result in a "tourniquet effect" and impede venous return.

19. Apply a sterile dressing over the site.

a. **Transparent dressing**

Carefully remove adherent backing. Apply one edge of dressing and then gently smooth remaining dressing over IV site (Figure 29-9).

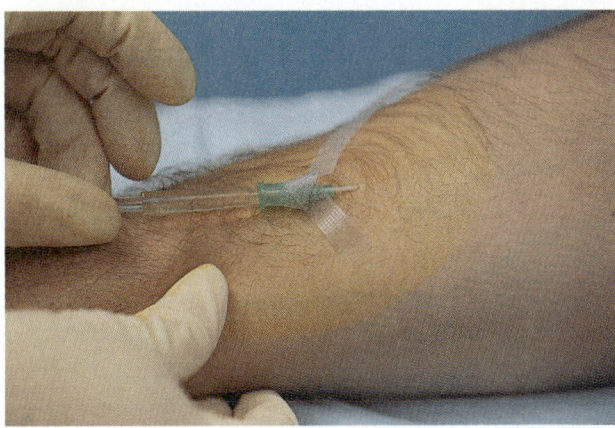

Figure 29-8 Tape the catheter.

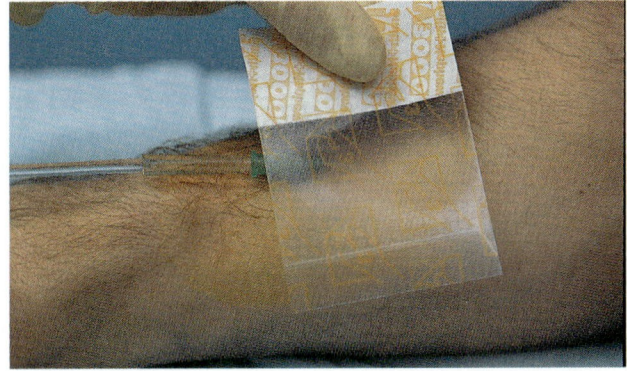

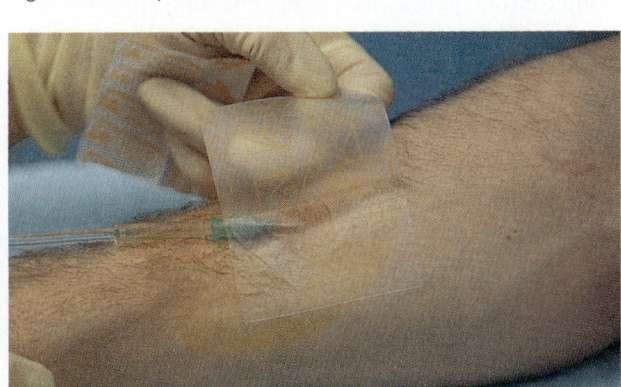

A

B

Figure 29-9 **A,** Apply transparent dressing, holding onto backing. **B,** Apply dressing smoothly over IV site.

Steps	Rationale
b. Sterile gauze dressing Apply Betadine ointment to insertion site. Place 2 × 2 gauze pad over venipuncture site and catheter hub. Do not cover connection between IV tubing and catheter hub. Secure with tape. **20.** Label the dressing, including the date, time, catheter gauge size and length, and nurse's initials.	Allows for easy recognition of type of device and time interval for site rotation. Intravenous Nursing Society's (INS) standard for site rotation of IV access devices is every 48 hours (INS, 1990). Check agency policy.
21. Instruct client on how to move about in and out of bed without dislodging IV line. Dispose of uncapped needle(s) and stylet in appropriate "sharps" container as soon as device is secured. **22.** See Completion Protocol (Chapter 1, p. 6).	

nurse alert   If venipuncture is unsuccessful, always obtain a new catheter before a second attempt. Never reinsert the stylet into the catheter, since this may cause injury to the catheter and potential catheter embolism.

Evaluation

1. Monitor client's intake and output, daily weights as indicated, skin turgor, mucous membranes, and vital signs for evidence of normal fluid volume.
2. Inspect client's IV site and extremity every 2 to 4 hours for the absence of pain, swelling, or redness during the infusion. Aspirate for blood return if necessary.
3. On completion of IV insertion and during IV infusion, ask if client is comfortable. Observe client during activity for restrictions to mobility.
4. Ask client to describe one symptom of infiltration, phlebitis, and occluded infusion device complications (e.g, swelling, pain, tenderness, reduced flow).
5. Monitor therapeutic drug levels, ensuring appropriate timing of laboratory specimens and infusions of medications.

UNEXPECTED OUTCOMES AND RELATED INTERVENTIONS

1. *Phlebitis:* Client complains of pain and tenderness at IV site with erythema at site or along path of vein. Insertion site is warm to touch, and rate of infusion may stop.
   a. Discontinue existing IV and restart in another site, preferably in opposite extremity, with new IV tubing and fluids.
   b. Document degree of phlebitis and nursing interventions per agency policy and procedure.

2. *Infiltration:* Client's rate of infusion slows; site of insertion becomes swollen, cool to touch, pale, and painful.
   a. Discontinue existing IV line and restart in another site, preferably in opposite extremity.
   b. Monitor previous insertion site every 4 hours until resolution of swelling.
3. Client experiences burning, irritation, redness, or pain during infusion without phlebitis or infiltration.
   a. Slow the infusion to deliver in maximum time for best therapeutic response.
   b. Assess client's tolerance to prescribed therapy. Discuss with client and physician insertion of midline or peripherally inserted central catheter as an option if duration of therapy and venous access permit.
4. Client's therapeutic drug levels are out of normal range.
   a. Notify physician with laboratory results.
   b. Change medication delivery schedule as ordered.
5. Infusion is completed before or after appropriate time frame.
   a. Evaluate access device for position and patency, and restart as necessary.
   b. Monitor client for too rapid infusion or fluid overload. Check vital signs, respiratory status, and intake and output.
   c. Monitor client for signs and symptoms of drug toxicity.

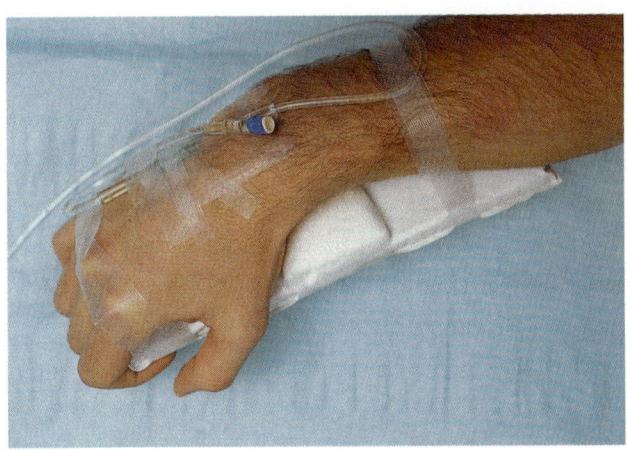

Figure 29-10 IV armboard.

c. Continue hourly monitoring for proper rate of infusion.
7. *Infection:* Client complains of chills, fever, and malaise; IV site may show purulent drainage.
   a. Discontinue IV site by prepping first with alcohol (removes resident bacteria). Allow to dry. Then place dry sterile gauze over insertion site and remove catheter.
   b. Retain previous IV catheter for possible culture, and notify physician.
   c. Document nursing intervention as delineated in agency policy and procedure.

DOCUMENTATION

Documentation may be recorded on an IV Maintenance Record (see pp. 516 to 517).

1500 After procedure explained and site prepped with alcohol and Betadine, left median antebrachial vein accessed with 20-gauge 1¼" Insyte catheter. Positive blood return after full advancement. Catheter flushed with 1 ml NS, and saline lock attached for IV antibiotics. Client stated insertion was nonpainful and "felt fine" after insertion.

d. Notify physician.
e. Reregulate remainder of infusion to infuse over prescribed time.
6. *Positional IV infusion:* Client's flow rate is altered and changes with position of extremity.
   a. Apply arm board (Figure 29-10).
   b. Remove dressing, reprep with prepping agents, and resecure devices.

Skill 29.2 | Regulating Flow Rates

The ability to establish accurate infusion rates in IV therapy is essential to deliver prescribed infusion volumes and medications. Complications associated with IV therapy (e.g., infiltration, phlebitis, clotting of device, circulatory overload) can be reduced or eliminated with a properly regulated IV infusion. Various factors can interfere with infusion rates (Table 29-2). Observation of the flow rate and IV system should occur hourly to achieve the desired therapeutic response.

Numerous methods are used to ensure an accurate hourly infusion rate for IV therapy. Fluids that run by gravity are adjusted through use of a flow control/regulator clamp. Fluids infused by an electronic infusion device or rate controller are regulated by a mechanical pump set at the prescribed rate. Physicians usually order the volume of fluid a client is to receive within a specific time frame. For example, "Administer 1 liter of D₅NS over 8 hours." The nurse must be able to calculate hourly flow rates to ensure the prescribed amount of fluid infuses over 8 hours. Regardless of gravity infusion or infusion via an electronic device, the nurse must assess infusion rates hourly.

When infusing high volumes of IV fluids (more than 150 ml/hour) to clients with impaired renal clearance, older adults, or pediatric clients, or when infusing drugs

or IV fluids that require specific hourly volumes, electronic infusion pumps permit accurate, on-time infusion. Electronic infusion devices deliver the infusion via positive pressure. A rate controller used on gravity infusions regulates the infusion but, unlike the electronic pump,

Table 29-2 **Alterations in Flow Rates**

Client factors	Mechanical factors
Change in client position	Height of parenteral container (should be higher than 36 inches [90 cm] above heart)
Flexion of involved extremity	Positional access device
Partial or complete occlusion of IV device	Viscosity or temperature of IV solution
Venous spasm	Occluded air vent
Vein trauma (phlebitis)	Occluded in-line filter
Manipulated by client or visitor	Improperly placed restraints
	Crimped administration set tubing
	Tubing dangling below bed
	Low battery of an electronic device

ST. JOHN'S HOSPITAL
Springfield, Illinois
I.V. MAINTENANCE RECORD

I.V. FLUID & I.V. MEDICATION

Site Code

R.J. or L.J. – Right or Left Jugular
R.S.V. or L.S.V. – Right or Left Subclavian Vein
R.L.L. or L.L.L. – Right or Left Lower Leg
R.H. or L.H. – Right or Left Hand
R.F.A. or L.F.A. – Right or Left Forearm
R.U.A. or L.U.A. – Right or Left Upperarm
R.F. or L.F. – Right or Left Foot
R.S., L.S. or M.S. – Right, Left or Mid Scalp
R.F.V. or L.F.V. – Right or Left Femoral Vein
R.A.C. or L.A.C. – Right or Left Antecubital
R.W. or L.W. – Right or Left Wrist

K.V.O. – Keep Vein Open
H.L. – Heparin Lock
P.B. – Piggyback
P. – Push

Triple Lumen Catheter

Proximal - 18 gauge (White) Draw blood, Blood Adm, Medications
Middle - 18 gauge (Blue) TPN Medications
Distal - 16 gauge (Brown) Blood Adm. Colloids Viscous Fluids CVP Monitoring Medications

Allergy:

No. of last I.V. _____ Letter of last expander _____

No. of last Blood/Component _____

Signature:

	DATE		
	Night Nurse		
	Day Nurse		
	Evening Nurse		

Order Date		Amount, Solution, Infusing Time or Rate, Medication, Dose, Time	Site(s)			Pump	Time	Time
		One Time I.V. Meds.						
	No.	I.V. Fluids						
		I.V. TUBING CHANGE. (Indicate I.V. No. & Time)						
	Stop Date	Intermittent & PRN I.V. Meds.						
		I.V.P.B. TUBING CHANGE (Indicate Drug & Time)						

#1005
(1 of 2)

I.V. MAINTENANCE RECORD

I.V. SITE ASSESSMENT

SITE CODE		TYPE CODE	
R.J. or L.J. – Right or Left Jugular		M.C. – Medicut	H.C. – Hickman Catheter
R.S.V. or L.S.V. – Right or Left Subclavian Vein	K.V.O. – Keep Vein Open	A.C. – Angiocath	B.C. – Broviac Catheter
R.L.L. or L.L.L. – Right or Left Lower Leg	H.L. – Heparin Lock	S.V. – Scalpvein	M.L.C. – Multi-lumen Catheter
R.H. or L.H. – Right or Left Hand	P.B. – Piggyback	A.S. – Angio-set	M.L.P. – Multi-lumen Proximal
R.F.A. or L.F.A. – Right or Left Forearm	P. – Push	C.D. – Cutdown	M.L.M. – Multi-lumen Middle
R.U.A. or L.U.A. – Right or Left Upperarm	Cath – Catheter	I.C. – Intracath	M.L.D. – Multi-lumen Distal
R.F. or L.F. – Right or Left Foot		I.P. – Infuse A Port	I. – Introducer
R.S., L.S. or M.S. – Right, Left or Mid Scalp			
R.F.V. or L.F.V. – Right or Left Femoral Vein			
R.A.C. or L.A.C. – Right or Left Antecubital			
R.W. or L.W. – Right or Left Wrist	NA – Not Applicable		

Document on each site once each shift & P.R.N.   No space is to be left blank.   Place "NA" in spaces which do not apply.

Date	Time	I.V. Site Start	d/c	Site Code	Cath Size	Type Code	Site Day	Cap Change	Dressing Change	I.V. Site: s̄ tenderness redness, edema, drainage	Signature

(Courtesy St. John's Hospital, Springfield, Ill.)

can be affected by many mechanical and client factors. Recent advances in infusion technology have resulted in a variety of devices available for use to ensure accurate delivery.

Many devices have sophisticated operating and programming capabilities that allow for single- and multiple-solution infusions at different rates. A variety of detectors and alarms respond to air in IV lines, completion of infusion, high and low pressure, low battery power, occlusion, and the inability to deliver at a preset rate. An anti–free flow safeguard (preventing bolus infusion in the event of machine malfunction) is an important element of an electronic infusion pump. Most pumps may be used for IV infusions. Manufacturer's recommendations for specific device features should always be checked.

Nursing Diagnosis

Nursing diagnoses associated with clients receiving medications and solutions include **Fluid Volume Deficit** related to fluid and electrolyte imbalance and **Risk for Fluid Volume Excess** related to excessive IV infusion or to alterations in regulatory mechanisms of hydration.

EQUIPMENT

Watch with a second hand
Paper, pencil (or calculator)
IV tubing, macro drip or micro drip, depending on rate ordered by physician
Electronic infusion control device (optional)
Volume control device (optional)
Tape
Label

Assessment

1. Identify client's risk for fluid imbalance (e.g., pediatric, older adult, history of heart failure or renal failure). **Strict control of infusion volumes may be required.**
2. Review client's medical record for physician's order, stating type, amount, and rate or duration of IV fluid order or IV medications.
3. Assess client's understanding of purpose of therapy and knowledge of how positioning affects flow rate.
4. Determine the presence of any client or mechanical factor that may alter ordered fluid rates (confusion, noncompliance, electrolyte imbalance). **This increases the risk of IV infusion complications.**
5. Obtain information from pharmacology references about specific infusion requirements of IV medication, admixture, or device.
6. Assess patency of IV device.

Planning

Expected outcomes focus on administration of IV fluids at the prescribed rate.

EXPECTED OUTCOMES

1. Client receives prescribed volume of fluid.
2. Client's IV fluids and medications are administered over appropriate time frame with achievement of therapeutic response.
3. Client describes factors that alter rate of flow.

Implementation

Steps	Rationale

1. See Standard Protocol (Chapter 1, p. 5).
2. Obtain IV fluid and appropriate tubing.
   a. *Macro drip:* Delivers rates *greater than* 100 ml/hr. (Drip factor is 10 to 15 gtt/ml depending on equipment used. Drop factor is printed on box.)
     Travenol Laboratories: 10 gtt/ml
     Abbott Laboratories: 15 gtt/ml
     McGraw Laboratories: 15 gtt/ml
   b. *Micro drip:* Delivers rates *less than* 100 ml/hr.
     Micro drip: 60 gtt/ml
3. Calculate desired flow rate (hourly volume) of prescribed infusion:.
	Use of correct tubing ensures more accurate infusion delivery. Macro drip tubing allows for higher infusion volumes. Micro drip tubing is used for slow delivery and lower volumes.

Steps	Rationale

Flow rate (ml/hr) =

$$\frac{\text{Total infusion (volume in ml)}}{\text{Hours of infusion (time to be infused)}}$$

Example: $\dfrac{1000\ ml}{8\ hr} = \dfrac{125\ ml}{1\ hr}$

4. Calculate the drop rate based on drops per minute.

$$\frac{\text{gtt factor}}{60} \times \frac{\text{Flow rate}}{1} = \text{Drop rate}$$

Examples: Infuse 120 ml/hr via 10 gtt/ml drop factor:

$$\frac{10}{60} \times \frac{120}{1} = 20\ \text{gtt/ml}$$

Via 15 gtt/ml:

$$\frac{15}{60} \times \frac{120}{1} = 30\ \text{gtt/ml}$$

Via 20 gtt/ml:

$$\frac{20}{60} \times \frac{120}{1} = 40\ \text{gtt/ml}$$

Via 60 gtt/ml (microgtt):

$$\frac{60}{60} \times \frac{120}{1} = 120\ \text{gtt/ml}$$

5. Optional method for calculation:
If drop factor is 10 gtt/ml, take ordered rate per hour and divide by 6.
 ✳ If drop factor is 15 gtt/ml, take ordered rate per hour and divide by 4.
If drop factor is 20 gtt/ml, take ordered rate per hour and divide by 3.
If drop factor is 60 gtt/ml, take ordered rate per hour and divide by 1.

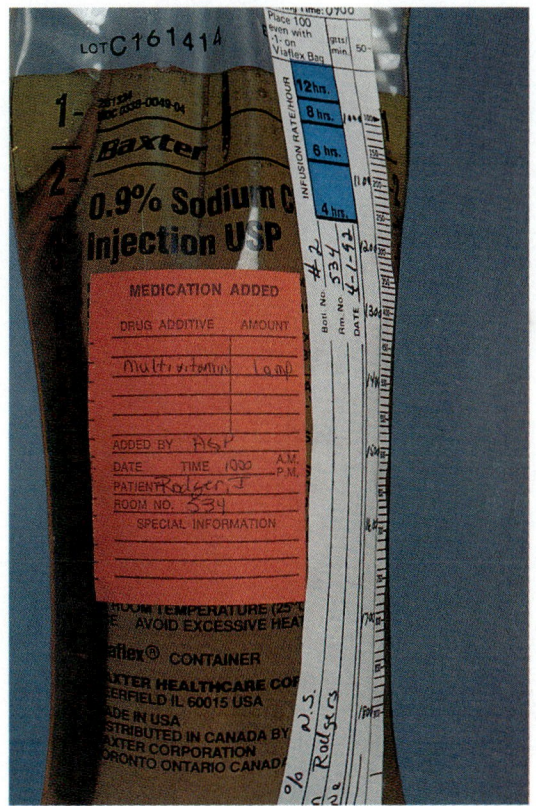

Figure 29-11 Apply time tape to IV bag.

6. Time-tape the IV bottle or bag by securing adhesive tape or fluid indicator tape along side of fluid container (Figure 29-11). Document each IV fluid bag sequentially, and note type of fluid, client's name, infusion span, and beginning and expected end of infusion.

Gives a visual scale to assess progress of infusion hourly. Avoid use of felt-tip pens or permanent markers on plastic bag; these can contaminate IV solutions (Milliam, 1992). In some agencies all fluids, including those on pumps, should be labeled and time-taped (see agency policy).

7. Close rate controlling clamp on IV tubing.

8. Insert infusion set into fluid bag. Remove protective cover from IV bag without touching opening. Remove cap from spike and insert spike into opening of IV bag (Figure 29-12). Hang bag from IV pole.

Maintains sterility of solution.

9. Fill drip chamber of tubing until half full by gently squeezing and releasing.

Creates vacuum, allowing fluid to enter drip chamber.

10. Open-rate controlling clamp and fill remainder of tubing (Figure 29-13). Invert Y connector sites to displace air. Most tubings can be fully filled or primed

Tubing must be fully filled with fluid before connecting to client to avoid air embolus.

Steps	Rationale

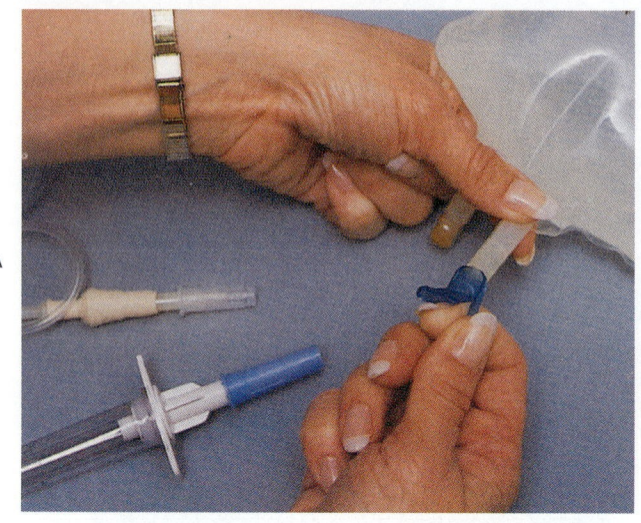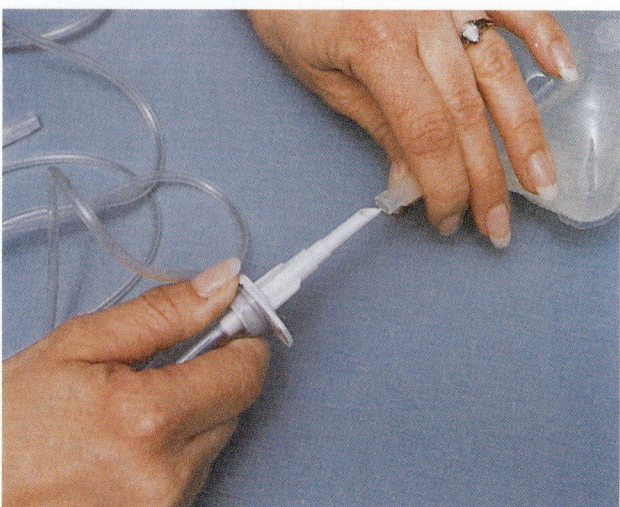

Figure 29-12 Insert spike of IV tubing into bag.

without removing the cover on the end of the IV tubing.

11. Close rate-controlling clamp on tubing.

12. Perform venipuncture (see Skill 29.1) and attach catheter to end of IV tubing, maintaining sterility.

13. With IV fluid bag a minimum of 36 inches (90 cm) above IV insertion site, adjust rate-controlling clamp to deliver drops per minute.

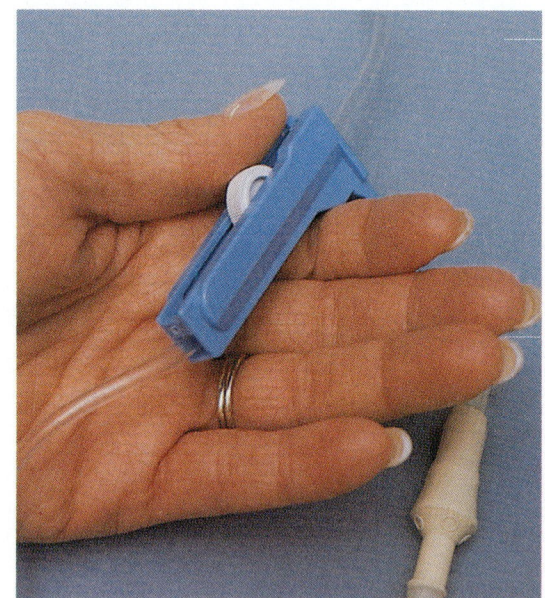

Figure 29-13 Open roller clamp to fill tubing.

14. *Option:* Attach to electronic infusion device or rate controller.

   a. Place electronic eye on half-filled drip chamber above fluid line (Figure 29-14).

Positioning necessary for accurate drip count.

   b. Insert IV tubing into chamber of control mechanism (Figure 29-15). (Consult manufacturer's instructions for use of pump.)

   c. Secure portion of IV tubing through "air in line" alarm system.

Allows for detection of air in tubing, which can enter vascular system, causing an embolus.

   d. Turn on pump, and select rate per hour and total volume to be infused (VTBI).

   e. Open rate-controlling clamp if closed and press start (Figure 29-16).

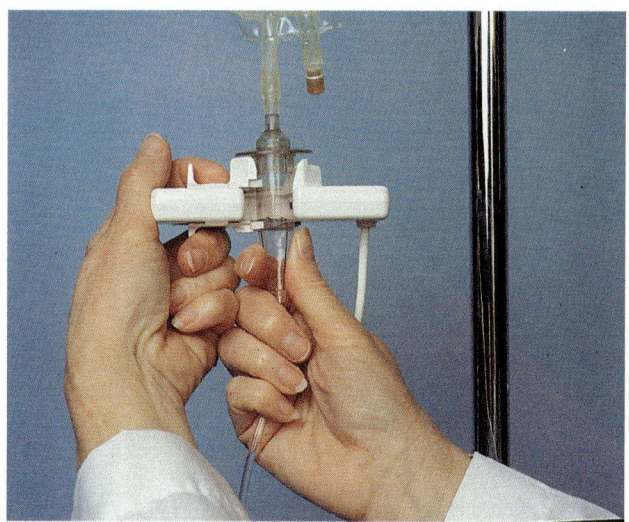

Figure 29-14 Place electronic eye on half-filled drip chamber.

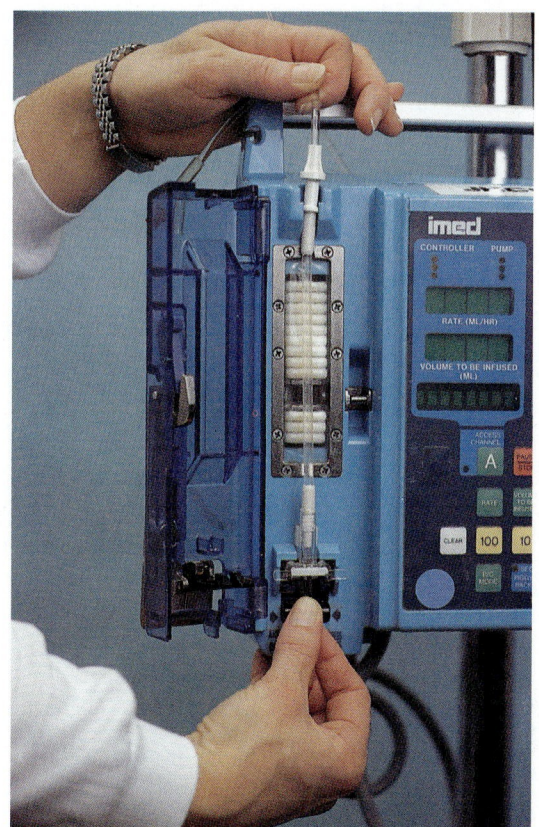

Figure 29-15 Insert tubing into pump chamber.

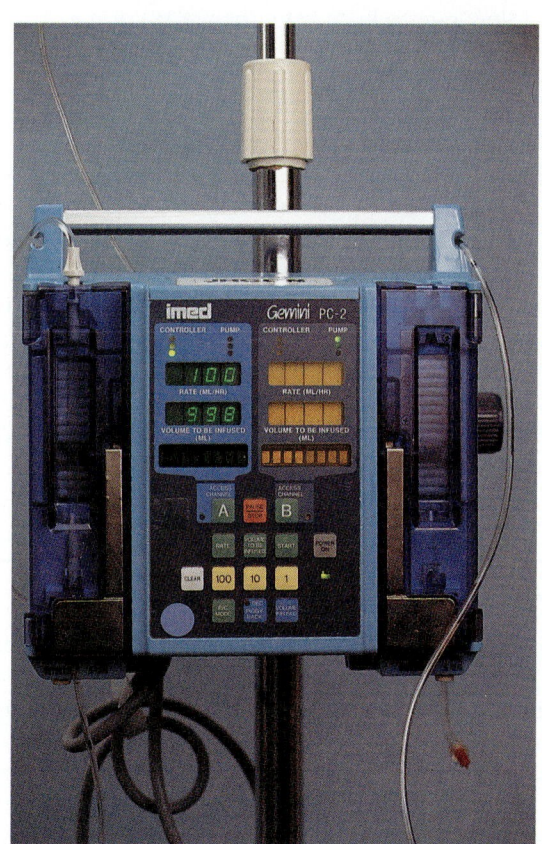

Figure 29-16 Press start button on IV pump.

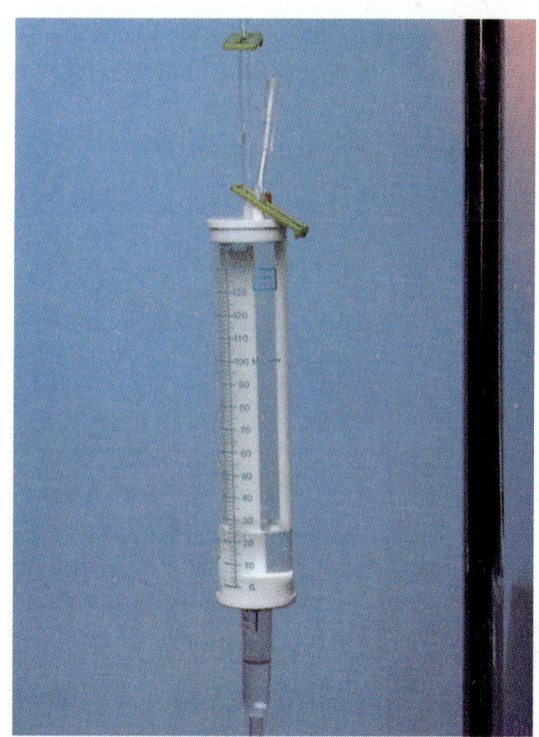

Figure 29-17 Volume control device.

Steps	Rationale
f. Monitor infusion hourly to assess patency of system when in alarm mode, and monitor for proper infusion rate and infiltration.	
15. *Option:* Attach IV tubing to volume control device.	
a. Place volume control device between IV bag and insertion spike of infusion set, using sterile technique (Figure 29-17).	
b. Fill IV tubing with fluid by opening regulator clamp.	
c. Place 2 hours of fluid allotment in chamber device.	This prevents infusion from running dry if 60 minutes elapses before nurse returns. Should infusion rate accidentally increase, will only allow 2 hours of fluids to infuse.
16. Instruct client about the following:	
a. To avoid raising hand or arm to a position that will affect flow rate.	
b. To avoid manipulation of rate control clamp.	
c. Purpose and significance of alarms.	
17. See Completion Protocol (Chapter 1, p. 6).	

Evaluation

1. Monitor client's IV infusion hourly for proper rate of infusion.
2. Observe client and client's laboratory values for signs and symptoms of overhydration or dehydration during infusion, observing for restoration of fluid and electrolyte balance and therapeutic response.
3. Evaluate client during ADLs for proper positioning of extremity and care of infusion tubing during activity.

UNEXPECTED OUTCOMES AND RELATED INTERVENTIONS

1. During hourly check, infusion is found to be behind. Recalculate remainder of infusion and confer with physician before reregulating.
2. Client experiences sudden onset of shortness of breath, tachycardia, restlessness, and confusion. Assessment of lung sounds reveals inspiratory crackles.

Client has received more than prescribed infusion volume.
   a. Evaluate for proper function of IV access device.
   b. Slow rate to keep vein open (KVO).
   c. Place client in high Fowler's position and notify physician.

DOCUMENTATION

Routine documentation is included on the IV Maintenance Record (see pp. 516 to 517).
1700 Client complaining of SOB. Lungs auscultated with inspiratory crackles in rt lower lobe. Dr. Lee notified. Order noted to decrease IV to 25 ml/hr. Positive blood return noted via 20-gauge IV right cephalic vein. Changed to IMED Gemini infusion at 25 ml/hr via pump. Purpose of fluid restriction and symptoms of pulmonary edema reviewed with client and wife with verbalized understanding.

Skill 29.3 | Administering IV Medications

Technological advances have resulted in the increase of drug delivery by the IV route. IV administration of medications is often preferred to oral or intramuscular (IM) administration because of efficacy of concentration, absorption, and rapid onset. The IV route is often required if the client is unable to take oral medications. Some drugs can only be administered by the IV route. Because of the principles that make IV administration the preferred route (rapid onset, improved serum drug concentrations), it also requires greater knowledge and skill by the nurse to prevent potentially dangerous complications when administering any IV medication. Parenteral administration of any drug is invasive and poses greater risk to the client.

When administering IV medications, the principles associated with delivery of any medication remain the same. The nurse should ensure it is the right client, right drug, right dose, right time, and right route. Drugs are documented immediately after administration. In addition to these basic rights, the nurse must also apply principles of IV therapy. Physical incompatibilities of IV medications, osmolality of drug admixtures, and potential for IV therapy–related complications must be considered before administering any medication intravenously.

A variety of methods are available for IV medication delivery. Since drugs given by the IV route are delivered directly into the vascular system, dosages are usually lower than for those given orally (LaRocca and Otto, 1994). Dosages and admixtures vary and are usually calculated based on the client's weight, drug distribution and absorption, safety of administration, excretion, and solubility in solution. IV medications can be mixed in large admixture volumes (e.g., addition of 40 mEq KCL to 1000 ml IV fluid), by "piggyback" infusion (e.g., administration of an antibiotic concurrently with an IV infusion), or by bolus injection (delivery of a small volume admixture through an existing IV access device). In all three methods of IV medication administration, the client is required to have an IV access device.

The nurse also must know the absorption, metabolism, and excretion of IV medications. Because the liver and kidneys metabolize and excrete by-products of the IV drug, systemic diseases such as liver and renal impairment affect absorption. Older adults usually have diminished renal and liver function and are more likely to experience toxicity related to IV drug administration than individuals with normal liver and kidney function. Clients with lower plasma proteins have more adverse effects when receiving IV medications, since therapeutic response to the drug is related to the amount of drug not bound to a plasma protein or tissue. Drug binding influences both the effectiveness of the drug given as well as the duration of the effect (LaRocca and Otto, 1994).

Some drugs such as heparin are required to be given by continuous infusion to maintain a therapeutic action. The efficacy of other drugs (e.g., antibiotics) and their therapeutic response are determined by therapeutic drug monitoring. Serum drug levels such as peak and trough aminoglycoside levels (gentamicin, vancomycin, amikacin) are performed at specific intervals during IV medication therapy to monitor response as well as protect the client from adverse effects if excretion of the metabolized drug is reduced. Blood levels reveal if drug doses are too high or low. Dosages are adjusted by increasing or decreasing the time between administration or by increasing or decreasing the drug amount to provide therapeutic levels within a narrow range. Monitoring therapeutic drug levels is an additional responsibility of the nurse when administrating IV medications and is crucial in safe and effective delivery of care to the client.

When giving IV medications, the nurse also assesses clients for hypersensitivity (allergic) reactions. The rapid absorption of IV medications, if the client has an allergic response or delayed hypersensitivity, occurs quickly and can be exhibited by a mild skin rash to anaphylaxis. The extent of the reaction is related to the hypersensitivity to the drug and the amount actually infused. If an allergic reaction occurs, the nurse should stop the medication, keep the IV line open with a plain fluid infusion, monitor the client for respiratory distress and changes in vital signs, notify the physician, and be prepared to administer

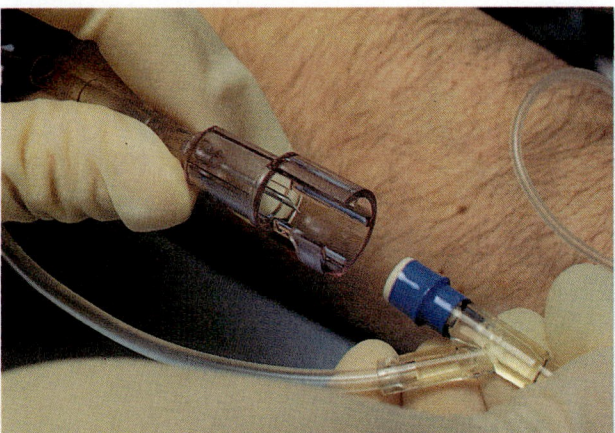

A

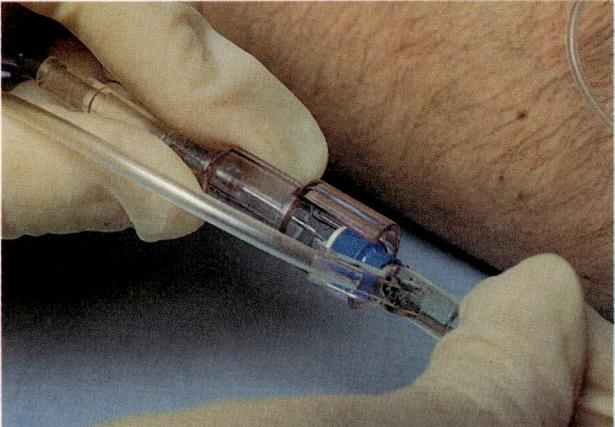

B

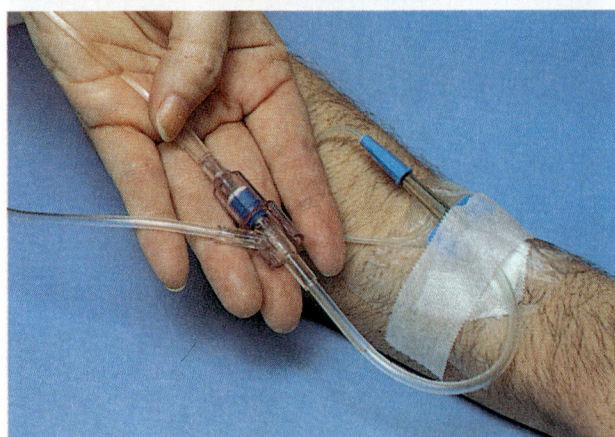

C

Figure 29-18 Needleless device; piggyback needle-lock device connected to injection port of main IV line.

emergency medications and resuscitative measures if necessary.

The Centers for Disease Control and Prevention (CDC) and the Occupational Safety and Health Administration (OSHA) have made recommendations that all intermittent infusions be administered via a needleless system. This can be achieved by the addition of stopcocks or use of a manufactured needleless system. Needleless infusion lines allow a direct connection with the IV line via a recessed connection port or a blunt-ended cannula or shielded needle device (Figure 29-18). The risk of exposure to an IV needle is eliminated when using these devices.

Nursing Diagnosis

Because of the use of IV access in the delivery of IV medications, **Risk for Infection** related to the invasive IV device may be an appropriate diagnosis. Potential for **Fluid Volume Excess** may also be considered because of the admixture volumes and medication regulated during IV infusion administration. **Risk for Injury** related to toxicity or hypersensitivity reaction should also be considered when giving IV medications. **Knowledge Deficit** related to drug therapy would be a consideration if assessment data reveal a lack of information with regard to side effects and purpose, or if a new drug is added to the client's therapeutic regimen. When a client receives an uncontrolled volume of fluid during medication administration, the nurse should be alert for **Decreased Cardiac Output** and **Ineffective Breathing Patterns.**

EQUIPMENT
IV Medication
  Vial or ampule of prescribed medication
  Small-volume admixture (NS, D_5W, or sterile water) in either syringe or 50 to 250 ml IV fluid bag
  Container for admixture diluent (Volutrol)
Sterile 19- to 21-gauge needle, 1 to $1\frac{1}{2}$ inches (20-gauge, 1-inch needle typically used) if system is not needleless
Label, if needed (Many small-volume admixtures are premixed and dispensed from pharmacy.)
Syringe pump, if applicable
Secondary administration set, if needed
Disposable gloves
Two 3 ml syringes filled with NS 0.9%

One 3 ml syringe filled with dilute heparin (10 U/ml) (optional)
Antiseptic swabs
Tape (optional)
IV pole
Medication administration record or computer printout

Assessment

1. Check physician's orders to determine type of IV solution, medication, dose, and route and frequency of administration.
2. Review information about drug, including action, purpose, peak onset, normal dose, side effects, and nursing implications. Note appropriate time for infusion (e.g., mg/min).
3. If administering aminoglycosides, assess baseline laboratory values (e.g., blood urea nitrogen [BUN] and creatinine, aminoglycoside peak and trough). **This determines drug efficacy and toxicity.**
4. Assess existing IV line for patency (see Skill 29.1), and note rate of main IV line.
5. Assess IV insertion site for signs of infiltration or phlebitis (pain, tenderness, redness, swelling, heat on palpation). **Administration of hyperosmolar drugs by IV route increases risk of phlebitis.**
6. Assess client's history of drug allergies. **This ensures a contraindicated medication is not administered.**
7. Assess client's understanding of purpose for drug therapy.

Planning

Expected outcomes of IV medication administration focus on ensuring therapeutic response of drug with minimum adverse reactions.

EXPECTED OUTCOMES
1. Drug infuses within desired period.
2. Client's IV site remains free of phlebitis or infiltration.
3. Client's laboratory values of therapeutic drug monitoring reveal desired response without renal toxicity.
4. Client does not show evidence of hypersensitivity or allergic reaction to IV medication.
5. Client or family is able to explain drug's purpose, action, side effects, and dosage.

Implementation

Steps	Rationale

1. See Standard Protocol (Chapter 1, p. 5).

2. Assemble medications in medication room using aseptic technique (see Chapter 14).

3. Check client identification, look at armband, and ask client to state name. — Identification of client is required before any medication administration.

4. Explain procedure, and encourage client to report any symptoms of discomfort at IV site during infusion.

5. IV push (bolus) (through existing line)

a. Select injection port closest to client. If add-on 0.22 μ filter is used, give IV push medications below the filter next to client, preventing medication from being absorbed in filter. — Ensures small-volume bolus enters vein quickly and directly.

b. Prepare injection site or cleanse connection port with antiseptic swab. Allow to dry.

c. Connect syringe to IV line.

(1) Needleless system

Remove cap of needleless injection port. Connect tip of syringe directly (Figure 29-19).

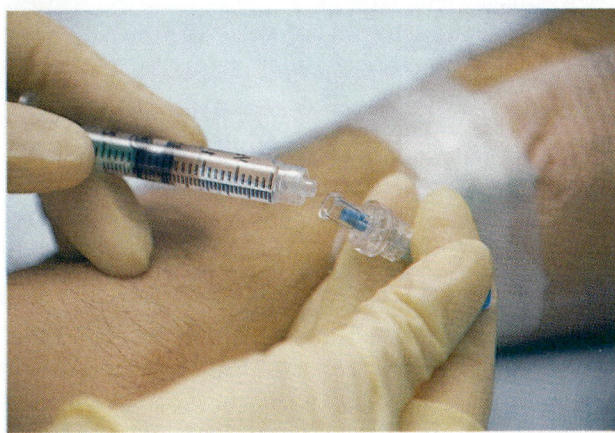

Figure 29-19 Connect tip of syringe directly to needleless port.

(2) Needle system

Insert small-gauge needle through center of injection port (Figure 29-20).

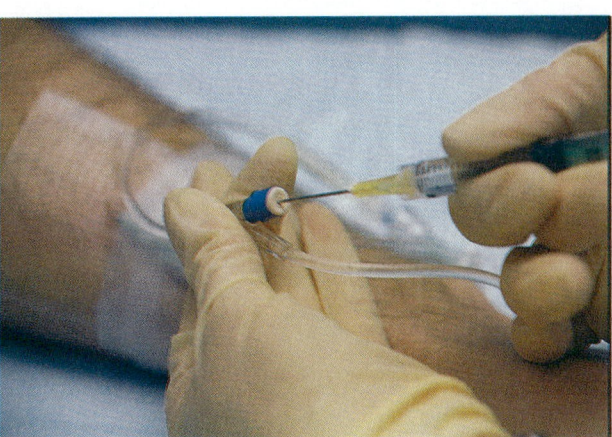

Figure 29-20 Needle system. Insert needle through port of main IV line.

Steps	Rationale
d. Occlude IV system by pinching tubing above injection port (Figure 29-21).	Prevents reflux of medication up tubing and inadvertent bolus when infusion resumed.
e. Aspirate gently on syringe plunger, observing for blood return.	Ensures drug will be delivered intravascularly.
f. After observing for blood return, continue to occlude IV tubing and inject medication slowly over appropriate time. Use watch to time administration (Figure 29-22).	

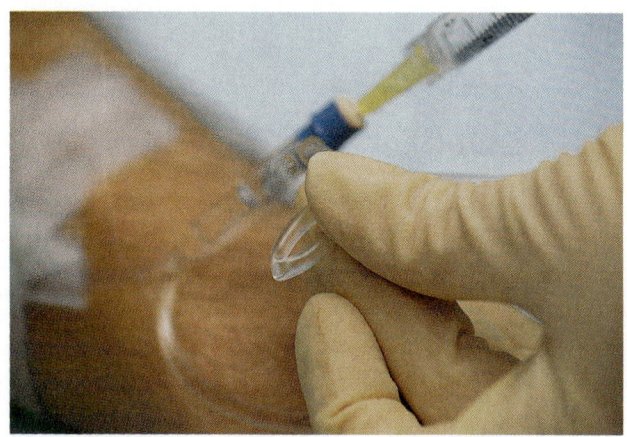

Figure 29-21 Occlude IV tube while injecting medication.

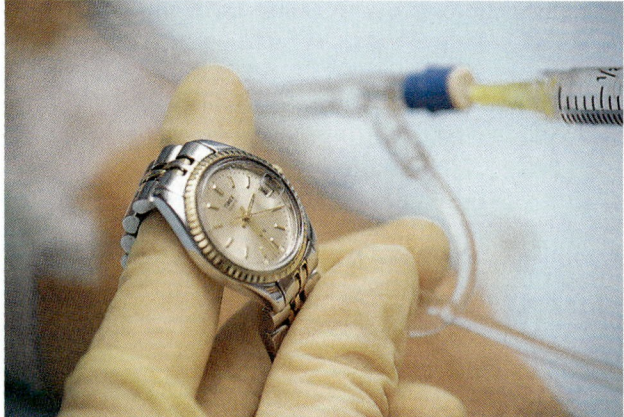

Figure 29-22 Inject medication and use watch to time administration.

Steps	Rationale
g. Release tubing, withdraw syringe, and recheck fluid infusion rate.	Fluid infusion may need to be readjusted if injection changed drip rate.
h. If using a needleless system, replace injection port cap with new sterile cap.	
i. Remove gloves and wash hands.	
j. Dispose of needles and syringes in appropriate container. *Do not* recap needles.	Prevents contaminated needle stick injury.

6. IV push (through IV lock)

Steps	Rationale
a. Prepare 2 to 3 1-ml syringes with 1 ml NS 0.9%. Attach small-gauge needle to syringe.	Flush will be used to clear lock before medication administration.
b. Cleanse injection port of IV lock with antiseptic swab.	
c. Insert syringe of NS 0.9% through injection port of IV lock (Figure 29-23). Remove needle if using a needleless system.	

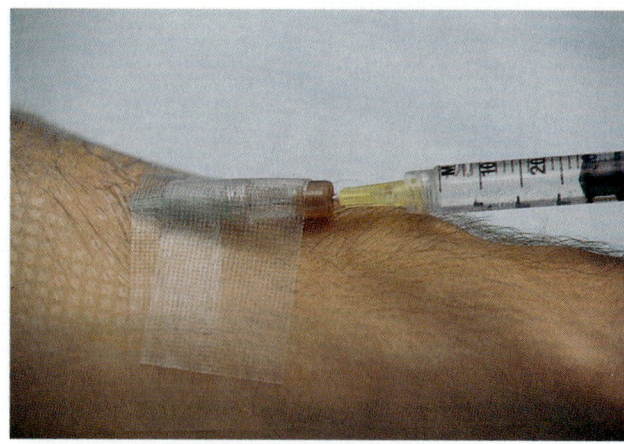

Figure 29-23 Insert syringe thru saline port.

Steps	Rationale

d. Aspirate gently and observe for blood return.

e. Flush with 1 ml NS after verifying blood return. If blood return is absent, assess for IV complications (see Skill 29.1).

f. Detach NS syringe, reprepare with antiseptic swab, and attach syringe filled with medication (see Step 6c).

g. Inject medication slowly over appropriate time, using a watch to ensure proper time of delivery.

h. Remove medication syringe.

i. Recleanse cap or port with antiseptic swab and attach syringe with 1 ml 0.9% NS. Inject NS flush.

j. *Option* (if agency protocol): Inject 1 ml dilute heparin, maintaining positive pressure in IV access device.

Ensures IV catheter is correctly positioned in vein.
Ensures medication is given IV and prevents incompatibility if heparin is used to maintain catheter patency.

Irrigation with NS prevents occlusion of IV access device.
Using SASH:
 *S*aline
 *A*dministration
 *S*aline
 *H*eparin
Prevents incompatibility of heparin with drug administered because 0.9% NS is isotonic.

---

nurse alert NS effectively maintains patency of peripheral IV lines (Goode et al., 1991). To maintain positive pressure in IV access device when flushing, clamp extension tubing if present or withdraw syringe during the final 0.2 to 0.4 ml of injection, creating a splash of NS (or dilute heparin if used) on the gloved hand when withdrawing syringe. This prevents reflux of blood in the IV catheter and prolongs patency of the access device. Some needleless system injection ports have an antireflux valve in injection port.

---

k. Remove gloves and wash hands.

l. Dispose of all needles and syringes in proper container. *Do not* recap needles.

Prevents accidental needle stick injury with contaminated needle.

7. IV piggyback (IVPB) through existing line

a. Attach tubing of administration set to prepared admixture container.

 (1) *Tandem (piggyback) infusion:* Small-volume admixture (50 to 100 ml) in a minibag that dilutes and administers drug. Insert spike of tubing into port of minibag (Figure 29-24).

 (2) *Syringe pump:* Small-volume admixture in a syringe (10 to 60 ml) to dilute and administer drug. Attach tubing to end of syringe.

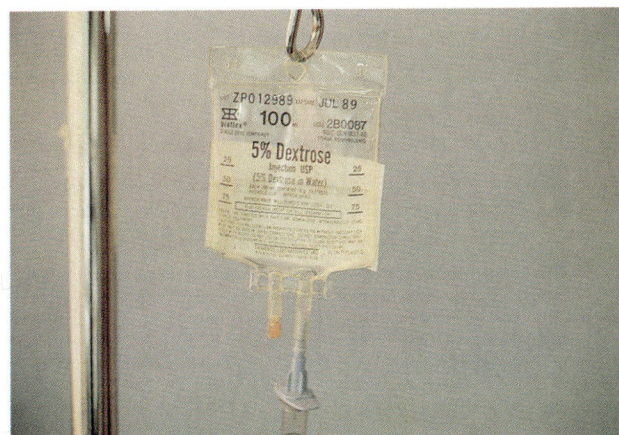

Figure 29-24 IVPB small-volume bag.

Steps	Rationale

b. Fill tubing with IV fluid.
   (1) *Tandem (piggyback) infusion:* Close roller clamp, squeeze chamber, and fill half full. Open roller clamp and prime remaining tubing.
   (2) *Syringe pump:* Gently push plunger of syringe to fill tubing completely.

Infusion tubing should be fluid filled and free of air bubbles to prevent air embolism.

c. Administer IVPB (tandem infusion). Attach needle to end of IV minibag tubing and insert into injection port farthest away from client after cleansing port with antiseptic swab. For needleless system, attach tubing to recessed connection port above backcheck valve (Figure 29-25).

Use of injection port closest to drip chamber of primary IV line allows piggyback to infuse while stopping the flow of primary IV line through backcheck valve.

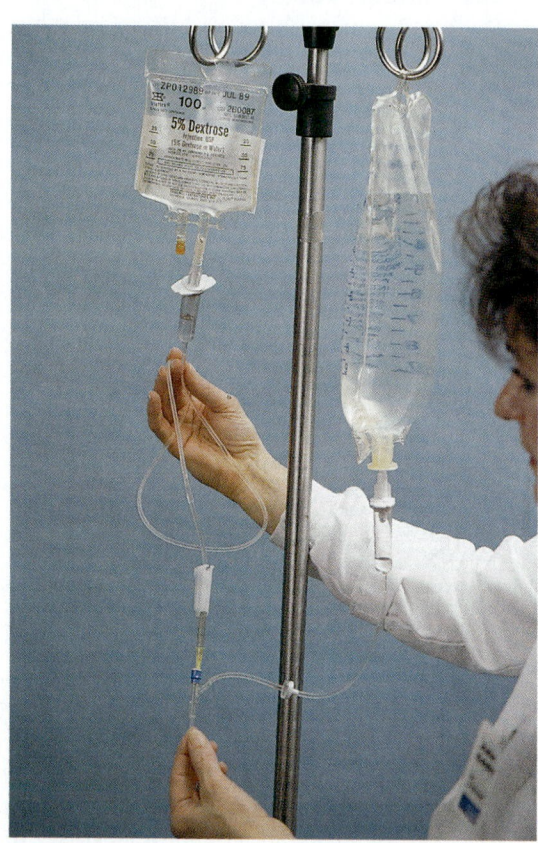

Figure 29-25 Attach IVPB to main line through injection port away from client.

   (1) Lower primary IV line. (Hook may be used to lower primary IV line.)

Allows infusion of minibag and prevents infusion of primary line.

   (2) Open regulator or clamp on minibag infusion.
   (3) Regulate flow rate of infusion to deliver medication over 20 to 90 minutes (see agency policy).
   (4) After medication has infused, check flow rate of primary infusion.

Backcheck valve prevents infusion of primary line while medication is infusing. Primary infusion will automatically begin to flow when tandem (piggyback) infusion is empty.

   (5) Reregulate primary infusion to desired IV rate.

Prevents infusion of excess fluid.

Steps	Rationale

    (6) Leave secondary bag and tubing in place for future drug administration or discard in appropriate container. Discard needle in sharps container.

Establishment of secondary line produces route for microorganisms to enter main line. Repeated changes in tubing increase risk of infection. Check agency policy and procedure for frequency of administration set tubing change.

8. Mini-infusion or syringe pump

  a. Place prefilled syringe with primed tubing into mini-infusor pump (follow manufacturer's directions) (Figure 29-26).

  b. Attach end of tubing to designated port *or* insert sterile needle into injection port of existing IV line after cleansing injection port with antiseptic swab.

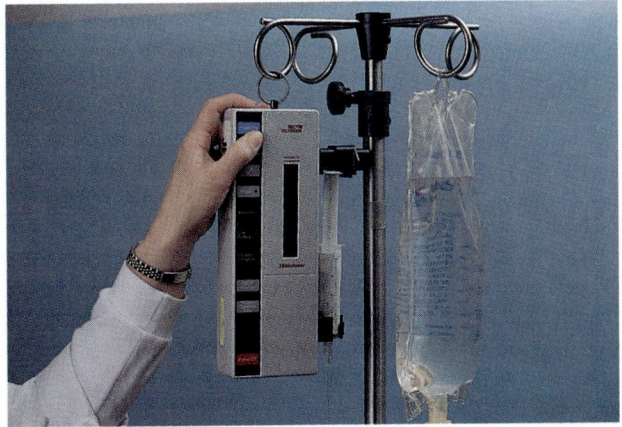

Figure 29-27 Hang mini-infusor pump on IV pole with syringe and primary IV.

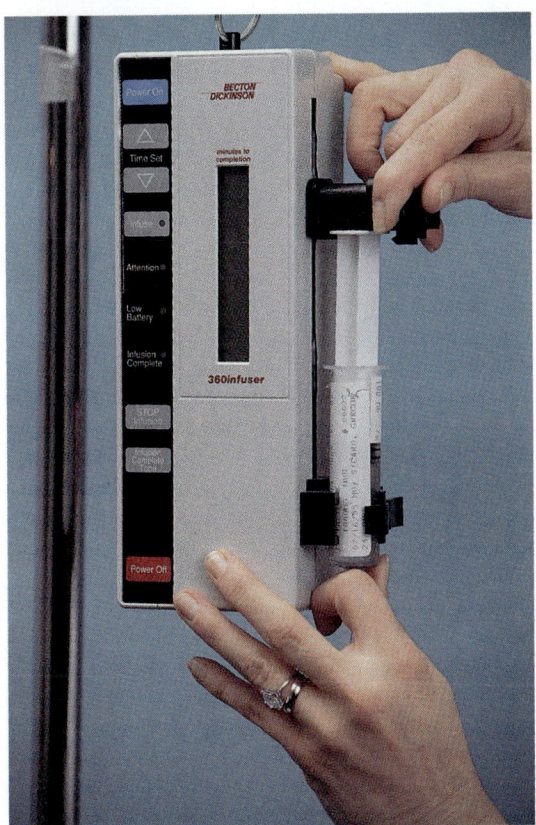

Figure 29-26 Place prefilled syringe into spring loaded mini-infusor pump.

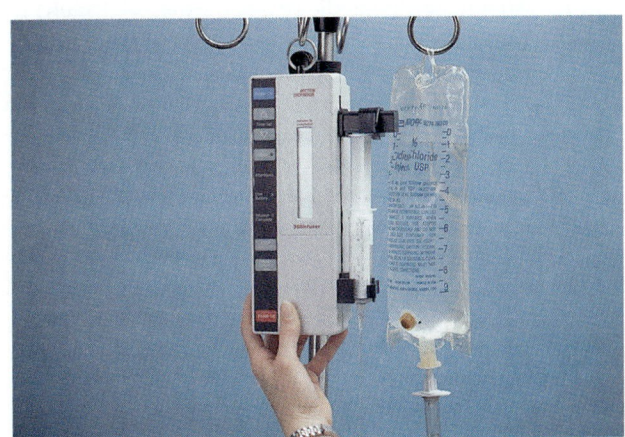

Figure 29-28 Press button on pump to "on."

  c. Hang mini-infusor pump with syringe on IV pole with primary IV line (Figure 29-27). Press button to "on" position (Figure 29-28). The infusion-complete alarm in "on" position should be used if available and if infusing via saline/heparin lock.

Prevents delay in flushing after completion of infusion, maintaining patency of access device.

  d. After medication infuses, turn off pump. Check flow rate of primary IV infusion and regulate to desired rate. (If stopcock is used, turn to "off" position after infusion is complete and cap.)

Prevents infusion of excess fluid.

  e. Leave infuser tubing in place or discard in appropriate container.

Maintains sterility of system.

Steps	Rationale

9. IVPB: saline or heparin lock (Figure 29-29)

a. Take minidrip (60 gtt/ml) IV tubing and insert spike into minibag.

Minidrip used to regulate small-volume infusion.

b. Close roller clamp and squeeze drip chamber to fill half full.

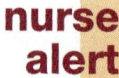 **nurse alert** If client complains during infusion of hyperosmolar drugs (e.g., erythromycin, vancomycin), assess IV site for symptoms of chemical phlebitis. IV infusion of drug greater than 650 mOsm/L is known to cause chemical phlebitis. If client is symptom free, slow infusion and decrease rate to infuse over maximum time allowed.

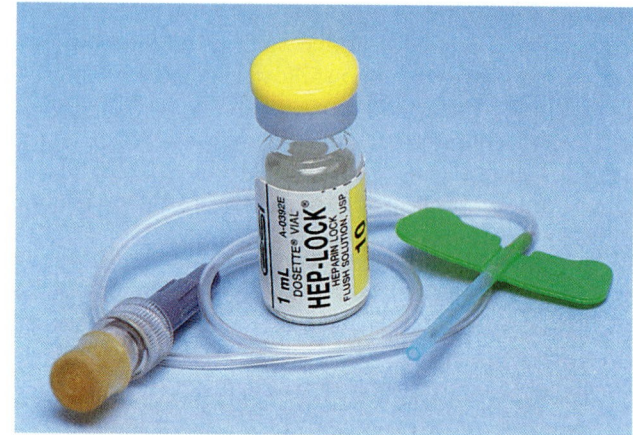

Figure 29-29 Saline lock and butterfly IV with flush solution.

c. Open roller clamp and fill remaining tubing.

Flushes air from tubing.

d. Attach sterile needle (e.g., 20 gauge × 1 inch) to tubing. Attach sterile cap to end of primed tubing if using needleless system.

Needle should be changed with each administration.

e. Prepare injection port of needleless system or heparin stopper with antiseptic swab.

f. Insert 3 ml syringe filled with 1 ml NS 0.9% and gently aspirate. Check for blood return, then flush NS slowly. Note any pain, swelling, or burning at IV site.

Ensures placement of IV in vein. Symptoms may suggest phlebitis or infiltration and the need to restart peripheral IV line.

g. Reprepare port or stopper with antiseptic swab. Attach end of tubing to port or insert sterile needle.

h. Open flow clamp and regulate IV medication to infuse 20 to 90 minutes. (Refer to agency policy.)

i. Continue to observe infusion periodically until complete. When complete, disconnect, maintaining aseptic technique.

j. Prepare injection port with antiseptic swab, insert syringe with 1 ml NS, and gently flush, maintaining positive pressure in IV access device (see Step 6j).

Always use SASH to flush port and prevent drug incompatibilities.

k. Reprepare and inject dilute heparin concentration (per agency and procedure), repeating procedure and using positive pressure.

l. Apply new sterile needle and cap to minibag tubing and retain for next administration.

Maintains sterility of IV tubing for future reuse.

m. Dispose of syringe and needles in appropriate container.

Steps	Rationale

nurse alert Prompt flushing after IVPB via saline/heparin lock prevents fibrin sheath formation or clotting when infusion is completed. Should IV access device clot after IVPB administration, do not forcefully flush. INS standards prohibit declotting of peripheral IV access (INS, 1990). If blood collects in IV tubing, clear tubing with remaining solution or change tubing. Blood retained in IV tubing promotes bacterial growth and predisposes client to risk of infection.

10. See Completion Protocol (Chapter 1, p. 6).

Evaluation

1. Observe client's infusion for proper rate of administration, and note time of completion.
2. Inspect client's IV site and tubing for symptoms of IV complications (e.g., swelling, pain, tenderness, redness at site).
3. Monitor therapeutic drug levels of aminoglycosides.
4. Monitor client during infusion for allergic response or adverse reaction (e.g., urticaria, respiratory distress, tachycardia, hypotension).
5. Ask client to name IV medication, purpose, side effects, dosage, and frequency.

UNEXPECTED OUTCOMES AND RELATED INTERVENTIONS

1. Client experiences burning, irritation, redness, or pain during infusion.
   a. Reinspect site and check for blood return.
   b. If phlebitis present, discontinue infusion and reinsert if IV therapy still necessary.
2. Client experiences adverse reaction or allergic reaction during infusion of drug.
   a. Stop the infusion.
   b. Maintain existing IV line.
   c. Notify physician.
   d. Monitor vital signs and respiratory status.
   e. Administer medications as ordered.
   f. Be prepared to perform cardiac or respiratory resuscitation.
   g. After acute episode subsides, advise client of allergy and necessity for future reporting to health care personnel; advise client of significance of allergy; advise client as to the availability of Medic Alert identification tags.

3. Client is unable to state purpose of drug, significance to treatment of current illness, side effects, or health management related to drug.
   a. Reinforce information, giving simple instructions, written if necessary.
   b. Communicate to other health personnel, particularly if client is to continue IV therapy in home setting.
   c. Include family or care provider during instruction.

SAMPLE DOCUMENTATION

1. Record drug dose and route and time of administration on medication administration record or computer printout. (See Medication and Administration Record, Appendix A.)
2. Record volume of fluid on client's intake and output record. (See Intake and Output Summary, p. 109.)

0810 During first 5 minutes of infusion of 100 ml NS and 1 g Ampicillin, client complained of sudden onset of "can't catch my breath," clutching at throat; high-pitched inspiratory stridor noted. Macular rash generalized over face and upper extremities noted. Ampicillin stopped immediately and IV fluids maintained at 125 ml hr. VS 98/60, 120, 26. MD notified. Epinephrine 0.5 mg IVP given, with inspiratory distress subsiding within 30 seconds of administration. Allergy band applied.

0830 VS 120/84, 96, 18. Client states breathing is normal. Expressing some fear over "how fast it came on." Significance of allergy, implications for future administration, and notification of dentists, physicians, and other health care providers discussed. States will apply for Medic Alert tags. Aware that vital signs will continue to be monitored and to notify immediately for any signs of respiratory distress.

Skill 29.4 | Transfusions with Blood Products

Technological advances in transfusion therapy now allow administration of various blood components specifically needed by the client. These technological advances also create an increased responsibility for nurses to have expanded knowledge of transfusion therapy, allowing for safe administration.

Blood and blood component transfusion is a major factor in restoring and maintaining quality of life for the client with hematological disorders, cancer, injury, or surgical intervention (LaRocca and Otto, 1994). Caring for the client receiving blood or blood components may be a routine nursing responsibility, but overlooking a minor detail could be dangerous to the client.

Transfusions of blood and blood products are closely regulated and monitored. Standards of operations for all blood bank centers are set by the American Association of Blood Banks (AABB), OSHA, Food and Drug Administration (FDA), and the American Red Cross. These standards include the collection of donor blood, distribution of the product, and standards for transfusion. Always verify specific agency or institutional policy as to specific procedural requirements before any transfusion.

Blood and blood component therapies treat and restore hemodynamic homeostasis. A written physician's order to transfuse should always include which component to transfuse and the duration of the transfusion. If more than one blood product is to be given, the sequence or order of transfusion should be specified. Any additional medications, such as antihistamine (given when history shows previous allergic response), antipyretics (given when history shows previous febrile nonhemolytic response), or diuretics (given when history shows potential for CHF or pulmonary edema), or any other special treatment of the components should also be given by the physician when ordering the transfusion (Harovas and Anthony, 1993).

Three blood identification systems, ABO, Rh, and most recently HLA typing, are used to ensure transfusion products match the recipient's blood as closely as possible (Table 29-3). Autologous transfusion (client's own blood) is the ideal method, but ensuring compatibility through blood typing keeps transfusion reactions to a minimum (Table 29-4). Before transfusion in nonemergent situations, the client's blood type and Rh factor *must always* be verified to be compatible with the donor transfusion.

The skill of transfusing blood or blood products requires the nurse to know thoroughly the policy and procedure of the agency or institution. The nurse must ensure the safe administration of the product and closely monitor before, during, and after the transfusion.

There is an increasing public awareness of the possible transmission of human immunodeficiency virus (HIV) and hepatitis B virus (HBV) through blood transfusion. Nurses and physicians must be prepared to answer thoroughly questions as to the benefits and risks of the transfusion and must reassure the client that every effort has been taken to ensure a safe blood supply. Clients should know that there is never a completely risk-free transfusion unless the blood is autologous. The nurse may discuss transfusion options available to the client and assist the client in reviewing risks and benefits to facilitate a decision and obtain consent.

Nursing Diagnosis

A client receiving blood transfusions requires careful monitoring. Because of the risk of receiving a transfused volume of blood, the client may be diagnosed with potential for **Fluid Volume Excess** related to the infusion of the product. **Fluid Volume Deficit** or **Risk for Fluid Volume Deficit** related to the loss of blood volume applies to clients requiring blood replacement. The client may also experience **Decreased Cardiac Output** related to reduced red blood cell (RBC) count and oxygen (O_2) transport capacity. Because of the potential risks of transfusion therapy, **Risk for Infection** related to contamination of blood or blood products, **Risk for Injury**

Table 29-3 Blood Type Identification

Client	Transfusion
Type A	A or AB plasma
	A or O RBCs
Type B	B or AB plasma
	B or O RBCs
Type AB	AB plasma
	A, B, AB, or O RBCs
Type O	A, B, AB, or O plasma
	O RBCs
Rh⁻	Must receive Rh⁻ blood
Rh⁺	Can receive Rh⁻ or Rh⁺ blood
O⁻	Universal donor for RBCs
AB⁻	Universal donor for plasma

RBCs, Red blood cells.

Table 29-4 ABO-Compatible Blood Products

Client's ABO Group	Compatible Whole blood	Compatible Red blood Cells	Compatible Plasma
O	O	O	O
A	A	A, O	A, AB
B	B	B, O	B, AB
AB	AB	AB, A, B, O	AB

related to the possibility of allergy or air embolism, and **Risk for Altered Body Temperature** related to possible allergy are alternative diagnoses. In the event of a massive transfusion or febrile reaction, the diagnosis of **Hyperthermia** could be considered. In the client who has never had a transfusion, **Knowledge Deficit** regarding side effects of transfusion reaction related to inexperience should be considered.

EQUIPMENT

Blood administration set with standard 170 μ filter
Ordered blood product
IV solution: NS 0.9%
Disposable gloves
Tape
Optional equipment
Infusion pump (Verify that infusion pump can be used to deliver blood or blood products.)
Leukocyte-depleting filter
Blood warmer (used mainly when massive transfusion is needed)
Pressure bag (used for rapid infusion in acute blood loss)

Assessment

1. Assess physician's order for type of blood product, length of transfusion (up to 4 hours for whole blood), and pretransfusion or posttransfusion medications to be given.
2. Assess client's transfusion history, including previous transfusion reaction. Verify that type and crossmatch has been completed within 72 hours of transfusion and, if applicable, that consent for transfusion is signed. **Clients with recent transfusion, pregnancy (within 3 months), or uncertain history are at high risk because of potential antibody response.**
3. Establish that client has a patent large-gauge IV set with positive blood return. **Whole blood and packed RBCs should be transfused through a**

large-bore catheter to prevent hemolysis of cells. Smaller gauges may be used for other blood components.

> **nurse alert** IV medications cannot be added to a blood bag or infused through a transfusion administration set. An additional IV site may be required if IV medications cannot be delayed or adjusted during blood transfusion(s).

4. Assess pretransfusion, baseline vital signs (blood pressure, pulse, respiration, temperature). If client is febrile (greater than 100° F or 37.8° C), notify physician before initiating transfusion (check agency policy). **This provides comparison to detect change in client's condition during transfusion.**
5. Assess client's medication schedule.

Planning

Expected outcomes focus on safe complication-free transfusion therapy, restoration of normal cell count, and improvement in oxygenation and tissue perfusion.

EXPECTED OUTCOMES

1. Client is free of signs and symptoms of transfusion reaction or fluid volume overload, evidenced by normal temperature and blood pressure and absence of chest pain, dyspnea, dizziness, or tachydysrhythmias.
2. Client demonstrates normal fluid balance, evidenced by normal urine output, improved hemoglobin (Hgb) and hematocrit (Hct), and normal RBC indices.
3. Client lists two benefits and risks of transfusion therapy.
4. Client experiences lessened stress or fear, evidenced by verbalized understanding and acceptance of transfusion therapy.
5. Client does not experience signs and symptoms of blood or blood product infiltrate or phlebitis.

Implementation

Steps	Rationale
1. See Standard Protocol (Chapter 1, p. 5).	
2. Obtain blood bag from laboratory following agency protocol. Blood transfusions must be initiated 15 to 30 minutes after release from laboratory.	Agencies differ as to personnel who can release a blood bag from a blood bank, but they always require two witnesses and some form of client identification. Only one unit is usually released at a time.
3. Open blood administration set and prime the tubing with NS 0.9% (Figure 29-30), completely filling filter with saline. Maintain sterility of system and close lower clamp.	If filter is not completely primed with saline, transfusion will slow because of coagulation of debris in partially primed filter. Saline is prepared to infuse in event of transfusion reaction.

Steps	Rationale

4. Have client void or empty urinary drainage collection container.

5. With another registered nurse or licensed nurse, correctly verify blood product and identify client (check agency policy):
  a. Client's name and identification number
  b. Client's name and identification number with forms from blood bank and with physician's order in client's record
  c. Client's blood group and Rh type
  d. Crossmatch compatibility
  e. Donor's blood group and Rh type
  f. Unit and hospital number

If transfusion reaction occurs, urine specimen obtained must be recent and preferably taken after transfusion is initiated to assess for presence of red blood cells from a hemolytic reaction.

If possible, have client identify self. Correct product must be administered to right client to avoid transfusion reaction.

nurse alert   Since most severe transfusion reactions occur from identification error (Harovas and Anthony, 1993), verification of client, product, product type, and crossmatch may be the *most* important step of the entire procedure.

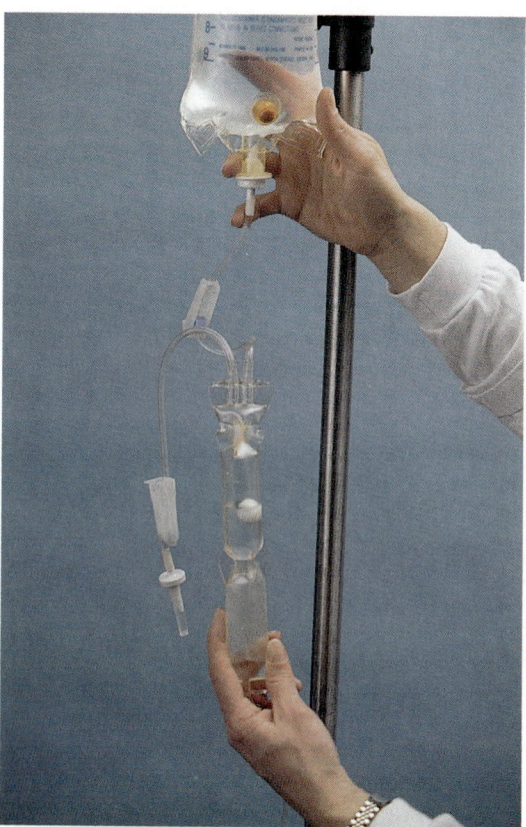

Figure 29-30 Prime tube with normal saline.

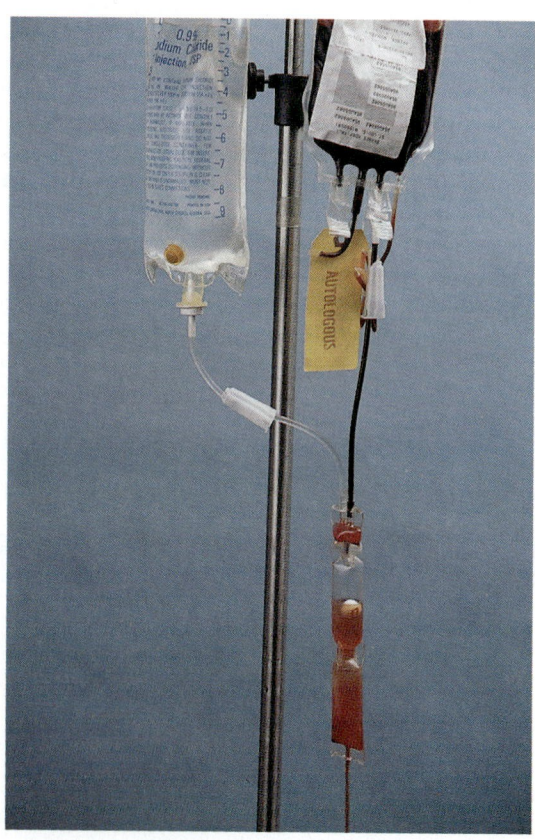

Figure 29-31 Attach blood tubing to unit of blood and fill tubing. Clamp to NS is closed.

Steps	Rationale

g. Expiration date and time on blood unit

h. Type of blood component is correct component ordered by physician

6. Inspect blood product for signs of leakage or unusual appearance, including clots, bubbles, or purplish color.

If signs of contamination are present, return blood product to laboratory.

7. Attach blood product by inserting spike of Y tubing located next to NS 0.9% tubing (Figure 29-31). Close NS clamp above filter and open clamp above filter to blood product. Clamp to NS 0.9% is closed.

8. Review with client the purpose of transfusion. Ask client to report immediately any signs and symptoms (during or after transfusion), including chills, low back pain, shortness of breath, nausea, excessive perspiration, rash, or even a vague sense of uneasiness.

Once transfusion reaction occurs, staff must respond immediately with treatment.

9. Connect NS-primed blood administration set directly to client's IV site.

10. Open lower clamp and regulate blood infusion to allow only 10 to 24 ml to infuse in the first 15 minutes. Remain with client.

If a reaction occurs, infusion of this amount minimizes the amount of incompatible blood transfused.

11. Obtain vital signs (temperature, pulse, respiration, blood pressure) 15 minutes after initiation of transfusion.

Change from baseline vital signs may indicate transfusion reaction.

12. Reregulate flow clamp if there is no transfusion reaction, and infuse the remaining volume of blood as ordered by physician. Packed RBCs are usually infused over 2 hours and whole blood over 3 to 4 hours. Drop factor for blood tubing is 10 gtt/ml (see Skill 29.2).

Careful regulation prevents adverse response. Client's condition and physician's orders dictate rate of blood infusion.

> **nurse alert** Blood must be transfused within 4 hours of spiking the blood bag. Even if infusion is not complete, blood must be discontinued. This reduces the potential for exposure to bacterial infection from blood.

13. Continue to monitor vital signs per agency and procedure during transfusion.

Ensures early identification of adverse response.

14. After blood has infused, close roller clamp above filter to blood and open NS.

15. Infuse NS until blood administration is completely clear.

Ensures all blood cells infused.

16. Discontinue transfusion and blood administration set.

17. Follow standard precautions and agency protocol for disposal of old blood bags and tubing.

Steps	Rationale
18. Blood transfusion increases risk of phlebitis. Apply injection cap and flush existing IV line or restart IV fluids as ordered only after assessing IV site for patency and signs and symptoms of phlebitis. If transfusing more than one unit of blood or blood product, maintain NS via blood administration set at KVO (keep vein open) rate until second unit is started. Verify with blood bank the number of units that can be transfused through the same administration set, based on tubing manufacturer's recommendation.	
19. See Completion Protocol (Chapter 1, p. 6).	

Evaluation

1. Observe for chills, flushing, itching, hives, dyspnea, tachycardia, drop in blood pressure or any sign of transfusion reaction.
2. Monitor intake and output and laboratory values (Hgb, Hct, prothrombin time [PT], partial thromboplastin time [PTT], platelet count) after transfusion. (In the hematologically stable adult, one unit of PRBCs should increase the Hgb by 1 g/dl and Hct by 3%. Each unit of random donor platelets should increase the platelet count by 5000 to 10,000/μL and each unit of single donor platelets by 50,000 to 100,000/μL [Harovas and Anthony, 1993].)
3. Ask client to describe purpose, benefit, and risk of transfusion.
4. Observe that client's behavior or appearance does not demonstrate signs of physical or emotional stress during the transfusion and that client can verbalize understanding of the need for transfusion.
5. Monitor IV site and status of infusion every time vital signs are taken.

UNEXPECTED OUTCOMES AND RELATED INTERVENTIONS

1. Client experiences pain, swelling, or discoloration at the IV site.
   a. Stop the transfusion and discontinue the IV infusion.
   b. Restart the IV infusion in another site.
2. Client complains of pain at infusion site when blood first initiated, but IV site is patent and not infiltrated.
   Apply warm pack to arm to prevent venous spasm from infusion of cold blood products.
3. Transfusion slows and client is not receiving proper volume.
   a. Check patency of set.
   b. Ensure blood bag is elevated to proper height.
   c. Verify that all clamps and stopcocks are open.
   d. Ensure filter is completely primed.
   e. Gently agitate blood bag.
   f. Close primary clamp (below the filter). Lower blood bag and open NS roller clamp. Dilute blood with 25 to 50 ml NS to facilitate infusion.
   g. Place unit to be infused in an electronic infusion device that permits blood transfusion.
   h. Apply pressure bag and inflate to a maximum of 300 mm Hg.
   i. Restart IV infusion with a large-gauge catheter.
4. Client expresses sudden temperature spike (greater than 100° F or 38.7° C), tachycardia, fall in blood pressure, low back pain, or dyspnea during transfusion.

nurse alert   Because symptoms of transfusion reaction are similar to those of life-threatening acute hemolytic transfusion reaction, assume any transfusion reaction to be hemolytic (Westphal, 1990). The initial management of any transfusion reaction is the same.

   a. Stop the transfusion.
   b. Keep the IV open with NS 0.9% via new infusion set.
   c. Notify physician and blood bank.
   d. Follow agency protocol for reporting and intervention.
5. Client's laboratory values fail to normalize after transfusion.
   Notify physician and continue to monitor client for active bleeding.

SAMPLE DOCUMENTATION

1000 Early AM CBC noted. MD aware of Hct 22. TxC drawn with two witnesses per phlebotomy.
1230 Voided 320 ml clear, amber urine. 18 angiocath inserted left cephalic vein. NS 0.9% initiated at KVO. 1 unit PRBCs started at 40 ml/hr, after witnessed by J. Doe, RN,

and M. Smith, RN. Client identified signs/symptoms of transfusion reaction to report (low back pain, dyspnea, chills). VS pretransfusion: T 37, P 88, R 16, BP 120/80. 1245 Free of back pain, dyspnea, chills, itching, or flushing. Transfusion rate increased to 90 ml/hr, infusion w/o pain, tenderness, or discoloration at site. VS: T 37.0, P 90, R 18, BP 120/80. Call light in reach.

1530 Transfusion 1 unit PRBCs completed. VS monitored q30min without change. Denies shortness of breath, chills, or back pain. IVF NS 0.9% maintained at 20 ml/hr via left cephalic vein. 18 gauge without redness, pain, or swelling. Stated "can't wait till I have more energy." Expressed relief transfusion completed without problems.

Skill 29.5 | Managing Central Lines

The central venous access device (CVAD) or central venous catheter (CVC) provides reliable, long-term access to a client's central veins. This replaces repetitive peripheral IV insertions. Used first in the 1970s for home parenteral nutrition, advances in technology of the CVC now allow for a multiplicity of therapies via a variety of approaches. The current trend in IV therapy is to place an appropriate venous access device early in therapy and has led to an estimated 5 million CVCs being placed in the United States annually (Maki, 1991). The nurse, actively involved in care, management, and education of the client with a CVC, is challenged to know the types of catheters, features, and management requirements.

The CVC is a reliable method of providing venous access for therapies requiring central vein hemodilution (total parenteral nutrition [TPN], vesicant chemotherapy, hyperosmolar drug infusions), for therapies requiring long duration (IV antibiotic therapy for subacute bacterial endocarditis, osteomyelitis, or other infectious diseases), and for clients who have limited peripheral venous access because of extensive peripheral IV therapy.

CVCs are placed under sterile technique via the infraclavicular subclavian vein, the internal jugular or external jugular vein, the femoral vein, or the basilic or cephalic vein in the upper extremity. Each location carries risks and benefits during and after insertion. The nurse completes an extensive assessment and evaluation when providing information to the client about CVCs. The length and type of therapy; client's venous status, life-style, body image, and physical abilities; and support and availability of family members or significant others to assist in catheter care are important factors when determining the best access device. The risk/benefit and cost/benefit are best communicated when selecting a CVAD before insertion.

CVCs can be categorized into four types, and all are suitable for clients receiving IV fluids and medications. Each provides for different lengths of therapy, short or long term. Some require surgical insertion, some are placed peripherally, and others exit on the thorax. Table 29-5 describes features of the different types of short-term percutaneous CVCs, tunneled CVCs, implanted venous access devices (IVADs), and peripherally inserted central catheters and features unique to each. All CVCs are radiopaque, allowing for x-ray verification of catheter tip placement if malposition is suspected, and are made of a variety of materials that are biocompatible. Regardless of the type of CVC, nurses play a vital role in maintaining patency, preventing infection, and educating the client with regard to care.

Complications associated with CVC require vigilance by health care professionals and can occur during insertion or at any point during the catheter's dwell time. Reports of CVC complications to the FDA through the Medical Device Reporting Act include (but are not limited to) infection, pneumothorax, hemothorax, hydrothorax, vessel and cardiac perforation, cardiac tamponade secondary to pericardial effusion, dysrhythmias, air embolism, and sheared catheters.

Except in emergencies, placement of a CVC requires adherence to strict aseptic technique. Infection, a potentially serious complication, has been shown to decrease 25% when a maximum sterile barrier (MSB) is used during insertion (Mermel, Stolz, and Maki, 1991). Catheters placed under nonsterile conditions should be replaced as soon as medically feasible. Any care given to a client with an indwelling CVC should be performed with strict asepsis. Ongoing assessment for CVC complications is a prime responsibility of the nurse delivering care.

Optimum placement of any CVC is the superior vena cava (SVC). Blood flow in the SVC reaches 1.5 L per minute and results in improved hemodilution of irritating drugs and IV fluids. Thrombosis is noted to be higher when tips of CVC devices are located in the subclavian or brachiocephalic vein (Ryder, 1993). SVC placement is necessary when infusing TPN to minimize the associated risk of thrombosis.

To manage and educate the client with a CVC effectively, the nurse must be familiar with basic anatomy of the central venous system. When the client has a peripherally inserted central catheter (PICC), knowledge of the upper arms' venous system is important. The nurse also must know the particulars of catheter care and management.

This skill addresses insertion of a CVC, care of an indwelling CVC, and care of the client when removing a CVC. When effectively managed, CVCs can provide reliable long-term venous access with limited complications to the client needing long-term IV therapy.

Table 29-5 **Types of Central Venous Access Devices**

	Percutaneous	Tunneled	Implanted port	PICC
LUMENS	Single Multilumen	Single Multilumen	Single Dual	Single Dual
DURATION	Short term	Long term	Long term	Long term
INSERTION	By M.D.	By M.D.	By M.D. in operating room	By M.D. or trained RN
FEATURES	Sutured Dwell time limited Sterile dressing change Daily flush with heparin Activity restrictions External catheter breakage possible	Secured by dacron cuff Clean dressing once healed Daily flush with heparin (except Groshong) Can be repaired if broken Requires surgical removal	Costly due to surgical insertion Requires needlestick to access Monthly flushing Intact body image and no activity restrictions when not accessed	Low cost Sterile dressing change Routine daily flushing External catheter breakage possible Nonsurgical insertion Smaller gauge inadequate for blood sampling

Nursing Diagnosis

Nursing diagnoses for clients with CVCs are based in part on risks associated with type, duration, and insertion of CVADs and the type of IV therapy the client will receive. **Risk for Infection** related to catheter insertion or potential break of aseptic technique during catheter management and site care is a primary focus in the client with a CVC. If the client has an externally placed catheter, **Body Image Disturbance** related to external placement of the device may be considered. In the client who transitions from acute care to home care with an indwelling CVC and becomes responsible for management and care of the catheter, **Knowledge Deficit** related to self-management must be considered. In the client with an accessed IVAD or tunneled catheter, **Impaired Skin Integrity** related to possible erosion of the skin at the exit site or to hub or needle movement during access should be a consideration.

EQUIPMENT (Figure 29-32)

Insertion
Alcohol and povidone-iodine prep swabs
Sterile towels, gloves, gowns, and masks
Vial of sterile saline
Heparin solution (10 U/ml or 100 U/ml depending on institutional policy)

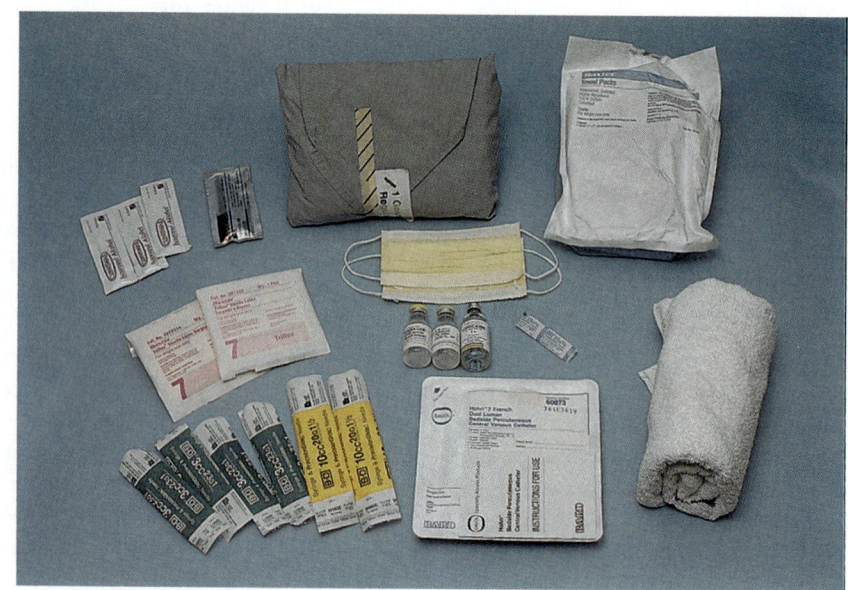

Figure 29-32 Equipment for central venous catheter (CVC) insertion.

Four 3 ml syringes
Two 10 ml syringes
25-gauge × 1-inch needle
Sterile CVC catheter (short-term percutaneous or PICC)
Lidocaine (1% or 2% with or without epinephrine) or ELMA (topical prilocaine, lidocaine) for topical anesthesia
Towel roll (for subclavian percutaneous catheter insertion)

Dressing change
Disposable gloves
Sterile gloves, gown, and mask
Sterile ½-inch Steri-Strips
Alcohol and povidone-iodine prep swabs
Povidone-iodine ointment (for use with gauze dressings only)
Dressing supplies (tape, transparent 4 × 6 membrane dressing or 4 × 4 sterile gauze)
Extension set with slide clamps (for PICC line dressing change)

Heparinization/tubing change
Alcohol and Betadine swabs
One to three 10 ml syringe(s)
One to three 5 ml syringe(s)
Vial of sterile saline
Heparin solution (10 U/ml or 100 U/ml depending on institutional policy)
Luer lock heparin injection cap(s) (one for each catheter lumen)
IV tubing for use in electronic infusion device
Extension set with slide clamp (PICC line only)

Blood sampling (Figure 29-33)
Blood tubes, labels, and requisitions
Alcohol and Betadine swabs
Disposable gloves
Three to five 10 ml syringes (for saline flush)
5 ml syringes (total number depends on aspirate volume required for laboratory sampling)
Vial of sterile saline
Heparin solution (10 U/ml to 100 U/ml depending on institutional policy)
One to three 3 ml syringes (for heparinization)
Sterile capped needle or sterile cap

Removal of percutaneous CVC or PICC
Disposable gloves
Sterile gloves
Alcohol and Betadine prep swabs
Betadine ointment
Sterile 2 × 2 gauge pads
Tape
Sterile container (one or two) (if tip and/or intracutaneous segment culture required)

Assessment

INSERTION

1. Assess client's disease state and need for IV therapy by reviewing the medical records.
2. Assess client's life-style, ability to care for catheter, availability of family member or significant other for support, and impact of CVC on body image.
3. Assess client's awareness and knowledge level of length of therapy, type of therapy, and management of CVC.

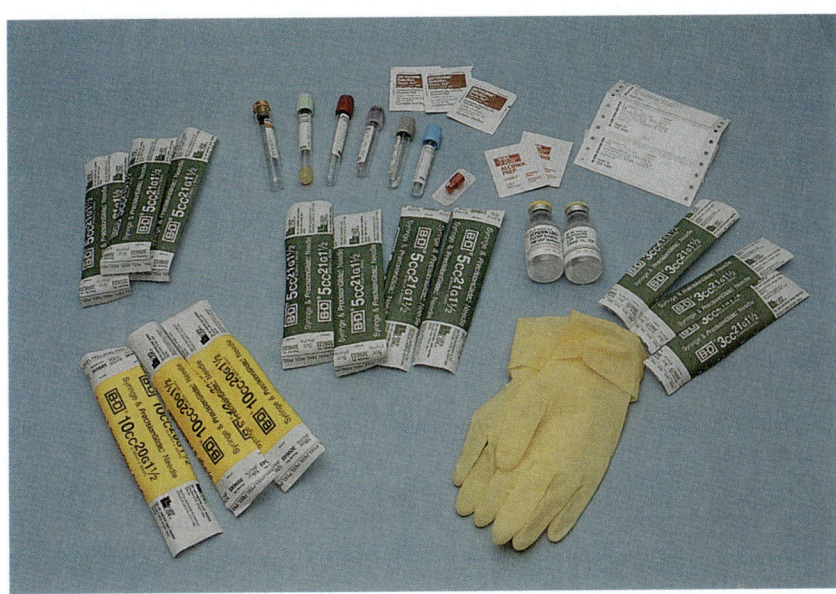

Figure 29-33 Equipment for blood sampling from CVC.

4. Assess required treatment schedule and physician's orders: IV fluid administration, blood sampling, blood products, and nutrition. **This may indicate the need for long-term IV therapy.**
5. Assess for drug allergies. **Local lidocaine will be applied to skin.**
6. Confer with physician on type of central access device to be inserted.
7. Assess potential insertion site or catheter exit site (if tunneled) for signs of infection (redness, tenderness, swelling, exudate). Assess tunnel by palpation if tunneled catheter.

DRESSING CHANGE

1. Assess occlusiveness of dressing. Refer to institutional policy and manufacturer's recommended guidelines for care.
2. Assess client's knowledge level of purpose, care, and management of CVC. Ask client to discuss or demonstrate care and management of catheter.
3. Assess for symptoms of CVC complications: pain on irrigation of infusion; loss of blood return or presence of intermittent blood return related to client's position; swelling or discomfort in neck, shoulder, or ipsilateral arm on insertion side; and elevated temperature.

BLOOD SAMPLING

1. Assess need to use CVC for blood sampling. Check for peripheral vein collapse.
2. Assess function of CVC by inspecting integrity of catheter and noting presence of leakage, mobility, and integrity of IVAD. Check ability to irrigate or infuse fluid and presence of blood return on aspiration.

DISCONTINUATION

1. Assess physician's order for discontinuing short-term percutaneous catheter or PICC.
2. Assess for symptoms of CVC complications (see Dressing Change).

Planning

Expected outcomes focus on minimizing risks of complications of central lines, prevention of infection, client education with regard to self-care management, and recognition of complications associated with CVCs.

EXPECTED OUTCOMES

1. Client tolerates positional changes during insertion of CVC or PICC line.
2. Site is free of bleeding or hematoma. Client is free of respiratory distress.
3. Client's CVC insertion site is free of redness, tenderness, swelling, or exudate. Client remains afebrile with normal white blood count (WBC).
4. Client's chest x-ray studies show proper tip placement of CVC. Catheter shows positive blood return and flushes with ease.
5. Client is free of symptoms of thrombosis and demonstrates no catheter tip migration or malposition.
6. Client explains purpose and type of CVC and lists or demonstrates proper management of infusion, flushing, and dressing change (if applicable).
7. Client lists three signs and symptoms of infection, thrombosis, and air embolism and necessary interventions for each.

Implementation

Steps	Rationale
1. See Standard Protocol (Chapter 1, p. 5).	
2. Assisting with central line insertion	
a. Cleanse insertion site with soap and water if excessively dirty. Clip excess hair with scissors.	Shaving can cause microabrasions and predisposes to infection.
b. Position client for insertion.	Straightens vein for cannulation.
(1) PICC: Supine with arm at 45-degree angle	
(2) Jugular: Trendelenburg with head turned to side	Trendelenburg position causes venous distention, aiding in cannulation of jugular system.
(3) Subclavian: Trendelenburg with towel roll vertical to spine between scapula (Figure 29-34).	Although Trendelenburg position will not distend subclavian vein, it reduces risk of air embolism during insertion.
c. Assess preinsertion vital signs.	Provides baseline for comparison if complications occur.

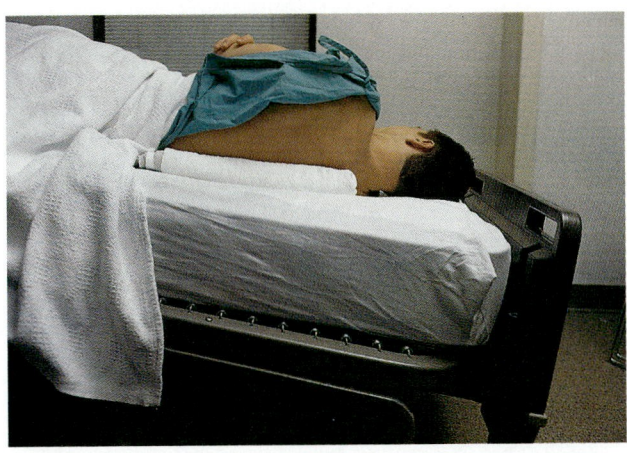

Figure 29-34 Client positioned in Trendelenburg position for subclavian placement; towel roll is placed vertical to spine between scapula.

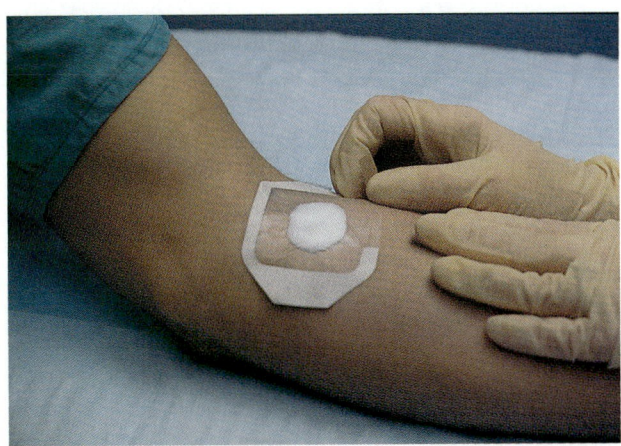

Figure 29-35 Apply topical lidocaine to peripherally inserted central catheter (PICC) site and cover with Tegaderm.

Steps	Rationale

d. Open supplies and prepare sterile field (see Skill 14.2).

e. Draw up lidocaine, NS, and heparin for flushing. **(For PICC insertion:** ELMA may be used for topical anesthesia. Apply to insertion site ½ to 1 hour before venipuncture, then cover with Tegaderm dressing) (Figure 29-35).

ELMA provides anesthesia but prevents obliteration of ACF vessels when using subcutaneous lidocaine. Aids in palpation.

f. Remain with client and assist with maintaining sterile field and proper positioning of client during insertion.

g. Instruct client to report pain, respiratory distress, or dizziness during catheter insertion.

h. After insertion, put on sterile gloves and mask, remove excess blood with sterile 4 × 4 pad, and cleanse skin with Betadine-soaked 4 × 4 pad, taking care not to cause bleeding at insertion site (Figure 29-36). Apply occlusive pressure dressing over site.

Could signify presence of complications of pneumothorax, perforation of great vessels, or nerve plexus injury. Occlusive dressing prevents entrance of microorganisms.

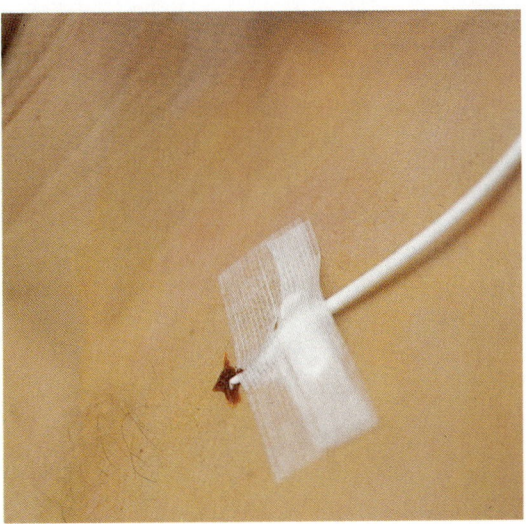

Figure 29-36 Secure CVC with Steri-Strips.

Steps	Rationale

i. Flush lumen with 5 to 10 ml NS after aspirating for blood return, then flush with 2.5 ml heparin solution. Maintaining positive pressure, close slide clamp if applicable and ensure Luer lock injection caps are tight.

Ensures integrity and patency of each lumen. Flushing with NS clears blood of blood return from each lumen. Heparin prevents clotting until lumen is used.

j. Assist in positioning client for chest x-ray study.

Radiographic verification of tip placement of CVC is required before use.

k. After insertion, assess vital signs, presence of respiratory distress, or complaints at area of insertion site.

Change in client's status may indicate pneumothorax or other complications.

3. Dressing Changes

a. Apply nonsterile gloves and mask.
b. Carefully remove old dressing and Steri-Strips if present.

Prevents catheter dislodgement.

> **nurse alert**
> In the older adult or the immunocompromised and nutritionally impaired client, the risk of a skin tear is a concern. Remove any tape and transparent membrane dressing (TMD) carefully. Alcohol, if skin is intact, will assist in breaking adhesive bond of some TMDs.

c. Assess catheter exit site or site (if nontunneled) for symptoms of infection. Note length of external catheter present (Figure 29-37). (Apply sterile gloves if necessary to palpate site.)

Change in amount of external catheter showing may indicate catheter migration, which predisposes to catheter sepsis or infection.

> **nurse alert**
> PICCs are sometimes unsutured. Extreme care must be used when removing old dressings. Assessment of catheter length is essential to ensure consistent tip placement. If necessary, put on sterile gloves to aseptically secure the catheter when removing old dressing.

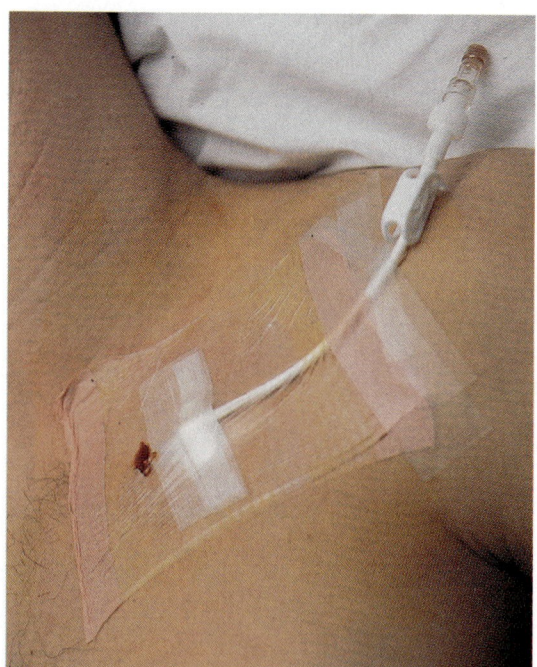

Figure 29-37 Apply transparent dressing over CVC site, covering catheter.

Steps	Rationale

d. Remove gloves and dispose of in container. Apply sterile gown and gloves.

Ensures sterile technique.

e. Prepare site with 70% alcohol in concentric circles away from the site. Repeat twice. Allow to air dry. Prepared area should exceed size of dressing.

Alcohol must remain in contact with skin for 30 seconds (INS, 1990).

> **nurse alert** Acetone has been shown to be an ineffective preparation agent in care of CVCs. It is associated with increased pain and skin irritation and can cause breakdown of some catheter material (Maki, 1991).

f. Repeat with povidone-iodine prep three times in same fashion. Allow to air dry. Prepared area should exceed size of dressing. (If client is allergic to Betadine, use alternative cleansing solution based on institutional policy.) Povidone-iodine must remain in contact with skin for 2 minutes and should not be wiped off (INS, 1990).

g. Remove gloves and put on new sterile gloves.

Gloves should be removed after preparation (INS, 1990).

h. Secure catheter with Steri-Strips if unsutured or if catheter migration is a concern (see Figure 29-37).

Securing catheter prevents migration. Application of Steri-Strips on jugular percutaneous catheters and PICC catheters is often done to reduce migration from movement of neck and arm.

i. Apply skin preparation or benzoin agent to area where tape or TMD is applied. Allow to air dry. (PICC line: Extension set is changed weekly with dressing change [see Heparinization/Tubing Change].)

Aids in securing dressing.

j. Apply sterile 4 × 4 Betadine ointment pad or TMD to sites covering catheter (and catheter extension set connection) (see Figure 29-37).

Betadine ointment is not used under TMDs on PICC lines.

k. Dispose of all soiled equipment in appropriate receptacle.

l. Remove gloves and wash hands.

4. Heparinization/tubing change

a. Prime new IV tubing with IV fluids (see Skill 29.1). Electronic infusion devices are recommended for use on all central lines (INS, 1990).

b. Prepare hub and tubing connection of old tubing with alcohol swab followed by Betadine swab. Allow to air dry.

Studies have shown that hubs of catheters can also become contaminated and cause catheter-related bacteria (Maki, 1991).

c. Change tubing every 48 to 72 hours (INS, 1990). TPN tubing is changed every 24 hours. Verify injection cap change per agency policy and procedure.

d. For tubing change

(1) Close slide clamp on catheter. If no clamp is available, have client perform Valsalva maneuver by holding breath or bearing down when old tubing is disconnected and new tubing is changed. If client is unable to perform Valsalva maneuver, position client in Trendelenburg position and change tubing while client forcibly exhales.

Reduces risk of air embolism when catheter is open to air.

(2) Grasp catheter hub and old tubing, remove end of old tubing, and immediately apply sterile end of new tubing.

Steps	Rationale
e. Secure tube connections with tape, open slide clamp, and resume infusion.	Prevents accidental disconnecting of tubing.
f. For injection cap change	
(1) Prepare one 10 ml syringe with sterile NS and one 5 ml heparin solution for each lumen of CVC. Follow agency policy and procedure.	Volume of heparin should be at least two times the internal volume of catheter (INS, 1990). Literature is inconsistent when describing optimum volume.
(2) Cleanse hub/injection port connection with alcohol swabs, followed by Betadine swabs. Allow to air dry.	Reduces risk of infection.
(3) Close slide clamp or have client perform Valsalva maneuver during injection cap change. If unable to perform Valsalva maneuver, place client in Trendelenburg position and change cap on forced expiration.	Reduces risk of air embolism.
(4) Quickly attach saline-filled syringe to hub, aspirate and verify presence of blood return, then flush with NS. Repeat procedure for each lumen.	
(5) Attach heparin-filled syringe to hub. Inject heparin using positive pressure or closing clamp slide. Positive pressure is achieved when delivering last 0.5 ml of solution by closing slide clamp or withdrawing needle of syringe while continuing to flush. (Exception: Groshong catheter is saline flush only.)	Prevents reflux of blood at catheter tip and fibrin sheath formation.
(6) Repeat heparin flush for each lumen.	

5. Blood sampling

a. Prepare 10 ml syringe of NS, 3 ml syringe of heparin flush (one for each lumen), and enough empty 5 ml syringes equal to volume of blood needed for laboratory sampling.

b. Prepare catheter hub or injection cap with alcohol and Betadine. Allow to dry.

c. Turn off all IV fluids for 1 minute and/or TPN fluids for 10 minutes.	Prevents hemodilution of sample and inaccurate laboratory results. All fluids being delivered should be turned off.
d. Blood sampling through injection port	
(1) Flush most proximal port of CVC with 10 ml NS, then with same syringe, aspirate 3 to 5 ml blood for discard.	Flushing catheter before sample withdrawal aids in obtaining blood return from CVC.
(2) Insert consecutive 5 ml syringes and aspirate blood to fill laboratory tubes.	Number of syringes and volume of sample depend on type of tests to be performed (check agency policy).
(3) Insert syringe with 20 ml NS and flush vigorously.	Clears inner lumen of catheter and prevents intraluminal fibrin collection in catheter, reducing risk of clotting.
(4) Follow with heparin solution and flush each lumen (see Heparinization/Tubing Change), maintaining positive pressure. Close clamp.	Prevents reflux of blood at catheter tip.
e. Dispose of all soiled supplies in proper receptacle. Dispose of any needles in sharps container. Wash hands.	

Steps	Rationale

6. Removal of CVCs

CVCs are removed when (1) therapy is completed, (2) sepsis is suspected, (3) there is external catheter breakage, (4) an occlusion cannot be cleared, or (5) thrombosis is present. A physician's order for catheter tip culture or intracutaneous segment culture (portion of catheter that exits skin) should be verified before removal.

a. Prepare sterile 2 × 2 swabs, Betadine ointment, alcohol, Betadine swabs, and suture removal kit.

b. Put on disposable gloves, remove dressing, and dispose of in proper container.

c. Inspect catheter site for signs of infection.

d. Remove and dispose of gloves. Apply sterile gloves.

e. Prepare catheter site with alcohol prep swabs, moving in concentric circles away from insertion site. Repeat twice.
> Eliminates resident bacteria lying on skin that may attach to catheter tip during catheter withdrawal.

f. Repeat preparation with Betadine swabs three times. Allow to dry. (Betadine is omitted if culturing catheter.)
> Alters culture results by destroying or minimizing bacterial count.

g. Carefully remove any external sutures anchoring catheter. While client performs Valsalva maneuver (or exhales on expiration), gently retract catheter. (Never forcefully remove catheter.)
> Forcefully removing catheter could cause breakage and catheter embolism.

h. After complete catheter removal, apply pressure over site with sterile 2 × 2 pads and Betadine ointment.

i. Observe for hemostasis. Secure sterile 2 × 2 pads and ointment with tape for occlusive dressing.
> Minimizes risk of air embolism until insertion site is healed. Provides occlusive dressing until epithelium covers insertion site.

j. Instruct client to leave dressing intact for 24 to 48 hours.

k. Dispose of all soiled supplies in appropriate receptacle and any needles or syringes in sharps container.

7. See Completion Protocol (Chapter 1, p. 6).

Evaluation

1. Observe client and inquire about comfort level during insertion.
2. Inspect CVC site immediately after insertion for hematoma or bleeding. Note respiratory status.
3. Inspect insertion site during dressing changes for redness or exudate. Ask if client notes tenderness. Monitor for increased temperature spike and increased WBC.
4. Verify with radiology the position of CVC tip, and aspirate every 8 hours for presence of blood return. Note patency of CVC.
5. Monitor for loss of blood return, complaints of neck pain, arm swelling, or sensation of flushing in the ear on the same side of the body.
6. Ask client to describe or demonstrate IV infusion and dressing change. Observe use of aseptic technique.
7. Ask client to list three symptoms associated with in-

fection (pain at site), air embolism (swelling or discomfort on neck, shoulder, or arm on insertion side), and thrombosis (loss of blood return).

UNEXPECTED OUTCOMES AND RELATED INTERVENTIONS

1. Client has temperature spike to 102.2° F (39° C). CVC insertion site is red and tender.
   a. Notify physician. Obtain peripheral blood culture and blood culture from CVC.
   b. Remove CVC if ordered, obtaining tip culture and intracutaneous segment culture if ordered.
   c. Establish peripheral IV site if appropriate and ordered for IV fluids and antibiotics.
2. When going to bathroom, client's proximal lumen is disconnected from IV fluids. Client complains of dizziness, shows respiratory distress, and is tachycardiac and tachypneic.
   a. Close clamp on proximal line.
   b. Place immediately in left lateral Trendelenburg position and notify physician immediately. Stay with client.
   c. Administer oxygen and be prepared to institute resuscitative measures if needed.
   d. Secure all connections and use only Luer lock devices.
3. Client's catheter loses blood return and cannot be flushed.
   a. Do not force irrigation.
   b. Obtain chest x-ray study to verify placement (INS, 1990) before declotting.
   c. Assess medication schedule for drug incompatibility.
   d. Obtain order for urokinase, 5000 IU, to declot catheter if not chemical precipitate.

e. Slowly instill volume equal to internal volume of catheter. Do not create pressure.
f. Complete declotting based on institutional policy and procedure and manufacturer's recommendations for declotting CVCs.
g. Remove volume of urokinase by aspirating 5 ml blood for discard. Flush with 10 ml NS and then heparinize.
4. Previously normal blood levels of PTT, gangcyclovir, or aminoglycoside are abnormal after withdrawal from CVC.
   a. Ensure IV fluids are turned off before laboratory sampling.
   b. Verify results by repeat sampling via peripheral venipuncture.
5. Blood return during laboratory sampling through PICC is sluggish, and catheter begins to clot.
   a. Use only 5 ml syringes during withdrawal.
   b. Stop aspirating, flush immediately with 10 ml NS, obtain discard, and resume withdrawal.
   c. Verify that PICC is 20 gauge or larger before laboratory sample is drawn from catheter.

SAMPLE DOCUMENTATION

1600 Left subclavian triple-lumen percutaneous central line dressing changed with aseptic technique. Insertion site not reddened, no tenderness or exudate. Sutures intact. Catheter remains at 19 cm. Cleansed with alcohol × 3 and Betadine × 3. Cath secured with Steri-Strips and sterile TMD. All connections secured. Proximal, middle, and distal lumen with positive blood return; flushed with 5 ml NS and 2 ml 100 U/ml heparin. Client denies pain; states, "I think this is much better than getting stuck."

Skill 29.6 | Administering Chemotherapy

Chemotherapy is the administration of drugs recognized as effective in the treatment of cancer. The purpose of chemotherapy administration is to prevent cancer cells from multiplying, invading adjacent tissues, and metastasizing to other organs or body systems. Cancer is the second most common cause of death in the United States after heart disease and affects individuals without regard to race, gender, socioeconomic class, or culture. Different types of cancer, however, are seen with increased incidence at specific ages and in select ethnic or gender groups with varying frequency and severity. Cancer morbidity and mortality increases rapidly with age; some researchers believe anyone who lives long enough will develop cancer (Belcher, 1992). Some cancers are seen with an increased familial tendency. It is unknown if a genetic susceptibility exists or if family members share a common exposure to risk factors.

General principles that guide the use of cancer chemotherapeutic agents are listed in the box (p. 547). Once a function of the physician, administration of chemotherapy is now considered a function of competent, qualified nurses with advanced training and skill. Because of the highly toxic nature of chemotherapeutic agents, the nurse must be aware of the purposes of treatment, the type of drug, and the client's pretreatment condition, stage of disease, response to therapy, and allergies or sensitivities. A baseline assessment is essential to evaluate the client's condition and response to and tolerance of therapy.

There are five major types of antineoplastic agents (Table 29-6). Effects of antineoplastic agents and their classification are determined primarily by the effect on the cell cycle. Specific research protocols govern the use of medications and chemotherapy according to cell time

General Principles That Guide Use of Cancer Chemotherapeutic Agents

1. Combination chemotherapy (multiple drugs), when carefully designed, has been consistently superior to single-agent therapy.
2. Complete remission is the minimum requirement to achieve cure or even significantly prolong survival.
3. The best chance for a significant response is with the first attempt; thus the type of treatment should be the approach with maximum effectiveness.
4. Drugs should be used in the highest possible doses to attain maximum tumor cell kill.
5. Drug dosage reduction to minimize toxicity is itself the most toxic side effect of chemotherapy.
6. Adjuvant chemotherapy is now well established in the treatment of breast cancer and holds promise for other types of cancer.
7. Various therapeutic approaches are used to lessen toxicity (e.g., doxorubicin is much less toxic when given by 96-hour infusion than when given as a bolus).
8. "Neoadjuvant," or induction, chemotherapy is the initial use of drugs to reduce a tumor's bulk and lower its stage, making it amenable to cure with local therapy (e.g., as in osteogenic sarcoma).
9. Chemoprevention of cancer is becoming a reality (e.g., 13-*cis*-retinoic acid has produced marked regression of leukoplakia, a premalignant lesion in the oral cavity).

Modified from Belcher AE: *Cancer nursing,* St Louis, 1992, Mosby.

Table 29-6 Five Major Types of Antineoplastic Agents

Type/Action	Examples
ALKYLATING AGENTS	
Interfere with normal process of cell division; cell cycle nonspecific	Cisplatin (Platinol) Cyclophosphamide (Cytoxan) Nitrogen mustard Carmustine (BCNU) Lomustine (CCNU)
ANTIMETABOLITES	
Cell cycle–specific agents with main chemotherapeutic activity in S phase	Vytosar 5-Fluorouracil (5-FU) Methotrexate
ANTIBIOTIC ANTITUMOR AGENTS	
Most believed to be cell cycle nonspecific; doxorubicin believed cycle specific for S phase; mitomycin most active in G and S phases	Bleomycin (Blenoxane) Daunorubicin (Cerubidine) Doxorubicin (Adriamycin) Mitomycin (Mutamycin) Mitoxantrone (Novantrone)
MITOTIC INHIBITORS	
Cell cycle specific for M phase; block mitosis in metaphase	Vinblastine (Velbane) Vincristine (Oncovin) Etoposide (VePesid)
HORMONAL DRUGS	
Specific mechanism of action unclear	Adrenocorticosteroids Androgens Estrogens Tamoxifen/progestins

sequences or cycles. Cycles are planned to provide maximum exposure of cancer cells to the drug while allowing the client to recover from drug-induced side effects. Cycles vary according to the type of cancer and the client's tolerance and response.

Chemotherapy, usually given in combination drug therapy, can be administered by a variety of routes (oral, IV, intracavitary, subcutaneous, intraarterial, intrathecal). However, the IV route is used most often. In recent years, venous access has become increasingly important because of the ease of access, safety, reduction of vein wasting, client comfort, and the ability to deliver continuous infusion. Continuous infusion of lower doses of some drugs is associated with lower toxicity (Belcher, 1992).

Most nursing implications for clients receiving chemotherapy involve safety. Safe handling of any chemotherapeutic agent is essential because the drugs are toxic not only to the cancer cells but to normal cells as well (see box on p. 548). Always refer to specific agency policy and procedure for "chemo spills." Safe administration is essential. When infused outside the venous system, many drugs can cause cellular damage, tissue necrosis, and loss of function. Extreme care is always exercised when administering vesicant agents such as dactinomycin, doxorubicin, epirubicin, and vincristine. A

vesicant can cause tissue necrosis if it extravasates. If a vesicant infiltrates, treatment of extravasations should be prompt to effectively minimize tissue damage. Chemotherapy should only be administered by registered nurses specifically trained to perform this procedure, since potential injury to the client is increased because of the nature of drug toxicity.

Chemotherapy, whether for reducing tumor size or for palliation, is most effective when complications and side effects are minimized and the client receives safe and effective therapy. Subjective assessment of the client's response, when described by client, and objective monitoring of laboratory values are essential. Tolerance and response are individual reactions, and the nurse plays a vital role in communicating side effects and adverse reactions as well as providing psychological support during a difficult time. Nurses must be prepared to assist clients with common side effects of chemotherapy: nausea, vomiting, anorexia, stomatitis, alopecia, leukopenia, anemia, and thrombocytopenia.

Precautions for Handling Antineoplastic Agents

All persons handling cytotoxic (hazardous) drugs such as antineoplastic agents should be properly trained in safety procedures and have access to policies and procedures that follow current government and professional practice standards.

DRUG PREPARATION AND ADMINISTRATION
Wash hands thoroughly, then wear a disposable gown, surgical latex gloves, and eye protection when preparing or administering cytotoxic drugs.

Whenever possible, it is highly recommended that preparation of injectable antineoplastic agents be performed in a clean-air work station (Hepa filter in BSC or biohazard cabinet).

Use areas for the preparation of drugs only for that purpose. Limit access to that area.

Remove only the required amount of the drug into the syringe. If more is withdrawn accidentally, inject the excess back into the vial and dispose of it properly.

Vent vials with a 20-gauge needle to avoid the creation of aerosol particles.

Nurses should not prepare or administer IV chemotherapy if they are pregnant because of suspected risk to the fetus from these agents.

DISPOSAL OF ANTINEOPLASTIC DRUGS AND EQUIPMENT
All antineoplastic drugs and all vials, needles, syringes, tubing, and equipment used in their administration need to be discarded with caution. Special leak-proof, puncture-proof, dou-

ble-bagged containers should be used and labeled BIOHAZARD for disposal by incineration.

Needles and syringes should not be broken and/or separated before disposal because leakage of the medication may occur.

SPILLAGE OR ANTINEOPLASTIC DRUG CONTACT WITH NURSE OR CLIENT SPILLAGE
Wear two pairs of gloves when cleaning up an antineoplastic drug spill. Wash hands before and after.

Wear a mask and eye protection if the medication is powdered.

Place the spilled substance in a plastic bag. Wipe up the remainder with a damp cloth and also place in the plastic bag.

Seal the bag and place it inside of a second bag, and seal the second bag. Label it BIOHAZARD and send it for disposal by incineration.

DRUG CONTACT WITH NURSE OR CLIENT
Thoroughly wash the affected area with soap and water. If clothing was contaminated, remove clothing immediately.

If eye contact was made, flush the eyes with copious amounts of water, holding the eyelids open during flushing.

DISPOSAL OF CLIENT EXCRETA
Urine, vomit, and other body fluids from clients receiving antineoplastic drugs should be handled with caution. Flush excreta down the toilet; wear gloves to avoid contact. Wash containers thoroughly.

Modified from McKenry LM, Salerno E: *Mosby's pharmacology in nursing,* ed 19, St Louis, 1994, Mosby.

Nurses have a major responsibility when planning and delivering care to the client receiving chemotherapy. The nurse who administers the drug is the resource for the client and client's family for safe and effective care. This skill focuses on the safe administration of antineoplastic agents by the IV route, whether by push, piggyback, or continuous infusion. The skill also reviews care of the client who experiences side effects as a result of chemotherapy.

Nursing Diagnoses

Potential nursing diagnoses associated with the administration of IV chemotherapy are specific to the combination drug therapies that are given and side effects of drugs, such as **Fluid Volume Deficit** related to nausea and vomiting, **Constipation** related to impaired intestinal motility, and **Altered Oral Mucous Membrane** related to stomatitis. Other diagnoses may be revealed as the client experiences "nadir" (time frame when peak of cell kill from chemotherapy occurs), such as **Diarrhea** related to destruction of gastrointestinal mucosa, **Sen-**

sory/Perceptual Alterations (auditory, tactile) related to drug-induced neurotoxicity, **Risk for Infection** related to drug-induced neutropenia from bone marrow suppression, and **Activity Intolerance** related to anemia.

The client experiencing cancer and the stress of chemotherapy may also have the diagnosis of **Ineffective Coping** related to stress of dealing with diagnosis and chemotherapy and **Body Image Disturbance** related to hormone therapy and alopecia.

For clients receiving chemotherapy for the first time, **Knowledge Deficit** regarding chemotherapy effects related to inexperience is appropriate.

EQUIPMENT (Figure 29-38)
IV needles: 21- or 23-gauge butterfly (IV push) or 22- or 20-gauge peripheral catheter if receiving continuous infusion (Use the smallest gauge possible to allow for improved blood flow around catheter.)
Tourniquet
Alcohol swabs
Betadine (povidone-iodine)

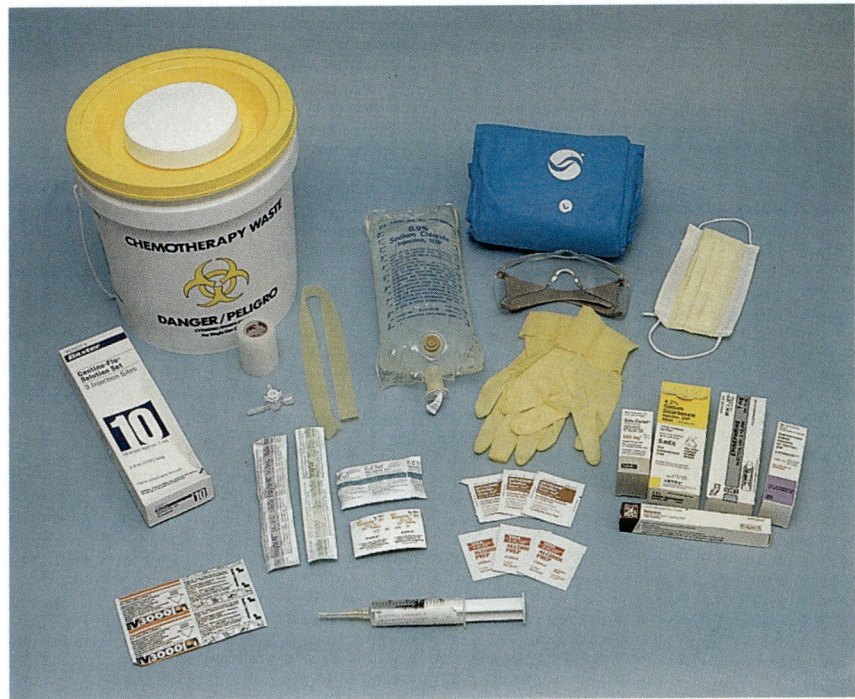

Figure 29-38 Equipment for administering chemotherapy.

Appropriate IV solution
IV tubing
Stopcock
Tape
Transparent dressing or Band-Aid
Long-sleeved isolation or disposable gown
Polyvinylchloride gloves
Mask (depending on agency policy)
Goggles
Chemotherapy waste disposal container
Emergency medications: epinephrine (Adrenalin), diphenhydramine (Benadryl), dopamine (Intropin), levarterenol bitartrate (Levophed), sodium bicarbonate, aminophylline, hydrocortisone, sodium succinate (for use in treatment of anaphylaxis or extravasation)
Any special equipment (chemo spill kit)
Syringes or small admixture volume of chemotherapeutic agents

> **nurse alert** Drugs should be prepared by specially trained pharmacists and are reconstituted under special conditions (reverse laminar flow hood). Some drugs must be given within a specified time after admixture. Ensuring that IV access is established, that laboratory values are adequate, and that client is ready for administration prevents time delays and waste of medications.

Assessment

1. Review medical orders and obtain information on drug, dosage, and specifics of administration.
2. Review client's medical and nursing history, assessing current status, medications taken, surgeries, and responses to previous treatments. **Review of past medical and nursing history assists in obtaining accurate information and may reduce the need for the client to repeat information (Edmunds, 1991).**
3. Review client's allergy history, specifically allergic response to chemotherapeutic drugs known to cause anaphylaxis, if previously administered.
4. Determine if laboratory data (complete blood count [CBC], platelet count) and any applicable pulmonary functions, electrocardiogram [ECG], and cardiac enzymes have been obtained. **This establishes a baseline to measure if toxicity develops after administration.**
5. Assess cumulative dose from previous administration of dose-limiting agents. **This ensures that dosage is not administered in excess of therapeutic amount.**
6. Assess client's previous experiences with chemotherapy during treatment and period between treatments. Obtain information on client's needs, expectations, fear of side effects, and management of side effects. Encourage input from family members.

Establishing a Teaching Plan for Client Receiving Chemotherapy

The following objectives should guide the nurse in establishing a teaching plan for the client receiving chemotherapy.
1. Describe how particular regimen is given.
2. State common side effects of treatment.
3. State ways to cope with nausea, vomiting, alopecia, stomatitis, and bone marrow suppression.
4. State signs and symptoms of side effects after discharge.
5. State medications that client should receive physician approval before taking, emphasizing interaction of over-the-counter medications.
6. Discuss steps of procedure and review cyclical administration and necessity of laboratory monitoring during nadir.

The following are suggestions for instruction to the client to encourage self-care activities and recognition and management of common chemotherapy side effects. Specific interventions should be based on individual assessment, nursing diagnosis, and type of chemotherapy the client is receiving.
1. Instruct client to complete all dental work before beginning chemotherapy.
2. Teach optimum oral hygiene to prevent stomatitis.
3. Encourage soothing, bland foods, and cool or room-temperature liquids.
4. Consult with physician if oral pain persists.

5. Instruct client to report dysphagia or presence of ulcers in or around mouth.
6. Instruct client to read a thermometer, to take temperature daily in afternoon, and to report any temperature greater than 101° F (38.3° C).
7. Instruct client to avoid contact with anyone who has an infection.
8. Instruct client to report any signs of infection, such as cough, sore throat, or dysuria.
9. Instruct client to report easy bruising; bleeding of gums, mouth, or nose; melena; or hematuria.
10. Instruct client in use of soft toothbrush, avoidance of flossing, and safety when using razors or nail clippers.
11. Instruct client to avoid constipation and to eat high-fiber diet and use stool softeners if constipation present.
12. Encourage use of caution to prevent falls or injury.
13. Instruct client experiencing diarrhea to decrease roughage, to increase fluid intake, and to eat small frequent feedings.
14. Encourage client to obtain cap or hairpiece before treatment begins.
15. Reassure client that hair growth should begin 8 weeks after completion of therapy but that hair may be a different texture or color.

---

7. Assess venous access device or condition of upper extremity veins. Solicit client's desire with regard to site selection, avoiding previously used vessels if possible. Avoid placement of device in flexion joint if vesicants are to be given.
8. Obtain current vital signs and weight and document mental status.
9. Obtain informed consent, if applicable (varies based on agency policy and procedure).
10. Identify clients at risk for complications during or after treatment:
    a. Older adults may have decreased hepatic blood flow, decreased glomerular filtration, decreased hemopoietic cell reserve, decreased renal flow, and decreased ability to activate carcinogens and drugs (Bleschik, 1988).
    b. Clients with difficult venous access
    c. Clients with allergy history
    d. Clients with history of previous complications from chemotherapy
    e. Clients receiving high-dose chemotherapy
    f. Clients who are anxious
11. Assess client's acceptance of chemotherapy, knowledge of chemotherapy, and expectations of treatment.

Planning

Expected outcomes of chemotherapy administration focus on safe administration of medications, management of specific chemotherapeutic agents and side effects, client understanding of chemotherapy side effects and self-care needs, and psychological support.

EXPECTED OUTCOMES
1. Client states common side effects of therapy.
2. Client is free of swelling or pain at IV site, blood return is present, and IV line is patent during administration.
3. Client is able to tolerate a bland diet of small frequent feedings and 2 L of fluids (IV or orally) and is free of any complaints of nausea, vomiting, and diarrhea 48 hours after administration of medication(s).
4. Client describes symptoms of bone marrow suppression; lists three symptoms (each) of neutropenia, anemia, and thrombocytopenia; and describes safety measures to prevent injury and exposure to infection.
5. Client initiates self-care measures and uses available cosmetic aids (see box above).

Implementation

Steps	Rationale
1. See Standard Protocol (Chapter 1, p. 5).	
2. Apply gown, goggles, and mask (optional).	Reduces risk of nurse's exposure to toxic chemotherapeutic agent.
3. Prepare premedication from vial or ampule (see Chapter 17).	
4. Verify prepared medications with physician's order.	
5. Establish IV access with smallest gauge possible and stopcock extension tubing (see Skill 29.1).	Improves hemodilution and administration of chemotherapy without risk of accidental needle puncture.
6. Prehydrate and premedicate client as ordered.	Adequate antiemetic control is essential in minimizing client's discomfort and alterations in hydration. Some chemotherapy agents require prehydration to minimize nephrotoxicity.
7. Examine syringes or small admixture volumes of chemotherapy agents for clarity.	Medications that are cloudy or have visible precipitate should not be given.
8. Verify labeling of drugs with physician's order in chart.	
9. Test venous integrity and IV flow by opening roller clamp on primary infusion line. Observe for free-flowing IV line and symptoms of infiltration.	Determines client's sensation of comfort at IV site and integrity of IV access.
10. Review potential adverse reactions with client, and encourage client to report burning and pain at IV site immediately.	May indicate beginning of extravasation.
11. Place absorbent pad under client's arm.	
12. Administer chemotherapy through stopcock.	
IV push	
a. Follow institutional policy regarding sequence of drugs if combination therapy contains a vesicant.	
b. Administer drug by attaching syringe to stopcock, aspirate for blood return, and open stopcock to allow simultaneous administration of medication and IV infusion flow.	Giving chemotherapy with infusion of fluids may lessen discomfort to client by increasing the dilution during administration.
c. Administer drug slowly over specified time. Pull back on syringe, aspirating for blood every 3 to 4 ml of medication administered.	Continued assessment of blood return during administration reduces risk of extravasation.
d. Observe site throughout administration for symptoms of infiltration, swelling, or redness at site or along tract.	If present, could indicate adverse or allergic reaction.
e. Continue to assess client's sensation at IV site during administration.	
f. Flush IV line with 10 to 15 ml of IV fluids between drugs.	Prevents incompatibility by preventing mixture of medications in IV line.
g. At completion of administration of all drugs, turn off stopcock to syringe and continue to infuse 20 to 30 ml of IV fluids.	Reduces venous irritability and clears IV tubing of all drugs, preventing drug leakage when discontinuing IV infusion.
IV piggyback infusion	
a. Attach small admixture volume of chemotherapeutic agent (Figure 29-39) to IV tubing suitable for electronic infusion device (EID) (see Skill 29.2).	All small admixtures that are given other than IV push should be placed on an EID to minimize too rapid infusion.
b. Open clamp and fill tubing, avoiding spillage of any fluid.	

Steps	Rationale

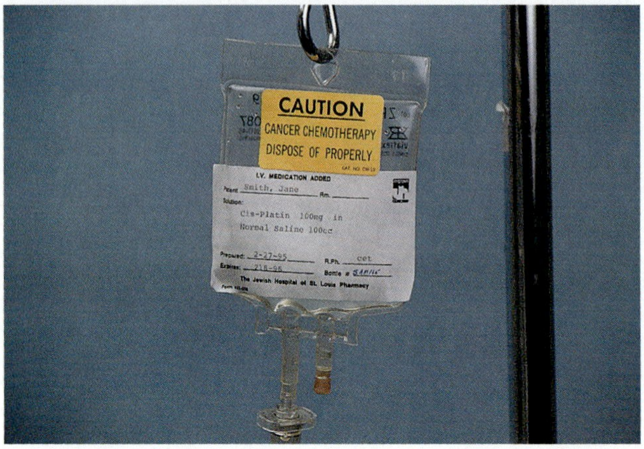

Figure 29-39 Small admixture of chemotherapy agent.

nurse alert High-dose etoposide (VP-16, 60 mg/kg) should be given via glass bottle with nitroglycerine tubing to prevent melting of routine chemotherapy tubing and chemotherapy spill.

c. Attach chemotherapy tubing to stopcock of primary IV line and secure with Luer lock device.

Prevents accidental disconnection.

d. Program EID for rate specified by physician.

e. Open stopcock and begin infusion.

f. Stay with client during first 10 to 15 ml of infusion.

Allows early assessment of signs and symptoms of adverse reactions and IV site complications.

g. Continue to observe client's IV site frequently during infusion. Ensure call light is within reach and client's arm is positioned comfortably before leaving.

h. When infusion is complete, turn off stopcock and stop infusion. Flush IV line with 20 to 30 ml of IV solution.

Infuses any residual medication.

13. Based on physician's order and client's need, IV line may be discontinued or remain in place. If IV access is to remain in place, ensure IV dressing is applied and intact and regulate IV fluids per order (see Skill 29.2). If IV site is to be discontinued, remove device and apply pressure until hemostasis is observed. Cover with sterile dressing or Band-Aid.

14. Dispose of equipment (IV bags, syringes, tubing, alcohol pads, absorbent pad) in chemotherapy waste container according to institutional policy.

Prevents exposure of personnel to toxic substances.

15. See Completion Protocol (Chapter 1, p. 6).

Evaluation

1. Ask client to state side effects from chemotherapy and the time after treatment when side effects will most likely occur.

2. Inspect IV access site during administration for blood return and after administration for pain or tenderness.

3. Observe client's tolerance to diet, and monitor intake and output every 8 hours. Maintain IV hydration, if ordered, or if client experiences nausea, vomiting, or diarrhea.

4. Have client list complications of bone marrow suppression and necessary management of complications.

5. Ask client to identify available community resources for self and family and available cosmetic aids, and observe for evidence of self-care.

UNEXPECTED OUTCOMES AND RELATED INTERVENTIONS

1. Client describes pain at IV site, blood return from IV access is absent, and swelling is present at the site during administration of vesicant. Extravasation of vesicant chemotherapeutic agent is suspected or confirmed. The nurse should:
   a. Stop administration of chemotherapeutic agent.
   b. Confirm extravasation.
   c. Leave needle in place.
   d. Aspirate any residual drug and blood in IV tubing, needle, and infiltration site.
   e. Instill IV antidote specific to agent administered.
   f. Remove IV needle.
   g. Inject antidote subcutaneously around site of extravasation, moving clockwise and using new 25-gauge needle with each injection. Avoid applying pressure to site.
   h. Photograph suspected area of extravasation according to hospital policy.
   i. Apply topical ointment if ordered.
   j. Cover with occlusive sterile dressing, which is changed twice daily for 7 days.
   k. Apply warm or cold compresses according to institutional policy.
   l. Notify physician of incident.
2. Client complains of uneasiness, dizziness, nausea, agitation, crampy abdominal pain, desire to urinate or defecate, generalized itching, chills, tightness in chest, urticaria, respiratory distress, hypotension, or cyanosis during administration of chemotherapy. Signs and symptoms of anaphylaxis are present. Guidelines for prevention of and intervention for anaphylaxis include the following:
   a. When administering drug with increased incidence of hypersensitivity, administer test dose before ordered dose.
   b. Monitor client for at least 15 minutes after test dose. Observe client for 15 to 30 minutes after medication administration.
   c. Stop administration if any of the symptoms listed above occur.
   d. Notify physician.
   e. Leave needle in place and maintain IV line with NS or ordered fluid.
   f. Place client in supine position.
   g. Monitor vital signs every 2 minutes until stable, then every 5 minutes for 30 minutes, then every 15 minutes.
   h. Maintain airway.
3. Chemotherapeutic agent is spilled during administration to client. Obtain a spill kit. Follow institutional policy and procedure for spill containment.
   a. Apply two pair of latex gloves used for chemotherapy administration, goggles, and gown (made of disposable, low-permeability fabric with long cuffed sleeves and closed front). Tuck cuffs of sleeves under gloves.
   b. Wipe up small (less than 5 ml or 5 g) spills with absorbent pads; contain larger (greater than 5 ml or 5 g) spills with absorbent pads.
   c. Clean spill area three times with detergent. Rinse with clean water.
   d. Dispose of all items used to clean spill in a chemotherapy disposal container. Wash hands thoroughly.
   e. Notify appropriate personnel (usually specially trained from housekeeping) that reusable items need further cleaning.
   f. If chemotherapy drug is spilled on client and/or nurse:
      (1) Remove contaminated items (gown, gloves) immediately and dispose of in chemotherapy disposal container.
      (2) Wash contaminated skin with soap (not a germicidal agent) and water.
      (3) If an eye is involved, flush with water for 5 minutes. Follow hospital procedure to obtain medical examination immediately.
      (4) Immediately following exposure, document the incident.

SAMPLE DOCUMENTATION

Record administration of drug on medication administration record or computer printout. Record the following in nurse's notes:

1600 CBC, creatinine, and BUN obtained and noted—WNL. IV started with 22-gauge butterfly in left cephalic after aseptic prep. Positive blood return noted. IVF NS 0.9% initiated at KVO. Procedure and side effects of chemotherapy reviewed, client verbalized understanding. Adriamycin 58.4 mg IVP given over 10 minutes without adverse reaction with free-flowing IV; positive blood return noted throughout administration when aspirated every 3 ml. Client denied c/o burning pain during IVP; no swelling or redness noted. Flushed with 30 ml NS without complication. IV site prepped and DC'd. Sterile dressing and Betadine applied. No hematoma noted. Received 150 ml NS during treatment. Reviewed with client side effects of Adriamycin; written teaching plan given with follow-up appointment. Expressed relief that "This one went well."

Skill 29.7 | Total Parenteral Nutrition

Total parenteral nutrition (TPN) is the administration of nutrients via the central circulation. Designed to support increased metabolic demands and replace enteral nutrition when the gastrointestinal (GI) tract is incapable of providing adequate nutritional absorption, TPN is a sophisticated field of high technology and has its own body of established knowledge. Standards of care for the client receiving TPN have been developed by the Intravenous Nursing Society (INS) and American Society for Parenteral and Enteral Nutrition (ASPEN). These standards guide the care of the client as well as the client's CVC during administration of TPN.

First used in the 1960s after researchers discovered that hyperosmolar solutions could be infused via a CVC, TPN can supply all the calories, dextrose, amino acids, fats, trace elements, and other essential nutrients needed for growth, weight gain, wound healing, convalescence, immunocompetence, and other health-sustaining functions (McKenry and Salerno, 1992). Exactly which conditions improve by TPN is controversial (LaRocca and Otto, 1994); however, TPN is indicated for clients with malnutrition or nonfunctional GI absorption (see box below).

Although different types of TPN solutions are available for clients with renal or liver impairment, and although solutions specific to the client with pulmonary impairment are available, the basic elements of TPN are similar. Carbohydrates in the form of glucose are the major source for metabolism and the only source for the central nervous system (CNS). Each gram of carbohydrate yields 3.4 kcal, and solutions are available in 5% to 70% dextrose in water. Concentrated dextrose is the primary caloric source in TPN.

Fat is the chief storage source of energy in the body and provides a concentrated caloric source because 1 g of fat yields 9 kcal. Fat emulsions, or lipids, can be administered to provide 40% to 60% of daily calories. One liter of 10% fat supplies 1100 calories. Lipids are a source of essential fatty acids and can prevent or correct fatty acid deficiencies. When lipids are added to the existing dextrose and amino acid solution, it is referred to as a 3-to-1 solution.

Protein is also provided in TPN in the form of amino acids. Since excess protein is metabolized and not stored in the body, maintenance of adequate protein is a major goal of nutritional support. Available preparations contain varying amounts of 3.5% to 10% amino acids. The client is monitored to achieve a positive nitrogen balance and anabolic state and is monitored throughout TPN by laboratory sampling and creatinine clearance.

Other additives typically found in TPN are vitamins, trace elements, fluids, and electrolytes. Addition of these elements is necessary for enzymatic activity and normal metabolism and is a requirement when the client is on long-term TPN. Medications may also be added to TPN (e.g., regular insulin, heparin, corticosteroids, H2 antagonists). Fluids and electrolytes are adjusted to each specific client's needs based on serum electrolytes and monitoring of daily weight and intake and output.

Because of complex admixtures and the potential for problems in solubility and pH, TPN solutions should be mixed only by a registered pharmacist in a controlled setting (laminar flow hood) to reduce the incidence of contamination and physical incompatibilities. The role of the nurse in caring for the client with TPN is nutritional assessment, monitoring of client response, and care and maintenance of the CVAD. When the client will continue on home TPN, the nurse educates the client about self-management.

Nutrition assessment is a critical step in initiating TPN. This baseline assessment guides the determination of TPN solution and caloric intake and is the basis for monitoring the client's response throughout TPN.

TPN is not without complications (Table 29-7). The most common complication is CVC sepsis. The hyperosmolar, high-glucose concentration found in the TPN solutions predisposes the client to higher risk of infection. Strict adherence to aseptic technique is essential when caring for the client with TPN (see Skill 29.4). Optimum management of CVCs may reduce the number of catheterizations per client and therefore the cost. Several

---

Indications for Total Parenteral Nutrition (TPN)

Client is unable to ingest or absorb sufficient nutrients through GI tract because of:
  Intestinal obstruction
  Mucositis from chemotherapy
  Nausea and vomiting
  Ileus
  Lack of enzymatic digestion
  Malabsorption
Client's oral intake is inadequate because of :
  Anorexia
  Elevated metabolic demands related to trauma, tumor, infection, or sepsis
Client is at risk for malnutrition because of:
  Gross underweight (> 80% below standard)
  Gross overweight (> 120% above standard)
  Recent weight loss of > 10%
  Alcoholism
  NPO for > 5 days
  Hypermetabolism because of disease state or condition

From Perry AG, Potter PA: *Clinical nursing skills and techniques,* ed 3, St Louis, 1994, Mosby.

Table 29-7 **Complications of Total Parenteral Nutrition (TPN)**

Problem	Cause	Symptoms	Immediate action	Prevention
Air embolism	IV tubing disconnected; part of catheter system open or removed without clamp on	Sudden respiratory distress; shortness of breath, coughing, chest pain	Clamp catheter; position client in left lateral Trendelenburg position; call physician.	Make sure all catheter connections are secure; clamp catheter.
Infection	Poor aseptic technique; contaminated tubing or infusate; secondary contamination from septicemia	Unexplained hyperglycemia, redness at infection site, fever, chills	Call physician.	Use proper aseptic technique.
Hyperglycemia	Client receiving solution too quickly; too little insulin in solution; infection	Excessive thirst, urination, blood sugar > 160 mg/ml	Call physician; may need to slow infusion rate (physician order).	Review medical history for glucose intolerance or diabetes; keep rate as ordered, never increase to "catch up"; use aseptic technique and routine blood glucose monitoring.
Hypoglycemia	TPN abruptly discontinued; too much insulin	Client shaky, dizzy, nervous, anxious	Call physician; if TPN discontinued abruptly, may need to restart $D_{10}NS$ at previous TPN rate; if client has oral intake, give ½ cup fruit juice; perform blood glucose monitoring; retest in 15 to 30 minutes.	Decrease TPN, "tapering" gradually until discontinued; blood glucose monitoring is used to ensure adequate insulin.

From Perry AG, Potter PA: *Clinical nursing skills and techniques,* ed 3, St Louis, 1994, Mosby.
Modified from Davis CL: Nursing care of total parenteral and enteral nutrition. In Fischer JE, editor: *Total parenteral nutrition,* ed 2, Boston, 1991, Little, Brown; Hickey MS: *Handbook of anteral, parenteral, and ARC/AIDS nutritional therapy,* St Louis, 1992, Mosby; Pennington CR: Review article: Toward safer parenteral nutrition, *Aliment Pharmacol Ther* 4(5):427, 1990.

studies have shown improved quality of care and lower sepsis rate when TPN clients are followed and managed by a group of specially trained nurses as members of a nutritional support team (Gianino, Brunt, and Eisenberg, 1992).

The three major parenteral systems for nutritional support are protein-sparing nutrition, peripheral parenteral nutrition, and central-line (total) parenteral nutrition (TPN). This skill involves care of the client with TPN. The client with TPN requires intense assessment, monitoring, and education. Complications associated with TPN, central venous catheter monitoring, and management of electrolyte imbalance, as well as physical and psychological needs of a client receiving TPN, can challenge the nurse.

Infusion of TPN is usually via a CVC inserted under stringent aseptic techniques and placed in the superior vena cava (SVC). The nurse may assist with placement (see Skill 29.5) and must ensure sterile conditions on insertion. The CVC should not be used for infusion until after x-ray verification has occurred. All TPN should be in-

fused through a 0.22 μ filter. Solutions with lipids, consisting of larger molecules, require a 1.2 μ filter for infusion (INS, 1990).

When initiating TPN, rates are gradually increased. "Tapering" allows pancreatic adjustment to the high-glucose infusion and allows for the increased insulin production necessary. A rate of 60 to 80 ml per hour is an approximate initial rate for the average-weight adult, but glucose tolerance may be compromised by sepsis, shock, hepatic and renal failure, diabetes, starvation, or administration of medications such as steroids. Older adults and very young persons are particularly susceptible to glucose intolerance, and thus insulin administration is sometimes necessary. Serum glucose greater than 200 compromises the immune response and increases susceptibility to infection. During the completion of TPN, rates are also tapered to prevent hypoglycemia.

The nurse continually evaluates the client's response to therapy. Physical parameters of positive nitrogen balance are monitored, as well as the client's psychological adjustment. The intake of food is associated with many

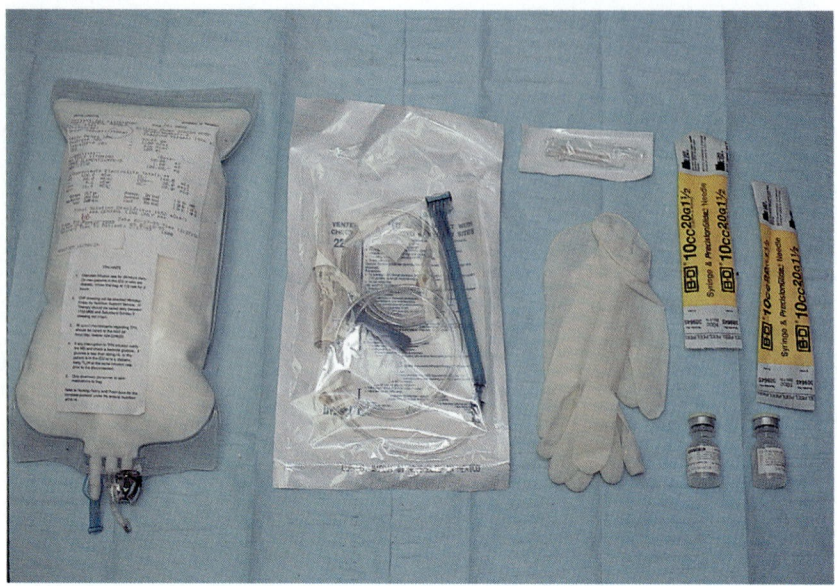

Figure 29-40 Equipment for total parenteral nutrition (TPN) infusion.

social events, and the client may feel socially isolated while on TPN. The nurse can assist in supporting and educating the client about the condition, prognosis, length of therapy, and response to therapy and can help to alleviate many fears and concerns.

Nursing Diagnosis

Nursing diagnoses associated with the client receiving TPN may include **Altered Nutrition: Less Than Body Requirements** related to inadequate protein intake, increased metabolic demands, or muscle wasting. Because of the high dextrose content of TPN and potential break in sterile technique when managing the CVC, **Risk for Infection** is an appropriate consideration. Assessment data may also reveal a **Knowledge Deficit** related to catheter management and possibly home care management of TPN related to the client's inexperience. If client has an external central access device, **Body Image Disturbance** should be considered. Finally, because TPN is costly and may involve temporary changes in family processes, **Ineffective Family Coping: Compromised** may be evidenced when assessing roles, financial resources, and stresses associated with TPN management.

EQUIPMENT (Figure 29-40)

Electronic infusion device (EID)
TPN bag labeled with solution, additives, and bag number
Tubing for EID
Alcohol and Betadine swabs
1 to 10 ml syringe
1 vial sterile NS
0.22 μ filter (solution without lipids)

1.2 μ filter (solution with lipids)
Tape

Assessment

1. Assess client's nutritional status, including (but not limited to) height, weight, anthropometric measurements, diet history, and baseline laboratory sampling of electrolytes, blood glucose, and creatinine. **This allows monitoring of client's progress during long-term TPN.**
2. Assess placement of CVC in superior vena cava and status of existing line.
3. Assess the CVC distal lumen for use or administration of any other parenteral infusion. **Distal lumen is usually "TPN designated" to minimize infection.**
4. Review physician's order for TPN, components of solution, and infusion rate.
5. Assess CVC for occlusiveness of dressing and patency before, during, and after infusion.
6. Assess solution for clarity, separation, oily appearance, and precipitation. (If present, do not use.) **This indicates solution is contaminated.**
7. Assess client/care giver for knowledge of self-management (willingness to learn, compliance with treatment regimen, availability of equipment, ability to assume self-care). **This determines client's/family's ability to manage TPN infusion in the home.**

Planning

Expected outcomes for TPN focus on improvement in client's nutritional status, prevention of infection, maintenance of fluid balance, and support to client requiring extended nutritional support in an alternative setting.

EXPECTED OUTCOMES

1. Client maintains laboratory values within normal limits and achieves weight gain.
2. Client's blood sugar remains within normal limits.
3. Client does not show signs and symptoms of CVC infection.
4. Client is free of fluid and electrolyte imbalance.
5. Client describes purpose and side effects of TPN.
6. Client demonstrates self-care management of CVC and TPN infusion.

Implementation

Steps	Rationale
1. See Standard Protocol (Chapter 1, p. 5).	
2. Verify CVC tip position and locate most distal lumen of CVC or assist physician with placement of CVC using maximum sterile barrier (see Skill 29.5). CVC should have positive blood return and SVC placement, with "TPN designated" port.	Break in sterile technique during insertion of CVC increases risk of infection.
3. Insert spike of IV tubing into TPN solution.	
4. Attach 0.22 or 1.2 μ filter to EID tubing (Figure 29-41). Prime according to manufacturer's recommendations.	Filters reduce possible microemboli through infusion.

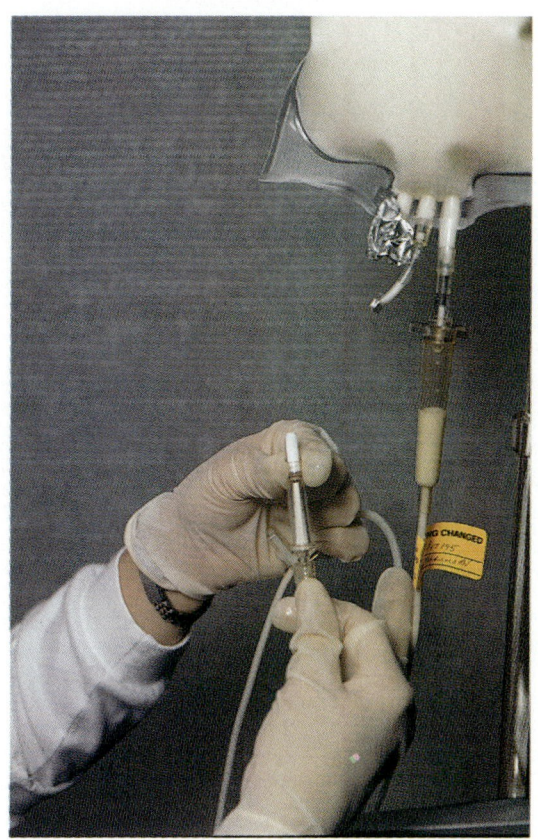

Figure 29-41 Attach filter to electronic infusion device (EID) for TPN.

5. Cleanse catheter and old tubing connection first with alcohol and then with Betadine swab. Allow each to dry.	Minimizes potential skin flora contamination at catheter/hub junction.

Steps	Rationale
6. Close clamp on distal lumen of CVC and disconnect old tubing. (If clamp is not present, client must perform Valsalva maneuver during opening of catheter hub.)	Minimizes potential for air embolism.
7. Attach syringe of 10 ml NS, open clamp, aspirate for blood return, then flush with NS.	Verifies patency of line.
8. Close clamp, disconnect syringe, and attach EID tubing with filter.	All TPN is infused via EID to ensure constant rate.
9. Open clamp, regulate pump for specified infusion to "taper on" TPN, and initiate infusion (Figure 29-42).	TPN infusion started gradually to ensure adequate insulin response.

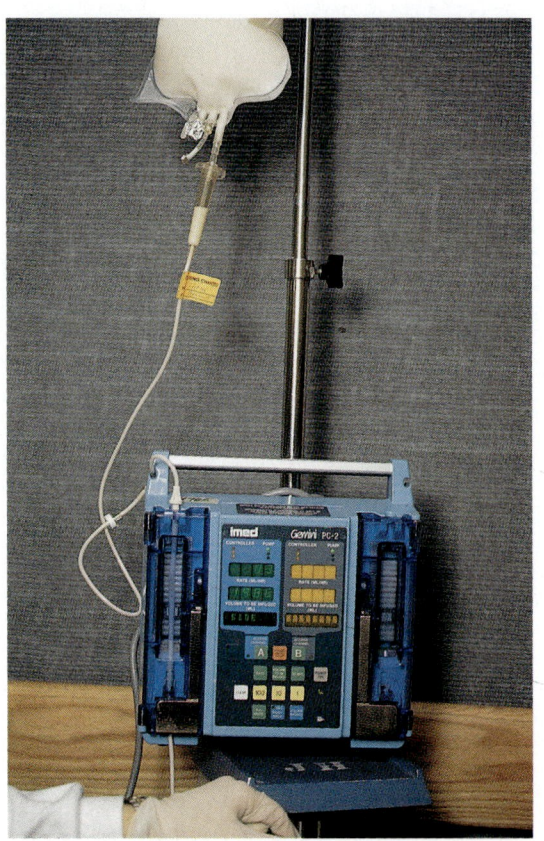

Figure 29-42 TPN solution infusing via IV pump.

Steps	Rationale
10. Secure all connections with tape. Connection to catheter hub should be Luer-lock.	Prevents inadvertent disconnection at junction. Minimizes air embolism and contamination.
11. Verify proper infusion rate until "tapering on" or "off" is completed.	"Tapering on" and "off" prevents hypoglycemia or hyperglycemia from high-dextrose concentration.
12. Continue to monitor TPN throughout infusion.	
13. Dispose of all contaminated equipment in appropriate receptacle.	
14. See Completion Protocol (Chapter 1, p. 6).	

Evaluation

1. Monitor client's daily weights and laboratory values.
2. Evaluate client's blood sugar with blood glucose monitoring device (see Skill 13.2) every 6 hours for 48 hours, then every morning while client is receiving TPN.
3. Monitor client's temperature and vital signs every 4 hours. Evaluate CVC insertion site for evidence of redness, tenderness, or exudate.
4. Monitor client's intake and output and serum electrolytes.
5. Ask client to describe purpose of TPN and side effects.
6. Have client demonstrate ability to change TPN solution bags, regulate infusion device, and change dressing.

UNEXPECTED OUTCOMES AND RELATED INTERVENTIONS

1. Client experiences chills and fever and complains of tenderness at CVC insertion site.
   a. Remove dressing and inspect site. Culture any exudate if present.
   b. Notify physician. Obtain culture of CVC tip and intracutaneous segment if ordered when discontinued (see Skill 29.5).
   c. Initiate peripheral infusion of 10% dextrose at same rate of TPN infusion for 2 to 4 hours if CVC is discontinued.
   d. Ensure sterile technique with all tubing and CVC dressing changes.
2. Client's blood sugar is not in the normal range.
   a. Assess for signs and symptoms of catheter infection, hepatic and renal failure, or stress.
   b. Notify physician. Administer insulin as ordered.
   c. Monitor blood glucose monitoring values every 6 hours for signs and symptoms of hyperglycemia or hypoglycemia.
3. Client suddenly becomes confused and lethargic, skin turgor is poor, and oral mucous membranes are not moist and pink.
   a. Monitor vital signs and intake and output, observing for intake greater than output or output greater than intake.
   b. Obtain and assess chemistry laboratory values, including glucose, magnesium, fluid and electrolytes, and hepatic and renal function parameters (see Appendix D).
   c. Notify physician with laboratory sampling results. Adjust TPN solutions if ordered.
   d. Provide safety measures to prevent injury. Explain to client and family that confusion may be related to metabolic intolerance.
   e. If ordered, discontinue TPN, aggressively treat with fluid and electrolyte replacement infusion, and correct hyperglycemia or hypoglycemia.

SAMPLE DOCUMENTATION

1800 #1 3-in-1 (2937 ml) initiated via distal port of Hickmann catheter after aseptic prep. Rate set at 43 ml for first hour, infusing via IMED Gemini pump. Positive blood return obtained from distal lumen, flushed with 10 ml NS before initiation of TPN. Accu-Chek 95. Instructed in importance of accurate intake and output and glucose monitoring during TPN. Hickmann dressing occlusive; client denied pain or tenderness at site. Verbalizes signs and symptoms of hypoglycemia/hyperglycemia with accuracy and stated would call if present.

2400 TPN rate as ordered, now infusing at 142 ml/hr via IMED Gemini pump. Client voided 380 ml clear, amber urine. Accu-Chek 105.

CRITICAL THINKING EXERCISES

1. Interpret each of the following:
   a. Mrs. Smith is receiving a continuous intravenous infusion.
   b. Mr. Harris's IV appears inflamed.
   c. Mrs. Levy's IV has been positional; be sure to check for infiltration.
2. Mr. Lou is to receive 1000 cc of IV fluid over the next 8 hours. How many drops of fluid per minute will Mr. Lou receive if your tubing delivers 10 gtts per cc? How many cc per hour?
3. Mr. Leon is to receive an IV piggyback infusion of Ancef, an antibiotic. The nurse instructs you to use SAS via his peripheral IV line.
   a. How will you proceed?
   b. What if the nurse had told you to use SASH?
4. Pepé is to receive 500 cc of whole blood. Upon inspecting Pepé's IV site you note that he has a 22-gauge intravenous catheter in place. What should you do, and why?
5. You are to administer 40 cc of IV Lasix to Mr. Leonard through his central line. You will begin by flushing the central line with normal saline. You will then give the Lasix over 1 to 2 minutes as prescribed. How quickly should you flush the central line after giving the Lasix? Explain.
6. How does the nurse's preparation of chemotherapy drugs differ from the preparation of other drugs?
7. Mr. Gill is receiving total parenteral nutrition. When you enter his room he requests a glass of water. Ten minutes later he again requests a glass of water, stating that he is really thirsty. How should you respond to Mr. Gill's request?

REFERENCES

Belcher AE: *Cancer nursing,* St Louis, 1992, Mosby.

Bleschik S: The normal physiologic changes of aging and their impact on the response to cancer treatment, *Semin Oncol Nurs* 4(3):178, 1988.

Edmunds MW: *Introduction to clinical pharmacology,* St Louis, 1991, Mosby.

Gianino MS, Brunt M, Eisenberg P: The impact of a nutritional support team on the cost and management of multilumen central venous catheters, *J Intravenous Nurs* 15(6):327, 1992.

Goode CJ et al: A meta-analysis of effects of heparin flush and saline flush: quality and cost implications, *Nurs Res* 40(6):324, 1991.

Harovas J, Anthony H: Your guide to troublefree transfusions, *RN* 56(11):26, 1993.

Intravenous Nursing Society: *Intravenous nursing standards of practice,* Philadelphia, 1990, Lippincott.

LaRocca JC, Otto SE: *Pocket guide to intravenous therapy,* St Louis, 1994, Mosby.

Maki DG: Infection caused by intravascular devices: pathogenesis, strategies for prevention. In Maki DG, editor: *Improving catheter site care,* New York, 1991, Royal Society of Medicine Services.

McKenry LM, Salerno E: *Mosby's pharmacology in nursing,* ed 19, St Louis, 1994, Mosby.

Mermel L, Stolz S, Maki DG: Epidemiology and pathogenesis of infection with Swan Ganz catheters: a prospective study using molecular epidemiology, *Am J Med* 91(3B):197, 1991.

Milliam PA: Starting IVs: how to develop your venipuncture expertise, *Nursing '92* 22(9):33, 1992.

Perry AG, Potter PA: *Clinical nursing skills and techniques,* ed 3, St Louis, 1994, Mosby.

Ryder M: Peripherally inserted central venous catheters, *Nurs Clin North Am* 28(4):937, 1993.

Westphal RG: *Handbook of transfusion medicine,* Washington, DC, 1990, American Red Cross Blood Services.

ADDITIONAL READINGS

Ahrens T, Wiersema L, Weilitz PB: Differences in pain perception associated with intravenous catheter insertion, *J Intravenous Nurs* 14(2):85, 1991.

American Society of Parenteral and Enteral Nutrition (ASPEN): Standards of practice: nutrition support nurse, *Nutr Clin Pract* 3(2):78, 1988.

Baranowski L: Central venous access devices: current technologies, uses, and management strategies, *J Intravenous Nurs* 16(3):167-194, 1993.

Belcher AE: *Blood disorders,* St Louis, 1993, Mosby.

Camp-Sorrell D: Advanced central venous access: selection, catheter devices and nursing management, *J Intravenous Nurs* 13(6):361, 1990.

Camp-Sorrell D: Implantable ports: everything you always wanted to know, *J Intravenous Nurs* 15(5):262, 1992.

Eisenberg PE, Howard MP, Gianino MS: Improved long-term maintenance of central venous catheters with a new dressing technique, *J Intravenous Nurs* 13(5):279, 1990.

Freedman SE, Bosserman G: Tunneled catheters: technologic advances and nursing care issues, *Nurs Clin North Am* 28(4):851, 1993.

Hadaway LC: Evaluation and use of advanced IV technology. Part I. Central venous access devices, *J Intravenous Nurs* 12(2):73, 1989.

Haire WD, Lieberman RP: Thrombosed central venous catheters: restoring function with a 6-hour urokinase infusion after failure of bolus urokinase, *J Parenter Enter Nutr* 16(2):129, 1991.

Hickey MS: *Handbook of enteral, parenteral, and ARC/AIDS nutritional therapy,* St Louis, 1992, Mosby.

Howard P, Eisenberg P, Gianino S: Dressing a central venous catheter a better way, *Nursing '92* 22(3):60, 1992.

Kim MJ, McFarland GK, McLane AM: *Pocket guide to nursing diagnoses,* ed 5, St Louis, 1993, Mosby.

LaRocca JC: *Handbook of home care IV therapy,* St Louis, 1994, Mosby.

Maki DG, McCormack KN: Defatting catheter insertion sites in total parenteral nutrition is of no value as an infection control measure, *Am J Med* 83:833, 1987.

Ryder M: Parenteral nutrition. In Kennedy-Caldwell C, Guenter P, editors: *Nutrition support nursing: core curriculum,* Silver Springs, Md, 1988, Aspen.

Shivnan JC et al: A comparison of transparent adherent and dry sterile gauze dressings for long-term central catheters in patients undergoing bone marrow transplant, *Oncol Nurs Forum* 18(8):1349, 1991.

Shizgall HM: Parenteral and enteral nutrition, *Ann Rev Med* 42:549, 1991.

Silberman H: Fat emulsions as major source in total parenteral nutrition, *Nutrition* 7(5):333, 1991.

Strand C, Wajsbort R, Sturmann K: Effect of iodophor vs. iodine tincture skin preparation on blood culture contamination rate, *JAMA* 269(8):1004, 1993.

Weinstein SM: *Plumer's principles and practice of intravenous therapy,* Philadelphia, 1993, Lippincott.

William SR: *Basic nutrition and diet therapy,* ed 9, St Louis, 1992, Mosby.

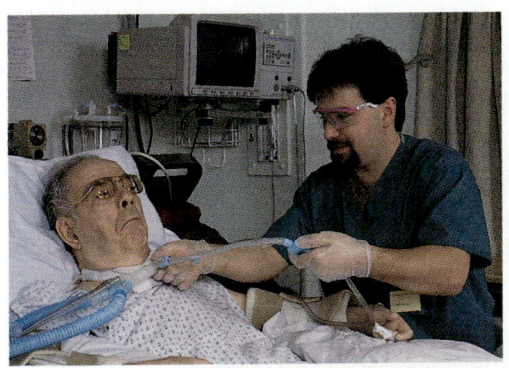

chapter 30

Promoting Oxygenation

Skill 30.1
Oxygen Administration

Skill 30.2
Airway Maintenance

Skill 30.3
Suctioning

Skill 30.4
Artificial Airway Management and Tracheostomy Care

Skill 30.5
Managing Closed Chest Drainage Systems

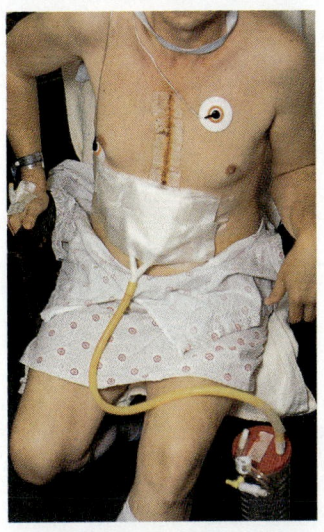

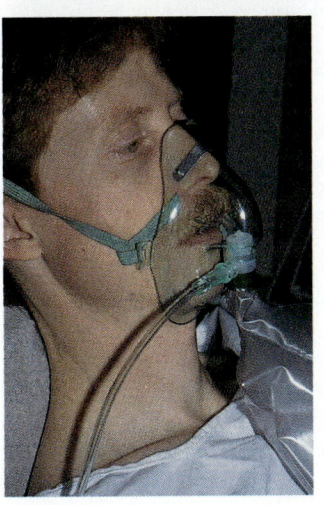

P hysiological needs, such as food, water, and air, are the primary stimulus for behavior according to Maslow's hierarchy of human needs. It is only when these needs are met that humans may attempt to reach higher levels of needs, such as safety, intimacy, and the need for knowledge and understanding. Preoccupation with breathing stifles the emergence of behaviors motivated by higher needs (Kersten, 1989). Until dyspnea is relieved, the client will not be able to focus on other areas of concern identified by the nurse.

Respirations are effective when sufficient oxygenation is obtained at the cellular level and when cellular waste and carbon dioxide are adequately removed via the bloodstream and lungs. When this system is interrupted, such as by lung tissue damage, obstruction of airways by inflammation and excess mucus, or impairment of the mechanics of ventilation, intervention is required to support the client or death may occur.

Nursing Diagnosis

Nursing diagnoses directly related to promoting optimum oxygenation include **Ineffective Airway Clearance** resulting from an ineffective cough or excessive secretions, **Ineffective Breathing Pattern** exhibited by clients with respiratory muscle weakness and fatigue or abnormal breathing pattern, **Impaired Gas Exchange** resulting from altered oxygen supply or alveolar hypoventilation, and **Inability to Sustain Spontaneous Ventilation** for those clients who exhibit an imbalance between ventilatory capacity and demand because of decreased ventilatory capacity and increased ventilatory demand.

Clients with oxygenation problems may be at risk for **Impaired Thought Processes** from inadequate oxygenation and carbon dioxide retention, **Activity Intolerance** related to imbalance between oxygen supply and demand, and **Risk for Infection** as a result of the damaged defense systems of the lungs. Psychosocial factors such as **Fear** and **Hopelessness** may be related to dyspnea and feelings of suffocation as well as the fear of dying or being a burden. **Care Giver Role Strain** related to the chronicity of many pulmonary diseases and **Impaired Verbal Communication** when the client receives a tracheostomy or is intubated may also be appropriate.

Skill 30.1 | Oxygen Administration

Oxygen therapy refers to the administration of oxygen to a client to prevent or relieve hypoxia. *Hypoxia* is a condition in which insufficient oxygen is available to meet the metabolic needs of tissues and cells. Hypoxia results from *hypoxemia,* which is a deficiency of oxygen in the arterial blood. Supplemental oxygen for the relief of hypoxemia may be temporary, until the cause of the problem is corrected, or long term, when it is required for a chronic condition. The delivery method utilized depends on the amount of supplemental oxygen required (Table 30-1), hospital or home use, and the portability desired (see Chapter 39).

EQUIPMENT
Delivery device ordered by physician
Oxygen tubing (consider extension tubing)
Humidifier
Sterile water
Oxygen source
Flow meter
"Oxygen In Use" sign

Table 30-1 Oxygen Delivery Systems

Delivery system	F_iO_2* delivered	Advantages	Disadvantages
Nasal cannula	1-6 L/min: 24%-44%	Safe and simple Easily tolerated Effective for low concentrations Does not impede eating or talking Inexpensive, disposable	Unable to use with nasal obstruction Drying to mucous membranes Can dislodge easily May cause skin irritation or breakdown Client's breathing pattern will affect exact F_iO_2
Oxymizer	1-15 L/min: 24%-60%	Higher concentrations without mask Releases O_2 only on inhalation Conserves O_2, increased portability Does not require humidification	Interferes with drinking from cup May be cosmetically unappealing Potential reservoir membrane failure Client's breathing pattern will affect exact F_iO_2
Venturi mask	4-10 L/min: 24%-50%	Delivers exact preset F_iO_2 despite client's breathing pattern Does not dry mucous membranes Can be used to deliver humidity	Hot and confining, mask may irritate skin F_iO_2 may be lowered if mask does not fit snugly Interferes with eating and talking
Partial rebreather	6-10 L/min: 35%-60%	Delivers increased F_iO_2 Easily humidifies O_2 Does not dry mucous membranes	Hot and confining, may irritate skin, tight seal necessary Interferes with eating and talking Bag may twist or kink; should not totally deflate
Nonrebreather	6-10 L/min: 60%-100%	Delivers highest possible F_iO_2 without intubation Does not dry mucous membranes	Requires tight seal, difficult to maintain and uncomfortable May irritate skin Bag should not totally deflate

*F_iO_2, Fraction of inspired oxygen concentration.

Assessment

1. Observe for signs and symptoms associated with hypoxia: apprehension, anxiety, decreased ability to concentrate, decreased level of consciousness, increased fatigue, dizziness, behavioral changes, increased pulse rate, increased depth and rate of respirations, cardiac dysrhythmias, pallor, cyanosis, clubbing, dyspnea, and use of accessory muscles of respiration. **Early detection of the signs and symptoms of hypoxia may result in earlier treatment and avoidance of the complications associated with hypoxia. Left untreated, hypoxia is life-threatening.**

2. If available, note client's most recent pulse oximetry readings and arterial blood gas (ABG) results. **Pulse oximetry is the noninvasive measurement of oxygenation but has limitations (see Chapter 10). ABGs objectively document hypoxemia and the carbon dioxide response (see Chapter 36).**

3. Perform a complete assessment of the respiratory system (see Chapter 12).

Planning

Expected outcomes focus on optimum oxygenation, safe application of oxygen therapy, and an understanding of and compliance with the oxygen prescription.

EXPECTED OUTCOMES

1. Client's oxygen saturation and ABGs return to or remain within normal limits or baseline levels.
2. Client's pulse; respirations; color; and subjective experiences of anxiety, fatigue, and decreased oxygenation status return to normal by discharge.
3. Client is able to state the indications for supplemental oxygen by discharge.
4. Client follows safety guidelines for supplemental oxygen therapy by discharge.
5. Client uses supplemental oxygen as prescribed by discharge.

Implementation

Steps	Rationale
1. See Standard Protocol (Chapter 1, p. 5).	
2. Explain to client purpose of oxygen administration and safety precautions (Table 30-2) and demonstrate correct application.	Patient may continue to have dyspnea while receiving oxygen because of other etiology (e.g., narrowed airways). Understanding of need and safety guidelines increases compliance and safety.
3. Attach delivery device to oxygen tubing. Consider extension tubing for clients who are not confined to bed.	Avoids complications of bed rest.
4. Attach appropriate flow meter to oxygen source.	Flow meters with smaller calibrations may be safer for clients requiring low-dose oxygen when larger doses may be harmful, as in client with chronic obstructive pulmonary disease (COPD).
5. Attach tubing to flow meter.	
6. Adjust oxygen flow rate to prescribed dosage. If humidifier is used, verify that water is bubbling (Figure 30-1).	Humidifier prevents drying of mucosa and airway secretions but may not be necessary for flow rates less than 3 L/min. Presence of bubbling indicates that oxygen is humidified before delivery to client.
7. Observe for proper fit and function of delivery device (Lewis and Collier, 1992).	
a. Nasal cannula Place tips of cannula into client's nares and adjust headband or plastic slide until cannula fits snugly and comfortably (Figure 30-2).	Effective mechanism of oxygen delivery up to 4 L/min.
b. Reservoir nasal cannula Fit as for nasal cannula. Reservoir is located under nose or as a pendant (Figure 30-3).	Able to deliver higher flow of oxygen than cannula without changing to a mask, which is claustrophobic for some clients. Delivers a 2:1 ratio (e.g., 6 L nasal cannula is approximately equivalent to 3 L reservoir device or Oxymizer).

Table 30-2 **Oxygen Safety Guidelines**

Guideline	Explanation
Make sure oxygen is set at prescribed rate.	Oxygen is a medication and should not be adjusted without a physician's order.
Smoking is not permitted. Avoid electrical equipment that may result in sparks.	Oxygen supports combustion. Delivery systems must be kept 10 feet from open flames and at least 5 feet from electrical equipment.

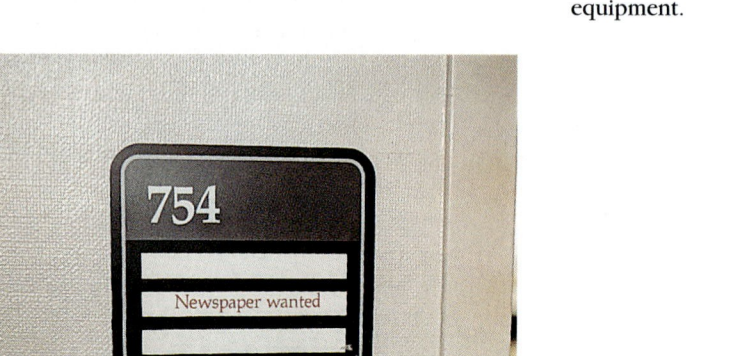

Guideline	Explanation
Store oxygen cylinders upright. Check oxygen available in portable cylinders before transporting or ambulating clients.	Secure with chain or holder to prevent tipping and falling. Gauge on cylinder should register in green range, indicating oxygen is available for transport and ambulation. Have back-up supply available if level is low.

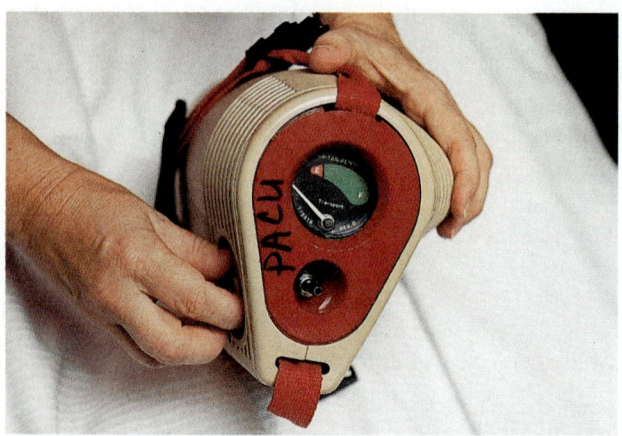

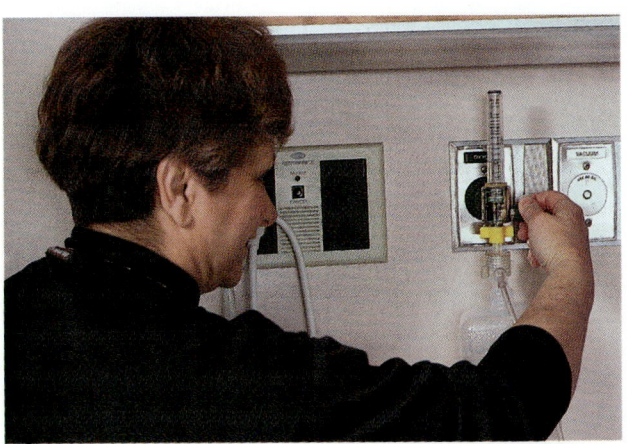

Figure 30-1 Flow meter attached to oxygen source.

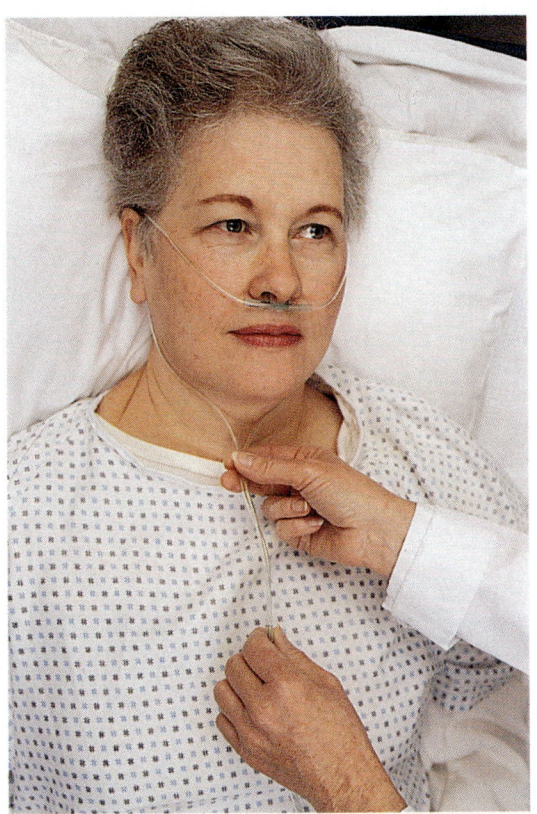

Figure 30-2 Nasal cannula is useful for low oxygen concentrations (2 L/min) for clients with chronic lung disease.

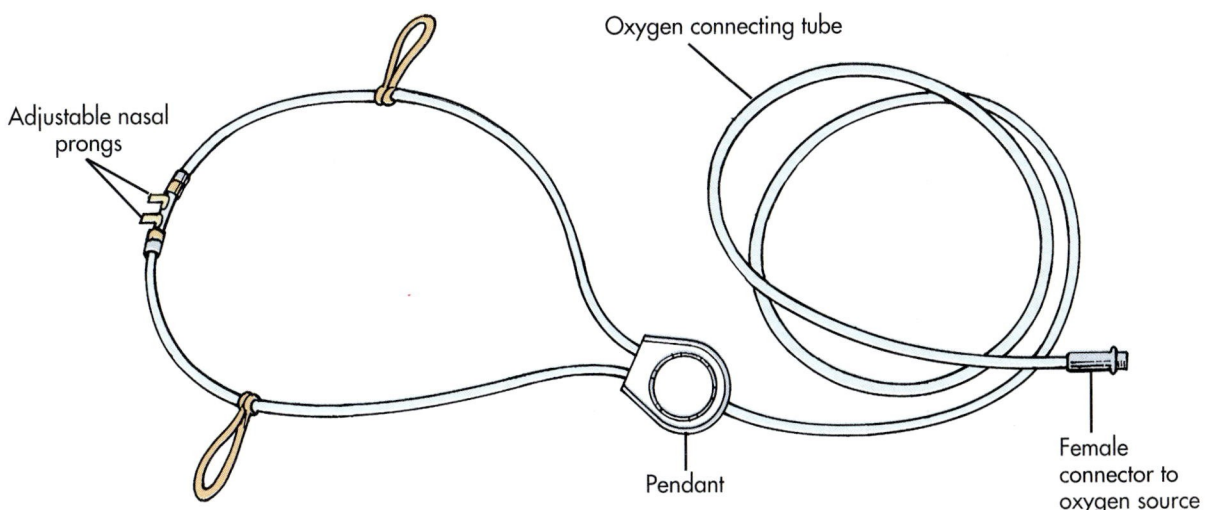

Figure 30-3 Oxygen-conserving device includes pendant-type cannula.

Steps	Rationale

c. Venturi mask

Rate set on flow meter will determine fraction of inspired oxygen concentration (F_iO_2). Low and high concentration adapters are available. Setting should correlate with prescribed dosage (Figure 30-4).

Delivers exact oxygen concentration despite respiratory pattern.

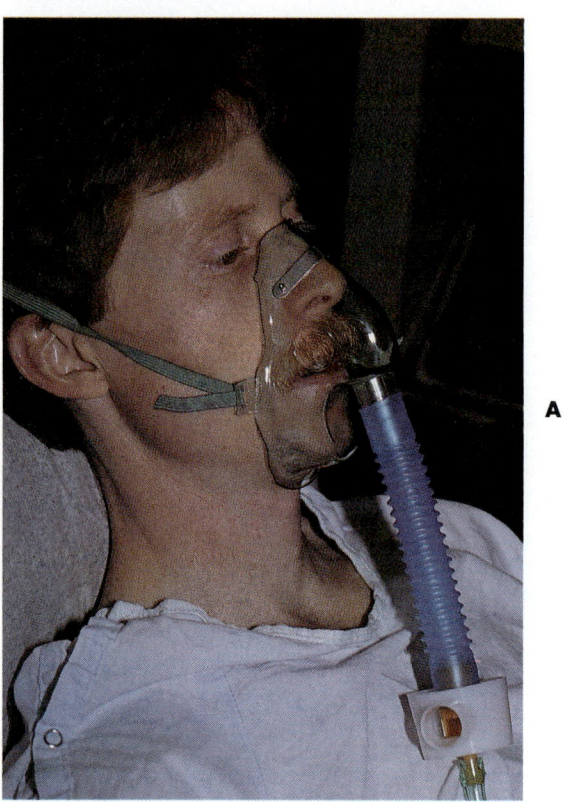

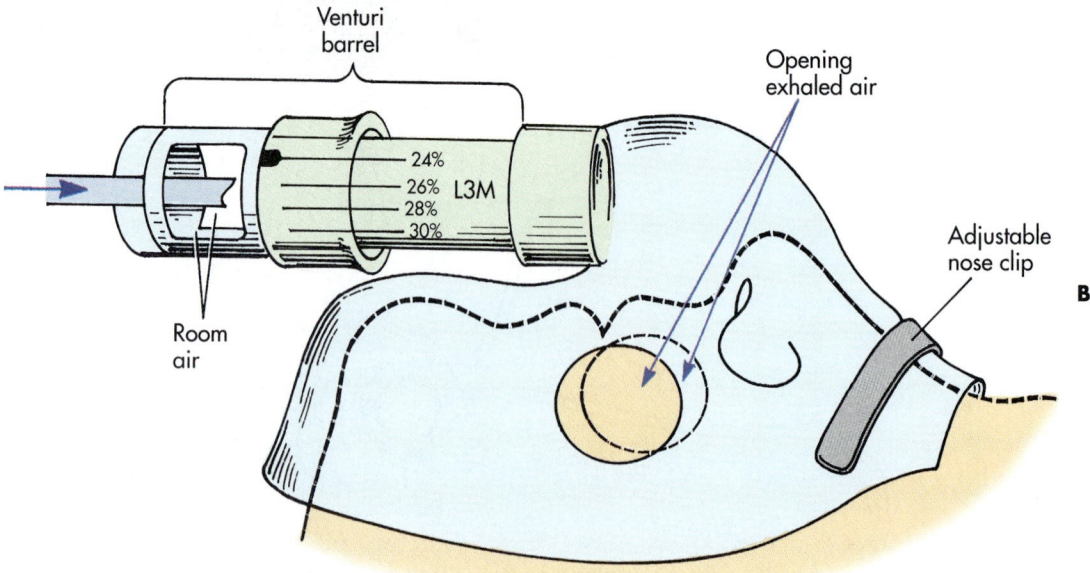

Figure 30-4 Turning Venturi barrel sets percentage of oxygen delivered from 24% to 40% at preset intervals.

Steps	Rationale

d. Partial rebreather mask
Reservoir should fill on exhalation and almost collapse on inhalation (Figure 30-5).

Effectively delivers higher oxygen concentrations.

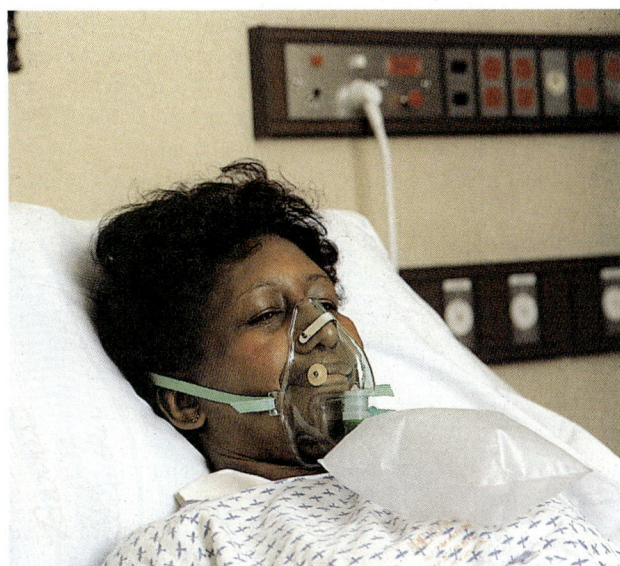

Figure 30-5 Partial rebreather mask can deliver concentrations of 40% to 60% using flow rates of 6 to 10 L/min.

e. Nonbreathing mask
Reservoir should fill on exhalation and should never totally collapse on inhalation.

f. Simple face mask
Place securely over client's nose and mouth (Figure 30-6).

Delivers highest possible oxygen concentration for non-intubated clients.

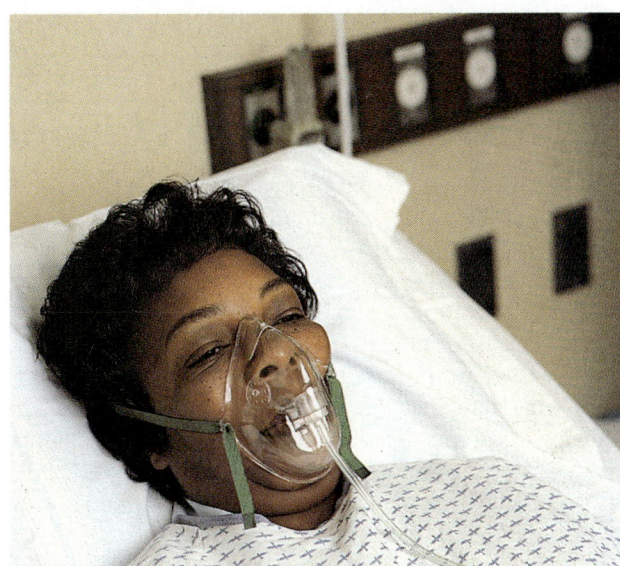

Figure 30-6 Simple face mask can deliver 35% to 50% using flow rates of 6 to 10 L/min for short time.

8. Ask physician to consider ABGs 10 to 15 minutes after initiation of therapy or change in oxygen concentration.

ABGs provide objective data regarding blood oxygenation and acid-base status (see Chapter 36).

9. Consult with physician regarding the need for pulse oximetry if client's oxygen level may be unstable.

Oximetry provides objective data regarding blood oxygenation and is used for trending (see Chapter 10).

10. See Completion Protocol (Chapter 1, p. 6).

Evaluation

1. Observe repeat ABGs and/or pulse oximetry for objective measurement of improvement.
2. Observe client for improved oxygen saturation, as demonstrated by decreased anxiety, improved level of consciousness and cognitive abilities, decreased fatigue, and absence of dizziness. Assess pulse and respirations, decreased pulse with regular rhythm, decreased respiratory rate, and improved color. These are signs that oxygenation is improving.
3. Ask client to verbalize indications for supplemental oxygen.
4. Observe if client follows safety guidelines in present setting, and ask client to verbalize safety guidelines for home use.
5. Observe for compliance to oxygen prescription.

UNEXPECTED OUTCOMES AND RELATED INTERVENTIONS

1. Client experiences nasal irritation, drying of nasal mucosa, sinus pain, or epistaxis.
   a. Apply a water-soluble lubricant to areas of irritation around nares.
   b. Recommend use of an isotonic saline nasal spray.
   c. Determine if a reservoir cannula is appropriate; obtain order.
2. Client develops irritation of the face or posterior surfaces of the ear.
   Apply ear protectors or reposition nasal cannula so that it does not come into contact with irritated areas.
3. Client has continued hypoxia.
   a. Monitor ABGs and/or pulse oximetry.
   b. Perform a complete respiratory assessment.
   c. Notify physician.
   d. Identify methods to decrease oxygen demand (e.g., total bed rest).
4. Client develops carbon dioxide retention, as demonstrated by confusion, headache, decreased level of consciousness, flushing, somnolence, carbon dioxide narcosis, or respiratory arrest.
   a. Monitor ABGs.
   b. Notify physician.
   c. Assist in maintaining oxygen pressure (Po_2) at 55 mm Hg. (Hypoxia must be treated, but Po_2 levels that exceed 60 to 70 mm Hg may worsen hypoventilation.)

SAMPLE DOCUMENTATION

0800 Client alert and oriented. Respirations even and easy. Color pink. O_2 4 L nasal cannula. Productive cough of yellow sputum. Fluids encouraged.

1000 Reddened areas are noted behind right ear, without breakdown. Foam ear protector added to nasal cannula tubing.

1200 No further redness noted behind ears. Client denies discomfort from cannula.

Skill 30.2 | Airway Maintenance

The respiratory system is comprised of a system of airways that must remain open and free of obstruction in order to decrease resistance of airflow to and from the lung. Hydration, nutrition, and positioning are noninvasive techniques for maintaining a patent airway. Positioning is an effective measure in reducing respiratory distress by promoting maximum lung expansion, improving effectiveness of the client's cough, and enhancing clearance of airway secretions. Select clients may require continuous positive airway pressure (CPAP) to prevent airway and alveolar collapse during spontaneous breathing. Sleep apnea is one indication for CPAP. CPAP maintains positive airway pressure above atmospheric pressure during the inspiratory and expiratory phases of the respiratory cycle. Increased alveolar surface area is made available for oxygen transport, and the client's work of breathing is reduced, thus improving the client's level of oxygenation.

Medications such as antibiotics, bronchodilators, steroids, decongestants, antihistamines, and expectorants may also be used. The peak expiratory flow rate (PEFR) may be used to determine the effectiveness of therapy in patients with chronic airflow obstruction using objective data. The PEFR is the maximum flow rate that can be generated during a forced expiratory maneuver, expressed in liters.

EQUIPMENT

Application of CPAP (Figure 30-7)
   Mask with straps, face or nasal
   CPAP valve (2.5, 5, 7.5, or 10 cm water)
   Oxygen source
   CPAP generator
   Appropriate signs
PEFR measurements (Figure 30-8)
   Peak flow meter
   Patient diary, if appropriate

Assessment

1. Assess for possible impairment of airway clearance: increased work of breathing or inability to clear copious or tenacious secretions by coughing.

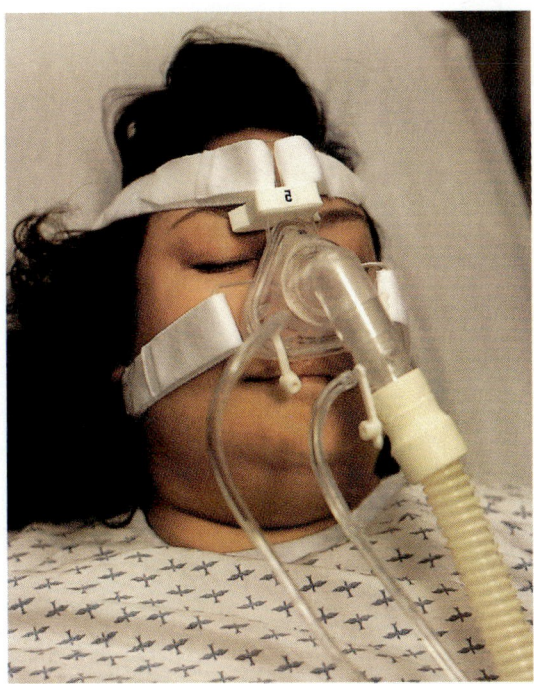

Figure 30-7

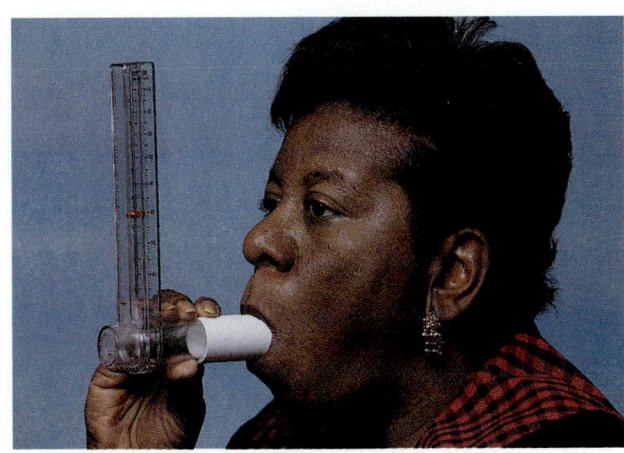

Figure 30-8

2. Observe for signs of airway obstruction: shortness of breath, wheezing, use of accessory muscles of respiration, pallor or cyanosis, nasal flaring, snoring respirations, or sleep apnea.

3. Assess client's baseline knowledge of positioning, CPAP, and PEFR.

4. Review physician's order for CPAP and predicted values for PEFR.

Planning

Expected outcomes focus on client's airway patency, comfort, and knowledge and ability for self-care.

EXPECTED OUTCOMES

1. Client maintains a position that promotes maximum lung expansion and comfort.
2. Client's airways are cleared of retained secretions.
3. Client's periods of sleep apnea are reduced to fewer than two episodes in 6 hours.
4. Client's objective measures of oxygenation improve or remain normal (ABGs, pulse oximetry).
5. Client expresses comfort while CPAP is in place by discharge.
6. Client and family demonstrate correct use of CPAP or PEFR by discharge.
7. Client and family verbalize an appropriate action plan based on PEFR values obtained by discharge.
8. Client verbalizes the benefits of positioning, CPAP, and/or PEFR by discharge.

Implementation

Steps	Rationale
1. See Standard Protocol (Chapter 1, p. 5).	
2. Teach correct positioning of client **a. Sitting** Semi-Fowler's or high Fowler's, sitting on side of bed, or in chair with elbows resting on knees (Figure 30-9, *A*). Clients with COPD may benefit by leaning over table with arms propped up (Figure 30-9, *B*). *Effective cough:* High Fowler's with knees bent and a small pillow or hand to support the abdomen and augment expiratory pressure.	Promotes optimum lung expansion and maximizes use of accessory muscles.

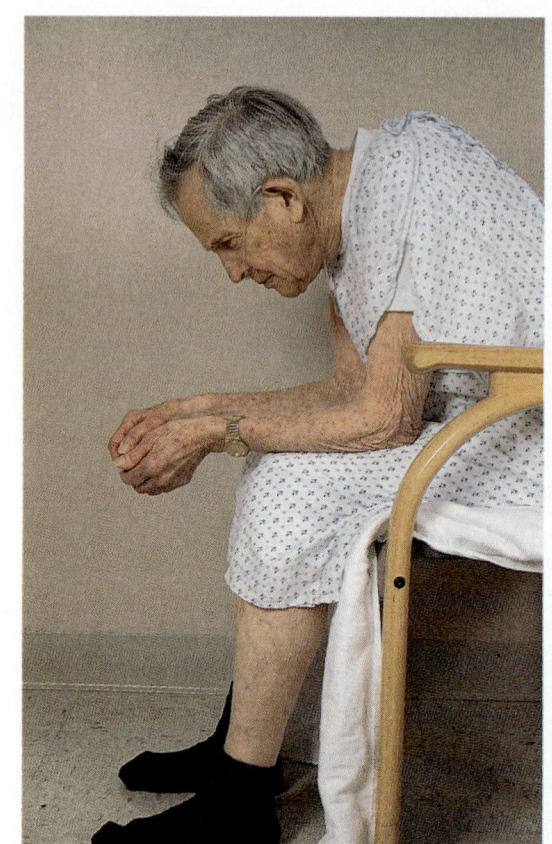
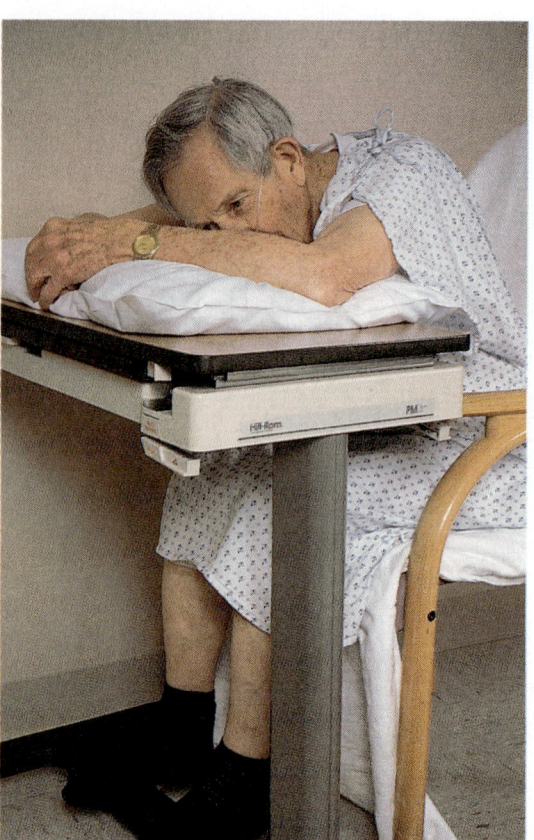

A B

Figure 30-9

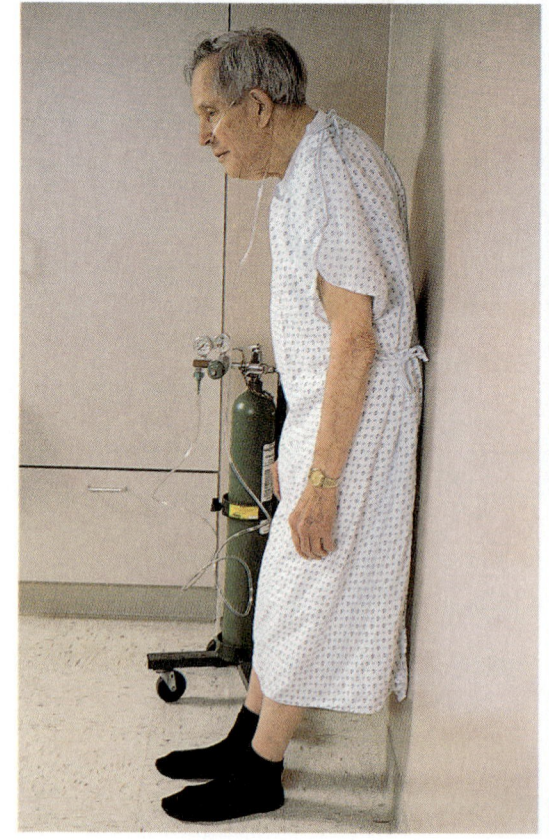
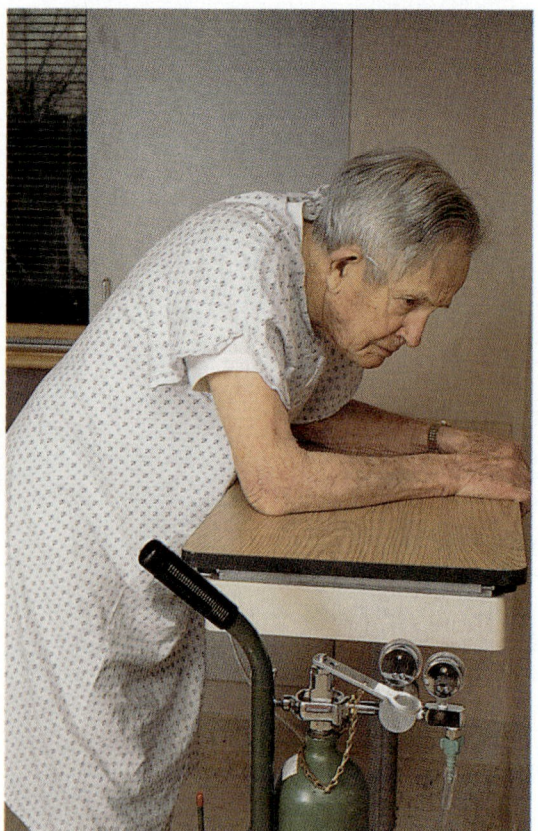

A B

Figure 30-10

Steps	Rationale

b. Standing

When client who is ambulating experiences shortness of breath or the need to cough, encourage a position that supports client (Figure 30-10).

c. Supine

Determine if two pillows or flat is more comfortable for client. Turn at least every 2 hours to encourage secretion drainage. Consider maneuvers to drain areas of lungs with retained secretions by gravity if tolerated by patient. If unilateral reexpansion is needed (e.g., after surgery), have client lie with side requiring expansion up: "good side down, affected lung up."

Decreases orthopnea. Obese clients may experience decreased abdominal interference of full lung expansion when lying flat.

Promotes lung expansion on the affected side. Exchange of respiratory gases is improved.

3. Apply CPAP

a. Explain purpose and rationale. Explain need for tight seal with resulting improvement in symptoms.

b. Position client in semi-Fowler's or high Fowler's, if appropriate.

c. Position face mask or nasal mask tightly, and adjust head strap until seal is maintained and client is able to tolerate (see Figure 30-7).

d. Instruct patient to breathe normally.

e. Apply at ordered setting for prescribed length of time.

Client may experience claustrophobic sensations and feelings of discomfort from continuous pressure. Support and education help client develop tolerance.

Promotes optimum lung expansion.

Ensures maintenance of CPAP.

Reduces hyperventilation and fatigue.

4. Obtain PEFR measurements

a. Instruct client about purpose and rationale.

b. Place client in an upright position.

c. Slide indicator to base of the numbered scale.

d. Instruct client to take a deep breath.

e. Have client place meter mouthpiece in the mouth and close lips, making a firm seal (see Figure 30-8).

f. Have client blow out as hard and fast as possible through the mouth only.

g. This maneuver should be repeated two additional times, with the highest number recorded.

h. If client is to record PEFR at home, have client demonstrate PEFR technique independently and assess ability to record PEFR accurately in a diary. Assist client in developing an appropriate action plan as prescribed by physician.

5. See Completion Protocol (Chapter 1, p. 6).

Promotes optimum lung expansion.

Tight seal ensures all expired breath will be measured for accurate reading.

Maximum effort is required for an accurate reading. Air expelled through nares will not be measured and will decrease PEFR readings.

Enables client to know when to contact physician or take prescribed medications. Reassure client of good airflow when normal readings are obtained.

Evaluation

1. Observe client's body alignment and position whenever in visual contact with client. Reposition as needed, at least every 2 hours.

2. Auscultate and examine chest at least every 8 hours.

3. Assess client's respiratory status during sleep to determine response to CPAP. Ask if client subjectively feels more rested after arising.

4. Observe repeat ABGs and/or pulse oximetry for objective measure of improvement.

5. Assess client's tolerance of CPAP mask and compliance to therapy.
6. Observe a return demonstration by client/family to determine if correct technique is being used with CPAP or PEFR.
7. Ask client to explain the appropriate response to different PEFR values he or she may obtain.
8. Ask client to explain purpose and benefits of positioning, CPAP, and PEFR.

UNEXPECTED OUTCOMES AND RELATED INTERVENTIONS

1. Client is unable to maintain a patent airway.
   a. Evaluate positioning. Consider suctioning.
   b. Monitor ABGs/pulse oximetry.
   c. An artificial airway may be considered, if not present.
2. Client experiences worsening dyspnea with bronchospasm and hypoxemia.
   a. Monitor ABGs/pulse oximetry.
   b. Medicate as ordered.
   c. Evaluate for methods to decrease oxygen demand.
3. Client is unable to tolerate CPAP because of feelings of suffocation, shortness of breath, and discomfort related to pressure applied during CPAP.
   a. Check fit of delivery device. Consider alternate if difficulties continue.
   b. Provide client with encouragement, support, and education.
4. Client is unable or unwilling to give maximum effort for PEFR.
   a. Provide client with encouragement and education.

b. If unable to achieve adequate readings, contact physician immediately, medicate as ordered, and give support.

SAMPLE DOCUMENTATION

Positioning

0300 Dyspneic at rest. O_2 saturations 88%-90%. Respiratory rate 26 and shallow with use of accessory muscles. States he is unable to tolerate supine position. Assisted to chair, leaning forward with head and shoulders resting on pillow on stationary table. Pursed-lip breathing encouraged.

0315 States he is breathing easier. Color pink. O_2 saturations 90%-92%. Respiratory rate 28 with good pursed-lip breathing technique. Remains in chair.

CPAP

2400 Appears to sleep restfully. Respirations even and easy without snoring. No jerking movements noted. CPAP continues per face mask with good seal at 7.5 cm H_2O.

0800 No change noted in assessment during night. CPAP applied for 10 hours. No areas of irritation noted from mask. States she slept well without awakening.

PEFR

1000 Instructed on use of PEFR and able to give independent return demonstration without error. PEFR 300 ml (60% of predicted) with increase to 450 ml postbronchodilator.

1400 Achieved reading of 375 ml on PEFR and correctly identified need for bronchodilator. PEFR returned to 450 ml after Rx. Correct recording of both readings made in diary without difficulty.

Skill 30.3 | Suctioning

For some clients, use of noninvasive techniques, along with medications, is not sufficient to maintain a patent airway. In these cases, suctioning is considered. The method of suctioning used depends on the level of the secretions to be removed, the presence of an artificial airway, and the client's condition. Oropharyngeal (Yankauer) suctioning is performed by using a rigid plastic catheter with one large and several small eyelets (Figure 30-11) through which mucus enters when suction is applied. Alert clients can easily be taught this suction method to control the secretions in the oral cavity.

Endotracheal (ET; Figure 30-12) and tracheostomy (trach; Figure 30-13) tubes allow direct access to the lower airways for suctioning. These artificial airways may be inserted to create a route for mechanical ventilation, to allow easy access of suctioning, to relieve mechanical airway obstruction, or to protect the airway from aspiration because of impaired cough or gag reflexes.

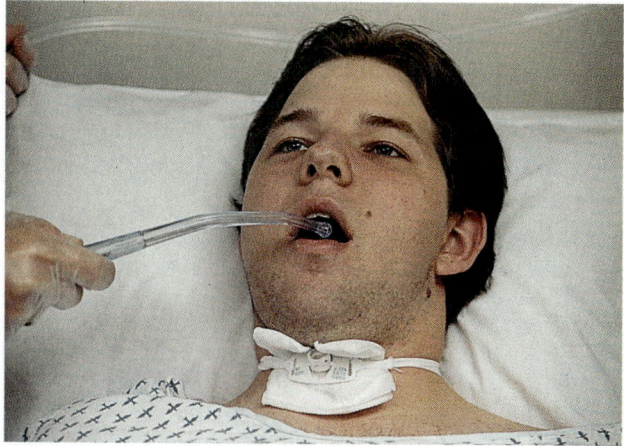

Figure 30-11 Oropharyngeal suctioning.

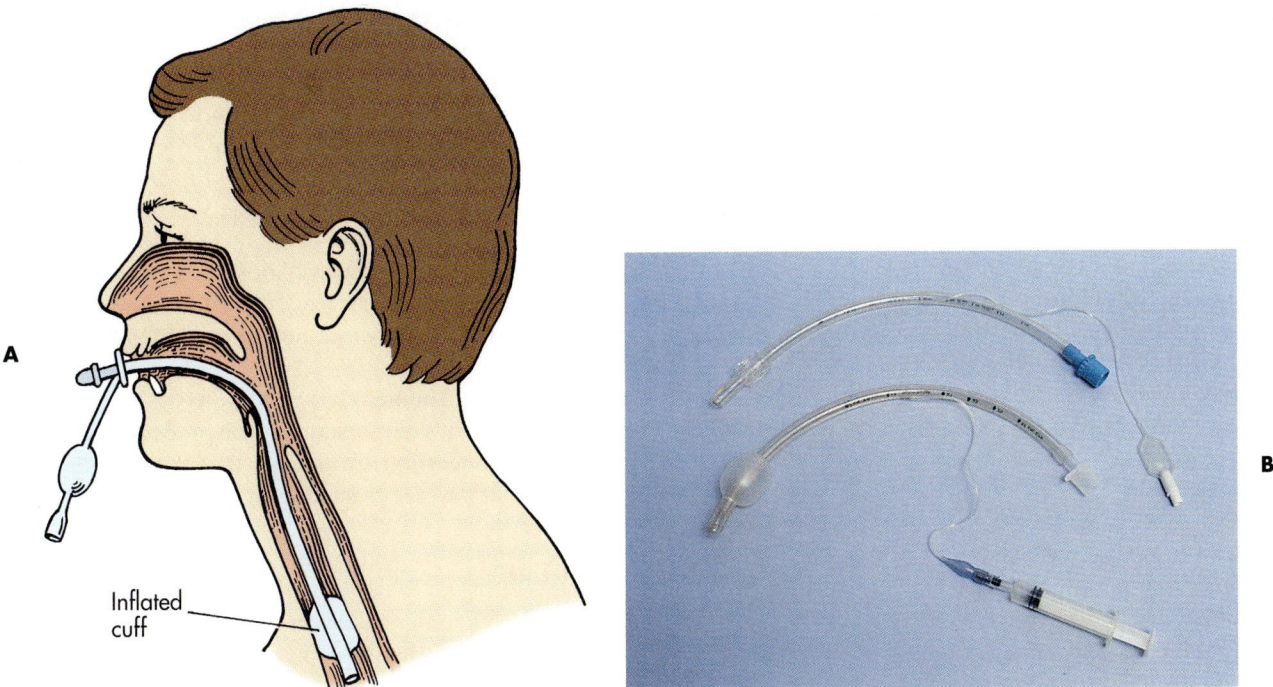

Figure 30-12 **A,** Endotracheal (ET) tube with inflated cuff. **B,** ET tubes with uninflated and in-flated cuffs and syringe for inflation. Client is unable to speak.

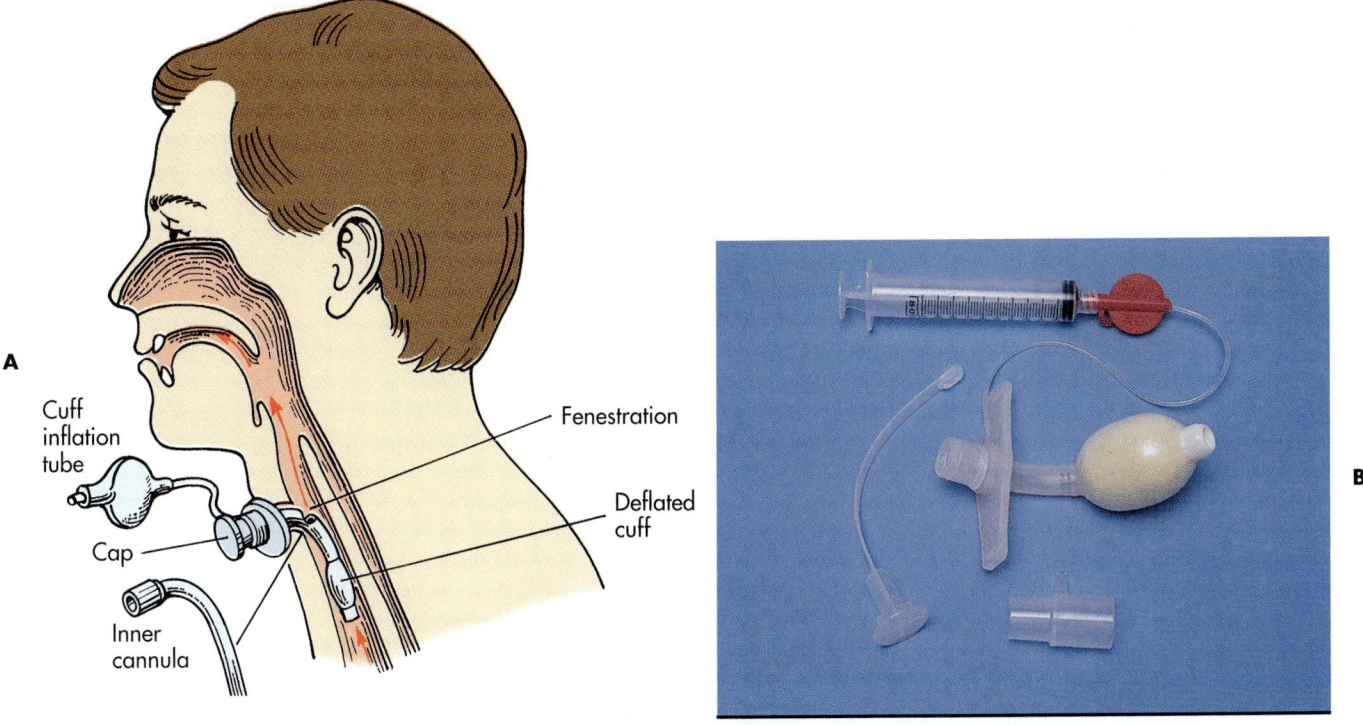

Figure 30-13 **A,** Tracheostomy tube (fenestrated) with inner cannula removed and cap in place to allow speech (Lewis and Collier, 1992). Tubes without opening interfere with speech. **B,** Tracheostomy tube with obturator for insertion and syringe for inflation of cuff.

EQUIPMENT

Oropharyngeal suctioning

Oropharyngeal suction catheter or Yankauer suction tip

Nonsterile gloves

Nonsterile basin (e.g., disposable cup)

Water (about 100 ml)

Portable or wall suction machine

Connecting tubing (6 feet)

Face shield, if indicated

Endotracheal or tracheostomy suctioning

12 to 16 French catheter (Adult)

Bedside table

Two sterile gloves or one sterile and one nonsterile glove

Sterile basin

Sterile normal saline (NS) (about 100 ml)

Clean towel or sterile drape

Portable or wall suction machine

Connecting tubing (6 feet)

Face shield, if indicated

Closed-system or in-line suctioning

Closed-system or in-line suction catheter

5 to 10 ml NS in syringe or vials

Portable or wall suction apparatus

Connecting tubing (6 feet)

Two clean gloves (optional)

Assessment

1. Observe for signs and symptoms of excess secretions.
   a. Assess oral cavity: Gurgling on inspiration or expiration, obvious oral secretions, drooling, gastric secretions or vomitus in mouth, and productive cough without expectorating secretions from the oral cavity.
   b. Assess for lower airway obstruction: coughing, secretions in the airway, labored breathing, or ineffective cough before deflation of ET tube or trach cuff.
2. Assess lung sounds.
3. Assess client's understanding of procedure and feeling of congestion to indicate that the oral cavity or lower airway needs suctioning.

Planning

Expected outcomes focus on airway patency, avoidance of infection, and client's comfort and understanding.

EXPECTED OUTCOMES

1. Client's airways are cleared of secretions. No sounds of congestion can be detected, and lung sounds are improved.
2. Client indicates easier breathing and decreased congestion.
3. Client performs correct oropharyngeal suctioning technique.

(See also Skill 30.1.)

Implementation

Steps	Rationale
1. See Standard Protocol (Chapter 1, p. 5).	
2. Oropharyngeal suctioning	
a. Fill basin or cup with approximately 100 ml of water.	
b. Connect one end of connecting tubing to suction machine and other to suction catheter.	
c. Turn suction device on. Set regulator to appropriate negative pressure: Wall suction, 80 to 120 mm Hg; portable suction, 7 to 15 cm Hg for adults.	Elevated pressure settings increase risk of trauma to mucosa.
d. Check that equipment is functioning properly by suctioning a small amount of water from basin.	
e. Remove oxygen mask, if present. Insert catheter into mouth. With suction applied, move catheter around mouth, including pharynx and gum line, until secretions are cleared. Encourage patient to cough. Replace oxygen mask (if used).	If catheter does not have a suction control to apply intermittent suction, take care not to allow suction tip to invaginate oral mucosal surfaces with continuous suction. Coughing moves secretions from lower and upper airways into mouth.

Steps	Rationale

f. Suction water from basin through catheter until catheter is cleared of secretions.

Clearing secretions before they dry reduces probability of transmission of microorganisms and enhances delivery of preset suction pressures.

g. Place catheter in a clean dry area for reuse with suction turned off or within client's reach, with suction on, if client is capable of suctioning self.

h. Discard water if not used by client. Clean basin or dispose of cup. Remove gloves and dispose.

3. Endotracheal or tracheostomy tube suctioning

a. Connect one end of connecting tubing to suction machine and place other end in a convenient location near client. Turn suction device on and set vacuum regulator to appropriate negative pressure: wall suction, 80 to 120 mm Hg; portable suction, 7 to 15 cm Hg for adults.

Excessive negative pressure damages tracheal mucosa and can induce greater hypoxia.

b. If indicated, increase supplemental oxygen to 100% or as ordered by physician. Encourage cough and deep breathing.

c. Prepare suction catheter.

  (1) Open suction kit or catheter using aseptic technique.
    If sterile drape is available, place it across client's chest. Do not allow suction catheter to touch any nonsterile surfaces.

Prevents contamination of clothing. Prepares catheter and prevents transmission of microorganisms.

  (2) Unwrap or open sterile basin and place on bedside table. Be careful not to touch inside of sterile basin. Fill with about 100 ml sterile NS (Figure 30-14).

NS is used to rinse catheter after suctioning.

d. Apply one sterile glove to each hand, or apply nonsterile glove to nondominant hand and sterile glove to dominant hand. Attach nonsterile suction tubing to sterile catheter, keeping hand holding catheter sterile (Figure 30-15).

Reduces transmission of microorganisms and allows nurse to maintain sterility of suction catheter.

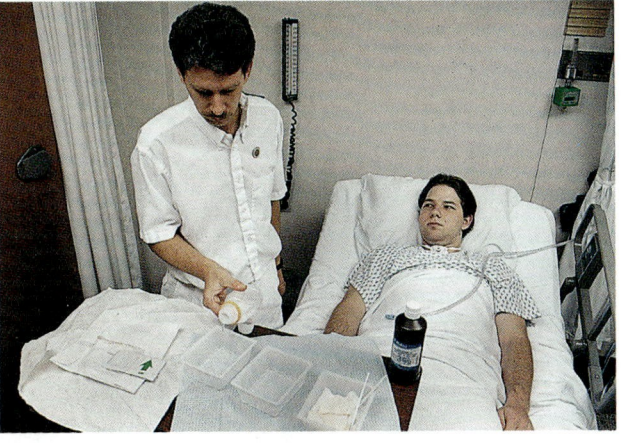

Figure 30-14

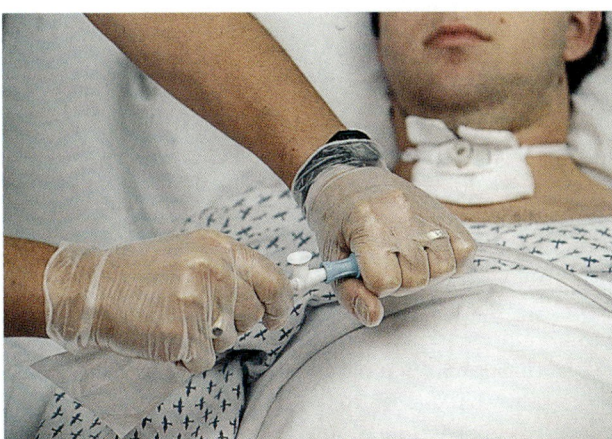

Figure 30-15

Steps	Rationale
e. Check that equipment is functioning properly by suctioning small amounts of saline from basin.	Lubricates catheter and tubing.
f. Hyperinflate and/or hyperoxygenate client before suctioning, using manual resuscitation Ambu bag or sigh mechanism on mechanical ventilator.	Hyperinflation decreases atelectasis caused by negative pressure. Preoxygenation converts large proportion of resident lung gas to 100% oxygen to offset amount used in metabolic consumption while ventilator or oxygenation is interrupted, as well as to offset volume lost out of suction catheter.
g. Open swivel adapter, or if necessary, remove oxygen or humidity delivery device with nondominant hand.	Exposes artificial airway.
h. Without applying suction and using dominant thumb and forefinger, gently but quickly insert catheter into artificial airway (best to time catheter insertion with inspiration) until resistance is met or client coughs, then pull back 1 cm (Figure 30-16).	Application of suction pressure while introducing catheter into trachea increases risk of damage to tracheal mucosa. Stimulates cough and removes catheter from mucosal wall.

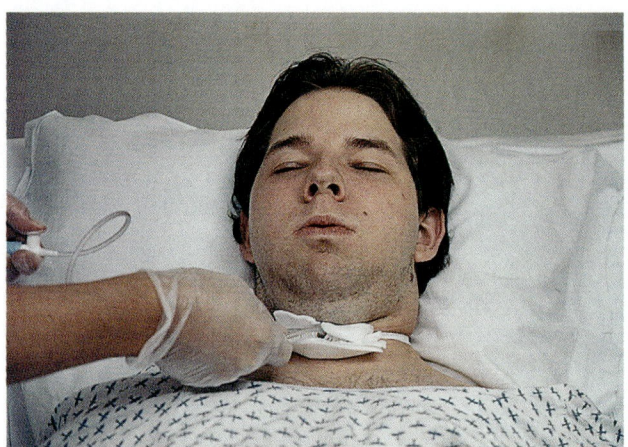

Figure 30-16

Steps	Rationale
i. Apply intermittent suction by placing and releasing nondominant thumb over vent of catheter, and slowly withdraw catheter while rotating it back and forth between dominant thumb and forefinger. The maximum time catheter may remain in airway is 10 seconds. Encourage client to cough.	Intermittent suction and rotation of catheter prevent injury to tracheal mucosal lining. If catheter "grabs" mucosa, remove thumb to release suction. Increased hypoxia related to removal of oxygen in airways and blockage of airways will occur during suctioning procedure.
j. Close swivel adapter or replace oxygen delivery device. Encourage client to deep breathe. Some clients respond well to several manual breaths from the mechanical ventilator or Ambu bag.	Reoxygenates and reexpands alveoli. Suctioning can cause hypoxemia and atelectasis.
k. Rinse catheter and connecting tube with NS until clear. Use continuous suction.	Removes catheter secretions. Secretions left in tubing decrease suction and provide environment for growth of microorganisms.
l. Assess client's cardiopulmonary status for secretion clearance and complications. Repeat Steps f through l once or twice more to clear secretions. Allow adequate time (at least 1 full minute) between suction passes for ventilation and reoxygenation.	Suctioning can induce dysrhythmias, hypoxia, and bronchospasms. Repeated passes with suction catheter clear airway of excessive secretions and promote improved oxygenation.

Steps	Rationale
m. Perform nasopharyngeal and oropharyngeal suctioning to clear upper airway of secretions. After these suctionings are performed, catheter is contaminated; do not reinsert into ET or trach tube.	Removes upper airway secretions. Upper airway is considered "clean," whereas lower airway is considered "sterile." Therefore, same catheter can be used to suction from sterile to clean areas, but not from clean to sterile areas.
n. Disconnect catheter from connecting tube. Roll catheter around fingers of dominant hand. Pull glove off inside out so that catheter remains in glove. Pull off other glove in same way. Discard into appropriate receptacle. Turn off suction device.	Reduces transmission of microorganisms. Clean equipment should not be touched with contaminated gloves.
o. Place unopened suction kit on suction machine or at head of bed.	Provides immediate access to suction catheter.

4. Endotracheal or tracheostomy tube suctioning with a closed-system (in-line) catheter

a. Attach suction.

Steps	Rationale
(1) In many institutions, catheter is attached to mechanical ventilator circuit by personnel from respiratory therapy (Figure 30-17). If not already in place, open suction catheter package using aseptic technique, attach closed-suction catheter (Figure 30-18) to ventilator circuit by removing swivel adapter and placing closed-suction catheter apparatus on ET or trach tube, and connect Y on mechanical ventilator circuit to closed-suction catheter with flex tubing.	Catheter becomes part of the circuit and is often changed by respiratory therapist to each circuit change or every 24 hours.
(2) Connect one end of connecting tube to suction machine and connect other to end of closed-system or in-line suction catheter if not already done. Turn suction device on and set vacuum regulator to appropriate negative pressure (80 to 120 mm Hg for adults).	Prepares suction apparatus. Excessive negative pressure damages tracheal mucosa and can induce greater hypoxia.

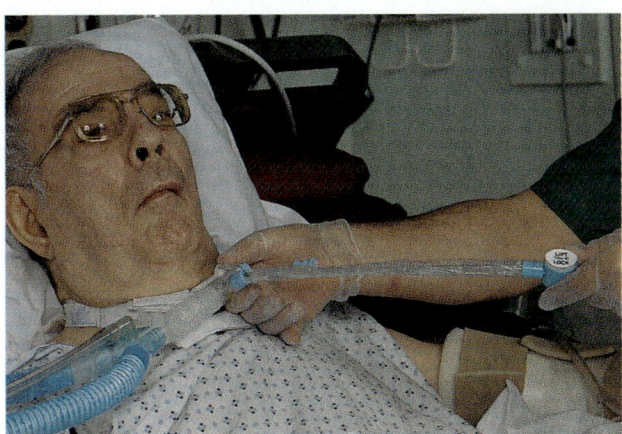

Figure 30-17

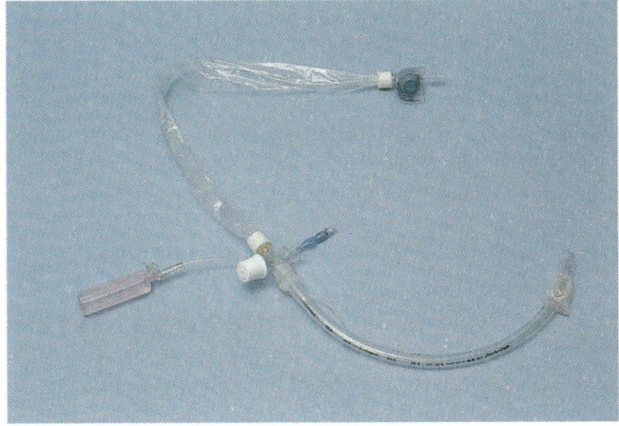

Figure 30-18 Closed system suction catheter attached to endotracheal tube.

Steps	Rationale
b. Hyperinflate and/or hyperoxygenate client using Ambu bag or manual breathing mechanism on mechanical ventilator according to institution protocol and clinical status (usually 100% oxygen).	Decreases atelectasis caused by negative pressure and increases oxygen available to tissues during suctioning.
c. Unlock suction control mechanism if required by manufacturer. Open saline port and attach saline syringe or vial.	
d. Pick up suction catheter enclosed in plastic sleeve with dominant hand. From 2 to 3 ml NS may be instilled to attached port to stimulate cough if secretions are thick and tenacious.	Saline travels down suction catheter and into airway. Timing NS with inhalation allows it to be delivered into lung rather than blown into ventilatory circuit.
e. Wait until client inhales NS or mechanical ventilator delivers a breath to dispense NS, then quickly but gently insert catheter on next inhalation. To insert catheter, use a repeating maneuver of pushing catheter and sliding (or pulling) plastic back between thumb and forefinger until resistance is felt or client coughs. (NOTE: Some catheters contain depth markings that are useful in positioning catheter.)	Catheter sterility and secretion containment are provided by plastic sheath. Mechanical ventilator breaths, oxygen, and positive end-expiratory pressure (PEEP) are not interrupted during suctioning. Catheter slides within plastic sheath. Coughing occurs or resistance is felt when catheter touches carina.
f. Encourage client to cough and apply suction by squeezing on mechanism while withdrawing. Be sure to withdraw catheter completely into plastic sheath so it does not obstruct airflow.	Removes secretions from airway. Catheter left in ET or trach tube limits airflow.
g. Reassess cardiopulmonary status, including pulse oximetry, to determine need for subsequent suctioning or complications. Repeat Steps c through f one to two more times to clear secretions. Allow adequate time (at least 1 full minute) between suction passes for ventilation and reoxygenation.	Repeated passes clear airway of secretions to promote ventilation and oxygenation. Suctioning can cause complications such as dysrhythmias, hypoxia, and bronchospasm.
h. When airway is clear, withdraw catheter completely into sheath. Be sure black line on catheter is visible in sheath. Squeeze vial or push syringe while applying suction to rinse inner lumen of catheter. Use at least 5 to 10 ml of NS. Lock suction mechanism, if applicable, and turn off suction.	Black line is reference point to determine correct position of catheter when not in use. Inability to see black line suggests catheter is in airway and may be impeding airflow. Interior of catheter must be rinsed to prevent bacterial growth. Failure to lock mechanism can result in inadvertent continuous suction and serious complications.
i. Client may require suctioning of oral cavity.	Catheter is continuously connected to ET or trach tube. Separate suction catheter is necessary for oral cavity.

5. See Completion Protocol (Chapter 1, p. 6).

Evaluation

1. Compare client's respiratory assessments before and after suctioning.
2. Ask client if breathing is easier and if congestion is decreased.
3. Observe client's technique and compliance with suctioning procedures.

UNEXPECTED OUTCOMES AND RELATED INTERVENTIONS

1. Client becomes cyanotic or restless or develops tachycardia, bradycardia, or other dysrhythmia.
   a. Discontinue attempt at suctioning until stabilized, unless client's condition is deteriorating because of secretions in airway.
   b. Monitor vital signs and pulse oximetry.

c. Preoxygenate for repeated attempts.
2. Bloody secretions are returned, which may indicate trauma.
   a. Evaluate technique and frequency of suctioning.
   b. If bleeding continues, notify physician of potential hemorrhage and monitor vital signs.
3. Client has paroxysms of coughing.
   a. Reassure client.
   b. Instruct client about relaxation techniques. Medicate as needed.
4. No secretions are obtained.
   a. Reassess respiratory system for presence of secretions.
   b. Stimulate client's cough.
   c. Check that suction system is functioning.

5. Thick secretions are present and difficult to suction.
   a. Stimulate client's cough.
   b. Notify physician if signs and symptoms of infection are present.
   c. Provide increased fluids if not contraindicated. Inadequately hydrated clients may have thick secretions.

SAMPLE DOCUMENTATION

1200 Occasional productive cough. Client requires hourly suctioning per ET tube of moderate amount (1 tsp or less) of thick yellow sputum. Able to use Yankauer catheter to suction mouth with good technique. Lungs clear after cough and suctioning. O_2 saturation 92% to 94%. Respirations nonlabored.

Skill 30.4 | Artificial Airway Management and Tracheostomy Care

The presence of an artificial airway places the client at high risk for infection. Correct care of the artificial airway will help to prevent infection from occurring. Artificial airways also make the client susceptible to airway injury. When artificial airways are used, it is essential that they be maintained in the correct position, or damage may occur.

Endotracheal tubes are used as short-term artificial airways to administer mechanical ventilation, relieve upper airway obstruction, protect against aspiration, or clear secretions (see Figure 30-12). ET tubes are generally removed within 14 days. If the client requires continued assistance from an artificial airway, a tracheostomy is considered for long-term use. A surgical incision is made into the trachea, and a short artificial airway (a trach) is inserted (see Figure 30-13, A).

EQUIPMENT

Endotracheal tube care
  Towel
  ET and oropharyngeal suction equipment
  1 to 1½-inch adhesive or waterproof tape (not paper tape) or commercial ET holder (follow manufacturer's instructions for securing)
  Two pairs of nonsterile gloves
  Adhesive remover swab or acetone on a cottonball
  Mouth care supplies (e.g., toothbrush, toothpaste, mouth swabs)
  Face cleanser (e.g., wet washcloth, towel, soap, shaving supplies)
  Clean 2 × 2 gauze
  Tincture of benzoin or liquid adhesive
  Face shield (if indicated)

Tracheostomy care
  Bedside table
  Towel
  Tracheostomy suction supplies
  Sterile tracheostomy care kit, if available, *or*
    Three sterile 4 × 4 gauze pads
    Sterile cotton-tipped applicators
    Sterile trach dressing
    Sterile basin
    Small sterile brush (or disposable cannula)
    Tracheostomy ties (e.g., twill tape, manufactured trach ties, Velcro trach ties)
  Hydrogen peroxide
  Normal saline (NS)
  Scissors
  Two sterile gloves
  Face shield, if indicated

Assessment

1. Assess client for signs and symptoms of need to provide airway management/tube care.
2. Identify factors that increase risk of complications from artificial airways.
3. Observe for factors that influence airway functioning.
4. Assess client's knowledge and comfort with procedure.
5. If applicable, assess client's understanding of and ability to perform own tracheostomy care.

Planning

Expected outcomes should focus on the prevention of infection and breakdown around the artificial airway.

EXPECTED OUTCOMES

1. Client's artificial airway/tube is in correct position and properly secured.
2. Client remains afebrile without signs and symptoms of infection.
3. Client's oral mucous membrane/stoma remains free of breakdown or accumulation of secretions.
4. Client's artificial airway is intact without persistent dried secretions.
5. Client understands purpose and is cooperative with care.
6. Client is able to demonstrate correct technique of tracheostomy care when appropriate.

Implementation

Steps	Rationale
1. See Standard Protocol (Chapter 1, p. 5).	
2. Endotracheal tube care	
nurse alert — Instruct client that it is important to resist biting or moving ET tube with tongue or pulling on tubing; removal of tape can be uncomfortable.	
a. Initiate suction.	Removes secretions. Diminishes client's need to cough during procedure.
b. Leave Yankauer suction catheter connected to suction source.	Prepares for oropharyngeal suctioning.
c. Prepare tape. Cut piece of tape long enough to go completely around client's head from nares to nares plus 15 cm (6 inches): adult, about 30 to 60 cm (1 to 2 feet). Lay adhesive side up on bedside table. Cut and lay 8 to 16 cm (3 to 6 inches) of tape, adhesive side down, in center of long strip to prevent tape from sticking to hair.	Adhesive tape must be placed around head from cheek to cheek below ears.
d. Have an assistant to apply a pair of gloves and hold ET tube firmly so that tube does not move.	Reduces transmission of microorganisms. Maintains proper tube position and prevents accidental extubation.
e. Carefully remove tape from ET tube and client's face. If tape is difficult to remove, moisten with water or adhesive tape remover. Discard tape in appropriate receptacle if nearby. If not, place soiled tape on bedside table or on distant end of towel.	Provides nurse with access to skin under tape for assessment and hygiene. Reduces transmission of microorganisms.
f. Use adhesive remover swab to remove excess adhesive left on face after tape removal.	Promotes hygiene. Unremoved adhesive can cause damage to skin and prevent poor adhesion of new tape.
g. Remove oral airway or bite block if present.	Provides access and complete observation of client's oral cavity.
h. Clean mouth, gums, and teeth opposite ET tube with mouthwash solution and 4×4 gauze, sponge-tipped applicators, or saline swabs. Brush teeth as indicated. If necessary, administer oropharyngeal suctioning with Yankauer catheter.	

Steps	Rationale
i. Oral ET tube only: Note "cm" ET tube marking at lips or gums. With help of assistant, move ET tube to opposite side or center of mouth. Do not change tube depth.	Prevents pressure sore formation at sides of client's mouth. Ensures correct position of tube.
j. Repeat oral cleaning as in Step h on opposite side of mouth.	Removes secretions from mouth and oropharynx.
k. Clean face and neck with soapy washcloth, rinse, and dry. Shave male client as necessary.	Moisture and beard growth prevent adhesive tape adherence.
l. Pour small amount of tincture of benzoin on clean 2 × 2 gauze and dot on upper lip (oral ET tube) or across nose (nasal ET tube) and cheeks to ear. Allow to dry completely.	Protects and makes skin more receptive to tape.
m. Slip tape under client's head and neck, adhesive side down. Take care not to twist tape or catch hair. Do not allow tape to stick to itself. It helps to stick tape gently to tongue blade, which serves as a guide. Then slide tongue blade under client's neck. Center tape so that double-faced tape extends around back of neck from ear to ear.	Positions tape to secure ET tube in proper position.
n. On one side of face, secure tape from ear to naris (nasal ET tube) or edge of mouth (oral ET tube). Tear remaining tape in half lengthwise, forming two pieces that are ½ to ¾ inch wide. Secure bottom half of tape across upper lip (oral ET tube) or across top of nose (nasal ET tube) (Figure 30-19, A). Wrap top half of tape around tube (Figure 30-19, B).	Secures tape to face. Using top tape to wrap prevents downward drag on ET tube.

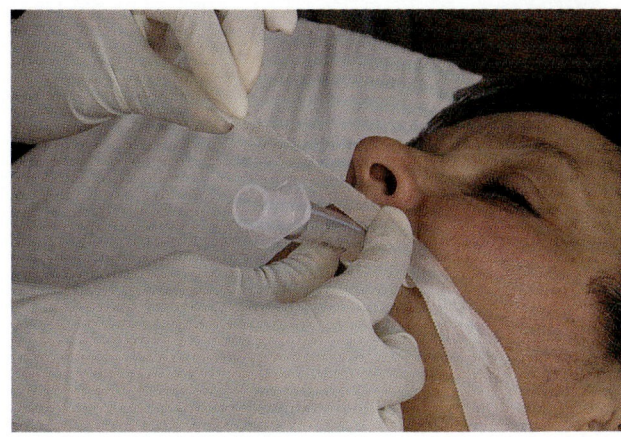

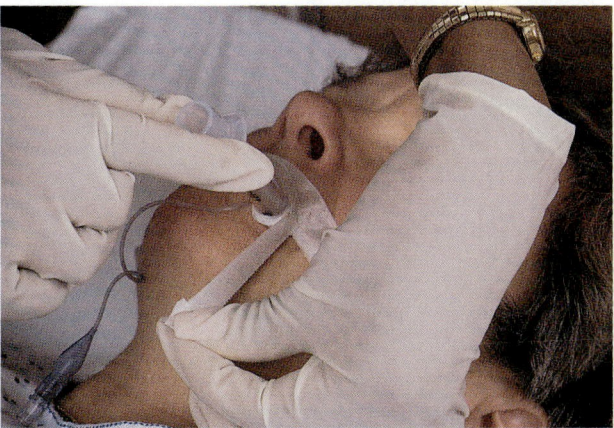

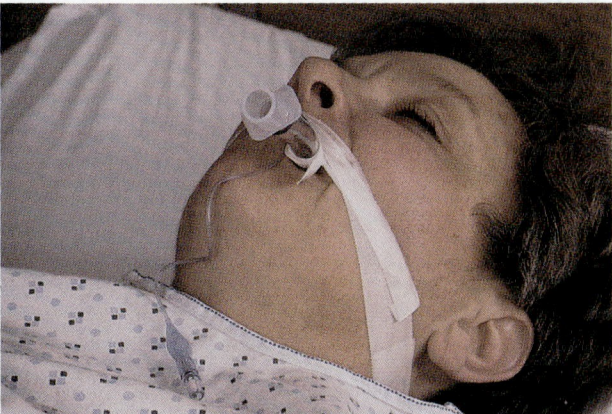

Figure 30-19

Steps	Rationale

o. Gently pull other side of tape firmly to pick up slack and secure to remaining side of face (Figure 30-19, *C*). Assistant can release hold when tube is secure. Nurse may want assistant to help reinsert oral airway.

Secures tape to face and tube. ET tube should be at same depth at the lips. Check earlier assessment for verification of tube depth in centimeters.

p. Clean oral airway in warm soapy water and rinse well. Hydrogen peroxide can aid in removal of crusted secretions. Shake excess water from oral airway.

Promotes hygiene. Reduces transmission of microorganisms.

q. Reinsert oral airway without pushing tongue into oropharynx.

Prevents client from biting ET tube and allows access for oropharyngeal suctioning.

3. Tracheostomy care

a. Suction trach (see Skill 30.3). Before removing gloves, remove soiled trach dressing and discard in glove with coiled catheter.

Removes secretions so as not to occlude outer cannula while inner cannula is removed. Reduces need for client to cough.

b. While client is replenishing oxygen stores, prepare equipment on bedside table. Open sterile trach kit. Open three 4×4 gauze packages using aseptic technique and pour NS on one package and hydrogen peroxide on another. Leave third package dry. Open two cotton-tipped swabbed packages and pour NS on one package and hydrogen peroxide on the other. Open sterile trach package. Unwrap sterile basin and pour about 2 cm (¾ inch) hydrogen peroxide into it (Figure 30-20). Open small sterile brush package and place aseptically into sterile basin. If using large roll of twill tape, cut appropriate length of tape (see Step 2c) and lay aside in dry area. Do not recap hydrogen peroxide and NS.

Allows for smooth, organized completion of trach care.

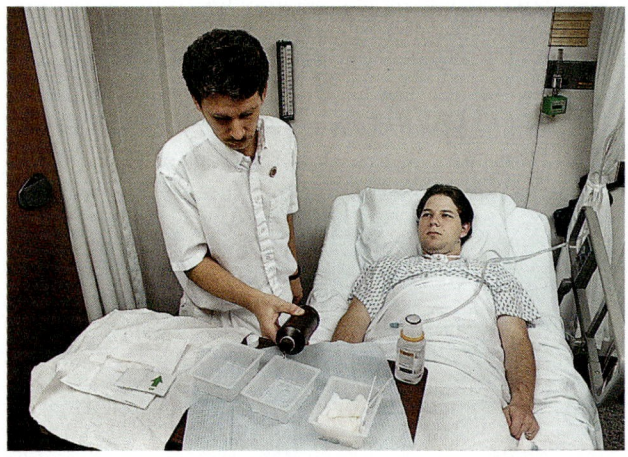

Figure 30-20

c. Apply gloves. Keep dominant hand sterile throughout procedure. Remove oxygen source.

Reduces transmission of microorganisms.

d. If a nondisposable inner cannula is used:

  (1) Remove with nondominant hand. Drop inner cannula into hydrogen peroxide basin.

Removes inner cannula for cleaning. Hydrogen peroxide loosens secretions from inner cannula.

  (2) Place trach collar or T tube and ventilator oxygen source over or near outer cannula. (NOTE: T tube and ventilator oxygen devices cannot be attached to all outer cannulas when inner cannula is removed.)

Maintains supply of oxygen to client.

  (3) To prevent oxygen desaturation in affected clients, quickly pick up inner cannula and use small brush to remove secretions inside and outside cannula (Figure 30-21).

Trach brush provides mechanical force to remove thick or dried secretions.

  (4) Hold inner cannula over basin and rinse with NS, using nondominant hand to pour.

Removes secretions and hydrogen peroxide from inner cannula.

Steps	Rationale

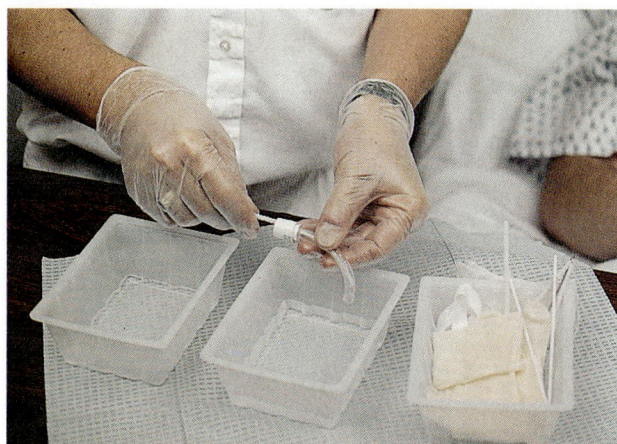

Figure 30-21

(5) Replace inner cannula and secure "locking" mechanism (Figure 30-22). Reapply ventilator or oxygen sources.

e. If a disposable inner cannula is used:

(1) Remove cannula from manufacturer's packaging.

(2) Withdraw inner cannula and replace with new cannula. Lock into position.

(3) Dispose of contaminated cannula in appropriate receptacle.

f. Using hydrogen peroxide–prepared cotton-tipped swabs and 4×4 gauze, clean exposed outer cannula surfaces and stoma under faceplate, extending 5 to 10 cm (2 to 4 inches) in all directions from stoma (Figure 30-23). Clean in circular motion from stoma site outward, using dominant hand to handle sterile supplies.

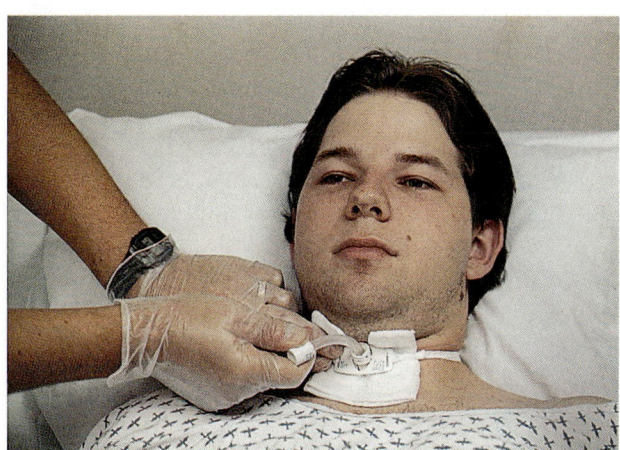

Figure 30-22

Aseptically removes secretions from stoma site.

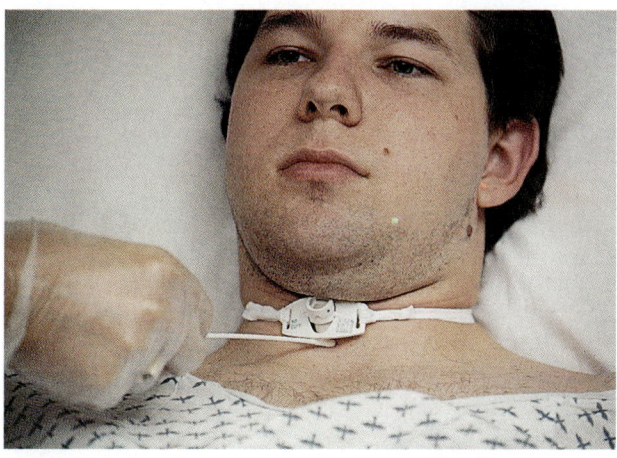

Figure 30-23

Steps	Rationale
g. Using NS-prepared cotton-tipped swabs and 4×4 gauze, rinse hydrogen peroxide from trach tube and skin surfaces.	Rinses hydrogen peroxide from surfaces, preventing possible irritation.
h. Using dry 4×4 gauze, pat lightly at skin and exposed outer cannula surfaces.	Dry surfaces prohibit formation of moist environment from growth of microorganisms and skin excoriation.
i. Instruct assistant, if available, to hold trach tube securely in place while ties are cut.	Promotes hygiene, reduces transmission of microorganisms, and secures trach tube.

nurse alert Assistant must not release hold on trach tube until new ties are firmly tied to reduce risk of accidental extubation. If no assistant present, do not cut old ties until new ties are in place and securely tied. (Follow manufacturer's guidelines for Velcro ties.)

Steps	Rationale
(1) Cut length of twill tape long enough to go around client's neck two times, about 60 to 75 cm (24 to 30 inches) for an adult. Cut ends on a diagonal.	Cutting ends of tie on a diagonal aids in inserting tie through eyelet.
(2) Insert one end of tie through faceplate eyelet and pull ends even (Figure 30-24).	
(3) Slide both ends of tie behind head and around neck to other eyelet, and insert one tie through second eyelet.	
(4) Pull snugly.	

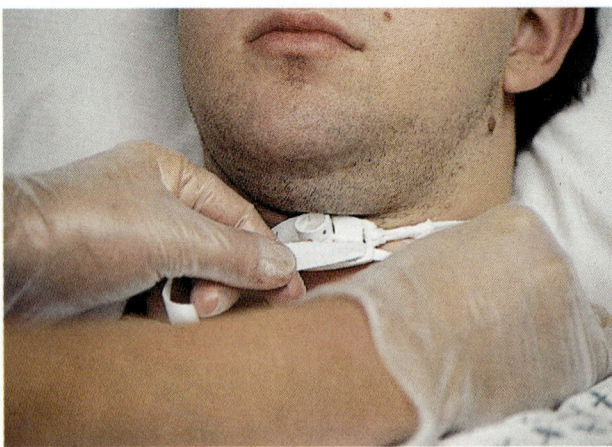

Figure 30-24

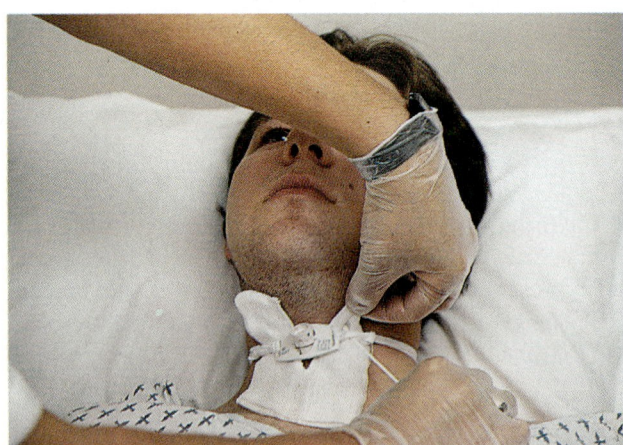

Figure 30-25

Steps	Rationale
(5) Tie ends securely in double square knot, allowing space for only one finger in tie.	One-finger slack prevents ties from being too tight when trach dressing is in place.
j. Insert fresh trach dressing under clean ties and faceplate (Figure 30-25).	Absorbs drainage. Dressing prevents pressure on clavicle heads.
k. Position client comfortably and assess respiratory status.	Promotes comfort. Some clients may require posttrach care suctioning.

4. See Completion Protocol (Chapter 1, p. 6).

Evaluation

1. Observe that airway is in proper position with tape/ties secure and comfortable for patient. ET tube should be at the same depth as before care (as per physician order), with the same centimeter marking at lips and equal bilateral breath sounds.
2. Measure client's temperature; observe stoma for signs of infection.
3. Observe client's oral mucosa.
4. Compare assessments before and after artificial airway care. Observe for signs of tissue breakdown or persistent dried secretions.
5. Observe client's actions to determine compliance with the procedure.
6. Have client indicate when trach care is required and independently demonstrate the technique for trach tube care.

UNEXPECTED OUTCOMES AND RELATED INTERVENTIONS

1. Tube is not secure, and artificial airway moves in or out or is coughed out by client.
   a. Secure trach ties with one-finger slack.
   b. For accidental extubation, call for assistance and manually ventilate client with Ambu mask, if necessary. Obtain replacement tube.
2. Breath sounds are unequal with ET tube.
   a. Evaluate ET tube for proper depth. If incorrect, arrange for ET tube to be repositioned as allowed by institution.
   b. Obtain order for chest x-ray study to verify placement if applicable.
   c. Evaluate for mucous plugs.
3. Breakdown or pressure areas are observed.
   a. Increase frequency of tube care.
   b. Make sure skin areas are clean and dry.
4. Hard, reddened areas with or without excessive or foul-smelling secretions are observed.
   a. Indicates infection. Notify physician.
   b. Increase frequency of tube care.
5. Respiratory distress is caused by mucous plug.
   Remove inner cannula, if applicable, for cleaning and suctioning.

SAMPLE DOCUMENTATION

0800 Routine ET tube care done. Size 7.5 cm tube remains with 22 cm marking at lips. No irritation or skin breakdown noted. Mouth care given. Respirations even and easy at a rate of 16/min. Clear breath sounds bilaterally.

| Skill 30.5 | **Managing Closed Chest Drainage Systems (Including Managing Postoperative Autotransfusions)** |

Trauma, disease, or surgery can interrupt the closed negative-pressure system of the lungs, causing lung collapse. Air (pneumothorax) or fluid (hemothorax) may leak into the pleural cavity. A chest tube is inserted and a closed chest drainage system is attached to promote drainage of air and fluid (Figure 30-26). Suction may be added to assist gravity in draining the lung. Lung reexpansion and improved oxygenation occurs as the fluid or air is removed.

The location of the chest tube indicates the type of drainage expected. Because air rises, apical and anterior chest tube placement (Figure 30-27, *A*) promotes removal of air. Chest tubes are placed low and posterior or lateral (Figure 30-27, *B*) to drain fluid. A mediastinal chest tube is placed just below the sternum (Figure 30-28) and drains blood or fluid, preventing its accumulation around the heart (e.g., after open heart surgery).

Although single-bottle systems are available, single-unit water-seal or waterless systems are most often used. The water-seal system is composed of two or three compartments or chambers (Figure 30-29). Fluid is drained into the first chamber. The second chamber contains the water seal, which allows air to escape because of the force of expiration but not to reenter on inspiration. If suction is to be used, a third chamber is used. The amount of suction depends on the amount of sterile water in the suction chamber.

The waterless system (Figure 30-30) follows the same principles, except sterile water is not required for setup. The water seal is replaced by a one-way valve located near the top of the system. Most of the single unit is the drainage chamber. The suction chamber contains a suction control float ball that is set by a suction control dial after the suction source is turned on.

Autotransfusion can be linked with chest drainage after open heart surgery or thoracic surgery to replace mediastinal blood lost and allow lung reexpansion (Figure 30-31). It is a relatively risk-free, inexpensive, and easy method that enables the client to avoid other-donor blood transfusion. The client's own blood is drained from the chest and reinfused.

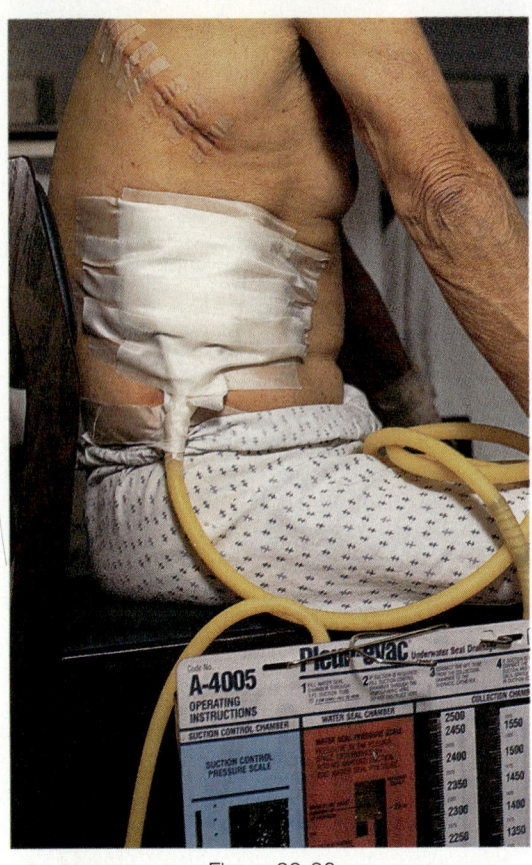

Figure 30-26

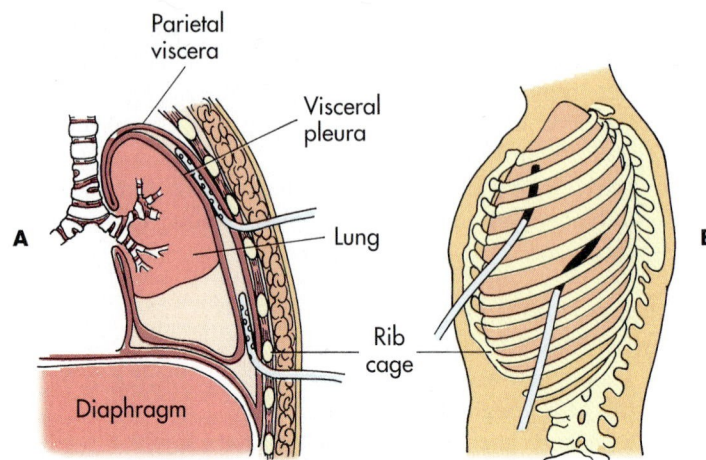

Parietal viscera

Visceral pleura

Lung

Rib cage

Diaphragm

A

B

Figure 30-27

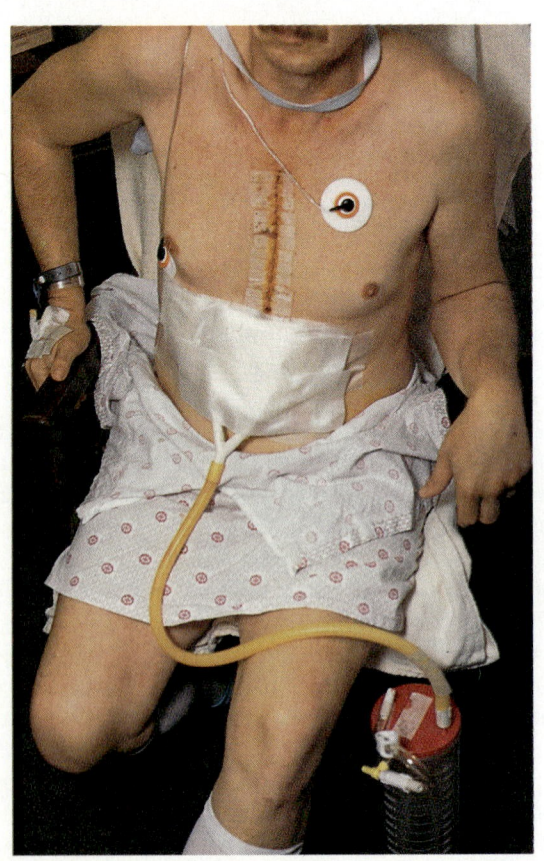

Figure 30-28

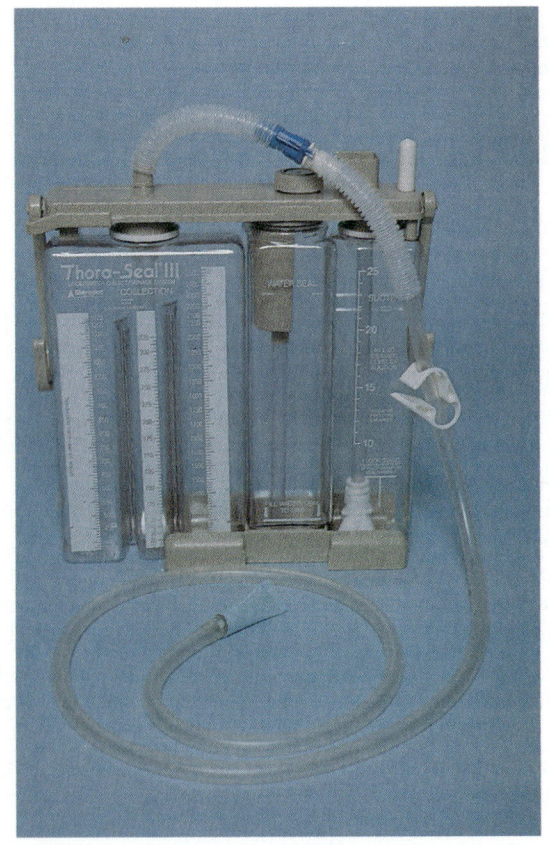

Figure 30-29

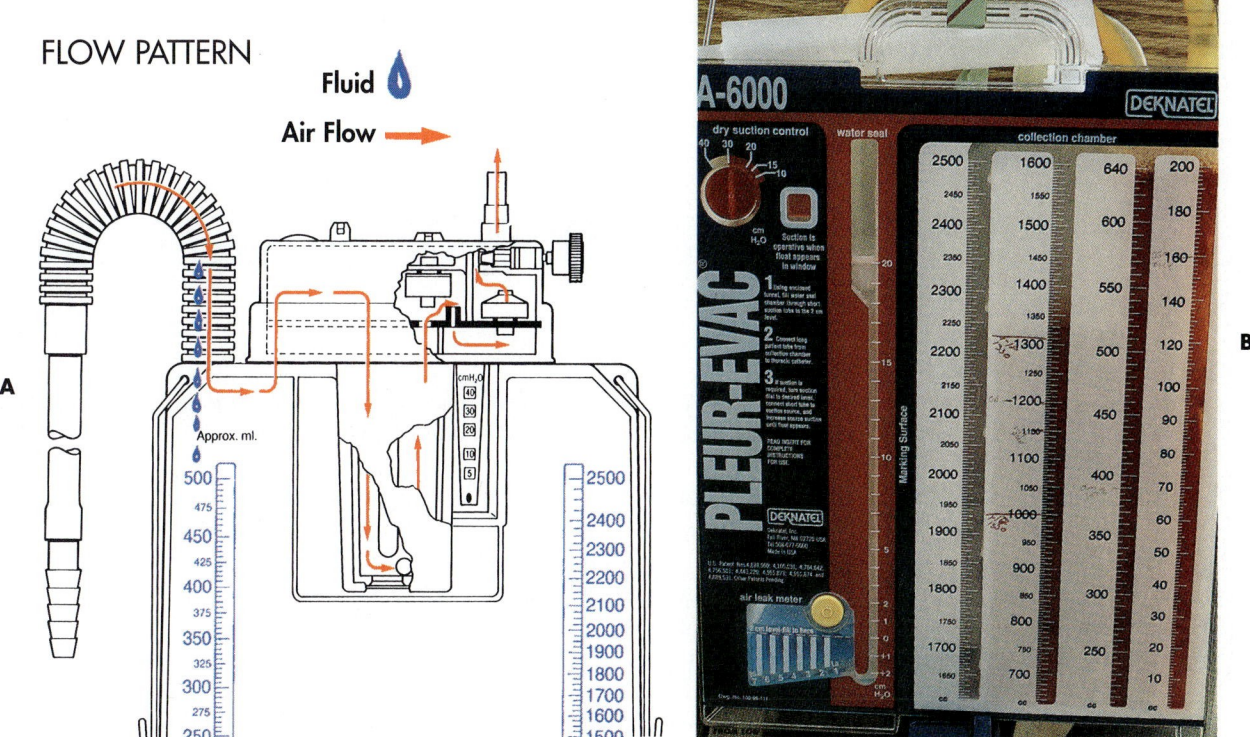

Figure 30-30 **A,** Suction-regulating device. **B,** Collection chamber is marked at specified intervals to monitor amount of drainage.

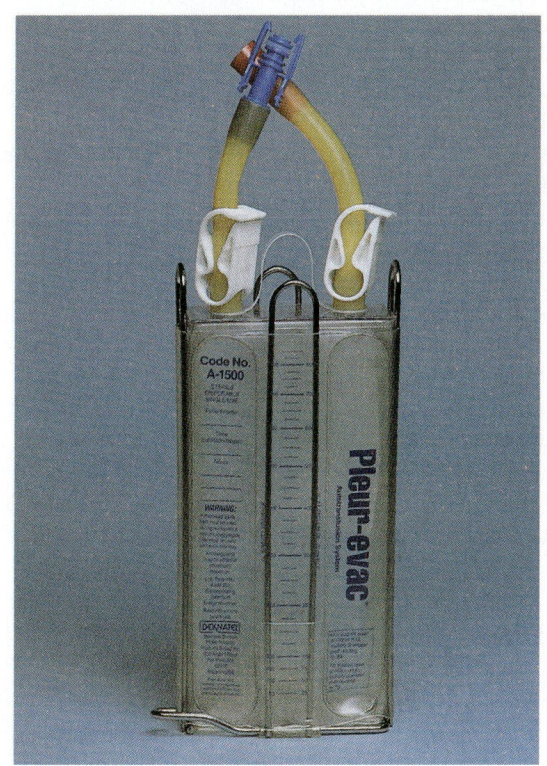

Figure 30-31

EQUIPMENT

Prescribed drainage system

Water-seal system

Sterile water or normal saline (NS) to fill 2.5 cm (1 inch) of water-seal U tube

Suction control chamber, if used

Waterless system

30 ml vial of injectable sodium chloride (NaCl) or water

20 ml syringe

21-gauge needle

Two shodded hemostats for each chest tube

1-inch adhesive tape for taping connections

Assessment

1. Perform a complete respiratory assessment.
2. Obtain vital signs.
3. Assess client's breathing pattern.
4. Ask if client is able to breathe deeply and comfortably.

Planning

Expected outcomes should focus on air and fluid drainage and reexpansion of the lung with maximum patient comfort.

EXPECTED OUTCOMES

1. Client's respirations are nonlabored.
2. Client's breath sounds are present in all lobes, and lung expansion is symmetrical.
3. Client's vital signs, hemoglobin, and hematocrit are within normal ranges by discharge.
4. Client uses breathing exercises and remains comfortable.
5. Chest tube remains in place, and chest drainage system remains airtight and functioning properly.
6. Client's oxygen saturation is greater than 94%.

Implementation

Steps	Rationale
1. See Standard Protocol (Chapter 1, p. 5).	
2. Set up water-seal system	
a. Obtain a chest drainage system. Remove wrappers and prepare to set up as a two- or three-chamber system.	Maintains sterility of system for use under sterile operating room conditions.
b. While maintaining sterility of the drainage tubing, stand system upright and add sterile water or NS to appropriate compartments.	Reduces possibility of contamination.
c. For a two-chamber system (without suction), add sterile solution to water-seal chamber (second chamber), bringing fluid to the required level as indicated.	Maintains water seal.
d. For a three-chamber system (without suction), add sterile solution to the water-seal chamber (second chamber). Add amount of sterile solution prescribed by physician to the suction control (third) chamber, usually 20 cm (8 inches). Connect tubing from suction control chamber to suction source.	Depth of rod below fluid level dictates highest amount of negative pressure that can be present within system. For example, 20 cm of water is approximately -20 cm of water pressure. Any additional negative pressure applied to system is vented into atmosphere through suction control vent. This safety device prevents damage to pleural tissues from an unexpected surge of negative pressure from suction source.
3. Set up waterless system	
a. Remove sterile wrappers and prepare to set up.	Maintains sterility of system for use under sterile operating room conditions.
b. For a two-chamber system (without suction), nothing is added or needs to be done to system.	Waterless two-chamber system is ready for connecting to client's chest tube after opening wrappers.
c. For a three-chamber waterless system with suction, connect tubing from suction control chamber to suction source.	Suction source provides additional negative pressure to system.
d. Instill 15 ml sterile water or NS into diagnostic indicator injection port located on top of system.	This is not necessary for mediastinal drainage because there will be no tidaling. Also, in an emergency, this is not necessary because system does not require water for setup.
4. Tape all connections in a spiral fashion using 1-inch adhesive tape. Then check both systems for patency:	Prevents atmospheric air from leaking into system and client's intrapleural space. Provides chance to ensure airtight system before connecting it to client. Allows correction or replacement of system if it is defective before connecting it to the client.
a. Clamp from drainage tubing that will connect client to system.	
b. Connect tubing from float ball chamber to suction source.	
c. Turn on suction to prescribed level.	

> **nurse alert**   Bubbling will be seen at first because there is air in tubing and system initially. This should stop after a few minutes unless other sources of air are entering system. If bubbling continues, check connections and locate source of air leak as described in Table 30-3.

Table 30-3 **Problem Solving With Chest Tubes**

Problem	Solution
Air leak is present.	Locate leak.
• Continuous bubbling is seen in water-seal bottle/chamber, indicating that leak is between client and water seal.	Tighten loose connections between client and water seal. Loose connections cause air to enter system. Leaks are corrected when constant bubbling stops.
• Bubbling continues, indicating that air leak has not been corrected.	Cross-clamp chest tube close to client's chest. If bubbling stops, air leak is inside client's thorax (client centered) or at chest tube insertion site.* *Unclamp tube and notify physician immediately.* Reinforce chest dressing. Leaving chest tube clamped with client-centered leak can cause collapse of lung, mediastinal shift, and eventual collapse of other lung from buildup of air pressure within pleural cavity.
• Bubbling continues, indicating that leak is not client centered.	In alternating fashion, gradually move clamps down drainage tubing away from client and toward suction-control chamber, moving one clamp at a time. When bubbling stops, leak is in section of tubing or connection that is between two clamps. Replace tubing or secure connection and release clamps.[†]
• Bubbling continues, indicating that leak is not in tubing.	Leak is in drainage system. Change drainage system. *[,†]
Tension pneumothorax is present.	Determine that chest tubes are not clamped, kinked, or occluded. Obstructed chest tubes trap air in intrapleural space when air leak originates within client.
• Severe respiratory distress	
• Chest pain	Notify physician immediately.
• Absence of breath sounds on affected side	Prepare immediately for another chest tube insertion; obtain a flutter (Heimlich) valve on large-gauge needle for short-term emergency release of air in intrapleural space; have emergency equipment (e.g., oxygen and code cart) near client.
• Hyperresonance on affected side	
• Mediastinal shift to unaffected side	
• Tracheal shift to unaffected side	
• Hypotension	
• Tachycardia	
Dependent loops of drainage tubing have trapped fluid.	Drain tubing contents into drainage bottle. Coil excess tubing on mattress and secure in place.
Water seal is disconnected.	Connect water seal and tape connection.
Water-seal bottle is broken.	Insert distal end of water-seal tube into sterile solution so that tip is 2 cm below surface level[‡], and set up new water-seal bottle. If no sterile solution is available, double-clamp chest tube while preparing new bottle.
Water-seal tube is no longer submerged in sterile fluid.	Add sterile solution to water-seal bottle until distal tip is 2 cm under surface level[‡], or set water-seal bottle upright so that tip is submerged.

* Data from Paulau D, Jones S: *RN* Oct. 1986.
† Data from Erickson R: *Nurs 81* 11(6):62, 1981.
‡ Data from Carroll PF: *Nurs 86* 16(12):26, 1986.

Steps	Rationale
5. Turn off suction source and unclamp drainage tubing before connecting client to system.	Having client connected to suction when it is initiated could damage pleural tissues from sudden increase in negative pressure. Suction source is turned on again after client is connected to three-chamber system.
6. Position the client	
a. Use semi-Fowler's to high Fowler's position to evacuate air (pneumothorax).	Permits optimum drainage of fluid and/or air. Air rises to highest point in the chest.
b. Use high Fowler's position to drain fluid (hemothorax).	Permits optimum drainage of fluid.

Steps	Rationale

7. Help physician attach drainage tube to chest tube.

Connects drainage system and suction (if ordered) to chest tube.

8. Tape tube connection between chest and drainage tubes. One method: one long strip of tape on each side with an overlapping tape wrapped spirally enables connections to be observed and remain secure.

Secures chest tube to drainage system and reduces risk of air leaks causing breaks in airtight system.

9. Check patency of air vents in system.
   a. Water-seal vent must have no occlusion.
   b. Suction control chamber vent must have no occlusion when using suction.
   c. Waterless systems have relief valves without caps.

Permits displaced air to pass into atmosphere.
Provides safety factor of releasing excess negative pressure into atmosphere.

10. Coil excess tubing on mattress next to client. Secure with a rubber band and safety pin or system's clamp.

Prevents excess tubing from hanging over edge of mattress in a dependent loop. Drainage could collect in loop and occlude drainage system.

11. Adjust tubing to hang in a straight line from top of mattress to drainage chamber.

Promotes drainage.

12. Provide two shodded hemostats for each chest tube. Shodded hemostats are usually attached to top of client's bed with adhesive tape or clamped to client's clothing during ambulation.

Chest tubes are double-clamped under specific circumstances: (1) to assess for an air leak (see Table 30-3), and (2) to empty or change collection bottle or chamber or disposable systems.
Have new system ready to be connected before clamping tube so that transfer can be rapid and drainage system reestablished.

13. Care for client with chest tube
   a. Monitor vital signs, drainage, and insertion site every 15 minutes for first 2 hours.

Provides immediate information about procedure-related complications.
Provides baseline for continuous assessment of type and quantity of drainage.

   (1) If chest tube has drainage fluid, indicate date and time (e.g., 0900) that drainage was first collected on drainage chamber's write-on surface.
   (2) Postoperative assessment is done every 15 minutes for first 2 hours. This assessment interval then changes based on client's status. Mark time and level of drainage on calibrated write-on strip periodically.

Permits timely and efficient amount of drainage from chest tube. Drainage is marked at specified periods and documented on nurse's notes and intake and output sheet. Ensures early detection of complications.

   b. After first 2 hours, assess client's physical and psychological status as indicated.

Detects early signs and symptoms of complications: apprehension, respiratory distress, and subcutaneous emphysema.

   c. Assess client's continued participation in care, as appropriate. Medicate as needed.

Chest tubes do not inhibit deep breathing, continued positioning and ambulation, and full range of motion.

   d. Observe the following:
   (1) Chest tube dressing: Note any drainage.

Ensures that dressing is occlusive.

   (2) Tubing: Ensure it is free of kinks and dependent loops.
   (3) Chest drainage system: Ensure it is upright and below level of tube insertion. Note presence of clots or debris in tubing.

System must be in this position to function properly.

   (4) Water seal
   (a) Observe for constant bubbling in water-seal chamber (see Table 30-3).

Fluid should rinse in the water seal or diagnostic indicator with inspiration and fall with expiration. This indicates that system is functioning properly.

Steps	Rationale

(b) Check for fluctuation with client's inspiration and expiration.

(5) Waterless

    (a) Check diagnostic indicator for fluctuations with client's inspirations and expirations.

    (b) Observe for left-to-right bubbling in diagnostic indicator.

When system is initially connected to client, bubbles are expected from chamber as air that was present in system and in client's intrapleural space is released. After a short time, bubbling stops. Fluid continues to fluctuate in water seal on inspiration and expiration until lung is reexpanded unless system becomes occluded.

e. Type and amount of fluid drainage: Note color and amount of drainage, vital signs, and skin color.

  (1) Less than 50 to 200 ml/hr is expected immediately postoperatively from a mediastinal chest tube, approximately 500 ml in first 24 hours. Drainage changes from dark red early in postoperative period to serous.

Sudden gush of drainage may be retained blood and not active bleeding. This increase in drainage can result from client's position change. Reexpansion of lungs forces drainage into tube. Coughing can also cause large gushes of drainage.

  (2) Between 100 and 300 ml of fluid may drain in a posterior chest tube during first 2 hours after insertion. This rate decreases after 2 hours; 500 to 1000 ml can be expected in first 24 hours. Drainage is grossly bloody during first several hours after surgery and then changes to serous.

Excess amounts and continued presence of frankly bloody drainage first several hours after surgery should be reported to physician, along with client's vital signs and respiratory status.

14. Obtain Specimen

a. Cleanse resealing diaphragm or tubing with an antiseptic.

Reduces transmission of microorganisms.

b. Insert needle with bevel in the fresh drainage.

c. Gently aspirate appropriate amount of fluid and place into properly labeled container.

d. Recleanse diaphragm with antiseptic swab.

15. Assist in chest tube removal

a. Administer prescribed medication for pain relief about 30 minutes before procedure.

Reduces discomfort and relaxes client.

b. Assist client to sit on edge of bed or to lie on side without chest tubes.

Physician prescribes client's position to facilitate tube removal.

c. Support client physically and emotionally while physician removes dressing and clips sutures.

Reduces anxiety and promotes cooperation.

d. Physician prepares an occlusive dressing of petroleum gauze on a pressure dressing and sets it aside on a sterile field.

Essential to prepare in advance for quick application to wound on tube withdrawal.

e. Physician asks client to take a deep breath and hold it or exhale completely and hold it.

Prevents air from being sucked into chest as tube is removed.

f. Physician quickly pulls out chest tube.

Prevents entry of air through chest wound.

g. Physician quickly applies prepared dressing over wound and firmly secures it in position with elastic bandage (Elastoplast) or wide tape. Physician sometimes uses skin clips or draws purse string sutures together before applying dressing.

Keeps wound aseptic. Prevents entry of air into chest. Wound closure occurs spontaneously. Clips or sutures aid in skin closure.

Steps	Rationale
16. Perform postoperative autotransfusion (ATS)	
a. Set up the Pleur-evac autotransfusion system (ATS) using technique that maintains the sterility of unit and following three steps printed on front of unit (Deknatel, Inc.) (see Figure 30-31).	Contamination of unit provides a ready source of infection to client.
b. Make sure all connections are tight and all clamps are open.	Tight connections ensure an airtight system, and open clamps allow chest drainage to enter the ATS bag.
c. A 200 μ double-sided mesh filter is located in the ATS bag to filter drainage.	Filtering drainage removes extraneous materials and microemboli.
d. ATS collection bag has a capacity of 1000 ml, marked in increments of 25 ml, and an area for marking times and amounts.	
e. Continue collection.	
(1) Open Pleur-evac A-1500 replacement bag using proper technique and close two white clamps.	Contamination of unit provides a ready source of contamination to client. Closed clamps maintain a closed system during replacement.
(2) Use high-negativity relief valve to reduce excessive negativity.	Eases removal of initial collection bag from metal support stand.
(3) Perform bag transfer.	
(a) Close clamp on chest drainage tubing.	Prevents air from entering chest cavity through tube and collapsing lung.
(b) Close two white clamps on top of initial ATS collection bag.	Maintains a closed system for reinfusion, preventing contamination of blood.
(c) Connect chest drainage tube to new ATS bag using red containers. Make certain that all connections are tight.	
(d) Open all clamps on chest drainage tube and replacement bag.	Reestablishes an autotransfusion collection system.
f. Connect red and blue connectors on top of initial collection bag, and remove it by lifting it from side hook and then from foot hook.	Maintains a closed system within bag and removes it for use in autotransfusion.
g. Secure replacement bag by connecting foot hook, replacing metal frame into side hook of Pleur-evac unit, and pushing down to secure frame into hook.	
h. Replacement bag is removed by placing the thumbs on top of metal frame and pushing up with fingers to slide bag out.	
i. Initiate Pleur-evac autotransfusion reinfusion.	
(1) Use a new microaggregate filter to reinfuse each autotransfusion bag.	Prevents infusion of microemboli and provides maximum filtration for each bag.
(2) Access bag by inverting it, spiking it through spike port with microaggregate filter, and twisting.	Connects autotransfusion bag to transfusion tubing.
(3) With bag upside down, gently squeeze it to remove the air and prime the filter with blood.	Gentle pressure is used to prevent hemolysis.
(4) Hang bag on an intravenous (IV) pole and continue to prime tubing until all air is gone. Clamp tubing, attach it to client's IV access, and adjust clamp to deliver the reinfusion at the appropriate rate.	Removes all air from transfusion tubing and establishes the reinfusion. Gravity, a blood cuff (not to exceed 150 mm Hg pressure), or a blood-compatible IV pump may be used.

Steps	Rationale
(5) If ordered, anticoagulants (i.e., heparin) can be added to the reinfusion through self-sealing port in autotransfusion connector.	Prevents clotting in the autotransfusion.
j. Discontinue autotransfusion.	
(1) Clamp chest drainage tube and connect it directly to Pleur-evac unit using red and blue connectors.	Prevents air from entering chest cavity through tube and collapsing lung.
(2) Open chest drainage tube clamp.	All drainage will be collected directly in Pleur-evac unit and must be appropriately discarded.
17. See Completion Protocol (Chapter 1, p. 6).	

Evaluation

1. Assess client for decreased respiratory distress and chest pain.
2. Auscultate client's lungs and observe chest expansion.
3. Monitor vital signs, hematocrit, and hemoglobin.
4. Evaluate client's ability to use deep-breathing exercises while maintaining comfort.
5. Monitor continued functioning of system, as indicated by reduction in the amount of drainage, resolution of the air leak, and complete reexpansion of the lung.
6. Monitor client's oxygen saturation.

UNEXPECTED OUTCOMES AND RELATED INTERVENTIONS

1. Air leak is unrelated to client's respiration.
   See Table 30-3 for determining the source of an air leak and problem solving.
2. Chest tubes become obstructed by a clot or kinked tube.
   a. Observe client for mediastinal shift or respiratory distress, which may constitute a medical emergency.
   b. Determine source of obstruction, as noted by lack of flow through tube or clot detected in system. If kinked, straighten tubing and adjust to prevent continued problems.
   c. If clot identified, notify physician. Stripping or milking the chest tube is controversial and should be performed according to hospital policy. Stripping creates a high degree of negative pressure

and potentially may pull lung tissue or pleura into drainage holes of chest tube (Duncan, Erickson, and Weigel, 1987).
3. Chest tube becomes dislodged.
   a. Immediately apply pressure over chest tube site with anything that is within immediate reach (e.g., several layers of client's hospital gown, bed sheet, or towel).
   b. Have assistant obtain a sterile petroleum dressing. Apply as client exhales. Secure dressing with a tight seal.
   c. Notify physician.
4. Substantial increase in bright-red drainage is observed.
   a. Observe for tachycardia and hypotension.
   b. Report to physician, since this may indicate client is actively bleeding.
5. Drainage system is knocked on side or damaged.
   a. Observe for signs of increasing pneumothorax, which would indicate that water seal is not being maintained. Notify physician.
   b. Obtain a second unit and change system after following setup guidelines.

SAMPLE DOCUMENTATION

0800 Client resting comfortably, denies complaint. Respirations even and easy. Lungs clear with breath sounds heard over all lung fields. Posterior chest tube and dressing remain intact with oscillation present in water-seal chamber. No air leak noted. 50 ml serous drainage collected in last 8 hours. Continues to take deep breaths without complaints of discomfort as instructed.

CRITICAL THINKING EXERCISES

1. Referring to the advantages and disadvantages of various oxygen delivery devices outlined in Table 30-1, make a recommendation for each of the following clients requiring supplemental oxygen. Give a rationale for your recommendations.

   a. A 42-year-old client requiring short-term, low-flow oxygen therapy after abdominal surgery.

   b. A 20-year-old client with a fractured nose and multiple chest contusions. The physician has prescribed F_iO_2 of 90% to 100%.

   c. An 80-year-old female who is extremely anxious and restless requires an F_iO_2 of 50% to 60%.

2. Critique the following sample documentation.

   0900 Client in bed with HOB elevated 30°. Correctly placed PEFR mouthpiece and exhaled slowly and completely. Recorded PEFR of 350 ml. Requested bronchodilator.

   a. Is there sufficient information to evaluate the client's ability to appropriately use PEFR? If not, what additional data should be recorded?

   b. Is there sufficient information to evaluate the effectiveness of this procedure?

   c. Identify data indicating the client does not understand the procedure.

3. How would you determine whether Yankauer or endotracheal suctioning would be most beneficial for a client without an artificial airway?

4. After entering a client's tracheostomy with a suction catheter, the client begins to cough and his face turns red. What should you do?

5. Many experts advocate intermittent suction to prevent tracheal mucosal injury. Others advise continuous suction. Can you think of a reason for this second approach?

6. You are viewing a video of yourself performing in-line suction for a simulated client on a mechanical ventilator. You observe the following:

   Turned suction device on and set at 100 mm Hg; unlocked suction control mechanism, waited for ventilator to deliver a breath, and inserted catheter on next inhalation while applying suction via the squeeze mechanism; withdrew catheter completely into plastic sheath checking for the black mark; rinsed the catheter with normal saline.

   a. Identify actions that do not meet the standards for proper in-line suctioning.

   b. What might be the possible consequences of each of the errors identified?

7. After performing tracheostomy care, you notice that when the client coughs the trach tube moves out.

   a. What would your priority nursing action be?

   b. Fifteen minutes later you enter the client's room and observe the client in respiratory distress. What should you do first?

8. While caring for a client with a chest-tube to water-seal drainage and 20 cm of wall suction, you note excessive bubbling in the water-seal bottle. The client has had the chest tube for 24 hours, after undergoing lung surgery.

   a. What should you do, and why?

   b. During ambulation you note that the drainage is serous and the volume for the last 8 hours is approximately 500 ml. What should your response be?

REFERENCES

Duncan C, Erickson R, Weigel RM: Effect of chest tube management on drainage after cardiac surgery, *Heart Lung* 16(1):1, 1987.

Kersten L: *Comprehensive respiratory nursing,* Philadelphia, 1989, Saunders.

Lewis SM, Collier IC: *Medical-surgical nursing: assessment and management of clinical problems,* ed 3, St Louis, 1992, Mosby.

Perry AG, Potter PA: *Clinical nursing skills and techniques,* ed 3, St Louis, 1994, Mosby.

ADDITIONAL READINGS

Clark AP et al: Effects of endotracheal suctioning on mixed venous oxygen saturation and heart rate in critically ill adults, *Heart Lung* 19(suppl):552, 1990.

Cross D, Nelson HS: The role of the peak flow meter in the diagnosis and management of asthma, *J Allergy Clin Immunol* 87(1):120, 1991.

Czarnik RE et al: Differential effects of continuous versus intermittent suction on tracheal tissue, *Heart Lung* 20(2):144, 1991.

Dettenmeier PA: *Pulmonary nursing care,* St Louis, 1992, Mosby.

Gunderson LP, Stone KS, Hamlin RL: Endotracheal suctioning–induced heart rate alterations, *Nurs Res* 40(3):139, 1991.

Janson-Bjerklie S, Shnell S: Effect of peak flow information on patterns of self-care in adult asthma, *Heart Lung* 17(5):543, 1988.

Kacmarek R, Mack CW, Dimas S: *Essentials of respiratory care,* ed 3, St Louis, 1990, Mosby.

Macey BA, Landstrom LL: Replacing a chest tube drainage collection device, *Am J Nurs* 93(3):95, 1993.

McPhersen SP, Spearman CB: *Respiratory therapy equipment,* ed 4, St Louis, 1990, Mosby.

National Institutes of Health: *Guidelines for the diagnosis and management of asthma,* pub no 91-3042, Bethesda, Md, 1991, US Department of Health and Human Services.

Noll ML, Hix CD, Scott G: Closed tracheal suction systems: effectiveness and nursing implications, *AACN Clin Issues Crit Care Nurs* 1(2):318, 1990.

Phipps WJ et al, editors: *Medical-surgical nursing: concepts and clinical practices,* ed 5, St Louis, 1995, Mosby.

Rudy EB et al: Endotracheal suctioning in adults with head injury, *Heart Lung* 20(6):667, 1991.

Shapiro BA et al: *Clinical application of respiratory care,* ed 4, St Louis, 1991, Mosby.

Taft AA et al: A comparison of two methods of preoxygenation during endotracheal suctioning, *Respir Care* 36(11):1195, 1991.

Taggart JA, Dorinsky NL, Sheahan JS: Airway pressures during closed suctioning, *Heart Lung* 17(5):536, 1988.

Weilitz PB: *A pocket guide to respiratory care,* St Louis, 1991, Mosby.

Wilson SF, Thompson JM: *Respiratory disorders,* St Louis, 1991, Mosby.

Wilson T: *Mosby's clinical nursing series: Respiratory disorders,* St Louis, 1990, Mosby.

Witmer MT, Hess D, Simmons M: An evaluation of the effectiveness of secretion removal with the Ballard closed-circuit suction catheter, *Respir Care* 36(8):844, 1991.

chapter 31

Gastric Intubation

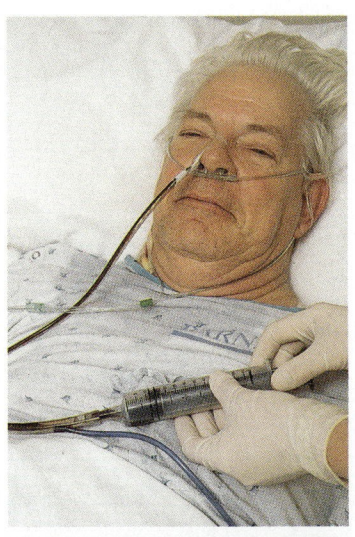

Skill 31.1
Inserting Nasogastric Tube

Skill 31.2
Irrigating Nasogastric Tube

Skill 31.3
Removing Nasogastric Tube

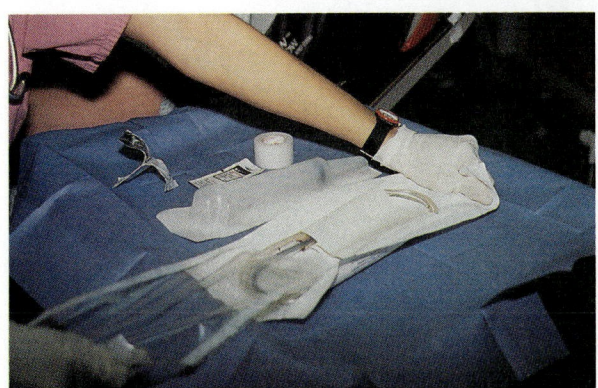

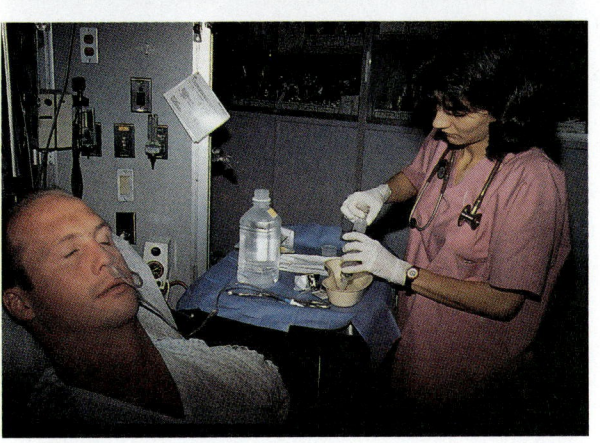

Intubation of the stomach with a flexible tube passed through the client's nares, nasopharynx, and esophagus and into the stomach (Figure 31-1) is sometimes performed after surgical procedures, when vomiting and gastric distention occur, and for irrigation of the stomach. Decompression of the stomach with removal of fluids and gas promotes abdominal comfort, decreases the risk of aspiration, and allows surgical anastomoses to heal without distention. When used for decompression, the tube is usually attached to low intermittent suction to facilitate the removal of secretions. For clients who are unable to swallow, the nasogastric (NG) tube is frequently used for the administration of medications. The tube can also be used to irrigate the stomach and to remove toxic substances, such as in poisoning.

NG tubes are typically of a larger diameter (12 to 18 Fr) than feeding tubes to enhance the removal of thick secretions or to instill fluids rapidly. Their stiffer composition and larger diameter make these tubes more uncomfortable for the client, and these tubes cause more irritation of the sensitive nasopharyngeal mucosa. NG tubes are constructed of a single lumen (Levin tube) or a central lumen and a separate air vent lumen (Salem sump tube). Important nursing measures for the client with an NG tube include measures to maintain patency of the tube, such as irrigation, and measures to promote comfort, such as positioning the tube to prevent pressure on the nares, cleansing around the nares, and lubrication of the oral and nasal membranes.

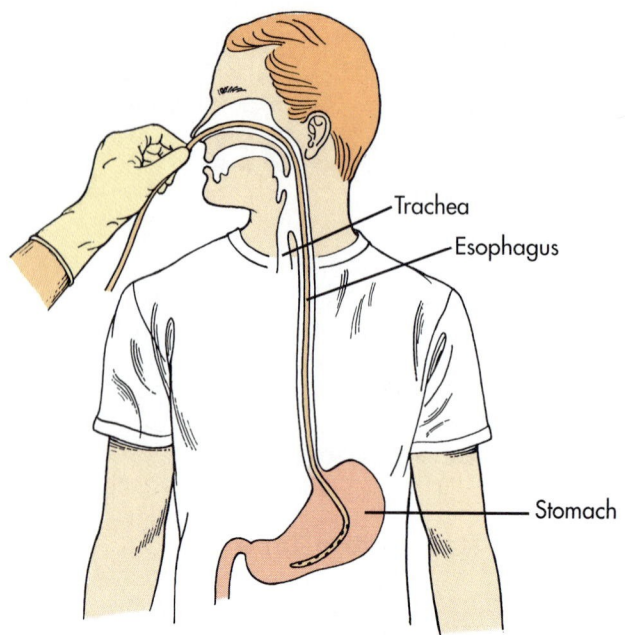

Figure 31-1 Placement of NG tube.

Trachea

Esophagus

Stomach

Nursing Diagnosis

Nursing diagnoses for clients who may undergo nasogastric intubation include **Risk for Aspiration,** in which clients are at risk of aspiration related to nausea and vomiting or delayed gastric emptying and this risk is a primary reason for placement of the tube. The presence of an NG tube can lead to the diagnosis of **Altered Oral Mucous Membranes,** because NG tubes typically cause irritation, drying, and crusting of secretions. Removal of gastric secretions can produce **Fluid Volume Deficit** associated with altered electrolyte imbalance (see Chapter 36).

| Skill 31.1 | ## Inserting Nasogastric Tube (Includes Checking Placement of Nasal Tube) |

This skill includes insertion of a large-bore flexible tube into the client's nares, nasopharynx, esophagus, and stomach. Placement of an NG tube requires a physician's order. The tube can be accidentally displaced into the pulmonary system, lie in the distal esophagus or gastric antrum rather than well into the stomach, or kink upon itself in the stomach. In addition to displacement, other complications of NG tubes include erosion of the tip of the nose, sinusitis, earache, esophagitis, gastric or esophageal ulceration and bleeding, and pulmonary aspiration (Metheny, 1993).

Care must be taken to reduce the discomfort related to an NG tube and to ensure that it remains correctly positioned and patent.

EQUIPMENT
Nasogastric tube (Figure 31-2)
Water-soluble lubricant
60 ml catheter tip syringe
Emesis basin
Towel
Clean gloves
Stethoscope
Cup of water and straw
Tongue blade
Tissues
Safety pin and rubber band

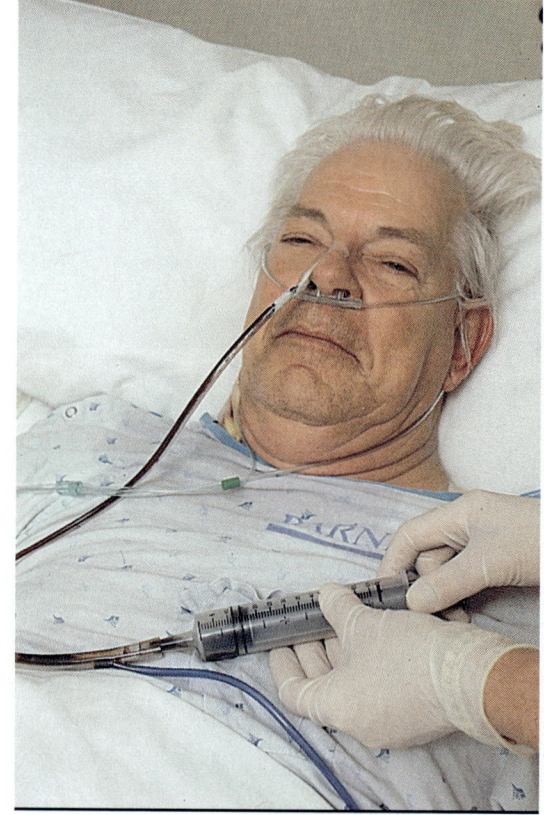

Figure 31-2

pH test strip

Indelible marker

Hypoallergic tape and tincture of benzoin (or tube fixation device)

Suction source

Assessment

1. Assess client's nares and oral cavity for deviated nasal septum, nasal surgery, inability to breathe well when either nasal opening is occluded, and nasal or oral irritation or bleeding. **This information determines which nares the tube should be inserted through and the need for special measures for oral hygiene or comfort after the tube is inserted.**

2. Assess client's ability and willingness to cooperate or assist with the procedure and the need for special positioning during insertion.

3. Assess client's abdomen for distention or pain and the presence or absence of nausea.

4. Assess client's need for specialized nutrition support.

Planning

Expected outcomes focus on decompression of the stomach, comfort, adequacy of fluid volume, adequacy of nutrition, and prevention of complications related to nasogastric intubation.

EXPECTED OUTCOMES

1. Client has no abdominal distention or pain.

2. Client's NG tube remains patent.

3. Client verbalizes enhanced comfort after nursing measures to promote oral and nasal hygiene and after lubrication of mucous membranes.

4. Client maintains good skin turgor, adequate urine output, and normal electrolyte balance.

5. Client's nasal membranes remain clear of abrasions, excoriation, or erosion, and membranes remain moist.

6. Client maintains within 10% of body weight or has nutritional support initiated if expected to have inadequate nutritional intake for more than 6 days (American Society for Parenteral and Enteral Nutrition, 1993).

Implementation

Steps	Rationale

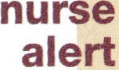 **nurse alert**   Client should be sitting upright in bed if possible. Have suction equipment and emesis basin within reach in case of vomiting.

1. See Standard Protocol (Chapter 1, p. 5).

2. Stand on side of bed closest to nostril chosen for insertion of tube.

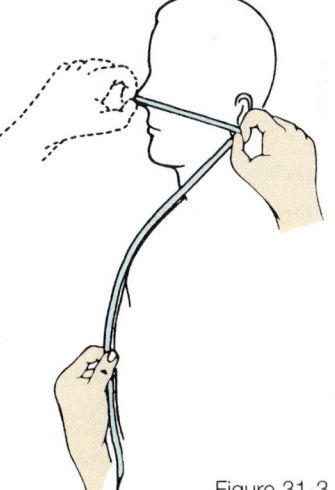

Figure 31-3

3. Measure estimated length of tube to reach well into stomach: measure distance from nose to earlobe to xiphoid process of sternum (Figure 31-3).

   Approximates distance from nares to stomach.

4. Mark this distance on tube with a removable piece of tape or an indelible marker.

5. Cut a piece of tape about 3 inches (8 cm) long, and split one half of it into two pieces to form a Y.

6. Lubricate about 4 inches (10 cm) of the distal end of the tube with a water-soluble lubricant.

Steps	Rationale

7. Tell client that insertion is about to begin, and ask client to keep head in neutral position looking straight ahead (Figure 31-4).

Promotes comfort and reduces friction during insertion.

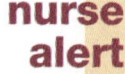 **nurse alert** Do not force tube past point of resistance, since force may cause trauma to nasal mucosa.

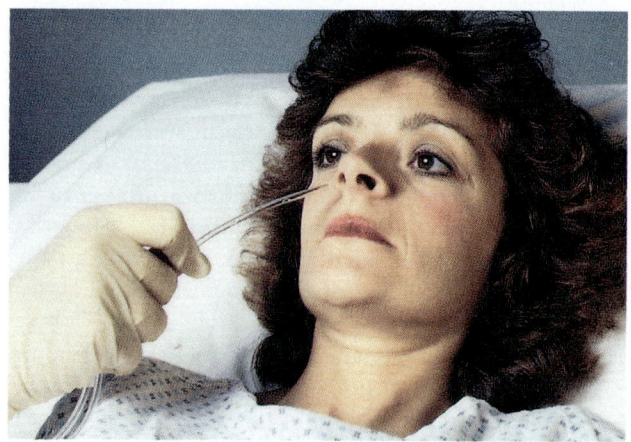

Figure 31-4

8. Gently insert tube along floor of nasal passage using gentle pressure. If resistance is met, gently rotate tube and try again. With continued resistance, withdraw tube, lubricate it again, and attempt insertion in opposite nostril.

Promotes comfort and reduces friction during insertion.

9. Insert tube to nasopharynx, rotate it toward the opposite nostril, then pass tube into oropharynx.

Helps to prevent coiling of tube in oropharynx.

10. Stop and allow client to relax. Provide tissues as needed to remove tears or excess lubrication around nares.

Mucosal irritation and discomfort can produce tearing.

11. Ask client to bend head forward and swallow small sips of water if allowed or to swallow without water as tube is advanced.

12. Advance tube 3 to 5 inches (7 to 12 cm) with each swallow. If coughing or gagging occurs, withdraw tube a bit and allow client to relax.

Tube may be displaced into larynx and produce coughing.

13. Ask client if tube feels as though it is coiling in back of throat, and check back of oropharynx using tongue blade to compress client's tongue. If tube has coiled, withdraw it until the tip is back in the oropharynx. Then reinsert with client swallowing.

14. Continue to advance tube with swallowing until tape or mark is reached.

Tip of tube must be well within stomach for adequate decompression.

15. Temporarily anchor tube to cheek with tape until placement is checked.

16. Ask client to speak.

Inability to speak can indicate that tube is through vocal cords onto the lungs.

17. Attach a large syringe to end of tube and place stethoscope over left upper abdominal quadrant. Flush tube with 20 ml of air. Listen for whooshing sound. Pull back on syringe to aspirate a sample of gastric secretions.

Insufflation of air into the stomach with auscultation may not be a totally reliable way to test for placement.

18. Test pH of secretions with a color-coded pH strip (Figure 31-5).

Gastric secretions are usually highly acidic with a pH of 4 or less.

Steps	Rationale

19. If pH of aspirate is not 4 or less, advance tube by about 2 inches (5 cm) and repeat Steps 15 and 16.
20. When gastric aspirates are obtained, anchor tube to nose and avoid pressure on nares.
    a. Apply tincture of benzoin sparingly to nose and allow it to become "tacky."
    b. Apply tube fixation device using shaped adhesive patch (Figure 31-6, *A*).
    c. Alternative: Apply tape to client's nose. Wrap two ends of tape around tube (Figure 31-6, *B*).
21. Fasten rubber band to end of NG tube in a slip knot, and pin rubber band to client's gown, allowing enough slack for movement of head.
22. Keep head of bed elevated at least 30 degrees unless physician orders otherwise.
23. Attach NG tube to suction source.
24. See Completion Protocol (Chapter 1, p. 6).

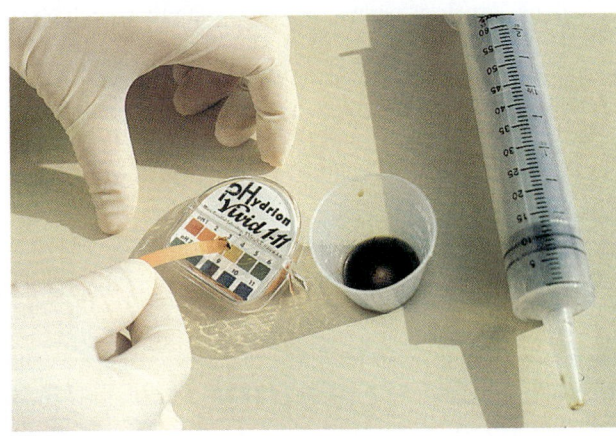

Figure 31-5

Presence of NG tube renders the pyloric sphincter incompetent and increases the risk of gastroesophageal reflux.

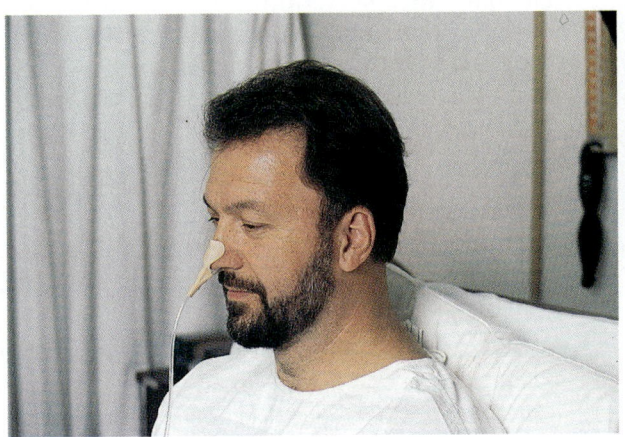

A

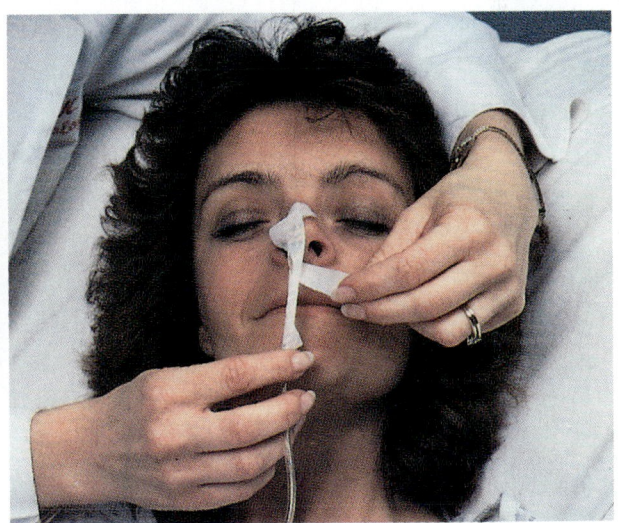

B

Figure 31-6

Evaluation

1. Palpate client's abdomen for distention and pain. Auscultate for bowel sounds.
2. Observe color of gastric secretions and patency of NG tube.
3. Ask client if oral and nasal hygiene measures have increased comfort.
4. Assess client's skin turgor. Measure urine output and specific gravity, and monitor client's laboratory studies.
5. Observe integrity or condition of nasal and oral mucosa.
6. Monitor client's body weight and length of time without adequate nutrition.

UNEXPECTED OUTCOMES AND RELATED INTERVENTIONS

1. Client develops abdominal distention, vomiting, or absence of drainage from tube.
   Assess patency of tube and irrigate tube as needed.
2. Client complains of discomfort from dry mucous membranes.
   a. Perform oral hygiene more frequently.

b. Ask physician whether client can suck on ice chips or throat lozenges or chew gum.
3. Client develops signs of fluid volume deficit (see Chapter 36).

Report decreased urine output, poor skin turgor, or excessive loss of secretions to physician.

1000 Inserted 16 Fr Salem sump tube into left nares and advanced it to 50 cm mark. Client assisted with insertion by swallowing and states he is comfortable following procedure. 50 ml of light-green gastric secretions were aspirated from tube with a measured pH of 3. Tube secured with tape and attached to low intermittent suction.
1200 Client given moistened swabs to lubricate oral mucosa. Stated increased comfort after use of swabs.

Skill 31.2 | Irrigating Nasogastric Tube

This skill involves irrigation of the NG tube with an isotonic saline solution to maintain patency of the tube. Irrigation should be performed when the tube's patency is in question, such as when the volume of gastric secretions has decreased or the client is experiencing symptoms such as abdominal pain or nausea, or if the client's abdomen is distended. The NG tube should also be irrigated before and after its use for the administration of medications.

EQUIPMENT (FIGURE 31-7)
60 ml catheter tip syringe
Normal saline
Towel
Disposable gloves

Assessment

1. Assess the volume, color, and character of gastric secretions. **Thick secretions and a reduced volume of secretions indicate the need to irrigate the NG tube.**
2. Assess client's abdomen for distention or pain.
3. Assess bowel sounds and passage of flatus.

Planning

Expected outcomes focus on maintenance of tube patency to ensure adequate decompression of the stomach.

EXPECTED OUTCOMES
1. Client's NG tube remains patent.
2. Client denies abdominal discomfort or nausea.

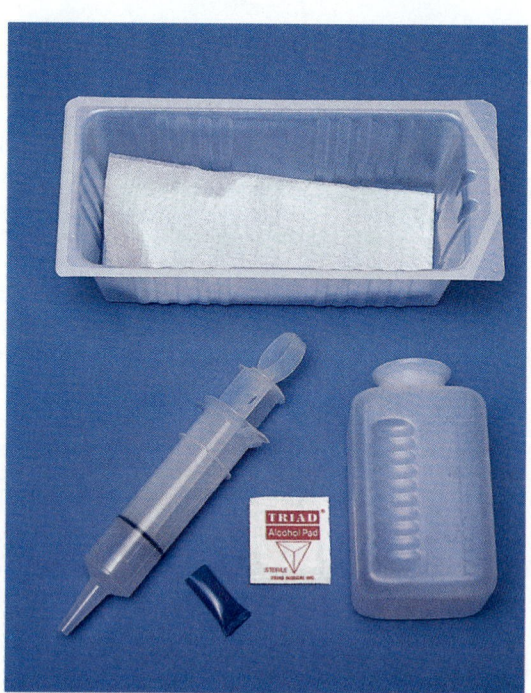

Figure 31-7

Implementation

Steps	Rationale

> **nurse alert** Client should be sitting upright in bed if possible.

1. See Standard Protocol (Chapter, 1, p. 5).

2. Draw up 30 ml of normal saline into large syringe.
3. Kink NG tube and remove from suction source. Lay end of suction tubing on towel.
4. Insert tip of irrigation syringe into end of NG tube and unkink tubing (see Figure 31-2).
5. Determine that NG tube is properly placed (see Skill 31.1, Steps 17 to 19). Inject saline steadily; do not force.
6. If unable to instill fluid, reposition client on left side and try again.
7. When saline has been instilled, withdraw fluid by pulling back gently on syringe.
8. Record difference in volume instilled and volume withdrawn. If equal, no documentation is required.
9. Reconnect NG tube to suction.
10. See Completion Protocol (Chapter, 1, p. 6).

Rationale:

Prevents soiling of client's gown and bed by drainage of gastric secretions.
Avoid use of pigtail vent on Salem sump for irrigation.

Tip of tube may be against stomach wall. Notify physician if unable to instill fluid.

Maintains accurate intake and output records.

Evaluation

1. Measure client's abdominal girth and inspect the color, volume, and character of NG secretions.
2. Assess client for abdominal pain, nausea, or bloating.

UNEXPECTED OUTCOMES AND RELATED INTERVENTIONS

1. Client's NG tube cannot be irrigated and is no longer patent.
   Contact physician. The buildup of secretions poses a risk for aspiration.
2. Client's NG tube can be irrigated, but irrigation fluid cannot be withdrawn and the tube continues to drain poorly.
   Contact physician. Position of tube may need to be confirmed.

SAMPLE DOCUMENTATION (See Intake and Output Summary, p. 109.)

0800 NG tube draining scant amounts. Irrigated with 30 ml normal saline. Initially, NG tube irrigated sluggishly, but became easier to irrigate. Withdrew 20 ml light-green fluid at end of irrigation. Client stated he had been feeling mild nausea.

1000 Increased volume of light-green gastric secretions draining from NG tube. Client states he no longer feels nauseated.

Skill 31.3 | Removing Nasogastric Tube

This skill involves removal of the NG tube when it is no longer needed for decompression of the stomach. A physician's order is required for this procedure. Generally, an NG tube is no longer required when gastric secretions empty normally into the duodenum through the pyloric sphincter and when intestinal motility returns. The client's ability to handle gastric secretions is sometimes evaluated by removing the NG tube from suction and putting it to gravity drainage, or by clamping the NG tube for a specified number of hours per day. If the client has not had a return of gastric or intestinal motility, the symptoms of abdominal distention, discomfort, or nausea will return.

EQUIPMENT
Tissues
Towel
Disposable gloves
60 ml catheter tip syringe

Assessment

1. Assess client for abdominal distention and symptoms such as nausea or abdominal pain.
2. Assess client for signs of returning bowel function, such as bowel movements, flatus, and presence of bowel sounds.

Planning

The expected outcome focuses on minimizing the discomfort caused by removal of the tube.

EXPECTED OUTCOME
Client remains comfortable after removal of the tube.

Implementation

Steps	Rationale
nurse alert Client should be sitting upright in bed if possible.	
1. See Standard Protocol (Chapter, 1, p. 5).	
2. Place towel over client's chest to protect gown and cover tube.	
3. Turn off suction.	Avoids trauma to mucosa during removal.
4. Attach large syringe to tube and flush with 20 ml of air.	Clears gastric fluids from tube that could irritate esophagus and mouth during tube removal.
5. Remove tape from client's nose and unpin tube from gown.	
6. Tell client that removal of tube is about to begin and will not be as uncomfortable as insertion.	Reduces anxiety and enhances cooperation.
7. Ask client to take a deep breath and hold it as tube is removed.	Airway is partially occluded during removal of tube. Minimizes risk of aspirating gastric contents if spilled from tube during removal.
8. Kink tube and pull tube out quickly and steadily onto towel.	Kinked tube is less likely to expel gastric contents (if present) into throat or trachea.
9. Give tissues to client to clean nares or assist client as needed.	
10. Measure volume of drainage. Record on Intake and Output Summary (see p. 109). Dispose of NG tube.	Maintains accurate intake and output.
11. Provide mouth care.	Promotes comfort.
12. See Completion Protocol (Chapter 1, p. 6).	

Evaluation

Ask client about level of comfort after removal of the tube and after provision of mouth care.

UNEXPECTED OUTCOMES AND RELATED INTERVENTIONS

Client complains of pain after removal of the NG tube.

  a. Consult with physician about the use of topical anesthetics to reduce pain from irritated nasal mucosa.

  b. Encourage client to ingest warm, soothing liquids if able. Be alert for any swallowing problems that may indicate erosion of the esophagus.

SAMPLE DOCUMENTATION

1300 Removed NG tube without difficulty. Mouth care provided after the removal. Client stated throat was sore but mouth care provided some relief.

CRITICAL THINKING EXERCISES

1. You are observing another student insert a nasogastric tube into Mr. Lister's stomach. The student has placed lubricant on the tube, asked Mr. Lister to hyperextend his neck, and is proceeding to advance the tube through Mr. Lister's nasal passage. After the student advances the tube 6 to 7 inches, Mr. Lister begins to cough. What suggestion(s) can you give the student that will likely rectify the problem?

2. The nurse is attempting to irrigate Mrs. Sanders' nasogastric tube but is having difficulty instilling the solution. Evaluate the following actions on the part of the nurse.
  a. Gently but forcefully continues to attempt irrigation of the NG tube until it irrigates easily.
  b. Uses the pigtail vent on the salem sump to instill the fluid.
  c. Assists Mrs. Sanders to her left side and attempts to irrigate the NG tube again.

3. You have just explained to Mr. Gray that you are going to remove his nasogastric tube because it is no longer needed. When you instruct him to hold his breath while the tube is being removed, he asks you why. How will you answer his question?

REFERENCES

American Society for Parenteral and Enteral Nutrition Board of Directors: Guidelines for the use of parenteral and enteral nutrition in adult and pediatric patients, *J Parenter Enter Nutr* 17(4):1SA, 1993.

Metheny N: Minimizing respiratory complications of nasoenteric tube feedings: state of the science, *Heart Lung* 22(3):213, 1993.

ADDITIONAL READING

Camp D, Otten N: How to insert and remove nasogastric tubes quickly and easily, *Nursing* 20(9):59, 1990.

Enteral Nutrition

Skill 32.1
Administering Tube Feedings

Skill 32.2
Administering Medication Through a Feeding Tube

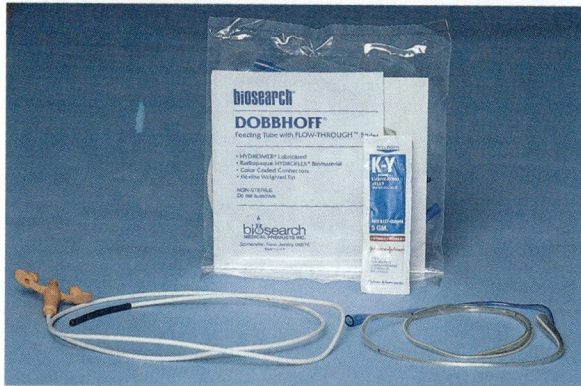

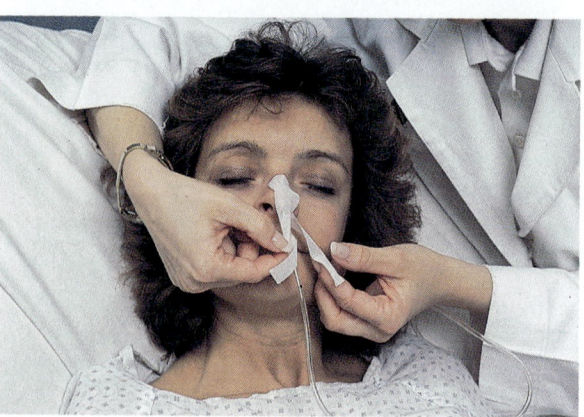

When clients have an intact and functional gastrointestinal (GI) tract but are unable to consume food or fluids orally, enteral nutrition is the preferred technique for nourishment. Enteral nutrition involves the provision of nutrients to the GI tract for digestion and absorption. Tube feedings are used for clients who cannot ingest food safely but who still have a functioning GI tract.

Tube feedings may be used for short-term management of nutritional problems during acute illness and recovery. The primary reason that clients receive tube feedings is to prevent or treat malnutrition related to diminished intake. Also, clients may require tube feeding because of ineffective swallowing or a weakened gag reflex causing aspiration. Some clients are "hypermetabolic" as a result of sepsis or burns and are unable to ingest enough nutrition to meet their bodies' needs. After the feeding tube is placed, clients are still at risk for aspiration and need careful nursing management to avoid this complication.

For short-term nutritional support, 6 weeks or less, enteral feeding tubes are usually placed nasally (or infrequently via the mouth) into the stomach, duodenum, or jejunum (Eisenberg, 1994). Feeding tubes may also be placed with an endoscope or surgically if prolonged need is expected.

Tube feedings may also be used to provide nutrition for clients who cannot swallow safely or those who are unable to eat enough to sustain daily function. These groups may include clients with brain injury or an altered or reduced level of consciousness and clients with neuromuscular diseases who have a high incidence of aspiration, such as those with amyotrophic lateral sclerosis (ALS) and muscular dystrophy (MD). In these clients, tubes may be placed endoscopically or surgically through the abdominal wall gastrostomy (into the stomach) or jejunostomy (into the small intestine) (Figure 32-1).

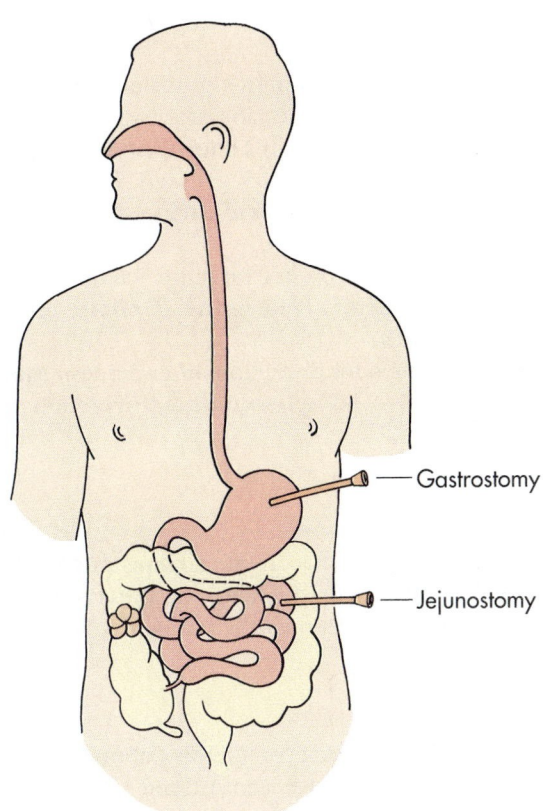

Figure 32-1 Placement for two types of feeding tubes.

- Gastrostomy
- Jejunostomy

Tube feeding formulas may consist of blended table food; commercial preparations that are of varying osmolarity, caloric, fat, protein, and lactose content; or elemental formulas that require no digestion to absorb. Some tube feedings are also designed for specific diseases, such as renal, respiratory, or hepatic failure. The choice of tube feeding depends on the client's clinical condition (Bockus, 1993).

Tube feedings may be administered in several ways. They can be given as a bolus amount via gravity, several times a day through a large-bore syringe; as a continuous gravity drip for ½ to 1 hour several times per day using a pouch to hang the feeding; or as a continuous drip per infusion pump, on whatever schedule best meets the client's needs: 8 or 12 or 24 hours per day.

Checking for placement of the feeding tube before administering medication or tube feeding is an integral part of the skill. Tubes may have been inadvertently misplaced or migrated into the esophagus and into the lung. Aspiration and pneumonia, or peritonitis, can develop from administering a tube feeding in a misplaced tube. Data show that auscultation alone is not a safe method to check tube placement. Aspiration of GI contents may confirm tube placement in the stomach, but straw-colored pleural fluid can look similar. Testing pH is a strong indicator for correct placement but is just beginning to enter general nursing practice. Using several methods to test placement is the safest way to be certain of tube placement.

Many potential complications may arise from tube feeding administration. The cost of managing the ensuing complications and infections is expensive. Complications may be related to the tube itself, such as placement of the tube in the lung, frequent tube clogging, or the tube inadvertently being pulled out. Complications may also occur when the administered tube feeding causes delayed gastric emptying, cramping, diarrhea, or aspiration (Young and White, 1992).

Medications may be administered through feeding tubes. Liquid medication is preferred, but some pills may be crushed, dissolved in water, and instilled. Never crush extended-release, sublingual, or slow-acting (SA) medications, or medications with a coating on them (enteric coated), because their absorption and effects will be altered. A pharmacist should be consulted before pills are crushed or before capsules are opened and dissolved for tube feeding administration. The pharmacist can also assist in determining the effectiveness of the medication depending on the location of the feeding tube (i.e., stomach, duodenum, or jejunum). Many medications are available in liquid form (Lehmann and Barber, 1991).

Nursing Diagnosis

Altered Nutrition: Less Than Body Requirements related to insufficient intake is appropriate when there is evidence of weight loss and/or inability to swallow. **Risk for Aspiration** is another indication for use of tube feedings. Clients may experience **Diarrhea** or **Constipation** related to altered intake associated with tube feedings.

Skill 32.1 | Administering Tube Feedings

This skill includes the administration of tube feeding via bolus, and continuous drip via gravity or infusion pump. It is very important to check placement of nasogastric and nasointestinal tubes before initiating feedings. Using good handwashing and clean equipment and hanging formula only for the recommended time to prevent spoiling are critically important for avoiding contamination of the system and subsequent infection in the client.

EQUIPMENT
Formula (Figure 32-2)

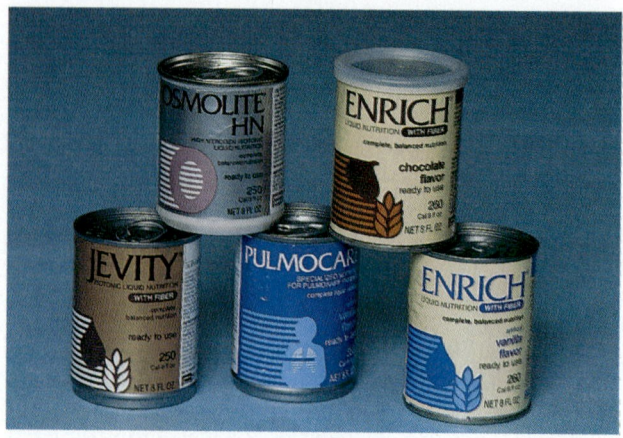

Figure 32-2

50 to 60 ml syringe
   Catheter tip for large-bore tubes
   Luer lock tip for small-bore tubes
Stethoscope
pH test strip (range 1.0 to 8.0)
Graduate container
Administration set
   Bolus: 60 ml bulb or plunger syringe
      or
   Gavage/Intermittent infusion: plastic feeding bag
      with drip chamber and tubing (see Figure 32-6)
      or
   Infusion pump: pump, plastic feeding bag with ap-
      propriate drip chamber and tubing for pumps (see
      Figure 32-7)
Tap water

Assessment

1. Identify signs and symptoms of malnutrition, including baseline weight and laboratory values (albumin,
   protein, lymphocyte, etc.). **Determine client's need
   for enteral nutrition: depressed level of consciousness, surgery, swallowing disorders, or
   trauma.**
2. Verify physician's orders for tube feeding formula,
   rate, and frequency. **Determine if client has any
   food allergies.**
3. Assess abdomen for distention or tenderness. **Auscultate for active bowel sounds before each feeding.**

Planning

Expected outcomes focus on safe administration of tube
feeding formula, client tolerance of the formula, and
avoidance of complications related to tube feeding administration.

EXPECTED OUTCOMES

1. Nutritional monitoring parameters (laboratory values,
   weight status, wound healing) trend toward normal
   by discharge.
2. Client voices no complaints during feeding.
3. Client experiences no aspiration by discharge.
4. Client has residual volume less than 100 ml before
   tube feeding.

Implementation

Steps	Rationale
1. See Standard Protocol (Chapter 1, p. 5).	
2. Elevate head of bed to high Fowler's, at least 30 degrees, or reverse Trendelenburg if spinal injury present.	Reduces risk of aspiration during feeding with head higher than stomach.
3. Check placement of feeding tube.	Radiographic evidence of placement is the most accurate, but cost and radiation exposure prohibit frequent checks many times per day (Metheny, 1993).
a. Aspirate intestinal contents with appropriate syringe inserted into end of tube (Figure 32-3).	Presence of green or yellow secretions indicates distal end of tube is in place. Use caution, since straw-colored pleural fluid can resemble GI fluid.
b. Place drop of GI contents on pH test paper for measurement (see Figure 31-5).	Gastric contents have a pH range of 1 to 4. Intestinal fluids range from 5 to 7. Pleural fluids range from 7 to 8 (Metheny et al., 1989).
c. Auscultate for gurgling sound with stethoscope over client's left upper quadrant while injecting 10 to 20 ml of air into tube.	Use caution, since gurgles may be heard from the esophagus or the distal lung. Gurgles are very soft if tube is in jejunum or duodenum.

Steps	Rationale

d. If tube is nasally inserted, inspect oral cavity for tube kinking or curling in back of the throat.

Indicates that tube may no longer be correctly positioned in the GI tract.

e. If unable to aspirate or inject air into tube, consider that tube is clogged or kinked, and attempt to flush with 30 ml of warm water.

Using a small syringe (3 to 6 ml) generates a large force and may rupture small-bore feeding tubes. Fluids other than water have not been found to be any more effective in unclogging tubes (Young and White, 1992).

4. Aspirate GI contents for residual volume; if client has a small-bore feeding tube, aspirate slowly to avoid collapse. Determine volume with graduate container if necessary.

Evaluates absorption and tolerance of last feeding, or may indicate delayed gastric emptying. Small-bore feeding tubes in the intestine may not have residual volumes.

nurse alert   If residual amount is greater than last hour's infusion or 100 ml, hold feeding 1 hour and recheck residual (Bockus, 1991).

5. Readminister residual volume to client by allowing it to flow from syringe into tubing. If large volume of residual, administer slowly.

Avoids fluid and electrolyte imbalance. Slow administration minimizes nausea.

6. Prepare formula for administration.
a. If pouring directly from a can, check expiration date and wipe off top of can (Figure 32-4).
b. If using premixed bags, check date and time of mixing, as well as correct strength (full, half strength, etc.).

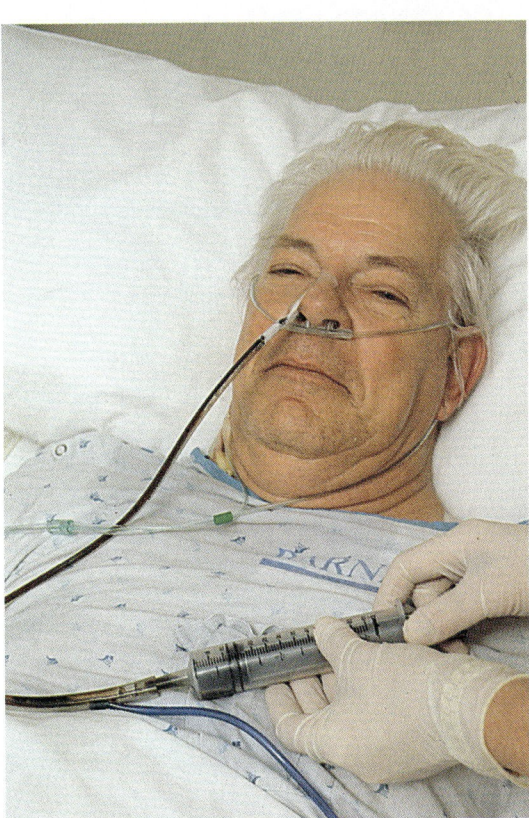

Figure 32-3

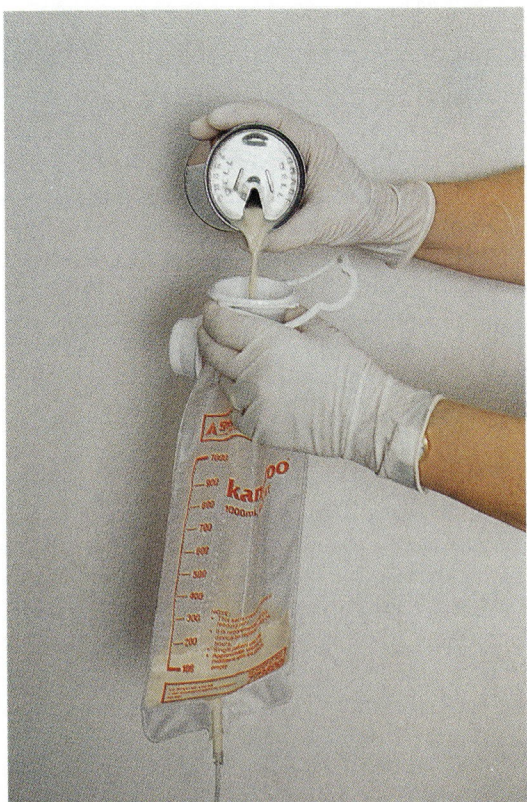

Figure 32-4

Steps	Rationale

7. Bolus feedings by gravity

a. Administer the tube feeding with **60 ml bulb or plunger syringe.**

b. Remove cap or plug from end of tube and pinch closed to prevent leakage.

c. Attach syringe by removing bulb or plunger and inserting tip into end of tube. Elevate to no more than 18 inches (45 cm) above insertion site (Figure 32-5).

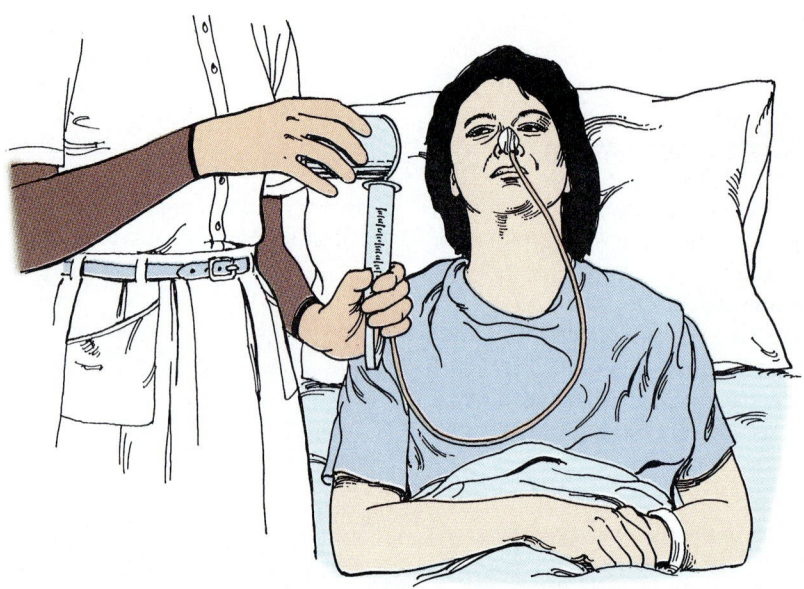

Figure 32-5

d. Fill syringe with formula, unpinch tube, and allow to empty gradually, refilling until ordered amount has been administered.

Slow delivery of tube feeding (50 to 100 ml/min) is better tolerated. Continuous draining from syringe avoids air entry and gas production.

e. Flush tube with 30 to 60 ml tap water (or ordered amount) when feeding complete.

Prevents tube clogging with thicker feeding.

f. Recap/plug tube.

8. Gravity drip over ½ to 1 hour

a. Administer the tube feeding with **gavage bag** (Figure 32-6).

Easily tolerated in the stomach. Allows periods for client to be unattached to a feeding system.

b. Prepare administration set: clamp tubing, prepare gavage bag with prescribed type and amount of formula, unclamp and prime tubing to remove air, then reclamp tubing.

c. Label bag with tube feeding type, strength, and amount. Include date, time, and initials.

d. Pinch end of feeding tube. Remove plug/cap.

Prevents air from entering stomach.

e. Securely attach gavage tubing to end of feeding tube.

f. Set rate by adjusting roller clamp on tubing. Usually this type of tube feeding infuses for 30 to 60 minutes three to six times per day.

Steps	Rationale

g. Flush tube with 30 to 60 ml tap water (or ordered amount) when feeding complete.

Prevents tube clogging.

h. Recap/plug tube.

9. Feeding via infusion pump

a. Administer the tube feeding as a **continuous drip via infusion pump** (Figure 32-7).

Allows a smaller volume of feeding to be delivered continuously. There is less risk of aspiration or missed feedings.

b. Prepare administration set, with type and amount of formula to last no more than 8 hours. Clamp tubing, spike bottle, and unclamp and prime tubing. Reclamp tubing.

Avoids spoilage. Prefilled vacuum packages are available from the manufacturer and are less likely to spoil.

c. Label bag with tube feeding type, strength, and amount. Include date, time, and initials.

d. Hang tube feeding set on intravenous (IV) pole with infusion pump. Connect tubing to pump and set rate.

e. Pinch end of feeding tube. Remove plug/cap. Connect infusion tubing to client feeding tube.

f. Open roller clamp on infusion tubing. Turn infusion pump on.

g. Check residual volumes every 4 hours by aspirating with 60 ml syringe.

Ensures that tube feeding is continuing to infuse through the GI system.

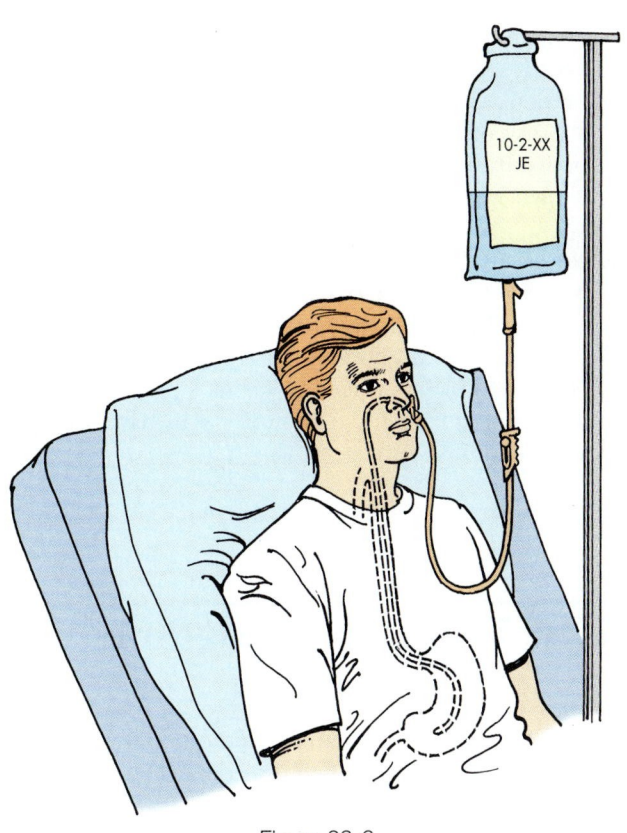

Figure 32-6

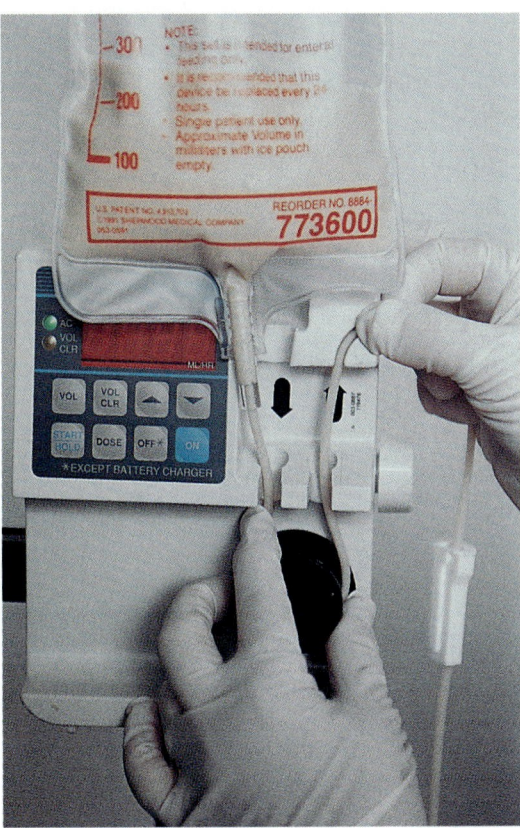

Figure 32-7

Steps	Rationale
10. Fill 60 ml syringe with ordered volume of water (generally 30 to 50 ml). Inject into feeding tube to flush after bolus, or as ordered with continuous drip.	Aids in avoiding a clogged tube. Water replacement is vital to help client maintain adequate fluid and electrolyte balance.
11. Flush tube with water every 4 to 8 hours as in Step 8g, and clamp end when no feedings are infusing.	
12. Rinse syringe or bag and tubing with warm water after all bolus and gavage feedings.	Rinsing removes formula left in equipment, reduces potential for bacterial growth, and allows for reuse of equipment. Most institutions require replacement with new equipment every 24 hours.
13. Ask if client is comfortable while the infusion is continuing.	Complaints of cramping may indicate tube feeding is too cold or is infusing too fast. Diarrhea should be reported to the physician. Client may need antidiarrheal agents (e.g., Kaopectate, Lomotil).
14. See Completion Protocol (Chapter 1, p. 6).	

Evaluation

1. Monitor weight and laboratory values daily.
2. Assess client's level of comfort with each tube feeding or at each shift if a continuous drip is given. Nausea or vomiting may indicate need for change in rate of administration.
3. Observe and assess client for shortness of breath, low oxygen saturation, and presence of liquid the color of feeding from airway. Blue dye may be added to feeding to confirm presence of feeding in lungs.
4. Monitor the amount of residual tube feeding aspirated to evaluate for absorption vs. decreased gastric motility.

UNEXPECTED OUTCOMES AND RELATED INTERVENTIONS

1. Client's feeding tube is unable to be aspirated or injected with air or water.
   a. Attempt to flush with large-bore syringe and warm water. (Avoid using a small-bore syringe because this exerts large amounts of pressure and may rupture tube.)
   b. Notify physician if unable to clear feeding tube.
   c. If tube cleared, keep tube patent by flushing every 4 hours, before clamping off each time, and before and after each feeding and medication infusion.

2. Aspirated residual appears straw colored with a pH of 7.0.
   a. Hold tube feeding.
   b. Contact physician. Consider chest x-ray film to evaluate tube placement.
3. Client vomits. Heart rate and respiratory rate are elevated, and client is coughing.
   a. Hold tube feeding; assess lungs.
   b. Notify physician of probable aspiration.
4. Client receiving a continuous-infusion tube feeding appears ashen. Respirations are rapid and shallow. Breath sounds are full of rhonchi. Client coughs up secretions that are very similar to the tube feeding.
   a. Turn off tube feeding.
   b. Notify physician. Prepare for supplemental oxygen, chest x-ray film, and probable tube removal.

SAMPLE DOCUMENTATION

0900 NG feeding tube placement confirmed via aspiration and pH 3.0. Full strength Osmolyte hung per infusion pump at 60 ml/hour. Head of bed elevated 30 degrees. No complaints voiced by client.
1200 Client had liquid stools times 3 in past 2 hours. Physician notified for orders.

Skill 32.2 | # Administering Medication Through a Feeding Tube

This skill involves the safe administration of oral medications through a feeding tube. Specific attention needs to be paid to proper placement of the tube and whether the medication can be crushed for administra-tion through the tube. Liquid medication is the best choice to administer through a feeding tube, but some medicines only come in tablet form. Most tablets may be crushed; however, those that are sublingual, enteric coated, or sustained release should not be given by tube, since their absorption, metabolism, and effectiveness will be unpredictable. Capsules may be emptied of powder or aspirated of gelatin, dissolved, and given through the feeding tube if they are not sustained release for the same reasons (Lehmann and Barber, 1991).

Medications should not be mixed in with tube feedings because of potential interruptions in tube feeding flow (e.g., turning feeding off while client in radiology department), spillage, delayed absorption of the medication, or possible drug precipitation. It is always best to consult with a pharmacist before administering medications through a feeding tube.

EQUIPMENT

50 to 60 ml syringe
   Catheter tip for large-bore tubes
   Luer lock tip for small-bore tubes
Stethoscope
pH test strip
Graduate container
Medication to be administered
Pill crusher if medication in tablet form
Syringe with needle if medication in gelatin form
Warm water (to dissolve dry/gelatin medication)
Tap water
Tongue blade or straw to stir dissolved medication

Assessment

1. Verify physician's order for medication type, dosage, frequency, and route of administration.
2. Assess client for active bowel sounds before giving medication.

Planning

Expected outcomes focus on administration of appropriate medication via the tube feeding route and avoidance of tube clogging from medication administration.

EXPECTED OUTCOMES

1. Medication is instilled followed by evidence of improvement in relation to desired effects.
2. Client's feeding tube remains patent after medication administration.

> **nurse alert** Verify that medications to be administered do not include any sublingual, enteric-coated, or sustained-release medications.

Implementation

Steps	Rationale
1. See Standard Protocol (Chapter 1, p. 5).	
2. Elevate head of bed to high Fowler's, at least 30 degrees, or in reverse Trendelenburg if spinal injury present.	Reduces risk of aspiration.
3. Prepare medication for instillation in feeding tube.	
a. Review five "rights" for administration of medication (see Skill 16.1).	
b. *Tablets:* Crush pill (in its package if possible) with pill crusher (Figure 32-8). Dissolve the powder in 15 to 30 ml warm water.	Crushing medication in its package prevents some from being lost (Lehmann and Barber, 1991).
c. *Capsules:* Open and dissolve the powder in 15 to 30 ml warm water.	

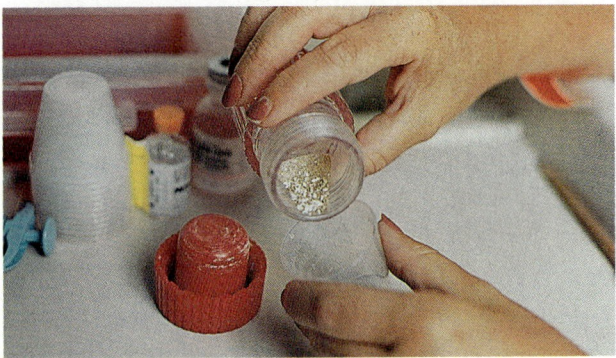

Figure 32-8

Steps	Rationale

d. *Gelatin capsules:* Aspirate with a syringe, or capsule may be dissolved in warm water (Figure 32-9) over several minutes. After capsule dissolves, remove its gelatin outer layer.

Less medication is wasted if capsule is dissolved in warm water, but this may require 15 to 20 minutes before administration.

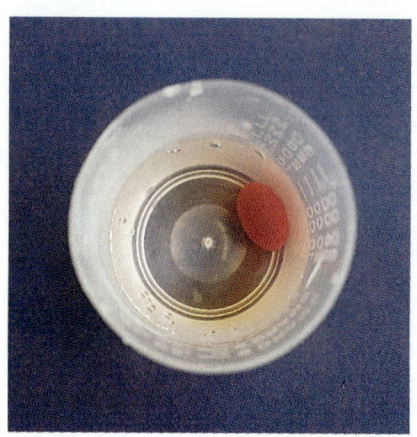

Figure 32-9

4. Check placement of feeding tube. (See Skill 32.1, Step 3 a to e.)
5. Aspirate stomach contents for residual volume, determine volume with graduate container if necessary, and reinstill to client (Figure 32-10).
6. Pour dissolved medication into syringe and allow to flow by gravity into feeding tube (Figure 32-11). Flush with 10 ml water after each medication.

If residual remains greater than 100 ml, hold medication and contact physician for further orders.

If a problem develops during medication administration (e.g., spillage, coughing, tube clogging), nurse can tell which medications have been lost and which are still available for later administration.

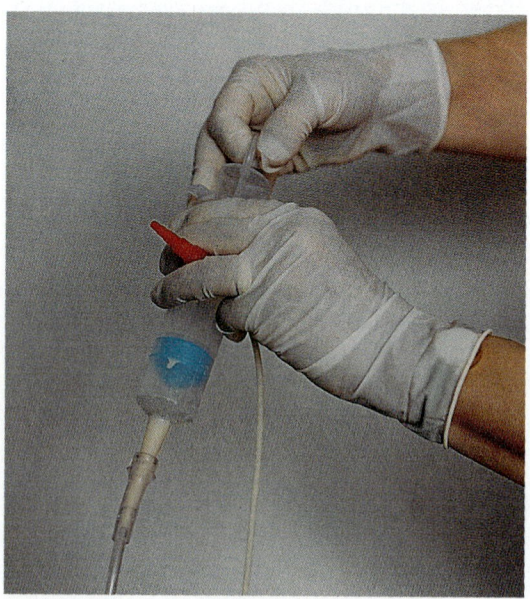

Figure 32-10

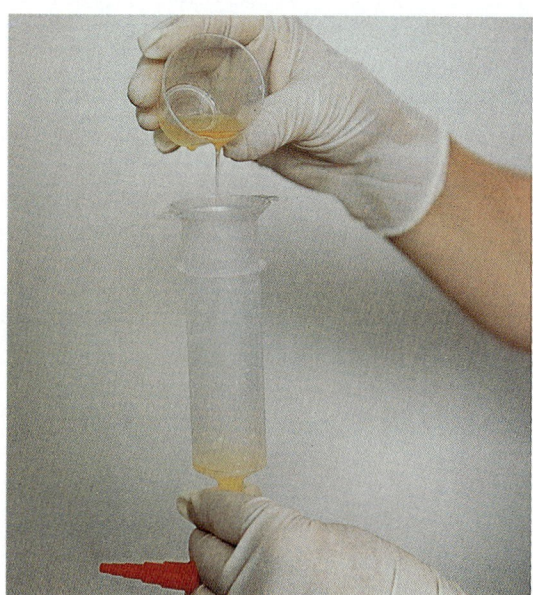

Figure 32-11

7. Follow medication with 30 to 60 ml of water to flush tube of medications.
8. See Completion Protocol (Chapter 1, p. 6).

Avoids tube clogging with medication and ensures medication enters stomach, where it can be absorbed.

Evaluation

1. Observe for desired effects within appropriate time frame depending on medication administered.
2. Observe tube patency before and after medication administration.

UNEXPECTED OUTCOMES AND RELATED INTERVENTIONS

1. Client has Theo-Dur 300 mg ordered bid per tube.
   a. Note that Theo-Dur is a sustained-release medication intended to break down and be absorbed slowly over 8 to 12 hours.
   b. Contact physician for orders to have client receive theophylline elixir every 4 to 6 hours for better tolerance.
2. Client is unable to receive medication because of blockage in tube.
   a. Attempt to flush tube with warm water to clear clog.
   b. If unable to flush clog, contact physician for replacement of tube and potential need to reroute medication if dose cannot be skipped or delayed until a new feeding tube is placed.

SAMPLE DOCUMENTATION

NOTE: Documentation for medications via feeding tube is usually done on the medication sheet, the same as for any other medication. Other documentation occurs only if a problem is noted.

1300 Unable to administer medication due to clogged tube, despite efforts to unclog. Physician notified, medications held pending placement of new tube.

CRITICAL THINKING EXERCISES

1. Unable to feed herself at this time, Carmen has been ordered to receive intermittent tube feedings. You have prepared the prescribed enteral feeding and have all the equipment ready in Carmen's room. What is the most important action you will take before beginning the tube feeding? Explain.
2. Mrs. Thomas is receiving continuous tube feedings via an infusion pump.
   a. What is the primary advantage of delivering a feeding by this method?
   b. An hour after starting the tube feeding, Mrs. Thomas complains of stomach cramps. What is your assessment of Mrs. Thomas's complaint, and how should you respond?
3. You are observing an RN administer medication to Mr. Redd, a client with an enteral feeding tube. The nurse turns off the feeding pump, disconnects the infusion tubing from the feeding tube, and connects a 60 cc syringe. She then aspirates for tube placement. The nurse then fills the syringe with the prescribed medication and slowly pushes it down the feeding tube. She follows the medication with a 20 cc flush of water and restarts the feeding tube. How would you evaluate the nurse's actions?

REFERENCES

Bockus S: Troubleshooting your tube feedings, *Am J Nurs* 91:24, 1991.

Bockus S: When your patient needs tube feedings: making the right decisions, *Nursing '93* 23(7):34, 1993.

Eisenberg PG: Nasoenteral tubes: a nurse's guide to tube feeding, *RN* 57(10):62, 1994.

Lehmann S, Barber JR: Giving medications by feeding tube: how to avoid problems, *Nursing '91* 21(11):58, 1991.

Metheny N: Minimizing respiratory complications of nasoenteric tube feedings: state of the science, *Heart Lung* 22(3):213, 1993.

Metheny N et al: Effectiveness of pH measurements in predicting feeding tube placement, *Nurs Res* 38:280, 1989.

Young, C, White S: Preparing patients for tube feeding at home, *Am J Nurs* 92:46, 1992.

ADDITIONAL READINGS

Adams CW: How tube feeding complications can develop, *Nursing '90* 20(3):59, 1990.

Eisenberg P: Enteral nutrition: indications, formulas, and delivery techniques, *Nurs Clin North Am* 24(2):315, 1989.

Kohn C, Keithley JK: Enteral nutrition: potential complications and patient monitoring, *Nurs Clin North Am* 24(2):339, 1989.

McConnell EA: Administering a bolus gastrostomy feeding, *Nursing '90* 20(11):102, 1990.

Metheny N et al: Effectiveness of inadvertent respiratory placement of small bore feeding tubes: a report of 10 cases, *Heart Lung* 19(6):631, 1990.

Metheny N et al: How to aspirate fluid from small-bore feeding tubes, *Am J Nurs* 93:86, 1993.

Petrosino BM et al: Implications of selected problems with nasoenteral tube feedings, *Crit Care Nurs Q* 12(3):1, 1989.

Walsh SM, Banks LA: How to insert a small-bore feeding tube safely, *Nursing '90* 20(3):55, 1990.

Webber-Jones J et al: How to declog a feeding tube, *Nursing '92* 22(4):62, 1992.

chapter
33

Altered Bowel Elimination

Skill 33.1
Removing Impactions

Skill 33.2
Pouching a Stoma

Skill 33.3
Irrigating a Colostomy

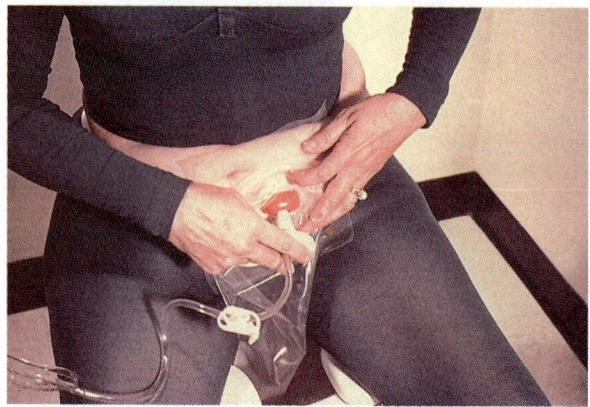

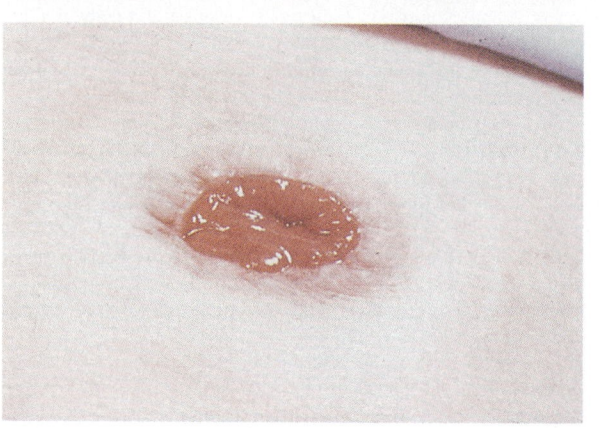

Many clients suffer from constipation, especially when illness requires an extended period of immobility. Left unrecognized, constipation can progress to fecal impaction, in which stool may block the intestinal lumen. Stasis of bowel contents produces distention and pain. In some cases liquid stool passes around the obstruction, which can be misinterpreted as diarrhea. If enemas and suppositories do not facilitate passage of stool, the impaction may need to be removed manually.

A stoma is a surgically created opening in the intestines to the outside of the client's body. It comes from the Greek word *stomat,* meaning opening or mouth. Depending on the reason for the surgery, an ostomy can be permanent or temporary. There are two types of ostomies in the gastrointestinal (GI) tract (Figure 33-1). The most common type is a *colostomy,* which is a stoma made from the large intestine or colon. The other ostomy, an *ileostomy,* is found in the small intestine (Fazio and Tjandra, 1992; Hampton and Bryant, 1992; Nadler, 1992).

Care of a client with an ostomy involves many dimensions. These include providing the physical care of the stoma, containing the ostomy output or effluent, protecting the skin around the stoma (peristomal skin), preventing peristomal irritation, and preventing fecal contamination of the surgical wound (Hampton and Bryant, 1992). Teaching the client self–ostomy care is critical (Fazio and Tjandra, 1992; Wilson, 1992). This includes pouch change techniques, colostomy irrigation, and diet management. Helping the client adjust to the change in body image can be facilitated by having an ostomy visitor meet with the client (Gloeckner, 1991; Krainski, 1994; Pieper, 1992; Quayle, 1994; Ramer, 1992). Many booklets and support groups are available that can help the client make the transition to living with an ostomy (Rheaume and Gooding, 1991).

Nursing Diagnosis

Nursing diagnoses associated with clients who have ostomies include **Altered Health Maintenance** related to the self-care of the ostomy, **Body Image Disturbance** related to presence of the ostomy, and **Risk for Impaired Skin Integrity** related to irritation of peristomal skin.

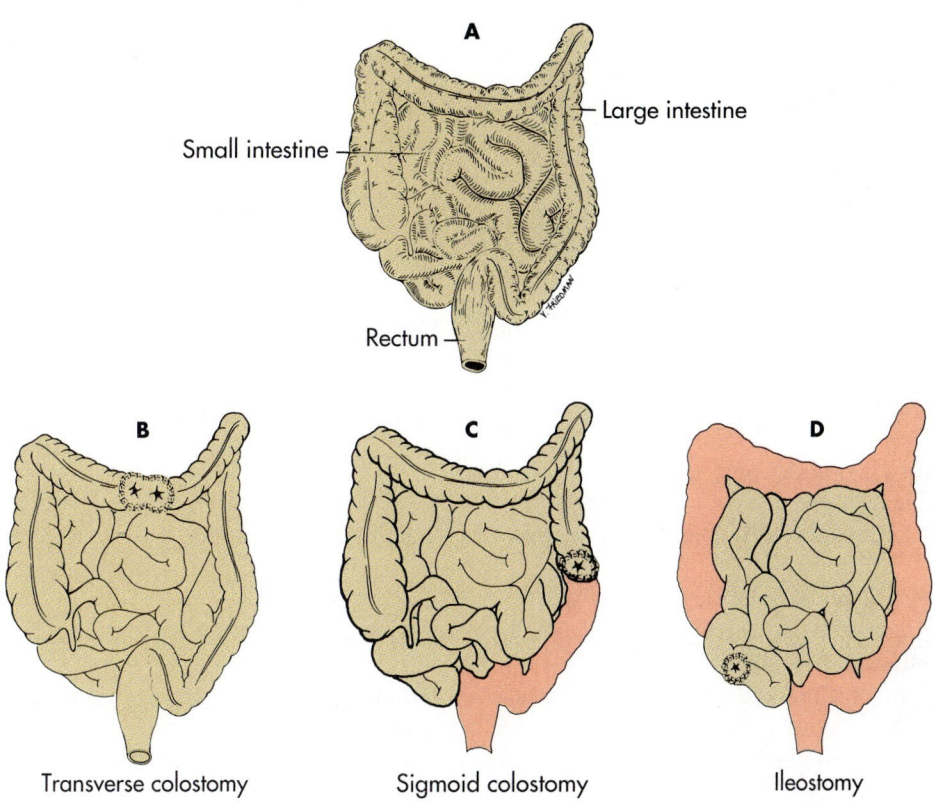

Figure 33-1 **A,** Normal intestinal structure. Types of colostomies: **B,** transverse (double barrel) colostomy; **C,** sigmoid colostomy; and **D,** ileostomy.

Skill 33.1 | Removing Impactions

This skill is usually performed when the administration of enemas or suppositories have been unsuccessful at removing hard or large stools. Digital removal of an impaction may be embarrassing and uncomfortable for the client. Excessive digital manipulation may cause trauma to the mucosa and subsequent bleeding or vagus nerve stimulation and subsequent slowing of the heart rate.

EQUIPMENT
Clean gloves
Water-soluble lubricant
Waterproof pad
Toilet tissue
Bedpan
Bedpan cover
Basin, washcloth, towel, and soap

Assessment

1. Assess client's normal and current bowel elimination pattern as to frequency, characteristics of stool, use of laxatives and other medications, urge to defecate but inability to do so, and abdominal discomfort, especially when attempting to defecate. **This information is valuable in determining contributing factors and preventing recurrence of this problem.**
2. Assess client's abdomen for distention, auscultate for the presence of bowel sounds, and palpate the abdomen for masses. **Distention may contribute to**

constipation. **Hyperactive bowel sounds may result from reduced patency of GI tract.**

3. Measure client's current vital signs to establish a baseline. **Vagus nerve stimulation may slow the heart rate.**

4. Check client's record for physician's order for digital removal of impaction. **A physician's order is necessary because of possible vagus nerve stimulation.**

Planning

Expected outcomes focus on removal of the impaction and prevention of further occurrences.

EXPECTED OUTCOMES

1. Client's rectum is free of stool.
2. Client's vital signs remain normal after procedure.
3. Client resumes normal defecation.
4. Client experiences minimal discomfort.
5. Client/family verbalizes ways to prevent fecal impaction.

Implementation

Steps	Rationale
1. See Standard Protocol (Chapter 1, p. 5).	
2. Assist client to a left side-lying position with knees flexed.	Provides access to the rectum.
3. Place waterproof pad under buttocks.	
4. Place bedpan next to client.	
5. Instruct client to take slow, deep breaths during procedure.	Aids in relaxing smooth muscle of anal sphincter.
6. Lubricate gloved finger with lubricating jelly.	
7. Insert index finger into rectum and advance finger toward the umbilicus.	Follows course of rectum.
8. Gently rotate finger along side of the rectal wall. Work finger into hardened feces.	Removing small pieces of stool promotes less discomfort during procedure.
9. Work stool down toward end of rectum.	

nurse alert Periodically assess heart rate and for signs of fatigue. Stop for decrease in heart rate, rhythm changes, or fatigue. Vagus nerve stimulation slows heart rate. Procedure may be painful and tiring for client.

10. Continue to clear rectum. Allow rest intervals as needed.	
11. After removal of impaction, assist with washing buttocks as needed.	
12. Review with client and family factors that promote normal peristalsis (e.g., activity, bulk-forming fluids, increased fluid intake).	
13. See Completion Protocol (Chapter 1, p. 6).	

Evaluation

1. Perform rectal examination to determine if rectum is clear of stool.
2. Reassess vital signs and compare with baseline values.
3. Monitor client for next defecation and inspect character of stool.
4. Ask client if relieved from rectal discomfort.
5. Ask client/family to describe preventive measures.

UNEXPECTED OUTCOMES AND RELATED INTERVENTIONS

1. Client has seepage of liquid fecal material after removal of impaction.
   a. Contact physician. An enema may be needed to remove hardened feces higher in the rectum.
   b. Increasing fluids, bulk in diet, and activity level may aid peristaltic activity.
2. Client experiences bradycardia, decrease in blood pressure, and decrease in level of consciousness as a result of vagus nerve stimulation.
   a. Stop procedure.
   b. Notify physician immediately.
   c. Take appropriate actions.
3. Client has trauma to the rectal mucosa, as evidenced by blood on the gloved finger.
   a. Assess rectal area every hour for bleeding.
   b. If bleeding continues, contact physician for further treatment measures.

SAMPLE DOCUMENTATION

1000 Digitally removed moderate amount of hard, dark-brown feces from rectum. No bradycardia, fatigue, rectal bleeding, or pain noted. Abdomen soft, nontender, with bowel sounds in all four quadrants.

Skill 33.2 | Pouching a Stoma (Including Skin Care)

This skill includes the physical inspection of the client's stoma and application of a skin barrier and pouch.

The purpose of a pouch over an ostomy is to contain the effluent or drainage and to protect the skin surrounding the stoma from irritation. Proper fitting of the pouch is imperative. The pouching system and skin barrier should not leak, cut into the stoma, cause any other trauma to the stoma, or expose peristomal skin to discharge. Pouches that allow visibility of the stoma help the clinician to see and assess the stoma easily but may decrease the client's initial acceptance of the stoma.

Immediately after surgery, the stoma is often edematous. The size and shape of the stoma will change. Measurement of the stoma size at each pouching system change is very important to assist in proper fitting of the skin barrier and pouch. A variety of pouching systems can be used. Some pouches are one piece and have a skin barrier already attached to it. Others are a two-piece system, in which the skin barrier with a flange is attached around the client's stoma first, and then the pouch is attached. During the postoperative period, the amount of pressure on the abdomen during the pouch changing procedure should be minimal. During this period, the client may also require analgesia prior to pouching. It is important to use the correct type of pouching system accurately for the client's particular stoma needs.

EQUIPMENT (Figure 33-2)

Skin barrier
Ostomy pouch with closure device
Belt (optional with some pouches)
Deodorant
Gloves
Washcloth
Scissors
Ostomy measuring guide
Printed ostomy instructions and booklets

Assessment

1. Identify the type of ostomy (e.g., colostomy or ileostomy) that client has (see Figure 33-1). **Type of**

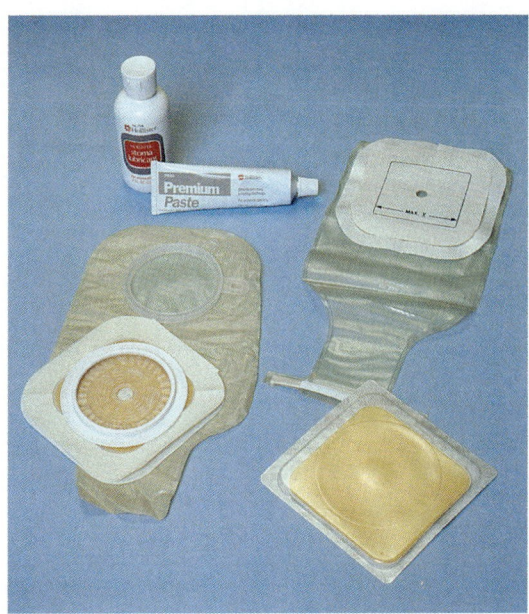

Figure 33-2 Ostomy pouches and skin barriers.

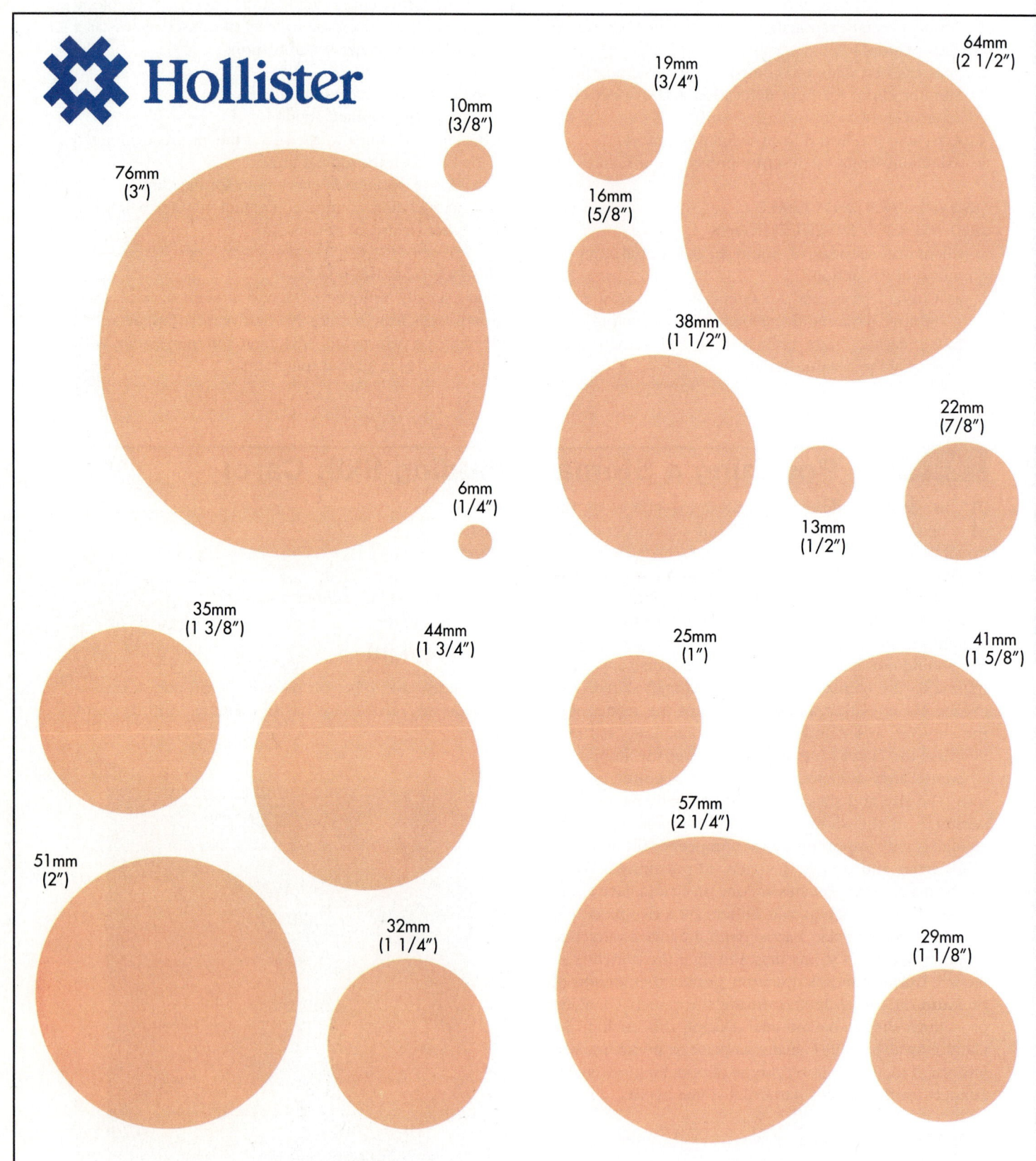

Figure 33-3 **A,** Measuring card. (Courtesy Hollister, Inc., Libertyville, Ill.)

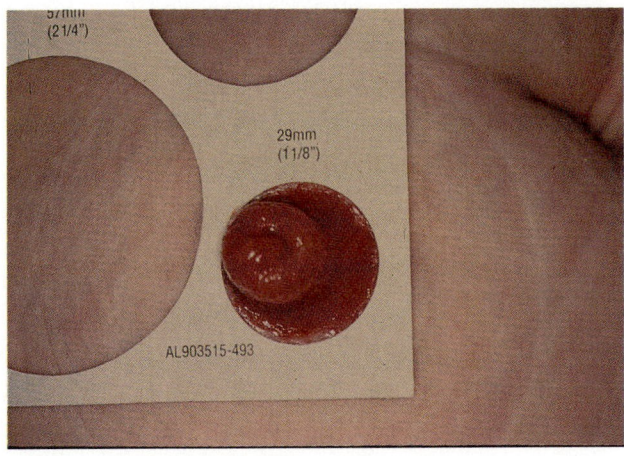

Figure 33-3, cont'd — **B,** Measuring an ostomy.

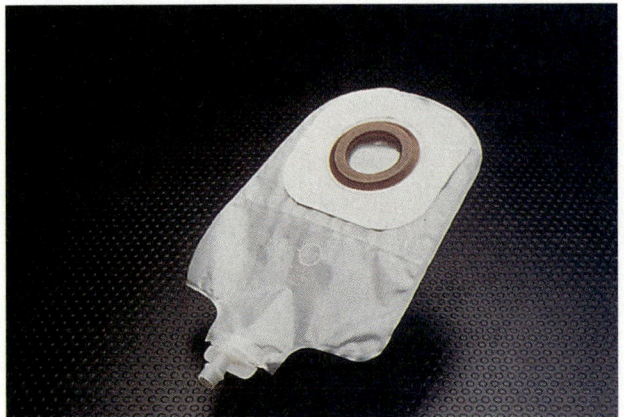

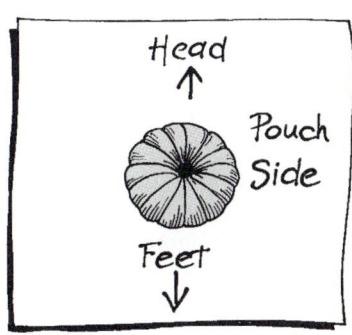

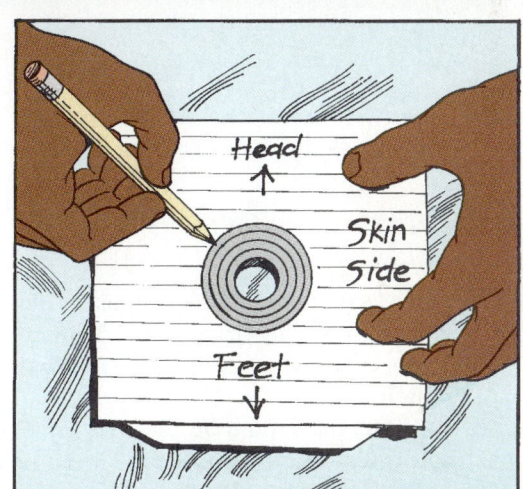

client ostomy is important when deciding on type of pouching system to use. Pouch type will vary as to amount and consistency of drainage and client's stoma characteristics.

2. Assess client's stoma for the following characteristics:
   a. *Size*: Use a measuring card to determine the correct size of the client's stoma (Figure 33-3). **Accurate stoma size is critical for planning and selecting ostomy pouch size.**
   b. *Shape:* If the stoma is round, use the precut, presized pouches as an option (Figure 33-4, *A*). **Irregularly shaped stomas require a custom cut shape made on the skin barrier to match the shape of the stoma** (Figure 33-4, *B* and *C*).

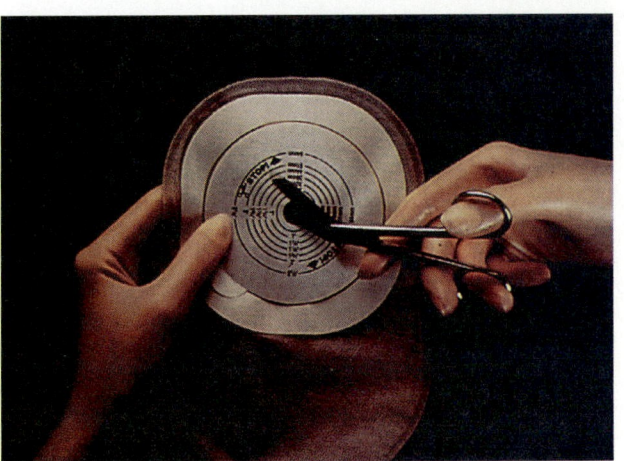

Figure 33-4 Steps for preparing skin barrier and pouch. (Courtesy Hollister, Inc., Libertyville, Ill.)

Table 33-1 **Characteristic Output of GI Stomas**

Type	Amount (ml)	Consistency	pH
Esophagostomy	1000-1500	Saliva	Slightly alkaline
Gastrostomy	2000-2500	Liquid	0.5-1.5
Jejunostomy	1000-3000	Liquid	Slightly acid
Ileostomy	750-1000	Toothpaste	Alkaline
Cecostomy and ascending colostomy	500-750	Toothpaste	Alkaline
Transverse colostomy		Mushy to semiformed	Alkaline
Descending and sigmoid colostomy		Semiformed to formed	Alkaline

Thelan LA, Davie JK, Urden LD: *Textbook of critical care nursing: diagnosis and management,* ed 2, St Louis, 1994, Mosby.

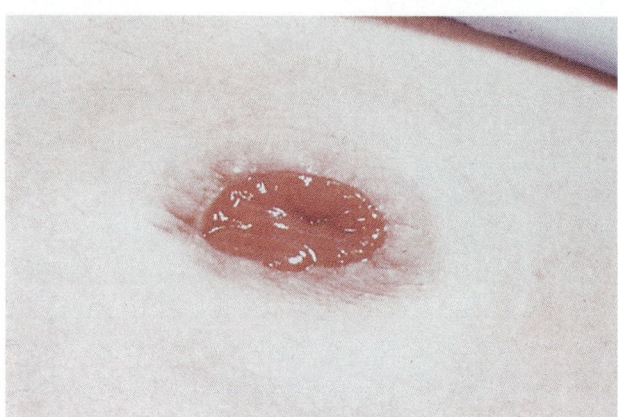

Figure 33-5 (Courtesy Hollister, Inc., Libertyville, Ill.)

c. *Type:* Determine whether stoma is flush to the skin or protruding (Figure 33-5). **Type of stoma is important when selecting skin barrier and pouch.**

d. *Color:* Stoma should be pink-red in color. **Dark-colored stoma can indicate stoma necrosis.**

e. *Effluent:* Determine amount and consistency of the fecal drainage from the stoma (Table 33-1). **Differences in drainage in the type of ostomies should be considered when selecting the ostomy pouch. Only a pouch designed for stool should be used.**

Planning

Expected outcomes focus on helping client adjust to life with an ostomy emotionally as well as physically when performing self–ostomy care, preventing peristomal skin breakdown, and containing effluent.

EXPECTED OUTCOMES

1. Client's skin remains intact.
2. Ostomy drainage is contained.
3. Client correctly demonstrates self-ostomy pouch and skin barrier change by discharge.
4. Client integrates the stoma into body image.

Implementation

Steps	Rationale
1. See Standard Protocol (Chapter 1, p. 5)	
2. Inspect pouch daily to see if it has to be emptied. **Empty ostomy pouch *before* pouch is half full.**	Minimizing leaking fosters a positive body image. A full, heavy ostomy pouch will break the seal and cause leakage.
3. For one-piece system	
a. Open end of drainable pouch and empty contents into bedpan or toilet.	Do not let effluent splash on client when emptying pouch. Observe effluent.
b. Rinse inside of pouch with a cup of warm water. Wipe and dry end of pouch.	Empties pouch of effluent and cleans the inside.

Steps	Rationale
c. Close end of pouch by applying the pouch closure device (or rubber band) according to manufacturer's instruction.	Lessens chance of pouch accidentally opening and stool coming out on client.
4. For two-piece system	
a. Hold one hand on skin barrier, and with other hand on pouch pull tab, remove pouch from skin barrier.	Avoid unnecessary removal of skin barrier.
b. Empty contents of pouch into toilet and observe effluent.	
c. Rinse pouch, clean, dry, and reattach to flange of skin barrier.	Some two-piece pouches can be reused. Others are disposable.
d. Close end of pouch by applying pouch closure device (or rubber band) according to manufacturer's instruction.	Lessens chance of pouch accidentally opening and stool coming out on the client.
Change ostomy pouch.	Only replace if pouch is leaking. Disposable pouches should not be routinely changed daily.
5. Remove pouch (one-piece system) or pouch and skin barrier (two-piece system) and discard according to hospital policy for universal precautions.	
6. Wash gently around stoma with warm water and washcloth.	Stoma may bleed slightly; this is normal.
7. Inspect stoma daily and peristomal skin for color (redness) and any trauma, such as ulceration, cuts, or necrosis (Table 33-2 and Figure 33-6).	

Table 33-2 **Peristomal Skin Damage**

Type or cause of damage	Appearance	Treatment principles
CHEMICAL DAMAGE Effluent in contact with skin Incorrect use of adhesives or solvents	Erythematous and denuded areas corresponding to leakage of effluent *or* areas of product use (adhesives, solvents)	Eliminate effluent contact with skin; allow adhesives to dry and remove solvents from skin. *Topical:* Skin barrier powder; sealants if needed
MECHANICAL DAMAGE (see Figure 33-6, *A*) Inappropriate skin care (scrubbing or "picking") Incorrect tape removal or fragile skin, resulting in "stripping" of epidermis	Patchy areas of erythema or denudation corresponding with areas subjected to trauma or "taped" areas	Eliminate cause; teach atraumatic skin care, appropriate tape removal, and use of sealants when indicated. *Topical:* Skin barriers (powder; with sealant as indicated; solid barriers until area has healed)
FUNGAL RASH (*CANDIDA*) (see Figure 33-6, *B*) Antibiotics resulting in fungal overgrowth Persistent skin moisture	Maculopapular rash with satellite lesions	Keep skin dry; eliminate pooled urine; restore normal flora. *Topical:* Antifungal powder and sealant as indicated
ALLERGIC REACTION Can be caused by any product	Areas of erythema or pruritus corresponding to area of skin exposed to allergen	Use patch test if needed to determine allergen; eliminate contact with allergen. *Topical:* Corticosteroid agent if needed for control of pruritus (cream or spray, not ointment, which would interfere with pouch adherence)

From Hampton BG, Bryant RA: *Ostomies and continent diversions: nursing management,* St Louis, 1992, Mosby.

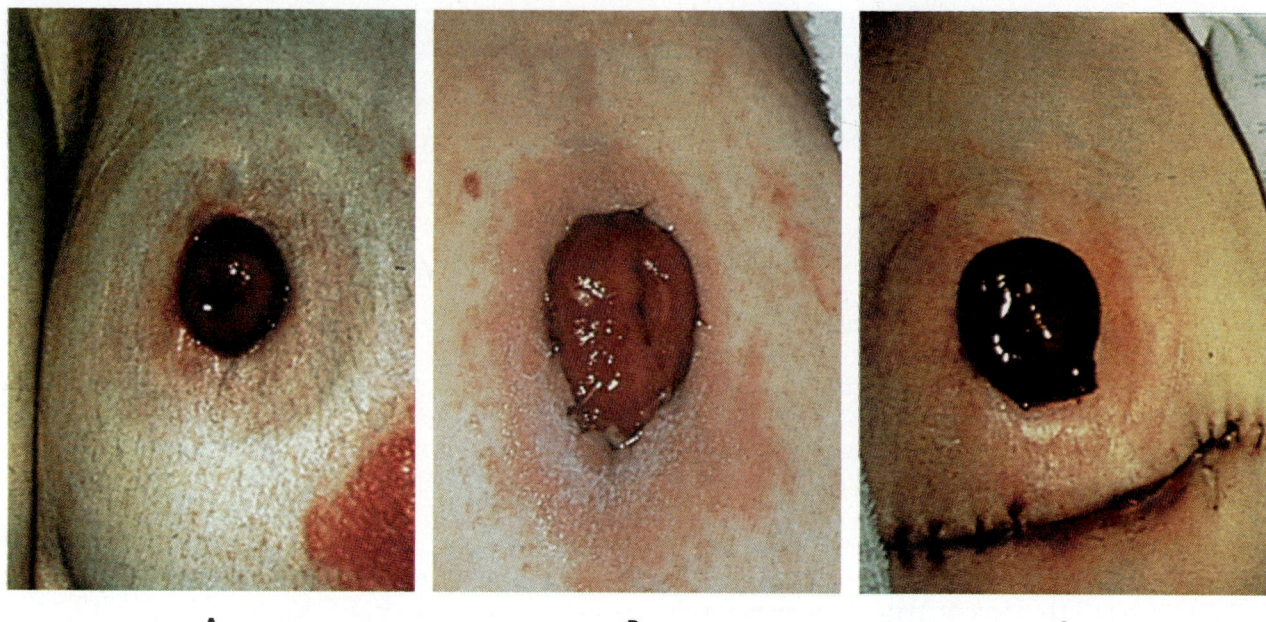

A   **B**   **C**

Figure 33-6 **A,** Mechanical injury. **B,** Candidiasis. **C,** Necrosis. (Courtesy Hollister, Inc., Libertyville, Ill.)

Steps	Rationale
8. Remeasure stoma using measuring card at each pouch change (see Figure 33-3).	Stoma will shrink postoperatively. Client's weight gain or loss can affect pouching needs.
9. Cut out ostomy pouch and attached skin barrier to proper stoma size (Figure 33-7). For two-piece system, apply skin barrier with flange first (Figure 33-8).	Leave $\frac{1}{8}$" for ileostomy and $\frac{1}{4}$" for colostomy of skin exposed around stoma when determining size to cut skin barrier (Hampton and Bryant, 1992). Prevents trauma to stoma.
10. Place skin barrier around stoma as single unit. Hold hand over it for a few minutes.	Enhances the sticking of skin barrier to peristomal skin.
11. Apply liquid deodorant to a small piece of tissue paper and drop in ostomy pouch or squirt a few drops directly into pouch.	Minimizes odor when emptying pouch.

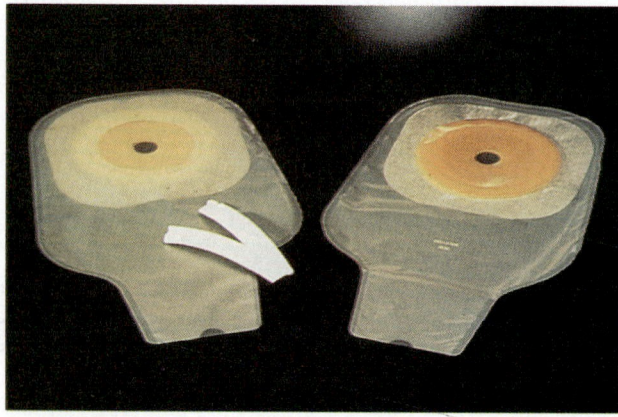

Figure 33-7 (Courtesy Hollister, Inc., Libertyville, Ill.)

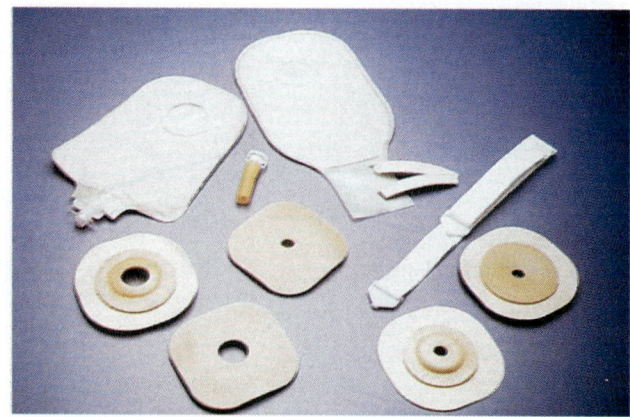

Figure 33-8 (Courtesy Hollister, Inc., Libertyville, Ill.)

Steps	Rationale
12. Close end of pouch using closure device. Gently tug on bottom of pouch to make sure it is closed properly.	
13. Reinforce skin barrier with tape on all four sides. Some pouches need a belt.	Gives added security.
14. Client and support person should be instructed in self-care of ostomy.	Client needs to have pouch care demonstrated.
15. Encourage client to touch stoma and refer to it by correct name of "stoma."	Nicknames for stoma may diminish the client's self-esteem.
16. Client should be encouraged to do own ostomy care on the second day or as early as feasible for individual client.	Learning is facilitated when learner is actively involved.
17. Give copy of printed ostomy literature/booklet to client. (See box for effects of food on output from stoma.)	This gives the opportunity to review diet and ostomy care and to assess level of understanding of printed materials.
18. Make referral for ostomy visitor to see client. Ideally these visits should be initiated before surgery.	Visit from another person with the same type of ostomy can help in client's acceptance of stoma.
19. Make arrangements for client to obtain supplies before discharge.	Client needs to know what ostomy supplies are needed and where to obtain them for self–ostomy care after discharge.
20. Make referral to a stoma specialist such as an enterostomal (ET) therapy nurse.	Specialists are an important resource in the care of clients with an ostomy.
21. See Completion Protocol (Chapter 1, p. 6).	

Effects of Food on Stoma Output

FOODS THAT THICKEN STOOL
Bananas
Rice
Bread
Potatoes
Creamy peanut butter
Applesauce
Cheese
Tapioca
Yogurt
Pasta
Pretzels
Marshmallows

FOODS THAT LOOSEN STOOL
Dried or string beans
Chocolate
Raw fruits
Raw vegetables
Highly spiced foods
Fried foods
Greasy foods
Prune or grape juice
Leafy green vegetables (lettuce, broccoli, spinach)

FOODS THAT COLOR STOOL
Beets
Red jello

FOODS THAT CAUSE STOOL ODOR
Fish
Eggs
Asparagus
Garlic
Some spices
Beans
Turnips
Cabbage family vegetables (onions, cabbage, brussel sprouts, broccoli, cauliflower)

FOODS THAT CAUSE URINE ODOR
Seafood
Asparagus

FOODS THAT CAUSE GAS
Dried and string beans
Beer
Carbonated beverages
Cucumbers
Cabbage family of vegetables (onions, brussel sprouts, cabbage, broccoli, cauliflower)
Dairy products
Spinach
Corn
Radishes

From Hampton BG, Bryant RA: *Ostomies and continent diversions: nursing management,* St Louis, 1992, Mosby.

Evaluation

1. Inspect peristomal skin for signs of skin breakdown and assess client's stoma status.
2. Monitor amount, color, consistency, and frequency of fecal elimination from the stoma. Check bag for leakage.
3. Observe client perform self-care of ostomy pouching.
4. Observe client's behavior when looking at stoma and handling equipment. Note whether client talks about stoma.

UNEXPECTED OUTCOMES AND RELATED INTERVENTIONS

1. Client's peristomal skin breaks down.
   a. Assess for causes of the skin breakdown.
   b. Remeasure the stoma size.
   c. Check if the selected pouch is correct for client's stoma size.
2. Client's skin barrier and pouch leak.
   a. Assess if client is waiting too long (e.g., if pouch is more than half full of stool) to empty pouch.
   b. Remeasure stoma and reevaluate pouch and skin barrier size.

   c. Determine if client is cutting out the correct size on the skin barrier (see Figure 33-4, *B*).
   d. Evaluate if stoma is in a skin fold or whether other irregularities exist (Figure 33-9).
   e. Assess for peristomal hernia (Figure 33-10).
   f. Determine whether a convex disk, skin barrier paste, or other measures are needed to prevent leakage (Young, 1992).
3. Client cannot do self-ostomy pouching change.
   a. Determine if client lacks the physical or mental ability to do self-ostomy care.
   b. Eliminate distractions and other factors (e.g., pain) that might interfere with client's performance of self-ostomy care.
   c. Reevaluate client's understanding of self-ostomy care.
   d. Reevaluate client's problems with self-image, coping skills, and support systems (Salter, 1992).

SAMPLE DOCUMENTATION

1600 Bud colostomy stoma is 1½", round, slightly swollen, and red in color. Peristomal skin is intact. Stoma is functioning × 3300ml of dark brownish liquid stool. Normal bowel sounds present. Two-piece ostomy pouching system with hydrocolloid skin barrier in place and intact. Client has not yet looked at stoma. Awaiting ostomy volunteer visitor. ET nurse began instruction of client's self-ostomy care technique.

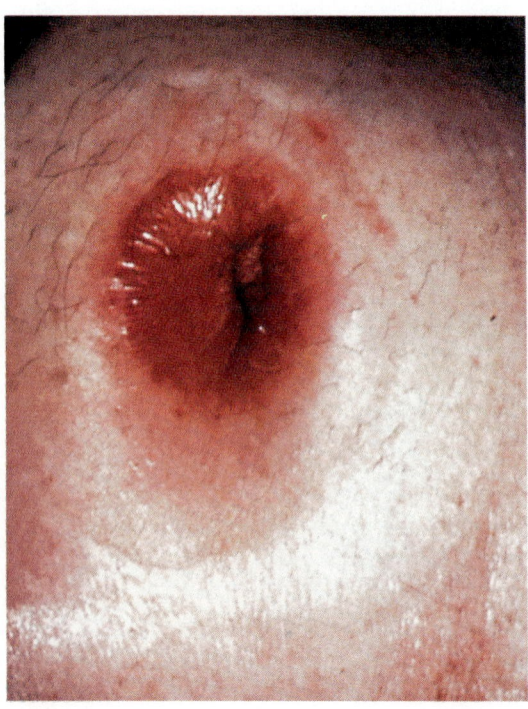

Figure 33-9 (Courtesy Hollister, Inc., Libertyville, Ill.)

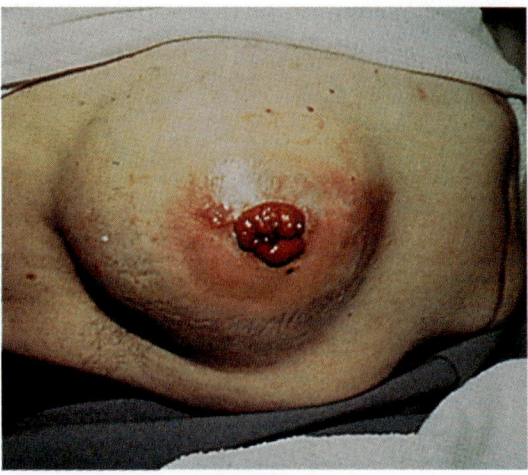

Figure 33-10 (Courtesy Hollister, Inc., Libertyville, Ill.)

Skill 33.3 | **Irrigating a Colostomy**

This skill includes the administration of an ordered irrigating solution into the colostomy stoma. Depending on the purpose of the irrigation, it can also include teaching the client how to perform the irrigation procedure.

The purpose of a colostomy irrigation is to cleanse the bowel of feces (e.g., before tests or surgical procedures or to relieve constipation) or to reestablish a pattern of regular bowel elimination after stoma surgery. The irrigation solution distends the bowel and stimulates it to empty the stool contents. Clients who choose this method of control over fecal elimination from the stoma need to learn the correct technique. Irrigations are usually only indicated for descending or sigmoid colostomies. Stomas more proximal in the intestine have more frequent and more liquid output, making the outcome of managing fecal elimination by irrigation not achievable. Another reason that clients with ileostomies do not irrigate is the possible additional problem of fluid and electrolyte imbalance. Not all clients will perform irrigation (Sanada, Kawashima, and Yamaguchi, 1992).

Other colostomy irrigation criteria to consider are the client's past history of bowel function (normal vs. irregular or diarrhea bowel elimination), ability to learn and perform the irrigation procedure, access to adequate toilet facilities and water, and personal preference. Irrigation is not usually recommended for children or young adults (potential bowel dependency problems) or clients having pelvic or abdominal irradiation, those with a temporary colostomy, clients with a poor prognosis, or those who have a stomal prolapse or peristomal hernia.

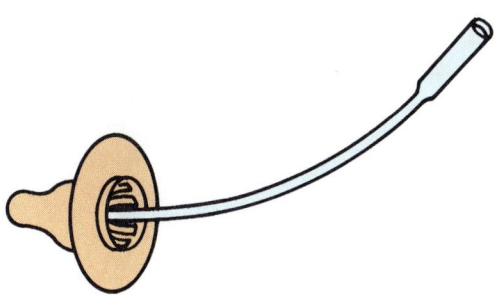

Figure 33-11

EQUIPMENT

Disposable clean gloves
Ostomy irrigation set
    Irrigation cone (Figure 33-11)
    Irrigation sleeve with appropriate closure device
    Ostomy belt (if needed for particular irrigation sleeve)
    Irrigation solution bag with attached tubing and flow
       control clamp
Water-soluble lubricant
Irrigating solution as ordered (warm water or normal
    saline)
Ostomy pouch
Toilet tissue
Bedpan or toilet
Documentation record

Assessment

1. Assess client's level of comfort (using a scale of 0 to 10) and need for pain management. **Administer pain medication and institute non-pharmacologic measures to control pain before procedure.**
2. Assess appropriateness of routine irrigation as a management option. **Only clients with a descending or sigmoid colostomy are appropriate candidates because the stool is more formed and less liquid.**
3. Assess client's ability to manipulate irrigation equipment and to understand concepts of bowel management. **Client must have the mental and physical capability to master the irrigation technique.**
4. Assess client's readiness to learn self–colostomy irrigation. **Client must decide if this management option of regulating fecal elimination is consistent with life-style and personal preferences.**

Planning

Expected outcomes focus on regular bowel evacuation and client learning to perform the colostomy irrigation.

EXPECTED OUTCOMES

1. Client achieves regular bowel movements from the stoma with no leakage between irrigations.
2. Client independently does the colostomy irrigation procedure.

Implementation

Steps	Rationale
1. See Standard Protocol (Chapter 1, p. 5).	
2. Teach client how to do self–colostomy irrigation. Start by having client do a few steps of the irrigation procedure.	Teaching is more effective when client is actively involved. Do not overwhelm client with amount of information taught at each session.
3. Determine specific time of day to do colostomy irrigation that fits into client's life-style.	To achieve predictable regulation of feces from colostomy, irrigation should be done at the same time of day. One hour after largest meal of the day, at client's convenience, and when client has a regular time for bowel movement each day are important factors to consider when planning.
4. Have client sit on toilet seat. Turn hospital gown around so that client's back is covered. If client cannot sit on toilet, have client sit on a chair next to toilet. If client cannot get out of bed, place a bedpan next to client on side that stoma is located.	Do not overexpose client because chilling may occur.
5. Remove client's pouch and dispose of according to hospital policy for universal precautions.	
6. Lubricate client's little finger and gently guide it into stoma for about 1 inch to learn the direction or angle of bowel from stoma. Have client hold finger in stoma for about 1 minute.	Teaches client the direction of the colon and helps dilate stoma. If bright-red blood is noted when client removes finger, reassure client that this will occasionally happen because mucosa bleeds readily because of higher vascularity in this area.
7. Place irrigation sleeve over client's stoma. Angle sleeve for appropriate flow of fecal returns (e.g., if client is using bedpan at 45 degrees). Angle of irrigation sleeve facilitates flow of fecal returns. Know particular use of the selected irrigation equipment. Some irrigation sleeves attach to flange of the two-piece skin barrier. Some sleeves require use of a belt. If so, adjust belt so it fits comfortably and is not too tight or too loose (Beare and Myers, 1994).	Make sure irrigation sleeve is correctly attached. End of sleeve *must* be in toilet or bedpan to prevent spillage of feces. 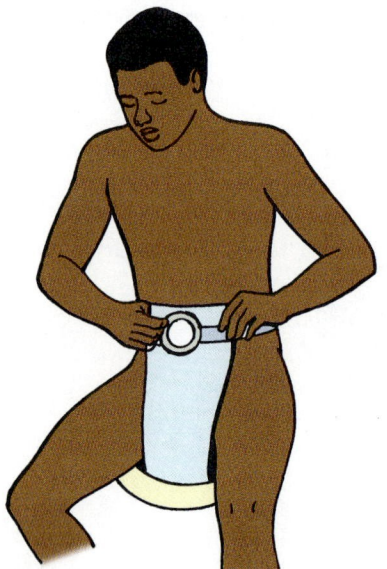
8. Use an irrigation cone (see Figure 33-11). Do not use a catheter or regular enema set.	Irrigation cone prevents backflow. Catheter or regular enema set can perforate bowel.
9. Prepare the irrigation solution bag. 　a. Close flow control clamp on irrigation solution bag.	

Steps	Rationale
b. Fill irrigation solution bag with appropriate amount and temperature of irrigation solution. Tepid water or normal saline are irrigation solutions used.	If solution is too hot, it can burn bowel. If too cold, it can cause cramps.
c. Hold irrigation solution bag up to check correct amount of irrigation solution.	Initially, 500 ml may be used. No more than 1000 ml should be used.
d. Open flow control clamp and allow solution to run through irrigation solution bag tubing so that all air is removed from tubing.	Prevents air from entering colon and causing cramping.
e. Close flow control clamp and apply water-soluble lubricant to irrigation cone.	Lubricant makes insertion of irrigation cone easier.

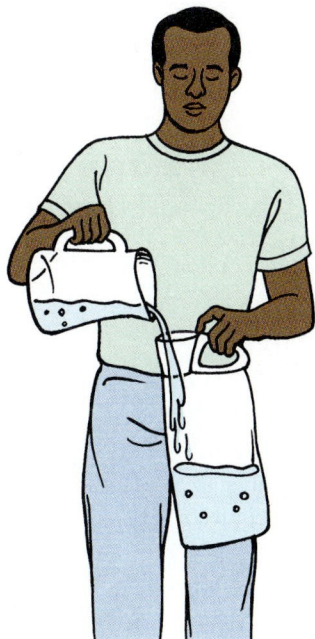

10. Place irrigation solution bag so that bottom of bag is at client's shoulder level when client is sitting.	This position prevents too high a pressure and reduces possibility of bowel damage.

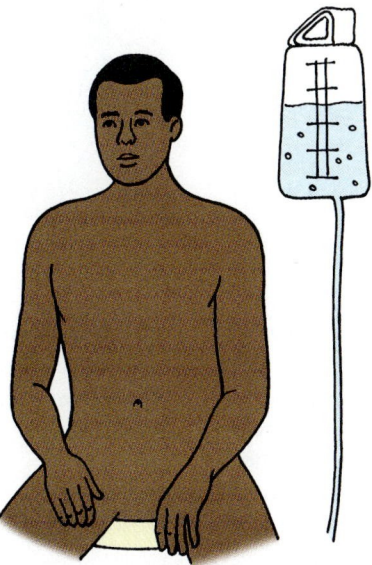

Steps	Rationale

11. Insert tip of irrigating cone into stoma (Figure 33-12). Gentle pressure should be used to hold tip in place in stoma.

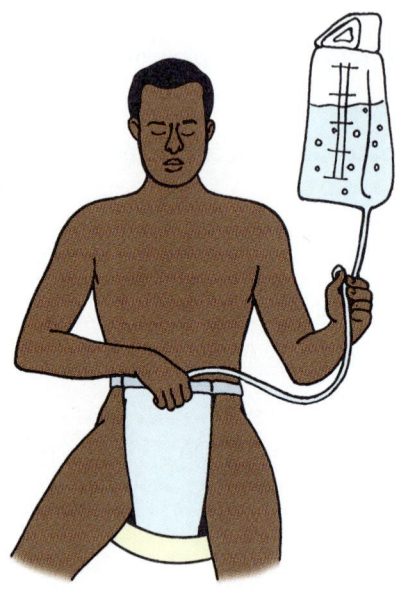

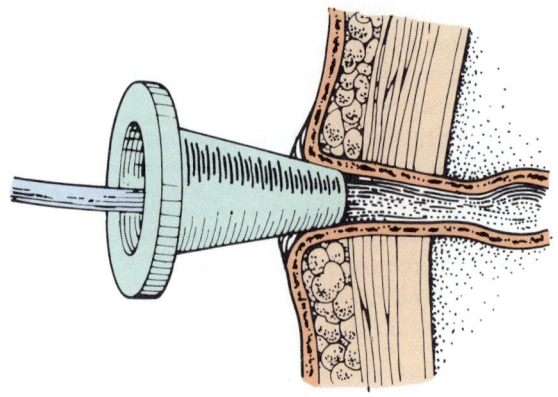

Figure 33-12

nurse alert To prevent damage to bowel, do *not* insert entire length of irrigation cone into stoma. Too little pressure will cause the irrigation to flow on side of cone and not into client. Too much pressure can block flow of irrigation solution into client.

12. Open flow control clamp and allow the solution to flow into client. This should take 5 to 10 minutes. If there is no flow, recheck direction of cone (Figure 33-13).

Too rapid instillation of irrigation solution can adversely affect client.

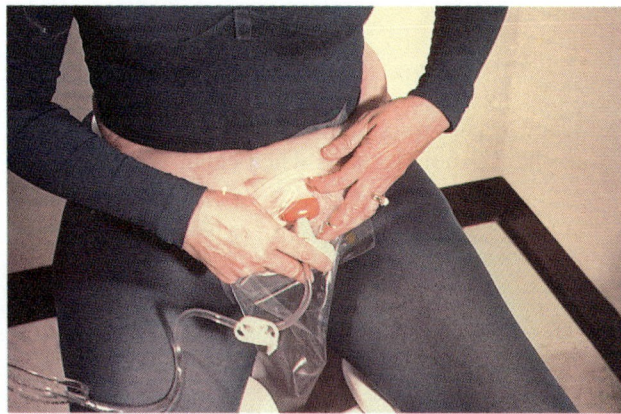

Figure 33-13

13. If cramping occurs, reduce or stop flow of irrigation fluid.

14. When all the irrigation fluid has been instilled into client's stoma, close flow control clamp and remove irrigation cone from stoma. For some irrigation sleeves, top should now be closed using the appropriate closure method (e.g., zip-lock top, clothespins).

Client's complaint of abdominal cramps indicates need to stop irrigating and wait until cramps subside.

Proper use of irrigation equipment will prevent spillage of feces.

Steps	Rationale

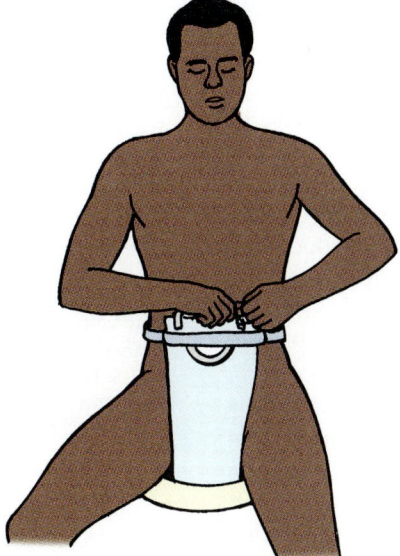

15. Initial evacuation of stool from stoma takes 10 to 20 minutes.

Make sure end of irrigation sleeve is in toilet or bedpan.

16. After initial evacuation of stool is over, close end of irrigation sleeve with the clip or closure device and await the secondary evacuation. Client may get off toilet and walk around at this time.

Client may walk around, shower, or shave. Exercise stimulates bowel.

17. When the secondary return flow stops (about 30 minutes), rinse irrigation sleeve with water to remove any stool, then remove sleeve. Hang washed irrigation sleeve up to dry.

Some irrigation sleeves are reusable.

18. Wipe stoma with toilet tissue to remove any stool. Put an appropriate colostomy pouch over stoma. If client is using a two-piece pouching system, place a new flange cap or closed-end pouch onto skin barrier (see Skill 33.2).

An appropriate pouch or cap may be worn to contain feces in case of elimination between irrigations.

19. See Completion Protocol (Chapter 1, p. 6).

Evaluation

1. Observe amount and character of fecal material and fluid that is returned after the irrigation. Assess degree to which regularity of bowel movements is being achieved. Does client have fecal drainage between irrigations?
2. Observe client's response to the irrigation procedure. Assess client's knowledge and ability to do the irrigation procedure.

UNEXPECTED OUTCOMES AND RELATED INTERVENTIONS

1. Client has feces from the colostomy stoma between irrigations.

   a. Reassess if client is an appropriate candidate for this management option.
   b. Evaluate whether anything has changed in client's treatment plan or life-style that could account for this finding.
   c. Evaluate whether client understands to follow the schedule for irrigation at the same time each day.
   d. Evaluate if sufficient time has occurred since beginning the irrigation routine (6 to 8 weeks) to allow the bowel time to react to the irrigation stimulus.

2. Client cannot independently perform the irrigation procedure correctly.

a. Reassess client's self-irrigation technique for accuracy.

b. Observe client perform the irrigation technique, and monitor for errors in technique that could account for this finding.

3. Client has no fecal returns after the irrigation.

a. Evaluate client for possible postoperative ileus or obstruction. More often, lack of fecal returns may indicate that client is dehydrated.

b. Encourage client to increase fluid intake, to alter diet intake if constipated, and to wear a pouch that can contain the expected fecal output until the next scheduled irrigation.

SAMPLE DOCUMENTATION

0800 Second colostomy irrigation done in bathroom by client with minimal nurse assistance. 500 ml lukewarm water instilled easily into stoma using cone applicator. Effective for large amount of brownish fluid and semisoft stool. Tolerated procedure well, no cramping or complaints. Correctly replaced ostomy pouch onto ostomy skin barrier at end of irrigation procedure. States, "Feels like I'm beginning to do this right."

CRITICAL THINKING EXERCISES

1. You suspect a fecal impaction in a 71-year-old female under your nursing care.
   a. Identify your first nursing action.
   b. What piece of data is important to obtain before beginning the digital examination? Explain.
   c. During the procedure you note the client's pulse is 54. What should you do?

2. During a routine change of a client's ostomy appliance you note that the peristomal skin is red and inflamed. How would you revise nursing care measures to address this problem?

3. You are in the process of irrigating a client's colostomy. After preparing the irrigant and placing the irrigation sleeve over the client's stoma, you begin infusing the irrigant via a cone applicator. The irrigant begins to leak around the cone.
   a. What should you do?
   b. Twenty minutes after instillation of 500 ml of lukewarm water, the client has no fecal return. What are your options at this point?

4. Velma is a 66-year-old female hospitalized for a respiratory tract infection. She has a descending colostomy and states she has been having trouble with loose stools and gas. She asks for your assistance in selecting the day's meals from the hospital menu. Which food selections would you encourage Velma to choose?

Breakfast	Lunch	Dinner
Scrambled eggs	Rice pilaf	Fried chicken
Bacon strips	Baked chicken	Baked potato
Cheese omelet	Hamburger	Noodles Alfredo
Apple sauce	French fries	Green beans
Prune juice	Corn	Broccoli
Banana	Tapioca pudding	Peas
Toast	Apple	Dinner roll
Milk	7-Up	Chocolate cake
Coffee	Milk	Vanilla yogurt

REFERENCES

Beare PG, Myers JL: *Principles and practice of adult health nursing,* ed 2, St Louis, 1994, Mosby.

Fazio VW, Tjandra JJ: Prevention and management of ileostomy complications, *J ET Nurs* 19(2):48, 1992.

Gloeckner M: Perceptions of sexuality after ostomy surgery, *J Enterostom Ther* 18 (1):36, 1991.

Hampton BG, Bryant RA: *Ostomies and continent diversions: nursing management,* St Louis, 1992, Mosby.

Krainski MM: The role of hardiness in adjustment to an ostomy, *Ostomy Wound Manage* 40 (4):52, 1994.

Nadler LH: General considerations and complications of the ileostomy, *Ostomy Wound Manage* 38 (4):18, 1992.

Pieper B: Persons who have stomas: violent injury versus disease, *J ET Nurs* 19 (1):7, 1992.

Quayle BK: Making positive choices: body image and the new ostomy patient, *Ostomy Wound Manage* 40 (4):16, 1994.

Ramer L: Self-image changes with time in the cancer patient with a colostomy after operation, *J ET Nurs* 19 (6):195, 1992.

Rheaume A, Gooding BA: Social support, coping strategies, and long-term adaptation to ostomy among self-help group members, *J Enterostom Ther* 18 (1):11, 1991.

Salter MJ: Aspects of sexuality for patients with stomas and continent pouches, *J ET Nurs* 19 (4):126, 1992.

Sanada H, Kawashima K, Yamaguchi A: Natural evacuation versus irrigation, *Ostomy Wound Manage* 38 (4):24, 1992.

Thelan LA, Davie JK, Urden LD: *Textbook of critical care nursing: diagnosis and management,* ed 2, St Louis, 1994, Mosby.

Wilson RE: Patient education sheets, *Ostomy Wound Manage* 38 (4):45, 1992.

Young MJ: Convexity in the management of problem stomas, *Ostomy Wound Manage* 38 (4):53, 1992.

ADDITIONAL READINGS

Kelly M: Mind and body: stoma body image, *Nurs Times* 90(42):48, 1994.

Klop A: Body image and self esteem among individuals with stomas, *J Enterostomal Ther* 17:98, 1990.

Paulford-Lecher N: Teaching your patient stoma care, *Nurs* 23(9):47, 1993

chapter 34

Altered Urinary Elimination

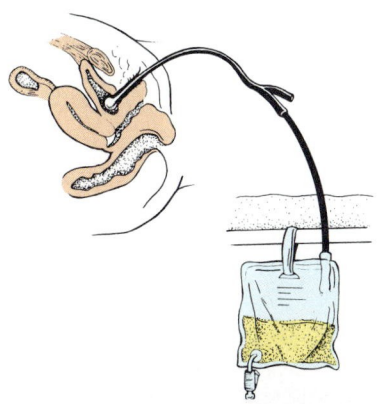

Skill 34.1
Urinary Catheterization

Skill 34.2
Urinary Diversions

Skill 34.3
Continuous Bladder Irrigation

Skill 34.4
Suprapubic Catheters

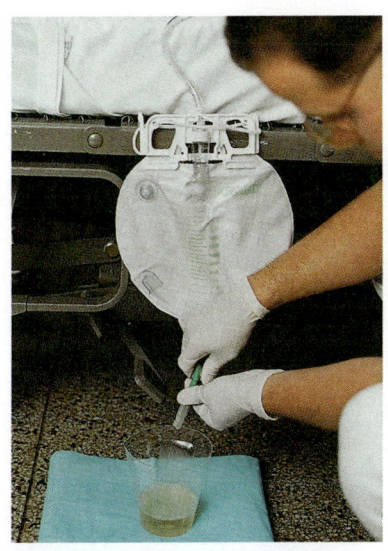

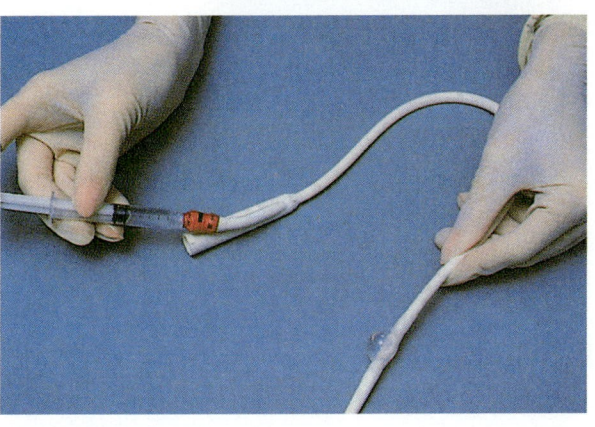

U rinary elimination, micturition, is a necessary natural process in clients. Clients normally urinate or void through the genitourinary system. When the urinary system fails to function properly, virtually all body systems can be affected. Normal urine output is at least 30 ml per hour or a total of 1 to 2 L per day.

The urinary system consists of two kidneys, where wastes are removed from blood to form urine. Urine passes through the two ureters and on into the bladder (Figure 34-1). Once the bladder has accumulated 250 to 300 ml of urine, a signal is sent to the central nervous system indicating fullness and the need to void. Once the bladder contracts, urine passes through the urethra to the urinary meatus (Figures 34-2 and 34-3).

If urine flow is altered, the client may have an indwelling catheter or suprapubic catheter to assist in correcting the body's inability to empty the bladder. At other times, urine must be redirected to another outlet, a urinary diversion. Urinary diversions are ostomies or openings coming from the bladder, ureters, or kidneys to the outer wall of the abdomen. Another intervention to correct altered urine flow may be irrigating the catheters to prevent obstruction of urine flow.

Clients may have altered body images with urinary system dysfunctions. The urinary system is a very private body part and one that is not seen or freely discussed. When an external device, such as a urinary diversion or an indwelling catheter, is used, the client's body image may be further altered. Privacy, confidentiality, and expla-

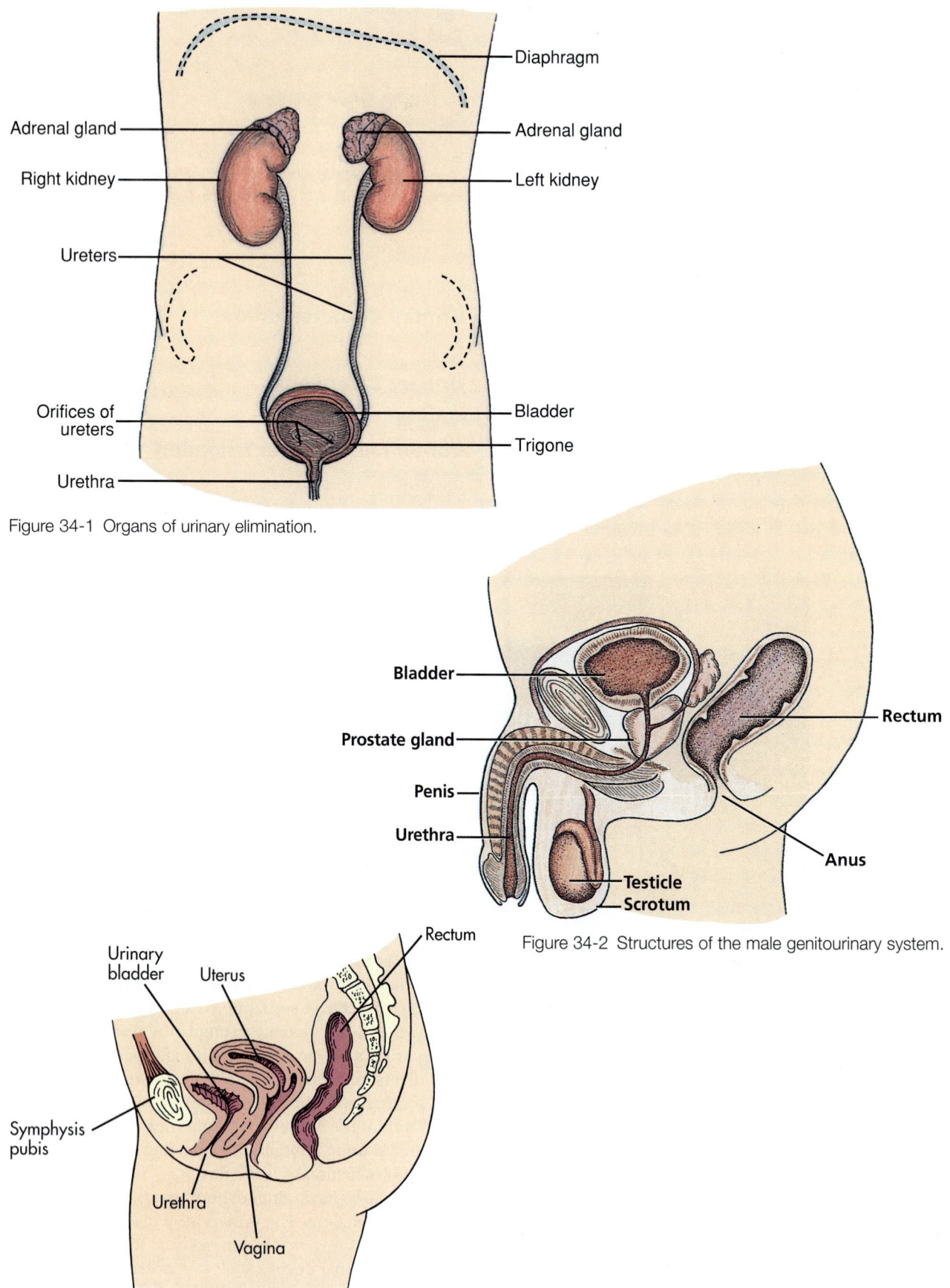

Figure 34-1 Organs of urinary elimination.

Figure 34-2 Structures of the male genitourinary system.

Figure 34-3 Structures of the female genitourinary system.

nations are necessary interventions when dealing with altered urinary elimination.

Nursing Diagnosis

Clients with altered urinary elimination may have a nursing diagnosis of **Risk for Infection** related to urinary retention, inadequate perineal hygiene, or lack of knowledge of care for the urinary catheter or urinary stomas. **Urinary Retention** may result from obstructions, paralysis, or inadequate muscle tone of the bladder. Several diagnoses pertaining to **Incontinence (Functional, Reflex, Stress, Total,** and **Urge)** are appropriate depending on whether the client has neurological deficits or bladder dysfunction. **Impaired Skin Integrity** related to inadequate knowledge of care for urinary stomas or to irritation from adhesive around the stoma may be appropriate.

Another possible nursing diagnosis is **Sexual Dysfunction** related to presence of a catheter for a prolonged time or to altered body image. **Social Isolation** may be appropriate when a client consciously or unconsciously believes that limited involvement with other people is imposed by physical changes or by anxiety related to altered body image. **Ineffective Family Coping** may be appropriate when family members are unable to support adaptation to artificial urinary devices.

Skill 34.1 | Urinary Catheterization (Male and Female)

Catheterization of the bladder involves introducing a rubber or plastic tube through the urethra and into the bladder. This provides a continuous flow of urine. Aseptic technique must be used when inserting a catheter into the urinary meatus because the urinary system is sterile. An indwelling or a straight catheter may be used to relieve the bladder of urine either because obstructions are present (e.g., from cancer or trauma), to obtain a urine specimen, to prevent the leakage of urine when performing a surgical procedure (e.g., a hysterectomy), or as a last resort, to assist the client who is incontinent of urine. Intermittent catheterization is preferable to indwelling catheterization (Davey, 1994), as the liklihood of a urinary tract infection is reduced.

EQUIPMENT
Catheter kit with appropriate catheter (size and type) (Figure 34-4)
Urinary drainage device
Extra sterile gloves and catheter
Clean gloves
Bath cloth, towel, soap and basin for water
Flashlight or lamp
Flat sheet or bath blanket
Measuring container

Assessment

1. Assess client's weight, age, level of consciousness, ability to cooperate, and mobility of lower extremities. **This determines how much assistance is needed holding client's legs in correct position.**
2. Assess client's prior experience with catheterizations. **History of previous catheterizations affects client's likelihood to cooperate.**
3. Palpate for bladder over the symphysis pubis.

4. Observe perineal region, observing for anatomical landmarks, erythema, drainage, or discharge.
5. Ask client to give the time of the last voiding and to describe urine (if nurse did not observe). **Determines if urinary retention is likely.**
6. Ask client to check chart for allergy to betadine.

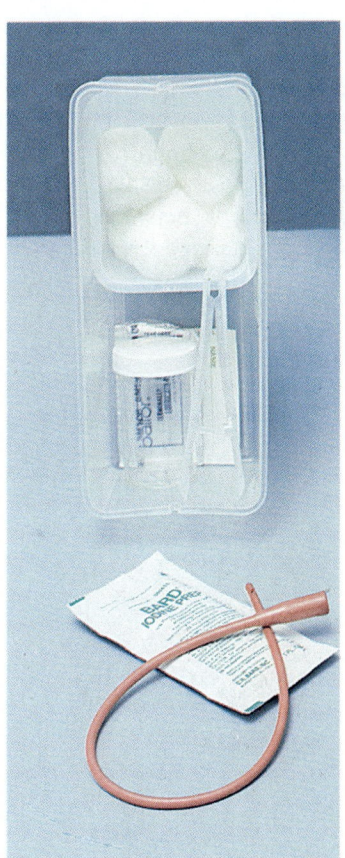

Figure 34-4

Planning

Expected outcomes focus on emptying bladder and client comfort.

EXPECTED OUTCOMES

1. After the catheter is inserted, no more than 750 ml is allowed to drain at one time.
2. Client has a urine output of at least 30 ml/hr.
3. Client's bladder is not distended.
4. Client verbalizes comfort following procedure.

Implementation

Steps	Rationale

> **nurse alert**   Check for history of urethral obstruction. Pathological conditions such as enlarged prostate gland (male) may impair passage of catheter and alter choice of catheter size.

1. See Standard Protocol (Chapter 1, p. 5).
2. Explain procedure to client and describe expected sensation of pressure/burning.
3. Assist female client into dorsal recumbent position (on back with knees flexed).
4. Drape with bath blanket so that only perineum is exposed (Figure 34-5).
5. Assist male client to lie flat, with legs abducted.
6. Drape upper body with small sheet or towel, and cover legs with sheet so that only genital area is exposed (Figure 34-6).
7. Place catheter kit on overbed table and open outer wrap using sterile technique.
8. Put on sterile gloves (see Skill 14.1).
9. Position equipment between or to the side of client's legs, maintaining sterility of gloves.

Anticipatory preparation may relieve anxiety.

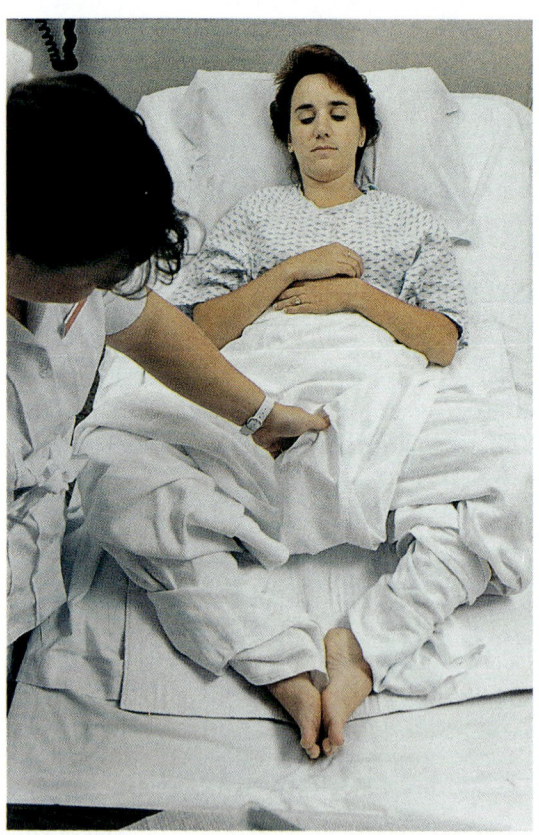

Figure 34-5

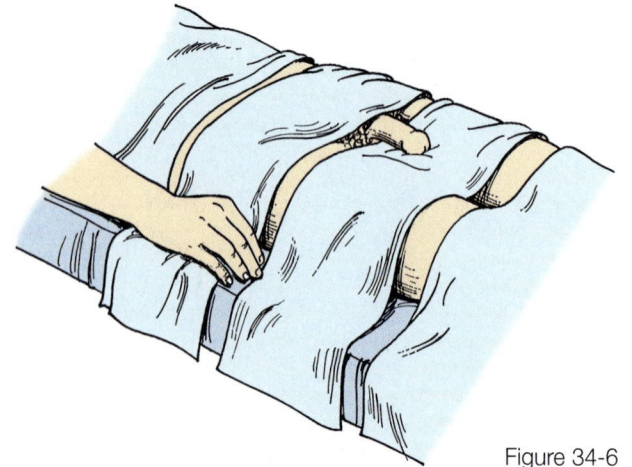

Figure 34-6

Steps	Rationale

10. Prepare equipment.
  a. Check bag clamp.
  b. Test balloon by injecting saline into balloon port (Figure 34-7). Withdraw if no leakage.
  c. Lubricate catheter with water-soluble gel.
  d. Open specimen container if needed.
  e. Pour antiseptic solution over all but one cotton ball.

Prevents urine leakage.
Ensures proper inflation and deflation.
Makes insertion easier.

Dry cotton ball is used to remove excess antiseptic solution from meatus.

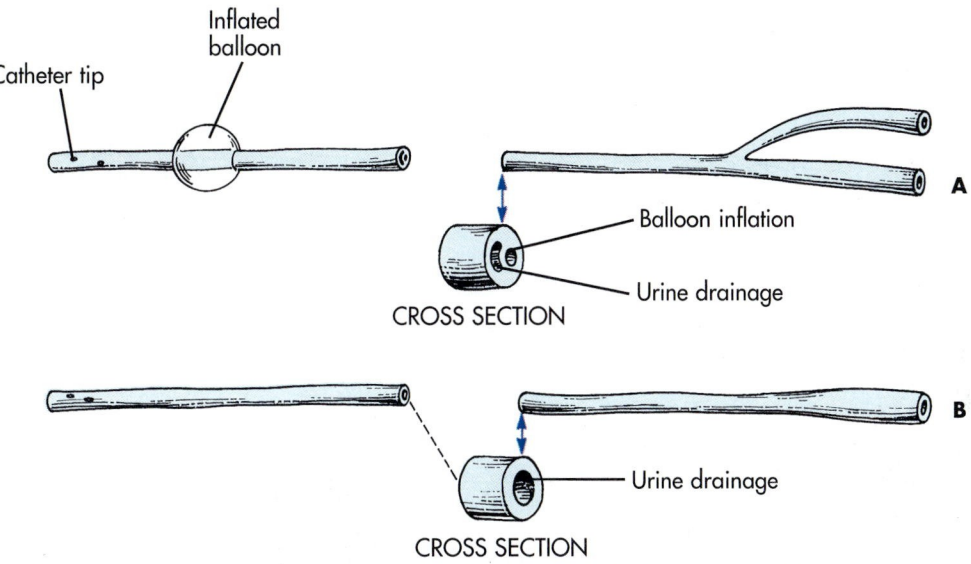

Figure 34-7 Types of urinary catheters: **A,** indwelling (Foley) catheter; **B,** straight catheter.

11. Cleansing and catheter insertion: female
  a. Place sterile drape under buttocks, touching only corners. Client's knees are flexed.
  b. Separate labia with fingers of nondominant hand (now contaminated). This hand remains in this position for remainder of the procedure.
  c. Cleanse labia and meatus.
  (1) With dominant hand (sterile), use forceps to hold cotton balls.
  (2) Use each cotton ball for one stroke.
  (3) Cleanse from anterior to posterior.
  (4) First stroke is on farthest side from nurse and closest to meatus.
  (5) Second stroke is on side of meatus closest to nurse (Figure 34-8).

Prevents labia from contaminating area being cleansed.

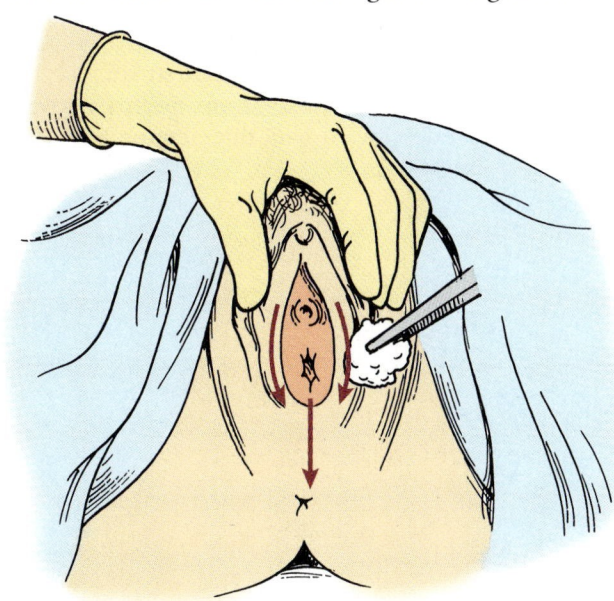

Figure 34-8

  (6) Third stroke is down center of meatus.

Cleanses from clean to dirty areas.

Steps	Rationale

d. If meatus is difficult to visualize, have a second person hold a flashlight or direct a lamp.

e. Insert catheter until urine flows, then advance another 1 to 2 inches (2 to 5 cm) for a total of 3 to 4 inches (7 to 10 cm) (Figure 34-9).

Female urethra is 2 to 3 inches (5 to 7 cm) long.

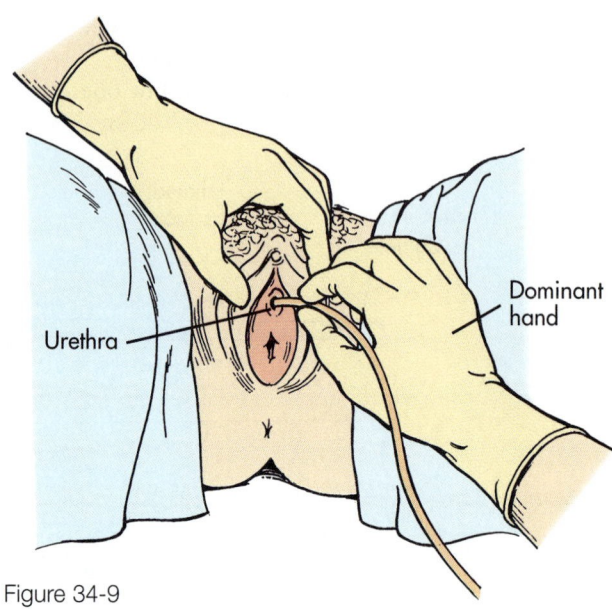

Figure 34-9

12. Cleansing and catheter insertion: male

a. Touching only corners, place sterile drape with hole centered over penis (optional).

Provides sterile field.

b. Hold penis at right angle to body with nondominant hand (now contaminated). This hand remains in this position for remainder of the procedure.

Opens urethra.

c. Use forceps to hold cotton balls and cleanse penis and meatus with dominant hand (sterile).

(1) Retract foreskin, if present, with nondominant hand.

(2) Use forceps to hold cotton balls.

(3) Use each cotton ball for one stroke.

(4) Use circular strokes from meatus outward and downward with three cotton balls (Figure 34-10).

Cleanses from clean to dirty areas.

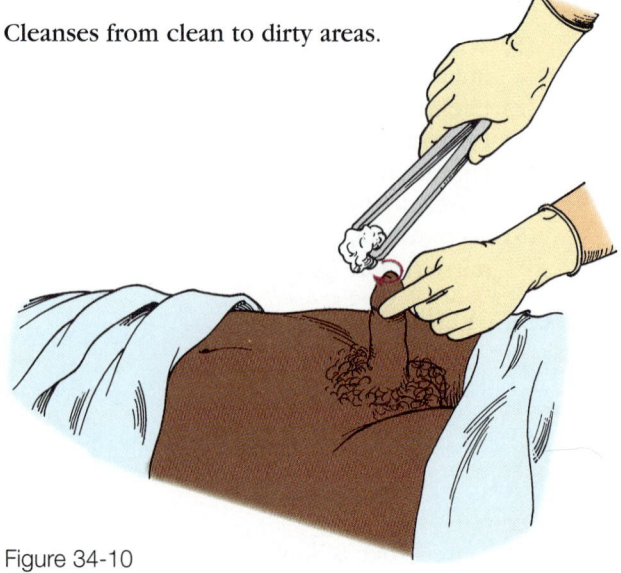

Figure 34-10

Steps	Rationale

d. Insert catheter with dominant hand until urine flows, then advance another 1 to 2 inches (2 to 5 cm) for a total of 7 to 9 inches (17 to 22 cm).

Male urethra is 6 to 8 inches (15 to 20 cm) long. Often only 2 to 3 inches of catheter is visible after insertion.

13. Hold catheter securely in place until:

a. Bladder is empty.

or

b. Inflate catheter balloon with normal saline, then pull gently on catheter until resistance is met (Figure 34-11). Nondominant hand may be used to hold syringe and plunger.

or

c. Urine specimen is obtained (volume depends on laboratory test ordered).

Allows catheter to settle against neck of bladder.

nurse alert After approximately 750 ml of urine has drained, clamp for 20 minutes, then unclamp. This prevents bladder spasms.

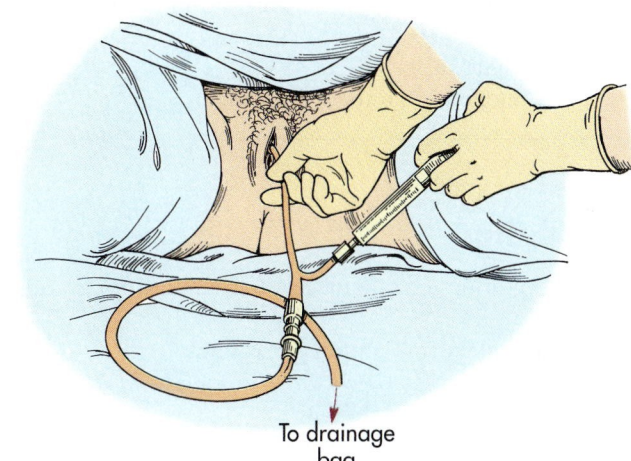

To drainage bag

Figure 34-11

14. Remove straight catheter, pulling slowly but evenly.

Reduces trauma to urethra.

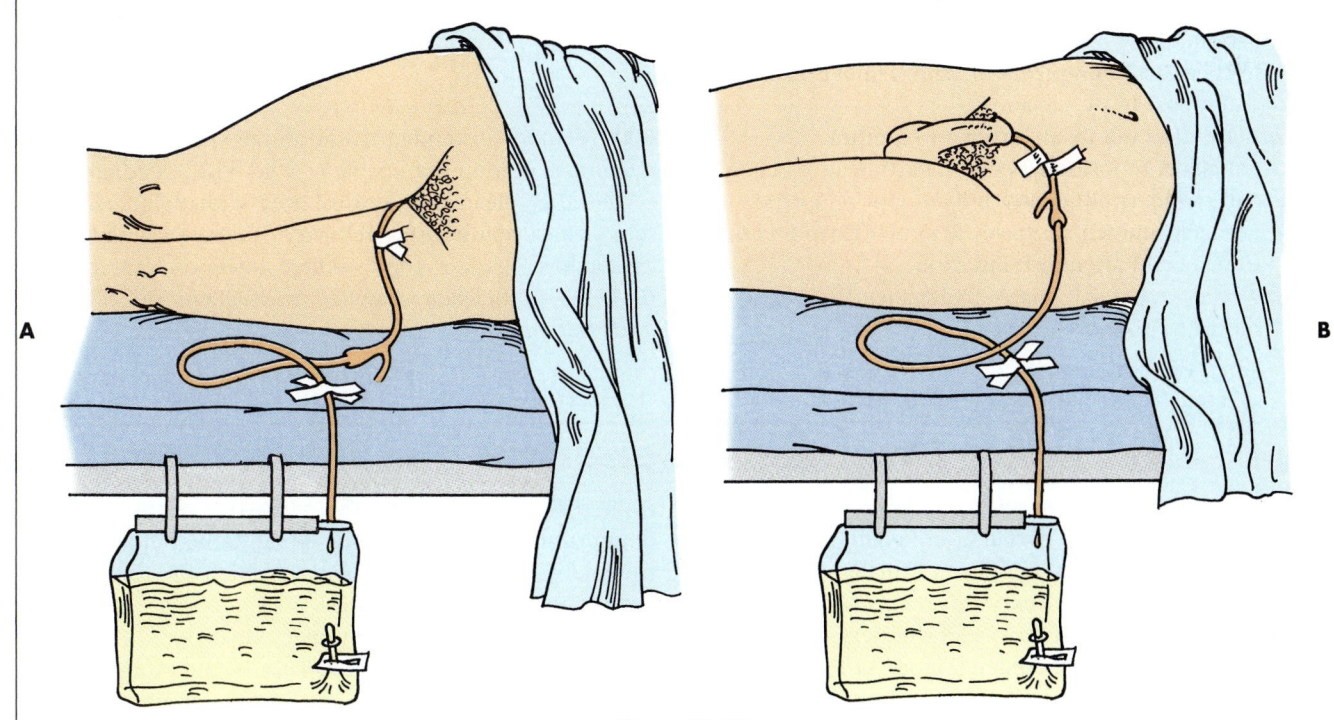

Figure 34-12

Steps	Rationale

15. Secure indwelling catheter and attach to drainage bag.
  a. **Female:** Secure to inner thigh with tape or catheter strap (Figure 34-12, *A*).
  b. **Male:** Secure to lower abdomen with tape or catheter strap (Figure 34-12, *B*). Replace foreskin if present.	

16. Position drainage bag lower than bladder and coil tubing on bed.	Prevents reflux of urine. Catheter drains by gravity.
17. Cleanse and dry perineal area. Position client for comfort.	Betadine is irritating to skin.
18. Measure urine.	Monitors output as baseline assessment.
19. See Completion Protocol (Chapter 1, p. 6).	

Evaluation

1. Observe urine in catheter bag for amount, color, and clarity.
2. Measure intake and output per routine.
3. Palpate bladder.
4. Ask client if comfortable.

UNEXPECTED OUTCOMES AND RELATED INTERVENTIONS

1. Client complains of discomfort during inflation of balloon.
   a. Stop immediately—if not advanced far enough in urethra, could cause serious trauma to urethra.
   b. Advance another 1 inch (2.5 cm) and reattempt inflation.
   c. If client still complains of pain, remove catheter and report to physician.
2. Catheter does not insert easily into urethra.
   a. For male, reposition penis toward head of client and retract (pull) gently and attempt reinsertion.
   b. For male and female, have client take deep breaths to relax and attempt reinsertion.
   c. Never force if still unable to advance. Remove and report to physician.

3. Catheter goes into vagina.
   a. Leave catheter in vagina.
   b. Reclean urinary meatus. With another sterile catheter, insert catheter into meatus.
   c. Remove catheter in vagina after inserting second catheter in bladder.
4. Sterility is broken during catheterization by nurse or client.
   a. Replace gloves if contaminated and start over.
   b. If client places foot or body part in sterile field, but not on equipment, do not use that part of the sterile field.
   c. If client touches equipment, nurse *must* replace with sterile items or replace with new kit and start over.

SAMPLE DOCUMENTATION

0800 Bladder distended 4 cm above symphysis pubis. C/O full sensation but unable to void. #18 Fr catheter inserted after cleansing perineal area with Betadine. 700 ml of clear yellow urine returned. Tolerated with "mild discomfort." Bladder nondistended, lower abdomen soft. Catheter to bedside drainage with client on rt. side with side rails up × 4.

Skill 34.2 | Urinary Diversions (Continent and Incontinent)

Urinary diversions are surgical procedures performed on clients who have partial or complete excision of the bladder (cystectomies) due to malignancies or trauma to the bladder. Urinary diversions are ostomies or openings coming from the bladder, ureters, or kidneys to the outer wall of the abdomen (Figure 34-13). Two examples are ureterostomies (openings from the ureter to the outer wall of the abdomen) and the ileal conduit (a ureter is transplanted into a closed-off portion of the ileum, which has one opening going to the outer wall of the abdomen). Urine is rerouted through the urinary diversion instead of the bladder.

There are two types of urinary diversions. The first type is a *continent* diversion. That is, the stoma has a muscular closure similar to the meatus sphincter, so a catheter is inserted to drain the urine. When the catheter

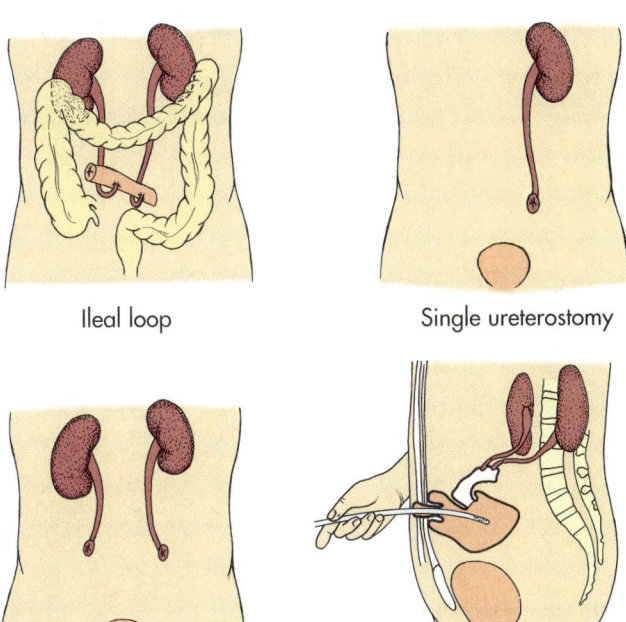

Ileal loop

Single ureterostomy

Double ureterostomy

Continent urinary diversion

Figure 34-13

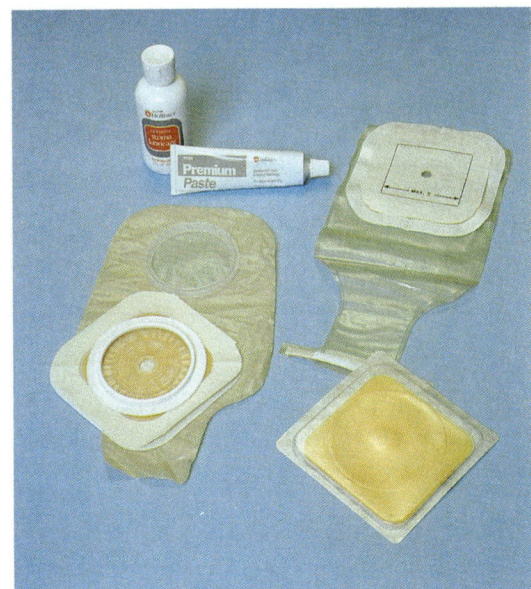

Figure 34-14

is not in use, a small gauze pad covers the stoma to protect client's clothes from mucous drainage.

The second type is an *incontinent* urinary diversion, such as the ileal conduit, which requires pouching continuously (see Skill 33.2). The pouch has to be emptied frequently, and the adhesive holding the pouch may cause skin irritation. Numerous products on the market are available for pouching and skin barrier protection. Check your agency's protocol and client preference.

Incontinent and continent urinary diversions affect the body image of clients. The nurse may have to help the client deal with psychological problems as well as care of the stoma. Clients should be informed that the stoma will continue to shrink for approximately 1 year.

EQUIPMENT (Figure 34-14)

Clean gloves
Washcloth, towel, soap and water
Underpad
Scissors with pointed end
Measuring guide
Tissue or toilet paper
New pouch and adhesive if required
For continent diversions: sterile gloves, catheter, and antiseptic

Assessment

1. Observe location of stoma and type of appliance in use. (If first time and no pouch selected, consider location and size of stoma, client's age and weight, activity level, and financial situation.)
2. Observe stoma site for color (pink with no erythema or necrotic tissue), moistness, and irritation.
3. Observe and palpate skin around stoma for erythema, excoriation, edema, and drainage. **Determines need for skin barrier.**
4. Assess client's ability and willingness to learn self-care. **The nurse must ensure that client or significant other can comprehend and follow directions and that he or she understands the importance of following protocol for care of urinary diversions to prevent infections, irritation of peristomal skin and stoma, and obstruction of urine flow.**

Planning

Expected outcomes focus on maintaining urine flow and stoma and skin integrity.

EXPECTED OUTCOMES

1. Client's urine output is maintained.
2. Client's stoma remains shiny, moist, and free of erythema and purulent drainage.
3. Client's peristoma skin is intact.
4. Client correctly cares for stoma, skin, and pouch by discharge.

Implementation

Steps	Rationale

> **nurse alert** Pouch should be changed every 3 to 7 days and emptied when one-third to one-half full. Apply protective barrier to healthy skin only, if used (contains alcohol).

1. See Standard Protocol (Chapter 1, p. 5).

2. Position client to allow for easy access to stoma so that abdomen is as smooth or flat as possible. Be sure client can view procedure.

3. Continent urinary diversion

a. Put on sterile gloves.

b. Apply antiseptic to three sterile gauze pads and cleanse the stoma in a circular motion, moving from the center outward.   Prevents nosocomial infections.

c. Insert catheter into stoma 2 to $2\frac{1}{2}$ inches (5 to 6 cm) to drain urine in a graduate container.

d. Cleanse around stoma with soap and water and pat dry.   Prevents skin irritation.

e. Apply gauze over stoma.   Prevents mucus from getting on clothes.

4. Incontinent urinary diversion

a. Prepare new pouch.

   (1) Use measuring guide to cut appliance ring so margin around stoma and pouch is $\frac{1}{8}$ to $\frac{1}{4}$ inch.   Protects skin.

   (2) Check drainage valve on pouch.   Prevents leakage.

   (3) Remove protective covering over adhesive ring (Figure 34-15).

   (4) Have all equipment ready to decrease leakage of urine when removing old pouch and applying new one.

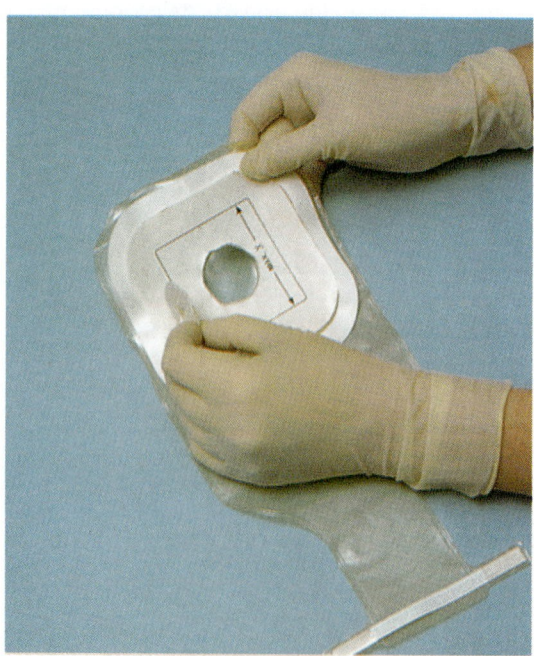

Figure 34-15

Steps	Rationale

b. Replace pouch.

(1) Remove old pouch and place in plastic bag.

(2) Remove any drainage and/or urine on stoma or around catheter (if in use) with tissue.

Prevents skin irritation.

(3) Roll gauze pad and hold over stoma while cleaning around stoma (Figure 34-16).

Wicking collects urine and prevents leakage on skin and bed linens.

(4) Cleanse area around stoma with soap and water, and pat dry.

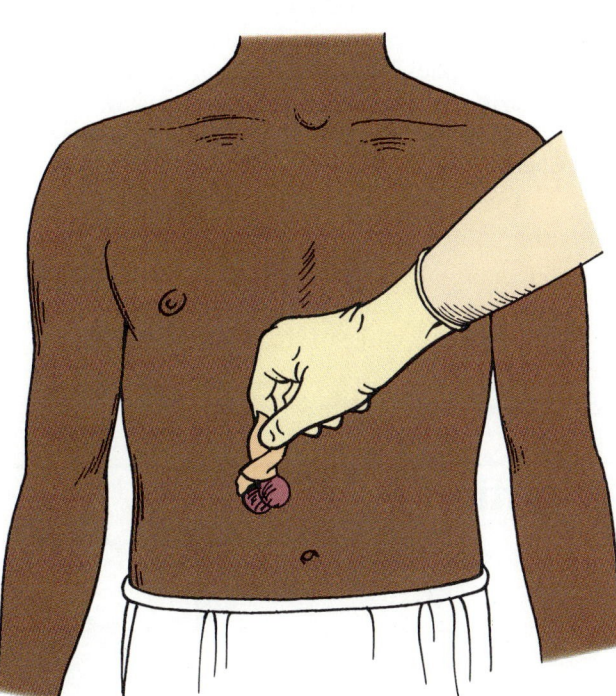

Figure 34-16

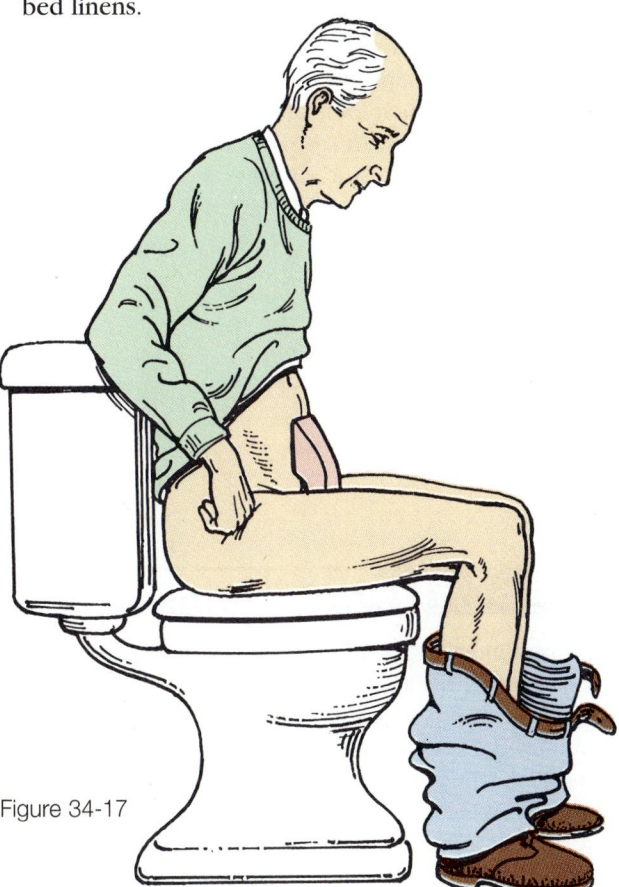

Figure 34-17

(5) Apply pouch over stoma or catheter and hold pressure for 5 minutes. If skin barriers or additional adhesives used, apply at this time.

Helps to adhere pouch to skin. Skin barriers help protect peristomal skin from breakdown.

c. Empty pouch.

(1) Place client on toilet or commode and put pouch valve end between legs or hold container under valve and empty (Figure 34-17).

(2) Rinse pouch with tepid tap water (may use perineal bottle) (Figure 34-18).

(3) After rinsing, pat valve dry and close.

5. Allow client time to ask questions regarding procedure.

6. See Completion Protocol (Chapter 1, p. 6).

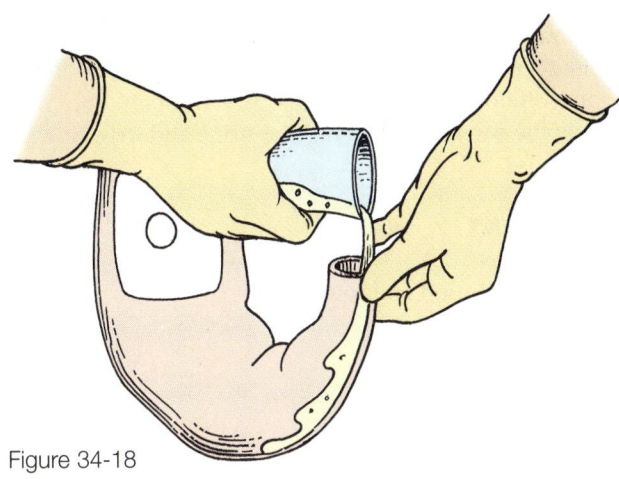

Figure 34-18

Evaluation

1. Observe urine output through stoma: urine is free flowing and greater than 240 ml every 8 hours.
2. Observe and palpate stoma for shine, moistness, erythema, edema, or tenderness.
3. Observe peristomal skin for excoriation or erythema.
4. Observe client demonstrate pouching care during next change.

UNEXPECTED OUTCOMES AND RELATED INTERVENTIONS

1. Skin irritation around stoma: itching and burning (usually from improperly fitted pouch).
   a. Remove pouch immediately.
   b. Cleanse area with soap and water and pat dry.
   c. If lotion or moisturizer used to ease irritation, use a dissolving base so adhesive will adhere.
   d. Apply new pouch.

2. Odors are coming from pouch.
   a. If pouch is leaking, change complete pouch.
   b. Increase intake of cranberry juice, ascorbic acid, protein, grains, and cereals. (This will acidify the urine and decrease odor and potential for infection.)
3. Client will not participate in care of stoma.
   a. Give psychological support to client's feelings.
   b. Contact local support group with physician's approval.
   c. Guard against displaying disapproval or repugnant behavior while caring for client.

SAMPLE DOCUMENTATION

0800 Pouch changed on ileal conduit, client assisted with handling supplies. Stoma is shiny, moist, and red. Peristomal skin has no excoriation, erythema, or drainage. 250 ml of clear yellow urine. Cleansed with soap and water. Client correctly reapplied pouch.

Skill 34.3 | Continuous Bladder Irrigation

Continuous bladder irrigation (CBI) requires a physician's order and must be performed using sterile technique. CBI is a continuous infusion of a sterile solution into the bladder, usually using a three-way irrigation set and a triple-lumen catheter, which has three ports. One port goes to the client to drain urine, one goes to the irrigation solution, and one is used to inflate the catheter balloon (Figure 34-19). The primary use of CBI is to keep an indwelling catheter patent and free of blood clots or sediment. CBI is frequently ordered after bladder surgeries.

The physician must order the solution, strength, and flow rate. If the physician only specifies solution, check your agency's protocol for strength and rate. The irrigation solution infuses continuously through one port while the second port drains the urine and irrigation solution.

EQUIPMENT
Clean gloves
Irrigation solution and tubing
IV pole

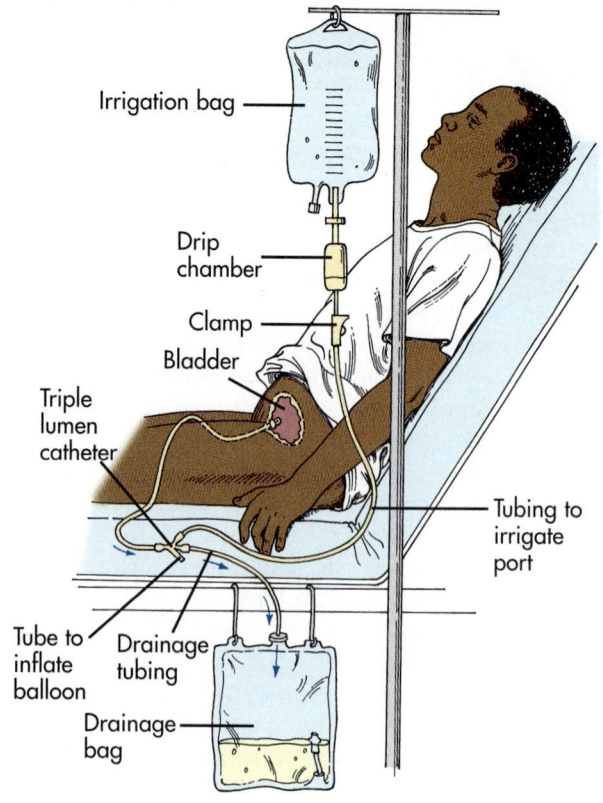

Figure 34-19

Assessment

1. Assess client's level of consciousness and ability to co-operate.
2. Palpate bladder for distention and tenderness.
3. Ask client about the presence of bladder pain or spasms. **Blood clots will cause bladder spasms and may be too large to come through the irrigation catheter lumen. This is one way the nurse can tell when the irrigation solution's rate should be increased.**
4. Observe urine for color, amount, and clarity.
5. Compare irrigation solution intake with urine output. **A blood clot may obstruct the opening of the catheter in the bladder and not allow urine and the irrigation solution to flow from the bladder, but may allow irrigation solution to still infuse into the bladder. If this happens, the bladder may become overdistended and rupture.**

Planning

Expected outcomes focus on continuous urine flow and client comfort.

EXPECTED OUTCOMES

1. Client's urine drains freely (at least 30 ml/hr).
2. Client's urine output has decreased blood clots and sediment.
3. Client does not complain of bladder pain or spasms.
4. Balance between bladder irrigation and output of irrigant is within 100 ml for an 8-hour period.

Implementation

Steps	Rationale
1. See Standard Protocol (Chapter 1, p. 5).	
2. Place label on irrigation solution bag with client's name, room number, date, and time. Mark bag for GU IRRIGATION ONLY in red, type of solution, and any additives.	Indicates fluid is not to be infused intravenously.
nurse alert Irrigation solution and tubing should be changed every 24 hours to decrease potential for infection.	
3. Prepare the solution (must maintain sterility). a. Close clamp on tubing and spike the bag with the tubing. b. Place on an IV pole. c. Fill the drip chamber one-half full by squeezing the chamber. d. Open the clamp and remove air. e. Close the clamp and maintain sterility.	Air will cause bladder fullness and spasms.
4. Maintaining sterility, connect tubing to irrigation port of catheter.	
5. Remove gloves.	
6. Adjust rate at roller clamp (according to physician's orders or agency protocol).	
7. If urine bright red or has clots, increase irrigation rate until clears.	Assists with clotting active bleeding in bladder and flushes clots out of bladder.
8. Change irrigation solution as needed.	
9. Put on gloves and empty catheter bag as needed.	
10. Compare urine output with irrigation solution's infusion every hour.	May overdistend bladder if irrigant and urine do not flow from bladder.
11. See Completion Protocol (Chapter 1, p. 6).	

Evaluation

1. Measure client's *urine* output by subtracting total irrigating solution used from total drainage in bag.
2. Observe client's urine for blood clots and sediment.
3. Ask client if lower abdomen is comfortable (over bladder).
4. Ensure urine output and irrigation solution from bladder are free flowing.

UNEXPECTED OUTCOMES AND RELATED INTERVENTIONS

1. Irrigation solution will not infuse or is slower than previous set.
   a. Check for kinks in the tubing.
   b. Assess for clots or sediment obstruction (may need to irrigate manually; follow agency protocol).
   c. Readjust height of IV pole and readjust clamp.
2. Irrigant going in but not being returned.
   a. Assess for clots and manually irrigate with 50 ml sterile normal saline "using gentle pressure" (or follow agency protocol).
   b. Assess client for bladder spasms and distended bladder (may need antispasmodics).
   c. Notify physician or charge nurse.
3. Bright-red bleeding occurs even with irrigation dripping wide open.
   a. Assess for hypovolemic shock (vital signs, color and moisture on skin, anxiety level).
   b. Leave irrigation dripping wide open and call physician or charge nurse.
4. Client has bladder spasms.
   a. Reassure and try methods to relax: apply warm cloth to lower abdomen, use heating pad (with order), flex knees to 45 degrees, and reposition catheter. Ensure catheter and tubing are not kinked and tubing is coiled on the bed to facilitate drainage by gravity.
   b. Administer ordered urinary antispasmodics.
   c. If unrelieved, call physician.

SAMPLE DOCUMENTATION

0800 Lower abdomen soft and flat, catheter to bedside drainage with 225 ml of bright-red urine with moderate size dark bloody clots passing. 3000 ml of normal saline to irrigation port infusing at 60 gtt per minute. Client rates spasms at a 5 on a 0 to 10 scale (with 10 the worst). Lying on lt. side, knees flexed.

Skill 34.4 | **Suprapubic Catheters**

Suprapubic catheters are inserted by physicians either at the bedside with the client under local anesthesia or while in surgery under general anesthesia. An incision is made through the abdominal wall above the symphysis pubis (Figure 34-20). Benefits of suprapubic catheters are (1) lower incidence of urinary infection, (2) client is able to void naturally when suprapubic catheter is clamped, and (3) client experiences more comfort when ambulating and can handle catheter easier.

Disadvantages of suprapubic catheters include (1) they require physician to insert through abdominal wall, and (2) they must be cleansed each day using sterile technique and supplies.

The nurse is responsible for maintaining the suprapubic catheter and teaching the client about the catheter before discharge. Numerous suprapubic catheters and appliances are available. They may be attached to the skin with sutures or adhesive material.

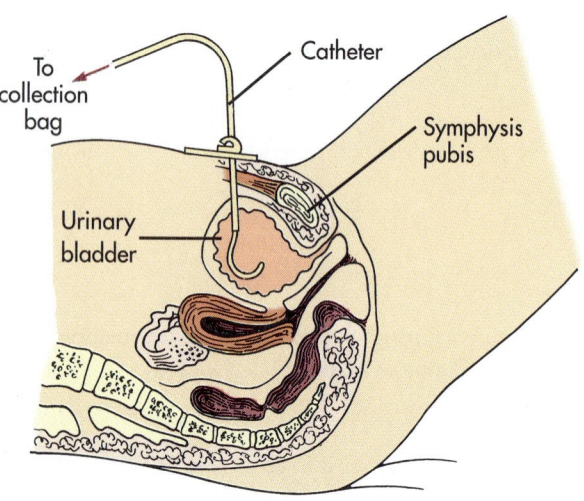

Figure 34-20

EQUIPMENT

Clean gloves
Sterile gloves
Gauze
Antiseptic solution
Split gauze
Nonallergenic tape
Plastic bag

Assessment

1. Assess client's level of consciousness and ability to cooperate.
2. Assess old dressing for drainage (color, odor, amount).
3. Assess catheter insertion site for erythema, edema, drainage, and odor.
4. Assess urine in catheter or bag for color, clarity, and odor.
5. Assess for increase in body temperature. **Infection at the suprapubic catheter site or of the urinary tract may cause an elevated body temperature.**

Planning

Expected outcomes focus on prevention of infection, maintaining the integrity of the client's urinary system, and maintaining client's level of comfort.

EXPECTED OUTCOMES

1. Client's urine is free from odor, sediment, and bacteria.
2. Client's urine culture remains free of bacterial infection by discharge.
3. Client remains afebrile.
4. Client's catheter site is free of erythema, edema, discharge, or tenderness.
5. Client's catheter is patent, and output is 30 ml or greater per hour.
6. Client verbalizes signs and symptoms of urinary tract infection and insertion site infection by discharge.
7. Client correctly demonstrates care for insertion site by discharge.
8. Client's level of discomfort is 4 or less (scale of 0 to 10).

Implementation

Steps	Rationale
nurse alert 1. Client must be able to cooperate and understand sterility concepts. 2. Change dressing every day and as needed per agency protocol. 3. Closed system must be maintained, and urine should flow freely through catheter at all times.	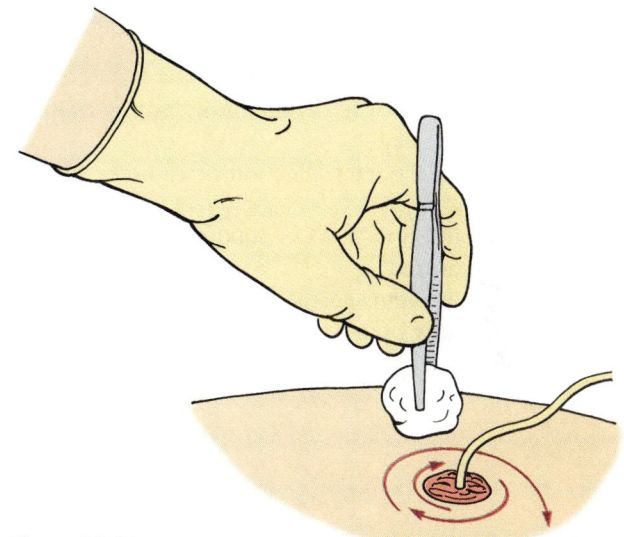 Figure 34-21
1. See Standard Protocol (Chapter 1, p. 5).	
2. Position client so that catheter site can be seen easily.	
3. Remove old dressing and place dressing and gloves in bag.	
4. Put on sterile gloves.	
5. Assess insertion site and patency of catheter.	
6. Maintaining sterility, place antiseptic on gauze and cleanse catheter insertion site. Beginning at the site, move the gauze in a circular motion around catheter, making larger and larger circles outward (Figure 34-21).	Going back over same area with same gauze contaminates area.
7. Perform Step 6 as many times as needed to cleanse site.	
8. Take one gauze pad and cleanse catheter from proximal to distal.	Cleanses organisms off catheter that could migrate to site.
9. With sterile gloved hand, apply split gauze around catheter and tape in place.	
10. Ensure bag and catheter junctions are securely in place.	Prevents leakage of urine or organisms from entering bladder.

Steps	Rationale
11. Ask client if there are any questions about catheter care. **12.** See Completion Protocol (Chapter 1, p. 6).	

Evaluation

1. Observe client's urine for sediment or unusual odor.
2. Review laboratory urine culture and sensitivity for presence of bacteria.
3. Monitor body temperature.
4. Observe catheter insertion site.
5. Monitor suprapubic catheter output.
6. Ask client to state signs and symptoms of urinary tract infection and insertion site infection.
7. Observe client demonstrate care of insertion site.
8. Ask client to rate discomfort (scale of 0 to 10).

UNEXPECTED OUTCOMES AND RELATED INTERVENTIONS

1. Urine through catheter is obstructed (may be caused by blood clots, catheter tip against wall of bladder, or sediment collection).
   a. Call physician for irrigation orders.
   b. Increase fluids (if not contraindicated) to 2000 to 3000 ml per day.
2. Client has urinary tract infection or catheter site infection.
   a. Increase fluids to 2000 to 3000 ml per day (if not contraindicated).
   b. Increase protein, cereal, and grain foods to increase acidity of urine, and increase intake of cranberry juice.
   c. Perform good handwashing and use sterile technique for catheter care.
   d. Monitor body temperature and notify physician for temperatures greater than 101° F (38.3° C).
   e. Follow agency or CDC protocol and culture drainage at site of catheter.
3. Catheter becomes dislodged.
   a. Apply sterile gauze to site.
   b. Apply pressure if bleeding.
   c. Reassure client.
   d. Notify physician.
4. When catheter clamped, client complaints of distended bladder before time to release clamp.
   a. Release clamp and drain no more than 750 ml of urine at one time.
   b. Recalculate time for clamping, if off schedule.

SAMPLE DOCUMENTATION

0800 Client alert and awake, old dressing removed from suprapubic catheter site with small amount dark-brown drainage on gauze with no unusual odor. Site has no redness, edema, or drainage. Cleaned with betadine swabs around site. Redressed with split gauze. Tolerated without complaints of discomfort. Side rails up × 4, in supine position.

CRITICAL THINKING EXERCISES

1. You have been informed that Mrs. Huddle needs a Foley catheter placed before her scheduled surgery. You have gathered all necessary supplies, gained Mrs. Huddle's permission, draped her, and have begun the procedure. You find that visualization of her urinary meatus is difficult, and you are concerned that you will contaminate the catheter.
   a. How should you proceed?
   b. After inserting the Foley catheter and taping it in place, you note that the urinary drainage bag has 650 cc of urine in it, and urine is still draining. Does this require any action on your part? If so, what?
2. What is the most appropriate action on the part of the nurse in each of the following situations?
   a. Client complains of severe pain when you start to inflate the balloon of the catheter.
   b. During the catheterization procedure, the client jerks her leg onto your sterile field, contaminating the catheter and your gloves.
   c. When checking the balloon before inserting the Foley catheter you note that you are unable to aspirate the fluid from the balloon.
3. You are caring for two clients. One has a continent urinary diversion and the other has an incontinent urinary diversion.
   a. Cite at least three examples of how the care of these clients is similar.
   b. Which client is at greater risk for the development of skin breakdown?
4. Your client, Mr. Price, has a suprapubic catheter. While assessing him you note that there is little urinary drainage from the catheter. What is the most appropriate action on your part?

REFERENCES

Davey F: Myths surrounding use of urinary catheters: a summary of key beliefs that inhibit acute care nurses from altering their use of indwelling catheters, *Can J Infect Control* 9(2):39, 1994.

Seidel H et al: *Mosby's guide to physical examination,* ed 3, St Louis, 1995, Mosby.

ADDITIONAL READINGS

Krasner D: Six steps to successful stoma care, *RN* 56(7):32, 1993.

MacKenzie J: Questioning the assumption that urinary catheterization is a pain free event for women, *J Clin Nurs* 2(2):64, 1993.

McConnell EA: How to use a urometer, *Nursing* 21(10):28, 1991.

Paulford-Lecher N: Teaching your patient stoma care, *Nursing* 23(9):47, 1993.

Petillo MH: The patient with a urinary stoma: nursing management and patient education, *Nurs Clin North Am* 22(2):263, 1987.

Razor BR: Continent urinary reservoirs, *Semin in Oncol Nurs* 9(4):272, 1993.

Roe B: Catheter associated urinary tract infection: a review, *J Clin Nurs* 2(4):197, 1993.

Smith DB: Continent diversions: an overview, *Dimensions in Oncol Nurs* 3(4):18, 1990.

chapter 35

Altered Sensory Perception

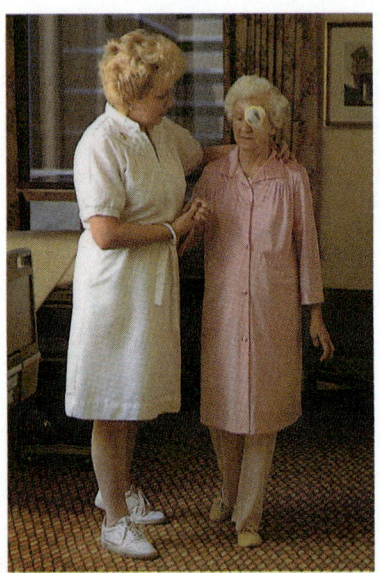

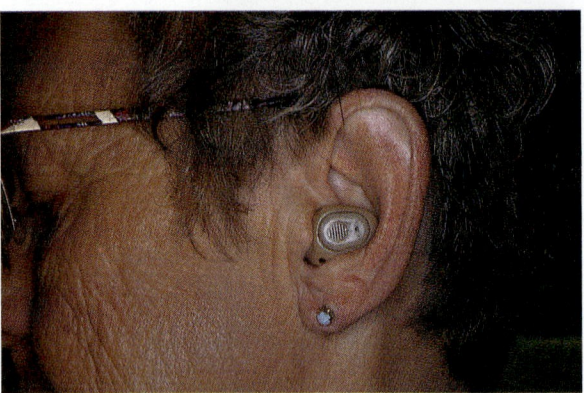

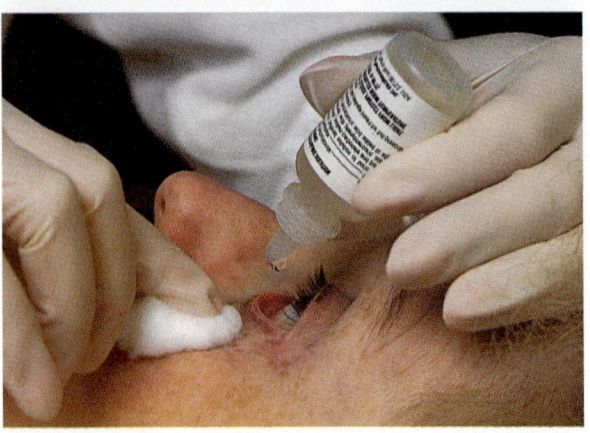

Eyeglasses and contact lenses help restore visual loss, and hearing aids help improve sound reception. Clients depend on these devices to improve sensory function without detracting from an attractive appearance. Artificial eyes, in particular, help clients maintain appearances when an eye has been lost because of injury or disease.

Clients with existing sensory loss must be protected from injury. A client with visual impairment needs to be oriented to the environment using touch. For example, feeling the walls establishes a sense of direction. Touching furniture establishes physical boundaries; therefore moving furniture may create a safety hazard. When assisting ambulation, the nurse should stand on the client's nondominant side approximately one step ahead. This permits use of the dominant hand to feel for barriers and landmarks. Location of key items (e.g., call light, telephone) may need to be described and placed within the client's reach. Side rails are also important, particularly if the client cannot walk alone.

A hearing deficit can cause a client to feel isolated. Clients deaf since childhood who cannot hear themselves speak are likely to have speech alterations. Sign language, lipreading, or writing are alternatives to facilitate communication. Face the client before beginning to speak, and make sure there is enough light for the client to visualize the lips. Speak slowly and articulate clearly using a normal tone of voice. It is not helpful to exaggerate lip movements. Talk toward the client's best ear, using gestures.

Clients can be extremely sensitive about lens or prosthesis care. Accidental breakage or malfunction can seriously impair sensory function and threaten self-esteem if the client is dependent on others for assistance.

Most clients have an established routine for cleaning their contact lenses or eye prostheses. If unable to care for these aids, clients usually show great interest in the manner in which the nurse performs cleaning and maintenance procedures. Careful handling of these devices is vital to avoid damage or injury.

Use techniques that facilitate interaction with the client when a sensory loss exists. For example, if a client wears a hearing aid, the nurse should use communication techniques that ensure the client's ability to hear and understand.

Encourage clients to express feelings about changes in body image, such as feeling unusual or different, because of reliance on an artificial device for function or appearance. Families become frustrated when they cannot communicate with the client whose hearing aid malfunctions. The nurse needs to demonstrate understanding of this frustration and teach families methods for interacting more effectively.

A visual or hearing impairment may be caused by the presence of foreign bodies, irritants, or secretions. Cerumen accumulation or impaction can cause discomfort and further hearing loss, particularly in the older adult and with clients wearing hearing aids. Inflammation or infection of the eyes can produce drainage or secretions that reduce vision. Irrigation of the eye or ear on a regular basis can help restore or maintain existing function. The presence of a foreign body or irritant in the eye or ear requires immediate intervention to restore function and prevent possible permanent loss.

Nursing Diagnosis

An appropriate nursing diagnosis associated with a visual or hearing impairment is **Sensory/Perceptual Alterations:** (specify) **(Visual/Auditory),** in which clients experience a change in how they perceive and respond to environmental stimuli. Clients with a hearing loss may also have **Impaired Verbal Communication,** depending on their ability to use and understand language. Clients requiring irrigations of the eye or assistance with contact lenses or prostheses may be at **Risk for Infection,** especially if proper technique is not used. A client with a sensory impairment in an unfamiliar environment, such as a hospital room, is especially at **Risk for Injury.** A nursing diagnosis of **Pain** may also apply when injury or infection involves the eye or ear. Clients who are unable to demonstrate proper care techniques may have a **Knowledge Deficit.** Visual or hearing impairments can also affect psychosocial status, resulting in **Impaired Social Interaction** or **Social Isolation.**

Skill 35.1 | Caring for Clients with Contact Lenses

There are three basic types of contact lenses: hard, soft, and rigid gas permeable (RGP), also known as oxygen permeable. They differ in size, material, and amount of oxygen flow to the eye's surface. Soft lenses are large enough to cover the cornea completely and can be easily torn because they consist primarily of water. Rigid lenses are smaller and made of firm, durable plastic. Hard lenses are becoming obsolete.

Contact lenses are also available as daily wear, extended wear, and disposable. All lenses must be removed periodically to prevent ocular infection and corneal ulcers or abrasions. Daily-wear lenses should be removed overnight for cleaning and disinfection and should not be worn more than 10 to 14 hours daily (Cohen and Krachmer, 1992; White et al., 1991). It is recommended that all extended-wear lenses be worn no longer than six consecutive nights without cleaning and disinfecting (Johnson & Johnson, 1994). Disposable lenses are available for daily and extended-wear and are usually replaced every 1 to 2 weeks (White et al., 1991). The following are some basic safety principles regarding care of contact lenses:

1. Use only lens care solutions recommended by the eye care practitioner.
2. Lenses should be removed according to a prescribed schedule. Every time they are removed, they must be cleaned, rinsed, and disinfected.
3. Lenses should not be worn overnight unless recommended by the eye care practitioner.
4. Disposable or planned replacement lenses should be thrown away after the prescribed wearing period.

As contact lenses are worn, they can accumulate secretions and foreign matter that can irritate the eyes, cause distorted vision, and increase the risk of infection. Burning, discomfort, tearing, and redness of the conjunctiva may be symptoms of lens overwear. Persistence of symptoms even after lens removal is abnormal, however, and may indicate serious ocular problems.

It is extremely important that nurses determine

whether clients wear contact lenses, particularly when clients are admitted to hospitals or agencies in unresponsive or confused states. If a seriously ill client is wearing contact lenses and this goes undetected, severe corneal injury can result.

EQUIPMENT

Clean lens storage container
Bath towel
Small lens suction cup (optional)
Sterile saline solution
Sterile lens cleaning solution
Sterile lens rinsing solution
Sterile lens disinfectant
Sterile enzyme solution (depends on care regimen)
Sterile rewetting solution (depends on care regimen)
Cotton ball or cotton-tipped applicator
Emesis basin
Disposable gloves

Assessment

1. Inspect the eye or ask client if contact lens is in place. **Lenses are generally comfortable to wear, and client may forget they are in place.**
2. Ask client the following questions:
   How long do you normally wear your lenses on an average day?
   Do you wear the lenses overnight?
   What method of lens care do you use?
   How frequently do you clean and disinfect the lenses? When did you last clean and disinfect them? **Determines client's compliance with lens care.**
3. Observe client's ability to manipulate and hold contact lens. **Determines level of assistance required in care.**
4. Assess the eyes for the following: redness, pain, reduced visual acuity (blurred vision or halos), photophobia, excess tearing, discharge, and swelling of the eyelids or conjunctivae (Cohen and Krachmer, 1992).

Planning

Expected outcomes focus on maintaining vision and prevention of complications.

EXPECTED OUTCOMES

1. Client verbalizes comfort after removal and reinsertion of lenses.
2. Client's eye shows no signs of ocular infection, such as redness, pain, swelling, discharge, blurred vision, or photophobia.
3. Client verbalizes improved visual perception after lens cleaning.
4. Client demonstrates no signs of eye injury, as evidenced by irritation, pain, foreign body sensation, redness, and tearing.
5. Client demonstrates the proper technique for removing, cleaning, and reinserting lenses.

Implementation

Steps	Rationale
1. See Standard Protocol (Chapter 1, p. 5).	
2. Place towel just below client's face.	Catches lens if one should accidentally fall from eye.
3. Removing soft lenses for a dependent client	
a. Add a few drops of sterile saline to client's eye.	Lubricates eye to facilitate lens removal.
b. Tell client to look straight ahead. Using middle finger, retract lower eyelid to expose lower edge of lens.	
c. With pad of index finger of same hand, slide lens off cornea onto white of eye.	Use of finger pads prevents injury to cornea and damage to lens.
d. Pull upper eyelid down gently with thumb of other hand and compress lens slightly between thumb and index finger.	
e. Gently pinch lens and lift out without allowing lens edges to stick together.	

Steps	Rationale

f. If lens edges stick together, place lens in palm and soak thoroughly with sterile saline. Gently roll lens with index finger in back-and-forth motion. If gentle rubbing does not separate edges, soak lens in sterile solution.

g. Follow procedure for cleansing and disinfecting lenses.

h. Repeat Steps a to g for other lens.

4. Removing rigid lenses for a dependent client

a. Be sure lens is positioned directly over cornea. If it is not, have client close eyelids, place index and middle finger of one hand beside the lens, and gently but firmly massage lens back into place.

b. Place index finger on outer corner of client's eye and draw skin gently back toward ear (Figure 35-1).

c. Ask client to blink. Do not release pressure on lids until blink is completed.

d. If lens fails to pop out, gently retract eyelid beyond edges of lens. Press lower eyelid gently against lower edge of lens.

e. Allow both eyelids to close slightly and grasp lens as it rises from eye. Cup lens in hand. A lens suction cup can be used for confused or unconscious clients. Gently apply suction cup to lens surface and lift lens out.

f. Follow procedure for cleansing and disinfecting lenses.

g. Repeat Steps a to f for the other lens.

5. Cleansing and disinfecting

a. Open lens storage case. Check expiration dates of solutions.

b. After removal of lens from eye, apply one or two drops of cleaning solution to lens in palm of hand (use cleanser recommended by lens manufacturer or eye care practitioner).

c. Rub lens gently but thoroughly on both sides for 20 to 30 seconds. Use index finger (soft lenses) or little finger or cotton-tipped applicator soaked with cleaner (rigid lenses) to clean inside lens. Be careful not to touch or scratch lens with fingernail.

d. Holding lens over a small basin, rinse thoroughly with manufacturer-recommended rinsing solution (soft lenses) or cold tap water (rigid lenses).

e. Place lens in proper storage case compartment: **R** for right lens and **L** for left lens (Figure 35-2). Center lens in storage case, convex side down. Fill with recommended disinfecting solution. Label case with client's name and room number.

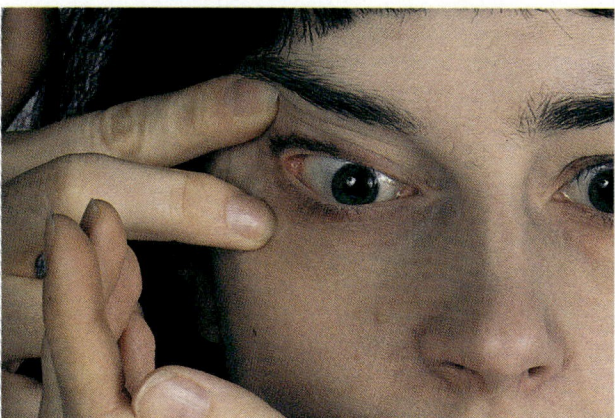

Figure 35-1 As done by client.

Maneuver should cause lens to dislodge and pop out. Lid margins must clear top and bottom of lens until the blink.

Lens suction cup helps reduce the risk of scratching the eye as lens is removed.

Removes tear components, including mucus, lipids, and proteins that collect on lens.

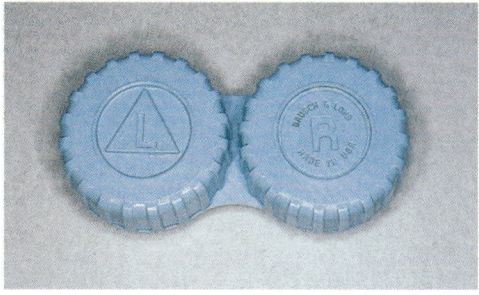

Figure 35-2

Lenses may be different prescriptions.

Steps	Rationale

nurse alert Follow instructions of manufacturer or eye care practitioner regarding the time and procedure for disinfection/neutralization, since they vary among products. Some disinfecting solutions can harm the eyes if used improperly.

6. Inserting soft lenses

a. Remove right lens from storage case and rinse with recommended rinsing solution; inspect lens for foreign materials, tears, or other damage.

b. Check that lens is not inverted (inside out). — Soft lens is inverted if bowl has lip; it is in proper position if curve is even from base to rim.

c. Using middle or index finger of opposite hand, retract upper lid until iris is exposed.

d. Use middle finger of the hand holding lens to pull down lower lid.

e. Tell client to look straight ahead; gently place lens directly on cornea; release lids slowly, starting with lower lid.

f. Tell client to close eyes slowly and roll them toward lens if not on the cornea.

g. Tell client to blink a few times.

h. Ask client to open eyes. Check for blurred vision or discomfort. — Ensures lens is centered, free of trapped air, and comfortable.

i. Repeat Steps a to h for left eye.

j. Discard used solution. Rinse case thoroughly and allow to air dry.

7. Inserting rigid lenses

a. Remove right lens from storage case; attempt to lift lens straight up (Figure 35-3). — Sliding lens out of case can cause scratches on the surface.

b. Rinse with cold tap water. — Hot water causes lens to warp.

c. Wet lens on both sides using prescribed wetting solution.

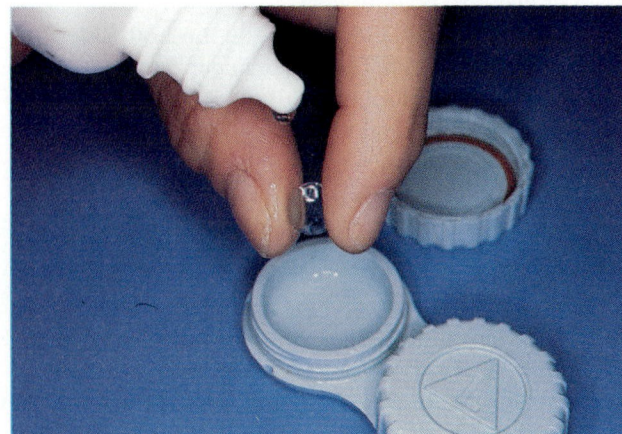

Figure 35-3 As done by client.

Steps	Rationale

d. Place right lens concave side up on tip of index finger of dominant hand (Figure 35-4, *A*).

Inner surface of lens should face up so that it is applied against cornea.

e. Instruct client to look straight ahead while retracting both upper and lower lids; place lens gently over center of cornea (Figure 35-4, *B*).

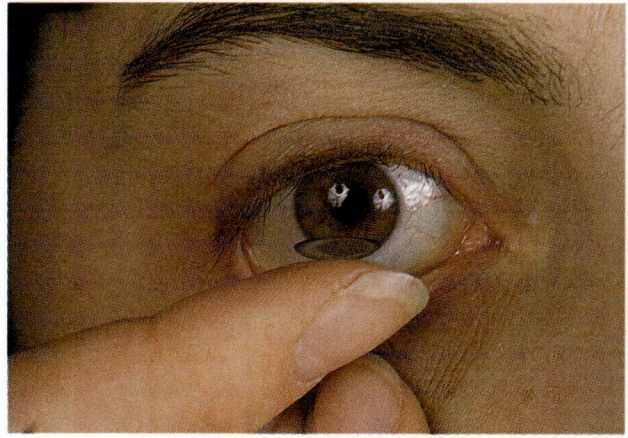 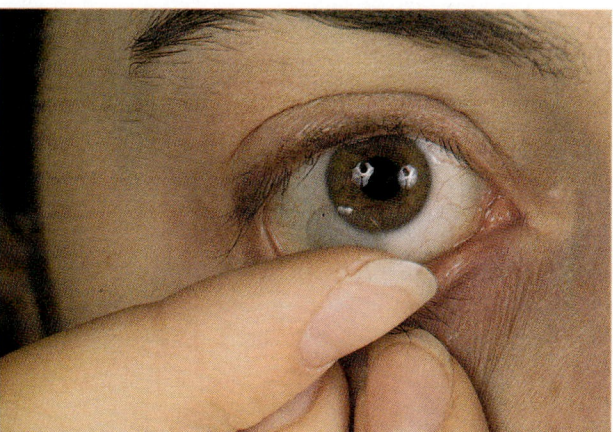

A   B

Figure 35-4 **A** and **B,** As done by client.

f. Ask client to close eyes briefly and avoid blinking.

Helps to secure position of lens.

g. Ask client to open eyes. Check for blurred vision or discomfort.

h. Repeat Steps a to g for left eye.

i. Discard used solution. Rinse case thoroughly and allow to air dry.

8. See Completion Protocol (Chapter 1, p. 6).

Evaluation

1. Ask client about comfort after removal and reinsertion of lenses.
2. Inspect eye for signs of ocular infection.
3. Ask client about visual perception after lens cleaning.
4. Observe client for signs of eye injury.
5. Observe client demonstrating technique for lens care.

UNEXPECTED OUTCOMES AND RELATED INTERVENTIONS

1. Client complains of burning, pain, or foreign body sensation.
   a. Remove lenses.
   b. If symptoms persist, notify physician.
2. Client complains of blurred vision.
   a. Retract eyelids and locate position of lens. Ask client to look in direction opposite of lens, and with index finger, apply pressure to lower eyelid margin and position lens over cornea.
   b. If lenses feel dry, apply a rewetting solution (if recommended) according to instructions.
   c. If symptoms persist, remove lenses and notify physician.
3. Client develops inflammation of conjunctiva, pain, discharge, excess tearing, or reduced vision.
   Remove lenses and notify physician.
4. Client is unable to perform lens care correctly.
   a. Demonstrate correct lens care.
   b. Observe return demonstration until correctly performed.

SAMPLE DOCUMENTATION

2000 Client complaining of eye discomfort. Slight redness of conjunctiva noted bilaterally. Contact lenses removed by client. Cleansing and disinfecting performed according to instructions. Client wearing glasses.

2200 No complaints of eye discomfort. Conjunctiva pink, no redness noted.

Skill 35.2 | Caring for an Eye Prosthesis

As a result of tumor, infection, congenital blindness, or severe trauma to the eye, clients may have to undergo an enucleation, a procedure involving the complete removal of the eyeball. All that remains is the socket and eyelids. For obvious cosmetic purposes, clients who have had an enucleation are often fitted with an artificial eye, or prosthesis.

Artificial eyes are made of glass and plastic and fit just behind the client's eyelids. Each prosthesis is designed to take on the appearance of the client's natural iris, pupil, and sclera. Prostheses are relatively easy to remove and insert and can be worn day and night. Cleansing with soap and water can be done daily or anytime up to several months based on client preference.

EQUIPMENT (FIGURE 35-5)
Soft washcloth or cotton gauze square
Wash basin with warm water or saline
4 × 4 gauze pads
Mild soap

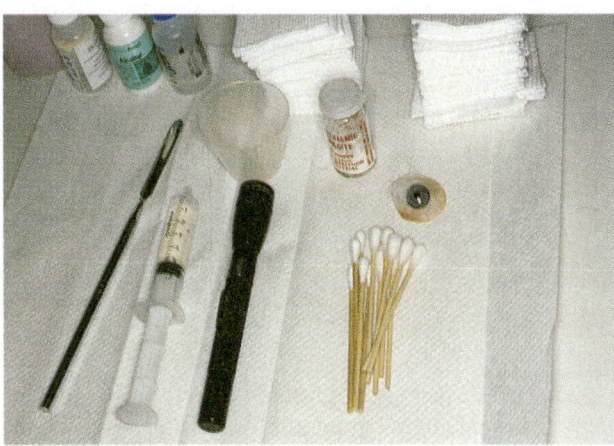

Figure 35-5

Facial tissues
Bath towel
Suction device (e.g., rubber bulb syringe or medicine dropper bulb) (Optional: syringe removes prosthesis by suction if manual removal is not successful.)
Disposable gloves
Covered plastic storage case

Assessment

1. Determine which eye is artificial (no movement or pupillary reaction to light).
2. Inspect surrounding tissues of eyelid and eye socket for inflammation, tenderness, swelling, or drainage after prosthesis removal.
3. Assess client's routines for prosthetic care: frequency and methods of cleaning. **Determines compliance with and knowledge of self-care.**
4. Assess client's ability to remove, clean, and reinsert prosthesis.

Planning

Expected outcomes focus on comfort and prevention of infection.

EXPECTED OUTCOMES
1. Client verbalizes feelings regarding prosthesis removal.
2. Client's eyelid margins and eye socket are clean and of normal pink color, with lashes turned away from prosthesis.
3. Client demonstrates no signs of infection, such as redness, tenderness, swelling, or discharge of socket or eyelid margins.
4. Client verbalizes that prosthetic eye fits comfortably.
5. Client demonstrates the proper technique for removing, cleaning, and reinserting prosthesis.

Implementation

Steps	Rationale
1. See Standard Protocol (Chapter 1, p. 5).	
2. With thumb, gently retract lower eyelid against lower orbital ridge (Figure 35-6, *A*).	
3. Exert slight pressure below eyelid (Figure 35-6, *B*). If prosthesis does not slide out, use bulb syringe or medicine dropper bulb to apply direct suction to prosthesis.	Maneuver breaks suction, causing prosthesis to rise and slide out of socket (Bocking et al., 1990).

Steps	Rationale

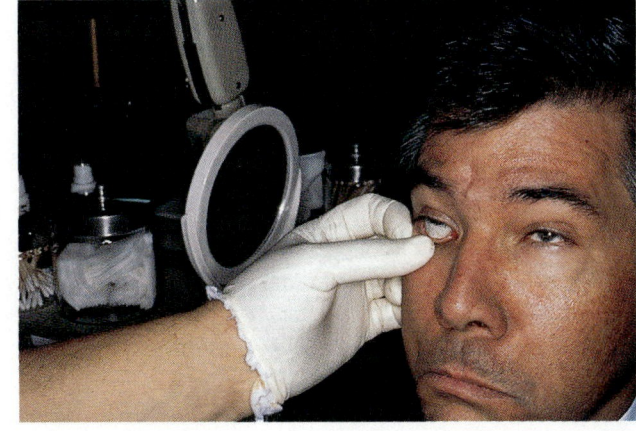 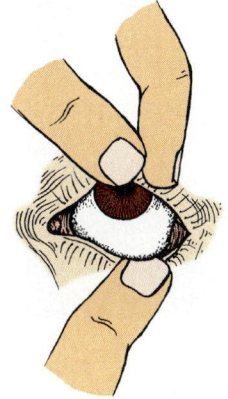 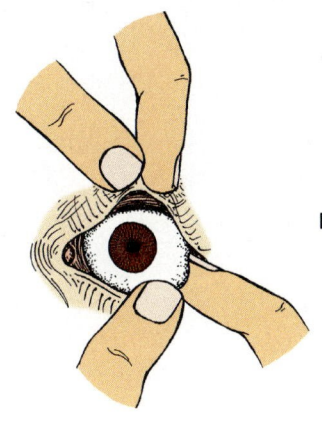

A   B

Figure 35-6

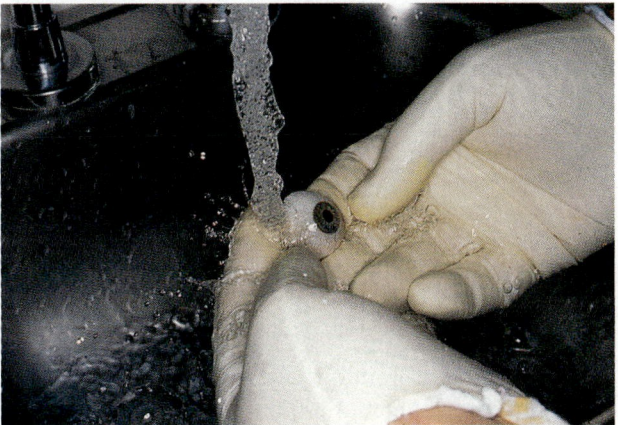

Figure 35-7

4. Place prosthesis in palm of hand and clean with mild soap and water or plain saline by rubbing between thumb and index finger.

5. Rinse well under running tap water and dry with soft washcloth or facial tissue (Figure 35-7).

6. If client is not to have prosthesis reinserted, store in sterile saline or water in plastic storage case. Label with client's name and room number.

7. Clean eyelid margins and socket.
   a. Retract upper and lower eyelids with thumb and index finger.
   b. Wash socket with washcloth or gauze square moistened in warm water or saline.
   c. Dry socket well with gauze pads.   **Removes moisture that can harbor microorganisms.**
   d. Wash eyelids with mild soap and water, wiping from inner to outer canthus, using a clean part of cloth with each wipe. Dry eyelids using the same method.

8. Moisten prosthesis with water or saline.   **Makes insertion easier because dry plastic would rub against tissue surfaces.**

9. Retract client's upper eyelid with index finger or thumb of nondominant hand (Figure 35-8).

10. With dominant hand, hold prosthesis so that notched or pointed edge is positioned toward nose. Iris faces outward.   **Correct positioning of prosthesis ensures proper fit (Bocking et al., 1990).**

11. Slide prosthesis up under upper eyelid as far as possible. Then push down lower lid to allow prosthesis to slip into place.

12. Gently wipe away excess fluid if necessary.   **Wipe toward nose to prevent dislodgement.**

13. See Completion Protocol (Chapter 1, p. 6).

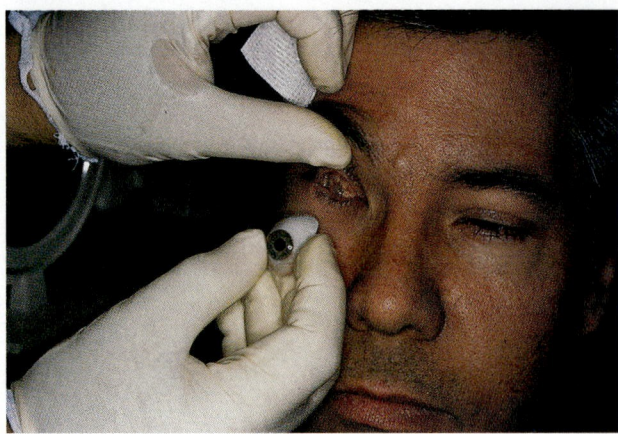

Figure 35-8

Evaluation

1. Ask client about feelings regarding prosthesis removal.
2. Inspect eyelids and eye socket for cleanliness, color, and position of eyelashes.
3. Inspect eyelids and socket for signs of infection.
4. Ask client if prosthesis fits comfortably.
5. Observe client demonstrating technique for prosthesis care.

UNEXPECTED OUTCOMES AND RELATED INTERVENTIONS

1. Client states prosthesis feels uncomfortable.
   a. Reposition prosthesis.
   b. Remove prosthesis. Inspect for any rough areas.
2. Client develops signs of inflammation in socket or eyelid.
   a. Remove prosthesis for a few days if necessary. Clean eyelid and socket.
   b. Provide client with an eye patch if desired.
3. Client develops excessive, purulent, or foul drainage.
   a. Remove prosthesis and clean area. Provide eye patch if desired.
   b. Evaluate temperature every 4 hours and as necessary.
   c. Notify physician of assessment findings.
4. Client is unable to perform prosthesis care correctly.
   a. Demonstrate correct prosthesis care.
   b. Observe return demonstration until correctly performed.

SAMPLE DOCUMENTATION

1400 Client complaining of tenderness at left artificial eye. Prosthesis removed. No scratches or rough edges noted. Slight redness and edema noted at outer canthus. Socket and eyelids cleaned with normal saline. Client agrees not to wear prosthesis until symptoms improve. Prosthesis cleaned and stored. Eye patch provided.

Skill 35.3 | Eye Irrigations

Eye irrigation is performed to relieve local inflammation of the conjunctiva, apply antiseptic solution, or flush out exudate or irritating solutions. It is a procedure typically used in emergency situations when a foreign object or some other substance has entered the eye (Perry and Potter, 1994). When a chemical or irritating substance contaminates the eyes, irrigate **immediately** with copious amounts of water for at least 15 minutes to prevent corneal burning (McConnell, 1991).

EQUIPMENT

Prescribed irrigating solution: volume usually varies from 30 to 180 ml at 98.6° F (37° C). (For chemical flushing, use tap water or prescribed IV fluid in volume to provide continuous irrigation over 15 minutes.)
Sterile basin for solution
Curved emesis basin
Waterproof pad or towel
Cotton balls
Soft bulb syringe, eyedropper, or IV tubing
Disposable gloves

Assessment

1. Assess reason for eye irrigation. **This information determines the amount and type of solution and the immediacy of treatment.**
2. Assess the eye for redness, excessive tearing, and discharge. Assess the eyelids and lacrimal glands for edema. Ask client about itching, burning, pain, blurred vision, or photophobia (McConnell, 1991). **Provides baseline for condition of eye.**
3. Assess client's ability to cooperate. Extra assistance may be needed.

Planning

Expected outcomes focus on physical and psychological comfort and improving vision.

EXPECTED OUTCOMES

1. Client verbalizes reduced burning/itching after eye irrigation.
2. Client demonstrates minimal anxiety during irrigation.
3. Client verbalizes improved visual acuity after eye irrigation.
4. Client maintains normal pupillary reaction and eye movement after irrigation.

Implementation

Steps	Rationale

1. See Standard Protocol (Chapter 1, p. 5).

2. Reassure client that eye can be closed periodically and that no object will touch eye.

Relieves client's anxiety.

> **nurse alert** Remove contact lenses (if possible) before beginning irrigation.

3. Assist client to side-lying position on the same side as the affected eye. Turn head toward affected eye.

Irrigation solution will flow from inner to outer canthus, preventing contamination of unaffected eye and nasolacrimal duct.

4. Place waterproof pad under client's face.

5. With cotton ball moistened in prescribed solution (or normal saline), gently clean eyelid margins and eyelashes from inner to outer canthus.

Minimizes transfer of debris from lids or lashes into eye during irrigation.

6. Place curved emesis basin just below client's cheek on side of affected eye.

7. Gently retract upper and lower eyelids to expose the conjunctival sacs. To hold lids open, apply pressure to lower bony orbit and bony prominence beneath eyebrow. Do not apply pressure over eye.

Retraction minimizes blinking and allows irrigation of conjunctiva.

8. Hold irrigating syringe, dropper, or IV tubing approximately 1 inch (2.5 cm) from the inner canthus.

If irrigator touches the eye, there is risk of injury.

9. Ask client to look up. Gently irrigate with a steady stream toward the lower conjunctival sac to the outer canthus (Figure 35-9).

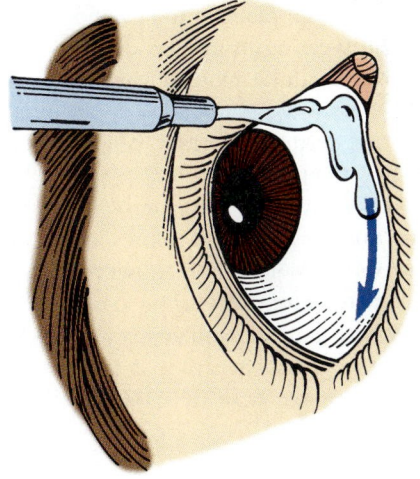

Figure 35-9

10. Allow client to close the eye periodically.

Lid closure moves secretions from upper to lower conjunctival sac.

11. Continue irrigation until all solution is used or secretions have been cleared. (NOTE: A 15-minute irrigation is needed to flush chemicals.)

12. Dry eyelids and facial area with sterile cotton ball.

13. See Completion Protocol (Chapter 1, p. 6).

Evaluation

1. Ask client about comfort level after eye irrigation.
2. Observe for verbal and nonverbal signs of anxiety during irrigation.
3. Ask client if vision is blurred after irrigation.
4. Observe pupillary reaction (to light and accommodation) and extraocular eye movement (see Skill 12.4).

UNEXPECTED OUTCOMES AND RELATED INTERVENTIONS

1. Client demonstrates extreme anxiety during irrigation.
   a. Reinforce the rationale for irrigation.
   b. Allow client to close eye periodically during irrigation.
   c. Instruct client to take slow, deep breaths.
   d. Seek extra assistance if needed to prevent injury.

2. Client complains of pain and foreign body sensation in the eye after irrigation. Excessive tearing and photophobia noted.
   a. Advise client to close the eye and avoid eye movement.
   b. Notify physician or eye care practitioner of findings.

SAMPLE DOCUMENTATION

0800 Client complaining of blurred vision and tenderness in left eye. Yellow, crusty drainage noted on eyelids with slight edema and redness of conjunctiva. Eyelids cleaned and eye irrigated with 30 ml warm, sterile, normal saline. Antibiotic ointment applied. Client tolerated procedure without difficulty.

0900 Client states that eye "feels better." Vision clearer. PERRLA. Normal eye movements noted. Conjunctiva remains red with slight edema.

Skill 35.4 | Caring for Clients with Hearing Aids

Hearing is vital for normal communication and orientation to sounds in the environment. For people with hearing loss, hearing aids amplify so that sound is heard at a more effective level. Following are the two most popular types of aids (Weinstock, 1990):

1. An in-the-canal (ITC) aid fits entirely in the canal (Figure 35-10). It has cosmetic appeal, is easy to manipulate and place in the ear, does not interfere with the wearing of eyeglasses or use of the telephone, and can be worn during most physical exercise. However, obtaining a proper fit is more difficult, and cerumen tends to plug this model more than the others.

2. An in-the-ear (ITE or intraaural) aid fits into the external auditory ear and allows more fine tuning (Figure 35-11). It is more powerful and can help with a wider range of hearing loss than the ITC aid. It is easy to position and adjust and does not interfere with eyeglass wearing. It is, however, slightly more noticeable than the ITC aid and is not rec-

ommended for persons with moisture or skin problems in the ear canal. It is the most common type of aid.

Three other less popular styles are available:

1. A behind-the-ear (BTE or postaural) aid hooks around and behind the ear and is connected by a short, clear, hollow plastic tube to an ear mold inserted into the external auditory canal (Figure 35-12). It is useful for clients with rapidly progressive hearing loss, those with manual dexterity difficulties, or those who find partial ear occlusion intolerable. Children are usually fitted with this type of aid because only the ear mold has to be changed as the child grows. Disadvantages are that it may be

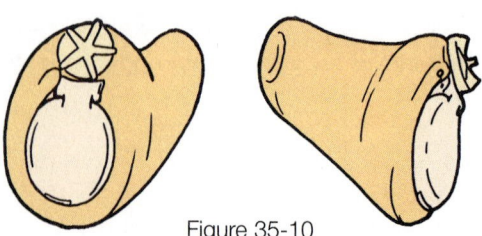

Figure 35-10

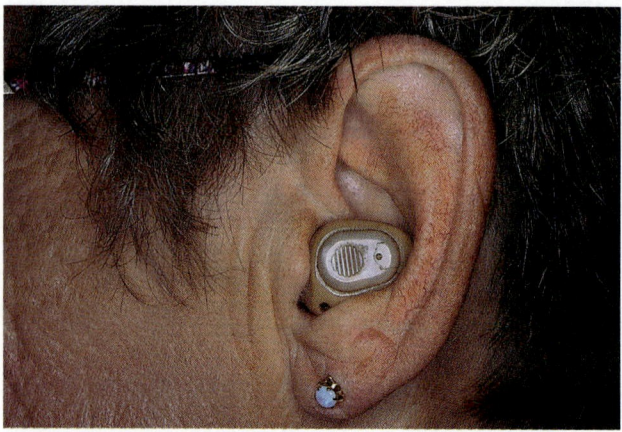

Figure 35-11

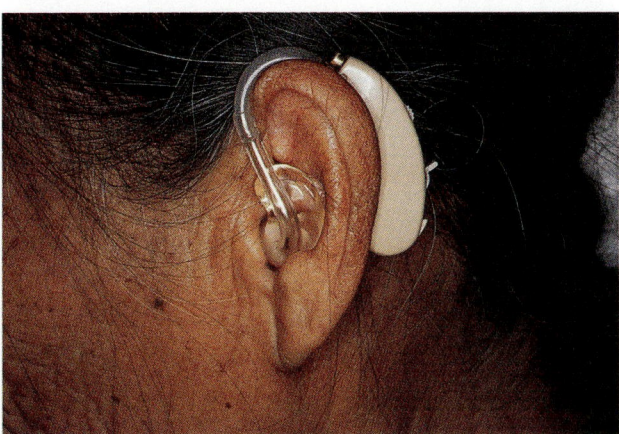

Figure 35-12

more visible, may interfere with eyeglasses and telephone use, and is more difficult to keep in place during physical exercise.

2. The eyeglass aid is a hearing aid that fits in the ear canal and attaches to a battery located on the arm of the eyeglass frame. The frame must be bulky to accommodate the equipment; therefore, style selection is limited.

3. The body aid is a bulky instrument used for severe hearing loss. A fitted ear mold attaches to a round receiver that connects to a transmitter the size of a cigarette case. The case may be hidden in the clothing, but the receiver and wire cannot. This type of aid is rarely used today.

The devices can be tailored to a client's specific amplification need. Anyone caring for a hearing aid should protect the device from moisture, heat, and breakage.

Newer systems offer special features that allow more precise hearing.

EQUIPMENT
Overbed table
Soft towel and washcloth
Brush or wax loop
Storage case
Disposable gloves

Assessment

1. Assess client's knowledge of and routines for cleansing and caring for hearing aid. **Determines compliance with and knowledge of self-care.**
2. Observe whether client can hear clearly with use of aid by talking slowly and clearly in normal tone of voice.
3. Inspect ear mold for cracked or rough edges.
4. Inspect for accumulation of cerumen around aid and plugging of opening in aid.

Planning

Expected outcomes focus on facilitating communication and promoting comfort and appropriate self-care.

EXPECTED OUTCOMES
1. Client hears conversation spoken in normal tone of voice and responds appropriately.
2. Client demonstrates proper care of the hearing aid.
3. Client responds appropriately to environmental sounds.
4. Client verbalizes that the aid fits comfortably.

Implementation

Steps	Rationale
1. See Standard Protocol (Chapter 1, p. 5). 	
2. Cleaning hearing aid a. Wipe aid with soft washcloth. Use wax loop or brush (supplied with aid) or tip of syringe needle to clean the holes in the aid; do not jam wax deeper into holes.	Wax prevents normal sound transmission (Brinkmann, 1991).
b. Open battery door and allow it to air dry.	Increases battery life and allows moisture to evaporate (Shimon, 1992).
c. Wash ear canal with washcloth moistened in soap and water. Rinse and dry.	Removes cerumen from ear canal.

Steps	Rationale
d. If hearing aid is to be stored, place in storage case labeled with client's name and room number. If more than one aid, note right or left. Turn off hearing aid when not in use.	
3. Inserting hearing aid	
a. Check batteries by closing battery case and turn volume slowly to high. Cup hand over hearing aid. If squealing or whistling sound is heard, it is working. If no sound heard, replace batteries over a soft surface and test again.	
b. Turn aid off and volume control down.	Protects client from sudden exposure to feedback sounds.
c. Hold aid so that the bore—the long portion with the hole(s)—is at the bottom.	
d. Insert bore into the canal first. Use other hand to pull up and back on outer ear. Gently twist and push aid into ear until it is in place and fits snugly.	
e. Adjust volume gradually to comfortable level for talking to client in regular voice 3 to 4 feet away. Rotate volume control toward nose to increase volume and away from nose to decrease volume.	For most people, hearing aids work best at lower volume settings.
4. See Completion Protocol (Chapter 1, p. 6).	

Evaluation

1. Converse with client in a normal tone of voice and observe response.
2. Observe client perform hearing aid care.
3. Observe client's response to environmental sounds.
4. Ask client about comfort after hearing aid insertion.

UNEXPECTED OUTCOMES
AND RELATED INTERVENTIONS

1. Client is unable to hear conversations or environmental sounds clearly. Client's verbal responses are inappropriate.
   a. Remove hearing aid and check battery for power and correct placement.
   b. Inspect ear mold for cerumen blockage.
   c. Change volume setting.
   d. If problems persist, contact audiologist or hearing aid specialist.

2. Client is unable to perform care of hearing aid.
   a. Demonstrate correct aid care.
   b. Observe return demonstration until correctly performed.
3. Client complains of ear discomfort and may complain of whistling sound.
   a. Remove aid and reinsert.
   b. Assess external ear for signs of inflammation.
   c. If problems persist, contact audiologist or hearing aid specialist.

SAMPLE DOCUMENTATION

1000 Client responding inappropriately to questions. Unable to hear normal conversation tone. Complains of hearing an "echo." Volume turned down on ITE aid in right ear. Daughter states that client frequently turns the volume up so he can "hear better." Reviewed proper volume settings and improved listening techniques with client and daughter.

Skill 35.5 | Ear Irrigations

The common indications for irrigation of the external ear are presence of a foreign body, discharge from local inflammation of the canal, and accumulation of cerumen. If irrigation is to be performed for impacted cerumen, a few drops of mineral oil or baby oil can be instilled three times a day for 1 week before irrigation to loosen the cerumen plug (Zivic and King, 1993). Precautions must be taken to avoid instilling hot or cold fluid into the ear because these may cause dizziness or nausea in clients. Never irrigate the ear if vegetable matter, such as a pea or bean, is occluded in the canal. The material can swell on contact with the irrigating solution, causing more pain and difficulty with removal (McConnell, 1992).

The greatest danger during administration of an ear irrigation is rupture of the tympanic membrane. Fluids must not be instilled under pressure or with the ear canal occluded by the irrigating device.

EQUIPMENT

Prescribed sterile irrigating solution warmed to 98.6° F (37° C)
Irrigation syringe (bulb or piston)
Sterile basin for solution
Curved emesis basin
Towel or waterproof pad
Cotton balls
Cotton-tip applicators
Disposable gloves

Assessment

1. Review medical history for ruptured tympanic membrane, myringotomy tubes, or surgery of auditory canal. **These factors contraindicate ear irrigation.**
2. Assess client's comfort level. **Provides baseline to evaluate changes in client's condition.**
3. Assess client's hearing ability in the affected ear.
4. Assess client's knowledge of proper ear care.
5. Inspect the pinna and external auditory meatus for redness, swelling, drainage, abrasions, and presence of cerumen or foreign objects. (If indicated, use an otoscope to inspect deeper portions of the auditory canal; see Skill 12.4).

Planning

Expected outcomes focus on comfort and improved auditory perception.

EXPECTED OUTCOMES

1. Client denies increased pain during instillation.
2. Client verbalizes increased comfort after irrigation.
3. Client demonstrates minimal anxiety during irrigation.
4. Client's ear canal is clear of discharge, cerumen, or foreign material after irrigation.
5. Client demonstrates improved hearing acuity in the affected ear after irrigation.

Implementation

Steps	Rationale
1. See Standard Protocol (Chapter 1, p. 5).	
2. Assist client to a sitting or lying position with head turned toward the affected ear. Place towel or waterproof pad under client's head and shoulder. Place basin under affected ear (Figure 35-13).	Solution will flow from ear canal to basin.
3. Pour prescribed irrigating solution into sterile basin.	
4. Gently clean auricle and outer ear canal with moistened cotton applicator. Do not force drainage or cerumen into ear canal.	

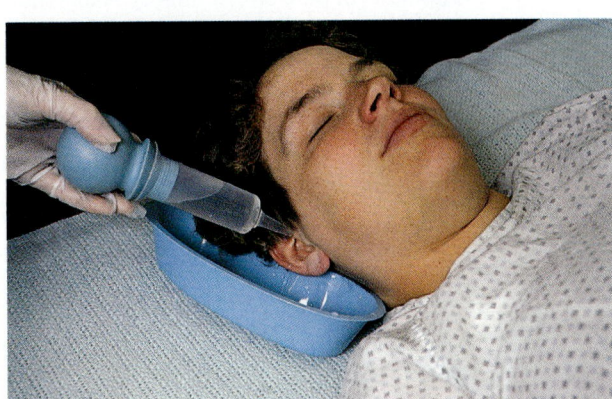

Figure 35-13

Steps	Rationale
5. Fill syringe with warmed solution (approximately 50 ml).	Warm solution prevents caloric response.
6. Gently grasp auricle and pull upward and outward for adults or down and back for children.	Straightens ear canal.
7. Hold tip of syringe ½ inch (1 cm) above the opening to ear canal. Slowly instill irrigating solution and allow fluid to drain out. Continue until canal is clean or solution is used. Do not occlude canal with tip of syringe.	
8. Dry outer ear canal with cotton ball. Leave cotton *loosely* in place for 5 to 10 minutes. Have client lie with affected ear down to drain excess fluid.	Cotton collects draining fluid.
9. See Completion Protocol (Chapter 1, p. 6).	

Evaluation

1. Ask client about pain level during irrigation.
2. Ask client about comfort level after irrigation.
3. Observe for verbal and nonverbal signs of anxiety during irrigation.
4. Inspect condition of external meatus and ear canal.
5. Assess hearing acuity in the affected ear after irrigation.

UNEXPECTED OUTCOMES AND RELATED INTERVENTIONS

1. Client complains of increased ear pain during irrigation.
   Discontinue irrigation and notify physician.
2. Client's ear canal remains occluded. Client's hearing acuity has not improved in the affected ear.
   a. Repeat irrigation if prescribed.
   b. If condition persists, notify physician.

SAMPLE DOCUMENTATION

1000 Client complaining of difficulty hearing in right ear. Cerumen plug noted in canal. Irrigated right ear with 50 ml warm normal saline. Return fluid clear with brown particles. No complaints of pain or discomfort. States that hearing "is fine." Responding appropriately to normal conversation tone. Right ear canal clear.

CRITICAL THINKING EXERCISES

1. Mary Beth is an 18-year-old female being seen in the day clinic for pain in the left eye. She states it feels like "there's something in my eye."
   a. What are some essential questions you should ask the client during nursing assessment?
   b. In preparing for eye irrigation you realize that Mary Beth has a cast on her left arm. She states it's too uncomfortable to lie on her left side. How will you adjust the procedure?
   c. How would you modify the irrigation procedure for a young child who is extremely afraid and crying?
2. You are giving morning care to Mr. Frazier, an 80-year-old client.
   a. Mr. Frazier's hearing aid begins to whistle and he states, "This darn thing doesn't seem to be working—I can't hear as well as I could several days ago." What nursing action(s) would you take?
   b. As you are cleaning the hearing aid you notice an excessive amount of cerumen on the device, in the auricle, and in the outer ear canal. What criteria would you use to determine if ear irrigation is necessary?
   c. The physician recommends irrigation. During the procedure Mr. Frazier begins to complain of dizziness and nausea. What should you do?
3. How would ear irrigation differ in an 8-year-old child who has inserted a kernel of corn into the ear?

REFERENCES

Bocking H et al: Artificial eyes, *Nurs Times* 86(18):40, 1990.

Brinkmann K: Why can't your patient hear you? *RN* 54(1):46, 1991.

Cohen E, Krachmer J: Red eyes and contact lenses, *Patient Care* 26(9):143, 1992.

Johnson & Johnson Vision Products: *Your guide to healthy contact lens wear,* New Brunswick, NJ, 1994, Johnson & Johnson.

McConnell E: How to irrigate the eye, *Nursing '91* 21(3):28, 1991.

McConnell E: How to irrigate the ear, *Nursing '92* 22(1):66, 1992.

Perry A, Potter P: *Pocket guide to basic skills and procedures,* ed 3, St Louis, 1994, Mosby.

Shimon D: *Coping with hearing loss and hearing aids,* San Diego, 1992, Singular Publishing Group.

Weinstock C: Hearing aids: a link to the world, *FDA Consumer* 24(1):18, 1990.

White G et al: Disposable contact lenses, *Am Fam Physician* 43(5):1643, 1991.

Zivic R, King S: Cerumen-impaction management for clients of all ages, *Nurse Pract* 18(3):29, 1993.

ADDITIONAL READINGS

Cunningham D, Ganzel T: Hearing aids: how they work and whom they help, *Hosp Med* 27(7):70, 1991.

Kim M, McFarland G, McLane A: *Pocket guide to nursing diagnoses,* ed 5, St Louis, 1993, Mosby.

Nelson J: Getting the 'max' from your new hearing aids, *Hear Instr* 45(2):44, 1994.

Ocular irrigation: normal saline is not the only choice, Emerg Med 23(18):60, 1991.

Perry A, Potter P: *Clinical nursing skills and techniques,* ed 3, St Louis, 1994, Mosby.

Phipps W et al, editors: *Medical-surgical nursing: concepts and clinical practice,* ed 2, St Louis, 1995, Mosby.

Potter P, Perry A: *Fundamentals of nursing: concepts, process, and practice,* ed 3, St Louis, 1993, Mosby.

chapter
36

Monitoring Fluid, Electrolyte, and Acid-Base Balances

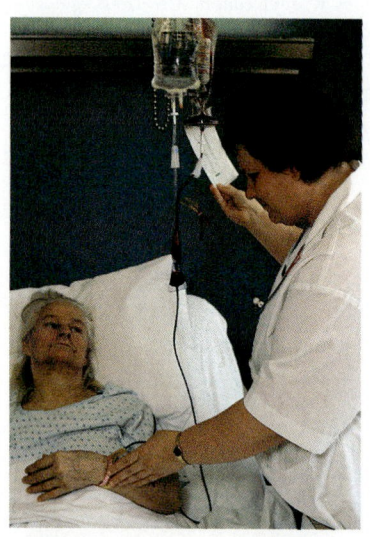

Skill 36.1
Dehydration and Fluid Volume Excess

Skill 36.2
Electrolyte Imbalances

Skill 36.3
Acid-Base Imbalances

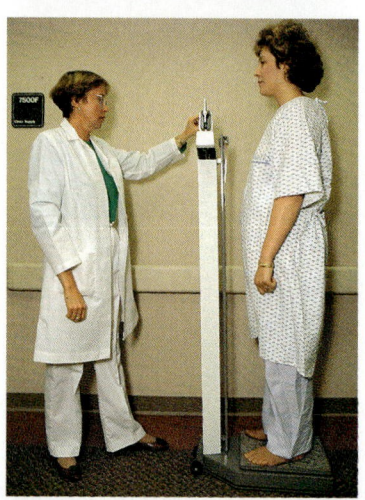

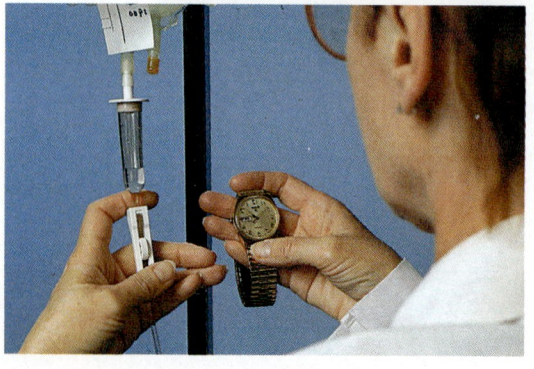

Fluid, electrolyte, and acid-base imbalances occur to some degree in most clients with a major illness or injury. The imbalances are commonly classified as deficits or excesses. In clinical situations several imbalances in the same client are common. Some fluid and electrolyte imbalances are directly related to the illness or disease, such as with diabetes, burns, or congestive heart failure. In some situations therapeutic measures such as major surgery, intravenous fluid therapy, diuretics, or mechanical ventilation can indirectly influence fluid, electrolyte, and acid-base balance (Lewis and Collier, 1992).

The fluid environment inside the cells (intracellular fluid, or ICF) must remain stable to maintain healthy cellular function. The fluid environment outside the cells (extracellular fluid, or ECF) interacts with the outside environment to protect that intracellular stability. The ECF environment provides the cells with the steady delivery of nutrients and removal of metabolic wastes so necessary for life.

Extracellular fluids include *intravascular fluid* or plasma, which is the fluid within the blood vessels, and *interstitial fluid,* which is fluid necessary for cellular metabolism between cells.

Fluid spacing is a term used to classify distribution of body water. Normal distribution of fluid in intracellular and extracellular spaces can be referred to as *first spacing*. When there is excess fluid in interstitial spaces (edema), it is called *second spacing*. An abnormal collection of fluid in potential spaces, such as with ascites, burns, septic shock, or peritonitis, is called *third spacing* (Horne et al., 1991).

Body fluids are composed of a greater percentage of water and smaller percentages of electrolytes and nonelectrolytes such as glucose, bilirubin, minerals, and urea. Electrolytes are major body fluid solutes. These substances dissociate in solution into negatively (anions) and positively (cations) charged ions that conduct weak electrical currents. The numbers of positive and negative charges must be equal in body fluids. The body enzyme systems require electrolyte balance to function well.

Permeable membranes maintain the unique makeup of each body fluid compartment by permitting the movement of water and electrolytes while also allowing the movement of nutrients and wastes. Fluids and solutes move across these membranes by means of osmosis (Figure 36-1), diffusion (Figure 36-2), filtration (Figure 36-3), and active transport (Figure 36-4). The body expends a significant amount of energy maintaining the proper fluid and solute concentrations in its various compartments.

Changes in ECF osmolarity (number of solutes in solution) produce changes in ICF volume because of osmotic water movement. Water seeks an equilibrium by moving osmotically toward the greater concentration of particles. Thus, if a hypertonic or hypotonic solution is

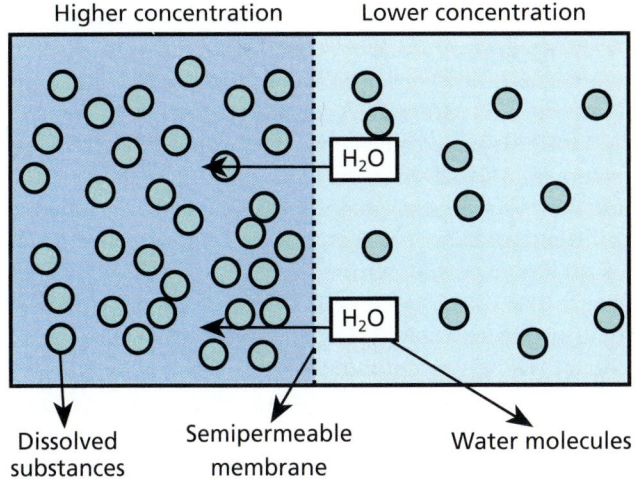

Figure 36-1 In osmosis, **water molecules** move from the less concentrated area to the more concentrated area in an effort to equalize the concentration of solutions on two sides of a membrane.

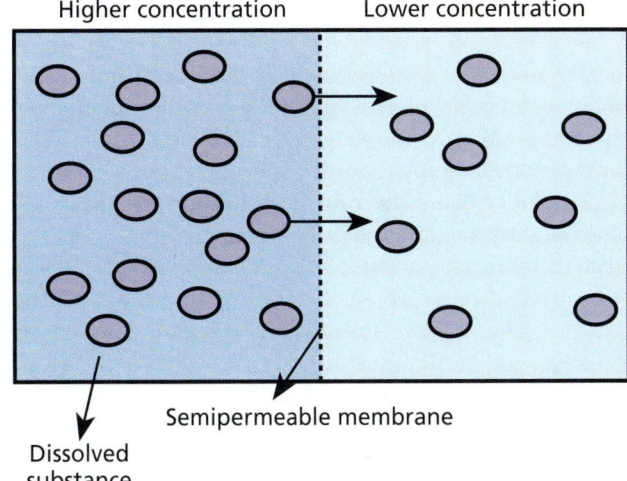

Figure 36-2 Diffusion is the movement of **dissolved substances** across a semipermeable membrane from an area of higher concentration to an area of lower concentration (along its concentration gradient).

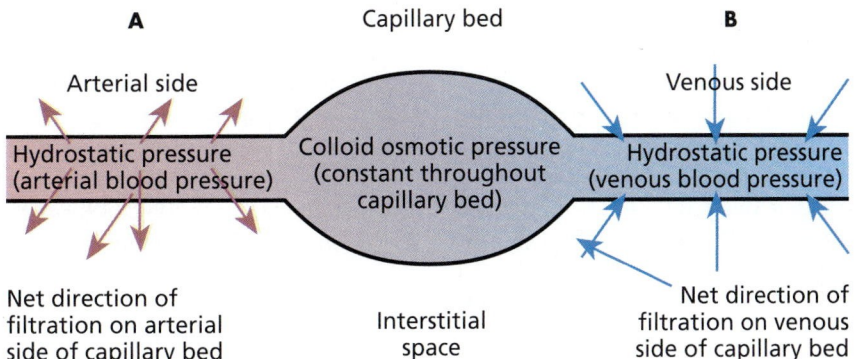

Figure 36-3 An example of **filtration** pressure changes within a capillary bed. **A,** Arterial blood pressure exceeds colloid osmotic pressure, resulting in the movement of water and dissolved substances out of the capillary into the interstitial space. **B,** Venous blood pressure is less than colloid osmotic pressure, resulting in the movement of water and dissolved substances into the capillary.

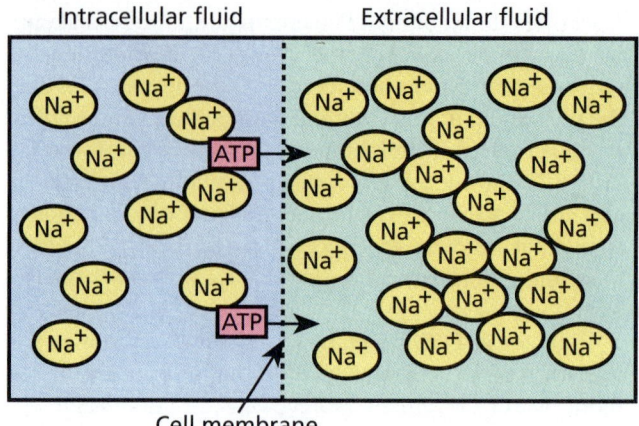

Intracellular fluid   Extracellular fluid

Cell membrane

Figure 36-4 An example of **active transport.** Energy (ATP) is used to move sodium molecules across a semipermeable membrane against sodium's concentration gradient (i.e., from an area of lesser concentration to an area of greater concentration).

added to the ECF compartment, osmotic water movement will occur into the ECF or ICF compartments, respectively. If an isotonic solution is added to the ECF compartment, no fluid movement will occur.

The kidneys are the primary regulators of body fluid and electrolyte and acid-base balance. Fluid and electrolyte balance is accomplished by the renal reabsorption or excretion of water, electrolytes, and nonelectrolytes. The kidneys and lungs participate in acid-base balance. The kidneys reabsorb or excrete hydrogen ions (acidic component) and produce or excrete bicarbonate (the basic component). The lungs contribute to acid-base regulation by hypoventilation (elimination of less carbon dioxide) and hyperventilation (elimination of more carbon dioxide).

Nursing Diagnosis

Nursing diagnoses relating to fluid and electrolyte imbalance include two major categories: **Fluid Volume Deficit** (FVD) and **Fluid Volume Excess** (FVE). **Fluid Volume Deficit** may be related to vomiting, diarrhea, and fever. **Hyperthermia** associated with systemic infection or septicemia, draining wounds, and impaired skin integrity associated with burns also contributes to fluid loss and electrolyte imbalance.

As a result of insufficient fluid in the body, the client may have **Fatigue,** or dry or **Altered Oral Mucous Membranes.** Other difficulties caused by inadequate body fluids can be **Decreased Cardiac Output,** in which case the client may manifest **Impaired Thought Processes** or **Altered Tissue Perfusion.**

Fluid Volume Excess may be related to altered regulation of fluid as in the presence of congestive heart failure (CHF) and renal failure. Such clients may experience **Ineffective Airway Clearance** and **Fatigue** as a result of alterations resulting from the disease process. Another factor that increases the risk for fluid volume excess is fluid overload resulting from the client's intolerance of the rate of infusion of intravenous fluids.

| Skill 36.1 | # Monitoring for Dehydration and Fluid Volume Excess |

A fluid volume deficit (dehydration) is a decrease in ECF volume. A deficit develops when there is either inadequate fluid intake or an excessive fluid loss. Such a deficit may be accompanied by electrolyte or acid-base imbalances. The symptoms of dehydration are a direct result of decreased volumes of fluid in the tissues and/or the circulation (Weldy, 1992).

The sympathetic nervous system compensates for a fluid deficit with increased heart rate and contractility and increased vascular resistance. Also, there is increased antidiuretic hormone (ADH), aldosterone production, and thirst so that body water is conserved or increased. Hypovolemic shock and acute renal failure are possible complications of fluid volume deficits if homeostatic mechanisms fail or are not supported adequately by independent and collaborative nursing actions.

Fluid volume excess is an abnormal increase in ECF volume or a shift from the interstitial to the vascular compartment within the ECF compartment. The signs of fluid excess are a direct result of increased volumes of fluid in the circulation and/or a shift of fluid into the interstitial tissues. The body responds by releasing atrial natriuretic factor (ANF) and decreasing ADH and aldosterone production. All three of these processes lead to diuresis if kidney function is normal. If these mechanisms fail or are not supported by well-planned nursing care, one major complication of fluid volume excess can be congestive heart failure.

EQUIPMENT
Watch with sweep hand
Thermometer
Sphygmomanometer
Stethoscope
Body weight scale
Client's medical record

Assessment

1. Consult the medical record, client, and family to identify risk factors for fluid volume imbalances (Tables 36-1 and 36-2).
2. Check the medical record and interview client and family to discover data that manifest fluid imbalances.
3. Assess client's and family's understanding of the risk for fluid imbalances and the reason certain assessments need to be performed.

Planning

Expected outcomes focus on identifying a high risk for or an actual fluid deficit or excess. Treatment should begin quickly to avoid complications such as shock, renal failure, and CHF.

EXPECTED OUTCOMES

1. Client/family identifies risk factors for fluid volume imbalances.
2. Client's vital signs, laboratory values, intake and output measures, weight, and other physical assessments are consistent with normovolemia.
3. Client and family state what assessments need to be performed and why.

Table 36-1 **Risk Factors for Fluid Volume Deficit (Decreased Intake or Excess Loss)**

Factor	Comment
Infants	Dependent on others to supply fluids
Older adults	Decreased thirst mechanism, immobility
Head injury	Decreased antidiuretic hormone (ADH), diabetes insipidus
Fever	Increased fluid loss through skin, lungs
Gastric suction	Fluid and electrolyte loss
Wound drainage	Plasma, blood, and electrolyte loss
Burns	Plasma, blood, and electrolyte loss
Hemorrhage	Direct fluid loss from circulation
IV line	Incorrect solution or rate
Addison's disease	Sodium and water loss
Diuretics	Water and electrolyte loss
Vomiting/diarrhea	Water and electrolyte loss

Table 36-2 **Risk Factors for Fluid Volume Excess (Increased Intake or Fluid Retention)**

Factor	Comment
Head injury	Increased antidiuretic hormone (ADH), water retention
IV line	Incorrect solution or rate
Steroids	Sodium and water retention
Bowel surgery	Fluid shift into bowel lumen
Bowel obstruction	Fluid shift into bowel lumen
Ascites	Fluid shift (e.g., with CHF)
Congestive heart failure (CHF)	Fluid shift into third spaces

Implementation

Steps	Rationale
1. Review the chart for laboratory values and assess vital signs, intake and output (I&O), and body weight.	
2. Explain rationale for assessments to client and family.	Improves cooperation

Assessment	FVD	FVE	Rationale FVD	FVE
Temperature	Increased			
Pulse	Increased, then decreased, weak	Bounding	Pulse may be irregular if potassium (K), calcium (Ca), and magnesium (Mg) at low levels.	
Respiration	Increased rate	Increased rate, orthopnea		

Steps			Rationale		
Assessment			**Rationale**		
	FVD	FVE		FVD	FVE
Blood pressure (BP)	Decreased, then normal	Increased, then decreased	BP decrease from low cardiac output.		
Weight	Decreased	Increased	Fast weight loss.		Fast weight gain.
I&O	I < O	I > O			
Serum osmolarity	Increased	Decreased	Higher concentration of electrolytes with fluid loss.		Excess fluid volume reduces concentration of electrolytes.
Hematocrit (Hct)	Increased	Decreased	Hct and BUN increase from hemoconcentration (FVD).		Hct and BUN decrease from hemodilution (FVE).
Blood urea nitrogen (BUN)	Increased	Decreased			
Potassium ions (K^+)	Decreased with gastrointestinal (GI) losses	Decreased			
Sodium ions (Na^+)	Decreased with most losses	Decreased			
Urine specific gravity	Increased	Decreased	Measure of kidneys' ability to conserve water in deficit situation. Measure of concentration of nitrogenous wastes.		Measure of kidneys' ability to excrete excess water. Measure of dilution of nitrogenous wastes.
Urine color	Dark	Pale			
Osmolarity	Increased	Decreased			

3. Conduct history and physical examination of client.

Assessment			Rationale		
	FVD	FVE		FVD	FVE
Level of consciousness (LOC)	Dizziness, restlessness, confusion, lethargy, psychosis, coma		Most symptoms are caused by decreased cardiac output. Agitation and psychosis may result from increased Ca^{++} levels with hemoconcentration in FVD. Rapid loss of Na^+, as with GI losses, contributes to coma.		
Eyes	Sunken, dry, less tearing	Blurred vision, periorbital edema			
Fontanels	Depressed	Bulging			
Mouth	Dry mucous membranes, sticky saliva	Swollen tongue, tongue furrows			
Thirst	Late sign		Thirst occurs with severe loss.		

Steps			Rationale	

Assessment			Rationale	
	FVD	FVE	FVD	FVE
Skin	Dry, warm, flushed, inelastic turgor; with shock: pale, cool, clammy	Edema		Pitting edema indicates significant fluid excess or 10 pounds (20 L) of extra fluid in body.
Jugular venous distension (JVD)	<3 cm or flat with bed down	>3 cm even sitting upright		
Capillary refill	>3-4 seconds			
Hand vein filling	>3-5 seconds to fill	<3-5 seconds to empty		
Lungs		Crackles		
GI	Sunken abdomen; anorexia, nausea, abdominal cramps, constipation	Increased girth (ascites); vomiting, diarrhea	These symptoms can occur with both FVD and FVE.	
Renal	Oliguria	Oliguria or diuresis		Diuresis occurs if kidneys are functioning.

Evaluation

1. Review medical record to determine if underlying risk factors for fluid volume imbalances have been controlled or corrected.
2. Conduct ongoing examination of client to determine whether the fluid imbalance has been corrected.
3. After teaching, ask client and family to state what assessments are being performed and why.

UNEXPECTED OUTCOMES AND RELATED INTERVENTIONS

1. After treatment, client remains either hypovolemic or hypervolemic.
   a. Analyze the data supporting the persistent fluid imbalance.
   b. In collaboration with other health team members, administer ordered fluids either orally or intravenously or medications such as diuretics.

2. Client or family cannot state why assessments for body fluid balance are being done.
   a. Assess client or family to determine the cause for the knowledge deficit.
   b. Develop a new or modified teaching plan.
   c. Explain rationale for assessments as measurements are taken.

SAMPLE DOCUMENTATION

1000 Client admitted per stretcher. States nausea, vomiting × 3 days at home. Vital signs: T 98.4, P 100, R 12, supine BP 118/80, standing BP 90/60. Alert, oriented to person, place, time. Complains of dizziness, thirst, nausea. Oral mucous membranes dry, jugular veins flat with head of bed down, inelastic skin turgor, capillary refill <3 seconds. Dr. Miller called. Orders received.

Skill 36.2 | Monitoring Electrolyte Imbalances

Assessment of electrolyte imbalances includes data about risk factors and signs and symptoms of imbalances gathered by interviewing the client and family and by performing a physical assessment. These data include information on serum electrolyte levels that is available in the client's record.

EQUIPMENT
Watch with sweep hand
Thermometer
Sphygmomanometer
Stethoscope
Client's medical record

Table 36-3 **Risk Factors for Electrolyte Imbalances**

Hypernatremia (with water loss)	Hyponatremia (with less ECF volume)
Diaphoresis	Diuretics
Hypercapnia	CHF
Diabetes insipidus	Renal disease
Osmotic diuresis	Cirrhosis
	GI losses

Hyperkalemia	Hypokalemia
IV potassium	Diuretics
Renal disease	Stress
Hyperglycemia	Diaphoresis
Acidosis	Diabetes mellitus
Burns	Cortisone therapy
Trauma	GI losses

Hypercalcemia	Hypocalcemia
Vitamin D overdose	Diuretics
Hyperparathyroidism	Diarrhea
Malignancy	After gastrectomy
Immobility	Poor intake
Paget's disease	Hypoparathyroidism
Bone tumors	High phosphorus
Renal failure	Low magnesium

Hyperphosphatemia	Hypophosphatemia
Renal failure	Protein deficiency
Respiratory acidosis	Glycosuria
Catabolic state	Hypokalemia
Cytotoxic treatments	Hypomagnesemia
Renal retention	Hyperparathyroidism
Phosphoric acid (PO_4) laxatives	Vomiting
PO_4 enemas	Diarrhea
	Respiratory alkalosis
	Alcoholism

Hypermagnesemia	Hypomagnesemia
Renal failure	Colitis
Magnesium (Mg) laxatives	GI cancer
Mg enemas	Laxatives
Mg antacids	Purgatives
	Diuretics
	Vomiting
	GI suction
	Malnutrition
	Alcoholism

Assessment

1. Consult the medical record, client, and family to identify risk factors for electrolyte imbalances (Table 36-3).
2. Check the medical record to identify normal, high, or low electrolyte levels.
3. Assess client's and family's understanding of the risk for electrolyte imbalances and the reason certain assessments need to be performed.

Planning

Expected outcomes focus on identifying a high risk for or an actual electrolyte imbalance. Treatment should begin quickly to avoid complications that can be life-threatening.

EXPECTED OUTCOMES

1. Client has normal serum electrolyte levels.
2. Client and family state why assessments of electrolyte imbalance need to be performed.

Implementation

Steps

1. Assess client's physical and mental status to discover signs and symptoms of electrolyte imbalance.
2. Explain rationale for assessments to client and family.

Electrolyte imbalance	Rationale	Imbalance	Rationale
HYPERNATREMIA (>147 mEq/dl) **With water loss** Thirst Low fever Hypotension Edema Weight gain	Symptoms caused by fluid shift into ECF.	**HYPONATREMIA** (<137 mEq/dl) **With less ECF volume** Nausea Vomiting Hypotension Irritability	Symptoms caused by fluid shift into ICF and ECF.
With Na⁺ gain Flushed skin Fatigue Restlessness Agitation Coma		**With more ECF** Edema Weight gain Hypertension Muscle spasm Weakness, coma	
HYPERKALEMIA (>5.0 mEq/dl) Irritability Anxiety Abdominal cramps Diarrhea Paresthesia Bradycardia	Symptoms caused by effect of hyperkalemia on neuromuscular function and conduction system of heart.	**HYPOKALEMIA** (<3.5 mEq/dl) Fatigue Leg cramps Nausea Vomiting CHF Ileus Paresthesia Bradycardia Flaccidity	Symptoms caused by effect of hypokalemia on neuromuscular function and conduction system of heart.
HYPERCALCEMIA (>10.5 mEq/dl) Lethargy Confusion Depression Nausea Fractures Dysrhythmia Coma	Many symptoms caused by changed neuromuscular action potential.	**HYPOCALCEMIA** (<8.5 mEq/dl) Numbness Cramps Tetany Convulsions Fractures Irritability Depression	Many symptoms caused by changed neuromuscular action potential.
HYPERPHOSPHATEMIA (>4.5 mEq/dl) Cramps Tetany Oliguria Dysrhythmia	Symptoms result from low calcium levels.	**HYPOPHOSPHATEMIA** (<2.5 mEq/dl) Confusion Seizures Chest pain Muscle pain Numbness Memory loss Bone pain	

Steps			
Electrolyte imbalance	Rationale	Imbalance	Rationale
HYPERMAGNESEMIA ($>$2.5 mEq/dl) Nausea Vomiting Flushing Diaphoresis Hypotension Hyporeflexia Drowsiness Coma		**HYPOMAGNESEMIA** ($<$1.5 mEq/dl) Nausea Vomiting Agitation Mood changes Confusion Hyperreflexia Convulsions Dysrhythmia Tremors	

Evaluation

1. Check the laboratory values in the medical record to determine whether an electrolyte imbalance has been corrected.
2. Ask client and family to state why the assessments of electrolyte imbalance are being performed.

UNEXPECTED OUTCOMES AND RELATED INTERVENTIONS

1. After treatment, client has a persistent electrolyte imbalance.
   a. Analyze the available data supporting the imbalance.
   b. In collaboration with other health team members, administer electrolyte supplements or replacements, IV solutions, and/or enemas to restore electrolyte balance.

2. After teaching, client and family cannot state why assessments for electrolyte imbalance are being performed.
   a. Assess client and family to determine the cause for the knowledge deficit.
   b. Develop a new or modified teaching plan.
   c. Explain rationale for assessments as measurements are taken.

SAMPLE DOCUMENTATION

1100 Client admitted. Temperature 98, pulse 110 weak and irregular, respirations 28. Supine BP 124/86, standing BP 98/70. States increasing shortness of breath $\times$ 2 weeks, fatigue, weakness, nausea, anorexia—"I haven't eaten much the last 3 days." Dozing, rouses easily, states, "My legs ache—that started yesterday." Serum Na 135, K 3.2. Call in to Dr. Johnson's service. Orders received.

Skill 36.3	**Monitoring Acid-Base Imbalances**

The normal pH range for the body is 7.35 to 7.45, where pH is the concentration of hydrogen ions (H^+). Values in the normal range indicate that there is balance or equality between the acids and the bases in the body (Figure 36-5). The kidneys and the lungs are the major systems regulating acid-base balance.

The lungs rapidly correct for a change in the H^+ concentration. If the concentration is low (*alkalosis*), the respiratory rate is decreased so the body retains carbon dioxide (CO_2). Carbon dioxide combines with water to form carbonic acid (H_2CO_3), which corrects for the alkalosis. If the concentration of H^+ is high (*acidosis*), the respiratory rate increases to excrete carbon dioxide. This corrects for the acidosis by preventing the formation of carbonic acid.

The kidneys reabsorb or excrete bicarbonate (HCO_3^-) to contribute to a normal acid-base balance or a normal level of H^+. They also can excrete H^+ ions by combining them with phosphate ions and ammonia. The H^+ ions are then excreted as phosphoric acid (PO_4) and ammonium (NH_4). These processes take more time to restore acid-base balance than do the respiratory homeostatic mechanisms.

To assess acid-base balance, a specimen of arterial blood is analyzed for the pH, the amount of oxygen (arterial oxygen tension, Pao_2) and the oxygen saturation of

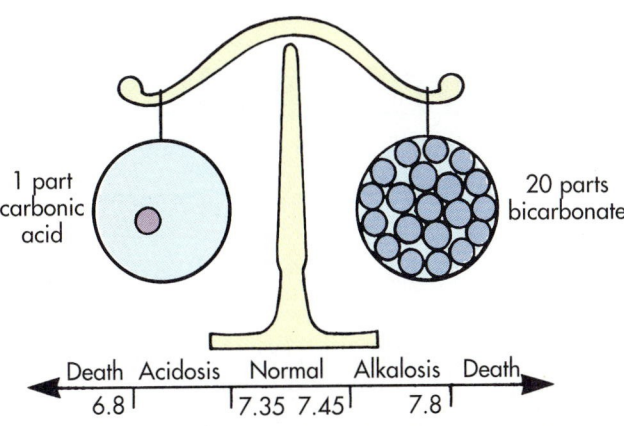

Figure 36-5 Carbonic acid-bicarbonate ratio and pH.

hemoglobin (Sao_2), the amount of carbon dioxide (arterial CO_2 tension, $Paco_2$), and the amount of HCO_3^-. The test is called *arterial blood gases* (ABGs). The test yields information as to whether acid-base balance is normal, acidotic, or alkalotic. It also gives information about whether the cause of the imbalance is a respiratory or a metabolic change in the body and whether the imbalance is being corrected or compensated by the respiratory or renal systems (Mims, 1991).

EQUIPMENT

ABGs laboratory report
Client's medical record

Assessment

1. Consult the medical record, client, and family to identify risk factors for acid-base imbalances (Table 36-4).
2. Assess client's and family's understanding of the risk for acid-base imbalance and the reason the ABG assessment needs to be done.

Planning

Expected outcomes focus on identifying any high risk for or actual acid-base imbalance. Treatment should begin quickly to avoid any life-threatening complications.

EXPECTED OUTCOMES

1. Client will have an acid-base balance evidenced by ABGs within normal limits.
2. Client/family will verbalize understanding of factors that alter acid-base balance.

Table 36-4 **Risk Factors for Acid-Base Imbalances**

Acid-Base Imbalance	Comments
RESPIRATORY ACIDOSIS Chronic obstructive pulmonary disease (COPD) Head injury Oversedation Anesthesia Drug overdose Neuromuscular diseases Mechanical ventilation Cardiac arrest Pulmonary edema Smoke inhalation Pneumothorax Hemothorax Pneumonia Adult respiratory distress syndrome (ARDS)	Hypoventilation is the basic problem. It causes excretion of fewer H^+ ions than are being produced. May also result from tidal volume set too low.
RESPIRATORY ALKALOSIS Hypoxia Pulmonary embolism Anxiety Pregnancy High altitude Severe anemia CHF Pain Mechanical ventilation Fever Pneumonia	Hyperventilation is the basic problem. It causes excretion of more H^+ ions than are being produced. May also result from tidal volume set too low.
METABOLIC ACIDOSIS Diabetic ketoacidosis Lactic acidosis Renal failure Diarrhea	Accumulation of acids or loss of HCO_3^- is the basic problem.
METABOLIC ALKALOSIS Vomiting Nasogastric drainage Diuretic therapy Steroid therapy Cushing's disease Aldosteronism Massive blood transfusion	Loss of H^+, a shift of H^+ into the cells, or retention of HCO_3^- is the basic problem.

Implementation

Steps	Rationale
1. Explain purpose of ABG testing to client.	

2. Review the pH value.
    Normal: 7.35 to 7.45
    pH > 7.40: alkalosis
    pH > 7.55: critical
	The higher the pH, the lower the H^+ concentration.

pH < 7.40: acidosis pH < 7.20: critical	The lower the pH, the higher the H^+ concentration.

3. Check the $Paco_2$.
    Normal: 35 to 45 mm Hg
    Respiratory acidosis (Figure 36-6)
        $Paco_2$ > 45 mm Hg
        pH < 7.40
	$Paco_2$ is the partial pressure of CO_2 in the blood. When client is ventilating adequately, CO_2 is being eliminated in proper amounts; thus, pH is normal. With hypoventilation, not enough CO_2 is eliminated; acidosis results.

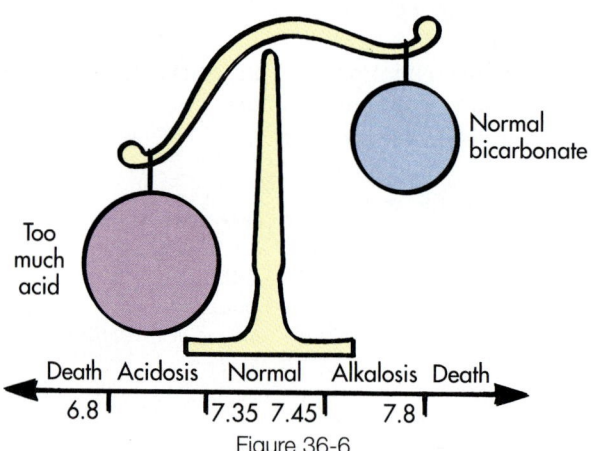

Figure 36-6

Respiratory alkalosis (Figure 36-7)
    $Paco_2$ < 40 mm Hg
    pH > 7.40
	With hyperventilation, too much CO_2 is eliminated (alkalosis).

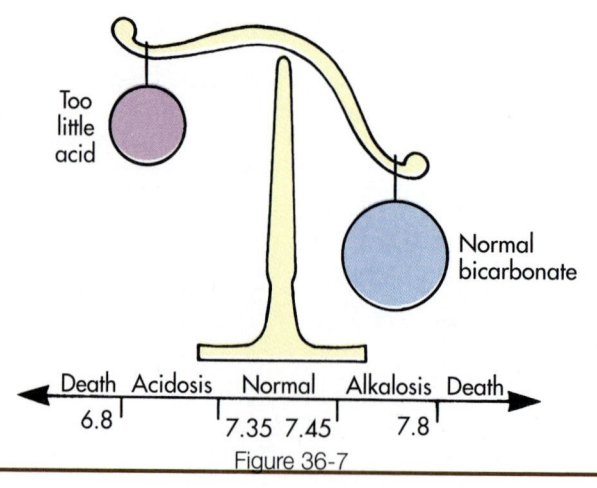

Figure 36-7

Steps	Rationale

4. Check the HCO_3^- value.
   Normal: 22 to 26 mEq/L
   Metabolic acidosis (Figure 36-8)
      $HCO_3^- < 24$ mEq/L
      pH < 7.40

Acidosis results when acid load exceeds the HCO_3^- available for buffering.

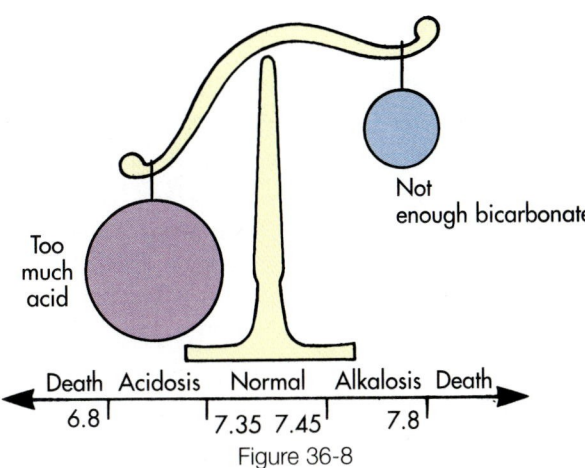

Figure 36-8

Metabolic alkalosis (Figure 36-9)
   $HCO_3^- > 24$ mEq/L
   pH > 7.40

Alkalosis results when acid loss occurs.

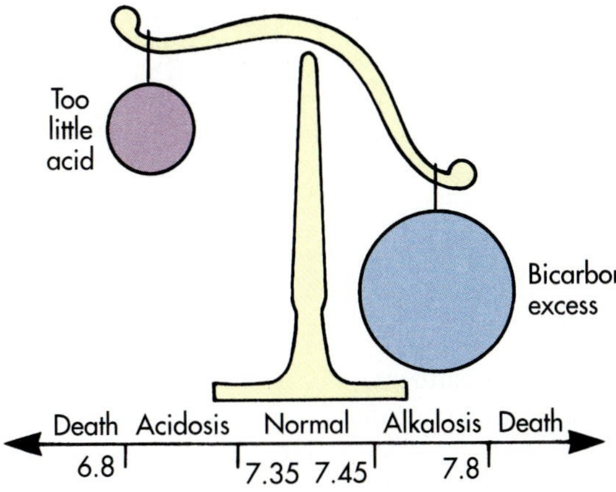

Figure 36-9

5. Analyze the Pa_{CO_2} and HCO_3^-.
   Respiratory acidosis
      Pa_{CO_2} up 10 mm Hg (from 40 to 50 mm Hg)
      pH down 0.08 (from 7.40 to 7.32)

   Respiratory alkalosis
      Pa_{CO_2} down 10 mm Hg (from 40 to 30 mm Hg)
      pH up 0.08 (from 7.40 to 7.48)

   Metabolic acidosis
      HCO_3^- down 10 mEq/L (from 24 to 14 mEq/L)
      pH down 0.15 (from 7.40 to 7.25)

For every 10 mm Hg change in Pa_{CO_2}, a 0.08 change in pH occurs in the opposite direction.

If the Pa_{CO_2} changes in the opposite direction as pH and is a larger deviation than that of the HCO_3^-, the cause of the acid-base change is respiratory.

For every 10 mEq/L change in HCO_3^-, a 0.15 change occurs in pH in the same direction.

Steps	Rationale
Metabolic alkalosis HCO_3^- up 10 mEq/L (from 24 to 34 mEq/L) pH up 0.15 (from 7.40 to 7.55)	If the HCO_3^- changes in the same direction as the pH and is a larger deviation than that of the $Paco_2$, the cause of the acid-base change is metabolic. If both the $Paco_2$ and HCO_3^- are in the normal range, the pH should be interpreted as normal even if it deviates from 7.40.
6. Check the Pao_2 and the Sao_2. Normal Pao_2: 80 to 100 mm Hg	Normal Pao_2 has no bearing on acid-base balance.
Low Pao_2: hypoxemia (Pao_2 of 50 to 60 mm Hg)	Hypoxemia can result in hypoxia (low tissue O_2).
Hypoxia can result in metabolic acidosis.	Hypoxia can exist even with ABG normality, that is, when hemoglobin (Hgb) is low or cardiac output is low, resulting in low tissue oxygenation.
Normal Sao_2: 95% to 99% (at sea level)	Sao_2 is the percentage of Hgb that is saturated by O_2.
7. Check for compensation. Respiratory acidosis (chronic or compensated) pH is down. $Paco_2$ is up. HCO_3^- is up.	Increased renal reabsorption of HCO_3^- begins in 8 hours and is maximal in 3 to 5 days.
Respiratory alkalosis (chronic or compensated) pH is normal. $Paco_2$ is down. HCO_3^- is down.	Decreased renal absorption of HCO_3^- begins in 8 hours and is maximal in 3 to 5 days.
Metabolic acidosis (chronic or compensated) pH is down. $Paco_2$ is down. HCO_3^- is down.	Hyperventilation occurs immediately to excrete CO_2.
Metabolic alkalosis (chronic or compensated) pH is up. $Paco_2$ is up. HCO_3^- is up.	Hypoventilation occurs immediately to prevent excretion of CO_2.

Evaluation

1. Analyze client's recent ABG reports, after treatment, to see whether an acid-base imbalance has been corrected.
2. Ask client and family to explain why the ABG is needed.

UNEXPECTED OUTCOMES AND RELATED INTERVENTIONS

1. After treatment, client demonstrates a persistent acid-base imbalance.
   a. Analyze the available data supporting the persistent imbalance.
   b. In collaboration with other health team members, improve client's ventilation or administer IV sodium bicarbonate to correct for acidosis. To correct for alkalosis, administer chloride and saline fluids or assist client to breathe slowly into a paper bag.
2. After teaching, client and family cannot state why ABG assessments are being done.
   a. Assess client and family to determine additional factors related to the knowledge deficit.
   b. Develop a new or modified teaching plan.

SAMPLE DOCUMENTATION

0900 Client admitted. Vital signs: P 102-112, R 36, BP 148/84. Alert, conversational, dyspnea at rest. Skin pale, diaphoretic, cool. States cough productive of thick yellow sputum, lung sounds with coarse crackles throughout. ABGs: pH 7.32, $Paco_2$ 50, HCO_3^- 24. Dr. Lindsay called. Orders received.

CRITICAL THINKING EXERCISES

1. Consider the following client situations. Indicate which individuals are at risk for developing a fluid volume deficit or excess.

   a. A 78-year-old female who is confused and confined to bed.

   b. A 50-year-old male admitted to the emergency room after a car accident. He has a head injury and has lost blood from multiple traumatic wounds.

   c. A 45-year-old male on long-term steroid therapy.

   d. A 38-year-old female who is post-op following abdominal surgery. She has a nasogastric tube to low Gomco suction and an open abdominal wound.

   e. An 88-year-old male admitted to the hospital with congestive heart failure.

   f. A 50-year-old client admitted with a history of alcoholism and cirrhosis of the liver. His abdomen is grossly distended with ascitic fluid.

2. You are assigned to a medical-surgical unit. At 1400 the postanesthesia care nurse calls and advises you that you will be receiving Mr. Mathews, who has just had a bowel resection. The nurse gives you the following report: Alert and oriented in all spheres. Capillary refill 3 seconds, lungs clear to auscultation. Abdominal dressing dry and intact. Estimated blood loss 300 cc; BP 148/82, P 92, R 16. NG tube and Foley catheter in place.

   a. To get a better picture of the client's fluid and electrolyte status, what additional questions should you ask the recovery room nurse?

   b. After the client returns from the postanesthesia care unit, what assessments will you make at the bedside in relation to the client's hydration status?

   c. The following morning you note the client's daily lab values are as follows: Hematocrit 38% (high), BUN 30 mg/dl (high), Na+ 132 mEq/dl (low), K+ 3.1 mEq/dl (low), urine specific gravity 1.030 (high), serum osmolarity 298 mOsm (high), calcium 8.8 mEq/dl (normal), glucose 120 mg/dl (high/normal). Identify lab values that are congruent with a fluid volume deficit. What does each abnormal value indicate in this situation?

   d. What factors may have contributed to these abnormal lab values?

   e. Of the available lab values, which causes you the most concern, and why?

3. An 84-year-old woman is brought to the emergency room with a history of carcinoma of the breast with metastasis to the bone. According to her family, she had become confused, weak, and immobile. She was frequently incontinent of large amounts of urine. On assessment it was evident she had vomited en route to the ER; she had poor skin turgor, hypoactive bowel sounds, BP 92/48, P 140 and irregular, R 24; she was lethargic but responsive to painful stimuli. Stat electrolytes were drawn. Based on this data, offer a conclusion regarding the client's condition.

4. Analyze the following arterial blood gas values. Determine the source of the acid-base change (i.e., respiratory or metabolic), and determine whether the opposite system is compensating for the imbalance.

   a. $PaCO_2$ 55 mm Hg, pH 7.37, HCO_3 24 mEq/L

   b. $PaCO_2$ 50 mm Hg, pH 7.60, HCO_3 36 mEq/L

   c. $PaCO_2$ 40 mm Hg, pH 7.30, HCO_3 18 mEq/L

   d. $PaCO_2$ 30 mm Hg, pH 7.48, HCO_3 20 mEq/L

REFERENCES

Horne M, Heitz U, Swearingen P: *Fluid, electrolyte, and acid-base balance,* St Louis, 1991, Mosby.

Lewis SM, Collier IC: *Medical-surgical nursing,* ed 3, St Louis, 1992, Mosby.

Mims B: Interpreting ABGs, *RN* 54:3, 1991.

Weldy NJ: *Body fluids and electrolytes,* ed 6, St Louis, 1992, Mosby.

ADDITIONAL READINGS

Anderson S: ABGs—Six easy steps to interpreting blood gases, *Am J Nurs,* August, 1990.

Angelucci D, Todaro A: Reversing acute dehydration, *Nurs* 23(6):33, 1993.

Bove LA: How fluids and electrolytes shift after surgery, *Nursing '94* August, 1994.

Ciocon JD, Fernandez BB, Ciocon DG: Leg edema: clinical clues to the differential diagnosis, *Geriatrics* 48(5):34, 1993.

Kositzke JA: A question of balance: dehydration in the elderly, *J Gerontol Nurs* 16(5):4, 1990.

Martin JH: Dehydration in the elderly surgical patient, *AORN J* 60(4):666, 1994.

Raimer R: How to identify electrolyte imbalances on your patient's EKG, *Nursing '94* June, 1994.

Romanski SO: Interpreting ABGs, *Nursing '86* September, 1986.

Stringfield YN: Back to basics—acidosis, alkalosis, and ABGs, *Am J Nurs* November, 1993.

Tasota FJ, Wesmiller SW: Assessing ABGs: maintaining the delicate balance, *Nursing '94* May, 1994.

chapter 37

Emergency Measures for Life Support in the Hospital Setting

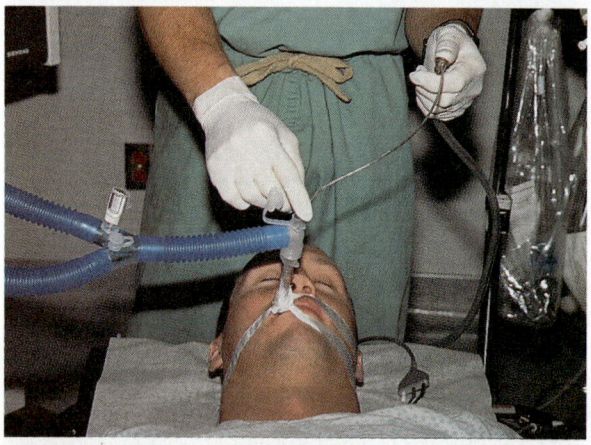

Skill 37.1
Resuscitation

Skill 37.2
Code Management

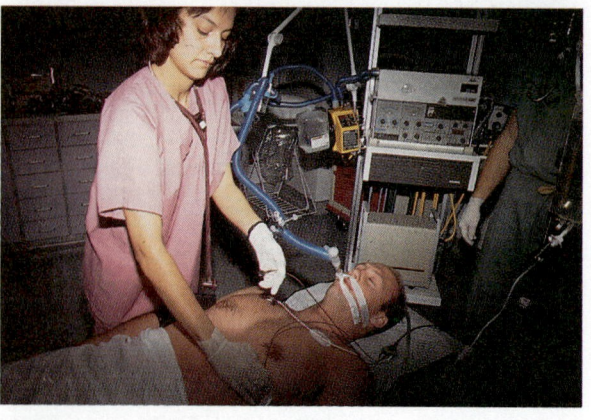

The cardiovascular and pulmonary systems work together to transport oxygen to the tissues and remove carbon dioxide and other waste products of metabolism. The amount of oxygen delivered to the tissues depends on several physiological components. These components are ventilation (amount of oxygen entering the lungs), perfusion (circulation of blood to lungs and tissues), ability of oxygen to diffuse to the tissues and the oxygen-carrying capacity of the blood, and tissue oxygen requirements. Also, the heart must be able to pump adequate amounts of blood for circulation throughout the body. The carrying capacity of the blood depends on hemoglobin present and its ability to carry oxygen, as well as the amount of oxygen dissolved in the blood. Oxygen dissolved in the blood accounts for approximately 3% of the inspired oxygen. Ventilation, or gas exchange, allows for the diffusion of oxygen from inspired air to the capillary beds and movement of carbon dioxide to be expired during exhalation. This exchange occurs at the alveolar level.

The brain and kidney are the two organs that are most affected by decreases in circulating oxygen. Respiratory arrest or cardiac arrest are considered to be emergency situations that the nurse must be prepared to handle at any time. Respiratory arrest, or absence of breathing, results in no oxygen exchange and buildup of carbon dioxide and waste products in the tissues. Cardiac arrest results in cessation of circulating blood, eliminating oxygen transport.

Predisposing factors to a cardiac or pulmonary arrest may include illnesses involving the cardiopulmonary system, presence of an airway obstruction, fluid and electrolyte imbalances, and ingestion of toxic substances. Unless otherwise indicated, such as a client having DNR (do not resuscitate) status, all clients receive cardiopulmonary resuscitation (CPR) in the event of an arrest. Individual hospital policy and procedure define methods of identification of clients' resuscitation status. Advanced directives offer valuable information concerning resuscitation status and individual client determinations regarding life-prolonging measures (see Chapter 38). Determination of resuscitation status may have been accomplished before a client's hospital admission. However, resuscitation status may need to be discussed with the client after diagnostic tests or severe accident or illness preclude a full recovery to prehospitalization status. The physician initiates discussion with the client and family. Family members may not agree with the client's wishes regarding resuscitation status, or they may disagree among themselves regarding status determination when the client is physically unable to decide. Many hospitals or institutions have a mechanism to assist the client and/or family members regarding this issue. Social service or an ethics committee may be of assistance to the client.

Nursing Diagnosis

Nursing diagnoses that apply when clients undergo CPR include **Ineffective Breathing Pattern,** in which a client who is not breathing (respiratory arrest) is unable to achieve adequate gas exchange of oxygen and carbon dioxide. This may be related to injury or paralysis affecting the diaphragm or phrenic nerve. It may also be related to a collapsed lung (pneumothorax) or chest trauma with blood accumulated in the chest (hemothorax). **Ineffective Airway Clearance** related to copious secretions associated with pneumonia or airway obstruction can also result in respiratory distress.

Impaired Gas Exchange can be associated with cardiac or pulmonary disorders that interfere with the body's ability to exchange carbon dioxide and oxygen at the cellular level. **Decreased Cardiac Output** occurs when there is a cardiac arrest and when there are cardiac disorders such as dysrhythmias, blockage of the coronary arteries, or congestive heart failure (CHF). Finally, **Altered Tissue Perfusion** of vital organs (brain, kidney, heart) occurs if cardiopulmonary function is not maintained or restored.

Skill 37.1 | Resuscitation

Cardiopulmonary arrest is identified by the absence of pulse or respiration. Once this is assessed, the nurse must immediately begin CPR. CPR is an emergency procedure that combines artificial breathing techniques and external cardiac massage. This technique is accomplished in an established and orderly pattern known as the ABCs. Resuscitation efforts include (A) establishing an *a*irway, (B) initiating *b*reathing, and (C) maintaining *c*irculation. Early CPR followed by immediate electrical defibrillation of the heart (when indicated) and advanced cardiac life support can improve the survival of cardiopulmonary arrest victims. Tissue damage, including permanent heart and brain damage, occurs within 5 minutes of cessation of oxygen delivery to the tissues.

Proper positioning of the head is essential for artificial respiration to be adequate and to avoid obstruction of the airway by the tongue. When a cervical spine injury is suspected, the jaw thrust maneuver is used to avoid hyperextension of the neck and to minimize the risk of causing further damage. External cardiac compression must be performed with the client's spine supported by a hard surface and compressive efforts applied in the correct anatomical position.

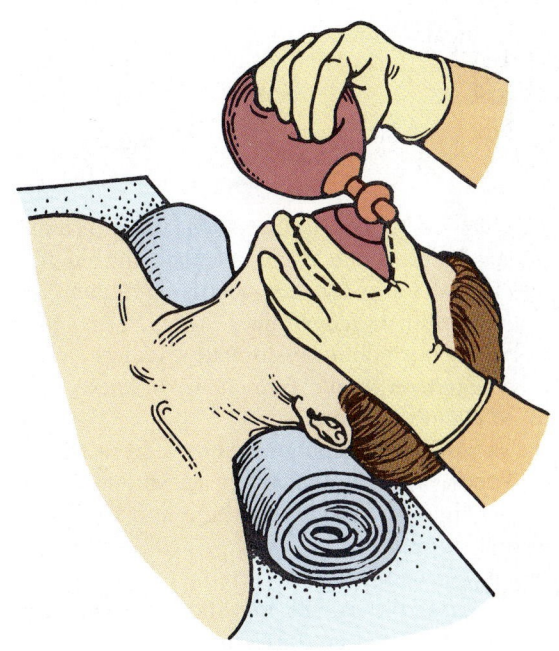

Figure 37-1

EQUIPMENT

Bag valve mask device (Figure 37-1)
CPR pocket mask (see Figure 37-5)
Chest compression board
Resuscitation cart
Suction apparatus
Pulse oximetry monitoring equipment (optional)

Assessment

1. Assess the client's unresponsiveness by shaking the client and shouting, "Are you OK?" **This information assists the nurse in determining if the client is unconscious, rather than intoxicated, sleeping, or hearing impaired.**
2. Activate the emergency medical services according to hospital policy and procedure (call a code 99, 555, etc.).

3. Assess the presence of respirations and carotid or brachial (in children) pulse. **In children under age 1 year, the brachial site is the easiest anatomical location to assess the presence of a pulse.**

Planning

Expected outcomes focus on the goals of care, which are restoration of cardiac and pulmonary function before onset of irreversible brain or other organ damage.

EXPECTED OUTCOMES

1. Adequate oxygenation and tissue perfusion is maintained during artificial resuscitation.
2. Client regains spontaneous respirations during resuscitation.
3. Client regains an adequate cardiac output as a result of resuscitation.

Implementation

Steps	Rationale

nurse alert This skill requires that CPR be performed immediately on discovery of a client with cardiopulmonary arrest and that electrical defibrillation equipment be obtained as soon as possible.

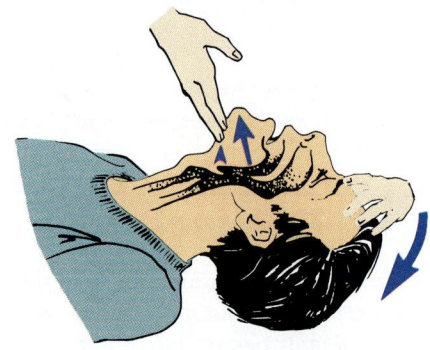

Figure 37-2

1. See Standard Protocol (Chapter 1, p. 5).

2. Call for assistance.

Effective CPR cannot be continuously maintained by one person. The helper can also obtain resuscitation cart or equipment.

3. Place victim on hard surface, such as floor, ground, or a backboard. If the client must be moved to the supine position, use the logrolling technique to maintain spinal precautions.

External cardiac compressions are most effective when the heart is compressed between the sternum and a hard surface (American Heart Association, 1993).

4. Correctly position for resuscitative efforts.
   a. One-person rescue: face client, on knees, parallel to client's sternum.
   b. Two-person rescue: one person faces client, on knees, parallel to client's head. Second person is on opposite side facing client and is parallel to the sternum.

Allows rescuer to move quickly between head and sternum.
Allows one rescuer to perform artificial breathing while the other rescuer performs chest compressions.

5. Open the airway.
   a. Use head-tilt, chin-lift method (no head or neck trauma is suspected) (Figure 37-2).

Tongue is the most common cause of airway obstruction in unconscious client. If necessary, remove foreign body.

Steps	Rationale

b. Jaw thrust maneuver: grasp angles of client's lower jaw and lift with both hands, displacing the mandible forward (Figure 37-3).

If head or neck injury is present or suspected, this maneuver allows opening of airway without disrupting head and neck alignment, therefore preventing any further damage.

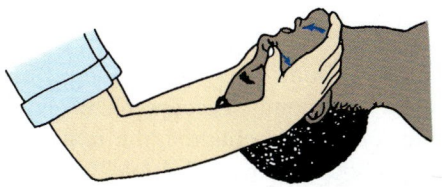

Figure 37-3

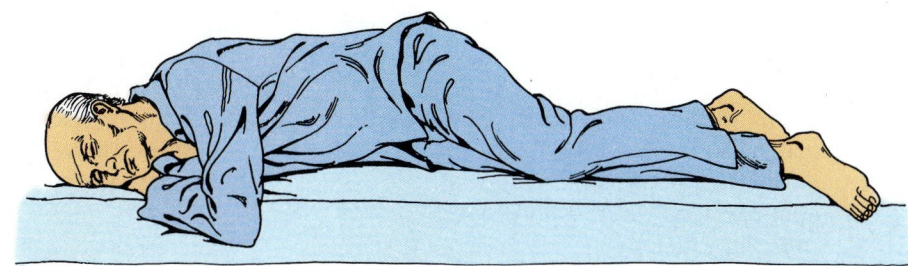

Figure 37-4

6. Observe for chest movement, listening for breaths and feeling for breaths.

Indicates client has spontaneous respirations.

7. If client is breathing and no trauma is present, place client in the recovery position (Figure 37-4).

Place client on the side using the arm and leg for stabilization.

8. If client is not breathing, administer artificial respiration.

a. *Adult:* Pinch client's nose with fingers and occlude mouth with nurse's mouth or use CPR pocket mask (Figure 37-5). Give two slow breaths ($1\frac{1}{2}$ to 2 seconds). Continue with 10 to 12 breaths per minute. Allow the lungs to deflate between breaths (American Heart Association, 1993).

Forms an airtight seal around client's mouth and prevents air from escaping through the nose. An excess of air volume and rapid respiratory rates may force air into the stomach, resulting in gastric distention.

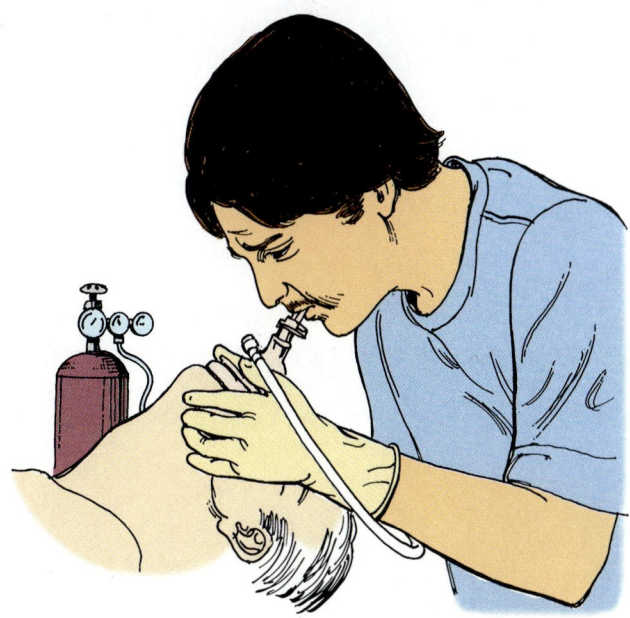

Figure 37-5

Steps	Rationale

b. *Infant and child:* Place nurse's mouth or CPR pocket mask over nose and client's mouth forming an airtight seal. Give two slow breaths (1 to 1½ seconds). Continue with 20 breaths per minute (American Heart Association, 1993).

Give breaths with only enough force to make chest rise and fall. Slow breaths deliver air at the lowest possible pressure to reduce the risk of gastric distention.

9. If lungs do not inflate, check for visible airway obstruction. Remove foreign body (if visible). Perform Heimlich maneuver if airway remains obstructed.

Vomitus or other foreign body may obstruct the airway, preventing air from entering the lungs. Blind finger sweeping of the mouth is acceptable in adults to clear airway. In infants and children, the mouth is opened and foreign body removed if visible. Do not use blind finger sweeping.

10. Suction secretions as needed or turn client's head to the side if no obvious trauma is present.

Suctioning secretions assists in preventing airway obstruction. Turning the head to one side allows the secretions to drain by gravity.

11. Check for presence of carotid pulse in adult or brachial pulse in infant. Feel for 3 to 5 seconds (American Heart Association, 1993).

Carotid pulse is present when other peripheral pulses are not. Delivering external cardiac compressions in the presence of a pulse may cause serious injury.

12. If no pulse, initiate chest compressions.
   a. *Adult:* Place hands on lower third of the sternum (Figure 37-6). Lock elbows and maintain shoulders in line with the sternum (Figure 37-7).
   b. *Child:* Place the heel of one hand on the lower third of the sternum (Figure 37-8).
   c. *Infant:* Place first and second fingers of one hand on sternum about ½ inch (1 cm) below nipple line (Figure 37-9).

Correct positioning of the hands decreases chance of injury.

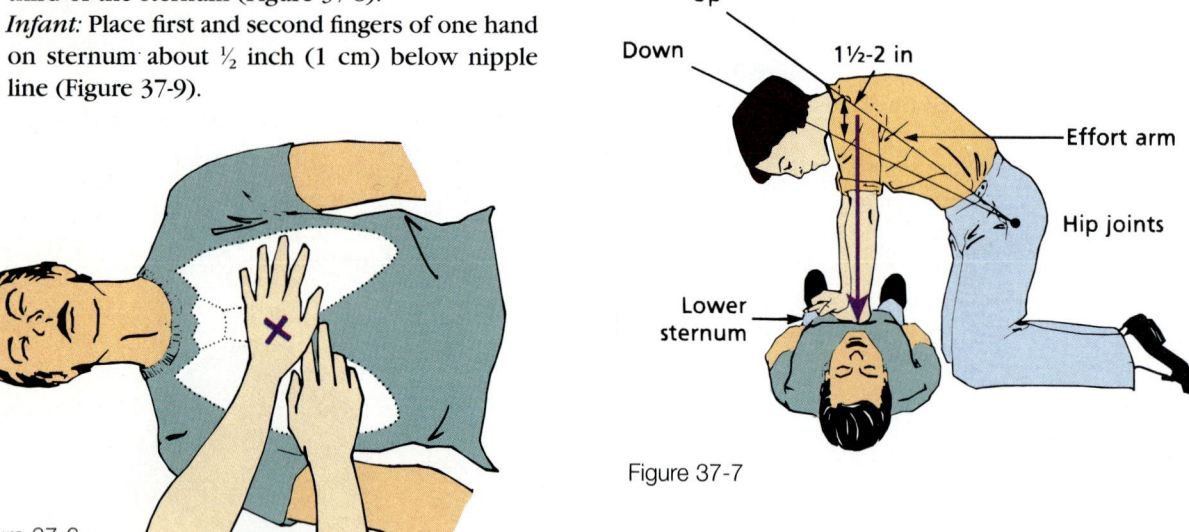

Figure 37-6

Figure 37-7

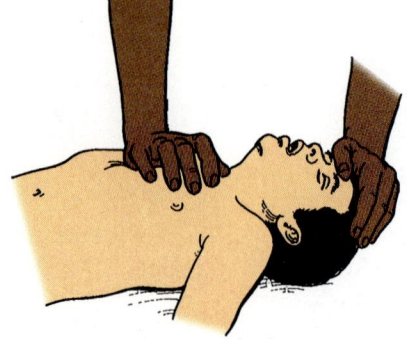

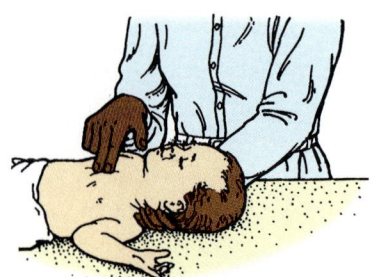

Figure 37-8

Figure 37-9

Steps	Rationale

13. Compress chest downward to proper depth and release.
   a. *Adult:* 1½ to 2 inches (4 to 5 cm)
   b. *Child:* 1 to 1½ inches (2.5 to 4 cm)
   c. *Infant:* ½ to 1 inch (1 to 2.5 cm)
	Compression on the sternum squeezes the heart between the sternum and the spine. The heart fills on release of compression.

14. Maintain correct ratio proportionate to number of rescuers (American Heart Association, 1993).
One rescuer: 15 compressions, 2 breaths
Two rescuers: 5 compressions, 1 breath
   a. *Adult:* 80 to 100 compressions per minute
   b. *Child:* 100 compressions per minute
   c. *Infant:* At least 100 compressions per minute
	Number of compressions per minute determines the cardiac output.

15. Monitor the adequacy of the compressions during two-rescuer CPR, with palpation of the carotid pulse during compressions. Have the rescuer performing the breathing palpate the carotid pulse during compression. (Do not delay compression.)	If the carotid pulse is not palpable, compressions may not be strong enough or hand position on the sternum may be incorrect. CPR cannot be interrupted for more than 5 seconds. Interruption of CPR for intubation should be closely monitored to avoid prolonged cessation of life support measures.
16. Continue CPR until nurse is relieved, client regains cardiopulmonary function independently, or physician directs that CPR be discontinued. 17. See Completion Protocol (Chapter 1, p. 6).	Artificial respirations and cardiac function are provided.

Evaluation

1. Inspect client's chest wall for rise and fall during administration of artificial breathing. Monitor for adequate seal over client's mouth.
2. After four complete cycles of compressions and breaths, palpate for the presence of a carotid or brachial (infant) pulse. Assess again at least every 5 minutes thereafter.
3. Assess the pupillary response to light. If there is adequate oxygenation to the brain, the pupils will constrict to light.

UNEXPECTED OUTCOMES
AND RELATED INTERVENTIONS

Client develops a fractured rib or sternum or laceration of an internal organ such as the lung or liver.

   a. Monitor correct hand placement during administration of CPR.
   b. Assess client for predisposing factors to injury, such as osteoporosis or other medical problems.

SAMPLE DOCUMENTATION

2230 Found client lying in bed and unresponsive. No breathing noted. Carotid pulse not palpable. Code and CPR immediately initiated.

2342 Client resuscitated by Code 99 team and transferred to the medical intensive care unit with respiratory care in attendance.

Skill 37.2 | Code Management

This skill includes the initial response and management of cardiopulmonary arrest in a client. Care must be taken to perform the basic skills of CPR immediately on discovery of an unresponsive client. In many hospital settings, a code team or cardiac arrest team is available to respond and assist in resuscitation of a client with cardiac arrest.

The team usually includes physicians, intensive care nurses, respiratory therapy personnel, laboratory technologists, and other personnel. A hospital chaplin from the pastoral care department also comes to be with the family. Until the team's arrival, the persons present initiate CPR. Excess furniture is moved out of the way, and resuscitation equipment (including a crash cart) is brought to the room. Family or visitors are asked to wait in a nearby area. If the client is in a two-bed room and the roommate can be assisted to leave, this is appropriate. If the roommate cannot leave, it is advisable for someone to remain with the person.

In most hospital settings, the head of the bed can be removed and used as a firm surface under the client. As soon as possible, an intravenous (IV) line is initiated if not already present. The client is intubated, and an ambu bag used for ventilation.

A cardiopulmonary arrest is approached in an orderly and organized fashion to ensure the most expedient care. The goal is to restore cardiopulmonary function without adverse outcome. The Committee on Emergency Cardiac Care (1992) has researched cardiac arrest outcomes and updated a set of detailed outlines to guide in the initial care of these clients. Specific recommendations for emergency cardiac drugs, electrical defibrillation, and supportive measures are included in the *Advanced Cardiac Life Support* guidelines (Cummins, 1994).

EQUIPMENT

Bag-valve mask device
CPR pocket mask, if available
Chest compression board
Resuscitation cart (Figure 37-10)
Defibrillator/monitor
Emergency cardiac medications (lidocaine, epinephrine, atropine, dopamine)
IV needles (16 and 18 gauge), IV fluids (0.9 % normal saline)
Endotracheal intubation equipment
Suction apparatus
Pulse oximetry monitoring (optional)

Assessment

1. Assess client's unresponsiveness (see Skill 37.1).
2. Activate the emergency medical service in accordance with hospital policy and procedure (call code 99, 555, etc.) (see agency policy).
3. Open client's airway.
4. Establish absence of breathing and carotid pulse (brachial with infants).

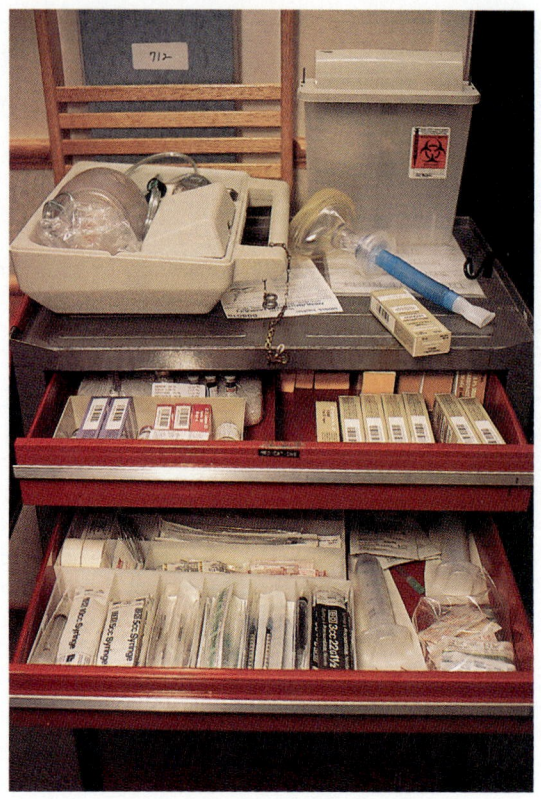

Figure 37-10

Planning

Expected outcomes focus on the establishment and maintenance of artificial breathing and circulation during client's resuscitation. Prevention of injuries as a result of CPR and vital organ damage as a consequence of inadequate tissue perfusion should also be considered.

EXPECTED OUTCOMES

1. Client regains cardiopulmonary function.
2. Client maintains adequate oxygenation to the vital organs, brain, and kidneys during resuscitation.

Implementation

Steps	Rationale

nurse alert — This skill requires application of the basic principles of CPR to maintain tissue perfusion until additional assistance or the cardiac arrest team arrives.

1. See Standard Protocol (Chapter 1, p. 5).

2. Call for assistance and additional nursing personnel (see agency policy).

3. First available person brings the resuscitation cart with emergency drugs, IV access supplies, and equipment.

Familiarity with location of supplies and equipment facilitates efficiency and teamwork.

4. If pulse is *present*, initiate the following:
  a. Provide artificial respiration (see Skill 37.1).
  b. Administer oxygen at high flow rate by mask and ambu bag (Figure 37-11).

Assists in increasing oxygen circulating to the tissues.

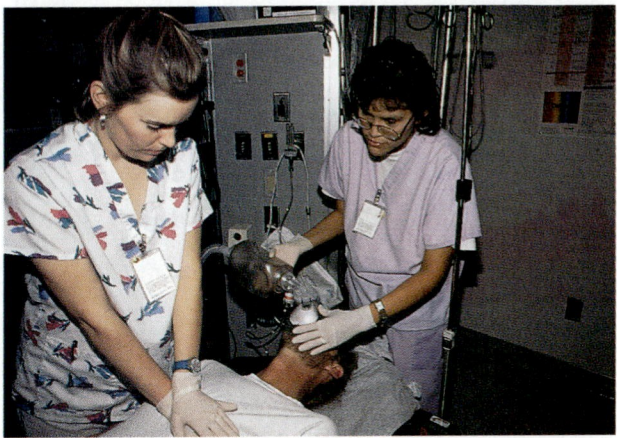

Figure 37-11

  c. Prepare for endotracheal intubation.

  Intubation provides a patent airway and increases pulmonary ventilation.

  d. Monitor vital signs.

  A cardiac dysrhythmia resulting in hypotension requires immediate intervention.

  e. Establish IV access with an 18-gauge or larger needle and infuse 0.9% normal saline.

  Provides a route for rapid drug administration, access for blood samples (laboratory), and fluid administration. Physiologic saline is isotonic.

  f. Obtain a 12-lead electrocardiogram (ECG).

  Assists with determination of dysrhythmia, if present.

  g. Review history for suspected causes.

  Hypotension, shock, pulmonary edema, acute myocardial infarction, and dysrhythmia are possible causes of a respiratory arrest. Treatment depends on the cause.

  h. Obtain arterial blood gases (ABGs) (Table 37-1) and keep samples on ice.

  Provides valuable information regarding oxygenation and information regarding ventilatory status.

Table 37-1 **ABG Measurements**

Measurement	Description	Normal values
Pao$_2$	Amount of oxygen in arterial blood	80-100 mm Hg
Paco$_2$	Pressure of carbon dioxide in arterial blood; measurement of how well lungs are eliminating carbon dioxide (CO_2 controlled by lungs)	35-45 mm Hg
pH	Acidity or alkalinity of arterial blood; measurement of hydrogen ion concentration	7.35-7.45
HCO$_3^-$	Amount of bicarbonate in arterial blood; controlled by kidneys	22-26 mEq/L
O$_2$ saturation	Percentage of hemoglobin that is carrying oxygen	94%-100%

Measurement	Abnormal values	Possible cause
Pao$_2$	<50 mm Hg	Hypoxia
pH	<7.35	Acidemia
	>7.45	Alkalemia
Paco$_2$	>45 mm Hg	Hypoventilation/CO_2 retention by lungs
	<45 mm Hg	Hyperventilation/excessive CO_2 excretion by lungs
HCO$_3^-$	<22 mEq/L	Renal excretion of excessive HCO$_3^-$
	>26 mEq/L	Renal retention of excessive HCO$_3^-$

Modified from Sheehy S, Jimmerson C: *Manual of clinical trauma care,* St Louis, 1994, Mosby.

Steps	Rationale

5. If pulse is absent, initiate the following:

a. Place client on hard surface or backboard and lay flat.

b. Initiate CPR (see Skill 37.1).

c. Determine presence or absence of dysrhythmia by obtaining an ECG, or place client on cardiac monitor (Figure 37-12).

Head portion of many hospital beds is removable to serve this purpose.

A quick ECG may be obtained by using the "Quick Look" function of a defibrillator or applying three ECG leads (lead II) and using the monitor on the defibrillator.

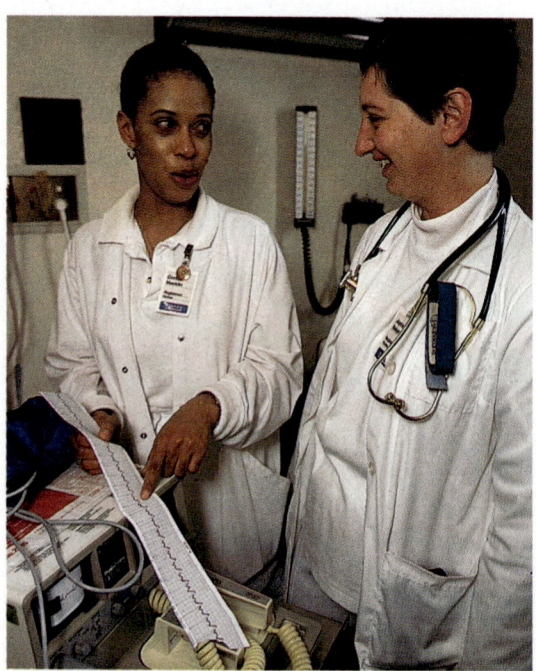

Figure 37-12

Steps	Rationale

d. If client pulseless, ventricular fibrillation or ventricular tachycardia is present, and use of defibrillation is treatment of choice. It is imperative that client be defibrillated as soon as possible after cardiac arrest.

In initial cardiac arrests that are nontraumatic, 80% to 90% are caused by a tachydysrhythmia. Most successful resuscitations depend on early defibrillation (Cummins, 1994).

> **nurse alert** No one should be in contact with client or any item in contact with client during defibrillation. A warning is called out before initiating the charge.

6. Defibrillation is performed only by personnel trained and certified to do so.
   a. Defibrillator is turned on and proper energy level selected.
   b. Conductive materials (saline pads, electrode gel, or defibrillator gel pads) are applied to client's chest, where defibrillator paddles will be placed.
   c. Paddles are charged and placed on the chest wall with one to the right of the sternum just below the clavicle and the other to the left of the precordium (Figure 37-13).

Output is in joules or watts per second. Shock may be delivered at 200 joules and increased if necessary.

Decreases electrical opposition and helps minimize or prevent burns.

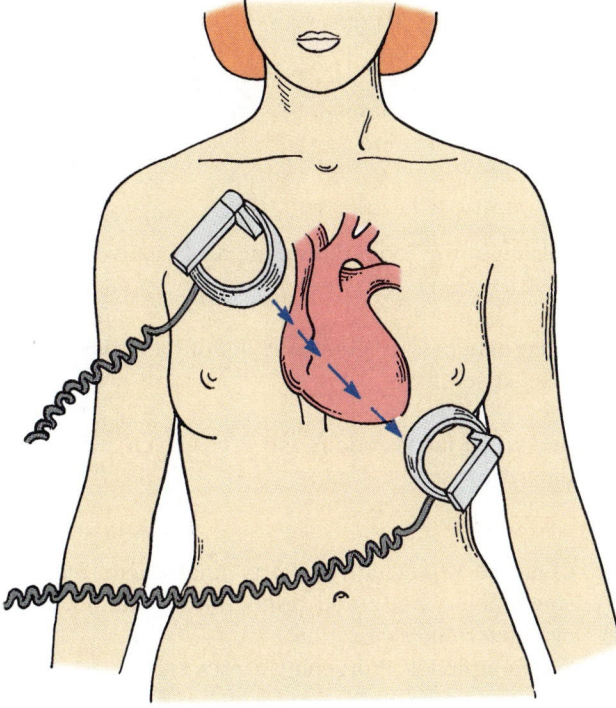

Figure 37-13

d. Operator applies 20 to 25 pounds of pressure to the paddles, then calls "all clear."
e. Operator depresses both buttons simultaneously to discharge the electrical current.
f. Check for return of carotid pulse after each intervention of defibrillation or medication administered.
7. If a different dysrhythmia is present, prepare for the following:
   a. Assist with endotracheal intubation by preparing suction apparatus.

Ensures that personnel are not touching the client, bed, or electrical equipment at the time of discharge.

Establish a patent airway and increase pulmonary ventilation.

Steps	Rationale

b. Determine the cardiac rhythm present and correct the cause. (Additional education and clinical experience in dysrhythmia recognition is required to interpret and intervene for cardiac dysrhythmias.)

8. If not involved in the performance of CPR, nurse should obtain supplies and drugs as requested from the resuscitation cart (Figure 37-14).

Code team members are specially trained in advanced cardiac life support techniques. Rapid location of supplies assists the code team in providing care to client.

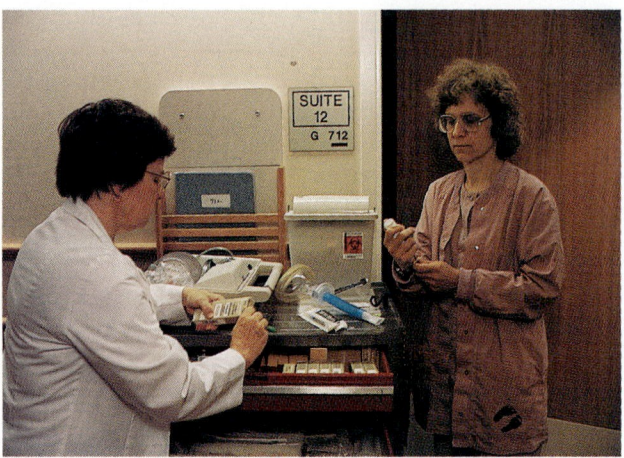

Figure 37-14

9. Remain in the room during the resuscitative phase.

Nurse caring for client is the person most familiar with client's medical history, which aids in diagnosis and treatment by the code team.

10. Keep unnecessary personnel out of room during resuscitative phase.

Cardiopulmonary arrest situations attract many hospital personnel. Too many people may interfere with rapid and expeditious delivery of care.

11. Record all interventions and drugs given, including time, route, and amount.

During a code situation, interventions are performed in a very rapid sequence. Accurate recording of the drugs and interventions assists the code team in planning the next intervention (see boxes on p. 689).

12. Continue resuscitative efforts until client regains spontaneous pulse and respirations or until physician determines cessation.

13. See Completion Protocol (Chapter 1, p. 6).

Evaluation

1. Assess presence of carotid pulse after the first set of four complete cycles of CPR and every 5 minutes thereafter or after every intervention as directed by the code leader.
2. Assess carotid or femoral pulse during compressions to determine the adequacy of compressions.

NOTE: CPR is not interrupted for more than 5 seconds. CPR is resumed between all interventions.

UNEXPECTED OUTCOMES AND RELATED INTERVENTIONS

1. Client experiences injury as a result of cardiac compressions, such as fracture of the rib or sternum or lacerated lung or liver.

   Monitor correct hand placement before cardiac compressions.
2. Client converts back to life-threatening dysrhythmia of ventricular tachycardia or ventricular fibrillation.

Critical Care Calculations

BASIC FORMULA

$$\frac{\text{Concentration}}{60} = \frac{\text{Total minute dose}}{\text{Rate}}$$

PRESENT RATE

$$\text{Rate} = \frac{60 \times \text{Total minute dose}}{\text{Concentration}}$$

DESIRED DOSE

$$\text{Total minute dose} = \frac{\text{Concentration} \times \text{Rate}}{60}$$

REMINDERS

1. Rates in cc/hr = microdrops/minute (μgtt/min)
2. Concentration of solution is in mg/ml or μg/ml.

$$\text{Concentration} = \frac{\text{Drug in solution (mg)}}{\text{Volume of solution (ml)}}$$

   To convert mg/ml to μg/ml, multiply by 1000.
   EXAMPLE: 0.2 mg/ml = 200 μg/ml
3. Total minute dose is in mg/min or μg/min, depending on solution strength. When prescribed as μg/kg/min, multiply by patient weight.
   EXAMPLE: Desired dose = 3 μg/kg/min for 50 kg person
   Total minute dose =
   $$3 \text{ μg/kg/min} \times 50 \text{ kg} = 150 \text{ μg/min}$$
4. Client's lean body weight is suggested reference weight for titration of potent medications. To convert lbs to kg, divide by 2.2.

From Keen JH, Baird MS, Allen JH: *Mosby's critical care and emergency drug reference,* St Louis, 1994, Mosby.

Common Vasoactive Infusions

dobutamine (Dobutrex)
Concentration: 250 mg/250 D$_5$W (1000 μg/ml)
  Usual dose: 2.5-20 μg/kg/min
  Initial dose: 60 kg: 9 ml/hr is 2.5 μg/kg/min
              80 kg: 12 ml/hr is 2.5 μg/kg/min
           100 kg: 15 ml/hr is 2.5 μg/kg/min

dopamine (Intropin)
Concentration: 400 mg/250 D$_5$W (1600 μg/ml)
  Usual dose: 2.5-20 μg/kg/min
  Initial dose: 60 kg: 6 ml/hr is 2.5 μg/kg/min
              80 kg: 8 ml/hr is 2.5 μg/kg/min
           100 kg: 9 ml/hr is 2.5 μg/kg/min

epinephrine (Adrenalin)
Concentration: 1 mg/250 D$_5$W (4 μg/ml)
  Usual dose: 2-10 μg/min
  Initial dose: 30 ml/hr is 2 μg/min

nitroglycerin (Tridil)
Concentration: 50 mg/250 D$_5$W (200 μg/ml)
  Usual dose: 10-200 μg/min
  Initial dose: 3 ml/hr is 10 μg/min

nitroprusside (Nipride)
Concentration: 50 mg/250 D$_5$W (200 μg/ml)
  Usual dose: 0.5-10 μg/kg/min
  Initial dose: 60 kg: 9 ml/hr is 0.5 μg/kg/min
              80 kg: 12 ml/hr is 0.5 μg/kg/min
           100 kg: 15 ml/hr is 0.5 μg/kg/min

norepinephrine (Levophed)
Concentration: 4 mg/250 D$_5$W (16 μg/ml)
  Usual dose: 0.5-30 μg/min
  Initial dose: 4 ml/hr is 1 μg/min
             15 ml/hr is 4 μg/min

From Keen JH, Baird MS, Allen JH: *Mosby's critical care and emergency drug reference,* St Louis, 1994, Mosby.

---

   a. Continuously monitor with ECG after resuscitative phase.
   b. Monitor vital signs and observe for hypotension.
3. Client is pronounced dead by physician member of the code team after all emergency life support interventions are unsuccessful.
   a. Support family/significant others during initiation of grieving process.
   b. Perform postmortem care (see Skill 38.2).
   c. Review resuscitation efforts with team members, and evaluate effectiveness of interventions (e.g., troubleshoot, streamline process).
   d. Discuss personal feelings regarding client's death and resuscitative efforts with team members, supervisor, or other professionals as needed.

SAMPLE DOCUMENTATION

0734 Found client unresponsive. Code 99 called. CPR initiated.

0738 Code team here. Monitor shows ventricular fibrillation.

0739 External defibrillation at 200 joules. No carotid pulse.

0741 External defibrillation at 300 joules. Faint carotid pulse present.

CRITICAL THINKING EXERCISES

1. You have just started your clinical rotation on the adult medical-surgery unit. You have been taught CPR and have been oriented to the facility's policies regarding emergency situations. As you leave your client's room you notice that the nurse in the next room is performing mouth-to-mouth resuscitation on her client.
   a. How should you respond?
   b. The nurse requests that you check the client's pupils before assisting with CPR. What will you be assessing for?
2. After the cardiac arrest team arrives, you are relieved of performing CPR and told you may remain in the room if you wish. Although you would like to stay and observe the process, why might it be best to leave?
3. The code cart is filled with supplies and equipment necessary to carry out cardiopulmonary resuscitation. Why is it essential that nursing personnel be very familiar with this cart?
4. The physician in attendance at the code requests a suction machine. You can anticipate that the suction will be used for what purpose?
5. What important interventions remain to be completed when cardiopulmonary resuscitative efforts fail and the client dies?

REFERENCES

American Heart Association: *Basic life support heartsaver guide,* Dallas, 1993, The Association.

Cummins R, editor: *Textbook of advanced cardiac life support,* Dallas, 1994, American Heart Association.

Committee on Emergency Cardiac Care: Guidelines for cardiopulmonary resuscitation and emergency cardiac care, *JAMA* 268(16), 1992.

Keen JH, Baird MS, Allen JH: *Mosby's critical care and emergency drug reference,* St Louis, 1994, Mosby.

Sheehy S, Jimmerson C: *Manual of clinical trauma care,* St Louis, 1994, Mosby.

ADDITIONAL READINGS

Bailey MM, Arbour R: Getting through your first code, *Nursing* 23(6): 60, 1993.

Braun AE: What to do when a patient needs defibrillation or cardioversion, *Nursing* 21(7): 50, 1991.

Ellstrom K, Bella LD: Understanding your role during a code, *Nursing* 20(5):36, 1990.

Shaffer RB, Lynn-McHale DJ: Action STAT! Responding quickly to asystole, *Nursing* 21(9):33, 1991.

Sommers MS: The shattering consequences of C.P.R.: how to assess and prevent complications, *Nursing* 22(7):34, 1992.

Willens JS: Strengthen your life-support skills, *Nursing* 23(4):54, 1993.

Facilitating Grief Work

Skill 38.1
Care of the Dying Client

Skill 38.2
Care of the Body After Death

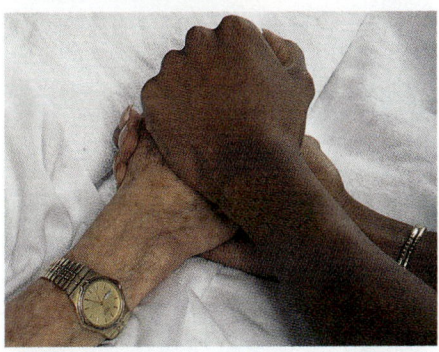

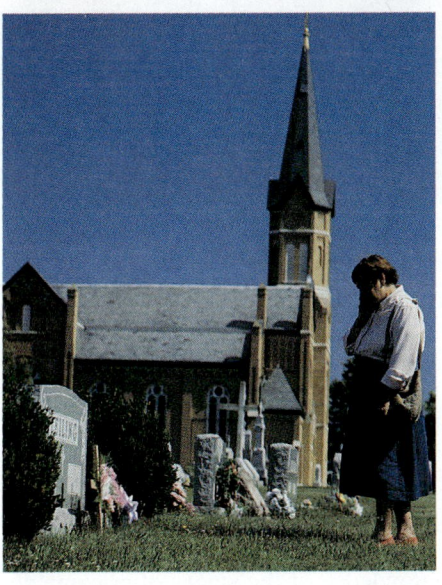

Death is an overwhelming experience that affects family, friends, and care givers in addition to the person who is dying. Feelings, values, and experiences influence the extent to which nurses can support clients and families during a loss or death. A nurse needs to be sensitive to the needs of dying clients, providing care that offers respect and dignity.

It is important for the nurse to recognize that care of the dying and the body after death has social, religious, cultural, and legal implications. Each client and family member needs to be cared for in a unique way on the basis of their reaction to the loss. Having the same nurse assigned as often as possible fosters development of a therapeutic relationship and promotes individualized care.

Every person has a spiritual dimension. *Spirituality* can be defined as that which gives meaning and purpose to life. Spirituality enables persons to reconcile with the past, accept the present, and achieve life satisfaction (Young, 1993). Nurses need to be aware that spiritual needs may be manifested in ways other than through specific religious practices. Spirituality and religious and cultural practices have a strong influence on the events surrounding dying and death. Religious groups may have customs that apply to cremation, autopsy, burial of amputated parts, or burial in consecrated ground (see box on p. 692). Some believe that a lifelong preparation for death can deepen the experience of living by not denying the inevitability of death, but by incorporating death into life (Swain, 1988). Involvement of the pastor, rabbi, or hospital chaplain can be very helpful in providing supportive care (Figure 38-1).

The nurse may find it possible to attend to physical symptoms associated with illness and death but find it difficult to become involved in meaningful interpersonal relationships to support a dying client and family members. To deal effectively with clients who are dying and their families, nurses must examine their own beliefs and feelings about death.

Some Religious Practices Related to Dying and Death

Orthodox Jews and some conservative and reform Jews oppose autopsy and cremation. The body may be ritually cleansed, and burial is carried out as soon as possible.

Islamics believe it is essential to confess sins and ask family for forgiveness before death. After death, the family washes the body and ties the hands and feet. No metal scissors can be used to prepare ties. Only relatives and friends may touch the body. There is no autopsy unless required by law.

Hindus view death and rebirth as nearly synonymous. The family of a *Buddhist* may want to have a priest provide last rites chanting at the bedside.

Christians usually require no rituals before or after death. *Episcopalians* and *Lutherans* may want the sacrament of the sick. *Eastern Orthodox Christians* and *Roman Catholics* consider this sacrament mandatory. Sacraments are for the living, according to these traditions.

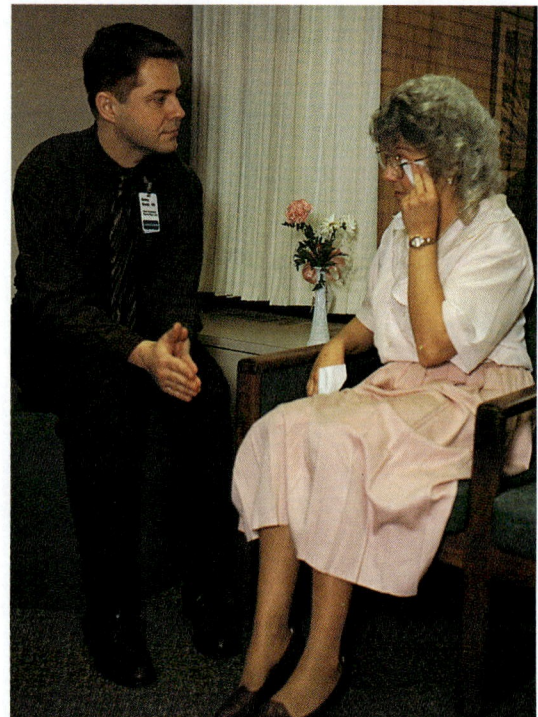

Figure 38-1 Referral to a chaplain can be a helpful nursing intervention for family members suffering an actual or anticipated loss.

Asking the following questions may assist in self-awareness:

- Do you believe it is part of your role as a nurse to talk with families about death?
- Are you comfortable with expression of intense emotions, suffering, and struggle?
- What are your personal experiences with significant loss?
- Do you have unfinished grief work?
- Are you prepared for tears?

It is acceptable for care givers to cry. Tears can communicate empathy and caring. It is less appropriate to lose control with sobbing. If this happens, the client or family may feel the need to stop crying and comfort the nurse (Ufema, 1991b). Nurses need the opportunity to mourn their losses (Figure 38-2). Unexpressed grief can lead to distress that results in inability to care for others. Some institutions provide opportunities for staff to gather for mutual support, closure, and grieving for the loss of clients.

Death can come suddenly and unexpectedly, as in cases of trauma or suicide. Often, however, death comes slowly and painfully with terminal illness. It is important to be aware that normal grief includes many feelings that tend to make people think they are ill or "crazy." Physical reactions associated with grief after a significant loss include fainting, diaphoresis, anorexia, nausea, diarrhea, rapid heart rate, restlessness, insomnia, fatigue, sensations of tightness in the throat, choking, shortness of breath, weakness, anxiety attacks, and pain without any physical cause. In addition, normal grief includes feelings of anger, guilt, anxiety, and numbness, as well as mood swings that vary in intensity and may continue for approximately 2

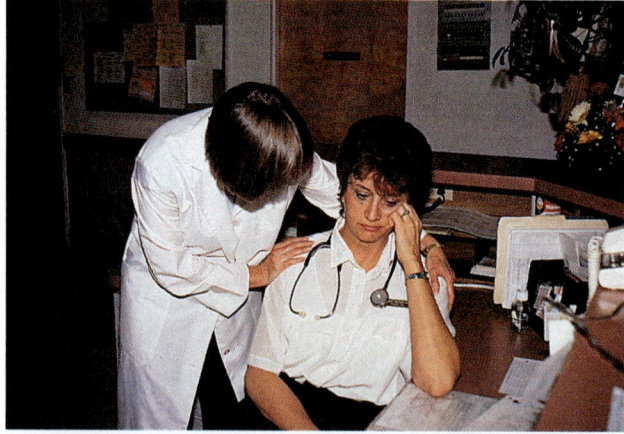

Figure 38-2 Nurses may need the opportunity to express grief when a client dies.

years after any significant loss. These tend to be intensified around anniversaries and holidays. Multiple losses increase the intensity of the grief response. In some cases, facilitating grieving of family members before the event of death shortens the length of time that grief is experienced after the loss.

Knowledge of the stages of grieving and dying helps nurses anticipate emotional needs of clients and families

Table 38-1 Behaviors of Kübler-Ross' Stages of Dying and the Grieving Process

Stage	Behaviors
Denial	Avoids reality, cannot deal with decisions about treatment; may attempt activities of which client is no longer physically capable; isolates self from sources of accurate information; fails to comply with medical therapy; uses considerable emotional energy to deny truth; may appear artificially happy.
Anger	May retaliate against family members, nursing staff, or physicians; becomes demanding and accusing; anger may arouse guilt because client is aware of dependence on care givers; guilt may foster feelings of anxiety and low self-esteem.
Bargaining	Is fearful of losing body functions, experiencing uncontrollable pain, and losing control; is willing to do anything to change prognosis or fate; accepts new forms of therapies.
Depression	Recognizes potential loss of loved ones; may withdraw from important relationships to avoid painful feelings; may become quiet and noncommunicative when feeling loss of control; may express feelings of loneliness; does little to maintain appearance; may become suicidal when unrealistic hopes of a cure fade.
Acceptance	Accepts terms of death; begins to make plans for death (e.g., writes a will, completes financial arrangements for the family, gives up personal possessions); is able to discuss feelings about death; reminisces about the past.

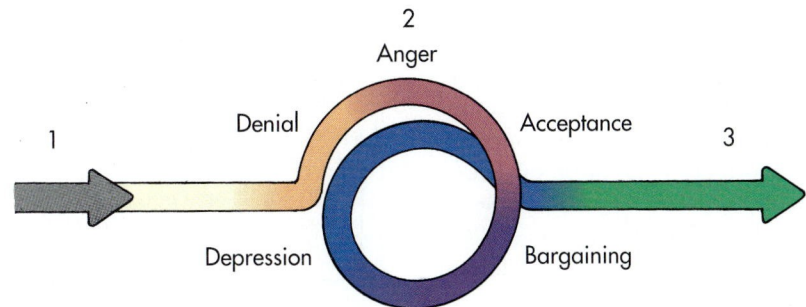

Figure 38-3 *1*, More or less stable time. *2*, Significant loss interrupts the pattern of living; abrupt change occurs whether loss is sudden or anticipated. Responses to the loss vasilate through stages. *3*, Loss is integrated and stable pattern can be resumed.

and plan interventions to help them understand and deal with their grief. These stages occur in individuals suffering losses such as death of a relative or close friend and in individuals facing their own death. In addition, the grief response is common after the loss of a body part or function, independence, home or familiar environment, and relationships, such as after divorce. The nurse's role is to assess grieving behaviors, recognize how grief is influencing behavior, and provide support. This assessment of grief behaviors can be used to support persons experiencing a significant loss.

Kübler-Ross (1969) provided a framework that identifies stages of the grieving process. This framework includes five stages: denial, anger, bargaining, depression, and acceptance (Table 38-1). Although the grieving process has predictable experiences and distinctive symptoms, no two persons react or progress through it in the same way. The process of normal grief follows no set sequence, and clients and families may pass back and forth, reexperiencing symptoms in unpredictable ways

and for varying periods, as shown in Figure 38-3 (Sunderland and Shelp, 1987).

Hospice care involves a philosophy that focuses on symptom management, relief of suffering, and palliative care rather than cure (Robb, 1994). To participate in a hospice program, clients, their families, and the physician must reach a shared decision not to participate in curative treatment. Generally, the prognosis is for 6 months or less (Gurfolino and Dumas, 1994). Clients who participate in hospice programs may be suffering with cancer; end-stage cardiac, lung, or renal disease; acquired immunodeficiency syndrome (AIDS); or other terminal illness. The goal is to enhance the quality of life with a holistic approach; it is not a decision to end life. The process involves an interdisciplinary team approach with nurses, social workers, volunteers, and pastoral care (Figure 38-4).

Hope is characterized by a confident yet uncertain expectation of achieving a future goal (Dufault and Martocchio, 1985). Hope is a complex series of thoughts,

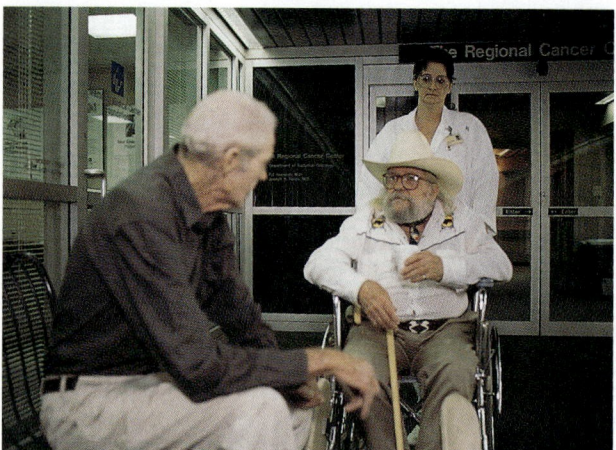

Figure 38-4 Volunteers provide important support to hospice clients.

Modified from Dufault K, Martocchio BC: Hope: its spheres and dimensions, *Nurs Clin North Am* 20:379, 1995.

Dimensions of Hope

AFFECTIVE

Sensations and emotions (i.e., feelings of confidence or an attraction to the desired outcome) that are part of hoping.

COGNITIVE

Processes by which persons wish, imagine, perceive, think, learn, or judge in relation to hope.

BEHAVIORAL

Actions a person takes to directly achieve hope. Actions may be physiologic, psychosocial, cultural, or spiritual.

AFFILIATIVE

A person's sense of involvement beyond self. Social interaction, mutuality, attachment, and intimacy compose affiliation. There is a relationship with others.

TEMPORAL

A person's experience of time (past, present, future) in relation to hoping.

CONTEXTUAL

Hope is perceived within the context of life as interpreted by the person. Life situations influence and are a part of hope. An actual or potential loss may be the context in which hope arises.

feelings, and actions that change often (see box at right). Awareness of the dimensions of hope helps relieve the grieving associated with terminal illness. When physician-assisted suicide is raised as a possibility, it is important to realize that the client has lost hope (Stempsey, 1994). When clients are told there is no hope of recovery, they may hear a message that there is no hope in their continued living. The hospital chaplain is a good resource for those who are searching for meaning in life in the face of dying.

Allowing expressions of *sadness* is a therapeutic measure. Crying is not a sign of weakness but a sign of strength. Tears testify being in touch with intense feelings, and this calls for great courage. Crying can remove chemicals that build up during emotional stress (Tengbom, 1990). As persons open themselves to grief and allow tears to flow, over time healing will come. Some clients cannot express emotions. If this is the case, they change the subject, withdraw from conversation, or leave the room.

Another helpful concept is *serenity*. Serenity is an inner peace that can be learned and requires effort to achieve. It is different from joy, which tends to be related to specific circumstances. It is different from contentment, which is happiness with what one has. Serenity is an inner peacefulness that exists even during difficult times. Serene persons are caring, active, involved, and responsible for their lives. The box (p. 695) lists characteristics of serenity (Roberts and Messenger, 1993).

ADVANCE DIRECTIVES

The issue of quality at the end of life has come under intensive judicial and public scrutiny. It is a client's legal right to determine the degree and kind of care desired. The U.S. Federal Patient Self-Determination Act of 1990 states that every institution receiving Medicare or Medicaid funds must advise all clients in writing of their right to refuse treatment and of their right to prepare an advance directive—a living will or power of attorney for health care. It is the nurse's responsibility to know the laws of the state and to learn of the client's wishes (Badzek, 1992; Law enlarges caregiver role, 1992). A *durable power of attorney* for health care designates an agent to make decisions in the event the client is unable to do so and expresses clearly the client's intentions. The *living will* declares a client's intentions in the event that a medical condition is terminal. This depends more on the physician's decision. The people taking care of the client are not to delay death if it is imminent and irreversible, even if it is impossible for the client to communicate with those providing the care.

These documents must be created as a voluntary act by adults of sound mind, must be signed by the client, and must be witnessed by two adults. Forms are available to clients on admission, and laws of the state must be followed carefully for the documents to be effective. Clients may amend, alter, or void these documents at any time by destroying the document or with a written statement that declares such intent to set them aside.

When the decision is made by a client and family not to initiate cardiopulmonary resuscitation (CPR) measures after the client's heart fails, written "Do not resus-

---

Serenity
1. Awareness of an inner haven that can be reached when the person wishes to do so.
2. Ability to detach from negative circumstances.
3. A sense of connectedness and belonging.
4. Ability to give of oneself without expecting anything in return.
5. A trust in a source of power and strength.
6. Ability to accept what one cannot change.
7. Ability to take responsibility to change what can be changed.
8. Ability to live in the present.
9. Capacity to forgive self and others.
10. Awareness of the larger picture and the insignificance of some transient events.

From Roberts KT, Messenger TC: Helping older adults find serenity, *Geriatr Nurs* 14(6), 1993.

Organs and Tissues that Can Be Donated	
ORGANS	**TISSUES**
Lung*	Skin
Liver*	Cornea
Pancreas*	Dura
Kidney†	Fascia
Stomach	Cartilage
Small bowel	Tendons
	Veins
	Heart valves
	Bone marrow
	Bones

*Segments may be from a living donor.
†Living donor can be used.

---

citate" (DNR) or no-code orders are required. The nurse is required to initiate and maintain CPR for all other clients (see Skill 37.1) until the client recovers or the physician pronounces the client's death.

The Uniform Determination of Death Act (UDDA) is recognized in all 50 states. This defines death as irreversible cessation of circulatory and respiratory functions or irreversible cessation of all functions of the brain, including the brainstem, with inability to maintain homeostatic functions without mechanical assistance.

The Omnibus Budget Reconciliation Act (OBRA) of 1986 mandates that families of potential donors be given the right to the option of organ and tissue donation. A national organization maintains a waiting list of clients in need of organs, which is increasing significantly. Potential donors include anyone whose time of death can be verified. "Brain-dead" clients are good candidates for donation, since their organs and tissues are likely to be healthy (see box above, right). The family must understand clearly that the client is dead before they are offered the option of organ donation. Early referral permits continued oxygenation and perfusion of organs until organ recovery can begin. Certain infections, such as AIDS, make organ donation inappropriate (Chabalewski and Norris, 1994). There is no cost to the family for organ donation, and it does not delay the funeral or disfigure the body.

A trained nursing staff member or a physician is required in most states to ask the family or client's guardian for organ or tissue donation. Institutional policies for required request procedures must encourage discretion and sensitivity in dealing with potential donor families. Nurses may feel uncomfortable making dona-tion requests, since families of deceased clients often undergo considerable grief. However, research has shown that families often are willing to donate if they are asked and if the requester feels comfortable making the request (Malecki and Hoffman, 1986). Local organ recovery organizations can provide more information about organ and tissue donation.

Nursing Diagnosis

Anticipatory Grieving is appropriate when the experience of the grieving process occurs before the actual loss. This may lessen the intensity of grief after the loss takes place. **Dysfunctional Grieving** is an appropriate nursing diagnosis when an individual does not proceed through normal grieving, as when emotional reactions are inhibited, exaggerated, or prolonged. Clients at risk for dysfunctional grieving include those with multiple losses, inadequate social support, or stressful and prolonged anticipated loss. **Hopelessness** is appropriate if the client feels that life cannot possibly improve and no one can do anything to help. **Powerlessness** is an appropriate nursing diagnosis when the client or family perceives solutions, but no way to do anything because of lack of control or resources. Powerlessness may lead to hopelessness. **Spiritual Distress** is appropriate when suffering or dying persons are having difficulty utilizing their belief system as a source of strength, hope, or meaning. **Fatigue** is appropriate when the client or family has an overwhelming and sustained sense of exhaustion that is not relieved by rest. In addition, nursing diagnoses may arise from a variety of physical symptoms related to the disease process.

Skill 38.1 | **Care of the Dying Client**

Nursing care of terminally ill clients can be demanding and stressful. A client and family may experience anticipatory grief for months before death occurs. A dying client must be cared for with respect and concern. Promoting comfort in the terminally ill client is important so that the dying person retains energy to maintain quality life activities.

A client may have dysfunction of any body system. The metabolic demands created by cancerous tumors and systemic chronic disease cause overwhelming weakness and fatigue. Adequate oxygenation, pain control, nutrition, elimination, and control of nausea and vomiting are major challenges for many clients. Physical changes that indicate that dying is imminent include a cooling down of body tissues, altered sleep patterns, disorientation, incontinence, altered breathing patterns, restlessness, and decreased food and fluid intake.

Dehydration may have beneficial effects during the dying process by decreasing urine output, abdominal distention, vomiting, lung congestion, coughing and choking, and edema of the extremities and tumor site. Dehydration may also decrease pain and discomfort by decreasing interpretation of sensation by the CNS (Zerwekh, 1983).

Assessment

1. Assess each symptom in terms of onset, precipitating factors, quality, severity, and factors that have promoted relief. **The nurse's primary role is to provide relief of symptoms.**
2. Identify usual decision-making patterns and persons whom client perceives as supportive in this process (e.g., family/friends or pastor/chaplain). **The nurse should rely on resources to provide client with a sense of security.**
3. Ask client what factors impose barriers in ability to express feelings. **Lack of privacy, pain, stress, and fatigue may create barriers.**
4. Listen for information that helps identify the stage of grief client is experiencing (see Table 38-1).

Planning

Expected outcomes focus on promoting comfort, autonomy, and integrity throughout the dying experience.

EXPECTED OUTCOMES

1. Client maintains symptom control (e.g., pain, nausea and vomiting, fatigue, anxiety), which allows optimal quality of life.
2. Client makes decisions regarding care as transitions toward end of life occur.
3. Client and family express feelings about changes as they occur.
4. Client and family express experience of being treated with dignity and respect.

Implementation

Steps	Rationale
1. See Standard Protocol (Chapter 1, p. 5).	
2. Relieve pain and promote comfort.	
a. Administer appropriate analgesics on a regular schedule rather than PRN.	Pain affecting terminally ill client may be acute or chronic.
b. Choose the most effective route for optimal pain relief.	Oral sustained-release pills or elixirs, transdermal patches, and patient-controlled analgesia (PCA) intravenously or by epidural catheter may be used.
c. Promote relaxation and slow breathing, and encourage expression of feelings (see Skills 2.1 and 9.2).	Tension, emotional distress, and fear can increase the experience of pain.
d. Position the client comfortably, and use pillows, special beds, or mattresses as indicated (see Chapter 24).	
e. Provide frequent skin care, including baths, skin lubrication, and massage. Dry, clean bed linens minimize irritants.	

Steps	Rationale
f. Provide oral care, at least every 2 to 4 hours, using a soft toothbrush or foam swab. Apply a light film of petroleum jelly to the lips and tongue.	As death approaches, a person's mouth remains open, the tongue becomes dry and swollen, and the lips become dry and cracked.
g. Remove crusts from eyelid margins. Artificial tears may be used to reduce corneal drying.	The blinking reflex diminishes near death, causing drying of the cornea.
3. Provide oral intake, if permitted.	
a. Encourage small, frequent feedings of foods requested by client.	
b. Plan menus, using small quantities of nutritious, odorless foods.	Strong odors may cause nausea. Small portions are more manageable.
c. Suggest home-cooked meals, which may be preferred by client when family is able to provide them.	This gives family a chance to participate.
d. Have food available on nursing unit at all times, including juice and milkshakes with nutritive value.	Promotes snacking when client feels like eating.
4. Relieve nausea and vomiting.	
a. Administer antiemetics before meals or on a regular schedule.	Preventing episodes of nausea promotes comfort.
b. Control environmental odors.	Odors often provoke nausea or vomiting.
c. Promptly clean up any emesis and provide mouth care.	Promotes comfort.
5. Provide for energy conservation.	Increased metabolism associated with tumor growth, chronic pain, altered nutrition, infection, and organ dysfunction can contribute to fatigue.
a. Identify valued and desired activities, and have client conserve energy for accomplishment of those tasks.	
b. Identify ways to modify tasks to conserve energy.	
c. Offer frequent rest periods in a quiet environment.	
d. Pace nursing care activities, alternating periods of activity and rest.	
6. Ensure maintenance of elimination (see Chapter 8).	Decreased activity, dehydration, and pain medications interfere with normal elimination.
a. Use stool softeners, laxatives, or suppositories on a regular basis.	
b. Encourage use of bedside commode rather than a bedpan when possible.	Normal position promotes elimination.
7. Promote oxygenation.	Lung pathology, excessive or thick secretions, CNS depression, and anemia are some of the factors that alter oxygenation.
a. Position in semi-Fowler's position.	Improves lung expansion.
b. Gently suction accumulated secretions from the mouth and throat only as needed.	Minimizes irritation of mucous membranes, which can increase secretions.
c. Provide oxygen therapy as ordered (see Chapter 30).	
8. Assist in client's grief work according to current stage.	
a. Denial: may selectively hear what client wants to believe.	Protects client from being overwhelmed.
b. Anger: may be directed toward staff, family, client, or God.	Indicates need for acceptance, concern, and support.

Steps	Rationale
c. Bargaining: may attempt to buy time or seek a different diagnosis.	Associated with trying new treatments and alternative therapies.
d. Depression: may withdraw or express feelings of sadness and despair.	Withdrawal allows time to process the real and anticipated losses.
e. Acceptance: may express feelings of tranquility and serenity, faith and readiness.	Client and family may reach this at different times and in different ways. It may or may not be sustained.
9. Encourage client and family to participate in decisions about physical and supportive care to the extent possible.	Stress, physical or mental fatigue, and fear interfere with ability to participate in decision making.
a. Assist client and family to recognize what the problem is and what decision needs to be made.	Decisions about treatment options, pain control, use of hospice care, funeral arrangements, organ donation, and legal and financial matters may be needed.
b. Discuss possible alternatives or options that client and family can identify.	
c. Identify resources, information, and options if client and family do not have the knowledge needed.	
d. Participate in discussion of probable outcomes of various alternatives based on actual or potential threats to values or belief system.	
e. Offer additional resources to assist in the decision.	
10. Promote hope.	Hope gives client meaning to the experience, ensuring more confidence in dealing with death.
a. Identify client and family strengths. Give positive feedback and encouragement appropriately.	
b. Clarify information about illness and circumstances and correct misinformation.	
c. Help client recognize experiences of love and caring and ways that these are important to others.	
d. Encourage discussion of desired goals, reminiscing, reviewing values, and reflecting on the meaning of suffering, life, or death.	
11. See Completion Protocol (Chapter 1, p. 6).	

Evaluation

1. Assess client's degree of relief from pain, nausea and vomiting, fatigue, anxiety, and other symptoms.
2. Ask about progress in decisions identified by client and family as essential during this time.
3. Ask about client's level of comfort with expression of feelings about changes as they occur.
4. Observe for evidence that client and family are treated with dignity and respect.

UNEXPECTED OUTCOMES AND RELATED INTERVENTIONS

1. Symptoms are not under control with prescribed treatment plan.

   a. Use alternative therapy, music, distraction, therapeutic touch, slow breathing, prayer, meditation, and other approaches deemed appropriate by client and family.
   b. Collaborate with physician for alternative medications.
2. Client and family disagree about major decisions.
   a. Support client's right to decide to the extent possible.
   b. Allow family to discuss issues without client present, and listen without agreeing or disagreeing.
3. Client or family is in denial regarding prognosis. Assess what they want to know, without confronting

them with information they are not ready for, by asking the following questions (Taylor and Ferszt, 1994):

a. What is your understanding of this illness?
b. What do you understand about the plan for treatment?
c. What adjustments are needed as a result of this illness?
d. How have you and your family dealt with stressful situations in the past?

SAMPLE DOCUMENTATION

1000 Client rates pain at 4 (scale 0 to 10) with transdermal patch. Denies nausea. Expresses extreme fatigue and appears restless when family is not at bedside. Talked with the chaplain for 40 minutes this morning.

1100 Asking about hospice care. Referred to coordinator for additional options. Family wants to have client at home if possible. Family tearful. Talking about plans for holiday and hoping family can be together. Encouraged to keep communications open and continue to support each other.

Skill 38.2 | Care of the Body After Death

When death occurs, the traditional clinical signs are cessation of the apical pulse, respirations, and blood pressure. Many clients, however, are maintained on mechanical ventilators, artificial pacemakers, and supportive intravenous (IV) medications that maintain respiration and blood circulation. Thus, identifying clinical death is often difficult. *Brain death* is an irreversible form of unconsciousness that is characterized by complete loss of brain function while the heart continues to beat. Institutions have brain death protocols to determine death. The legal definition of brain death varies from state to state and the provinces of Canada. The usual clinical criteria for brain death include the absence of reflex activity, movements, and respiration, with the pupils dilated and fixed. Before brain death is formally determined, a client usually undergoes two or three EEGs, which measure electrical brain activity, over 12 to 24 hours. A cerebral arteriogram, which measures circulation to the brain, may also be performed. The EEGs must show no electrical impulses for death to be confirmed.

When the physician pronounces the client dead, therapies or actions taken during CPR or code efforts are documented in the medical record. The time of death is documented, as determined by the physician. The physician may request permission from the family for an autopsy. An autopsy, or postmortem examination, is performed to confirm or determine the cause of death, gather data regarding the nature and progress of a disease, study the effects of therapies on body tissues, and provide statistical data for epidemiology and research purposes. A consent form must be signed by the appropriate family member and the physician or designated requestor. Autopsies are required in circumstances of unusual death (e.g., violent trauma, unexpected death in the home) as well as death occurring within a set time frame after hospitalization. Each state has guidelines for when autopsies are requested. Autopsies normally do not affect the client's appearance or delay burial. In some cases, removal of invasive tubes and appliances is pro-

hibited, especially in coroner's cases or cases requiring autopsies. Organ donation arrangements must be made in a timely fashion.

After all requests are made, it becomes the responsibility of the nurse to care for the client's body with dignity. Often the family members wish to view the body before final preparations are made. The nurse should give the family time needed to say good-bye to the deceased before the body is prepared for transfer to the morgue.

EQUIPMENT

Disposable gloves, gown, and other protective clothing
Plastic bag for hazardous waste disposal
Wash basin, washcloth, warm water, and bath towel
Clean gown or disposable gown for body (check agency policy)
Absorbent pads
Body bag or shroud kit (contains plastic sheet, gauze ties, and two identification tags for wrapping and identifying body)
Small pillow or towel
Adhesive tape, gauze dressings
Paper bag, plastic bag, or other suitable receptacle for client's clothing, belongings, and other items to be returned to family
Valuables envelope

Assessment

1. Assess for presence of family or significant others and whether they have been informed of client's death. Ask if they wish to view the body. Observe their response. Offer time to ask questions. **It is the physician's responsibility to notify family of client's death. Nurse provides emotional support and prepares body for viewing.**

2. Assess client's religious preference or cultural heritage. **May influence family's preference for viewing or preparation of the body.**

3. Determine if family wishes to have a chaplain, minis-

ter, or priest at the bedside. **Specific religions dictate ceremonies at time of death.**

4. Determine if client was under isolation precautions for an infectious disease. **Precautions must be taken to prevent spread of infection.**
5. Review agency policy for method of preparing the body, including removal of equipment, care of dentures or hairpieces, and wrapping of the body. **Procedure incorporates legal guidelines, especially if there will be an autopsy.**

Planning

Expected outcomes focus on facilitating grieving.

EXPECTED OUTCOMES

1. Family members express grief verbally and nonverbally.
2. Family discusses options for autopsy, funeral, and organ or tissue donation.
3. Client's body is prepared for viewing and transport.

Implementation

Steps	Rationale
1. See Standard Protocol (Chapter 1, p. 5).	
2. Explain to family that it will take a short time to prepare the body for viewing. Family members may wish to participate in this process, but it is usually done in private.	Promotes the expression of grief.
3. If another client is in the room, explain what has happened and offer the opportunity to leave room until procedure is completed.	Serves to relieve anxiety.
4. Position client supine with arms at sides, palms down, or arms across the abdomen. Do not place hands on top of one another.	Client appears natural and comfortable. Bottom hand will become discolored.
5. Place small pillow or folded towel under the head, or elevate head of bed 10 to 15 degrees.	Prevents pooling of blood in the face and subsequent facial discoloration.
6. Gently place fingers over the client's closed eyelids for a few seconds. (Optional: Place moistened cotton balls over closed eyelids.)	Holds eyelids in place to create a natural appearance.
7. If applicable, insert client's dentures into the mouth. If mouth fails to close, place a rolled-up towel under the chin.	It is difficult to insert dentures after rigor mortis occurs. Dentures maintain natural facial expression.
8. Remove all bottles, bags, or receptacles from urinary catheters, nasogastric tubes, IV lines, or drainage tubes.	Collection devices and contents are not needed for autopsy examinations.
9. Agency policy dictates tube care. For tubes remaining in the body, either remove, clamp, or cut to within 1 inch (2.5 cm) of the skin and tape in place.	Specific guidelines apply if an autopsy is to be performed.
10. Remove soiled dressings and replace with clean gauze dressings.	Controls odor caused by microorganisms.
11. Wash body parts soiled by blood, urine, feces, or other drainage. (A mortician will provide a complete bath.)	Prepares body for viewing and reduces odors.
12. Place an absorbent pad under client's buttocks.	Relaxation of sphincter muscles may cause release of urine or feces.
13. Brush and comb client's hair. Remove any clips, hairpins, or rubber bands.	Promotes well-groomed appearance. Hard objects such as pins can damage or discolor the face and scalp.
14. Remove all jewelry and give to family member. *Exception:* Family may request wedding band be left in place. Place a small strip of tape around client's finger over the ring.	Prevents loss of client's valuables.

Steps	Rationale
15. Place a clean gown on client (agency policy may require removal before body is wrapped).	Prepares body for viewing.
16. If family requests viewing, place a sheet or light blanket over the body with only the head and upper shoulders exposed. Provide soft lighting and offer chairs to family.	Maintains dignity and respect for client and family.
17. Prepare family members for client's appearance, including color, face, equipment, and tubes.	
18. Remain at bedside with family, then allow them time to view the body privately. Do not rush family. Offer a lock of hair as a keepsake.	Families need time to express their grief and say goodbye to their loved one.
19. After family has left the room, remove all linen and client's gown (refer to agency policy).	
20. Account for all personal items and valuables remaining in client's room. Label each. Use valuables list to inventory all items. Return valuables to immediate family members or store in locked container.	Nurse is responsible for safekeeping of client's personal valuables, such as jewelry, wallet, eyeglasses, or religious medals.
21. Complete identification tags and attach one to client's ankle. The remaining tag should be attached to the outside of the shroud. The identification bracelet on client's wrist remains in place.	Ensures proper identification of the body for eventual transfer to the morgue and mortician.
22. Then place body in body bag or shroud (check agency policy). Be sure the shroud completely encircles all body parts (Figure 38-5).	Prevents injury to skin and extremities. Avoids unnecessary exposure of body parts.

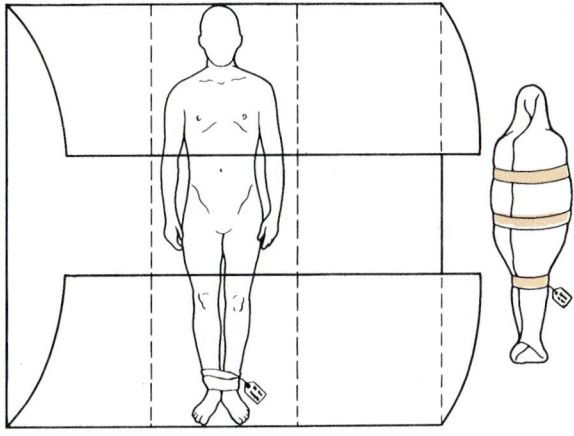

Figure 38-5

Steps	Rationale
23. Secure shroud with tape wrapped over the shoulders, waist, and legs. Do not use safety pins.	Keeps shroud secure. Protects body during transfer. Safety pins can damage skin.
24. Attach second completed label to outside of the body bag or shroud (check agency policy for location).	Ensures proper identification of the body.
25. If client had an infection, special labeling may be required.	Alerts health care workers and morticians who transport, store, and handle the body. Regulations regarding potentially infectious materials apply to any individual, living or dead, whose blood may be a source of occupational exposure to employees (OSHA, 1991).
26. Arrange transportation of the body to the morgue or mortuary. If delay is anticipated before the mortician arrives, the body should be cooled in the morgue.	Prevents further tissue damage.

Steps	Rationale
27. Carefully transfer the body to a stretcher. Keep body aligned. Cover with a clean sheet.	Prevents damage to body tissues. Stretchers that conceal the presence of a dead body promote denial that people die in hospitals (Ufema, 1991a).
28. Close doors to other clients' rooms. Arrange for an elevator to arrive on the floor, and transport the body as inconspicuously as possible according to agency policy.	Appearance of a body can be emotionally upsetting to other clients.
29. Remove remaining items and linen from client's room. Wash hands for at least 10 seconds.	Prevents transfer of microorganisms.
30. See Completion Protocol (Chapter 1, p. 6).	

Evaluation

1. Observe family's expression of grief.
2. Identify decisions concerning autopsy, funeral, and organ or tissue donation.
3. Ask if family has questions that need to be answered regarding viewing and transport.

UNEXPECTED OUTCOMES AND RELATED INTERVENTIONS

1. Family members are unwilling or unable to express grief during this initial phase.
   a. Respect where they are. Validate the loss.
   b. Encourage support of family, friends, or chaplain.
   c. Check back later.
2. Family expresses anger toward physician or staff.
   a. Listen without judgment or agreement.
   b. Offer opportunity to talk with patient representative.

SAMPLE DOCUMENTATION

See Expiration Flow Sheet (p. 703).

Expired at 0234 and pronounced dead by Dr. Avagio. Wife and son present and notified. Chaplain present. Reverend Hall notified at 0255. Family viewed body with chaplain. Questions answered and emotional support provided. Funeral arrangements to be with Memorial Funeral Home, notified at 0340. Autopsy refused by family. Body released to funeral home at 0430.

CRITICAL THINKING EXERCISES

1. Consider your personal beliefs about death and dying. What impact do your cultural background and religious beliefs have on your feelings about death?
2. Mr. Grover is a 68-year-old client with terminal cancer of the prostate. The cancer was diagnosed approximately 6 months ago, and Mr. Grover has had radiation and chemotherapy. During morning assessment you note that Mr. Grover is very quiet, and his wife confides that her husband seems to be pushing her away. She is concerned that he is no longer interested in bathing and shaving, since he has always been very neat and particular about his appearance. He refuses your offer to assist him with bathing.
   a. Analyze the above situation and determine the stage of grief Mr. Grover is experiencing.
   b. How would you revise your nursing care based on his behavior?
   c. While Mrs. Grover and her children are out for lunch, Mr. Grover begins to cry, stating he knows he is dying. He had hoped to be able to go home and be with his family, but he feels that would place too much burden on his family. His youngest daughter is getting married in 2 weeks. How would you respond?
   d. Identify nursing diagnoses that depict priorities in this situation.
3. Mrs. Steinfeld is a 50-year-old female brought to the emergency room by ambulance. She is experiencing severe chest pain and soon after arrival requires cardiopulmonary resuscitation. Emergency efforts are unsuccessful and Mrs. Steinfeld dies from a myocardial infarction. The family has not been located, and you realize that the client's name suggests she is Jewish. She has an endotracheal tube, Foley catheter, multiple IV lines, and defibrillator pads in place.
   a. Knowing very little about Jewish practices regarding death, what is your responsibility in this situation?
   b. What criteria should you use to determine if the endotracheal tube, Foley catheter, and IV lines can be removed?

Expiration Flow Sheet

Time of death _____   Pronounced dead by _____

Family notified: Name & Relationship _____

Family member responsible for funeral arrangements   Name: _____

_____   Relationship: _____   Time available: _____

Address: _____   # can be reached at _____

Physicians notified: _____

_____   Time _____

Hospital chaplain/family pastor notified _____   Time _____
Funeral home _____   Time notified _____
   Isolation Information: Infection Hazard?   YES   NO
Autopsy requested   YES   NO   Requested by: _____
Permission obtained for autopsy   YES   NO
Permission Experienced: Fall _____   Fracture _____
Security notified   Time: _____
Coroner notified (M-F [tel. no.] evening & weekends [tel. no.]) (if applicable)
  I. Time notified: _____
 II. Information the Coronary needs:
    Name of patient, time of death, age, address, physician, next of kin, autopsy (yes or no), procedure _____

ORGAN/TISSUE DONATION (**PLEASE COMPLETE I A&B, & II A BEFORE APPROACHING FAMILY**)
I. A. Is the patient 70 years old or older?   YES   NO
   B. Is the patient currently positive for HIV, Hepatitis A or B?   YES   NO
II. A. If you have answered "NO" TO THOSE TWO QUESTIONS, this patient may be a candidate for organ and/or tissue dona-
    tion. Please contact the ROBI Coordinator who is "On Call" at (tel. no.) (24 hours/day) to verify eligibility of patient to do-
    nate.
   B. Name of ROBI Coordinator: _____
   C. Patient is a candidate for donation.   YES   NO
    If yes, family permission obtained.   YES   NO
    Patient is not a candidate due to: _____

Disposition of chart   _____ To Laboratory (if autopsy)
                _____ To medical records (if no autopsy)

Disposition of body   _____ Morgue   Time _____
                _____ Funeral home
                _____ Pathology

Disposition of valuables _____

DATE _____

SIGNATURE _____

Courtesy Memorial Medical Center, Springfield, Ill.

REFERENCES

Badzek L: What you need to know about advance directives, *Nursing '92* 22(6):58, 1992.

Chabalewski F, Norris MK: The gift of life: talking to families about organ and tissue donation, *Am J Nurs* 94(6):28, 1994.

Dufault K, Martocchio BC: Hope: its spheres and dimensions, *Nurs Clin North Am* 20:379, 1985.

Gurfolino V, Dumas L: Hospice nursing: the concept of palliative care, *Nurs Clin North Am* 29(3):533, 1994.

Kübler-Ross E: *On death and dying,* New York, 1969, Macmillan.

Law enlarges caregiver role in end-of-life decisions, *Am J Nurs* 92(1):85, 1992.

Malecki M, Hoffman M: Personal level of discomfort among nurses and its effect on obtaining consent for organ and tissue donation, *It's News (Illinois Transplant Society)* 3:4, 1986.

Occupational Safety and Health Administration (OSHA): Occupational exposure to bloodborne pathogens, final rule, *Fed Register* 56(235):64, 1991.

Robb V: The Hotel Project: a community approach to persons with AIDS, *Nurs Clin North Am* 29(3): 1994.

Roberts KT, Messenger TC: Helping older adults find serenity, *Geriatr Nurs* 14(6), 1993.

Stempsey SJ: Another look at physician-assisted suicide, *Pastoral Care* 48(3), 1994.

Sunderland RH, Shelp EE: *AIDS and the Church,* Louisville, Ky, 1987, Westminster/John Knox Press.

Swain B: A Tibetan breathing approach to dying, *East/West,* April 1988.

Taylor PB, Ferszt GG: Letting go of a loved one: what you can do to support the family and promote a final healing, *Nursing '94* 24(1):55, 1994.

Tengbom M: Letting tears bring healing and renewal. In *Care notes,* St Meinrad, Ind, 1990, Abbey Press.

Ufema J: Helping loved ones say good-bye, *Nursing '91* 21(10):42, 1991a.

Ufema J: Meeting the challenge of a dying patient, *Nursing '91* 21(2):42, 1991b.

Young C: Spirituality and the chronically ill Christian elderly, *Geriatr Nurs* 14(6), 1993.

Zerwekh J: The dehydration question, *Nursing '83* 13(1):46, 1983.

ADDITIONAL READINGS

AIDS update: Examining the new OSHA regulation, *Nursing '92* 22(11):18, 1992.

Anthony M: No code: helping the family understands what it means, *Nursing '86* 16(8):55, 1986.

Geltman R, Paige R: Symptom management in hospice care, *Am J Nurs* 83(1):78, 1983.

Greve P: Legally speaking: advance directives—what the new law means for you, *RN* 54(11):63, 1991.

Lynch P et al: Implementing and evaluating a system of generic infection precautions: body substance isolation, *Am J Infect Control* 18(1):1, 1990.

Martocchio BC: Grief and bereavement: healing through hurt, *Nurs Clin North Am* 20:327, 1985.

Meyer C: Coming to new terms with death, *Am J Nurs* 92(8):19, 1992.

OSHA stiffens bloodborne rules, *Am J Nurs* 92(1):82, 1992.

Regs put new legal force behind universal precautions, *Am J Nurs* 92(1):82, 1992.

Wurzbach M: The dilemma of withholding or withdrawing nutrition, *Image—J Nurs Scholarship* 22(4):226, 1990.

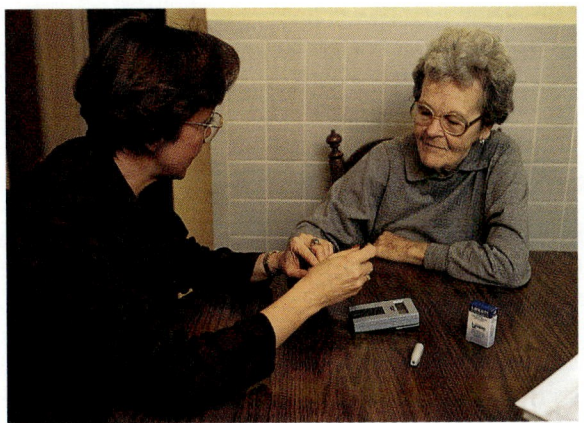

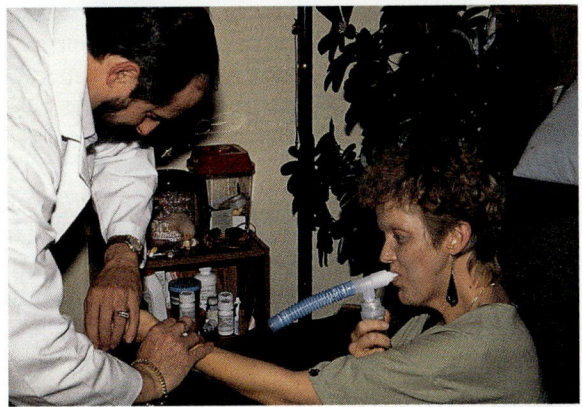

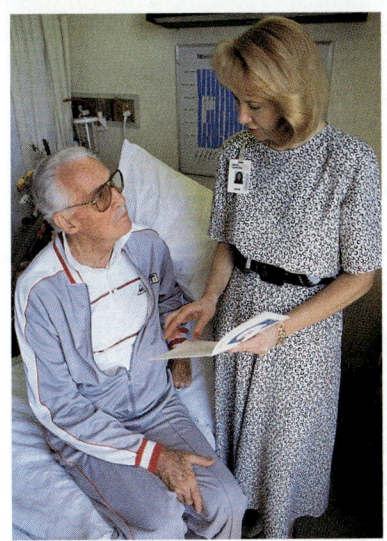

chapter 39

Discharge Teaching and Home Health Management

C lients must have the necessary knowledge, skill, and resources to meet self-care needs at home on discharge from a health care facility. Therefore, discharge teaching and planning are of utmost importance. Discharge planning is an organized, coordinated, interdisciplinary process that provides a plan of care for the client leaving the health care setting. The goal of discharge planning is to provide continuity of care, thereby ensuring a smooth transition for the client from the health care setting to the home environment.

The nurse's role in discharge planning follows the nursing process. The nurse must assess the biophysical, psychosocial, educational, self-care, environmental, and discharge needs of the client; for example, self-care, education, ability to perform a self–blood glucose test and read and interpret the results, ability to perform self-catheterization, ability to comply with home medication regimens. The discharge needs are determined from the analysis of the total assessment and nursing diagnoses then identified.

In the planning phase, the nurse and client jointly identify goals and expected outcomes. Achievement of these goals is based on selection of appropriate therapies and therapeutic services available. The nurse must know what community resources are available, the referral process, and the client's financial support.

Teaching is the major intervention in the implementation phase. Teaching strategies are based on assessment of the client's educational level and learning needs. Teaching is integrated throughout the client's stay in a health-care facility. For example, teaching clients how to self-administer medications or modify risk factors are teaching actions. Written and/or visual guidelines reinforce verbal instructions and should be provided to the client on discharge home.

When clients become actively engaged in the learning process, teaching/learning effectiveness is enhanced. Therefore, the best way for the nurse to evaluate a client's understanding of the material presented is to ask clients about the treatment regimen or to demonstrate a procedure that will be done by the client, family member, or significant other. Discharge instructions should reflect nursing actions of teaching, counseling, and appropriate referrals. Clear, concise, accurate documentation of the client's needs and abilities on the discharge plan

improves the continuity of care. The nurse should also document the client's and family's knowledge of and ability to comply with discharge instructions.

Finally, the discharge plan is confirmed with the client and family. The nurse can follow up several days after discharge to answer questions or may secure a follow-through from a referral agency.

Every client in a hospital requires discharge planning. Certain conditions, however, place a client at greater risk for being unable to meet continuing health care needs after discharge (see box below). When a client has one of these conditions, it is especially important to provide the necessary teaching or coordinate referrals to appropriate outside agencies.

Nursing Diagnosis

Health Seeking Behaviors is appropriate when the client is in stable health and is actively seeking to alter personal habits to achieve optimum health.

Knowledge Deficit is appropriate when the client has not been exposed to a new procedure, lacks recall, or verbalizes misinterpretation of previously learned information. This diagnosis can occur with any self-care requirement, such as drug administration or self-catheterization in the home environment. **Anxiety** results from the client's concern about how illness may change lifestyle, or the client may be unsure about learning a new behavior and performing it correctly in the home environment.

The aging process and chronic illnesses such as diabetes mellitus and cataracts may elicit a **Sensory/Perceptual Alterations** diagnosis. With these conditions, the client's sensory acuity is decreased and adaptations to the home environment may be needed. Psychological stress in relation to the disease state can also narrow the client's perceptual field. Therefore, the nurse must implement special approaches in helping the client adjust to home care requirements. **Impaired Physical Mobility** from activity intolerance, perceptual or cognitive impairment, disabilities, or age-related changes may limit the client's ability to take medications or perform self-care skills. Impaired physical mobility can also lead to **Risk for Injury,** which can occur as a result of potentially unsafe environmental conditions (e.g., physical set-up of the home). Clients who have sensory, cognitive, or motor disabilities are at highest risk.

Altered Health Maintenance is appropriate when a client or family is unable to identify, manage, or seek help to maintain health. This may be related to a wide variety of factors, including inadequate information, lack of awareness of threat to health, inadequate support systems, and lack of access to health care services.

Health beliefs, cultural influences, spiritual values, and the client-provider relationship may result in **Noncompliance** with self-care therapies. In many instances, non-

---

High-Priority Clients for Discharge Planning

- Clients in need of high-technology home therapy (intravenous therapy, hyperalimentation, chemotherapy, home ventilator)
- Diagnosis with long-term or terminal implications (positive for human immunodeficiency virus, cancer, cerebrovascular accident, chronic renal failure, traumatic brain or spinal cord injury)
- Medication management (complicated medication regimen, new insulin-dependent diabetic client, impaired vision, previous failure to follow prescribed medication regimen)
- Clients who require adaptive equipment at home (hospital beds, oxygen, wheelchairs, assistive devices)
- Clients who require postdischarge skilled nursing care follow-up (home health, special nurse clinic appointments, day care, nursing home)
- Clients who require rehabilitative therapy
- Older adult clients (65+ years) with additional chronic conditions (arthritis, pulmonary, cardiovascular, diabetes mellitus)
- Clients undergoing major surgical intervention

Modified from Beare P, Myers J: *Principles and practices of adult health nursing,* ed 2, St Louis, 1994, Mosby.

compliance is a result of the client "forgetting" to perform a certain task such as taking a medication on time or remembering to take it at all.

Risk for Infection is an appropriate diagnosis when clients are initiating an invasive procedure such as performing a clean, intermittent self-catheterization or doing a blood stick for glucose monitoring. This diagnosis may also exist if the home is not environmentally clean and the client does not follow aseptic technique when necessary. All clients after discharge may be at risk for **Impaired Home Maintenance Management.** This may be associated with client's disease or disability state, motor skills, inadequate support systems, decreased knowledge of available resources and ways to initiate contact, communication skills, and impaired cognitive or emotional functioning (Kim, 1995).

Skill 39.1 | Risk Assessment and Accident Prevention

This skill focuses on preparing the client to go home to a risk-free, safe environment. Discharge from an agency can be stressful if a client feels unprepared to resume normal activities or unable to adapt therapeutic regimens to living at home. Before being discharged, a client must know how to manage care in the home and what to expect in regard to any continuing physical problems. Without the necessary equipment and professional resources to care for continuing health problems, the client risks loss of any rehabilitation gains made before discharge. Failure to understand restrictions or implications of health problems may cause a client to develop complications after leaving the health setting. Inadequate discharge planning overlooks the client's needs within the home and increases the chance of the client reentering the health care system prematurely.

Unintentional injuries can occur at all ages of the life span. Many of these injuries result from hazards that are easy to overlook and also easy to fix. By taking steps to correct these hazards, many injuries can be prevented. Knowledge of specific motor and cognitive developmental changes enables the nurse to assess for potential injury for each client. Once the area of risk is identified, the nurse designs interventions to eliminate or reduce the threat to the client's safety.

EQUIPMENT
Assessment form(s)

Assessment

1. Assess client's health care needs for discharge, using nursing history, care plan, and ongoing assessments of physical and cognitive abilities.
2. Identify risk factors in relation to lifestyle patterns: smoking, stress, drug use, alcohol use, unplanned exercise habits, and personal hygiene. **Life-style habits frequently increase the risk for developing illnesses or disabilities during middle or older years.**
3. Obtain client's employment history to determine risks within the occupational setting. **Occupational inhalants such as asbestos, plastics, dusts, and gases have potential for causing chronic lung diseases or cancer.**
4. Assess client's and family's need for health teaching related to home therapies, restrictions resulting from health alterations, and possible complications. **This improves understanding of health care needs and ability to achieve self-care at home.**
5. With client and family, assess environmental risk factors within the home that might interfere with safe self-care (e.g., size of rooms, doorway clearances, steps, bathroom facilities, use of smoke detectors, disposal of in-home medical supplies). (A home health care nurse may be available on referral to assist with assessment.) **This provides the opportunity to decrease the risk of accidents in client's home.**
6. Determine actual or potential limitations resulting from sensory, motor, cognitive, or physical changes. **This provides the opportunity to identify factors that increase client's risk of injury.**
7. Assess client's acceptance of health problems and related restrictions. **Acceptance of health status can affect willingness to adhere to therapies and restrictions after discharge.**
8. Consult other health team members about needs after discharge (e.g., dietitian, social worker, home health care nurse). Make appropriate referrals. **Members of all health care disciplines should collaborate to determine client's needs and functional abilities.**

Planning

Expected outcomes focus on client's knowledge level, motivation to learn, identification of risk factors, and ability to perform self-care in the home environment.

EXPECTED OUTCOMES
1. Client explains how health care is to continue at home, including what treatments and medications are needed and when to seek medical attention for problems.

2. Client demonstrates self-care activities.
3. Client identifies safety risks in the home.
4. Client maintains a home environment that is adapted to client's motor, sensory, and cognitive developmental needs.

5. Client identifies three community resources available and how to initiate contact.

Implementation

Steps	Rationale
1. See Standard Protocol (Chapter 1, p. 5).	
2. Conduct teaching sessions with client and family as soon as possible during hospitalization (use time when giving a bath, passing medications, ambulating, or feeding client). Pamphlets or books may be given to client and family.	Gives client opportunity to practice new skills, ask questions, and obtain necessary feedback to ensure learning. Incorporating teaching during care activities maximizes use of available time.
3. Assemble teaching materials and provide a comfortable and quiet setting, free of distractions.	Comfortable environment enhances learning. Interruptions interfere with concentration.
4. Set up equipment and show skill to client. Utilize supplies and equipment that client will use at home. Employ teaching techniques of repetition, rephrasing, and summarizing. Have client demonstrate skill. Provide client with positive feedback.	Facilitates transfer of learning.
5. Teach health promotional activities in areas of nutrition, exercise, relaxation, and smoking cessation (if applicable).	Reduces risk of certain diseases (e.g., cardiopulmonary disease, cancer, obesity).
6. Teach client how to recognize stress and measures to deal effectively with psychophysiologic effects.	Prolonged stress response can increase client's risk of stress-related illnesses.
7. Reinforce illness prevention behaviors and information such as breast self-examination or warning signs for cancer (Figure 39-1).	Recognition of cancer warning signals can lead to early detection and cure.

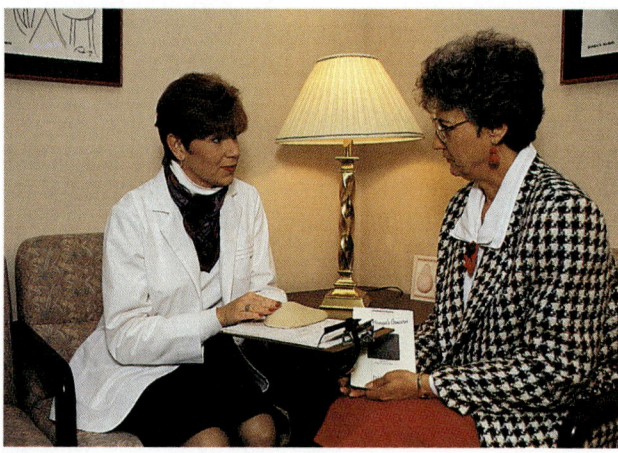

Figure 39-1

8. Suggest ways to make home environment safe.

   a. **Disposal of in-home medical supplies**
      (1) Place needles, syringes, lancets, or other sharp objects in a hard plastic or metal container such as soda bottles or laundry detergent containers with screw-on or tightly secured lid.

Client's level of independence and ability to retain function can be maintained within safe environment.

Prevents injury to self or others and prevents pollution.

Steps	Rationale

(2) Soiled bandages, disposable sheets, and medical gloves are placed in securely fastened plastic bag before placed in garbage can.

b. **Physical arrangements**

(1) *Stairs*

(a) Install treads with uniform depth of 9 inches (23 cm) and 9-inch risers (vertical face of steps).

    If stairs are of uniform size, older client need not continually adjust vision.

(b) Install uniform-textured or plain-colored surfaces on each tread, and mark edge of tread with contrasting color (orange, yellow).

    Uniform texture or color helps to decrease vertigo (Potter and Perry, 1993). Marking edge of tread provides obvious visual clue to end of step.

(c) Ensure proper lighting of each tread. Block sun or light bulb glare with translucent shades or screens, or use lower-wattage bulbs. Do not use fluorescent lighting.

    Older client's eyes are unable to adjust quickly to changes in lighting and are more sensitive to glare.

(d) Ensure adequate head room so that client does not have to duck to use stairs.

    Sudden changes in head position may result in dizziness.

(e) Remove protruding objects from staircase walls.

    Decreased peripheral vision may prevent client from seeing objects.

(f) Keep outdoor walkways and stairs in good condition (free of holes, cracks, and splinters) and well lighted.

    Decreased visual acuity can prevent client from seeing structural defect.

(2) *Handrails*

(a) Install smooth but slip-resistant handrails at least 2 inches (5 cm) from wall.

    Distance allows client to grasp handrail firmly for support.

(b) Secure handrail firmly so that client's weight can be supported, especially at bottom and top of stairway.

    Older client has greatest risk of falling at top and bottom of stairs because center of gravity is being shifted and balance is unstable.

(c) Install guardrails in bathroom near toilet and bathtub.

    Enables clients to have support while rising from sitting to standing position.

(3) *Floor coverings*

(a) Secure all carpeting, mats, and tile; place nonskid backing under area rugs.

    Sudden slip may cause dizziness and inability of client to regain balance. Decrease in muscle strength may decrease client's ability to adjust to slip and prevent fall.

(b) Provide unobstructed pathways.

c. **Prevention of fires and burns**

(1) Install smoke detectors.

    Prevents injury.

(2) Keep hot water temperature 120° F (48.8° C) or lower by adjusting water heater setting.

(3) Discourage smoking when sleepy or in bed (if applicable).

(4) Keep flammable objects away from stove when cooking.

9. Provide client and family with information about community health care resources.

    Community resources may offer services that client or family cannot provide.

10. See Completion Protocol (Chapter 1, p. 6).

Evaluation

1. Ask client to describe treatment regimens and physical signs and symptoms to be reported to physician.
2. Have client or family perform treatments and procedures to be continued at home.
3. Ask client to identify safety risks.
4. Ensure that family or a home health nurse inspects home environment so that it is free of obstacles and risks.
5. Ask client to identify resources available for a particular problem and how to initiate contact with that resource.

UNEXPECTED OUTCOMES AND RELATED INTERVENTIONS

1. Client is unable to identify safety risks.
   a. Reevaluate home environment with client and family members.
   b. Teach client the rationale for preventing and removing potential hazards from home environment.

2. Client demonstrates procedure incorrectly.
   a. Reassess client's knowledge level.
   b. Teach procedure, and reinforce areas of learning deficit.
   c. Demonstrate procedure, and have client return demonstration.
   d. Provide praise throughout learning session.

SAMPLE DOCUMENTATION

0900 Safety risks and hazards found in home environment discussed with client and family. Checklist completed with client and family members. Instructed family members to correct potential hazards of throw rugs and to install handrails in bathroom. Heartland Home Health Care Agency referral made with physician's order and discussed with client and family members.

1115 Client states family members will make necessary changes in home environment before discharge. Client able to correctly identify benefits of receiving home health nursing care to meet his needs.

Skill 39.2 | Teaching Self-Administration of Non-Parenteral Medications

This skill focuses on teaching techniques and strategies to ensure client compliance with home medication regimens. Every opportunity that the nurse has in the hospital setting to teach clients about their medications should be utilized.

Noncompliance with medication regimen is a common problem. Some clients tend to "forget" to take their medications, while others refuse to do so. Some individuals may have sensory or motor impairments that may make them unable to comply correctly with medication administration, and others fail to understand the necessity of taking their medications. Noncompliance may be aggravated in older adults by the lack of family support systems and by the varying degrees of physiological and psychological changes that accompany the aging process (Barry, 1993). In many instances, noncompliance accompanies the clients' lack of understanding about their own illness or injury; therefore, follow-up treatment with medications may be adversely affected. The nurse teaches and counsels clients to enhance their knowledge, safety, and compliance with their medication regimen. Teaching must be individualized for each client, since each person has unique characteristics and capabilities. Make sure that a client who has a sensory impairment is equipped with the appropriate appliances (i.e., hearing aid, glasses).

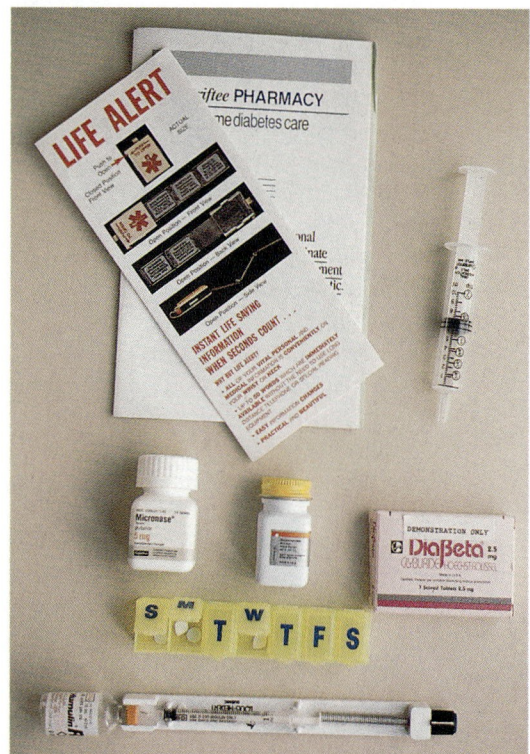

Figure 39-2

Review the discharge order and clarify any misinformation with the physician and, if necessary, consult with your facility's discharge planner. Also, arrange a time that the client's significant other may participate in the session(s).

EQUIPMENT (Figure 39-2)

Medication
Liquid to take with medication
Measuring devices (teaspoon, measuring cups)
Medication chart/record
Container for daily or weekly preparation

Assessment

1. Assess client's and significant other's knowledge related to medication therapy: names of drugs, action or purpose, daily dosages and time taken, potential side effects, and what to do if problems arise. **This determines how much teaching will be needed, providing the nurse with baseline information. Family members (or care givers) are important resources to help clients comply with therapy.**
2. Assess client's cognitive, sensory, and motor function: sight, hearing, touch, reading ability and comprehension, ability to swallow, ability to ambulate and tolerate activity, and willingness to cooperate. **Cognitive, sensory, and motor deficits may influence client's ability to comply with prescribed medication regimen.**

3. Assess client's belief in the need for drug therapy. Consider cultural values, religious beliefs, personal experiences with medications, and significant others' values about drugs. **These factors influence client's compliance with drug therapy.**
4. Check client's prescribed drugs. Has more than one physician prescribed medications? Are medications obviously inappropriate? Are labels clearly marked? Are time schedules confusing? Do different drugs look alike? Does client store medications together? **This assists nurse in determining sources of confusion affecting client's compliance.**

Planning

Expected outcomes focus on client's and care giver's knowledge level, self-care, motivation to learn, and ability to comply with medication regimen.

EXPECTED OUTCOMES

1. Client or significant other explains the purpose, action, and common side effects of each medication by discharge.
2. Client or significant other identifies by discharge whom to contact for questions or problems and what to do if a dose is missed.
3. Client explains how to self-administer medication.
4. Client prepares proper drug doses.
5. Client reads and interprets the drug label properly.
6. Client demonstrates self-administered medications by the prescribed route before discharge.

Implementation

Steps	Rationale
1. See Standard Protocol (Chapter 1, p. 5).	
2. Assemble teaching materials and provide a comfortable, quiet, well-lit setting, free of distractions.	Comfortable environment enhances learning. Interruptions interfere with concentration.
3. Present the information clearly and concisely in understandable terms in accordance with client's educational level and age.	
4. Allow client and care giver to ask questions.	Increases client's participation in learning process. Ongoing feedback ensures nurse that client is acquiring information.
5. Discuss the following information in relation to medication regimen: purpose, action, common side effects, significance of taking, dosage schedules, what to do if experiencing side effects, when and who to call for/with problems/concerns, drug safety guidelines, and implications when medications are not taken.	Content learned improves client's ability to self-medicate and comply with medication regimen.
6. Discuss additional information related to medication therapy as appropriate: always take the drug as prescribed for duration of course; consult physician be-	Minimizes chances of adverse or undesirable side effects. Older adults are at greatest risk for drug interactions because of physiological changes of aging.

Steps	Rationale
fore switching medications; follow the pharmacy directions on medication label; examine labels of other over-the-counter (OTC) drugs to prevent possible adverse reactions when drugs are inadvertently mixed; advise on storing medications.	
7. Provide frequent, short, teaching sessions.	Improves attention and retention of information discussed.
8. Provide learning aids, special charts, and devices to increase compliance (e.g., calendars, pill box with color-coded compartments) (see Figure 39-2).	
9. Demonstrate preparation of medication.	
10. Have client practice preparing medication(s). Offer assistance as necessary. Be sure client is wearing glasses and/or has hearing aid in place during session.	Nurse can observe client's ability to read labels correctly and prepare all medications for prescribed times.
11. Have client demonstrate steps in medication administration. Be sure to assess technique of swallowing.	Some clients do not drink enough water to swallow properly; the tablet could become lodged in the esophagus and cause esophageal lesions.
12. Provide client and family written instructions to take home (Figure 39-3).	While hospitalized, client may be anxious and easily distracted during teaching sessions. Written instructions help ensure compliance.

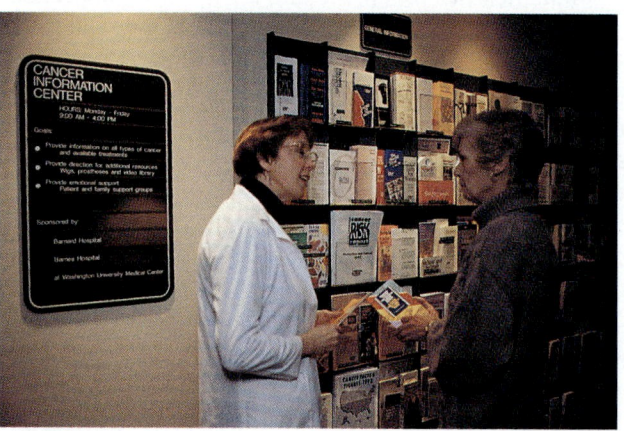

Figure 39-3

Steps	Rationale
13. Arrange for regular visits by home health nurse as deemed necessary.	Provides health care provider with knowledge of client's compliance with medication administration; early intervention then is possible.
14. See Completion Protocol (Chapter 1, p. 6).	

Evaluation

1. Ask client and significant other to explain purpose, action, and side effects of the prescribed medications.
2. Ask client and significant other to identify who to contact with concerns and what to do if a dose is missed.
3. Have client verbalize the steps in preparing the medication.

4. Have client prepare proper drug dosages.
5. Have client read and interpret the pharmacy label.
6. Observe client prepare and self-administer the medications.

UNEXPECTED OUTCOMES AND RELATED INTERVENTIONS

1. Client is unable to recall or explain information discussed in teaching session.

a. Determine what information client does have.

b. Determine what remaining information is essential for client safety and compliance, and provide additional teaching.

2. Client is unable to prepare medications as prescribed.

a. Reassess client's sensory and motor abilities to ensure safety and compliance.

b. Identify areas of concern in administering drugs. Provide emotional (positive) support of client's ability.

c. Have client demonstrate preparation of medications until successful.

d. Have family member prepare medications.

3. Client fails to comprehend the importance of information provided in the teaching session.

a. Observe client's emotional status and acceptance of the need for medication.

b. Enlist support of significant others to verify importance of medication regimen.

SAMPLE DOCUMENTATION

1000 Teaching regarding self-medication administration completed. Verbalized need to follow written instructions regarding medications while at home.

1200 Client administered own 1200 medications following appropriate guidelines.

Skill 39.3 | Teaching Self-Injections

Many drugs may be administered subcutaneously (e.g., narcotics, vaccines, insulin, heparin). Insulin and heparin are the medications most likely to be self-administered in the home environment. These medications must be administered subcutaneously because they are not absorbed by the oral route. Heparin should only be injected into the subcutaneous tissue of the abdomen. Several sites can be used for insulin injections. The client is instructed not to aspirate or rub the injection site after heparin administration. These actions could result in tissue damage and severe bruising. The client is also instructed to observe for signs of bleeding (e.g., bruising, bleeding gums, blood in stool).

This skill focuses on teaching clients how to administer insulin self-injections. Almost 3 million diabetic clients may require daily subcutaneous injections of insulin (ADA, 1993). The nurse is responsible for teaching clients how to give injections for the first time as well as for evaluating the injection techniques of clients administering their own insulin. Some diabetic clients are still trying to learn proper technique, and others do not realize they have been doing it incorrectly.

The ability of a diabetic client to learn how to administer injections depends in part on the progress of the disease. Diabetes is a chronic condition that can cause loss of vision and peripheral nerve damage. The nurse may need to adapt the equipment available to the client or educate only a family member. Special syringes with plunger locks ensure that only a specific dose is prepared. Syringes with large, numbered scales or magnifying glass adapters are available for clients with visual problems.

EQUIPMENT

Vial of insulin in correct concentration (U-100)

Two or three insulin syringes (0.5 to 1 ml, calibrated in units)

Bottle of sterile water or normal saline

Antiseptic swabs/alcohol swabs

Rotation chart

Assessment

1. Assess client's readiness and ability to learn: asks questions about disease, treatment, or injections; requests to learn how to give injections; is mentally alert; and participates in own care. Determine client's ability to read and see clearly. **This reflects client's ability to understand explanations and actively participate in teaching process. Mental or physical limitations affect client's ability to learn and alter nurse's method of instruction.**

2. Assess client's ability to hold and manipulate a syringe and hold insulin vial. **Peripheral neuropathy can alter diabetic client's sensation of touch and affect ability to handle syringe and vial safely.**

3. Assess client's visual ability by having client read numbers on insulin syringe or directions on a vial. If acuity is reduced, ask client to read numbers on syringe with enlarged numbers or to use magnifier with syringe. **Diabetic clients often experience swelling of the lens because of elevated blood glucose levels, causing reduction in visual acuity. It may be necessary to educate family members.**

4. Assess client's knowledge and understanding of diabetes, purpose and action of insulin, and reason insulin is required. **Client must know implications of too much or too little insulin, which can be fatal.**

5. Assess family members' interest in and ability to provide injections. **Family member may be principal administrator of injections; even if client can administer own injections, family member**

should be available as resource if client becomes ill.
6. Assess drug dosage and schedule client is ordered to receive at home.
7. If client administers own injections, assess client's techniques in giving injection. **Nurse's instruction may require only simple reinforcement, depending on client's level of skill.**

Planning

Expected outcomes focus on client and care giver's knowledge level, ability to perform self-care, motivation to learn, and ability to comply with procedure guidelines.

EXPECTED OUTCOMES
1. Client identifies the parts of the needle and syringe.
2. Client correctly manipulates the syringe and needle using aseptic technique.
3. Client uses aseptic technique throughout the procedure.
4. Client states which insulin is to be administered as well as the correct dosage.
5. Client correctly draws up the ordered insulin dose in corresponding insulin syringe.
6. Client selects injection sites recommended for insulin administration.
7. Client discusses the rationale for rotating sites.
8. Client correctly demonstrates an insulin self-injection.

Implementation

Steps	Rationale
1. See Standard Protocol (Chapter 1, p. 5).	
2. Assemble teaching materials and equipment needed. Provide a comfortable, quiet, well-lit setting, free of distractions. Have client sit at table where all equipment is displayed; make sure equipment is within easy reach and organized logically.	Comfortable environment enhances learning. Interruptions interfere with concentration. Enables client to visualize entire procedure.
3. Have client wash hands. Explain importance of handwashing.	
4. Have client manipulate syringe. Explain which parts must remain sterile and which can be touched.	Familiarity with aseptic technique in handling syringe ensures safe drug administration.
5. Have client compare syringe scale with insulin label concentration on insulin vial.	Concentration of insulin in units and number of units marked on syringe should match; for example, 100-unit syringe is used only with U-100 insulin.
6. Discuss client's ordered dose.	
7. Have client check expiration date on insulin and examine solution for color change, clumping, or other signs. If insulin has been refrigerated, allow to warm to room temperature.	Client should not take expired medication. Regular insulin should be clear. All other insulin types should be uniformly cloudy. A cold insulin injection can be painful and less effective than one at room temperature.
8. Demonstrate technique for mixing insulin vial by gently rolling bottle between the hands; then allow client to mix the vial. *Never* shake the vial.	After sitting, insulin forms crystal on bottom of vial. Mixing produces uniform solution. Shaking creates air bubbles.
Drawing up insulin	
9. Demonstrate and explain steps used to prepare syringe.	Demonstration is the most effective technique for teaching motor skill. Use simple step-by-step explanations so client may ask questions at any point during procedure.
a. Wipe off top of vial with alcohol and remove needle cover.	
b. Pull plunger out to same number of units to be removed from vial. This pulls air into syringe.	
c. Push needle slowly into rubber on top of vial while holding syringe barrel carefully. Do not bend needle (Figure 39-4).	
d. Push in plunger to push air into bottle; this prevents vacuum.	

Steps	Rationale

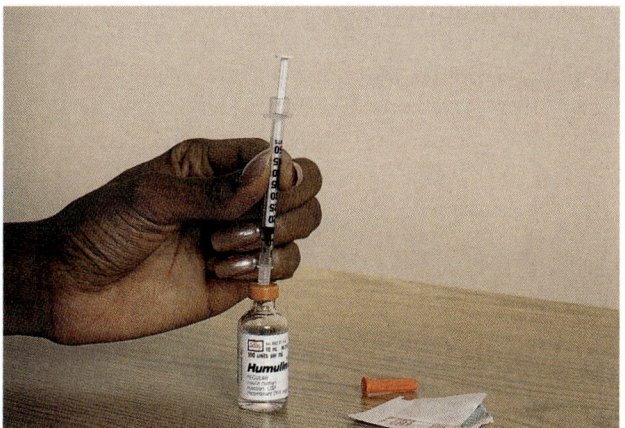

Figure 39-4

e. Hold vial and syringe together; turn both upside down. Hold vial between thumb and forefinger, supporting syringe with other hand (Figure 39-5).

f. Slowly pull back on plunger to number of units of insulin to be given. Be sure needle stays under fluid in vial.

g. Do not touch inside of plunger.

h. Check for clear air bubbles inside syringe. Small bubbles are not harmful but take up space in syringe. With bubbles present, correct amount of insulin may not be prepared.

i. Remove syringe from vial by pulling it straight out. If bubbles can be seen, tap side of syringe barrel sharply with middle finger while holding syringe upright. Have client gently push plunger back and forth three times; this usually purges syringe of air bubbles. When bubbles rise to top of syringe, pull back slightly on plunger, then push it back to correct number of units. This pushes air out through needle (Figure 39-6).

j. Check to be sure correct amount of insulin is in syringe and no air bubbles are present.

k. Put cap or sheath back without touching needle.

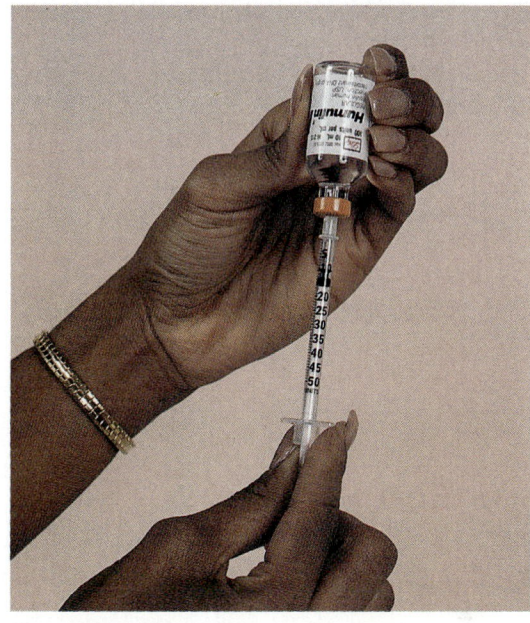

Figure 39-5

Explanation includes basic principles for syringe preparation: prevent vacuum in vial; prevent aspiration of air bubbles; keep syringe and needle sterile; remove air without ejecting fluid.

Many clients cannot see air bubbles.

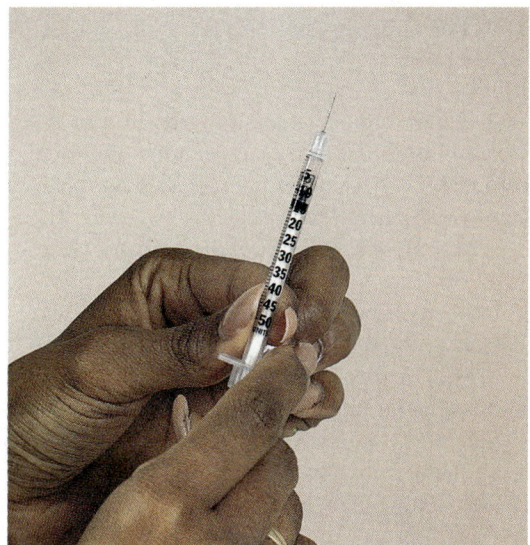

Figure 39-6

Steps	Rationale
10. Show chart of injection sites and find each accessible site on client's body (Figure 39-7).	Comparing body parts allows nurse to point out areas to be avoided, such as scars and bruises.
11. Discuss importance of rotating sites systematically, and provide client with injection record (Figure 39-8).	Insulin is absorbed differently in different parts of the body. Using the same area at the same time every day provides client with more consistent dosing and smoother control of diabetes.

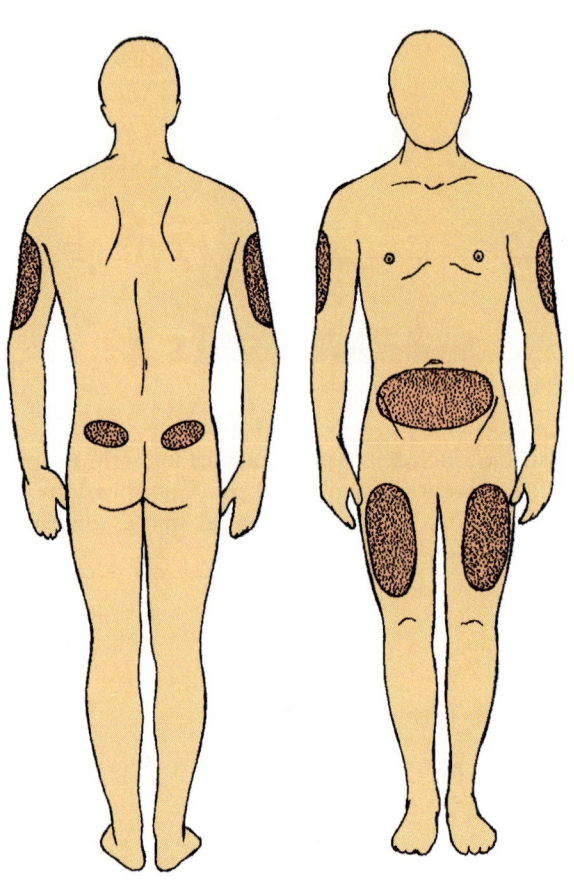

Figure 39-7

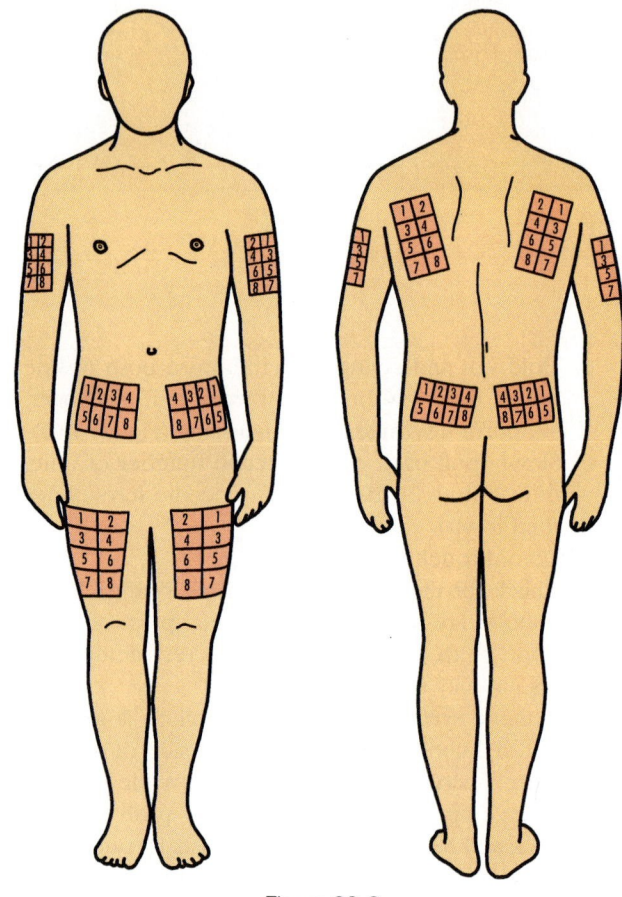

Figure 39-8

12. Have client choose injection site in abdomen or thigh where nurse can easily demonstrate injection.

13. Administer injection while explaining each step slowly, using simple terms.

   a. Wipe off site with alcohol swab to clean area; let dry.

   b. Take cover or sheath off needle.

   c. Hold syringe as you would a pencil.

   d. Grasp (or pinch up fold) injection site between thumb and fingers of free hand. To self-inject arm, press back of upper arm against wall or back of chair. "Roll" arm down to push up skin.

   e. With a quick jab, insert needle into cleansed area at a 90-degree angle. (A 45-degree angle may be used for children or thin adults.)

Nurse's instructions during demonstration should include principles for minimizing pain, injecting needle correctly, maintaining asepsis, and checking for insulin leakage.

Steps	Rationale

f. Do not push needle in; this may hurt. Gently insert needle and always hold onto syringe.

g. Let go of skin; push plunger in to administer insulin. Be sure to inject all the insulin.

nurse alert For children, thin adults, or those with superficial blood vessels, it may be necessary to aspirate before injection of insulin; teach how to assess for blood return.

h. Put alcohol swab over needle gently, and pull needle out quickly at same angle it was inserted. Check for insulin leakage at site.

i. Briefly hold alcohol swab over site.

j. Discard uncapped needle or needle enclosed in safety shield and attached syringe in a plastic receptacle.

k. Have client indicate on record chart where injection was given.

Prevents needle sticks.

Facilitates rotation of injection sites.

14. Have client ask questions about procedure.

Allows clarification of any misunderstanding and facilitates recall.

15. Provide client with written and, if possible, visual guidelines.

16. See Completion Protocol (Chapter 1, p. 6).

Evaluation

1. Ask client to identify the parts of the syringe and needle.
2. Observe client manipulating syringe.
3. Ask client to explain what is meant by aseptic technique. Observe client's ability to follow through with aseptic technique throughout procedure.
4. Have client verify physician orders for insulin type and insulin dosage. Have client explain which insulin to administer and the amount to give.
5. Observe client preparing insulin injection.
6. Have client point out on self the areas for site rotations.
7. Ask client why it is important to rotate sites.
8. Observe client's technique for self-administering an insulin injection in the proper location.

UNEXPECTED OUTCOMES AND RELATED INTERVENTIONS

1. Client is unable to meet one or more of the expected outcomes.
    a. Reassess client's readiness and ability to learn.
    b. Reassess client's sensory and motor capabilities.
    c. Determine if client is in pain or has other symptoms that can detract from learning and demonstrating.
    d. Identify areas of deficiencies.
    e. Reteach those areas in which client is deficient.
    f. Provide client with teaching booklet.
    g. Have client explain and demonstrate the self-injection technique several times in nurse's presence following procedural guidelines.

SAMPLE DOCUMENTATION

0900 Teaching self-injection of insulin started; client able to identify correct parts of syringe and basic principles of aseptic technique. Encouraged client to manipulate syringe and ask questions.

1000 Teaching continued; discussion and demonstration of drawing up insulin and injection technique completed. Chart shown of available injection sites; rationale provided for rotation of sites. Practiced drawing up normal saline in syringe.

0700 Administered own insulin injection following proper procedure with minimal assistance from RN.

Skill 39.4 | Teaching Self–Blood Glucose Monitoring

This skill focuses on teaching diabetic clients to perform self–blood glucose monitoring (SBGM) at home. SBGM has replaced urine testing as the preferred method to manage diabetes. Regular testing with this technique reveals daily patterns of blood glucose levels; thus the client and physician can use these readings to modify long-term insulin therapy, thereby keeping diabetes under control. The nurse must explain the purpose and the procedure to those clients and family members who will be performing SBGM. Self-testing of blood glucose is performed by two methods. Both methods require obtaining a large drop of blood by skin puncture. A hand-held, single-use lancet may be used, or one of many automatic lancet-holding devices are available on the market today. The blood is applied to a specially prepared chemical reagent strip.

The first method involves visually reading a reagent strip by comparing it to the color chart on the container. Examples of such strips include Chemstrip BG, Glucostix, and Trendstrips. If the color on the strip falls between two reference blocks on the chart, the results may need to be estimated. Thus, accurate results of blood glucose may not always be obtained.

The second type of SBGM is done by inserting a reagent strip into a reflectance meter. A variety of meters are on the market (Table 39-1). After applying a drop of blood from the skin puncture onto the reagent strip, the meter provides an accurate measurement of blood glucose in less than 5 minutes.

The meters use a wet-wash or dry-wipe method of testing. To perform a wet wash, the client flushes the blood-coated reagent strip with water before inserting the strip into the glucose meter. The dry-wipe method requires the client to wipe off the blood-coated reagent strip with a dry cotton ball (following manufacturer guidelines) before making a reading. Other products do not require blood to be wiped off before a reading is given. The methods allow measurement of blood glucose between 0 and 600 mg/dl, thus providing a sensitive measure of blood glucose. Talking glucose meter devices are available for visually impaired clients. When the nurse measures blood glucose or assists the client in measurement, gloves are worn per the Centers for Disease Control and Prevention (CDC) universal blood and body fluid precautions and Occupational Safety and Health Administration (OSHA) recommendations (OSHA, 1991). This skill describes the techniques to measure blood glucose with a meter using the dry-wipe method.

EQUIPMENT (Figure 39-9)

Antiseptic swabs
Cotton ball
Sterile lancet or blood-letting device
Paper towel
Glucose testing meter
Blood glucose reagent strips (brand determined by meter used)
Disposable gloves

Assessment

1. Assess client's and family members' understanding of procedure and purpose. Do they realize the importance of glucose monitoring? **Baseline information determines how much teaching will be needed. Family members are important resources to help client comply with therapy.**

Table 39-1 Glucose Meters Available on Market Today

Meters	Ranges measured (mg/dl)	Reagent strip	Timing	Memory
Accu-Chek III	20-500	Strip must be wiped correctly	Timing set manually	Yes, up to 20 values
One Touch Basic (instructions in English and Spanish)	0-600	No wiping	No timing; automatic	Stores last test
One Touch II (instructions in nine languages; symbolic for illiterate clients)	20-600	No wiping	No timing	250 readings
Companion 2 (large display window)	20-600	No wiping	No timing	20 readings
Pen 2 (small screen)	20-600	No wiping	No timing	20 readings
Accu-Chek Easy	20-500	No wiping	No timing	30 readings
Tracer II	20-500	Wiping required	Set timer	10 readings
Glucometer 3	20-500	Wiping required	Set timer	No memory

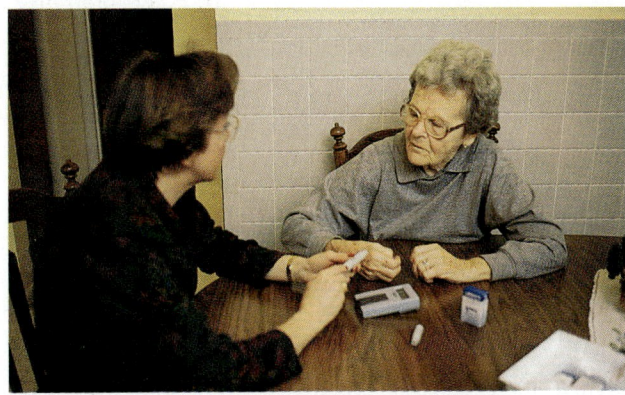

Figure 39-9

2. Assess client's sensory and motor function abilities: sight, touch, reading ability and comprehension, ability to handle skin-puncturing device, and ability to manipulate and calibrate meter. **Sensory and motor deficits may occur with diabetes and may prevent client from performing test correctly.**

Planning

Expected outcomes focus on client's knowledge level, motivation to learn, ability to perform procedure, and ability to monitor for complications.

EXPECTED OUTCOMES

1. Client obtains an accurate blood glucose reading.
2. Puncture site shows no evidence of continual bleeding or tissue damage.
3. Client explains the process of obtaining a blood specimen, completing the procedure and stating significance of test results.
4. Puncture site shows no evidence of infection (increased warmth, redness, tenderness).
5. The client demonstrates SBGM before discharge.

Implementation

Steps	Rationale
1. See Standard Protocol (Chapter 1, p. 5).	
nurse alert User error is the most common reason for inaccuracy (Kestel, 1993b).	
2. Have client wash hands with soap and **warm** water.	Establishes practice for client at home; ensures skin cleansing and vasodilation at selected puncture site.
3. Remove reagent strip from container and tightly seal cap.	Protects strips from accidental discoloration.
4. Turn glucose meter on.	Activates meter.
5. Insert strip into glucose meter (see manufacturer's directions) and make necessary adjustments.	Some machines must be calibrated; others require zeroing of timer. Each meter adjusts differently.
6. Remove unused reagent strip from meter and place on paper towel or clean, dry surface with test pad facing up.	Moisture on strip can change its color, altering reading of final results.
7. Choose puncture site on side of finger (if infant, outer aspect of heel).	Puncture site should be vascular.
8. Place finger in dependent position and gently massage finger toward puncture site.	Increases blood flow to area.
9. Clean site with antiseptic swab and **allow to dry completely.**	Wet alcohol can make the stick more painful and interfere with test results.
10. Remove cover of lancet or blood-letting device.	Cover keeps needle or lancet sterile.

Steps	Rationale
11. Place blood-letting device firmly against side of finger and push release button, causing needle to pierce skin (Figure 39-10). Hold lancet perpendicular to puncture site and pierce finger quickly in one continuous motion.	Perpendicular position ensures proper skin penetration.

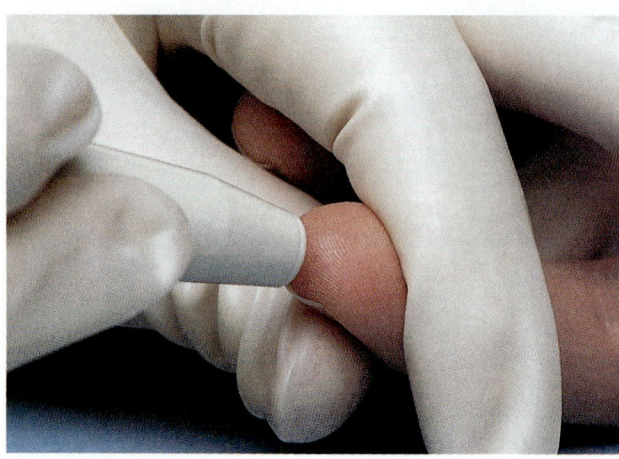

Figure 39-10

12. Wipe away first droplet of blood with cotton ball. (See manufacturer's directions for meter used.)	First drop of blood generally contains large portion of serous fluid, which can dilute specimen and cause false results.
13. Lightly squeeze puncture site until **large droplet of blood has formed without touching.**	Ensure proper coverage of test pad on reagent strip.
14. Hold reagent strip pad close to droplet of blood and lightly transfer droplet to test pad (Figure 39-11). **Do not smear blood.**	Droplet must be absorbed by test pad to ensure proper chemical reaction. Smearing causes inaccurate test results. Failure to get a large drop is a common mistake (Kestel, 1993a).

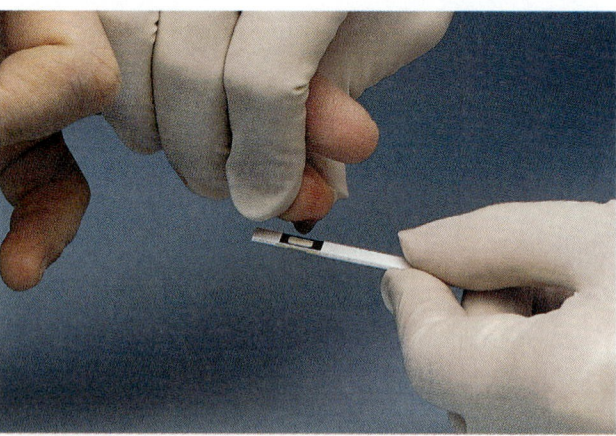

Figure 39-11

15. Immediately press timer on glucose meter and place reagent strip on paper towel or on side of timer. (See manufacturer's directions for meter used.)	Blood must be exposed to test strip for prescribed time to ensure proper results.
16. Apply pressure to skin puncture site.	Promotes hemostasis.
17. When timer displays 60 seconds (for Accu-Chek III model), use moderate pressure to wipe blood from test pad with cotton ball. No blood should remain on test pad for some meters. (See manufacturer's directions for meter used.)	For meters to read glucose levels, some strips must be dry. Refer to product directions for timing used with each type of meter.

Steps	Rationale
18. While timer continues to count, place reagent strip into meter (Figure 39-12). **19.** Read meter, noting reading on display (Figure 39-13).	Strip must be inserted correctly to obtain accurate reading. Each meter has specific time for reading glucose level.

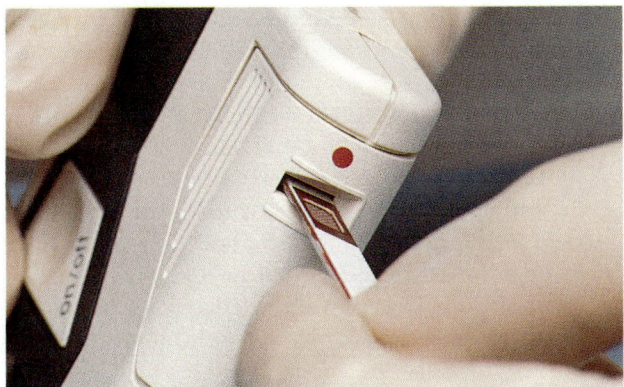

Figure 39-12

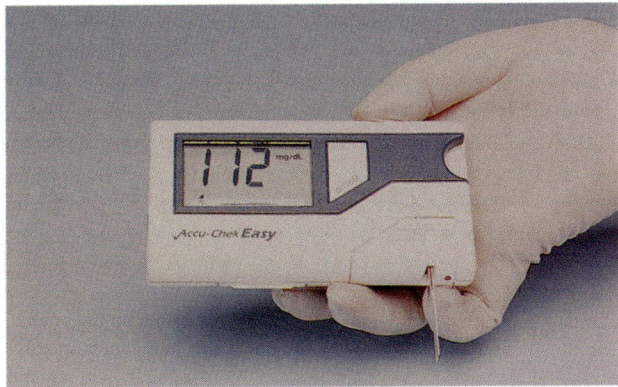

Figure 39-13

20. Turn meter off and dispose of test strip, cotton ball, uncapped lancet or autolet, and platform from lancet device (if indicated) in proper receptacle. **21.** Provide client with clear, concise, written directions for use at home. (Follow manufacturer's guidelines.) **22.** See Completion Protocol (Chapter 1, p. 6).	Meters are battery powered. Proper disposal reduces spread of microorganisms and ensures safety.

Evaluation

1. Observe client obtaining specimen and using glucose meter. Compare glucose reading obtained with normal glucose levels.
2. Inspect puncture site for bleeding or tissue damage.
3. Ask client to identify steps in performing an SBGM reading and why this is the preferred method for evaluating glucose levels.
4. Inspect puncture site for increased warmth, redness, or tenderness.
5. Have client demonstrate all steps in the procedure, including reading test results.

UNEXPECTED OUTCOMES AND RELATED INTERVENTIONS

1. Client did not collect an appropriate blood specimen.
   a. Observe client to see if blood is applied to strip correctly: one large hanging droplet that is distributed evenly. Teach not to smear blood on strip, which may cause inaccurate results.
   b. Encourage client to wash hands with warm water to induce vasodilation.
   c. Encourage client to hang hand down below level of the heart for several minutes, then perform a finger stick on side of the finger and squeeze the opposite side in a milking manner to produce a good-sized drop.
   d. Encourage client to use side of the finger, since this causes less pain and side contains more capillaries.
2. Client expresses misunderstanding of procedure and results.
   a. Assess areas of instruction that client does not understand.
   b. Assess client's anxiety level in relation to procedure performance.
   c. Provide additional teaching.
   d. Provide written instructions and visual guidelines in areas of misunderstanding.
3. Puncture site continues to bleed or is bruised.
   a. Apply pressure to puncture area.
   b. Instruct client not to use area until healing has occurred (until bruise and discomfort are gone).

SAMPLE DOCUMENTATION

0645 Skin puncture performed on left index finger by client. Results 76 per Accu-Chek III. Procedure performed correctly per procedure and manufacturer's guidelines. Results called to physician.

Skill 39.5 | Teaching Home Self-Catheterization

This skill addresses the proper way to teach a client to perform clean, intermittent self-catheterization. Many clients in the home environment utilize self-catheterization to manage acute or chronic bladder dysfunctions. Self-catheterization can be taught to clients with paraplegia, hemiplegia, or other illnesses that limit voluntary bladder control. When teaching self-catheterization to a client, the nurse must also teach a family member or significant other to complete the procedure.

Clients performing self-catheterization can choose to use either medical or sterile technique. Clients who are prone to infections should use sterile technique, whereas others can use medical asepsis (clean technique) without the risk of infection. For these clients, the bladder's natural resistance to microorganisms normally found in the home environment makes it unnecessary to use sterile technique.

Self-catheterization is an important component of a client's rehabilitation and return to a maximal level of functioning. Therefore, instruction is integrated into the rehabilitation program at an early stage and not merely tacked onto the end of the hospital stay.

EQUIPMENT
Catheter(s) (one or two, red rubber), size 14 or 16 French
Zephrin towelettes, "baby wipes," soap and water
Surgical lubricant that is water soluble (K-Y jelly or Surgilube)
Container with a cover to store catheter
Germicide solution
Toilet/container for draining urine

Assessment

1. Assess client's and significant other's knowledge base related to self-catheterization. Does client know why self-catheterization is the best technique? **This determines if client is ready and motivated to learn. Highly motivated people perform more successfully.**
2. Is client developmentally, cognitively, and physically able to do the procedure? Can client assume the position for self-catheterization? Can client manipulate the catheter? Is client able to care for the equipment used for the procedure? **The procedure may have to be adapted to individual needs.**
3. What is client's present knowledge base? **This aids in developing appropriate teaching strategies.**

Planning

Expected outcomes focus on client and care giver's knowledge level, ability to perform self-catheterization, motivation to learn the technique, and ability to comply with procedure guidelines.

EXPECTED OUTCOMES
1. Client and significant other provide reasons why self-catheterization is the best technique for managing bladder dysfunction.
2. Client correctly demonstrates self-catheterization before discharge.
3. Urine is clear, dilute, and odor free after self-catheterization.
4. Client verbalizes satisfaction with procedural technique.
5. Client demonstrates care of equipment following self-catheterization according to institutional recommendations.

Implementation

Steps	Rationale

1. See Standard Protocol (Chapter 1, p. 5).
2. Carry out individualized instruction, allowing client to ask questions or demonstrate each technique.
Reduction of microorganisms
  a. Teach and demonstrate handwashing and its significance.
  b. Explain and demonstrate opening catheter package, manipulating supplies, and handling catheter.
  c. Explain and demonstrate preparation of urethral meatus.
	Starting with simple concepts and working toward more complex ones facilitates learning. Return demonstration actively involves client in performing procedure on self, or client may need to start on model and work up to performing procedure on self with nurse's supervision.

Steps	Rationale

Insertion of catheter into bladder

   a. Identify possible positions for client to assume (sitting on toilet, frog leg, lying on bed with legs bent and knees apart).

   b. Review anatomical landmarks.

   c. Explain and demonstrate insertion of catheter: how to hold penis or separate labia, cleansing urethra, and distance to insert catheter.

   d. Explain normal sensations client will feel.

Care of equipment

Discuss and demonstrate principles of medical asepsis.

3. Explain that the following changes must be reported to health-care provider:

   a. Urine changes: color changes such as dark or cloudy appearance, bleeding or sediment, odor changes, or decrease in urine volume

   b. Pain or discomfort: In bladder area while performing procedure or at any time in bladder area with accompanying fever

   c. Inability to perform procedure, inability to pass catheter

4. Gather equipment: catheter, towelettes or soap and water, wet washcloth for rinsing, lubricant, container for urine collection if toilet unavailable, and container to store catheter.

5. Wash hands with soap and water.

6. Assume comfortable position (e.g., sitting on toilet, lying in bed).

7. **Female self-catheterization**

(Reinforce with written instructions and visual guidelines.)

   a. Wash urinary meatus (opening) with towelette or soapy washcloth. Spread vaginal folds to expose urinary meatus. Cleanse with front-to-back motion. Rinse with damp washcloth (Figure 39-14).

   b. Lubricate 1 to 3 inches (2.5 to 7.5 cm) of catheter, starting at the tip. Do not allow catheter to touch any other surfaces (Figure 39-15).

   c. Separate labia with nondominant hand.

Practicing psychomotor skills after cognitive learning allows client to apply and practice principles learned.

Proper care of equipment ensures maintenance of medical asepsis.

Indicates possible urinary tract infection. Antibiotic treatment may be required.

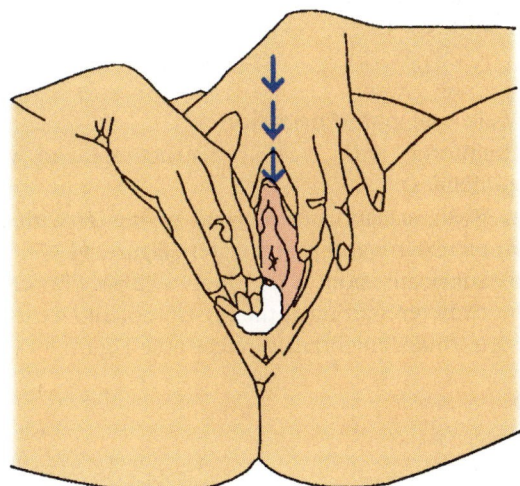

Figure 39-14 (Courtesy Methodist Medical Center of Illinois, Peoria, Ill.)

Front-to-back motion decreases chance of contamination.

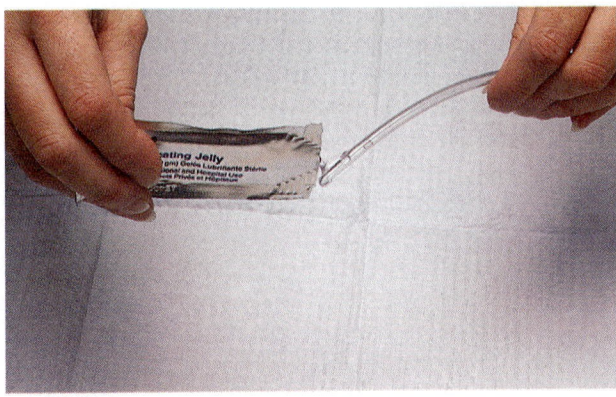

Figure 39-15

Steps	Rationale

d. Hold catheter in dominant hand, and slowly insert it into urinary meatus about 3 inches (7.5 cm) or until urine flows through (Figure 39-16).

Ensures catheter tip enters bladder.

e. Place other end of catheter into the container or toilet; allow all the urine to drain. Press on abdomen to be sure bladder is empty.

f. Slowly remove catheter after all urine has been drained.

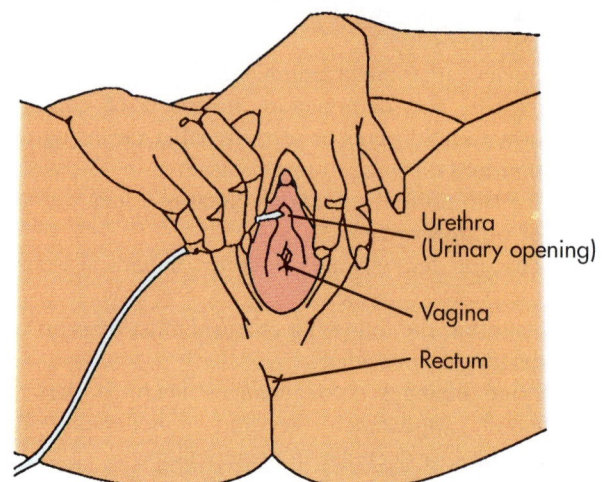

Figure 39-16 (Courtesy Methodist Medical Center of Illinois, Peoria, Ill.)

8. Male self-catheterization

(Reinforce with written instructions and visual guidelines).

a. Wash urinary meatus (end of penis) with towelette or warm soapy water (Figure 39-17).

b. Lubricate about 2 to 3 inches (2.5 to 7.5 cm) of catheter, starting at the tip. Do not allow catheter to touch any other surfaces (see Figure 39-15).

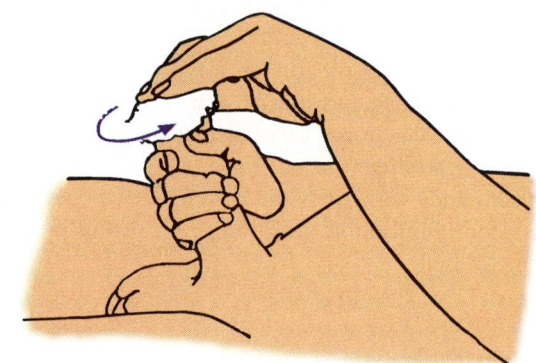

Figure 39-17 (Courtesy Methodist Medical Center of Illinois, Peoria, Ill.)

c. Hold penis with nondominant hand and at an angle "J" position.

Straightens urethra for easier catheter passage.

d. Insert catheter into urinary opening about 8 inches (20 cm) into bladder (Figure 39-18).

e. Let penis return to natural position after urine starts to flow. Allow urine to drain, making sure to hold catheter at all times; then slowly withdraw catheter after urine flow ceases.

9. Rinse catheter in cold water inside and out and place in covered container with a germicide solution (e.g., Detergicide, Sporiciden), or wash it in warm soapy water and allow to air dry. (Refer to agency policy.)

10. Discard catheter if it becomes difficult to clean. Catheters may be used for 7 to 30 days depending on cleansing of equipment and agency policy.

11. See Completion Protocol (Chapter 1, p. 6).

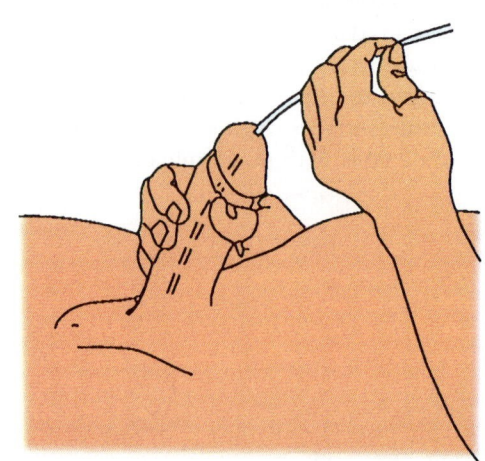

Figure 39-18 (Courtesy Methodist Medical Center of Illinois, Peoria, Ill.)

Evaluation

1. Ask client to state reasons self-catheterization is an appropriate choice for controlling bladder dysfunction.
2. Observe client performing catheterization on "like" model, then observe client's ability to perform self-catheterization using procedural guidelines.
3. Observe client's urine after self-catheterization.
4. Ask client for any questions or concerns about the procedure.
5. Have client explain proper care of the equipment, and evaluate ability to follow guidelines after self-catheterization.

UNEXPECTED OUTCOMES AND RELATED INTERVENTIONS

1. Client is unable to complete procedure.
   a. Reassess knowledge base.
   b. Assess for changes in cognition or psychomotor skill.
   c. Try different position for catheterization.
   d. Assess client's personal feelings about performing procedure.
   e. Reteach areas in which client is deficient.
2. Client develops a urinary tract infection. (Signs and symptoms include fever, cloudy foul-smelling urine, and back or flank pain.)
   a. Reevaluate client's technique for performing procedure and cleaning equipment.
   b. Assess home environment.
   c. Assess fluid intake. Encourage client to drink plenty of fluids.
   d. Instruct client to switch from clean to sterile catheter technique.

SAMPLE DOCUMENTATION

1400 Instructions regarding home self-catheterization given to client. Use of equipment, medical asepsis, and reasons for self-catheterization discussed. Catheterization demonstrated on model by nurse. Encouraged client to practice on model and ask questions.

1700 Client demonstrated procedure on model. Written and visual guidelines for self-catheterization given and explained to client.

Next day

1300 Client performed self-catheterization using aseptic technique in nurse's presence. 400 ml clear, yellow, odorless urine returned. Client praised on performance.

Skill 39.6 | Using Home Oxygen Equipment

Clients with alterations in oxygenation often require continuous oxygen therapy after discharge from the hospital. The duration of therapy may be from several weeks or months as clients recover from an acute lung injury or continuously for the remainder of their lives. Oxygen is a drug and is administered and monitored with the same care as any other medication. The box below lists oxygen safety measures to be followed.

Oxygen therapy is covered by Medicare and other third-party payors. Medicare has specific guidelines for reimbursement of oxygen therapy in the home. The box below outlines the Medicare guidelines to qualify for reimbursement for home oxygen therapy.

Three types of oxygen are available for home use: compressed oxygen, liquid oxygen, and oxygen concen-

---

Oxygen Safety Guidelines

- Oxygen is a medication and should not be adjusted without a physician's order.
- No smoking should be allowed in the client's room.
- A "No Smoking" sign is placed in a spot visible to visitors.
- Oxygen delivery systems must be kept 10 feet from any open flames.
- Oxygen supports combustion; however, it will not explode.
- When oxygen cylinders are used, they must be secured so that they will not fall over. Oxygen cylinders are stored upright, chained, or in appropriate holders.

Medicare Qualifications for Home Oxygen Therapy

$Pao_2 \leq 55$ mm Hg or $Sao_2 \leq 85\%$ or $Pao_2 = 56$ to 59 mm Hg *and*
Dependent edema suggesting congestive heart failure *or*
Cor pulmonale as evidenced on ECG *or*
Erythrocytosis as evidenced by hematocrit $> 56\%$

NOCTURNAL OXYGEN THERAPY
$Pao_2 \leq 55$ mm Hg during sleep *or*
Pao_2 falls more than 10 mm Hg during sleep *or*
$Sao_2 \leq 85\%$ during sleep or falls more than 5% during sleep

EXERCISE OXYGEN THERAPY
$Pao_2 \leq 55$ mm Hg during exercise *or*
$Sao_2 \leq 85\%$ during exercise

Pao_2, Arterial oxygen tension (partial pressure); Sao_2, oxygen saturation in blood; ECG, electrocardiogram.

trators. Liquid oxygen systems have smaller portable units that are filled from a larger stationary unit in the home. When at home, the client uses the stationary unit. The reservoir unit is refilled weekly or more often depending on the client's use. Liquid oxygen is the most portable and the most expensive. Table 39-2 lists the length of time a liquid oxygen system will last depending on the liter flow. Oxygen concentrators are moderate-sized units that extract oxygen from the room air, concentrate it, and deliver the prescribed liter flow to the client. Oxygen concentrators are the most economical but do not provide portability. Clients with an oxygen concentrator usually have small E cylinder tanks available for trips outside the home (Figure 39-19). Compressed oxygen is usually available in large H cylinders and in the small E cylinder tanks on carts, which are easily pulled along as the client walks. The large H cylinder tank will last approximately 50 hours at 2 L/min. Formulas for calculating the length of time an E or H cylinder will last depend on the liter flow (see box on p. 727).

Table 39-2 **Liquid Oxygen Timetable (in Hours)**

L/min	Stationary reservoirs		Portable units	
	17,000 L	25,000 L	500 L	1000 L
1	248	396	7	14
2	124	198	3	7
3	83	134	2	4½
4	61	99	1½	3½
5	40	80	—	—
6	—	—	1	2

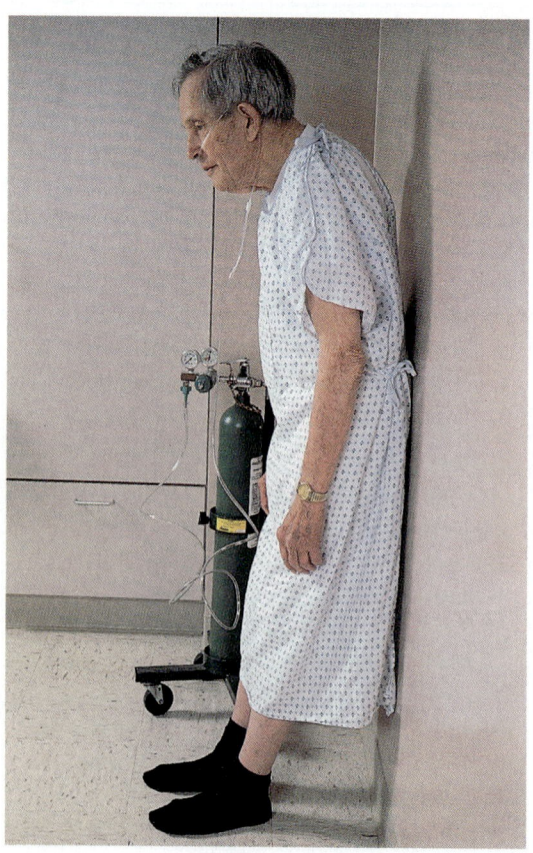

Figure 39-19

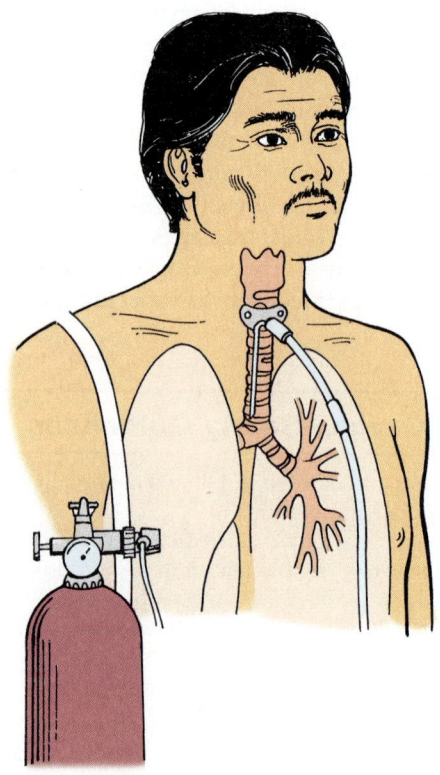

Figure 39-20

Calculating Length of Tank Time for E or H Cylinders

When oxygen cylinders are used, the following formulas are used to determine the length of time a tank will last.

FOR E CYLINDERS
Pressure on cylinder gauge (PSI): 500 psi (safety factor) $\times$ 0.3 (E cylinder factor) $\div$ L/min = minutes

FOR H CYLINDERS
Pressure on cylinder gauge (PSI): 500 psi (safety factor) $\times$ 3.1 (H cylinder factor) $\div$ L/min = minutes

EXAMPLE: E cylinder reads 1500 psi
        Liter flow rate is 4 L/min
        $(1500 - 500) \times 0.3 \div 4 = ?$
        $1000 \times 0.3 \div 4 = ?$
        $300 \div 4 = ?$
        75 minutes, or 1 hour 15 minutes

NOTE: Do not allow oxygen cylinder pressure to fall below 500 psi, or client may run out of oxygen.

The type of oxygen delivery is based on a thorough assessment of the client's needs. Criteria for determining the right oxygen delivery for the client include the client's activity level, the amount of oxygen prescribed for the client, the client's physical ability, the availability of assistance for activities such as refilling a liquid tank, and where the client lives. A client who is very mobile and active would benefit from a liquid oxygen system to encourage continuation of activities. A client who is homebound is best served with an oxygen concentrator and smaller E cylinder for infrequent trips outside the home. The nurse, physician, client, and home health company can determine the right system to meet a client's needs.

The client receiving home oxygen usually has the oxygen delivered via nasal cannula, although some clients may require the use of a simple face mask. Transtracheal oxygen is delivered directly into the trachea via a catheter (Figure 39-20). A T tube with reservoir or tracheostomy collar is used for clients with a permanent tracheostomy.

Nasal cannulas are changed weekly and cleaned with mild soap and water. Face masks, T tubes, and tracheostomy collars are cleaned daily with mild soap and water and allowed to air dry. Clients should have more than one delivery device so they can clean one and hang it to air dry while using the other.

This skill involves setting up and administering oxygen therapy to the client requiring oxygen administration in the home.

EQUIPMENT
Oxygen delivery device
    Nasal cannula
    Simple mask
    Tracheostomy collar
Oxygen tubing
Oxygen source
    Oxygen cylinders
    Liquid system
    Concentrator

Assessment

1. Assess client's and family's ability to use oxygen equipment while in the hospital or in the home. **Physical or mental impairment may indicate a need for assistance in the home.**
2. Assess client's and family's ability to determine the signs and symptoms of hypoxia.
3. Assess the availability of community resources for home oxygen therapy.

Planning

Expected outcomes focus on correct and safe use of the home oxygen equipment.

EXPECTED OUTCOMES
1. Client receives oxygen at prescribed rate.
2. Client and family verbalize the purpose and correct use of home oxygen by discharge.
3. Client and family demonstrate how to set up the oxygen system.
4. Client and family are able to verbalize safety guidelines for oxygen use.

Implementation

Steps	Rationale

1. See Standard Protocol (Chapter 1, p. 5).
2. Place oxygen delivery device in a clutter-free environment.
3. Check oxygen level remaining.
       Ensures adequate oxygen supply.
   a. Check liquid system by depressing button at lower right corner and reading the dial on the Liberator or Stroller (Figure 39-21).
   b. Check cylinders by reading amount on pressure gauge.
4. Connect oxygen delivery device (e.g., nasal cannula) to oxygen system.

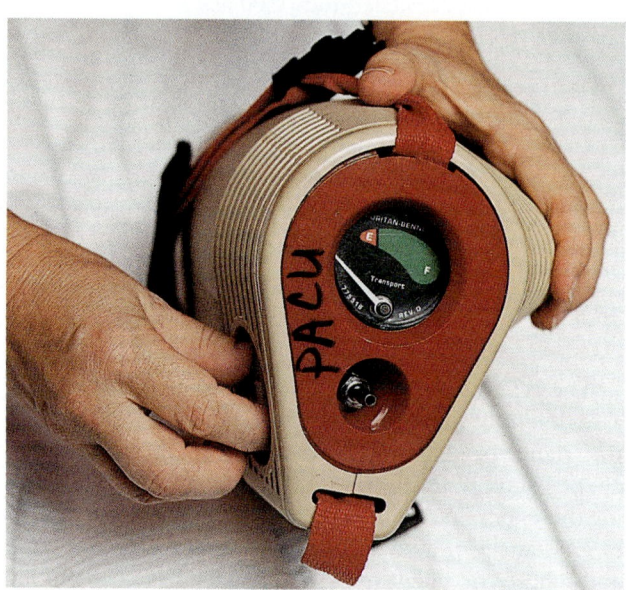

Figure 39-21

5. Determine and set correct liter flow rate.
6. Place oxygen delivery device on client (Figure 39-22).
7. When client is leaving the home and needs portability, the following steps are needed to prepare the portable units:

Ensures delivery of prescribed amount of oxygen.

Liquid system
   a. Refill Stroller by turning bayonet coupling lock on Stroller 45 degrees.

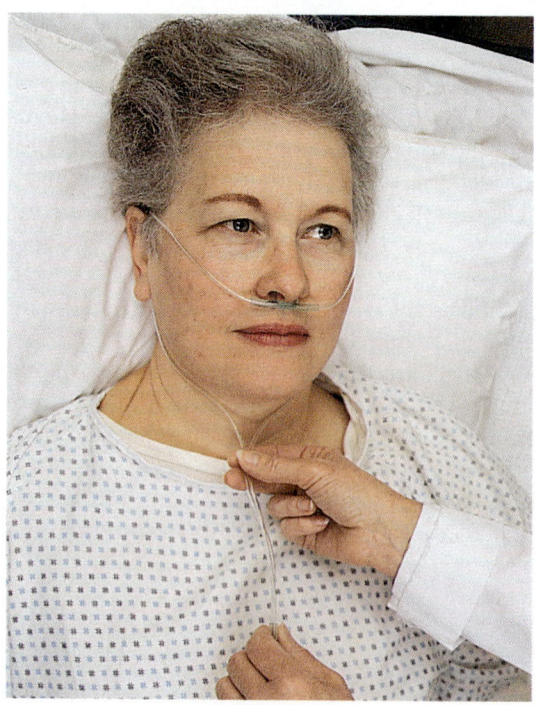

Figure 39-22

Steps	Rationale
b. Insert female adaptor on Stroller onto male adaptor on Liberator.	Allows secure connection between Liberator and Stroller to prevent leakage of liquid oxygen into the room.
c. Refill Stroller until indicator reaches full.	
d. Disconnect from Liberator.	
e. Return bayonet coupling lock to original position.	
f. Set prescribed flow rate and lock flow meter.	
g. Place Stroller on cart.	
h. Connect appropriate oxygen delivery device and oxygen tubing to Stroller.	
E tank oxygen source	
a. Place unused E tank in portable carrier.	
b. Turn valve at top of tank on for 1 second.	Removes dust particles and metal filings from fittings.
c. Attach regulator to E tank.	
d. Using oxygen key, open E tank.	
e. Determine level of oxygen in tank by reading gauge on regulator.	
f. Set prescribed flow rate.	
g. Connect appropriate oxygen delivery device and oxygen tubing to E tank.	
8. See Completion Protocol (Chapter 1, p. 6).	

Evaluation

1. Observe client's respiratory pattern and breathlessness to determine if client is receiving oxygen as prescribed.
2. Ask client and family to describe reasons for and correct setup for home oxygen use.
3. Observe client and family use home oxygen system to determine ability to deal with stressors associated with home use.
4. Ask client and family to describe safety guidelines for home oxygen use.

UNEXPECTED OUTCOMES AND RELATED INTERVENTIONS

Client develops signs and symptoms associated with hypoxemia.

   a. Determine if oxygen delivery device and source are delivering oxygen properly.
   b. Determine if prescribed oxygen flow rate is set correctly.
   c. Assess client for change in respiratory status, such as airway plugging, respiratory infection, or bronchospasm.

SAMPLE DOCUMENTATION

1600 Client and family able to return demonstrate appropriate use of liquid oxygen system, including refilling Stroller and monitoring oxygen level. Correctly stated signs and symptoms of hypoxemia and safety precautions for home oxygen use.

Skill 39.7 | Teaching Home Tracheostomy Care

The indications and procedure for performing tracheostomy care and suctioning in the home are similar to the care in the hospital except for the use of principles of medical asepsis or *clean technique* rather than surgical asepsis. In the hospital the client is more susceptible to infection because of the pathogenic microorganisms present. In the home setting the risk to the client is greatly reduced, and clean technique provides safe care for most clients.

Immunocompromised clients, clients with active infections, and clients living in unclean home environments are not appropriate candidates for clean technique. In these instances, surgical asepsis is indicated to reduce the client's risk of infection.

Home tracheostomy care actually begins in the hospital as the nurse teaches the client and family how to care for the tracheostomy. The client usually learns more easily when less invasive techniques such as stoma care precede more invasive techniques such as inner cannula care and suctioning.

Suctioning is done when the client feels resistance in the airways or coughs up mucus that cannot be expectorated. The client and family are taught how to assess for the need to suction based on the client's need to clear the airways. Tracheostomy care is performed at least daily but may be necessary as often as every 4 hours for clients with copious secretions. Hydration helps keep secretions thin and makes them easier to cough up and expectorate or suction.

This skill involves use of clean technique for suctioning and cleaning the tracheostomy tube in the home care setting. Care must be taken to provide safe and effective airway care with minimal disruption of the client's breathing pattern.

EQUIPMENT

Suction machine with connecting tubing (Figure 39-23)
Nonsterile gloves
Tracheostomy care set (Figure 39-24)
Small basin
Water that has been boiled and cooled to room temperature, or normal saline
4 × 4 gauze pads
Hydrogen peroxide
Appropriate size of sterile or clean and disinfected catheter
Small brush or pipe cleaner
Cotton-tipped swabs
Tracheostomy ties (twill tape, bias tape, nonelastic ribbon)
Mirror

Wet washcloth
Dry towel

Assessment

1. Assess client's and family's ability to perform tracheostomy care and suctioning properly while in the hospital.
2. Assess client's and family's knowledge and ability to observe for signs and symptoms of need to perform suctioning and tracheostomy care. Prompt response to airway obstruction is necessary.

Planning

Expected outcomes focus on correct assessment of need for suctioning, proper suction procedure, and proper tracheostomy care.

EXPECTED OUTCOMES

1. Client identifies signs and symptoms indicating need for tracheostomy care and suctioning.
2. Lower and upper airways are free of secretions.
3. Inner cannula of tracheostomy tube and dressings are free of secretions.
4. Client/family demonstrates clean technique for tracheostomy care and suctioning.

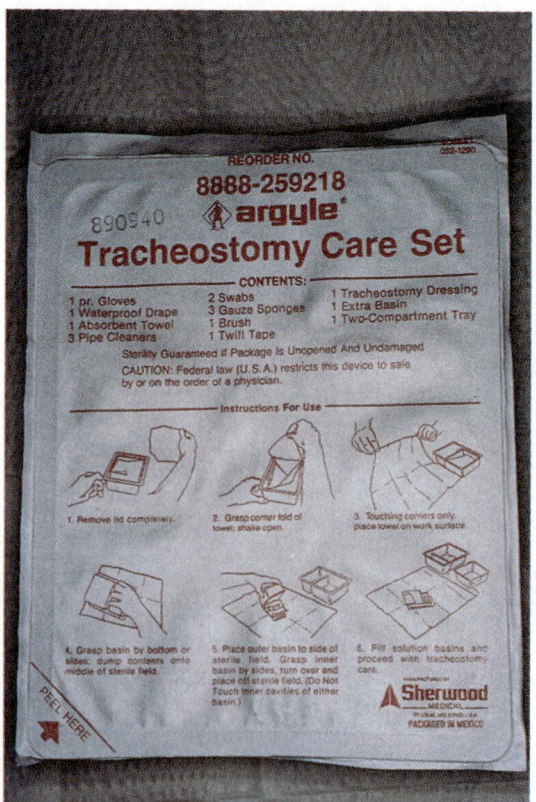

Figure 39-24

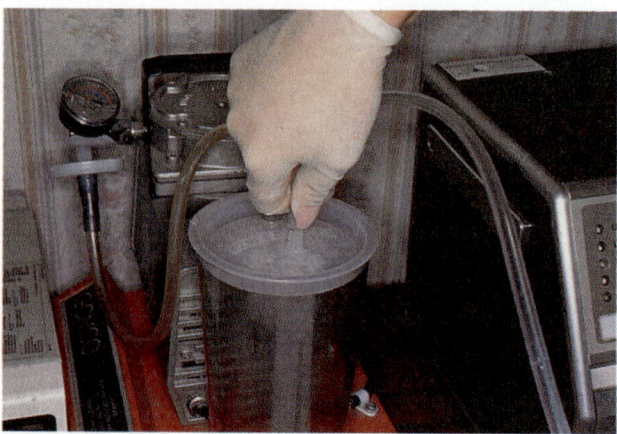

Figure 39-23

Implementation

Steps	Rationale

1. See Standard Protocol (Chapter 1, p. 5).

2. Tracheostomy suctioning

   a. Have client sit in chair or sit up in bed.

   b. Fill basin with ½ cup water or normal saline.

   c. Connect suction catheter to suction apparatus and check that equipment is functioning (Figure 39-25).

   d. Remove oxygen or humidity source from client.

   e. Insert catheter 6 to 8 inches (15 to 20 cm) without applying suction. If resistance is met, pull back catheter ½ inch (1 cm) (Figure 39-26).

Provides easier access to airway.

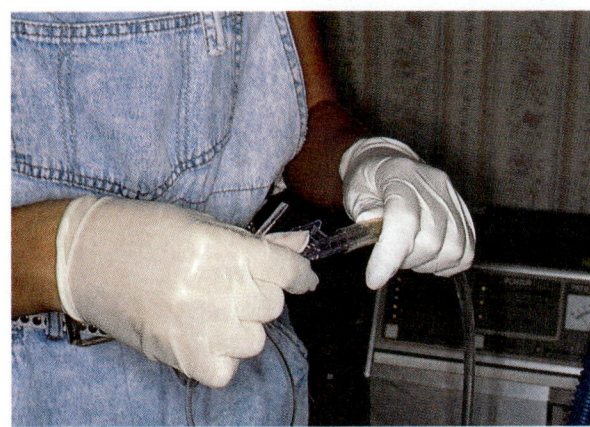

Figure 39-25

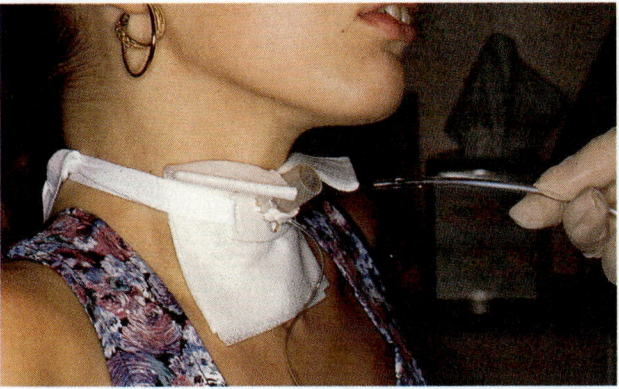

A

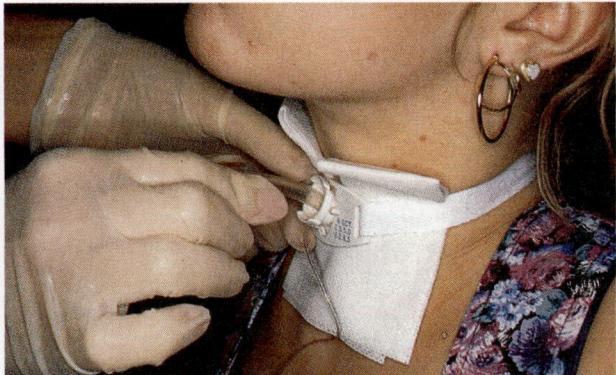

B

Figure 39-26

   f. Apply intermittent suction by placing and releasing thumb over catheter vent and slowly withdrawing catheter while rotating it between thumb and forefinger. (Explain that catheter will cause client to cough.)

   g. Reapply oxygen or humidity source.

   h. Repeat Steps e through g as needed to remove secretions.

   i. After suctioning is completed, rinse catheter with water in basin until clean.

   j. Disconnect suction catheter and coil around gloved hand.

     (1) If catheter is to be cleaned and disinfected, set aside.

     (2) If catheter needs to be discarded, pull glove over coiled catheter and discard.

Intermittent suction and rotation of catheter prevent injury to tracheal mucosal lining.

Removes secretions from catheter and reduces transmission of microorganisms.

Steps	Rationale

3. Tracheostomy care

a. Unlock safety lock and remove inner cannula of tracheostomy tube by pulling it straight out (Figure 39-27).
b. Hold over basin and pour hydrogen peroxide over and through inner cannula.
c. Use brush or pipe cleaner to remove crusted or adhering secretions.

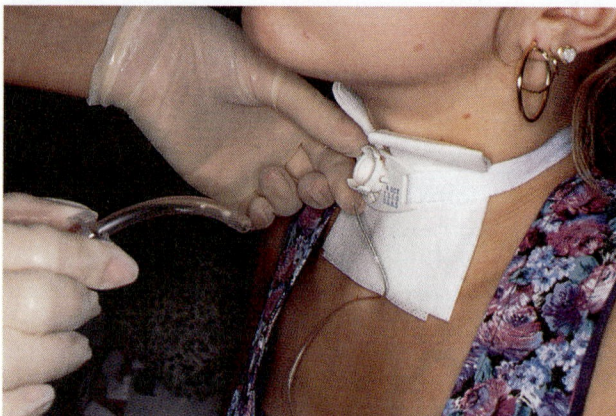

Figure 39-27

d. Rinse inner cannula with water or normal saline.

e. Replace inner cannula and lock into position.
f. Carefully remove soiled tracheostomy dressing. Hold outer cannula while slipping each side of dressing out from under the tracheostomy ties.
g. Wash around stoma site with soap and warm water, using cotton swabs (Figure 39-28).
h. Wash exposed outer cannula with wet washcloth.
i. Dry exposed outer cannula and skin sites.
j. Change tracheostomy ties. Have client hold faceplate of tracheostomy tube while removing old ties and applying new ones (Figure 39-29). Secure ties in a knot along the side of client's neck.
k. Gently slip edge of clean gauze under tie and around one side of tracheostomy tube. Repeat for other side (Figure 39-30).

Removes remaining hydrogen peroxide from inner cannula that could cause airway or stoma irritation.

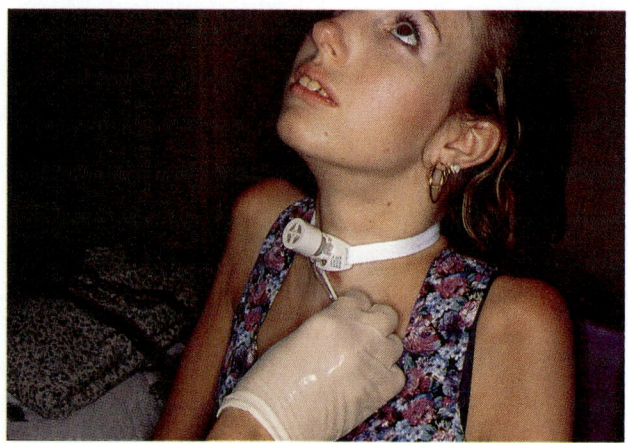

Figure 39-28

nurse alert   Client is at risk for tube coming out as ties are changed. Another tube may be needed, including a stylet for insertion.

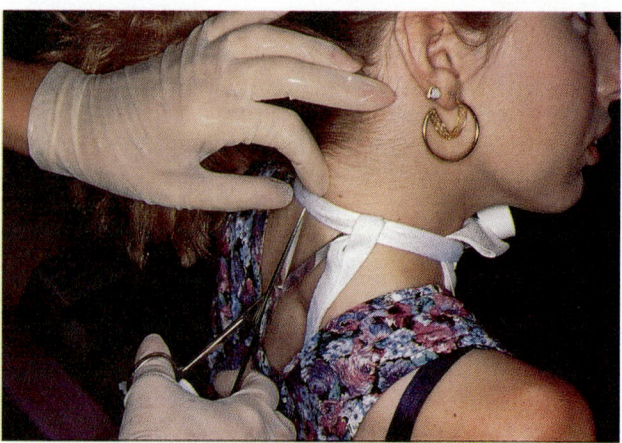

Figure 39-29

Steps	Rationale

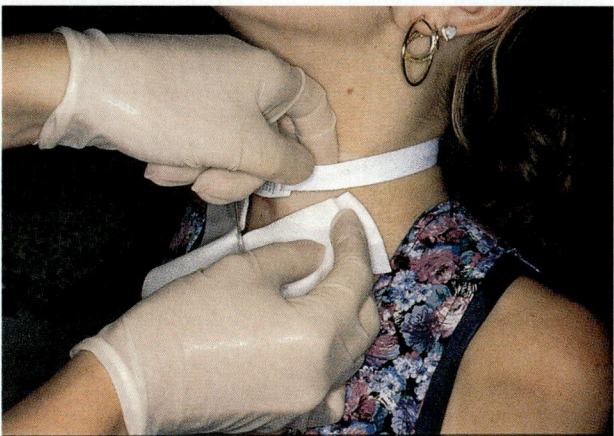

Figure 39-30

l. Clean reusable supplies in warm soapy water. Rinse thoroughly and air dry.

m. Store clean, dry supplies in loosely closed plastic bag.

Air must circulate, or humidity in bag can promote growth of microorganisms.

n. Place "button" on tracheostomy to facilitate speech (Figure 39-31).

4. Remove and discard gloves.

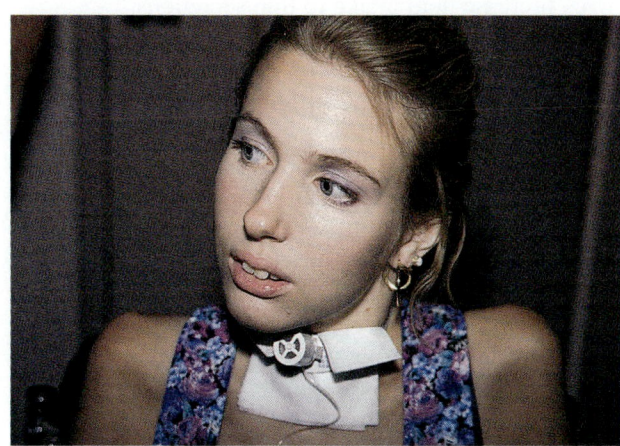

Figure 39-31

5. Disinfecting supplies

Method 1

a. Boil reusable supplies for 15 minutes.

b. Allow to cool, air dry, and store.

Method 2

a. Soak reusable supplies in equal parts of vinegar and water for 30 minutes.

b. Remove and rinse thoroughly.

c. Air dry and store.

Method 3

a. Soak reusable supplies in prepared disinfectant solution (quaternary ammonium chloride compounds) according to manufacturer's recommendations.

b. Rinse thoroughly.

c. Air dry and store.

6. See Completion Protocol (Chapter 1, p. 6).

Home environment is less likely to have pathogens to which the client is susceptible; therefore sterilization is not necessary.

Evaluation

1. Ask client to list signs and symptoms that indicate the need for suctioning, including difficulty breathing and continued coughing of secretions.
2. Auscultate lungs and airways.
3. Observe for signs of stomal or respiratory tract infections.
4. Ask client to demonstrate technique for tracheostomy care and suctioning.

UNEXPECTED OUTCOMES AND RELATED INTERVENTIONS

1. Client develops reddened or hard stoma site with or without drainage.
   a. Report finding to physician.
   b. Monitor for fever, malaise, or sputum color changes.
2. Client has copious colored secretions around stoma site or when suctioned.
   a. Notify physician.
   b. Increase suction frequency.
   c. Increase fluid intake to thin secretions.
3. Client is unable to perform skill.
   a. Review procedures with client and family.
   b. Assess need for home health nurse or aide to assist with care.
4. Tracheostomy tube comes out.
   a. Instruct client to remain calm and breathe slowly.
   b. Replace tube with new, clean tube, using stylet. Remove stylet and replace with inner cannula.
   c. Lock inner cannula into place.
   d. If unable to replace, notify physician immediately and support respirations as necessary.
5. Skin breakdown is present at stoma site.
   a. Clean around stoma site more frequently, and make sure area is kept clean and dry.
   b. Change tracheostomy dressing and ties when they become wet.

SAMPLE DOCUMENTATION

0800 Client able to suction adequately and performs tracheostomy care without difficulty. Secretions are white and thin. Stoma site is clean and dry without redness or evidence of infection.

CRITICAL THINKING EXERCISES

1. You are the home health nurse who has been assigned to follow Mrs. Reed's progress at home following her hip surgery. Mrs. Reed is able to perform most of her own care and walks with the assistance of a walker. While visiting Mrs. Reed you note that she lives alone in a small apartment with her two cats. She has several area rugs in the apartment. Her bathroom has a tub but no shower. Her kitchen cabinets are low and she can reach her food and utensils without difficulty. Her daughter visits her daily. Does Mrs. Reed have any safety hazards that she should be made aware of? If so, what?
2. Mr. Donnely is about to do a return demonstration of drawing up insulin into a syringe, and you are evaluating him. After washing his hands, Mr. Donnely cleans the vial rubber stopper with alcohol, uncaps the needle, and places it through the rubber stopper. He withdraws 10 units of regular insulin as prescribed and removes the needle. He finds that he has drawn up a large air bubble, so he holds the syringe in the upright position and expels the air. He then states that he is ready to administer the insulin. What is your evaluation of Mr. Donnely's demonstration?
3. You have been instructed to teach Mandy how to perform sterile self-catheterizations. Previously Mandy was allowed to do clean catheterizations. What conclusion can be drawn about the need to teach Mandy the new procedure?
4. Consider all the client teaching that you will be doing throughout your nursing career. Cite several teaching principles that will apply to all client teaching regardless of the subject.

REFERENCES

American Diabetes Association: Position statement: implications of the Diabetes Control and Complications Trial, *Diabetes Spectrum* 6(4):225, 1993.

Barry K: Patient self medication: an innovative approach to medication teaching, *J Nurs Care Q* 8(1):75, 1993.

Beare P, Myers J: *Principles and practices of adult health nursing,* ed 2, St Louis, 1994, Mosby.

Kestel F: Using blood glucose meters—what you and your patient need to know. Part I, *Nursing '93* 23(3):34, 1993a.

Kestel F: Using blood glucose meters—what you and your patient need to know. Part III, *Nursing '93* 23(5):51, 1993b.

Kim M, McFarland G, McLane A: *Pocket guide to nursing diagnoses,* ed 5, St Louis, 1995, Mosby.

Occupational Safety and Health Administration (OSHA), Occupational Safety and Health Act: blood-borne pathogens, *Fed Register* 56(235):64, 1991.

ADDITIONAL READINGS

American Diabetes Association: Consensus statement: self-monitoring of blood glucose, *Diabetes Care* 16(suppl 2):60, 1993.

American Diabetes Association: Position statement: insulin administration, *Diabetes Care* 16(suppl 2):31, 1993.

Carr P: Home care: beyond the hospital walls, *Am J Nurs* 93(8):14, 1993.

Dettenmeier PA: Home oxygen therapy. In *Pulmonary nursing care,* St Louis, 1992, Mosby.

Dettenmeier PA: Invasive techniques for improving oxygenation and ventilation airways. In *Pulmonary nursing care,* St Louis, 1992, Mosby.

Drass J: What you need to know about insulin injections, *Nursing '92* 22(11):40, 1992.

Hoffman LA: Novel strategies for delivering oxygen: reservoir cannula, demand flow, and transtracheal oxygen administration, *Respir Care* 39(4):363, 1994.

Jubeck ME: Teaching the elderly: a common sense approach, *Nurs* 24(5):70, 1994.

Kestel F: Using blood glucose meters—what you and your patient need to know. Part II, *Nursing '93* 23(4):50, 1993.

Manzetti JD, Hoffman LA: Nursing role in management of upper respiratory problems. In Lewis SM, Collier IC, editors: *Medical-surgical nursing: assessment and management of clinical problems,* ed 3, St Louis, 1992, Mosby.

McGovern K: 10 Golden Rules for administering drugs safely, *Nursing '92* 22(3):49, 1993.

Newman DK, Smith DA: Helping geriatric patients master self catheterization, *RN* 51(5):86, 1988.

Newton M, Newton D, Fudin J: Reviewing the Big Three injection routes, *Nursing '92* 22(2):34, 1992.

Peragalo-Ditko V: Buyer's guide to blood glucose meters, *Diabetes Self Manage* 8(3):34, 1991.

Petzinger RA: Diabetes aids and products for people with visual or physical impairment, *Diabetes Educ* 18(2):121, 1992.

Phillips C: Postdischarge followup care: effect on patient outcomes, *J Nurs Care Q* 7(4):64, 1993.

Pierson DJ: Controversies in home respiratory care: conference summary, *Respir Care* 39(4):294, 1994.

Proos M et al: A study of the effects of self-medication on patients' knowledge of and compliance with their medication regimen, *J Nurs Care Q* Special Report, 1992, p 18.

Rice R: *Home health nursing practice: concepts and applications,* St Louis, 1991, Mosby.

Roe C: The muddy waters of clinical teaching, *Am J Nurs* 92(7):20, 1992.

Ronczy NM, Beddome MAL: Preparing the family for home tracheostomy care, *AACN Clin Issues Crit Care Nurs* 1(2):367, 1990.

Safety For Older Consumers: *Home safety checklist,* 1986, US Consumer Product Safety Commission.

Stanhope M, Lancaster J: *Community health nursing: process and practice for promoting health,* ed 3, St Louis, 1992, Mosby.

Tirk J: Determining discharge priorities, *Nursing '92* 22(7):55, 1992.

Webber-Jones J: Performing clean, intermittent self-catheterization, *Nursing '91* 21(8):56, 1991.

Weilitz PB: Airway management. In *Pocket guide to respiratory care,* St Louis, 1991, Mosby.

Weilitz PB, Dettenmeier PA: Back to basics: test your knowledge of tracheostomy tubes, *Am J Nurs* 94(2):46, 1994.

Weilitz PB: Respiratory home care. In *Pocket guide to respiratory care,* St Louis, 1991, Mosby.

Williams M: Achieving patient compliance, *Nurs Times* 89(13):50, 1993.

appendix A

Sample Forms

738

ST. JOHN'S HOSPITAL
Springfield, Illinois

ADMISSION INFORMATION

Patient: _____ Doctor: _____ Date: _____

Room: _____	Height: _____ cm.	Date of previous admission:
Arrival Time: _____	Weight: _____ kg.	_____
From: _____	T.P.R. _____	Name patient prefers to be called:
How: _____	B.P. _____ (Circle) R L	_____

For female over age 20, date of last pap smear _____
Do you wish a Pap Smear during this admission? ☐ Yes ☐ No

(Circle) Lying, Sitting, Standing

Doctor's Orders with patient: ☐ Yes ☐

I.D. Band on: ☐ Yes ☐ Clear ☐ Green

VALUABLES: (List)   **DESCRIPTION:**   **DISPOSITION:**

Money: _____ _____

Credit Cards: _____ _____

Jewelry: _____ _____

_____ _____

Clothing: _____ _____

_____ _____

Who did you inform that the hospital is not responsible for valuables kept: _____

Admission Urine: ☐ Yes ☐ No   Artificial Eye: ☐ Yes ☐ No ☐ Rt ☐ Lt

Dentures: ☐ Yes ☐ No   Artificial Limb: ☐ Yes ☐ No _____

☐ Upper ☐ Lower ☐ Partial   Hearing Aid: ☐ Yes ☐ No _____
Description

Capped Teeth: ☐ Yes ☐ No   Appliances: _____
Description

Glasses: ☐ Yes ☐ No   Other: _____

Contact Lens: ☐ Yes ☐ No   _____

☐ Rt ☐ Lt ☐ Both   _____

All the above information obtained from: _____

PERSONS TO CONTACT:

Name   Phone   Information

_____

_____

_____

Admitted By: _____   *(Continued on reverse side)*

#317 (R 06/91)
(1 of 2)

ADMISSION INFORMATION

(Courtesy St. John's Hospital, Springfield, Ill.)

CHECKLIST FOR ORIENTATION OF NEW PATIENTS TO ENVIRONMENT*

☐ 1. Introduce Self

☐ 2. Introduce Roommate

☐ 3. Explain Nurse Call System

☐ 4. Demonstrate Electric Bed Controls

☐ 5. Explain Hospital Slide Rail Procedure *(Upper Rail Up)*

☐ 6. Caution Related to Sharps Disposal Box

☐ 7. Explain Telephone Operation

☐ 8. Demonstrate Room Light Operation

☐ 9. Explain T.V. Regulations

☐ 10. Explain Newspaper Service

☐ 11. Explain Mail Service

☐ 12. Explain Visiting Hours

☐ 13. Demonstrate Over Bed Tables and Patient Admission Kit

☐ 14. Show Appropriate Chest and Storage Area

☐ 15. Show Bathroom and use of Signal Light

☐ 16. Explain Patient's Valuable Policy *(Hospital **NOT** Responsible)*

☐ 17. Explain Discharge Time and Procedure

☐ 18. Present Patient Handbook - "Welcome To St. John's" To Patient or Family

*If Patient Unable to Understand - Please Explain Why

Explained By: _____ Time _____ Date _____

#317 (R 06/91)
(2 of 2)

740

ST. JOHN'S HOSPITAL
Springfield, Illinois

ADMISSION PATIENT PROFILE

*Asterisk markings identify those areas that have more detailed assessment forms that may be appropriate for this patient.

HEALTH PATTERNS ASSESSMENT (May be completed by RN or LPN)

Information Obtained From: ☐ Patient ☐ Family ☐ Friend ☐ Old Chart ☐ Transfer Sheet ☐ ER Record

Reason for Admission (as stated by patient): _____

_____

Previous Surgery(ies)/Hospitalizations: _____

_____

_____

Previous Transfusion(s)? ☐ No ☐ Yes Date _____

Known Food, Drug, Contact Allergies ☐ None *If yes, list and state reaction:* _____

_____

_____

_____

Latex Allergy: ☐ No ☐ Yes *(describe)* _____

MEDICATIONS: Patient is currently taking (include over-the-counter medications)				
Name	**Dose**	**Dosing Time**	**Day/Time of Last Dose**	**Brought to Hospital**
				☐ No ☐ Yes Disposition:
				☐ No ☐ Yes Disposition:
				☐ No ☐ Yes Disposition:
				☐ No ☐ Yes Disposition:
				☐ No ☐ Yes Disposition:
				☐ No ☐ Yes Disposition:
				☐ No ☐ Yes Disposition:
				☐ No ☐ Yes Disposition:
				☐ No ☐ Yes Disposition:
				☐ No ☐ Yes Disposition:
				☐ No ☐ Yes Disposition:
				☐ No ☐ Yes Disposition:
				☐ No ☐ Yes Disposition:
				☐ No ☐ Yes Disposition:

#4678 (R 04/95)
(1 OF 5)

ADMISSION PATIENT PROFILE

(Courtesy St. John's Hospital, Springfield, Ill.)

SYSTEMS ASSESSMENT (May be completed by RN or LPN)

NEURO/SENSORY

| | Additional Comments | Nursing Diagnosis Cues |

☐ CVA ☐ Side affected: ☐ Rt ☐ Lt ☐ Head injury _____

☐ Headache _____ ☐ Hx of Seizures _____ ☐ Stiff Neck

☐ Alert ☐ Oriented ☐ Confused ☐ Comatose ☐ Cooperative ☐ Withdrawn

☐ Anxious ☐ Hearing Difficulty ☐ P.E.R.L. ☐ Unsteady Gait

☐ Vision Difficulty Cataracts: ☐ Rt ☐ Lt Blind: ☐ Rt ☐ Lt Glaucoma: ☐ Rt ☐ Lt

☐ Syncope _____ ☐ Speech impairment (describe)

*Pain/Discomfort ☐ Yes ☐ No Describe _____

How is pain controlled? _____

☐ All above areas addressed

Nursing Diagnosis Cues: Sensory/Perceptual Alterations; Impaired Communication; Altered Thought Processes; Potential for Injury; Pain; Pain, chronic

PERFUSION

☐ Congenital Heart defects (describe) _____ ☐ CHF ☐ Anemia

☐ Heart Attack _____ ☐ Hypertension ☐ Perpheral Vascular Disease

☐ Pacemaker Check pt. I.D. Card for Model # _____ Manufacturer _____

☐ Automatic Implantable Cardioverter Defibrillator (AICD) Model # _____ Manufacturer _____

☐ Angina (describe) _____

☐ Stent (describe) _____ Apical Pulse: ☐ Reg. ☐ Irreg.

KEY: P = Pulse Present by Palpation Pulses: Radial ____ Rt. ____ Lt.

D = Pulse Audible with Doppler Posterior Tibial ____ Rt. ____ Lt.

A = Absent Pedal ____ Rt. ____ Lt.

☐ All above areas addressed

Nursing Diagnosis Cues: Decreased Cardiac Output; Fluid Volume Deficit; Fluid Volume Excess; Altered Tissue Perfusion; Pain

OXYGENATION

Respiration history: ☐ Asthma ☐ COPD ☐ Pneumonia ☐ TB ☐ Other _____

Smoking History: Do you smoke? ☐ Yes ☐ No Packs/day: ____ # of years ____

Have you ever smoked? ☐ Yes ☐ No Packs/day: ____ # of years ____

When did you quit? _____

Oxygen Therapy/Resp. Therapy used at home? ☐ Yes ☐ No Describe: _____

Breathing: ☐ Deep and regular ☐ Shallow ☐ Irregular ☐ SOB (describe) _____

Breath Sounds: ☐ Clear bilaterally ☐ Abnormal (describe) _____

Describe Cough: _____ Describe Sputum: _____

☐ All above areas addressed

Nursing Diagnosis Cues: Impaired Gas Exchange; Ineffective Airway Clearance; Ineffective Breathing Pattern; Activity Intolerance

*SKIN CONDITION

Indicate locations of any of the following by number:

1. Abrasion 5. Bruise
2. Burn 6. Laceration
3. Contusion 7. Rash
4. Decubitis 8. Scars
9. Sutures

Skin color _____
Skin temperature _____
Skin moisture _____
☐ Edema _____

☐ All above areas addressed

Nursing Diagnosis Cues: Impaired Skin Integrity; Altered Oral Mucous Membrane

MUSCULO-SKELETAL/PHYSICAL MOBILITY

☐ Arthritis ☐ Gout ☐ Fracture _____ ☐ Deformity noted (describe)

☐ Contractures: ☐ Rt. Arm ☐ Lt. Arm ☐ Rt. Leg ☐ Lt. Leg

☐ Previous limitations in mobility (specify)* _____

☐ Wheelchair** ☐ Bed Bound**

☐ History of falls (indicate frequency and reason) _____

Gait: ☐ Steady ☐ Unsteady ☐ Independent ☐ Needs ____ # of persons assist

Ambulatory devices: ☐ Cane ☐ Crutches ☐ Walker ☐ Other _____

☐ Assistance needed with bathing ☐ Assistance needed with dressing

☐ Amputations _____ ☐ Prosthesis _____

*☐ Pain Location _____ Describe _____

☐ All above areas addressed

Nursing Diagnosis Cues: Activity Intolerance; Self-care Deficit; Impaired Physical Mobility; Potential for Injury; Pain

** (NOTE: IF patient in wheelchair or bed bound complete "Pressure Ulcer Therapy" form)

#4678 (R 04/95)
(2 OF 5)

ST. JOHN'S HOSPITAL
Springfield, Illinois

ADMISSION PATIENT PROFILE

SYSTEMS ASSESSMENT (continued)   (May be completed by RN or LPN)

IMMUNE FUNCTION

Additional Comments — **Nursing Diagnosis Cues**

☐ Fever in last 48°   ☐ Transplant history _____

☐ Radiation therapy (date) _____   ☐ Chemotherapy (date) _____

☐ Venous access device _____   Site: _____

☐ Central Catheter _____   Site: _____

Malignancy history _____

☐ All above areas addressed

Potential for Infection

NUTRITIONAL/METABOLIC

Additional Comments — **Nursing Diagnosis Cues**

☐ Home Diet _____   ☐ Assistance with eating needed (describe) _____

☐ Recent Weight Changes ☐ Increase ☐ Decrease (reason) _____

Time Frame _____ Amount _____   ☐ Intentional ☐ Unintentional

☐ Nausea and vomiting ☐ Heartburn ☐ *Abdominal pain (describe) _____

☐ Diabetes: ☐ Insulin Dependent ☐ Diet Controlled ☐ Oral Meds _____

☐ Thyroid problems ☐ Hepatitis ☐ Alcohol use (Avg. number drinks/week) _____

☐ All above areas are addressed.

Altered Nutrition

Noncompliance

Self-Care Deficit, Feeding

Pain

ELIMINATION

Additional Comments — **Nursing Diagnosis Cues**

BOWEL: ☐ GI Bleed ☐ Colitis ☐ Diverticulitis ☐ Hemorrhoids Date of last BM _____

Bowel pattern (describe) _____   ☐ Stool changes (describe) _____

☐ Constipation ☐ Diarrhea Frequency _____   x/day ☐ Involuntary

Bowel Sounds: ☐ Present ☐ Absent   ☐ Abdominal Distention

URINE: ☐ Burning ☐ Hematuria ☐ Urgency ☐ Retention ☐ Renal disease

☐ Dysuria ☐ Incontinence (describe) _____

☐ Nocturia (_____ x/night)   ☐ Stream initiation difficulty

☐ Foley in place   Date inserted/changed _____

☐ Stent

☐ All above areas addressed.

Constipation

Diarrhea

Bowel Incontinence

Urinary Incontinence

Urinary Retention

Altered Patterns of Urinary Elimination

REPRODUCTIVE

Additional Comments — **Nursing Diagnosis Cues**

MALE: ☐ Prostate Problem (describe) _____

☐ History of Sexually Transmitted Disease: _____

FEMALE: ☐ Menstrual changes/problems (describe) _____

☐ History of Sexually Transmitted Disease: _____

☐ Breast changes/problems (describe) _____

☐ LMP _____   ☐ Pregnant _____ — EDD _____

For female over age 20, date of last pap smear: _____

☐ All above areas addressed

Sexual Dysfunction

Body Image Disturbance

ADMISSION PATIENT PROFILE

SYSTEMS ASSESSMENT (continued)   (May be completed by RN or LPN)

PSYCHO-SOCIAL/SPIRITUAL/CULTURAL	Additional Comments	Nursing Diagnosis Cues

☐ Lives with spouse ☐ Lives alone ☐ Lives with family
☐ Lives with friend ☐ Nursing Home ☐ Other _____
Do you plan to return to the same living arrangement? ☐ No ☐ Yes
Do you have close family members or significant others that are supportive to you if you
   need help? ☐ No ☐ Yes Name _____
               Relationship _____
☐ Are you the primary caregiver for someone at home? ☐ No ☐ Yes
	_____
	_____
	_____
	_____
	_____
		Ineffective Coping
		
		Altered Family Process
		
		Altered Health Maintenance
		
		Spiritual Distress

Do you have special religious/spiritual requests during this hospitalization? ☐ No ☐ Yes
Describe _____
_____
_____
_____
_____

What concerns you most about your hospitalization?
Describe _____
_____
_____
_____
_____

What concerns you most about your illness?
Describe _____
_____
_____
_____
_____

From an ethnic or cultural perspective, please describe any special habits, customs, beliefs or values that we
need to honor while you are a patient at St. John's Hospital. (For Example: Special food/dietary needs that
are based on your religion/culture.)
Describe _____
_____
_____
_____
_____

Signature of Data Collector: _____ Date: _____ Time: _____

ST. JOHN'S HOSPITAL
Springfield, Illinois

ADMISSION PATIENT PROFILE

ADVANCED DIRECTIVES

1. Do you want further information regarding advanced directives? ☐ Yes ☐ No
   - Patient received a copy of the patient handbook and was shown the advanced directive brochure. ☐ Yes ☐ No
     If no, (explain) _____

   - Notify Social Service as needed. ☐ Yes ☐ No
     If no, (explain) _____

2. If completed, do we have your current copy?
   ☐ Yes *(Nursing: Place in patient's chart and mark the front of the chart.)*
   ☐ Yes, placed in my record at a previous admission.
      (Nursing: Obtain copy from Medical Records and place copy in patient's current chart and mark the front of the chart.)
   ☐ No, Please advise patient to bring a copy to the hospital.
      (Nursing: Make a reminder note on the Patient Care Summary to follow-up.)

INITIAL TEACHING/DISCHARGE PLANNING / REFERRALS *(MUST be completed by RN)*

1. Patient/family teaching needs identified at this time:
   ☐ Medication _____ ☐ Pre-op_____ ☐ Other (specify)_____
   ☐ Dietary_____ ☐ Pre-Procedure _____
   ☐ Wound Care_____ ☐ Diabetic _____
   ☐ Ostomy Care _____ ☐ Pressure Ulcer Prevention _____

2. Does anyone from a community agency visit you at home? ☐ Yes ☐ No
   If yes, specify _____

3. Based on this Admission Patient Profile do you anticipate the patient needing any assistance when they are discharged from the hospital? ☐ No ☐ Yes
   If yes, specify _____
   _____

4. Screening Referrals to: Date/Time
   ☐ Cardiac Rehabilitation (ext. 4448 - order required)   _____
   ☐ Clinical Dietitian (ext. 4880)   _____
   ☐ Home Health Services (ext. 5641)   _____
   ☐ Oncology Clinical Nurse Specialist (ext. 4547)   _____
   ☐ Oncology Pain Management Service (ext. 4547)   _____
   ☐ Pastoral Care (ext. 4500)   _____
   ☐ Rehabilitation Department (ext. 4800 - order required)   _____
   ☐ Social Worker (ext. 4480)   _____
   ☐ Stoma Nurse (ext. 4035)   _____
   ☐ Other   _____

Signature _____ R.N. Date _____ Time: _____

***Asterisk markings identify those areas that have "more detailed" assessment forms that may be appropriate for this patient.**

ADMISSION PATIENT PROFILE

ST. JOHN'S HOSPITAL
Springfield, Illinois

CLINICAL RECORD

		A.M.	P.M.	A.M.	P.M.	A.M.	P.M.	A.M.	P.M.	A.M.	P.M.	A.M.	P.M.	A.M.	P.M.
DATE															
DAY OF HOSP															
TIME															

TEMPERATURE

105.8 = 41
104.0 = 40
102.2 = 39
100.4 = 38
98.6 = 37
96.8 = 36

PULSE	
RESPIRATION	
BLOOD PRESSURE — Systolic / Diastolic	
WEIGHT (Kg)	
URINATION	
DEFECATION	
SLEEP	
DIET	
APPETITE	
NURSES' SIGNATURE: NIGHT / DAY / EVENING	

#135 (R 04/92)

CLINICAL RECORD

(Courtesy St. John's Hospital, Springfield, Ill.)

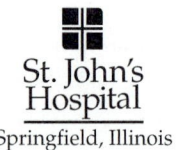

St. John's
Hospital
Springfield, Illinois

DIABETIC MANAGEMENT RECORD

DATE:	Time								
	Blood Glucose								
	Ketones								
	Medication Dosage								
	Comments								
	Initials								
DATE:	Time								
	Blood Glucose								
	Ketones								
	Medication Dosage								
	Comments								
	Initials								
DATE:	Time								
	Blood Glucose								
	Ketones								
	Medication Dosage								
	Comments								
	Initials								

INITIALS	SIGNATURE	INITIALS	SIGNATURE	INITIALS	SIGNATURE

DIABETIC MANAGEMENT RECORD

#700 (R 11/93)

(Courtesy St. John's Hospital, Springfield, Ill.)

An Affiliate of Hospital Sisters Health System

MEDICATION ADMINISTRATION
RECORD & PROFILE

MEMORIAL MEDICAL CENTER

START STOP	MEDICATION	00:01–07:00	07:01–15:00	15:01–24:00
START				
TC				
CS				
STOP				
START				
TC				
CS				
STOP				
START				
TC				
CS				
STOP				
START				
TC				
CS				
STOP				
START				
TC				
CS				
STOP				
START				
TC				
CS				
STOP				
START				
TC				
CS				
STOP				
START				
TC				
CS				
STOP				
START				
TC				
CS				
STOP				

INJECTION SITE CODES
RLA or LLA = RIGHT OR LEFT LOWER ABDOMEN
MA = MID ABDOMEN
RA or LA = RIGHT OR LEFT ARM
RAN or LAN = RIGHT OR LEFT ANTECUBITAL
RB or LB = RIGHT OR LEFT GLUTEUS MEDIUS
RD or LD = RIGHT OR LEFT DELTOID
RF or LF = RIGHT OR LEFT FOOT
RJ or LJ = RIGHT OR LEFT JUGULAR
RS or LS = RIGHT OR LEFT SUBCLAVIAN
RVG or LVG = RIGHT OR LEFT VENTROGLUTEAL
SCV = SCALP VEIN
RVL or LVL = RIGHT OR LEFT VASTUS LATERALIS
INP = INFUSION PORT
HCK = HICKMAN CATHETER

EYE CODES
OS = LEFT EYE
OD = RIGHT EYE
OU = BOTH EYES

TC / CS
TC = TUBING CHANGE
CS = CONTROLLED SUBSTANCE SCHEDULE

DOSAGE CODES
TC = TUBE CHANGE
▲ = CHANGE
INITIALS = DOSE ADMINISTERED
CIRCLED
INITIALS = DOSE NOT ADMINISTERED

PATIENT

PATIENT NO.

ROOM-BED NO.

DIAGNOSIS

PHYSICIAN

ADM. DATE

AGE

ALLERGIES

(Courtesy Memorial Medical Center, Springfield, Ill.)

```
CCHD -0410         ST. JOHNS DEVELOPMENT
03-26-XX  12:43        (QAB$$P)                    PAGE 001
::::::::::::::::::::::::::::::::::::::::::::::
DOE, JANE                    F W D  52
ACCT#: 93000775        MR#: 0895351      PATIENT CARE SUMMARY
SERV: MEDICAL          CCHD ..CH09
DR: EDISON, THOMAS MD  ADM: 03/26/XX
DR:                    DOB: 02/12/41
 ::::::::::::::::::::::::::::::::::::::::::::::
SUMMARY: 03/26 07:00    TO 15:15


PATIENT INFORMATION:
MEDICATION ALLERGIES:
    03/26           MEDICATION ALLERGY: NONE KNOWN
OTHER NURSING INFORMATION:
    03/26           ADMIT DX: DIABETIC ULCERS

ALL CURRENT MEDICAL ORDERS:

  MD TO NURSE ORDERS:
    03/26   8.   BLOOD: ACCUCHECK AC AND HS, (0009)
    03/26   9.   VITAL SIGNS, T-P-R, BP BID, (0009)
    03/26  10.   DRESSINGS: CHANGE DRESSING -- WET TO DRY --
                 L FOOT ULCER, (0009)

  DIET/I&O:
    03/26   1.   DIET: DIABETIC, 2000CAL, (0009)

  LABORATORY:
    03/26   2.   CBC, TODAY, (03/26/XX), (0009)
    03/26   3.   GLUCOSE, TOMORROW, (03/27/XX), (0009)

ALL CURRENT PHARMACY/INFUSION ORDERS:

  SCHEDULED MEDICATIONS:
    03/26   5.   INSULIN HUMAN REGULAR 100UNITS/ML INJ, 5
                 UNITS,SC, QAM,1/2HR AC/BKFST, (03/27/XX
                 0800-..), (0009)
    03/26   6.   INSULIN HUMAN REGULAR 100UNITS/ML INJ, 5
                 UNITS,SC, QPM,1/2HR AC/DINNR, (03/26/XX
                 1700-..), (0009)

  UNSCHEDULED MEDICATIONS:
    03/26   4.   INSULIN HUMAN REGULAR 100UNITS/ML INJ, 5
                 UNITS,SC, TODAY(IF APPROPRIATE),,(03/26/XX)
                 , (0009)

  PRN MEDICATIONS:
    03/26   7.   DARVOCET-N PROPOXYPHENE N 50MG/ACETAMINOPHEN
                 325MG TAB, #2, PO, Q4H, PRN, (0009)

                      LASTPAGE




::::::::::::::::::::::::::::::::::::::::::::::::::::::::::::::::::::::::
DOE, JANE                   0895351        PATIENT CARE SUMMARY
```

(Courtesy St. John's Hospital, Springfield, Ill.)

ST. JOHN'S HOSPITAL
Springfield, Illinois

PATIENT PROGRESS NOTES

DATE	TIME	PROGRESS NOTES	SIGNATURE

#299   PATIENT PROGRESS NOTES

(Courtesy St. John's Hospital, Springfield, Ill.)

750

This report is not a part of a patient's medical record. It is a Risk Management/Quality Improvement Tool.

"An incident is any happening which is not consistent with the routine operation of the hospital or routine care of a particular patient. It may be any situation, condition or event which could adversely affect the patient, visitor or the hospital."

HSHS
Hospital Sisters
Health System

Patient / Visitor
Incident Report
CONFIDENTIAL

Procedure:
A. Complete all applicable sections with facts
B. Do not complete shaded areas
C. Route according to hospital directive
D. Retain property and physical evidence involved

A) If patient, use addressograph; B) If no plate, give name/age/patient # and medical record #; C) If visitor, give name/age/address/phone #.

Facility/City/State

Incident Number:

Diagnosis

Incident Identification:
I ☐ Inpatient   O ☐ Outpatient   V ☐ Visitor

Type of incident: (check one only)

AM ☐	Against Medical Advice/Elopement	CN ☐	Consent		IV ☐	Intravascular
AD ☐	Adverse Reaction	CT ☐	Count		ME ☐	Medication
BE ☐	Behavioral	DE ☐	Delay		PP ☐	Policy/Procedure
BN ☐	Burn	EQ ☐	Equipment Related		PR ☐	Property
CO ☐	Complaint	FL ☐	Fall		TT ☐	Test/Treatment
		IN ☐	Infection		OT ☐	Other - Explain _____

Location of incident, be specific (eg., 5 North hallway, Radiology exam room, grounds, etc.):

Date of incident: / /

Time of incident: ☐ A.M. ☐ P.M.

Describe exactly what happened; why it happened; what causes were; use additional sheet of paper if needed.

_____

_____

_____

_____

_____

_____

_____

_____

☐ Property or equipment involved — describe:

Category:

☐ No apparent injury   If injury, state nature and part of body affected:

Injury:

Patient Factor:

Condition	Activity Orders	Bed Rails (Circle)	Bed Position	Restraints
A ☐ Alert	A ☐ Ambulatory with assistance	1 2 3 4 Raised	A ☐ Up	A ☐ YES
B ☐ Sedated	B ☐ Ambulatory w/o assistance	1 2 3 4 Lowered	B ☐ Down	B ☐ NO
C ☐ Confused	C ☐ Bed rest	**Call button within reach:**	**Floor condition:**	
D ☐ Sleeping	D ☐ _____	A ☐ Yes	A ☐ Wet	
		B ☐ No	B ☐ Dry	

Referred for Treatment:
☐ YES   ☐ NO   ☐ Refused

Was Physician Notified:
☐ YES   ☐ NO   Date: Time:

☐ A.M. ☐ P.M.   Physician's Name:

Was person seen by:
☐ Physician/Name_____

☐ Emergency Dept.
☐ Other _____

Employee Involved:

Witness (Name/Address/Phone):

Person Completing Report: Date:

Witness (Name/Address/Phone):

Supervisor Signature: Date:

RM-1 9/92

_____

(Courtesy Hospital Sisters Health System, Springfield, Ill.)

ST. JOHN'S HOSPITAL
Springfield, Illinois

PHYSICAL CARE/ACTIVITY — Medical/Surgical

Blank = no intervention needed at this time or N/A
CP = see care plan
NN = see nurses' notes   DC = discontinued
√ = performed/observed
∅ = no/none
     Dietary Intake: G = good
                     F = fair
                     P = poor

RA = right arm
LA = left arm
BA = both arms
RL = right leg
LL = left leg
BL = both legs

Date:														
Time:														
ELIMINATION Involuntary (Stool)														
Incontinent (Urine)														
HYGIENE Bed Bath														
Assist Bath														
Self Bath														
Oral Care / Skin Care														
Foley Catheter Care														
HS Care														
ACTIVITY Turn and Reposition #														
Dangle														
Chair #														
BRP #														
Ambulation #														
Range of Motion														
SAFETY Top Rails Up / All Rails Up														
Bed Position Low														
Call Bell Within Reach														
Vest Restraint														
Limb Restraint (See code)														
Circulation Checked q 30 min / Extremities Pink & Warm														
Restraints Released q 2 Hrs														
RESPIRATION Oxygen:														
Suction: Tracheostomy														
Oral / Pharyngeal														
Incentive Spirometry														
Cough & Deep Breathe														
Trach care														

#5003 (R 10/91)
(1 of 2)

PHYSICAL CARE/ACTIVITY — Medical Surgical

Date:													
Time:													

NUTRITION	NPO													
	Appetite:													
	Eats with assist / total feed													
	Nourishment													
	Feeding Tube													
	Tube Feedings:													
	Intermittent / Continuous													
	Bag and Tubing Change													
	Placement / Residual Check													
WOUND	Decubitis Location:													
	#1													
	#2													
	Dressing Location:													
	#1													
	#2													
	#3													
OTHER ASSESSMENTS	Isolation (type):													
	Eggcrate													
	Air Flow Mattress													
	Special Therapy Bed													
	K-Pad (location)													
	Ice Bag (location)													
	TED Hose													
	Anti-Embolism Device													
	NG Tube / Irrigation													
	Asleep													
	Visitors Present													
SIGNATURE														

```
ICUC -0284        ST. JOHNS DEVELOPMENT
04-01-XX  10:09        (QAY$$P)                              PAGE 001
:::::::::::::::::::::::::::::::::::::::::::
PATIENT, JANE              F W M 62
ACCT#: 93000811      MR#: 0895383
SERV: MEDICAL        ICUC ..IC02
DR: TYLER, ANN MD    ADM: 04/01/XX
DR:                  DOB: 10/06/30
:::::::::::::::::::::::::::::::::::::::::::               PLAN OF CARE

ADMIT DX:              DIABETIC ULCERS

CURRENT PROBLEMS:

04/01  IMPAIRED PHYSICAL MOBILITY
         R/T: WEAKNESS & FATIGUE
  EXPECTED OUTCOMES:                              DATE:
   04/01 PT WILL RESUME NORMAL ACTIVITIES    PRIOR TO DC
  NURSING APPROACHES:
   04/01 TURN & POSITION Q2HR
   04/01 INSTRUCT IN PROPER BODY MECHANICS
   04/01 INSTRUCT PT/S.O. IN PROPER TRANSFER
         TECHNIQUE
   04/01 INVOLVE PT/S.O. IN DEVELOPING PLAN FOR
         INCREASING MOBILITY
04/01  ALTERED TISSUE PERFUSION:  PERIPHERAL
         R/T: DECREASED ARTERIAL FLOW
  EXPECTED OUTCOMES:                              DATE:
   04/01 --IDENTIFY WAYS TO IMPROVE CIRCULATION
         TO FEET                             PRIOR TO DC
  NURSING APPROACHES:
   04/01 ASSESS PERIPHERAL PULSES, SKIN TEMP,
         COLOR, SENSATION, & MOTION
   04/01 DISCOURAGE PT FROM CROSSING LEGS
   04/01 AVOID PRESSURE TO POSTERIOR KNEE AREA
   04/01 AVOID PROLONGED SITTING OR STANDING
   04/01 ENCOURAGE TO WIGGLE:....TOES
   04/01 PERFORM ROM:....ACTIVE


04/01  FEAR
         R/T: POSSIBILITY ULCER WON'T HEAL
  EXPECTED OUTCOMES:                              DATE:
   04/01 PT WILL VERBALIZE &/OR DEMONSTRATE
         EFFECTIVE COPING MECHANISMS TO REDUCE
         OR ELIMINATE SOURCE OF FEAR        PRIOR TO DC
  NURSING APPROACHES:
   04/01 DISCUSS SITUATION & UNDERSTANDING OF
         SITUATION WITH PT & S.O.
   04/01 BE ACTIVE LISTENER TO PT CONCERNS
   04/01 ENCOURAGE EXPRESSION OF FEELINGS
   04/01 --DESCRIBE EVIDENCE OF HEALING AS
         OBSERVED

NURSES:  SIMMONS, TERRY       AIS

                    LASTPAGE
:::::::::::::::::::::::::::::::::::::::::::::::::::::::::::::::
PATIENT, JANE              0895383          PLAN OF CARE
```

(Courtesy St. John's Hospital, Springfield, Ill.)

ST. JOHN'S HOSPITAL
Springfield, Illinois
ROUTINE NURSING ASSESSMENT
Medical/Surgical

EDEMA: +1 = 0″ - ¼″
+2 = ¼″ - ½″
+3 = ½″ - 1″
∅ = Negative/No
✓ = observed or positive response
Blank = no assessment at this time
NN = see nurses notes
LE = lower extremity
UE = upper extremity
OTA = open to air

PU = purulent
SS = serosanguinous
B = brown
R = red
Y = yellow
G = green
P = pink
A = amber
C = clear
CL = cloudy

Date									
Time									
MENTAL STATUS	Alert								
	Oriented/Disoriented								
	Lethargic								
	Unresponsive								
BEHAVIOR	Agitated								
	Anxious								
	Restless								
MOTOR/SENSORY FUNCTION	Moves all extremities								
	Weakness UE LT/RT								
	LE LT/RT								
	Paralysis UE LT/RT								
	LE LT/RT								
	Numbness/Tingling								
	location								
SKIN/MUCOUS MEMBRANE	Temperature: warm/cool								
	Moisture: dry/moist								
	Skin: pink/pale								
	flushed/cyanotic								
	jaundiced								
	Mucous Membrane: pink/pale								
	flushed cyanotic								
	Edema:								
	location								
CARDIO-VASCULAR	Apical rate: reg./irreg.								
	Dorsalis pedis LT/RT								
	Posterior tibial LT/RT								

#4747 (R 10/91)
(1 of 2)

ROUTINE NURSING ASSESSMENT — Medical/Surgical

(Courtesy St. John's Hospital, Springfield, Ill.)

	Date									
	Time									
RESPIRATORY	Quality: unlabored/labored									
	deep/shallow									
	O₂ Therapy:									
	Sounds: clear LT/RT									
	diminished LT/RT									
	rales (crackles) LT/RT									
	rhonchi LT/RT									
	wheeze LT/RT									
	Cough: productive/nonproductive									
	Sputum: Color									
GASTROINTESTINAL/ ABDOMEN	Nondistended/Distended									
	Sounds: present/absent									
	Firm/Soft									
	Hyperactive/Hypoactive									
	Expelling flatus									
	Nausea									
WOUND	Location (✓ = no redness or edema)									
	#1									
	#2									
	#3									
DRESSING	Location (✓ = clean & dry)									
	#1									
	#2									
	#3									
DRAINAGE	Device and location:	description	description	description	description	description	description	description	description
	#1									
	#2									
	#3									
PAIN	Absent/Present									
	Location:									
	#1									
	#2									
	Severity scale (0-10) #1/#2									
	Intervention									
PATIENT TEACHING	Description									
	#1									
	#2									
	#3									
	Signature									

ST. JOHN'S HOSPITAL
Springfield, Illinois

VITAL SIGNS RECORD

KEY:
V = systolic	• = temperature	RA = right arm
Λ = diastolic	A = axillary	LA = left arm
LY = lying	O = oral	RL = right leg
ST = standing	R = rectal	LL = left leg
SIT = sitting	S = skin	
D = doppler	P = temperature probe	

Date																			
Time																			
Weight (kg)																			
Temp site																			
B/P site																			

Temperature / Blood pressure scale:
- 43.0 - 240
- 42.5 - 230
- 42.0 - 220
- 41.5 - 210
- 41.0 - 200
- 40.5 - 190
- 40.0 - 180
- 39.5 - 170
- 39.0 - 160
- 38.5 - 150
- 38.0 - 140
- 37.5 - 130
- 37.0 - 120
- 36.5 - 110
- 36.0 - 100
- 35.5 - 90
- 35.0 - 80
- 34.5 - 70
- 34.0 - 60
- 33.5 - 50
- 33.0 - 40

Pulse																			
Respiration																			

#284   (R 09/88)   **VITAL SIGNS RECORD**

(Courtesy St. John's Hospital, Springfield, Ill.)

appendix B

Abbreviations and Equivalents

Abbreviations and conversion from apothecary to metric

1 grain (gr) = 60 milligram (mg)
15 gr = 1 gram (g, gm)
15 minims = 1 milliter (ml, mL)
1 dram (dr) = 4 ml
1 ounce (oz) = 30 cubic centimeters (cc, ml)

Abbreviations for conversion using household measures

1 drop (gtt) = 1 minim
1 teaspoon (1 tsp) = 5 ml
3 tsp = 1 tablespoon (tbsp)
1 cup = 8 oz
16 oz = 1 pound (lb)

Standard equivalents, abbreviations, and conversions

1000 mg = 1 g
1000 ml = 1 liter (L)
2.2 lb = 1 kilogram (kg) = 1000 g
1 tsp = 5 ml (cc)
1 dr = 4 ml (cc)
mEq: millequivalent
mcg (μg): microgram

Symbols

/	Per
<	Less than
>	More than
≤	Equal to or less than
≥	Equal to or more than
≅	Approximately equal to
+ / −, ±	Plus or minus
♂	Male
♀	Female
1°	Primary; first degree
2°	Secondary; second degree
3°	Tertiary; third degree
↑	Up; increase
↓	Down; decrease
μ	Micron

Abbreviations related to types of intravenous (IV) fluids

D5W, D_5W: 5% dextrose and water
NS: normal saline
D5NS, D_5NS: 5% dextrose in 0.9% (normal) saline
LR: lactated Ringer's solution
D5 ½ NS, D_5½ NS: 5% dextrose in 0.45% saline
D5 ⅓ NS, D_5⅓ NS: 5% dextrose in 0.33% saline

Abbreviations

$\bar{a}$: before
abd: abdomen
ABGs: arterial blood gases
ac: before meals
ad lib: as desired
ADH: antidiuretic hormone
ADLs: activities of daily living
AFB: acid-fast bacillus (relates to tuberculosis)
AIDS: acquired immunodeficiency syndrome
ALL: acute lymphoblastic leukemia
AMB: ambulatory
AP (and lateral chest): anterior and posterior
ASA: aspirin
ASHD: arteriosclerotic heart disease
ax: axillary
BE: barium enema
bid: twice a day
BM: bowel movement
BP: blood pressure
BPH: benign prostatic hypertrophy
BR: bed rest
BRP: bathroom privileges
BSE: breast self-examination
BSI: body substance isolation
BUN: blood urea nitrogen
bx: biopsy
$\bar{c}$: with
C&S: culture and sensitivity
CA: cancer
CABG: coronary artery bypass graft
CAD: coronary artery disease
cap: capsule
CBC: complete blood count
CBI: continuous bladder irrigation
CBR: complete bed rest
CC: chief complaint
CDC: Centers for Disease Control
CHF: congestive heart failure
Cl: chloride

CN: cranial nerve
CNS: central nervous system
c/o: complains of
CO_2: carbon dioxide
COPD: chronic obstructive pulmonary disease
CPM: continuous passive motion
CPR: cardiopulmonary resuscitation
CSF: cerebrospinal fluid
CT: computed tomography
CVA: cerebrovascular accident (stroke)
CVP: central venous pressure
D/C: discontinue
DM: diabetes mellitus
DNR: do not resuscitate
DSD: dry sterile dressing
DTR: deep tendon reflex
dx: diagnosis
EC: enteric coated
ECG, EKG: electrocardiogram
EEG: electroencephalogram
elix: elixir
ER: extended release
ESR: erythrocyte sedimentation rate
ESRD: end-stage renal disease
ET: enterostomal therapist
FUO: fever of unknown origin
fx: fracture
g: gram
GI: gastrointestinal
gtt: drops
GU: genitourinary
Hb, Hgb: hemoglobin
HBV: hepatitis B virus
HCO_3^-: bicarbonate
Hct: hematocrit
HCV: hepatitis C virus
HEPA: high-efficiency particulate air
HIV: human immunodeficiency virus
h/o: history of
HOB: head of bed
HR: heart rate
hs: at bedtime
HTN: hypertension
I&O: intake and output
ICP: intracranial pressure
ICU: intensive care unit
IDDM: insulin-dependent diabetes mellitus
IM: intramuscular

IPPB: intermittent positive-pressure breathing
IV: intravenous
JVD: jugular vein distention
K: potassium
KUB: kidney, ureter, bladder
kvo: keep vein open (run IV very slowly)
LLQ: left lower quadrant
LMP: last menstrual period
LOC: level of consciousness
lytes: electrolytes
MAP: mean arterial pressure
MCHC: mean corpuscular hemoglobin concentration
MCV: mean corpuscular volume
MI: myocardial infarction
MRI: magnetic resonance imaging
N: nitrogen
Na: sodium
NaCl: sodium chloride
neg: negative
NG: nasogastric
NPO: nothing by mouth
NSAIDS: nonsteroidal antiinflammatory agents
O_2: oxygen
OD: right eye
OOB: out of bed
OR: operating room
OS: left eye
O.T.: occupational therapy
OTC: over the counter (medicine without prescription)
OU: both eyes
P: pulse
PACU: postanesthesia care unit
pc: after meals
PCA: patient-controlled analgesia
PE: physical education
PID: pelvic inflammatory disease
PMH: past medical history
PMI: point of maximum impulse
po: by mouth
postop: after surgery
preop: before surgery
prep: preparation
PRN: as needed
pt: patient
P.T.: physical therapy
PT: prothrombin time

PTT: partial thromboplastin time
PVD: peripheral vascular disease
q: each
qd: daily
q__h (fill in number of hours), e.g., q3h: every 3 hours
qid: four times a day
qod: every other day
qs: sufficient quantity
R: respirations
RA: rheumatoid arthritis
RBC: red blood cell
R/O: rule out (eliminate possibility of a condition)
ROM: range of motion
ROS: Review of systems
r/t: related to
RUQ: right upper quadrant
Rx: treatment
s̄: without
sc (SQ): subcutaneous
sl: sublingual
SOB: shortness of breath
sp gr: specific gravity
SR: sustained release
STAT: immediately
STD: sexually transmitted disease
supp: suppository
susp: suspension
sx: symptoms, signs
T: temperature
T&C: type and crossmatch
tab: tablet
TB: tuberculosis
TCDB: turn, cough, deep breathe
tid: three times a day
TPN: total parenteral nutrition
TPR: temperature, pulse, respirations
TURP: transurethral resection of prostate
UA: urinalysis
up ab lib: up as desired
URI: upper respiratory infection
US: ultrasound
UTI: urinary tract infection
VS: vital signs
VTBI: volume to be infused
WBC: white blood cell
WC: wheelchair
WNL: within normal limits
wt: weight

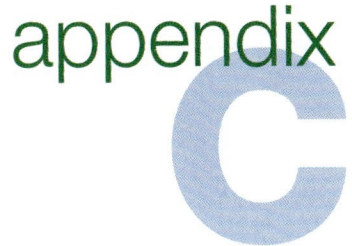

appendix C

Nursing Diagnoses:
(1994) North American Nursing Diagnosis Association (NANDA) and Functional Health Patterns

NANDA-Approved Nursing Diagnoses*

Activity Intolerance
Activity Intolerance, Risk for
†Adaptive Capacity, Decreased: Intracranial
Adjustment, Impaired
Airway Clearance, Ineffective
Anxiety
Aspiration, Risk for
Body Image Disturbance
Body Temperature, Altered Risk for
Bowel Incontinence
Breastfeeding, Effective
Breastfeeding, Ineffective
Breastfeeding, Interrupted
Breathing Pattern, Ineffective
Cardiac Output, Decreased
Caregiver Role Strain
Caregiver Role Strain, Risk for
Communication, Impaired Verbal
†Community Coping, Potential for Enhanced
†Community Coping, Ineffective
†Confusion, Acute
†Confusion, Chronic
Constipation
Constipation, Colonic
Constipation, Perceived
Coping, Defensive
Coping, Family: Potential for Growth
Coping, Ineffective Family: Compromised
Coping, Ineffective Family: Disabling
Coping, Ineffective Individual
Decisional Conflict (Specify)
Denial, Ineffective
Diarrhea
Disuse Syndrome, Risk for
Diversional Activity Deficit
Dysreflexia
†Energy Field Disturbance
†Environmental Interpretation Syndrome, Impaired
†Family Processes, Altered: Alcoholism
Family Processes, Altered
Fatigue

Fear
Fluid Volume Deficit (1)
Fluid Volume Deficit (2)
Fluid Volume Deficit, Risk for
Fluid Volume Excess
Gas Exchange, Impaired
Grieving, Anticipatory
Grieving, Dysfunctional
Growth and Development, Altered
Health Maintenance, Altered
Health-Seeking Behaviors (Specify)
Home Maintenance Management, Impaired
Hopelessness
Hyperthermia
Hypothermia
Incontinence, Bowel
Incontinence, Functional
Incontinence, Reflex
Incontinence, Stress
Incontinence, Total
Incontinence, Urge
†Infant Behavior, Disorganized
†Infant Behavior, Disorganized: Risk for
†Infant Behavior, Organized: Potential for Enhanced
Infant Feeding Pattern, Ineffective
Infection, Risk for
†Injury: Risk for Perioperative Positioning
Injury, Risk for
Knowledge Deficit (Specify)
†Loneliness, Risk for
†Management of Therapeutic Regimen, Community: Ineffective
†Management of Therapeutic Regimen, Families: Ineffective
†Management of Therapeutic Regimen, Individuals: Effective
Management of Therapeutic Regimen, Individuals: Ineffective
†Memory, Impaired
Mobility, Impaired Physical
Noncompliance (Specify)
Nutrition, Altered: Less Than Body Requirements
Nutrition, Altered: More Than Body Requirements
Nutrition, Altered: Risk for More Than Body Requirements
Oral Mucous Membrane, Altered

---

* It is appropriate to have "At Risk" nursing diagnoses; for example, a client with a history of lung disease may have a nursing diagnosis of **At Risk for Ineffective Airway Clearance,** or a client with a back injury may have a nursing diagnosis of **At Risk for Chronic Pain.** (Carpenito LJ: *Nursing diagnosis: application to clinical practice,* ed 6, Philadelphia, 1995, JB Lippincott, and Gordon M: *Nursing diagnosis: process and application,* ed 3, St. Louis, 1994, Mosby.)
†1994 additions.

Pain

Pain, Chronic

†Parent Infant/Child Attachment, Risk for altered

Parental Role Conflict

Parenting, Altered

Parenting, Risk for Altered

Peripheral Neurovascular Dysfunction, Risk for

Personal Identity Disturbance

Poisoning, Risk for

Post-Trauma Response

Powerlessness

Protection, Altered

Rape-Trauma Syndrome

Rape-Trauma Syndrome: Compound Reaction

Rape-Trauma Syndrome: Silent Reaction

Relocation Stress Syndrome

Role Performance, Altered

Self-Care Deficit, Bathing/Hygiene

Self-Care Deficit, Dressing/Grooming

Self-Care Deficit, Feeding

Self-Care Deficit, Toileting

Self-Concept, Disturbance in

Self-Esteem Disturbance

Self-Esteem, Chronic Low

Self-Esteem, Situational Low

Self-Mutilation, Risk for

Sensory/Perceptual Alterations (Specify) (Visual, Auditory, Kinesthetic, Gustatory, Tactile, Olfactory)

Sexual Dysfunction

Sexuality Patterns, Altered

Skin Integrity, Impaired

Skin Integrity, Risk for Impaired

Sleep Pattern Disturbance

Social Interaction, Impaired

Social Isolation

Spiritual Distress (Distress of Human Spirit)

†Spiritual Well-Being, Potential for Enhanced

Suffocation, Risk for

Swallowing, Impaired

Thermoregulation, Ineffective

Thought Processes, Altered

Tissue Integrity, Impaired

Tissue Perfusion, Altered (Specify Type) (Renal, Cerebral, Cardiopulmonary, Gastrointestinal, Peripheral)

Trauma, Risk for

Unilateral Neglect

Urinary Elimination, Altered

Urinary Retention

Ventilation, Inability to Sustain Spontaneous

Ventilatory Weaning Process, Dysfunctional (DVWP)

Violence, Risk for: Self-Directed or Directed at Others

Classification of Nursing Diagnoses by Functional Health Patterns

HEALTH PERCEPTION–HEALTH MANAGEMENT

Health-Seeking Behaviors (Specify)
Altered Health Maintenance
Ineffective Management of Therapeutic Regimen, Individual
Effective Management of Therapeutic Regimen, Individual
Ineffective Family Management of Therapeutic Regimen
Ineffective Community Management of Therapeutic Regimen
Noncompliance (Specify)
Risk for Infection
Risk for Injury
Risk for Trauma
Risk for Perioperative Positioning Injury
Risk for Poisoning
Risk for Suffocation
Altered Protection
Energy Field Disturbance

NUTRITIONAL–METABOLIC

Altered Nutrition: More than Body Requirements
Altered Nutrition: Risk for More than Body Requirements
Altered Nutrition: Less than Body Requirements
Ineffective Breastfeeding
Interrupted Breastfeeding
Effective Breastfeeding
Ineffective Infant Feeding Pattern
Impaired Swallowing
Risk for Aspiration
Altered Oral Mucous Membrane
Fluid Volume Deficit
Risk for Fluid Volume Deficit
Fluid Volume Excess
Risk for Impaired Skin Integrity
Impaired Skin Integrity
Impaired Tissue Integrity
Risk for Altered Body Temperature
Ineffective Thermoregulation
Hyperthermia
Hypothermia

ELIMINATION

Constipation
Colonic Constipation
Perceived Constipation
Diarrhea
Bowel Incontinence
Altered Urinary Elimination
Functional Incontinence
Reflex Incontinence
Stress Incontinence
Total Incontinence
Urge Incontinence
Urinary Retention

ACTIVITY–EXERCISE

Activity Intolerance
Risk for Activity Intolerance
Fatigue
Impaired Physical Mobility
Risk for Disuse Syndrome
Self-Care Deficit, Bathing/Hygiene
Self-Care Deficit, Dressing/Grooming
Self-Care Deficit, Feeding
Self-Care Deficit, Toileting
Diversional Activity Deficit
Impaired Home Maintenance Management
Ventilatory Weaning Response, Dysfunctional
Inability to Sustain Spontaneous Ventilation
Ineffective Airway Clearance
Ineffective Breathing Pattern
Impaired Gas Exchange
Decreased Cardiac Output
Altered Tissue Perfusion (Renal, Cerebral, Cardiopulmonary, Gastrointestinal, Peripheral)
Dysreflexia
Disorganized Infant Behavior
Risk for Disorganized Infant Behavior
Potential for Enhanced Organized Infant Behavior
Risk for Peripheral Neurovascular Dysfunction
Altered Growth and Development

SLEEP–REST

Sleep-Pattern Disturbance
Anxiety
Energy Field Disturbance
Fear
Dysfunctional Grieving
Relocation Stress Syndrome
(*See also* Self-Perception–Self-Concept)

COGNITIVE–PERCEPTUAL

Pain
Chronic Pain
Sensory/ Perceptual Alterations (Specify)
Unilateral Neglect
Knowledge Deficit (Specify)
Altered Thought Processes
Acute Confusion
Chronic Confusion
Impaired Environmental Interpretation Syndrome
Impaired Memory
Decisional Conflict (Specify)
Decreased Intracranial Adaptive Capacity

Modified from Gordon M: *Manual of nursing diagnosis, 1995-1996,* St Louis, 1995, Mosby.

SELF-PERCEPTION–SELF-CONCEPT

Fear
Anxiety
Risk for Loneliness
Hopelessness
Powerlessness
Self-Esteem Disturbance
Chronic Low Self-Esteem
Situational Low Self-Esteem
Body Image Disturbance
Risk for Self-Mutilation
Personal Identity Disturbance

ROLE–RELATIONSHIP

Anticipatory Grieving
Dysfunctional Grieving
Altered Role Performance
Social Isolation
Impaired Social Interaction
Relocation Stress Syndrome
Altered Family Processes
Altered Family Processes: Alcoholism
Altered Parenting
Risk for Altered Parenting
Parental Role Conflict
Risk for Altered Parent Infant/Child Attachment
Care Giver Role Strain
Risk for Caregiver Role Strain
Impaired Verbal Communication
Risk for Violence

SEXUALITY–REPRODUCTIVE

Altered Sexuality Patterns
Sexual Dysfunction
Rape-Trauma Syndrome
Rape-Trauma Syndrome: Compound Reaction
Rape-Trauma Syndrome: Silent Reaction

COPING–STRESS TOLERANCE

Ineffective Coping (Individual)
Defensive Coping
Ineffective Denial, or Denial
Impaired Adjustment
Post-Trauma Response
Defensive Coping
Family Coping: Potential for Growth
Ineffective Family Coping: Compromised
Ineffective Family Coping: Disabling
Ineffective Individual Coping
Ineffective Community Coping
Potential for Enhanced Community Coping

VALUE–BELIEF

Spiritual Distress (Distress of Human Spirit)
Potential for Enhanced Spiritual Well-Being)

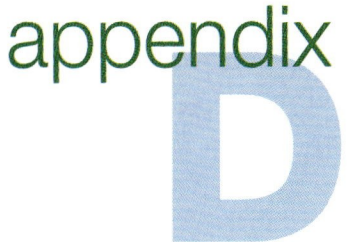

appendix D

Norms for Common Laboratory Tests

Serum: Complete Blood Count

Hemoglobin (Hgb)	Male: 13.5-18.0 g/dl	Female: 12-16 g/dl
Hematocrit (Hct)	Male: 40%-54%	Female: 38%-47%
Red blood cells (RBCs)	Male: 4.6-6.2 million/mm^3	Female: 4.2-5.4 million/mm^3
Leukocytes (white blood cells, WBCs)	5000-10,000/mm^3	
Neutrophils	54%-75% (3000-7500/mm^3)	
Bands	3%-8% (150-700/mm^3)	
Eosinophils	1%-4% (50-400/mm^3)	
Basophils	0%-1% (25-100/mm^3)	
Monocytes	2%-8% (100-500/mm^3)	
Lymphocytes	25%-40% (1500-4500/mm^3)	
T lymphocytes	60%-80% of lymphocytes	
B lymphocytes	10%-20% of lymphocytes	
Platelets	150,000-450,000/mm^3	

Serum: Clotting Indices

Prothrombin time (PT)	Male: 9.6-11.8 sec	Female: 9.5-11.3 sec
Partial thromboplastin time (PTT)	30-45 sec	
Bleeding time		
Duke	1-3 min	
Ivy	3-6 min	
Template	3-6 min	
Clotting time (Lee-White)	4-8 min	

Serum: Chemistry

Sodium (Na)	135-145 mEq/L
Potassium (K)	3.5-5.0 mEq/L
Chloride (Cl)	95-105 mEq/L
Bicarbonate (HCO_3^-)	19-25 mEq/L
Total calcium	9-11 mg/dl *or* 4.5-5.5 mEq/L
Phosphorus/phosphate	2.4-4.7 mg/dl
Magnesium	1.8-3.0 mg/dl *or* 1.5-2.5 mEq/L
Glucose	70-110 mg/dl
Osmolality	285-310 mOsm/kg

Liver Function Tests

Aspartate aminotransferase (AST, SGOT) (see also cardiac)	Male: 8-46 U/L	Female: 7-34 U/L
Alanine aminotransferase (ALT, SGPT)	10-30 IU/ml	
Total bilirubin	0.3-1.2 mg/dl	
Conjugated	0.0-0.2 mg/dl	
Unconjugated (indirect)	0.2-0.8 mg/dl	
Alkaline phosphatase	20-90 U/L	

Lipids

Cholesterol	120-220 mg/100ml
Total lipids	450-1000 mg/100ml
Triglycerides	40-150 mg/ml

Cardiac Enzymes Related to Myocardial Infarction

AST (SGOT; see also liver)	8-20 U/L (women slightly higher)	
Total creatine phosphokinase (CPK, creatine kinase)	Male: 12-70 U/ml	Female:10-55 U/ml
CPK-MB (muscle/brain)	0%	
Lactate dehydrogenase (LDH)	45-90 U/L	

Renal Function Tests

Blood urea nitrogen (BUN)	6-20 mg/dl	
Creatinine	Male: 0.6-1.3 mg/dl	Female: 0.5-1.0 mg/dl
Uric acid	Male: 4.0-8.5 mg/dl	Female: 2.7-7.3 mg/dl

Thyroid Function Tests

TSH	0.5-3.5μU/ml
T_3	25%-30%

Arterial Blood Gases (ABGs)

pH	7.35-7.45
Oxygen partial pressure tension (P_{O_2})	80-100
Carbon dioxide partial pressure tension (P_{CO_2})	35-45 mm Hg
Bicarbonate (HCO_3^-)	22-26 mEq/L
O_2 saturation (arterial)	95%+
Base Excess	+2/−2

Routine Urinalysis

pH	4.5-8.0
Specific gravity	1.010-1.025
Protein	None
Glucose	None
Ketones	Negative
RBCs	<2
WBCs	0-4/low-power field (LPF)
Casts	None or occasional epithelial
Crystals	Negative
Bacteria	Negative

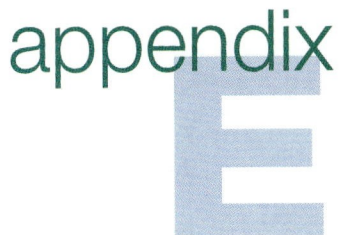

appendix E

Height and Weight Table:
Weights for Persons 29 to 59 Years According to Build*

| | Men | | | | | Women | | | |
| Height† | | Small frame | Medium frame | Large frame | Height† | | Small frame | Medium frame | Large frame |
Feet	Inches				Feet	Inches			
5	2	128-134	131-141	138-150	4	10	102-111	109-121	118-131
5	3	130-136	133-143	140-153	4	11	103-113	111-123	120-134
5	4	132-138	135-145	142-156	5	0	104-115	113-126	122-137
5	5	134-140	137-148	144-160	5	1	106-118	115-129	125-140
5	6	136-142	139-151	146-164	5	2	108-121	118-132	128-143
5	7	138-145	142-154	149-168	5	3	111-124	121-135	131-147
5	8	140-148	145-157	152-172	5	4	114-127	124-138	134-151
5	9	142-151	148-160	155-176	5	5	117-130	124-141	137-155
5	10	144-154	151-163	158-180	5	6	120-133	130-144	140-159
5	11	146-157	154-166	161-184	5	7	123-136	133-147	143-163
6	0	149-160	157-170	164-188	5	8	126-139	133-150	146-167
6	1	152-164	160-174	168-192	5	9	129-142	139-153	149-170
6	2	155-168	164-178	172-197	5	10	132-145	142-156	152-173
6	3	158-172	167-182	176-202	5	11	135-148	145-159	155-176
6	4	162-176	171-187	181-207	6	0	138-151	148-162	158-179

Source of basic data *Build study,* Society of Actuaries and Association of Life Insurance Medical Directors of America, 1980. Copyright 1983 Metropolitan Life Insurance Company.

*Indoor clothing weighing 5 pounds for men and 3 pounds for women.

†Shoes with 1-inch heels.

glossary

abduction Movement of a limb away from the body.

abnormal reactive hyperemia Hyperemia over a pressure site lasting longer than 1 hour after removal of pressure; surrounding skin does not blanch.

absorption Passage of drug molecules into the blood. Factors influencing drug absorption include route of administration, ability of the drug to dissolve, and conditions at the site of absorption.

accessory muscles Muscles in the thoracic cage that assist with respiration.

active transport Movement of materials across the cell membrane by means of chemical activity that allows the cell to admit larger molecules than would otherwise be possible.

adaptation Process by which changes occur in any of a person's dimensions in response to stress.

adduction Movement of a limb toward the body.

adventitious sounds Abnormal lung sounds heard with auscultation.

adverse reaction Harmful or unintended effect of a medication, diagnostic test, or therapeutic intervention.

afebrile Without fever.

afterload The resistance to ventricular ejection.

AHCPR Agency for Health Care Policy and Research, which synthesizes research and develops standards of practice.

Alzheimer's disease Disease of the brain parenchyma that causes a gradual and progressive decline in cognitive functioning.

analgesic Relieving pain; drug that relieves pain.

anaphylactic reaction Hypersensitive condition induced by contact with certain antigens.

angina pectoris Episodic chest pain caused most often by myocardial anoxia, resulting from atherosclerosis of the coronary arteries. Pain radiates down the inner aspect of the left arm and is often accompanied by a feeling of suffocation and impending death.

angiography Radiographic visualization of internal anatomy of the heart and blood vessels after the introduction of a radiopaque contrast medium.

anorexia Lack or loss of appetite resulting in the inability to eat.

antibodies Immunoglobulins, essential to the immune system, that are produced by lymphoid tissue in response to bacteria, viruses, or other antigens.

anticipatory grief Grief response in which the person begins the grieving process before an actual loss.

antiembolic stockings Elasticized stockings that prevent formation of emboli and thrombi, especially after surgery or during bed rest.

antipyretic Substance or procedure that reduces fever.

aphasia Abnormal neurological condition in which language function is defective or absent; related to injury to speech center in cerebral cortex, causing receptive or expressive aphasia.

apical pulse Heartbeat taken with the bell or diaphragm of a stethoscope placed on the apex of the heart.

apnea Cessation of airflow through the nose and mouth.

apothecary system System of measurement; basic unit of weight is a grain. Weights derived from the grain are the gram, ounce, and pound. The basic measure for fluid is the minim. The fluidram, fluid ounce, pint, quart, and gallon are measures derived from the minim.

approximate To come close together, as in the edges of a wound.

asepsis Absence of germs or microorganisms.

assessment First step of the nursing process; activities required in the first step are data collection, data validation, data sorting, and data documentation. The purpose is to gather information for health problem identification.

assimilation To become absorbed into another culture and to adopt its characteristics.

atelectasis Collapse of alveoli, preventing the normal respiratory exchange of oxygen and carbon dioxide.

atrioventricular (AV) node Portion of the cardiac conduction system located on the floor of the right atrium, it receives electrical impulses from the atrium and transmits them to the bundle of His.

auditory Related to, or experienced through, hearing.

auscultation Method of physical examination; listening to the sounds produced by the body, usually with a stethoscope.

auscultatory gap Disappearance of sound when obtaining a blood pressure; typically occurs between the first and second Korotkoff sounds.

autologous transfusion Collection of the client's blood for reinfusion after a surgical procedure.

autonomy Ability or tendency to function independently.

autopsy Postmortem examination performed to confirm or determine the cause of death.

autotransfusion Collection, anticoagulation, filtration, and reinfusion of blood from an active bleeding site.

bacteriuria Presence of bacteria in the urine.

bereavement Response to loss through death; a subjective experience that a person suffers after losing a person with whom there has been a significant relationship.

bioavailability Degree of activity or amount of an administered drug or other substance that becomes available for activity in the target tissue.

blanching Whitening of the skin from pressure, vasoconstriction, or hypotension.

bone resorption Destruction of bone cells and release of calcium into the blood.

bruit Abnormal sound or murmur heard while auscultating an organ, gland, or artery.

buccal Of or pertaining to the inside of the cheek or the gum next to the cheek.

buffer Substance or group of substances that can absorb or release hydrogen ions to correct an acid-base imbalance.

bundle of His Portion of the cardiac conduction system that arises from the distal portion of the AV node and extends across the AV groove to the top of the intraventricular septum, where it divides into right and left bundle branches.

cachexia Malnutrition marked by weakness and emaciation, usually associated with severe illness.

carcinogen Substance or agent that causes the development or increases the incidence of cancer.

cardiac output Volume of blood expelled by the ventricles of the heart, equal to the amount of blood ejected at each beat, multiplied by the number of beats in the period of time used for computation (usually 1 minute).

carotid pulse Rhythmical beating palpated over the carotid artery.

carriers Animals or persons who harbor and spread disease-causing organisms but who do not become ill.

cathartics Drugs that act to promote bowel evacuation.

catheterization Introduction of a catheter into a body cavity or organ to inject or remove fluid.

cerumen Yellowish or brownish waxy secretion produced by sweat glands in the external ear.

channels Method used in the teaching-learning process to present content: visual, auditory, taste, smell. In the communication process, a method used to transmit a message; visual, auditory, touch.

circadian rhythm Repetition of certain physiological phenomena within a 24-hour cycle.

collaboration The working together of health team members in the delivery of care to a client or group of clients.

colon Large intestine.

colonized Referring to the establishment of a mass of microorganisms, often nonpathogenic, in or on the body.

compliance Person's fulfillment of the prescribed course of treatment.

compress Soft pad of gauze or cloth used to apply heat, cold, or medications to the surface of a body part.

contaminated Process by which an object becomes unclean or unsterile.

contracture Permanent shortening of a muscle and the eventual shortening of associated ligaments and tendons.

core temperature Temperature of deep body tissues and organs.

crackles Fine bubbling sounds heard on auscultation of the lung; produced by air entering distal airways and alveoli, which contain serous secretions.

criteria Standards, principles, or requirements established for accomplishing or evaluating an activity or condition, such as formulating a nursing diagnosis.

culture Nonphysical traits, such as values, beliefs, attitudes, and customs, that are shared by a group of people and passed from one generation to the next.

cyanosis Bluish discoloration of the skin and mucous membranes caused by an excess of deoxygenated hemoglobin in the blood or a structural defect in the hemoglobin molecule.

death Cessation of life as indicated by the absence of heartbeat or respiration. Legally, death is total absence of activity in the brain and central nervous, cardiovascular, and respiratory systems.

débridement Removal of dead tissue from a wound.

defecation Passage of feces from the digestive tract through the rectum.

dehiscence Separation of a wound's edges, revealing underlying tissues.

dementia Irreversible mental state characterized by decreased intellectual function, changes in personality, impaired judgment, and often changes in affect as a result of permanently altered cerebral metabolism.

dermis Sensitive vascular layer of the skin directly below the epidermis; composed of collagenous and elastic fibrous connective tissues that give the dermis strength and elasticity.

diaphoresis Secretion of sweat, especially profuse secretion associated with an elevated body temperature, physical exertion, or emotional stress.

diastole Time between contractions of the atria or the ventricles during which blood enters the relaxed chambers.

diffusion Movement of molecules from an area of high concentration to an area of lower concentration.

diplopia Double vision caused by an abnormality of the extraocular muscles or nerves that innervate the muscles.

dorsalis pedis pulse Rhythmical beating palpated over the dorsalis pedis artery.

dorsiflexion Flexion toward the back.

dyspnea Sensation of shortness of breath.

dysrhythmia Deviation from the normal pattern of the heartbeat.

dysuria Painful urination resulting from bacterial infection of the bladder and obstructive conditions of the urethra.

ecchymosis Discoloration of the skin or a bruise caused by leakage of blood into subcutaneous tissues as a result of trauma to underlying tissues.

edema Abnormal accumulation of fluid in interstitial spaces of tissues.

effluent Discharge or drainage.

egocentricity Regarding of the self as the center, object, and norm of all experience and having little regard for the needs, interests, ideas, and attitudes of others.

endogenous infections Infections produced within a cell or organism.

endorphins Naturally occurring neuropeptides composed of amino acids and secreted within the central nervous system to reduce pain.

endoscope Instrument used to visualize the interior of body organs and cavities.

endotracheal tube Artificial airway inserted into a client's mouth or nose.

epidermis Outer layer of the skin that has several thin layers of skin in different stages of maturation; shields and protects the underlying tissues from water loss, mechanical or chemical injury, and penetration by disease-causing microorganisms.

eschar Scab or dry crust that results from excoriation of the skin.

ethnocentrism Tendency of members of one cultural group to view the members of other cultural groups in terms of the standards of behavior, attitudes, and values of their own group.

euthanasia Deliberately bringing about the death of a person who has an incurable disease or condition, either actively, by administering a lethal drug, or passively, by withholding treatment and allowing the person to die.

evisceration Protrusion of visceral organs through a surgical wound.

exacerbations Increases in the seriousness of a disease or disorder as marked by greater intensity in signs or symptoms.

exophthalmos Abnormal protrusion of one or both eyeballs.

exudate Fluid, cells, or other substances that have been slowly discharged from cells or blood vessels through small pores or breaks in cell membranes.

febrile Pertaining to or characterized by an elevated body temperature.

feces Waste or excrement from the gastrointestinal tract.

fibrin Protein product formed from the action of thrombin on fibrinogen in the clotting process.

fissures Cleft or groove on the surface of an organ, often marking division of the organ into parts.

fistula Abnormal passage from an internal organ to the body surface or between two internal organs.

flatus Intestinal gas.

gait Manner or style of walking, including rhythm, cadence, and speed.

gingiva Gum of the mouth; a mucous membrane with supporting fibrous tissue that overlies the crowns of unerupted teeth and encircles the necks of those teeth that have erupted.

glomerulus Cluster or collection of capillary vessels within the kidney involved in the initial formation of urine.

granulation tissue Soft, pink, fleshy projections of tissue that form during the healing process in a wound not healing by primary intention.

gurgles Abnormal coarse sounds heard during auscultation of the lung; produced by air entering large mucus-containing airways. Also called *rhonchi.*

gustatory Pertaining to the sense of taste.

health Dynamic state in which an individual adapts to his or her internal and external environments so that there is a state of physical, emotional, intellectual, social, and spiritual well-being.

health behaviors Activities through which a person maintains, attains, or regains good health and prevents illness.

hematemesis Vomiting of blood indicating upper gastrointestinal bleeding.

hematoma Collection of blood trapped in the tissues of the skin or an organ.

hematuria Abnormal presence of blood in the urine.

hemolysis Breakdown of red blood cells and release of hemoglobin that may occur after administration of hypotonic intravenous solutions, causing swelling and rupture of erythrocytes.

hemoptysis Coughing up blood from the respiratory tract.

hemorrhoids Permanent dilation and engorgement of veins within the lining of the rectum.

hemostasis Termination of bleeding by mechanical or chemical means or by the coagulation process of the body.

hemothorax Accumulation of blood and fluid in the pleural cavity between the parietal and visceral pleurae.

hernias Protrusions of an organ through an abnormal opening in the muscle wall of the cavity that surrounds it.

hirsutism Excessive body hair in a masculine distribution caused by heredity, hormonal dysfunction, or medication.

homeostasis State of relative constance in the internal environment of the body, maintained naturally by physiological adaptive mechanisms.

hospice System of family-centered care designed to help terminally ill persons be comfortable and maintain a satisfactory life-style throughout the terminal phase of their illness.

hypercapnia Greater than normal amounts of carbon dioxide in the blood; also called *hypercarbia.*

hypercarbia Greater than normal amounts of carbon dioxide in the blood; also called *hypercapnia.*

hyperemia Hyperemia over a pressure site lasting 1 hour or less after removal of pressure; surrounding skin does not blanch.

hyperextension Position of maximal extension of a joint.

hyperglycemia Elevated serum glucose levels.

hypertension Disorder characterized by an elevated blood pressure persistently exceeding 150/90 mm Hg.

hyperthermia Situation in which body temperature exceeds the set point.

hypertonic Situation in which one solution has a greater concentration of solute than another solution; therefore the first solution exerts greater osmotic pressure.

hyperventilation Respiratory rate in excess of that required to maintain normal carbon dioxide levels in the body tissues.

hypervolemia Increase in the amount of fluid in the circulating blood volume.

hypoglycemia Reduced serum glucose levels.

hypotension Abnormal lowering of blood pressure, which is inadequate for normal perfusion and oxygenation of tissues.

hypothalamus Portion of the brain that activates, controls, and integrates the peripheral autonomic nervous system, endocrine processes, and many body functions, such as body temperature, sleep, and appetite.

hypothermia Abnormal lowering of body temperature below 93°F or 35°C, usually caused by prolonged exposure to cold.

hypotonic Situation in which one solution has a smaller concentration of solute than another solution; therefore the first solution exerts less osmotic pressure.

hypoventilation Respiratory rate insufficient to provide carbon dioxide retention.

hypovolemia Abnormally low circulating blood volume.

hypoxia Inadequate cellular oxygenation that may result from a deficiency in the delivery or use of oxygen at the cellular level.

iatrogenic Caused by a treatment or diagnostic procedure.

idiosyncratic reactions Individual sensitivity to effects of a drug caused by inherited or other body constitution factors.

ileum Part of the small intestine.

immunity Quality of being insusceptible to or unaffected by a particular disease or condition.

induration Hardening of a tissue, particularly the skin, because of edema or inflammation.

infiltration Dislodging an intravenous catheter or needle from a vein into the subcutaneous space.

inflammation Protective response of body tissues to irritation or injury.

infusion Introduction of fluid into the vein, giving intravenous fluid over time.

inhalers Aerosol sprays, mists, or powders that penetrate lung airways, which the client inhales through the mouth.

injection Parenteral administration of medication; four major sites of injection: subcutaneous, intramuscular, intravenous, and intradermal.

insomnia Condition characterized by chronic inability to sleep or remain asleep through the night.

inspection Method of physical examination by which the client is visually and systematically examined for appearance, structure, function, and behavior.

instillation To cause to enter drop by drop, or very slowly.

integument Skin and its appendages: hair, nails, and sweat and sebaceous glands.

interstitial fluid Fluid that fills the spaces between most of the cells of the body and provides a substantial portion of the liquid environment of the body.

intonation Rise and fall in pitch of the voice in speech.

intracellular fluid Liquid within the cell membrane.

intractable pain Pain not easily relieved, such as that which occurs with some types of cancer.

intradermal Injection given between layers of the skin, into the dermis. Injections are given at a 5- to 15-degree angle.

intramuscular (IM) Injections given into muscle tissue. Intramuscular route provides a fast rate of absorption that is related to the muscle's greater vascularity. Injections are given at a 45- to 90-degree angle.

intravascular Fluid contained within the vessels of the circulatory system.

intravenous (IV) Injection directly into the bloodstream. Action of the drug begins immediately when given intravenously.

inversion Movement of a limb by turning inward toward the body.

irrigation Process of washing out a body cavity or wounded area with a stream of fluid.

ischemia Decreased blood supply to a body part such as skin tissue or to an organ such as the heart.

isolation Separation of a client from other clients to prevent the spread of infection or to protect the client from irritating environmental factors.

isometric Related to increased muscle tension without muscle shortening.

isotonic The situation in which two solutions have the same concentration of solute; therefore both solutions exert the same osmotic pressure.

jejunum Part of the small intestine.

kinesthesic Relating to perception of

position of body parts, weight, and movement.

Korotkoff sounds Sounds heard during the taking of blood pressure using a sphygmomanometer and stethoscope.

laceration Torn, jagged wound.

lactation Process and period in which the mother produces milk for a child.

leukocyte White blood cell.

leukocytosis Abnormal increase in the number of circulating white blood cells.

leukoplakia Thick, white patches observed on oral mucous membranes.

lipids Compounds that are insoluble in water but soluble in organic solvents.

lymphocyte One type of leukocyte developing in the bone marrow; responsible for synthesizing antibodies and T cells that attack antigens.

maceration Softening and breaking down of skin from prolonged exposure to moisture.

macrophages Large phagocytic cells of the reticuloendothelial system.

malignant hyperthermia Autosomal dominant trait characterized by often fatal hyperthermia in affected people exposed to certain anesthetic agents.

malnutrition Any nutritional disorder such as unbalanced, insufficient, or excessive diet or impaired absorption, assimilation, or utilization of food.

masticate To chew or tear food with the teeth while it becomes mixed with saliva.

medical asepsis Procedures used to reduce the number of microorganisms and prevent their spread.

melena Abnormal black, sticky stool containing digested blood; indicative of gastrointestinal bleeding.

metabolism Aggregate of all chemical processes that take place in living organisms, resulting in growth, generation of energy, elimination of wastes, and other functions concerned with the distribution of nutrients in the blood after digestion.

metered-dose inhaler Device designed to deliver a measured dose of an inhalation drug.

micturition Urination; act of passing or expelling urine voluntarily through the urethra.

milliequivalent per liter (mEq/L) Number of grams of a specific electrolyte dissolved in 1 liter of plasma.

mobility Person's ability to move about freely.

multicultural nursing Framework for broadening nurses' understanding of health-related beliefs, practices, and issues that are part of the lived experiences of people from diverse cultural backgrounds.

murmurs Blowing or whooshing sounds created by changes in blood flow through the heart or by abnormalities in valve closure.

NANDA North American Nursing Diagnosis Association, organized in 1973, which formally identifies, develops, and classifies nursing diagnoses.

narcolepsy Syndrome involving sudden sleep attacks that a person cannot inhibit; uncontrollable desire to sleep may occur several times during a day.

narcotic Drug substance, derived from opium or produced synthetically, that alters perception of pain and that, with repeated use, may result in physical and psychological dependence.

nebulization Process of adding moisture to inspired air by the addition of water droplets.

necrotic Of or pertaining to the death of tissue in response to disease or injury.

nephrons Structural and functional units of the kidney containing renal glomeruli and tubules.

neurotransmitter Chemical that transfers the electrical impulse from the nerve fiber to the muscle fiber.

nitrogen balance Relationship between the nitrogen taken into the body, usually as food, and the nitrogen excreted from the body in urine and feces. Most of the body's nitrogen is incorporated into protein.

nosocomial infections Infections acquired during hospitalization or stay in a health care facility.

NPUAP National Pressure Ulcer Advisory Panel.

nutrients Foods that contain elements necessary for body function, including water, carbohydrates, proteins, fats, vitamins, and minerals.

nystagmus Involuntary, rhythmical movements of the eyes; the oscillations may be horizontal, vertical, rotary, or mixed. May be indicative of vestibular, neurological, or vascular disease.

obesity Abnormal increase in the proportion of fat cells, mainly in the viscera and subcutaneous tissues of the body.

olfactory Pertaining to the sense of smell.

oncotic pressure Total influence of the protein on the osmotic activity of plasma fluid.

ophthalmic Drugs given into the eye, in the form of either eye drops or ointments.

organic brain syndrome Any psychological or behavioral abnormality associated with transient or permanent brain dysfunction caused by a disturbance of the physiological functioning of brain tissue.

orthopnea Abnormal condition in which a person must sit or stand up to breathe comfortably.

orthostatic hypotension Abnormally low blood pressure occurring when a person stands up.

osmolality Concentration of osmotic pressure of a solution expressed in osmols or milliosmols per kilogram of water.

osmoreceptors Receptors that are sensitive to fluid concentration in the blood plasma and regulate the secretion of antidiuretic hormone.

osmosis Movement of a pure solvent through a semipermeable membrane from a solution with a lower solute concentration to one with a higher solute concentration.

osmotic pressure Drawing power for water, which depends on the number of molecules in the solution.

ostomy Surgical creation of an artificial opening.

ototoxicity Having a harmful effect on the eighth cranial (auditory) nerve or the organs of hearing and balance.

oximeter, oximetry Device used to measure oxyhemoglobin in the blood.

oxygen saturation Amount of hemoglobin fully saturated with hemoglobin, given as a percent value.

pain Subjective, unpleasant sensation caused by noxious stimulation of sensory nerve endings.

palliative Relating to treatment designed to relieve or reduce intensity of uncomfortable symptoms but not to produce a cure.

pallor Unnatural paleness or absence of color in the skin.

palpation Method of physical examination whereby the fingers or hands of the examiner are applied to the client's body for the purpose of feeling body parts underlying the skin.

palpitations Bounding or racing of the heart associated with normal emotions or a heart disorder.

pathogens Microorganisms capable of producing disease.

pathological fractures Fractures resulting from weakened bone tissue; frequently caused by osteoporosis or neoplasms.

perception Person's mental image or concept of elements in his or her environment, including information gained through the senses.

perfusion (1) Passage of a fluid through a specific organ or an area of the body; (2) therapeutic measure whereby a drug intended for an isolated part of the body is introduced via the bloodstream.

peripheral Pertains to the outside, surface, or surrounding area of an organ, structure, or field of vision.

peristalsis Rhythmical contractions of the intestine that propel gastric contents through the length of the gastrointestinal tract.

pharmacokinetics Study of how drugs enter the body, reach their site of action, are metabolized, and exit from the body.

phlebitis Inflammation of a vein.

photophobia Abnormal sensitivity of the eyes to light.

pigmentation Organic material, such as melanin, that gives color to the skin.

placebo Dosage form that contains no pharmacologically active ingredients but may relieve pain through psychological effects.

plantar flexion Toe-down motion of the foot at the ankle.

pleural friction rub Adventitious lung sound caused by an inflamed parietal and visceral pleura rubbing together on inspiration.

pneumothorax Collection of air or gas in the pleural space.

popliteal pulse Pulse of the popliteal artery, palpated behind the knee of a person lying prone with the knee flexed.

posterior tibial pulse Pulse of the posterior tibial artery, palpated on the medial aspect of the ankle, just posterior to the prominence of the ankle bone.

postural drainage Use of positioning along with percussion and vibration to drain secretions from specific segments of the lungs and bronchi into the trachea.

postural hypotension Abnormally low blood pressure occurring when an individual assumes the standing posture; also called *orthostatic hypotension.*

preload Volume of blood in the ventricles at the end of diastole, immediately before ventricular contraction.

prescriptions Written directions for a therapeutic agent (e.g., medication, drugs).

pressure ulcer Inflammation, sore, or ulcer in the skin over a bony prominence.

primary intention Primary union of the edges of a wound, progressing to complete scar formation without granulation.

productive cough A sudden expulsion of air from the lungs that effectively removes sputum from the respiratory tract and helps clear the airways.

prolapse Falling, sinking, or sliding of an organ from its normal position or location in the body, such as a prolapsed uterus.

pronation Position of the hand in which the palm of the hand faces downward and backward.

prostaglandins Potent hormonelike substances that act in exceedingly low doses on target organs. They can be used to treat asthma and gastric hyperacidity.

protein Any of a large group of naturally occurring, complex, organic nitrogenous compounds. Each is composed of large combinations of amino acids containing the elements carbon, hydrogen, nitrogen, oxygen, usually sulfur, and occasionally phosphorus, iron, iodine, or other essential constituents of living cells. Protein is the major source of building material for muscles, blood, skin, hair, nails, and the internal organs.

proteinuria Presence in the urine of abnormally large quantities of protein, usually albumin. Persistent proteinuria is usually a sign of renal disease or renal complications of another disease, or hypertension or heart failure.

protocol Written and approved plan specifying the procedures to be followed during an assessment or in providing treatment.

ptosis Abnormal condition of one or both upper eyelids in which the eyelid droops, caused by weakness of the levator muscle or paralysis of the third cranial nerve.

ptyalin Digestive enzyme secreted by the salivary glands.

pulse deficit Condition that exists when the radial pulse is less than the ventricular rate as auscultated at the apex or seen on an electrocardiogram. The condition indicates a lack of peripheral perfusion for some of the heart contractions.

pursed-lip breathing Deep inspiration followed by prolonged expiration through pursed lips.

pyrexia Abnormal elevation of the temperature of the body above 37°C (98.6°F) because of disease. Same as *fever.*

pyrogens Substances that cause a rise in body temperature, as with bacterial toxins.

radial pulse Pulse of the radial artery palpated at the wrist over the radius. The radial pulse is the one most often taken.

radiation Method of temperature regulation used by the body to lower body temperature.

reactive hyperemia Condition characterized by increased blood flow to part of the body, as in the inflammatory response, local relaxation of arterioles, or obstruction of the outflow of blood from an area.

receptive aphasia Abnormal neurological condition in which language function is defective because of an injury to certain areas of the cerebral cortex;

specifically, language is not understood.

recommended daily allowances (RDAs) Suggested or recommended amounts of various nutrients used in planning diets.

reflex pain response Reflected, involuntary withdrawal of a body part away from a noxious or painful stimulus.

religious Relating to specific practices, rites, and rituals of one's professed religion.

reminiscence Recalling the past for the purpose of assigning new meaning to past experiences.

remissions Partial or complete disappearances of the clinical and subjective characteristics of chronic or malignant disease; remission may be spontaneous or the result of therapy.

renal calculi Calcium stones in the renal pelvis.

residual urine Volume of urine remaining in the bladder after a normal voiding; the bladder normally is almost completely empty after micturition.

respite care Short-term health services to the dependent older adult either in his or her home or in an institutional setting.

restraints Devices to aid in the immobilization of a client or client's extremity.

rhonchi Abnormal lung sound auscultated when the client's airways are obstructed with thick secretions.

sebum Normal secretion of the sebaceous glands of the skin; when combined with sweat, forms a moist, oily, acidic film that protects the skin from drying.

sensory deficit Defect in the function of one or more of the senses, resulting in visual, auditory, or olfactory impairments.

sensory deprivation State in which stimulation to one or more of the senses is lacking, resulting in impaired sensory perception.

sensory overload State in which stimulation to one or more of the senses is so excessive that the brain disregards or does not meaningfully respond to stimuli.

serum half-life Time needed for excretion processes to lower the serum drug concentration by half.

sexual response cycle Phases of biological sexual response: excitement, plateau, orgasm, and resolution as defined by Masters and Johnson.

sexuality "A function of the total personality . . . concerned with the biological, psychological, sociological, spiritual and culture variables of life . . . " (Sex Information and Education Council of the United States, 1980).

shearing force Friction exerted when a

person is moved or repositioned in bed by being pulled or allowed to slide down in bed.

shivering Process used by the body to raise body temperature.

sleep deprivation Condition resulting from a decrease in the amount, quality, and consistency of sleep.

sleep disorder Condition that interrupts the integrity of a normal sleep pattern, for example, the ability to fall or stay asleep.

sloughing Shedding of dead tissue cells.

socialization Process of being raised within a culture and acquiring the characteristics of the given group.

sterilization (1) Rendering a person unable to produce children; accomplished by surgical, chemical, or other means; (2) technique for destroying microorganisms using heat, water, chemicals, or gases.

stoma Artificially created opening between a body cavity and the body's surface; for example, a colostomy, formed from a portion of the colon pulled through the abdominal wall.

stressor Any event, situation, or other stimulus encountered in a person's external or internal environment that necessitates change or adaptation by the person.

stroke volume Amount of blood ejected by the ventricles with each contraction.

sublingual Route of medication administration in which the medication is placed underneath the client's tongue.

supination Position of the hand in which the palm of the hand faces upward.

surgical asepsis Procedures used to eliminate any microorganisms from an area. Also called *sterile technique.*

synapse Region surrounding the point of contact between two neurons or between a neuron and an effector organ.

synergistic effect When two drugs act synergistically, the effect of the two drugs combined is greater than the effect that would be expected if the in-

dividual effects of the two drugs acting alone were added together.

systole Contraction of the heart, driving blood into the aorta and pulmonary arteries. The occurrence of systole is indicated by the first heart sound heard on auscultation and by the palpable apex beat.

tachycardia Rapid regular heart rate ranging between 100 and 150 beats per minute.

tachypnea Abnormally rapid rate of breathing.

tactile Relating to the sense of touch.

tactile fremitus Tremulous vibration of the chest wall during breathing that is palpable on physical examination.

teratogens Chemical or physiological agents that may produce adverse effects in the embryo or fetus.

territoriality Persistent attachment of a person to a specific area or space.

thermoregulation Internal control of body temperature.

thoracentesis Surgical perforation of the chest wall and pleural space with a needle for the aspiration of fluid or to obtain a specimen for diagnostic or therapeutic purposes.

threshold Point at which a person first perceives a painful stimulus as being painful.

thrombosis Abnormal vascular condition in which a thrombus develops within a blood vessel of the body.

thrombus Accumulation of platelets, fibrin, clotting factors, and the cellular elements of the blood attached to the interior wall of a vein or artery, sometimes occluding the lumen of the vessel.

tinnitus Ringing heard in one or both ears.

tolerance Point at which a person is not willing to accept pain of greater severity or duration.

toxic effect Effect of a medication that results in an adverse response.

trochanter roll Rolled towel support placed against the hips and upper leg to prevent external rotation of the legs.

turgor Normal resiliency of the skin caused by the outward pressure of the cells and interstitial fluid.

urticaria Itchy skin eruption characterized by transient wheals of varying shapes and sizes with well-defined erythematous margins and pale centers.

Valsalva maneuver Any forced expiratory effect against a closed airway, as when an individual holds the breath and tightens the muscles in a concerted, strenuous effort to move a heavy object or to change positions in bed.

varicosities Abnormal conditions of a vein, characterized by swelling and irregular shape or course.

vasoconstriction Narrowing of the lumen of any blood vessel, especially the arterioles and the veins in the blood reservoirs of the skin and abdominal viscera.

vasodilation Increase in the diameter of a blood vessel caused by inhibition of its vasoconstrictor nerves or stimulation of dilator nerves.

venipuncture Technique in which a vein is punctured transcutaneously by a sharp, rigid stylet (e.g., a butterfly needle), a cannula (e.g., angiocatheter that contains a flexible plastic catheter), or a needle attached to a syringe.

ventilation Respiratory process by which gases are moved into and out of the lungs.

vertigo Sensation of dizziness, or clients feel as though they are spinning.

virulence Very pathogenic or rapidly progressive condition.

vital signs Temperature, pulse, respirations, and blood pressure.

vitamins Organic compounds essential in small quantities for normal physiological and metabolic functioning of the body. With few exceptions, vitamins cannot be synthesized by the body and must be obtained from the diet or dietary supplements.

wheezes Adventitious lung sound caused by a severely narrowed bronchus.

Index

H

O

U.S. Occupational Safety and Health Administration, 26, 27, 28, 31
    tuberculosis control and, 35
Universal precautions, 27
Unoccupied bed, making of, 74-76
UP; *see* Universal precautions
Upper body exercise, 52
Upper extremity, vitamin and mineral deficiencies and, 431
Ureterostomy, 638
    double, 639
    single, 639
Urethral obstruction, 634
Urge incontinence, 112, 633
Urinal, 111, 113-116
Urinalysis, norms for, 764
Urinary bladder; *see* Bladder, urinary
Urinary catheterization, 631, 633-638
Urinary catheters, types of, 635
Urinary diversions, 631, 638-642
Urinary elimination, 631
    in activities of daily living, 111-126; *see also* Elimination, assisting with
    altered, 111, 631-647
        abdominal assessment and, 168
        continuous bladder irrigation in, 631, 642-644
        nursing diagnosis in, 633
        pressure ulcer and, 416
        suprapubic catheters in, 631, 644-646
        urinary catheterization in, 631, 633-638
        urinary diversions in, 631, 638-642
    dying client and, 697
    organs of, 632
    patterns of, 111
Urinary incontinence; *see* Incontinence, urinary
Urinary retention, 112
    in abdominal disorders, 208
    in altered urinary elimination, 633
Urinary system, 631, 632
    infection of, 230
Urine
    collection of, for specimen, 229-238
        unit testing and, 239, 240-241
    color of, fluid volume excess or deficit and, 668
    containment devices for, 118
        specimen collection and, 229, 230
    drainage of, postoperative, 364, 369
    glucose testing of, 239, 240-241
    leakage of, 111
    measurement of, 106, 107
        clinical record form and, 745
    specific gravity of, fluid volume excess or deficit and, 668
Using air fluidized bed, 445, 450-452

Using air suspension bed, 445, 448-450
Using bariatric bed, 445, 454-455
Using disposable clean gloves, 30-31
    standard protocols for, 5
Using home oxygen equipment, 705, 725-729
Using mechanical lift, 51, 64-66
Using rotokinetic bed, 445, 452-454
Using support surface mattress, 445, 446-448
Utensils, adaptive, 98

V

Vaccination, 26
VacuDrain, 379
Vaginal cream, 306, 307
Vaginal douche, 307-308
Vaginal foam, 307
Vaginal irrigation, 307-308
Vaginal suppositories, 305, 306
Vagus nerve, 218
Vagus nerve stimulation, 616
Values, communication and, 15
Vascular assessment, 204-208
Vasoactive infusions, 689
Vasoconstriction, 405
Vasoconstrictors, as eye medication, 298
Vasodilation, 405
Vastus lateralis muscle, 326, 327-328
Vein site selection, 510-511
Velbane; *see* Vinblastine
Venous insufficiency, 173
Ventilation, 141, 678
    inability to sustain spontaneous, 562
Ventilator, pulse oximetry in, 154
Ventrogluteal muscle, 326, 327
Venturi mask, 562, 566
Vepesid; *see* Etoposide
Verbal communication, impaired, 17
Vertebral column, epidural analgesia and, 398
Vesicle, 162
Vest restraint, 41, 42
Vial, drawing up injections from, 317-318
Vibration, sensation of, testing for, 219
Vinblastine, 547
Vincristine, 547
Viscosity of blood, 405
Vision, 189-193
    communication and, 19
    impaired, feeding and, 99
Visual acuity, 189-193
Vital signs, 138-155
    baseline measurement of, 147

Index of Skills*

---

*Page numbers given indicate the beginning of the skill.